SUPPLEMENTS AND NEW

FOR INSTRUCTORS

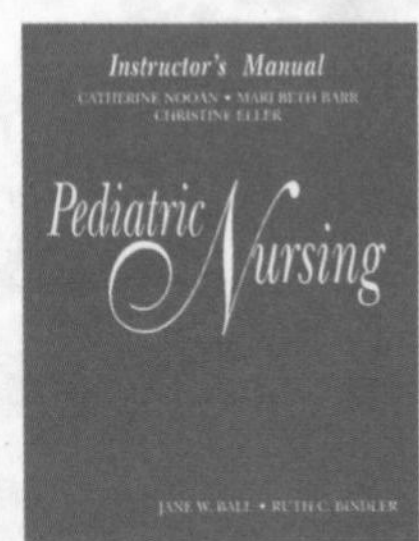

Instructor's Resource Manual ISBN: 0130452181
This manual contains a wealth of material to help faculty plan and manage the pediatric nursing course. It includes chapter overviews, detailed lecture suggestions and outlines, learning objectives, a complete test bank, teaching tips, and more for each chapter. The IRM also guides faculty how to assign and use the text-specific Companion Website, www.prenhall.com/ball, and the Student CD-ROM that accompany the textbook.

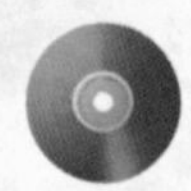

Instructor's Resource CD-ROM ISBN: 0130483583
This cross-platform CD-ROM provides several tools to aide faculty in teaching. It includes illustrations in PowerPoint from the new edition for use in classroom lectures. It also contains an electronic test bank, and animations from the Student CD-ROM. This supplement is available to faculty free upon adoption of the textbook.

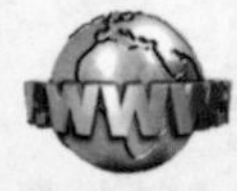

Companion Website Syllabus Manager
www.prenhall.com/ball
Faculty adopting this textbook have free access to the online Syllabus Manager feature of the Companion Website, www.prenhall.com/ball. It offers a whole host of features that facilitate the students' use of the Companion Website, and allows faculty to post syllabi and course information online for their students. For more information or a demonstration of Syllabus Manager, please contact your Prentice Hall Sales Representative.

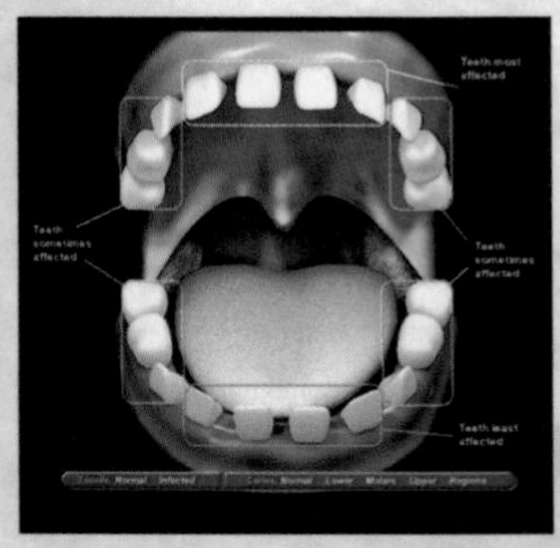

Online Course Management Systems
A variety of online course management companions are available. The online course management solutions feature interactive modules, electronic test bank, PowerPoint images, animations and assessments. For more information about adopting an online course management system to accompany Pediatric Nursing, 3rd Edition please contact your Prentice Hall Health Sales Representative or go online to www.prenhall.com/demo.

BRIEF CONTENTS

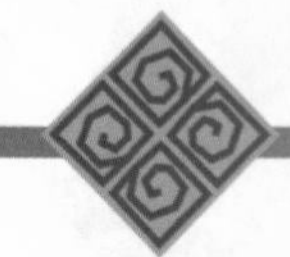

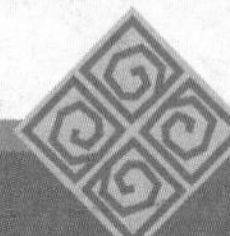
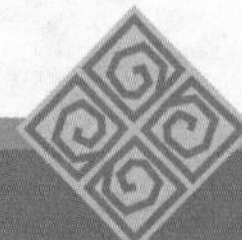
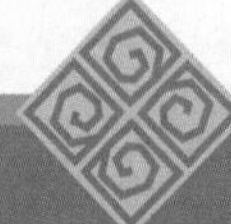

Third Edition

Pediatric Nursing

CARING FOR CHILDREN

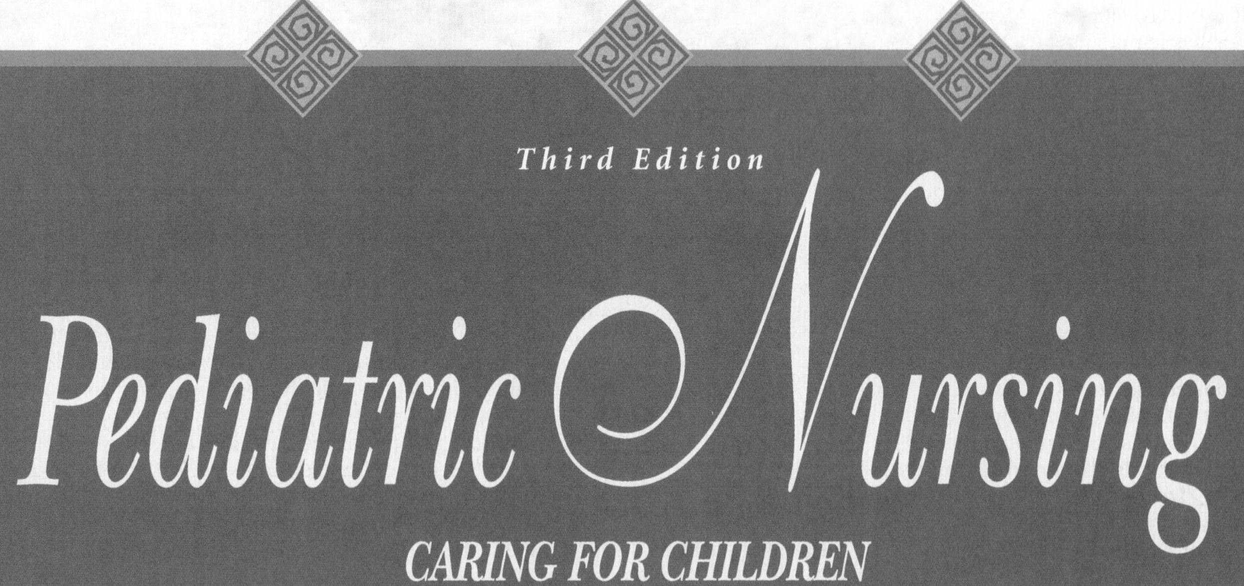

Third Edition

Pediatric Nursing

CARING FOR CHILDREN

Jane W. Ball, RN, CPNP, DrPH

Executive Director, Emergency Medical Services for Children National Resource Center, Children's National Medical Center, Washington, D.C.

Ruth C. Bindler, RNC, PhD

Associate Professor, Intercollegiate College of Nursing Washington State University Spokane, Washington

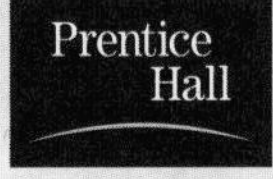

Upper Saddle River, New Jersey 07458

Library of Congress Cataloging-in-Publication Data

Pediatric nursing : caring for children/[edited by] Jane W. Ball, Ruth Bindler.—3rd ed.
p. ; cm.
Includes bibliographical references and index.
ISBN 0-13-099405-7
1. Pediatric nursing. I. Ball, Jane II. Bindler, Ruth McGillis.
[DNLM: 1. Pediatric Nursing—methods. 2. Nursing Assessment—methods. 3. Nursing Care—Child. 4. Nursing Care—Infant. WY 159 P3733 2003]
RJ245 .P4414 2003
610.73'62—dc21

2002066781

Publisher: Julie Levin Alexander
Assistant to Publisher: Regina Bruno
Executive Editor: Maura Connor
Senior Managing Editor: Marilyn Meserve
Development Editor: Kim Wyatt
Assistant Editor: Yesenia Kopperman
Editorial Assistant: Sladjana Repic
Director of Production and Manufacturing: Bruce Johnson
Managing Production Editor: Patrick Walsh
Production Liaison: Danielle Newhouse
Production Editor: Lori Dalberg, Carlisle Publishers Services
Manufacturing Manager: Ilene Sanford
Design Director: Cheryl Asherman
Design Coordinator: Maria Guglielmo
Interior Designer: Donna Wickes
Cover Designer: Cheryl Asherman
Electronic Art Creation: Precision Graphics
Photographers: Roy Ramsey & George Dodson
Manager of Media Production: Amy Peltier
New Media Project Manager: Stephen Hartner
New Media Production: Jack Yensen, Synergy
Marketing Manager: Nicole Benson
Marketing Coordinator: Janet Ryerson
Production Information Manager: Rachele Strober
Composition: Carlisle Communications, Ltd.
Cover Printer: Phoenix Color Corp.
Printing and Binding: Von Hoffmann Press

Notice: Care has been taken to confirm the accuracy of information presented in this book. The authors, editors, and the publisher, however, cannot accept any responsibility for errors or omissions or for consequences from application of the information in this book and make no warranty, express or implied, with respect to its contents.

The authors and publisher have exerted every effort to ensure that drug selections and dosages set forth in this text are in accord with current recommendations and practice at time of publication. However, in view of ongoing research, changes in government regulations, and the constant flow of information relating to drug therapy and drug reactions, the reader is urged to check the package inserts of all drugs for any change in indications of dosage and for added warnings and precautions. This is particularly important when the recommended agent is a new and/or infrequently employed drug.

Pearson Education, LTD
Pearson Education Australia PTY, Limited
Pearson Education Singapore, Pte. Ltd.
Pearson Education North Asia Ltd.
Pearson Education Canada, Ltd.
Pearson Educación de Mexico, S.A. de C.V.
Pearson Education—Japan
Pearson Education Malaysia, Pte. Ltd.

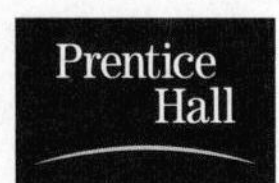

10 9 8 7 6 5 4 3 2 1
ISBN 0-13-099405-7

CONTENTS

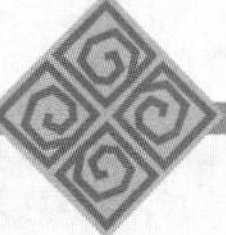
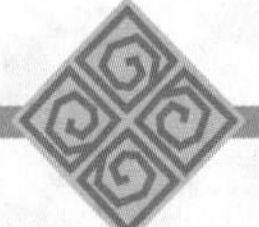

CHAPTER 8 The Child with a Life-Threatening Illness or Injury 263

CHAPTER 9 Pain Assessment and Management 287

CHAPTER 10 Alterations in Fluid, Electrolyte, and Acid-Base Balance 309

CHAPTER 14 Alterations in Cardiovascular Function 469

CHAPTER 15 Alterations in Hematologic Function 513

CHAPTER 16 Alterations in Cellular Growth 537

PREFACE

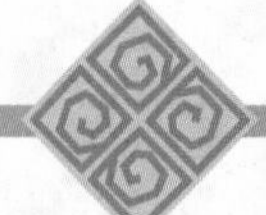
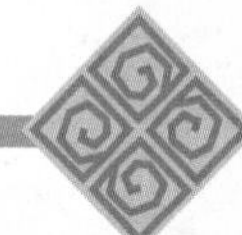

Pediatric nursing, like all of health care, is changing rapidly. Student nurses must learn what helps them to provide safe and effective care today, while integrating new knowledge and skills needed for nursing practice in the future. Faculty have the responsibility of teaching students to provide pediatric nursing care today, while equipping them to meet tomorrow's unknown health care challenges.

The goal of the third edition of this textbook is to provide core pediatric nursing knowledge that prepares students for practice, and to offer the tools of critical thinking needed to apply this learning to future challenges. Students must learn to question, to evaluate the research and experiences of others, to apply information in many settings, and to constantly adapt to changes while providing high-quality nursing care.

This textbook reflects a multitude of approaches to learning that can be helpful to all students. We acknowledge that many students learn pediatric nursing in a very short time period. Therefore, the approaches in this textbook are designed to help all students assess the child's needs and to make care decisions based on the standards of pediatric nursing practice.

Realities of Pediatric Nursing

The first edition of this textbook focused on the nursing care of children and their families in acute care environments. In the second edition, the focus was broadened to reflect the dramatic shift of pediatric health care out of the hospital and into ambulatory, home, and community settings. Many procedures are performed in short-stay units, and long-term care is often provided at home for children with complex health conditions. In the third edition, the trend for provision of care in a wide variety of settings is a continuing focus. Families are often the providers of care and case managers for children with complex health care challenges. Technological advances are resulting in earlier diagnoses and new therapies, and this content is integrated throughout the textbook.

Pediatric nursing care is provided within the context of a rapidly changing society. An examination of the major morbidities and mortalities of childhood guided the addition of new material and topics throughout the text. A new chapter on childhood nutrition addresses the influences of nutrition and associated conditions on long-term health of the individual. Another new chapter focuses on the common societal and environmental influences on health care that all nurses must understand when designing interventions to promote health. A continuing emphasis on the influence of injury is integrated throughout the book, with descriptions about the necessity of prevention and the impact of injury on mortality, hospitalization, disability, and health care needs.

Many graduating nurses practice in acute care facilities, and this textbook continues to emphasize the information necessary to prepare students for working in those settings. In addition, the information provided in this textbook will enable graduates to assume positions in ambulatory care facilities, home health nursing, schools, and a variety of other settings. Effective communication methods, principles of working with families, and knowledge of pathophysiologic, psychologic, and environmental factors found in this book can all be applied to a wide variety of settings.

Another major change in our society involves access to information and reliance on the Internet. In this edition, MediaLink icons send the student online to obtain the very latest information available on many topics. Nurses must learn to obtain information and then to analyze and judge the quality of information they find. Nurses must also assist children and family members to use the Internet wisely to help them in making health care decisions. Integration of websites throughout the book and exercises to examine and evaluate various sites assist the students applying this technology.

Organization and Integrated Themes

This book is organized by body system, as it is an easy approach for students to use when seeking information, studying, and preparing to care for children and families. This organizational framework also eliminates redundancy, which occurs when a developmental approach is used, thereby contributing to the concise approach in this textbook.

Several topics essential to comprehensive nursing care of children do not directly relate to body systems. Separate chapters with these important concepts provide foundational information for nursing care. These include growth and development, physical assessment, nutrition, societal and environmental influences on health, and mental health. Other chapters address care of the child in the hospital and in community settings, pain management, and needs of child and family during life-threatening conditions. Throughout the textbook, we integrate information that is pertinent to care for children related to age, culture, and family.

The nursing process is used as the framework for nursing care. **Nursing Management** is the major heading, with subheadings of **Nursing Assessment and Diagnosis, Planning and Implementation,** and **Evaluation.** When it is appropriate to focus on care in a specific setting, Care in the Community, Hospital-based Care, and Discharge Planning and Home Care Teaching are separated into sections. We feature **nursing care plans** throughout the text to help students approach care from the nursing process perspective. These nursing care plans include Nursing Intervention Classifications (NIC) and Nursing Outcome Classifications (NOC).

Several major concepts are integrated throughout the textbook to encourage the student to think creatively and critically about nursing care. These major themes are interwoven through narrative, margin boxes, art figures and captions, CD-ROM offerings, and Companion Website activities. This layout results in a comprehensive and unique presentation that engages students and makes them active participants in the learning process. The major concepts integrated throughout the learning materials are as follows:

- ***Nursing care*** is the critical and central core of this textbook. Nursing assessment and management are emphasized in all sections of the book, with nurses shown providing care in a variety of settings.
- ***Critical thinking and problem-solving principles*** are integrated in the organization, pedagogy, writing style, CD exercises, and art captions. Students practice critical thinking in their everyday lives, but need help to apply these concepts to the practice of nursing. This book and the accompanying learning materials help students understand how their normal curiosity and problem-solving ability can be applied to pediatric nursing. Students learn what questions to ask, how to ask them, where to find answers, and how to provide information to others.
- ***Communication*** is one of the most important skills that students need to learn. Effective communication with children is challenging because they communicate differently according to their developmental levels. Family members have communication needs in addition to those of their children. This book integrates communication skills by applied examples that help the student to communicate effectively with children and their families.
- ***Teaching*** about health care is an integral part of the pediatric nurse's responsibilities. Since hospitalizations are short and families increasingly care for children at home, information about health care needs and procedures have become even more important.

- ***Developing cultural competence*** is critical for all nurses in the increasingly diverse community of today's world. Students have all met people from different ethnic and cultural groups but they need help to understand, respect, and integrate differing beliefs, practices, and health care needs when providing care.
- ***Growth and development considerations*** and ***physical assessment*** are central to the effective practice of pediatric nursing. A separate chapter is devoted to each area, Chapters 2 and 4 respectively. In addition, both topics are integrated where appropriate in narrative, figures, captions, and on the CD.
- ***Legal and ethical considerations*** are provided throughout the text to sensitize students to thinking about the implications of nursing care. They are encouraged to learn the legal ramifications of actions, the ethical decision-making process in difficult situations, and their own personal and professional responsibilities.
- ***Home care considerations*** and ***community care considerations*** are an increasing part of nursing responsibilities. To assist students in transferring knowledge to caring for children in community settings, both narrative and boxes address this information in nursing management sections of chapters. In addition, an entire chapter is devoted to nursing care in the community and directly addressing the nurse's roles in these settings.

Features

Each chapter has undergone significant revision to update clinical information and resources. Content has been shifted and added to reflect current pediatric issues and care. New chapters include nutrition, and environmental and societal influences on health. There is an increased emphasis on home and community care, and families are integrated when possible.

Each chapter begins with a **chapter opening scenario** and photo illustrating a child with specific nursing care needs. This is accompanied by a list of **key terms.** A new feature, **MediaLink,** identifies specific content, animations, activities, and resources available to students on the accompanying student CD-ROM and Companion Website. Each chapter ends with a chapter review that consists of a summary of **chapter highlights,** a list of **references,** and a new section entitled **Explore MediaLink.** This last section encourages students to use the additional chapter-specific NCLEX review, exercises, and resources available on the accompanying free student CD-ROM and the Companion Website at *www.prenhall.com/ball.*

We have integrated features into the body systems chapters to enhance student learning. Based on feedback from prior users of the textbook, new **Pathophysiology Illustrated** boxes visually explain the pathophysiology of certain conditions in a format that the student can understand and apply. **As They Grow** boxes illustrate the anatomic and physiologic differences between children and adults. This enhances students' knowledge in association with a specific topic and helps them to apply theoretical information in practical situations. The **Clinical Manifestation** feature presents the etiology, clinical presentation, and clinical therapy for selected conditions. **Medications Used to Treat** boxes feature drug information for specific conditions when appropriate.

Numerous margin boxes relate directly to nursing care. These include **Clinical Tips, Safety Precautions,** and **Nursing Alerts.** To reflect the growing cultural diversity of the United States and Canada, **Culture** boxes are also integrated throughout the narrative, offering diverse perspectives and highlighting cultural variations in health care when appropriate. An added feature in this edition is the inclusion of boxes on **complementary and alternative practices,** which may be connected with cultural groups or other belief and practices, thus influencing health care practices. **Law and Ethics, Community Care, Research,** and **Home Care** boxes highlight the issues challenging nurses today, while **Growth and Development** boxes help to highlight nursing care at various stages of development.

Since nurses are frequent teachers of children and families, we are introducing the **Families Want to Know** feature, which offers information about the specific teaching that nurses will need to provide. This feature provides teaching that can benefit families as they care for children.

Art and Design

The first edition of this textbook pioneered a unique approach to narrative, figures, and captions that prevented duplication of information between the text and art. Many photographs prepared students for the realities of the clinical settings. This approach was continued in the second edition and has been enhanced even further in the third edition. The focus is on the child within a family and the many settings in which children are seen.

In the new edition, photographs reflect the changing society in which we all live, present realistic clinical situations, and challenge students to plan creative nursing approaches. Captions and margin material explain, question, and add to the students' learning. This approach ties explanations directly to the art rather than forcing the student to move back and forth between text and art. Figures and overlays on photos explain pathophysiology and demonstrate anatomical variations. This encourages students to think about what they are seeing and to test their knowledge, rather than passively absorbing information.

Special cross-reference icons are placed to refer students to further supplementary information found in the **Clinical Skills Manual**, the **CD-ROM**, the **Companion Website**, or in other sections of the textbook itself. These additional resources will enhance their knowledge even further and provide more experience in questioning resources and planning care. Students appreciate the variety in presentation techniques and readily engage with the material.

Comprehensive Teaching and Learning Package

Instructors and students alike value the in-text learning aids included in our textbook. We have developed a textbook that is easy to absorb and use as a reference. To enhance the teaching and learning process, the following supplements have been developed in close correlation with the new edition of *Pediatric Nursing: Caring for Children.* The full complement of supplemental teaching materials is available to all qualified instructors from your Prentice Hall Health sales representative.

Student CD-ROM. The student CD-ROM includes NCLEX-style multiple-choice questions that emphasize the application of nursing care. Students can test their knowledge and gain immediate feedback through rationales for right and wrong answers. The CD-ROM also provides several animations to help students understand and visualize difficult concepts in pediatric nursing care, as well as a comprehensive audio glossary of key terms. The CD-ROM also allows access to the Companion Website described later in this section. This CD-ROM is packaged free with every copy of the textbook.

Clinical Skills Manual. The full-color, highly visual, clinical skills manual describes several commonly performed pediatric nursing skills and clearly illustrates the steps to perform each skill. It is assumed that students have already had a basic skills course, so the material presented is designed to focus on techniques that are specific to pediatrics patients. Both hospital-based and community-based skills are included. Margin boxes emphasize material such as clinical tips and safety considerations. The protocols for performing skills contain rationales when needed to clarify recommended actions. This skills manual is available separately or at a special discount if packaged with the textbook.

Instructor's Resource Manual. This effective and timesaving aid has been revised and streamlined. It provides suggestions for covering important content and is organized by topics according to subject matter. It also includes an updated test bank that helps faculty quickly and easily create numerous unique examinations. Test items follow the NCLEX format and are classified by cognitive level, nursing process step, and client need. This manual also provides a guide to the instructor for using the accompanying CD-ROM and Companion Website.

Instructor's Resource CD-ROM. New to this package, the instructor's resource CD-ROM provides three resources in an electronic format. First, the CD-ROM includes testing software. Second, it includes a comprehensive collection of images from the textbook in PowerPoint format, so faculty can easily import these photographs and illustrations into their own classroom lecture presentations. Finally, it provides access to all animations and clips that are found on the student CD-ROM accompanying the textbook.

Companion Website and Syllabus Manager®. The new edition features a free Companion Website at *www.prenhall.com/ball.* This website serves as a text-specific, interactive online workbook to *Pediatric Nursing: Caring for Children, Third Edition.* The Companion Website includes modules for objectives, chapter outlines, audio glossary of key terms, discussion questions with essay responses, NCLEX review questions with automatic grading, links to other sites for student research, care map activities, and more. Instructors adopting this textbook for their courses have free access to an online syllabus manager with a whole host of features that facilitate the students' use of this Companion Website and allow faculty to post their syllabi online for their students. For more information or a demonstration of the syllabus manager, please contact your Prentice Hall Health sales representative or go online to www.prenhall.com/demo.

Online Course Management Systems. Online course companions are available for schools using course management systems. For more information about adopting an online course management system to accompany **Pediatric Nursing: Caring for Children, Third Edition,** please contact your Prentice Hall Health sales representative or go online to *www.prenhall.com/demo.*

In the third edition, we continued to make difficult choices about what to include and how extensively to cover each topic. Our decisions reflect feedback from faculty and students, the shifting challenges of pediatric health, and new technology available in both health care and education. We are confident that this book represents the very core of pediatric nursing and will help students prepare for and assume important roles as pediatric nurses.

Jane W. Ball
Ruth C. Bindler

REVIEWERS

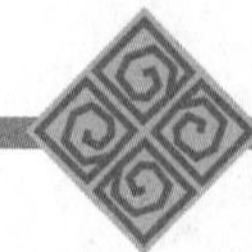

Marie Mangin Adorno, RN, MN
Assistant Professor of Nursing
Our Lady Holy Cross College
New Orleans, Louisiana

Kathleen Bush, RN
Mount Timpanogos Women's Health Care
Pleasant Grove, Utah

Jill Cash, RN, CS, MSN, FNP
Instructor, Nurse Practitioner
Southern Illinois University-Edwardsville
Edwardsville, Illinois

Barbara L. Coleman, MSN, RN, CPNP
Assistant Professor
Sinclair Community College
Dayton, Ohio

Nancy Copperman, MS, RP
Nutritionist
Schneider Children's Hospital
New Hyde Park, New York

Isabel Maria D. Couto, RN, BSN
Endocrinology Nurse
Children's National Medical Center
Washington, D.C.

Pamela S. Covault, RN, MS
Neosho County Community College
Chanute, Kansas

Cheryl DeGraw, RN, MSN, CRNP
Instructor
Florence–Darlington Technical College
Florence, South Carolina

Carol L. Doubblestein, MSN, RN, CPN
Nursing Faculty
Grand Rapids Community College
Grand Rapids, Michigan

Hobie Etta Feagai, BSN, MSN
Assistant Professor/Academic Coordinator, Undergraduate Programs
Hawaii Pacific University
Kaneohe, Hawaii

Margaret Fitzgerald
Nursing Faculty
Midwestern State University
Wichita Falls, Texas

Dawn Garzon, RN, CS, CPNP, PhD(c)
Barnes College of Nursing
University of Missouri
St. Louis, Missouri

Jane V. Harris, RN, MSN
Assistant Professor of Nursing
University of Southern Mississippi
Hattiesburg, Mississippi

Judith K. Hovey, PhD, RN, CPNP
Assistant Professor
Oakland University School of Nursing
Rochester, Michigan

Susan M. Mlynarczyk, RN, MS
Assistant Professor of Nursing
Hope College
Holland, Michigan

Kathy A. Russell, RNC, MSN
Nursing Faculty
Front Range Community College
Westminster, Colorado

Marsha Black Simpkins, RN, MSN, CPNP
Instructor
Southern Illinois University–Edwardsville
Edwardsville, Illinois

Jane Turek, RN, MSN, CDE
Diabetes Clinical Nurse Specialist
Children's National Medical Center
Washington, D.C.

Rochelle Williams, RN, MSN, CPNP
Clinical Instructor
Texas Women's University
Houston, Texas

ACKNOWLEDGMENTS

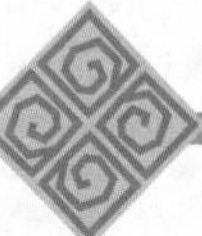 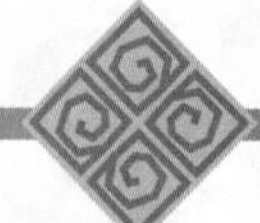 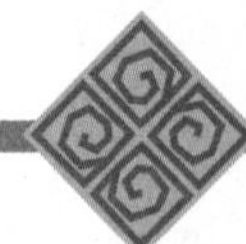

It is both exciting and challenging to have the opportunity to write a textbook. It is wonderful to observe the evolution of pediatric nursing practice, and to encourage nursing students to share our excitement and enthusiasm for working with children and their families. Although each edition carries its own unique set of challenges and circumstances, it is a privilege to contribute to the education of a new generation of student nurses.

This edition has undergone significant changes and integrates some style preferences and capabilities of our new publishing company, Prentice Hall Health. Maura Connor became our nursing editor, and she had a dream and vision of the potential for development of this textbook that matched our own. The vice president and publisher, Julie Alexander, enthusiastically supported this venture. Both have supported us in decisions regarding changes, updates, and features for the text.

Our developmental editor, Kim Wyatt, new to this edition, has been a tireless proponent for the approach, philosophy, and conceptual framework underlying the text. She explained our goals to others, and worked endlessly to enhance and organize the materials we provided. This effort could not have succeeded without her.

The Prentice Hall Health managing editor, Marilyn Meserve, was an important liaison for editorial consultation with Prentice Hall Health. Editorial Assistant Sladjana Repic was essential in facilitating communications with Prentice Hall; her pleasant and competent manners were outstanding. We thank Danielle Newhouse, production editor, Patrick Walsh, production managing editor, and Nicole Benson, senior marketing manager, for their expertise and valuable contributions. Our thanks also go to Cheryl Asherman, design director, for creating the fresh textbook design. Media editor Sarah Hayday helped bring our media ideas to fruition. At Carlisle Communications, we thank Lori Dalberg for coordinating production, and Carey Lange for her copyediting skills. Sharon Stoffels, from Boise State University, helped assemble content for the student CD-ROM, and the following people assembled the content for the Companion Website: Nancy Wagner, MSN, RN, Youngstown State University, Ohio; Kimberly Serroka, MSN, RN, Youngstown State University, Ohio; Bernadette Dragich, PhD, RN, FNP, Bluefield State College, West Virginia; and Tina Magers, MSN, RN, Mississippi College, Mississippi.

Other individuals made major contributions to this textbook. George Dodson and Roy Ramsey are dedicated and meticulous photographers who have worked with us for all editions. They have an amazing talent in capturing beautiful and creative images of children and families. Several agencies allowed us to photograph children. In Washington, D.C., they include Childrens National Medical Center, the Hospital for Sick Children, and Lafayette Elementary School. Wayne Neal, RN, MAT, was instrumental in helping us capture the children in these facilities. In Spokane, Washington, children were photographed at Shriners Hospital for Children, Sacred Heart Medical Center, All Seasons Child Care Center, and Central Valley Schools. Many students and parents agreed to have their children photographed in the practice laboratory of the Intercollegiate College of Nursing/Washington State College of Nursing. Connie Boleneus provided invaluable assistance in the photography of skills on children. Above all, we sincerely thank the children and families who allowed us to illustrate development, pediatric health care conditions, and nursing care by photographing children in hospital, home, and community settings. We also acknowledge the contributors from the first edition of this textbook:

Jan Dalby, RNC, MS
(Alterations in Geritourinary Function)

Linda Felver, RN, PhD
(Alterations in Fluid and Electrolyte and Acid–Base Balance)

Darla Gowan, RN, FNPC, MN
(Alterations in Skin Integrity)

Joyce Griffin, RN, OCN, PhD
(Alterations in Immune Function, Alterations in Hematologic Function)

Sandra Jo Hammer, RN, MPH, MSN
(Infectious and Communicable Diseases)

Linda Kinrade, RN, PNP, MN
(Alterations in Cellular Growth)

Katherine Morris, RN, CPNP
(Alterations in Endocrine Function)

Jean Moss, ARNP, CPNP, PhD
(Alterations in Eye, Ear, Nose, and Throat Function)

Ruth Novitt-Schumacher, RN, MSN
(Alterations in Gastrointestinal Function)

Nan Peterson, RN, MS
(The Child with a Life-Threatening Illness or Injury)

Deborah Thomas, RNC, MSN
(Alterations in Psychosocial Function)

Robert Wayner, MD
(Alterations in Neurologic Function)

Amy Weigelt-Leinweber, RN, BSN
(Alterations in Musculoskeletal Function)

Marcia Wellington, RN, MS
(Alterations in Neurologic Function, Atlas of Pediatric Procedures)

Rosemarie C. Westberg, RN, MSN
(Alterations in Respiratory Function)

Finally, our families once again have supported us tirelessly through the revision process. They sacrificed by allowing us to work on the book when we could have been with them. Yet, they show others the book with pride. We could not have accomplished this without their love and patience.

ABOUT THE AUTHORS

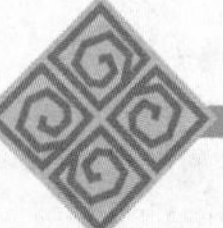

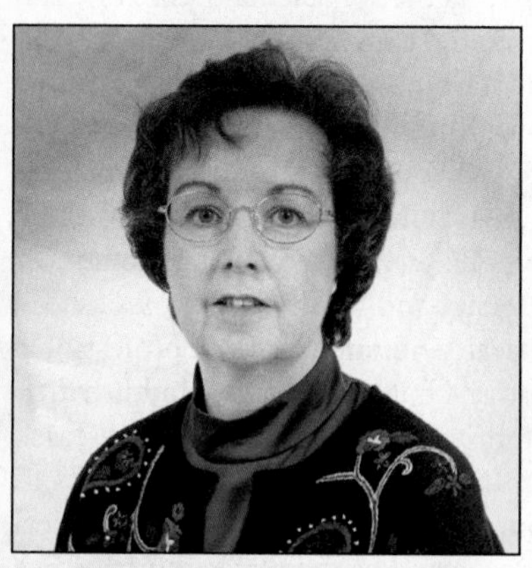

JANE W. BALL, RN, CPNP, DRPH Dr. Jane W. Ball graduated from the Johns Hopkins Hospital School of Nursing, and subsequently received a Bachelor of Science degree from the Johns Hopkins University. She worked in the surgical, pediatric emergency, and outpatient units of the Johns Hopkins Children's Medical and Surgical Center, first as a staff nurse and then as a pediatric nurse practitioner. This began her career as a pediatric nurse and advocate for children's health needs.

Jane obtained both Master of Public Health and Doctor of Public Health degrees from the Johns Hopkins University Bloomberg School of Public Health with a focus on maternal and child health. After graduation she became the chief of child health services for the Commonwealth of Pennsylvania Department of Health. In this capacity she oversaw the state-funded well-child clinics and explored ways to improve education for the state's community health nurses. After relocating to Texas, Jane joined the faculty at the University of Texas at Arlington School of Nursing to teach community pediatrics to registered nurses returning to school for a Bachelor of Science in Nursing degree. During this time she became involved in writing her first textbook, *Mosby's Guide to Physical Examination,* which is currently in its fifth edition.

After relocating to the Washington, D.C., area, she joined Children's National Medical Center to manage a federal project to teach instructors of emergency medical technicians from all states about the special care children need during an emergency. Exposure to the shortcomings of the emergency medical services system in the late 1980s with regard to pediatric care was a career-changing event. With federal funding, she developed educational curricula for emergency medical technicians and emergency nurses to help them provide improved care for children. A textbook, entitled *Pediatric Emergencies, A Manual for Prehospital Providers,* was developed from these educational ventures.

For the past 10 years, Jane has managed the federally funded Emergency Medical Services for Children National Resource Center. As executive director, she directs the provision of consultation and resource development for state health agencies, health professionals, families and advocates about successful methods to improve the health care system so that children receive optimal emergency care in all health care settings.

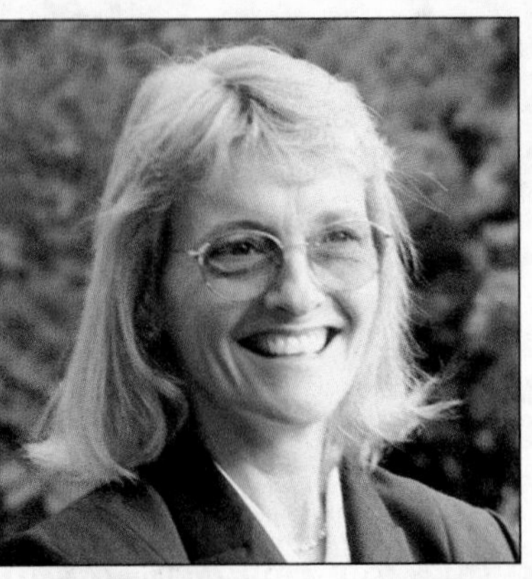

RUTH C. BINDLER, RNC, PhD Dr. Ruth Bindler received her Bachelor of Science in Nursing degree from Cornell University—New York Hospital School of Nursing in New York. She worked in oncology nursing at Sloan Kettering Cancer Center in New York, and then moved to Wisconsin and became a public health nurse there in Dane County. Thus began her commitment to work in pediatrics as she visited children and their families at home, and served as a school nurse for several elementary, middle, and high schools. Due to this interest in child health care needs, she earned a Master of Science degree in Child Development from the University of Wisconsin.

A move to Washington State was accompanied by a new job as a faculty member at the Intercollegiate Center for Nursing Education in Spokane. Ruth has been fortunate to be involved for 28 years in the growth of this nursing education consortium, which is a combination of public and private universities and colleges and is now the Intercollegiate College of Nursing/Washington State University College of Nursing. Presently she teaches the theory course in child health and a course on cultural diversity and health, and serves as lead faculty for the theory and clinical components of child health nursing. Her first professional book, *Pediatric Medications,* was published in 1981, and she has continued to publish articles and books in the areas of pediatric medications and pediatric health. Special research interests are cardiovascular risk factors and diabetes in children, topics that were the focus of her recent Doctor of Philosophy work in Human Nutrition at Washington State University. Ethnic diversity has been another theme in Ruth's work. She facilitates international and other diversity experiences for students, performs research with culturally diverse children, and works with underserved populations.

Ruth believes that her role as a faculty member has enabled her to learn continually, to foster the development of students in nursing, and to participate fully in the profession of nursing. In addition to teaching, research, publication, and leadership, she enhances her life by service in several professional and community organizations, and through activities with her family.

GUIDE TO *Pediatric Nursing*

THIRD EDITION

KEY TERMS

Key terms introduce each chapter with comprehensive definitions for each term. An Audio Glossary of each term is available on the Student CD-ROM and the Companion Website.

CHAPTER OPENING SCENARIO

Each chapter begins with a Chapter Opening Scenario and photo illustrating a child with specific nursing care needs that will be addressed later in the chapter.

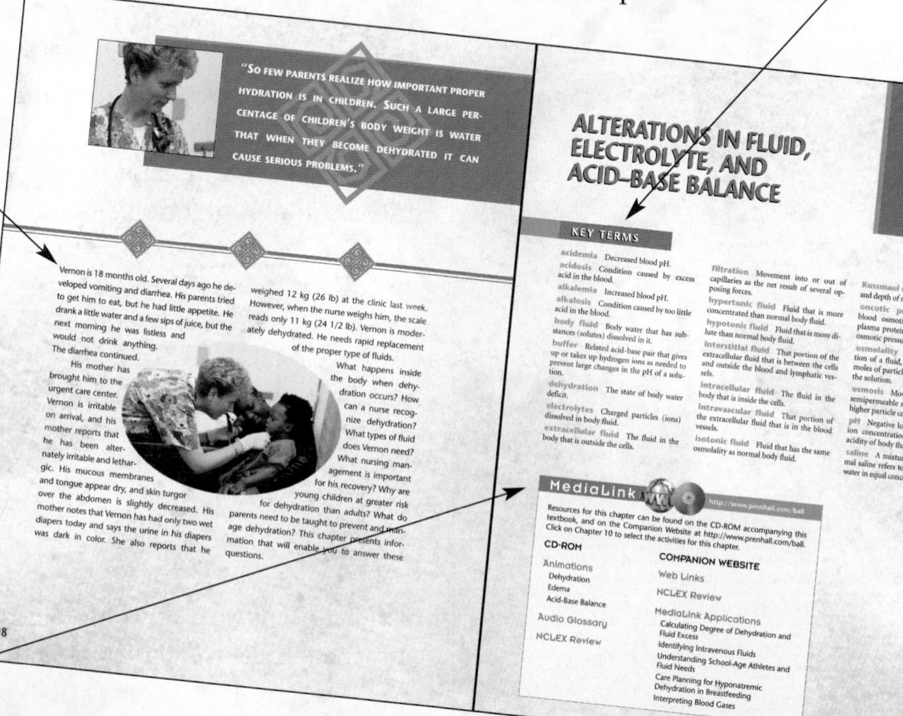

"SO FEW PARENTS REALIZE HOW IMPORTANT PROPER HYDRATION IS IN CHILDREN. SUCH A LARGE PERCENTAGE OF CHILDREN'S BODY WEIGHT IS WATER THAT WHEN THEY BECOME DEHYDRATED IT CAN CAUSE SERIOUS PROBLEMS."

Vernon is 18 months old. Several days ago he developed vomiting and diarrhea. His parents tried to get him to eat, but he had little appetite. He drank a little water and a few sips of juice, but the next morning he was listless and would not drink anything. The diarrhea continued.

His mother has brought him to the urgent care center. Vernon is irritable on arrival, and his mother reports that he has been alternately irritable and lethargic. His mucous membranes and tongue appear dry, and skin turgor over the abdomen is slightly decreased. His mother notes that Vernon has had only two wet diapers today and says the urine in his diapers was dark in color. She also reports that he weighed 12 kg (26 lb) at the clinic last week. However, when the nurse weighs him, the scale reads only 11 kg (24 1/2 lb). Vernon is moderately dehydrated. He needs rapid replacement of the proper type of fluids.

What happens inside the body when dehydration occurs? How can a nurse recognize dehydration? What types of fluid does Vernon need? What nursing management is important for his recovery? Why are young children at greater risk for dehydration than adults? What do parents need to be taught to prevent and manage dehydration? This chapter presents information that will enable you to answer these questions.

308

CHAPTER 10

ALTERATIONS IN FLUID, ELECTROLYTE, AND ACID–BASE BALANCE

KEY TERMS

acidemia Decreased blood pH.
acidosis Condition caused by excess acid in the blood.
alkalemia Increased blood pH.
alkalosis Condition caused by too little acid in the blood.
body fluid Body water that has substances (solutes) dissolved in it.
buffer Related acid-base pair that gives up or takes up hydrogen ions as needed to prevent large changes in the pH of a solution.
dehydration The state of body water deficit.
electrolytes Charged particles (ions) dissolved in body fluid.
extracellular fluid The fluid in the body that is outside the cells.
filtration Movement into or out of capillaries as the net result of several opposing forces.
hypertonic fluid Fluid that is more concentrated than normal body fluid.
hypotonic fluid Fluid that is more dilute than normal body fluid.
interstitial fluid That portion of the extracellular fluid that is between the cells and outside the blood and lymphatic vessels.
intracellular fluid The fluid in the body that is inside the cells.
intravascular fluid That portion of the extracellular fluid that is in the blood vessels.
isotonic fluid Fluid that has the same osmolality as normal body fluid.
Kussmaul respirations Increased rate and depth of respirations (hyperventilation).
oncotic pressure The part of the blood osmotic pressure that is due to plasma proteins; also called blood colloid osmotic pressure.
osmolality The amount of concentration of a fluid, technically, the number of moles of particles per kilogram of water in the solution.
osmosis Movement of water across a semipermeable membrane into an area of higher particle concentration.
pH Negative logarithm of the hydrogen ion concentration; used to monitor the acidity of body fluid.
saline A mixture of salt and water; normal saline refers to the mixture of salt and water in equal concentration in body fluids.

MediaLink http://www.prenhall.com/ball

Resources for this chapter can be found on the CD-ROM accompanying this textbook, and on the Companion Website at http://www.prenhall.com/ball. Click on Chapter 10 to select the activities for this chapter.

CD-ROM
Animations
Dehydration
Edema
Acid-Base Balance
Audio Glossary
NCLEX Review

COMPANION WEBSITE
Web Links
NCLEX Review
MediaLink Applications
Calculating Degree of Dehydration and Fluid Excess
Identifying Intravenous Fluids
Understanding School-Age Athletes and Fluid Needs
Care Planning for Hyponatremic Dehydration in Breastfeeding
Interpreting Blood Gases

309

MEDIALINK

MediaLink introduces each chapter of the text and lists additional specific content, animations, NCLEX Review, tools, and other interactive exercises, which appear on the accompanying Student CD-ROM and the Companion Website.

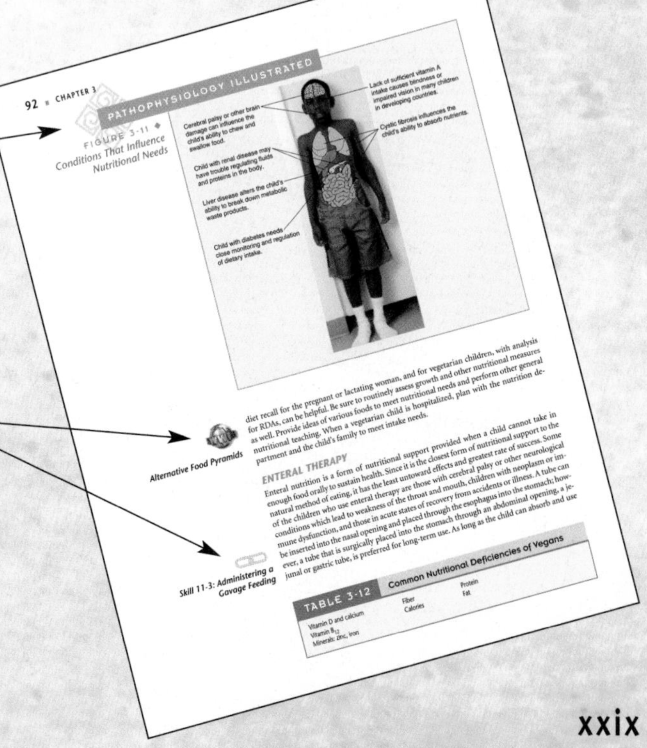

92 ▪ CHAPTER 3

PATHOPHYSIOLOGY ILLUSTRATED

FIGURE 3-11 ◆ Conditions That Influence Nutritional Needs

Alternative Food Pyramids

diet recall for the pregnant or lactating woman, and for vegetarian children, with analysis for RDAs, can be helpful. Be sure to routinely assess growth and other nutritional measures as well. Provide ideas of various foods to meet nutritional needs and perform other general nutritional teaching. When a vegetarian child is hospitalized, plan with the nutrition department and the child's family to meet intake needs.

ENTERAL THERAPY

Enteral nutrition is a form of nutritional support provided when a child cannot take in enough food orally to sustain health. Since it is the closest form of nutritional support to the natural method of eating, it has the least untoward effects and greatest rate of success. Some of the children who use enteral therapy are those with cerebral palsy or other neurological conditions which lead to weakness of the throat and mouth, children with neoplasm or immune dysfunction, and those in acute states of recovery from accidents or illness. A tube can be inserted into the nasal opening and placed through the esophagus into the stomach; however, a tube that is surgically placed into the stomach through an abdominal opening, a jejunal or gastric tube, is preferred for long-term use. As long as the child can absorb and use

Skill 11-3: Administering a Gavage Feeding

TABLE 3-12 Common Nutritional Deficiencies of Vegans

Vitamin D and calcium	Fiber	Protein
Vitamin B_{12}	Calories	Fat
Minerals: zinc, iron		

PATHOPHYSIOLOGY ILLUSTRATED

New Pathophysiology Illustrated boxes visually explain the pathophysiology of certain conditions as they affect children in a format that students can understand and apply.

CROSS-REFERENCE ICONS

There are three types of icons that appear regularly throughout the textbook margins. The CD and Website icons refer students to animations, additional content, resources or activities contained in the media supplements that will further enhance their clinical knowledge and critical thinking. The link icon [link icon] refers students to specific pediatric skills in the accompanying Clinical Skills Manual.

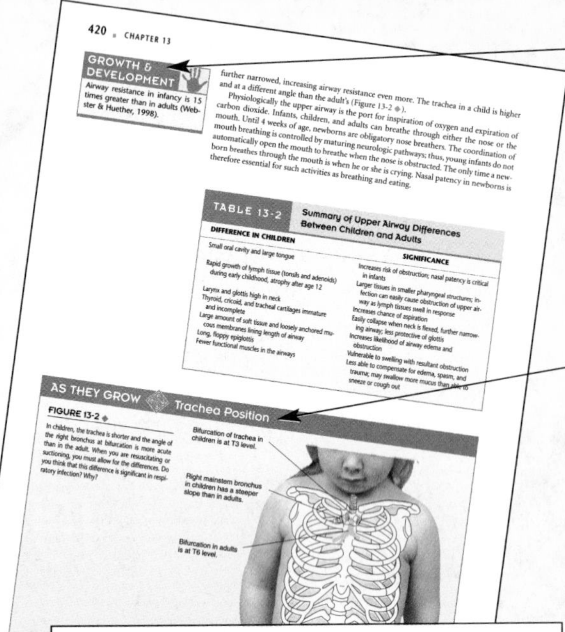

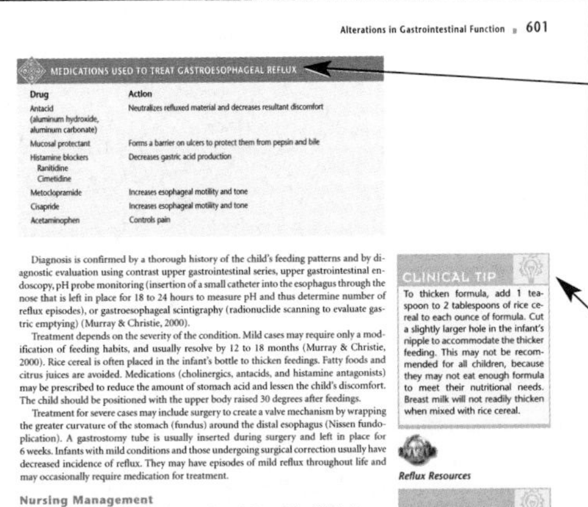

GROWTH & DEVELOPMENT

Growth and Development boxes help students focus nursing care at various stages of development.

AS THEY GROW

As They Grow boxes illustrate the anatomic and physiologic differences between children and adults. This enhances students' knowledge in association with a specific topic and helps them to apply theoretical information in practical situations.

MEDICATIONS USED TO TREAT

Medications Used to Treat boxes feature drug information for specific conditions when appropriate.

CLINICAL TIPS

Clinical Tips boxes throughout the margins offer practical hints for clinical practice.

HOME CARE

Home Care boxes throughout the margins assist students in applying to care for children in home settings, as well as preparing the family to care for the child at home.

CULTURE

Culture boxes are integrated throughout the narrative, offering diverse perspectives and highlighting cultural differences when appropriate.

FAMILIES WANT TO KNOW

These boxes offer information about the specific teaching that nurses will need to provide. This feature helps nurses provide teaching that can benefit families as they care for children.

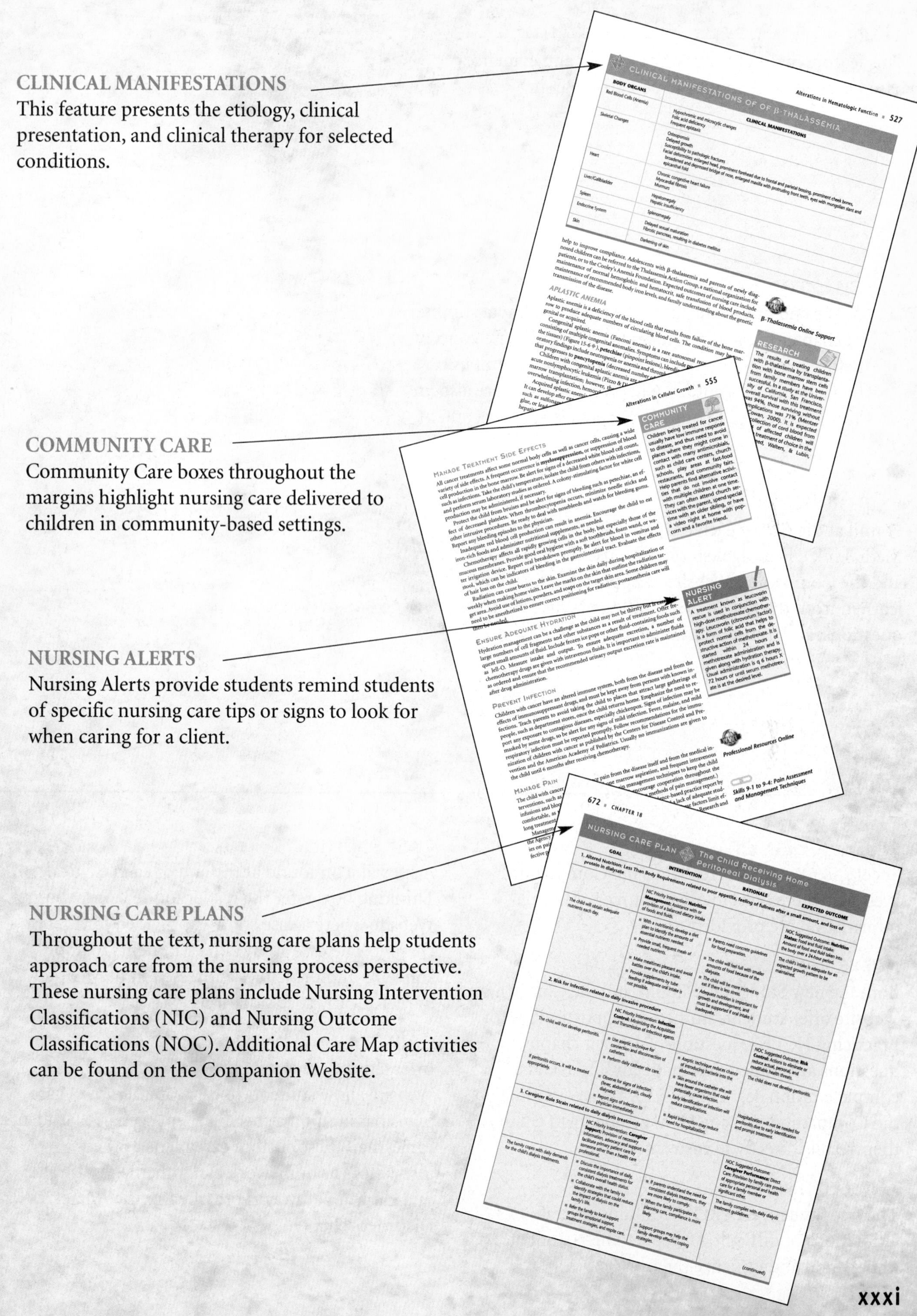

CLINICAL MANIFESTATIONS

This feature presents the etiology, clinical presentation, and clinical therapy for selected conditions.

COMMUNITY CARE

Community Care boxes throughout the margins highlight nursing care delivered to children in community-based settings.

NURSING ALERTS

Nursing Alerts provide students remind students of specific nursing care tips or signs to look for when caring for a client.

NURSING CARE PLANS

Throughout the text, nursing care plans help students approach care from the nursing process perspective. These nursing care plans include Nursing Intervention Classifications (NIC) and Nursing Outcome Classifications (NOC). Additional Care Map activities can be found on the Companion Website.

RESEARCH

This feature highlights nursing research and evidence-based practice as it applies to pediatric nursing.

CHAPTER HIGHLIGHTS

At the end of each chapter, students will find a summary of chapter highlights. Students who read these concepts before reading the chapter will find this helpful in focusing their attention. Chapter highlights are also an appropriate tool to quickly review the chapter content.

EXPLORE MEDIALINK

Found at the end of each chapter, the EXPLORE MediaLink encourages students to use the CD-ROM and the Companion Website to apply what they have learned from the text in case studies, practice NCLEX questions, and to use additional resources.

Alterations in Cellular Growth ▪ 557

FIGURE 16·10 ◆
A child in a pediatric oncology clinic giving injections to a doll. This type of play therapy helps the child deal with fear, thus lowering his or her stress level.

RESEARCH
Research has shown that two of the worst stressors for adolescents with cancer are (1) waiting for care and (2) dependence on parents. Nurses can devise interventions to minimize waiting for chemotherapy and other treatments or provide options such as meetings with other teens and computer use while waiting. When possible, enable the adolescent to make choices independently of parents (Enskar, Carlsson, & Golsater, et al., 1997).

Chapter Highlights

- Infants are at risk of heart failure because their immature heart is more sensitive to volume or pressure overload. The heart muscle fibers are less developed and the ventricles have less compliance so that stroke volume cannot increase substantially.
- Cardiac output depends almost completely on heart rate until the heart muscle is fully developed at 5 years of age.
- Congenital heart defects are the most common cause of congestive heart failure in infants and children.
- Signs of congestive heart failure may include tachypnea, tachycardia, pallor or cyanosis, nasal flaring, grunting, retractions, cough, crackles, periorbital and facial edema, jugular vein distention, and hepatomegaly.
- Congenital heart defects develop during the early weeks of pregnancy and are usually the result of a combined or interactive effect of genetic and environmental factors.
- In nonobstructive acyanotic heart defects, a left-to-right shunt allows extra blood volume to overload the pulmonary system and potentially cause congestive heart failure.
- An obstructive defect (i.e., aortic or pulmonic stenosis) causes pressure overload and hypertrophy of the closest ventricle.
- Cardiac catheterization provides a means for the evaluation of hemodynamics and pressure gradients within the heart, and for noninvasive correction of some heart defects.
- The child with a cyanotic heart defect may have life-threatening hypercyanotic spells requiring emergency treatment. Palliative or corrective surgery is often performed soon afterwards to prevent other life-threatening attacks.
- Heart transplantation is performed in infants and children for complex heart defects or cardiomyopathy in children.
- Pulmonary artery hypertension is a life-threatening complication of congenital heart disease with excessive pulmonary blood flow. Irreversible pulmonary vascular changes include inflammation, hypertrophy of pulmonary vessels, and fibrosis.
- Rheumatic fever is an inflammatory connective tissue disease following a streptococcal infection that may affect the heart, joints, skin, or central nervous system.
- Children who have a congenital heart defect, rheumatic heart disease, or a central venous catheter or who have had heart surgery are at risk for infective endocarditis.
- Two potentially life-threatening cardiac arrhythmias are supraventricular tachycardias and long QT syndrome.
- Kawasaki disease is the most common cause of acquired heart disease in children in the United States.
- Some children have familial or lifestyle-related hyperlipidemia that causes undesirable levels of cholesterol or triglycerides. These children should have dietary intervention to reduce the risk of coronary artery disease as an adult.
- All children with blood pressures in the 90th percentile for age are significantly more likely to develop hypertension as adults.
- Shock is an acute, complex state of circulatory dysfunction resulting in failure to deliver sufficient oxygen and other nutrients to meet cell and tissue demands.
- Signs that a child is in compensated hypovolemic shock include tachycardia, increased respiratory effort, delayed capillary refill, weak peripheral pulses, pallor, and cold extremities.
- Distributive shock is an abnormal pooling of blood in the extremities that may be caused by anaphylaxis, sepsis, or spinal cord injury.
- Myocardial contusion results from a strong, blunt force against the chest wall that injures the heart muscle, and may cause an arrhythmia.

EXPLORE MediaLink

- NCLEX review, case studies, and other interactive resources for this chapter can be found on the Companion Website at **http://www.prenhall.com/ball**. Click on Chapter 14 to select the activities for this chapter.
- For animations, more NCLEX review questions, and an audio glossary, access the accompanying CD-ROM in this textbook.

510

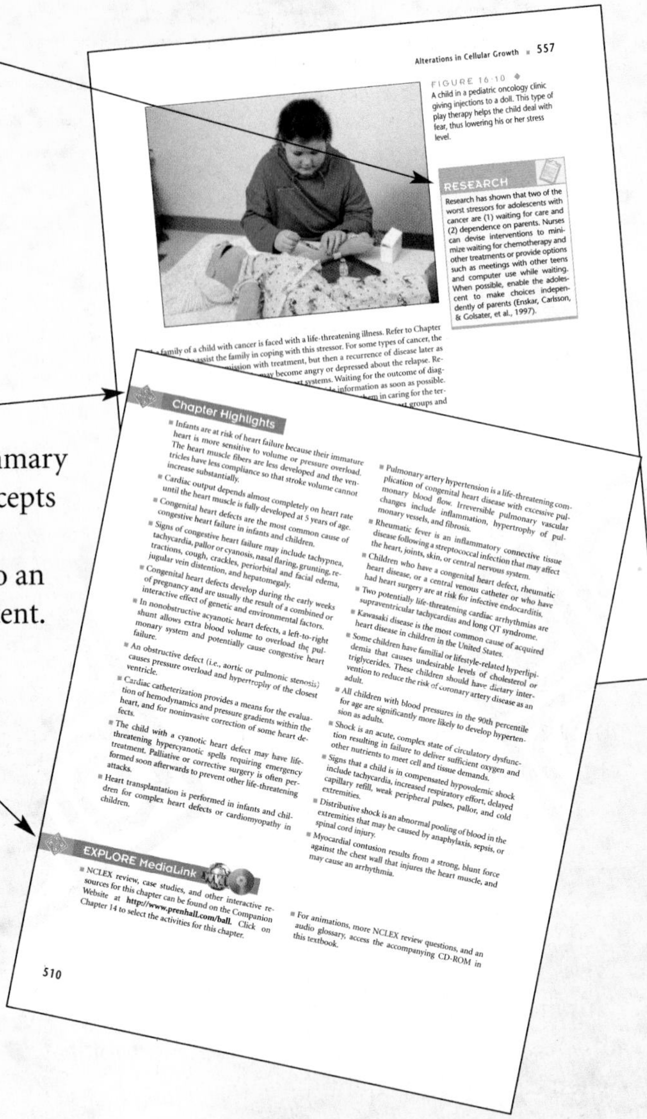

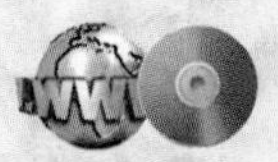

ADDITIONAL MEDIA RESOURCES

RESOURCE LINKS

Special icons refer the reader to the Companion Web site where links to other sources of useful information are provided.

NCLEX REVIEW

Both the new Student CD-ROM and the Companion Website offer students numerous opportunities for practicing NCLEX questions. For each chapter, questions are graded automatically and provide complete rationales. The NCLEX review module on the Companion Website allows students to email their results directly to instructors.

ANIMATIONS

The free Student CD-ROM contains several animations of difficult concepts to help students understand and visualize them.

CASE STUDIES

A special icon found at the end of each Critical Thinking box, refer the reader to the Companion Website where a case study is provided for that chapter. The case study allows students to apply concepts and principles addressed in the chapter to realistic practice situations.

CARE MAP ACTIVITIES

Interactive Care Map Activities on the Companion Website allow students to develop their own care plans based upon a specific client scenario. Students can e-mail these custom care plans to their instructors as homework assignments. A sample of a clinical pathway is provided in the Anxiety Disorders chapter.

SPECIAL FEATURES

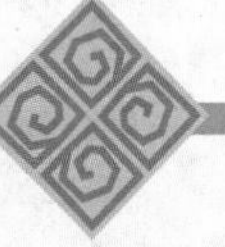
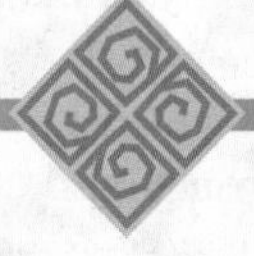
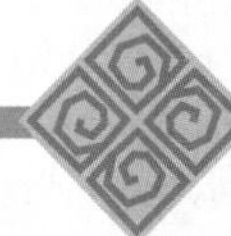

AS THEY GROW

PATHOPHYSIOLOGY ILLUSTRATED

MEDICATIONS USED TO TREAT

FAMILIES WANT TO KNOW

CLINICAL MANIFESTATIONS

CULTURE

COMMUNITY CARE

HOME CARE

GROWTH & DEVELOPMENT

SAFETY PRECAUTIONS

RESEARCH

NURSING CARE PLANS

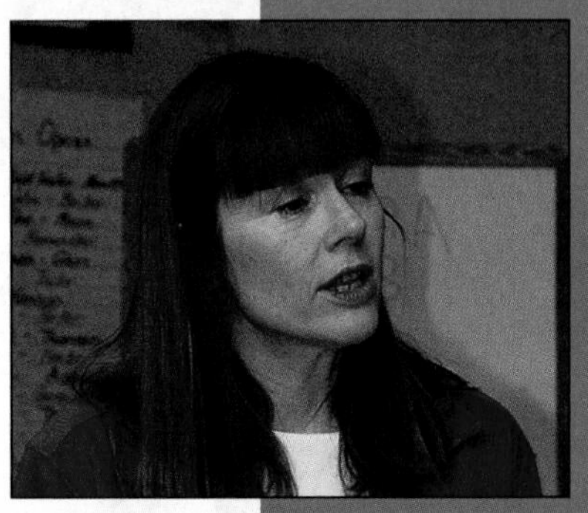

"THE ASTHMA CLUB HAS REALLY HELPED THESE CHILDREN BECOME MORE CONFIDENT IN MANAGING THEIR ASTHMA. IT HELPS THEM TO KNOW THAT THEY HAVE OTHER FRIENDS WITH THIS CONDITION."

Bethany and several of her classmates have asthma. If her asthma is not kept under control, Bethany has a difficult time concentrating in school because her attention centers on breathing. Several times over the past 2 years, she has gone to the doctor or the emergency department to obtain treatment for severe asthma attacks. These attacks have caused her to miss many days of school. Although Bethany has medications to help control her asthma, she does not always use them because of fear that the other children would view her as "different."

The number of children with asthma in the elementary school prompted the school nurse to start an asthma club. Her purpose in starting this club was to help the children with asthma learn more about their illness and ways to control the condition. She discovered that very few children understand how to recognize the early signs of an asthma attack. As a result, treatment often is not begun as soon as symptoms occur. Teaching the children about the condition has also enabled them to explain to peers why they sometimes have difficulty breathing and need to take medications.

Over the past few months, Bethany has learned to recognize signs of an asthma attack and when to use her inhaler. She has had to seek emergency treatment less often. She also enjoys knowing she has friends who are like her, working hard to "breathe easier."

CHAPTER

1

NURSE'S ROLE IN CARE OF THE ILL AND INJURED CHILD:

Hospital, Community Settings, and Home

KEY TERMS

advance directives A patient's living will or appointed durable power of attorney for health care decisions.

advocacy Acting to safeguard and advance the interests of another.

assent Voluntary agreement to participate in a research project or to accept treatment.

case management A process of coordinating the delivery of health care services in a manner that focuses on both quality and cost outcomes.

clinical practice guidelines Outlines detailing specific medical and nursing assessments and interventions during specific time intervals for a specific condition. This guideline is often adopted in an institution for all health care providers to follow so that quality of care is increased and costs of care are minimized.

continuity of care An interdisciplinary process of facilitating a patient's transition between and among settings based on changing needs and available resources.

continuum of care A system of care that includes each of the following elements: primary care, illness or injury prevention, acute care in the hospital, and restorative care in either the home or a rehabilitation center until the patient is reintegrated into family and community.

emancipated minors Self-supporting adolescents under 18 years of age not subject to parental control.

family-centered care A philosophy of care that integrates the family's values and potential contributions in the plans for and provision of care to the child.

informed consent A formal preauthorization for an invasive procedure or participation in research.

mature minors Adolescents of 14 and 15 years of age who are able to understand treatment risks and who in some states can consent to or refuse treatment.

moral dilemma A conflict of social values and ethical principles that support different courses of action.

morbidity An illness or injury that limits activity, requires medical attention or hospitalization, or results in a chronic condition.

quality assurance A process for monitoring the procedures and outcomes of care that uses indicators to measure compliance with standards of care.

quality improvement The continuous study and improvement of the processes and outcomes of providing health care services to meet the needs of patients by examining the system and processes of care and service delivery.

risk management A process established by a health care institution to identify, evaluate, and reduce the risk of injury to patients, staff, and visitors and thereby reduce the institution's liability.

MediaLink

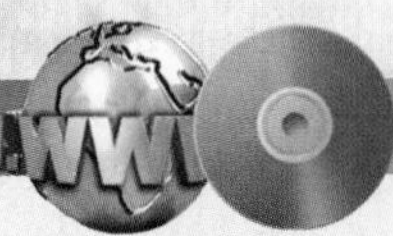

http://www.prenhall.com/ball

Resources for this chapter can be found on the CD-ROM accompanying this textbook, and on the Companion Website at http://www.prenhall.com/ball. Click on Chapter 1 to select the activities for this chapter.

CD-ROM	COMPANION WEBSITE
Audio Glossary	Web Links
NCLEX Review	NCLEX Review

Nurses in many settings come into contact with children who have asthma. Nurses are important members of the health care team during all phases of the **continuum of care,** a system of care that includes each of the following elements: illness or injury prevention, acute care in the hospital, and restorative care in either the home or rehabilitation center until the child is reintegrated into the family and community. In which of these roles did the school nurse help Bethany and her friends? In what other settings is pediatric nursing care provided? How many different roles for nurses can you identify for children with a health care problem throughout the continuum of care? This chapter reviews concepts important to pediatric nursing: the role of the nurse in pediatrics, the contemporary climate of pediatric health care, and legal and ethical issues.

What is the role of the nurse in working with children who have asthma? In how many different settings could you find nurses providing care to children with asthma? Does the type of nursing care provided to children by nurses differ among these settings? Regardless of the setting in which nurses work, assessment, nursing care interventions, and patient education are universal roles for nurses. This chapter defines the various roles and settings for the nursing care of children and the important challenges in providing that care.

ROLE OF THE NURSE IN PEDIATRICS

CLINICAL PRACTICE

Pediatric nursing focuses on protecting children from illness and injury, assisting them to attain optimal levels of health, regardless of health problems, and rehabilitation. This focus fits with the American Nurses Association (1998) definition of the scope of nursing practice: "the diagnosis and treatment of human responses to actual or potential health problems." The nursing roles in caring for children and their families include direct care, patient education, advocacy, and case management.

Direct Nursing Care

The primary role of pediatric nurses is to provide direct nursing care to children and their families. The nursing process provides the framework for delivery of direct pediatric nursing care. The nurse assesses the child, identifies the nursing diagnoses that describe the responses of the child and family to the illness or injury, and implements and evaluates nursing care. This care is designed to meet the child's physical and emotional needs. It is tailored to the child's developmental stage, giving the child additional responsibility for self-care with increasing age.

Nurses play an important role in minimizing the psychologic and physical distress experienced by children and their families. Providing support to children and their families is one component of direct nursing care. This often involves listening to the concerns of children and parents, being present during stressful or emotional experiences, and implementing strategies to help children and family members cope (see Chapter 8). Nurses can help families by suggesting ways to support their children in the hospital, in out-of-hospital settings, and in the home.

Patient Education

Patient education improves treatment results. In pediatric nursing, patient education is especially challenging, because nurses must be prepared to work with children at various levels of understanding and to change the behavior of family members.

As patient educators, nurses help children adapt to the hospital setting and prepare them for procedures (Figure 1-1 ◆). Most hospitals encourage a parent to stay with the child and to provide much of the direct and supportive care. Nurses teach parents to watch for important signs and responses to therapies, to increase the child's comfort, and even to provide advanced care. Taking an active role prepares the parent to assume total responsibility for care after the child leaves the hospital.

Counseling is another form of patient education. Counseling may involve provision of information, such as injury-prevention strategies and anticipatory guidance to promote de-

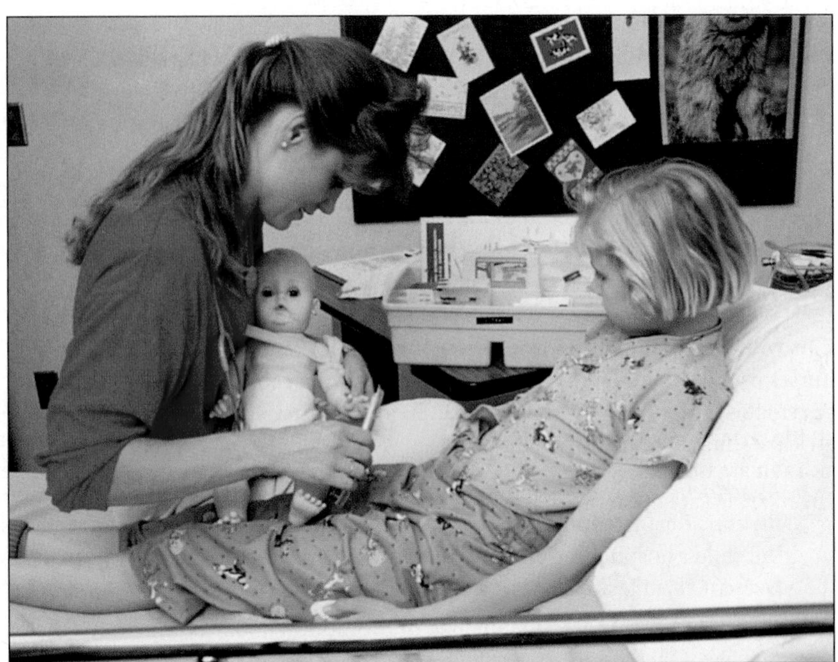

FIGURE 1-1 ◆ Explaining procedures can reduce the patient's and family's fears and anxieties about what to expect as well as teach procedures and proper home care.

velopment. Advance practice nurses or other experienced nurses are often responsible for counseling that is directed toward helping the child or family solve a problem.

Patient Advocacy

Advocacy—acting to safeguard and advance the interests of another—is directed at enabling the child and family to adjust to the changes in the child's health in their own way. To be an effective advocate, the nurse must be aware of the child's and the family's needs, the family's resources, and the health care services available in the hospital and the community. The nurse can then assist the family and the child to make informed choices about these services and to act in the child's best interests.

As advocates, nurses also ensure that the policies and resources of health care agencies meet the psychosocial needs of children and their families. The nurse must also protect the child and family by taking appropriate actions related to any incidents of incompetent, unethical, or illegal practices by any member of the health care team.

Case Management

What happens when a child has significant health problems? Can you handle it all?

When a child has a significant health problem or handicapping condition, health care professionals (physicians, nurses, social workers, physical and occupational therapists, and other specialists) create an interdisciplinary plan to meet the child's medical, nursing, developmental, educational, and psychosocial needs. Because nurses spend large amounts of time providing nursing care for the child and family, they often know more than other health care professionals about the family's wishes and resources. As a member of the interdisciplinary care plan team, the nurse serves as an advocate to ensure that the care plan considers the family's wishes and contains appropriate services. The nurse often becomes the child's case manager, coordinating the implementation of the interdisciplinary care plan. Sometimes the parent or a social worker becomes the case manager.

Case management is a process of coordinating the delivery of health care services in a manner that focuses on both quality and cost outcomes. This is often a collaborative practice with other health care providers that promotes **continuity of care,** an interdisciplinary process of facilitating a patient's transition between and among settings based on changing needs and available resources. The nurse case manager has control over the use of health care resources that are considered appropriate for the patient's condition and links the child and family to these services. The goal is to help the child and family have the best health care outcome and decrease fragmentation of care, while controlling the cost of health care services. Case management may be used for care of the patient when hospitalized as well as for long-term care of chronic conditions.

Discharge planning is a form of case management. Good discharge planning promotes a smooth, rapid, and safe transition into the community and improves the results of treatment begun in the hospital. To be a discharge planner, the nurse needs to know about community medical resources, home care agencies qualified to care for children, educational interventions, and services reimbursed by the child's health plan or other financial resources.

NURSING PROCESS IN PEDIATRIC CARE

Can you describe how the five steps of the nursing process relate to children? Pediatric nurses use the nursing process to identify and solve problems and to plan patient care. The systematic framework for practice that the nursing process provides is the same for pediatric patients as for other patients.

- *Assessment* involves collecting patient and family data and performing physical examinations during community-based health services, at admission, periodically during the child's hospitalization, and when home care services are provided. The nurse analyzes and synthesizes data to make a judgment about the patient's problems.
- *Nursing diagnoses* describe the health promotion and health patterns that nurses can manage. Once health patterns have been identified, specific nursing actions can be planned.
- *Nursing care plans* are based on goals that will improve the child's or family's dysfunctional health patterns. Specific expected outcomes should be realistic. The family and the nurse (and the child, when old enough) should agree with the care plan goals.

Standard care plans for specific diagnoses are often used in the pediatric unit of the hospital and by home health agencies. The nurse is responsible for individualizing standard care plans based on data collected from the child's assessment and from evaluation of the child's response to care. Individualized nursing action plans provide directions for nursing care.

- *Implementation* is the carrying out of interventions outlined in the nursing care plan. Interventions may be modified if the child's responses are undesirable.
- *Evaluation* is the use of specific objective and subjective measures (often called outcome measures or criteria) to assess the child's and family's progress in reaching the goals defined in the nursing care plan. Following the evaluation of their progress toward the goals, the nursing care plan may be modified. For example, as the child's condition improves and goals are attained, new goals and nursing action plans must be defined. Data from ongoing assessments are collected to guide the revision of the care plan.

Clinical practice guidelines and critical pathways are comprehensive interdisciplinary care plans for a specific condition, which describe the sequence and timing of interventions that should result in expected patient outcomes. The care plans are increasingly evidence based, using a synthesis of research, group consensus, and past medical decisions to identify the most effective practices for a patient's condition. They address nursing care, nutrition, diagnostic tests, medications and other treatments, mobility and activity, patient teaching, and discharge planning. (See Chapter 13 for an example.) Clinical practice guidelines or critical pathways are adopted within a health care setting to reduce variation in patient management, to limit costs of care, and to evaluate the effectiveness of care (Merritt, Palmer, Bergman, & Shiono, 1997; Melnyk, Fineout-Overholt, Stone, & Ackerman, 2000). Many nurses are engaged in research to identify cost-effective plans for care.

SETTINGS FOR PEDIATRIC NURSING CARE

Pediatric nurses function in a variety of settings. Within the hospital, acute care may be provided in the emergency department, observation or short-stay unit, postanesthesia unit, intensive care unit, general pediatric inpatient unit, and various outpatient clinics. Pediatric nurses working with children and families on a general pediatric hospital unit promote health improvement in the following ways:

- By gathering data and assessing the health of children and their families
- By providing ordered medical therapies
- By providing nursing care in a manner that preserves as many of the child's and family's normal routines as possible while maintaining the family unit
- By working with the family and health care team to develop an individualized health care plan and a discharge plan, or to implement a clinical practice guideline

The hospital stay is now integrated into a continuum that allows children to complete therapy at home, at school, or in other community settings. Pediatric nurses assist families in making the transition from the acute hospital setting to the following:

- The home, for a short recuperation or long-term management
- A rehabilitation center or long-term care hospital
- A nurse-managed home care or hospice program

Managing the child's transition from acute care to another setting involves planning the discharge, implementing interdisciplinary plans, helping the family to develop an emergency care plan in the event the child has an unexpected health care crisis, and collaborating with a broad range of health care professionals.

Pediatric nurses also work in several other health care settings:

- In *pediatricians' offices* and health care centers, nurses assess children, provide telephone counseling, and support and counsel families about growth and development and nutrition.
- In *clinic settings,* nurses assess children, assist with medical procedures, and educate families to ensure the continuous management of the children's health care problems.
- In *home health agencies,* nurses provide home care to children who require their services. Children need medical treatment and nursing care for acute, self-limited, chronic, and terminal conditions. This may involve visits for specific interventions such as medication administration or "private duty" (one-to-one) nursing care.
- In *rehabilitation centers,* nurses provide inpatient and ambulatory care to help restore children to an optimal state and plan for discharge management of chronic conditions.
- In *schools,* nurses assess children, monitor their health status, and provide health education to teachers and children. Many children who are assisted by technology or have chronic conditions attend school. The school nurse will develop, implement, and evaluate individual school health plans. In the case of Bethany and her friends from the asthma club, patient education helps them become more independent in managing their asthma.

LAW & ETHICS

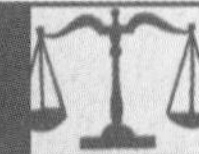

The Individuals with Disabilities Education Act (IDEA) provides free appropriate education to all handicapped children between infancy and 21 years of age. Provisions for needed medical care must be available in the school setting. States receive federal funding for IDEA services and bill Medicaid and other health plans with parental consent (Murray, 1999).

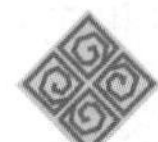

CONTEMPORARY CLIMATE FOR PEDIATRIC NURSING CARE

More than 85 million children under the age of 21 live in the United States. They account for 31.2% of the population (U.S. Census, 2001). (See Figure 1-2 ◆ for a distribution of the population by age group.) At one time, children were valued primarily as laborers. Over the past century, however, their unique needs and qualities have been recognized. In today's society, children are considered to have special value; they are vulnerable and need protection.

FAMILY-CENTERED CARE

Efforts to address and meet the emotional, social, and developmental needs of children and families seeking health care in all settings is a concept known as **family-centered care.** The importance of the family in helping the child recover from an illness or injury is recognized (Figure 1-3 ◆). Families are often considered partners in care, learning about children's conditions and participating in decisions regarding their care. Thus, families gain greater confidence and competence in caring for their children, which has become even more important as families play an ever increasing role in providing care for children's health care problems. The key elements of family-centered care are provided in Table 1-1.

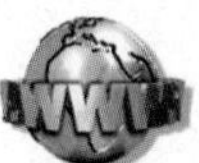

Family-Centered Care

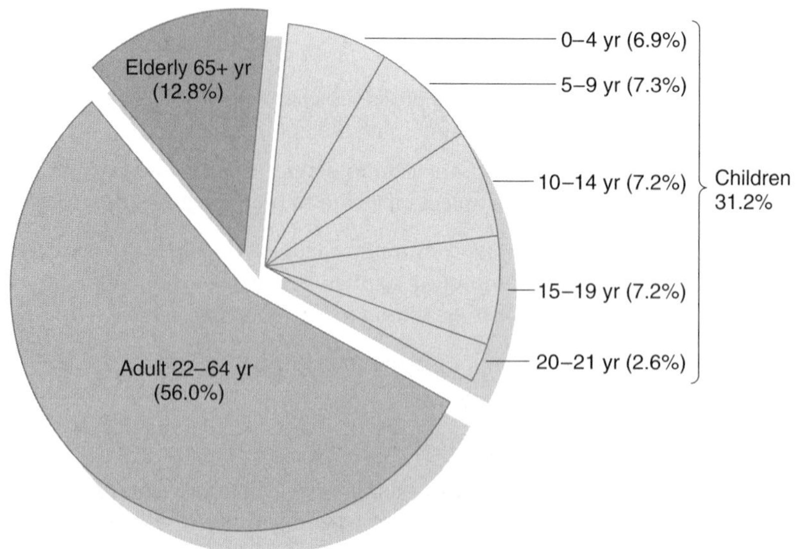

FIGURE 1-2 ◆
In 1999, children from birth to 21 years of age accounted for about one third of the population in the United States. NOTE: From U.S. Bureau of Census (2000). *Resident population estimates of the United States by age and sex, April 1, 1990 to July 1, 1999.* Washington, DC: U.S. Government Printing Office.

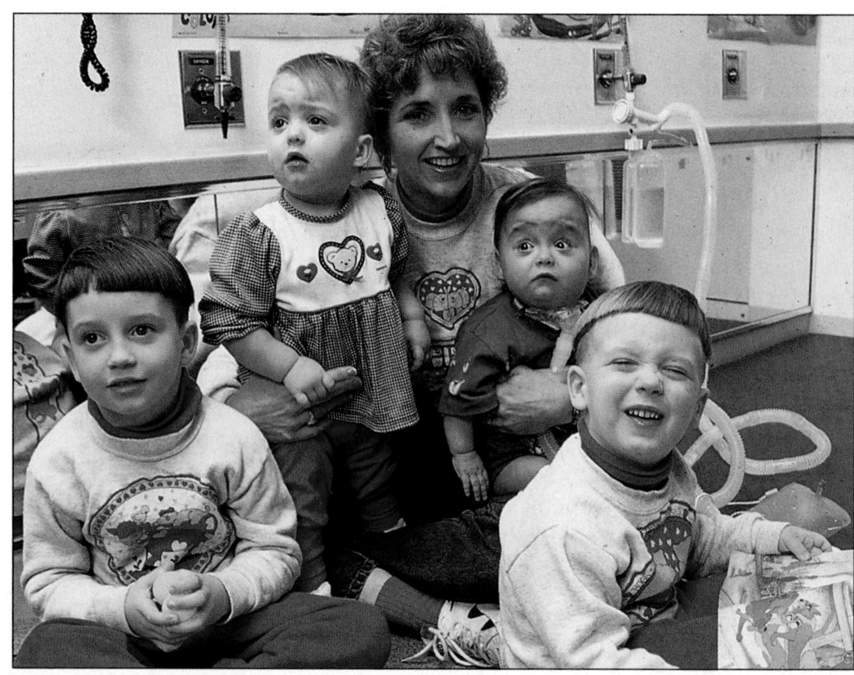

FIGURE 1-3 ◆
Many facilities now encourage family visitation for children with health problems that require long-term hospitalization. Extended family visits enable parents to learn about the child's care, and provide siblings with opportunities to interact with the hospitalized child.

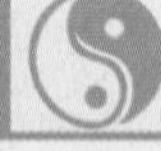

CULTURE

Conflicts can occur within a family when traditional rituals and practices of the family's elders do not conform with current health care practices. Nurses need to be sensitive to the potential implications for the child's health care, especially after the child is discharged from the hospital. When cultural values are not part of the nursing care plan, parents may be forced to decide whether the family's beliefs should take priority over the health care professional's guidance.

CULTURALLY SENSITIVE CARE

The U.S. population has a varied mix of cultural groups, with ever increasing diversity. More than 33% of all children less than 20 years of age are from families of minority populations (U.S. Census, 2001). Culture develops from socially learned beliefs, lifestyles, values, and integrated patterns of behavior that are characteristic of the family, cultural group, and community. The cultural background and values of children and their parents are often quite different from those of the nurse.

Specific elements that contribute to a family's value system include the following:

- Religion and social beliefs
- Presence and influence of the extended family, as well as socialization within the ethnic group
- Communication patterns
- Beliefs and understanding about the concepts of health and illness

TABLE 1-1 Key Elements of Family-Centered Care

- Incorporating into policy and practice the recognition that the family is the constant in a child's life, while the service systems and support personnel within those systems fluctuate.
- Facilitating family/professional collaboration at all levels of hospital, home, and community care:
  - care of an individual child
  - program development, implementation, evaluation, and evolution
  - policy formation
- Exchanging complete and unbiased information between family members and professionals in a supportive manner at all times.
- Incorporating into policy and practice the recognition and honoring of cultural diversity, strengths, and individuality within and across all families, including ethnic, racial, spiritual, social, economic, educational, and geographic diversity.
- Recognizing and respecting different methods of coping and implementing comprehensive policies and programs that provide developmental, educational, emotional, environmental, and financial supports to meet the diverse needs of families.
- Encouraging and facilitating family-to-family support and networking.
- Ensuring that home, hospital, and community service and support systems for children needing specialized health and developmental care and their families are flexible, accessible, and comprehensive in responding to diverse family-identified needs.
- Appreciating families as families and children as children, and recognizing that they possess a wide range of strengths, concerns, emotions, and aspirations beyond their need for specialized health and developmental services and support.

Note: From Shelton, T.L., & Stepanek, J.S. (1994). *Family-centered care for children needing specialized health and developmental services.* Child Life Council, 11820 Parklawn Dr. #202, Rockville, MD 20814, 301-881-7090.

- Permissible physical contact with strangers
- Education

Specific differences in beliefs between families and health care providers are common in the following areas:

- Help-seeking behaviors
- Causes of diseases or illnesses
- Death and dying
- Caretaking and caregiving
- Child-rearing practices

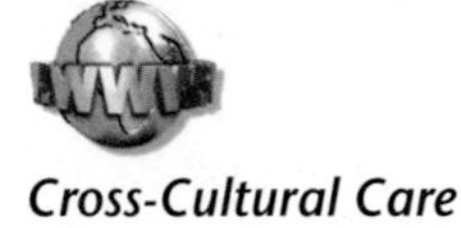

Cross-Cultural Care

These elements in differing degrees influence the cultural beliefs and values of an ethnic group, making the group unique. Misunderstandings may occur when the health care professional and the family come from different cultural groups. In addition, past experiences with care may have made the family angry or suspicious of providers. Nurses must be able to recognize, respect, and respond to ethnic diversity in a way that leads to a mutually desirable outcome. The nurse must identify culturally relevant facts about the patient to provide culturally appropriate and competent care.

When the family's cultural values are incorporated into the care plan, the family is more likely to accept and comply with the needed care, especially in the home care setting. Avoid imposing your personal cultural values on the children and families in your care. By learning about the values of the different ethnic groups in the community—their religious beliefs that have an impact on health care practices, their beliefs about common illnesses, and their specific healing practices—you can develop an individualized nursing care plan for each child and family.

PEDIATRIC HEALTH STATISTICS

Children have different health care problems than adults, and the problems may depend on age and development. For example, the leading causes of infant mortality (death occurring during the first year of life) vary according to the age of the infant (Figure 1-4 ◆).

The leading causes of death in neonates (birth to 28 days of age) are congenital anomalies, low birth weight, respiratory distress syndrome, and maternal complications of pregnancy. Sudden infant death syndrome accounts for nearly 28% of deaths to infants in the postneonatal period (between 1 and 12 months of age). Figure 1-4 shows the relative frequency of other major causes of death in the postneonatal period. The mortality rate for African-American infants is at least 2 times that of Caucasians for the leading causes of death, except for congenital anomalies (Health Resources and Services Administration, 2000). What could account for homicide as the fifth leading cause of death in infants? See Chapter 7 for an answer.

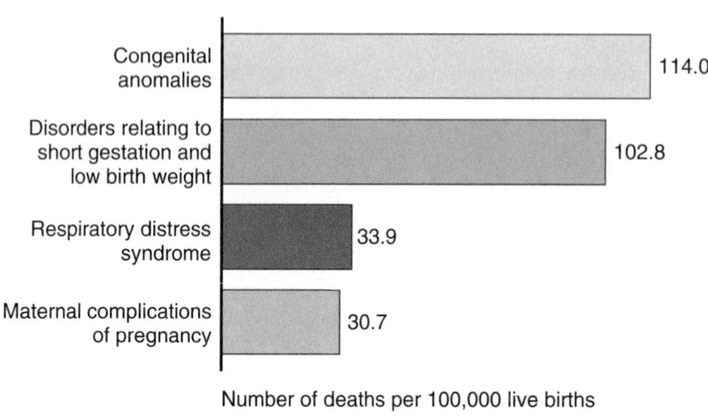

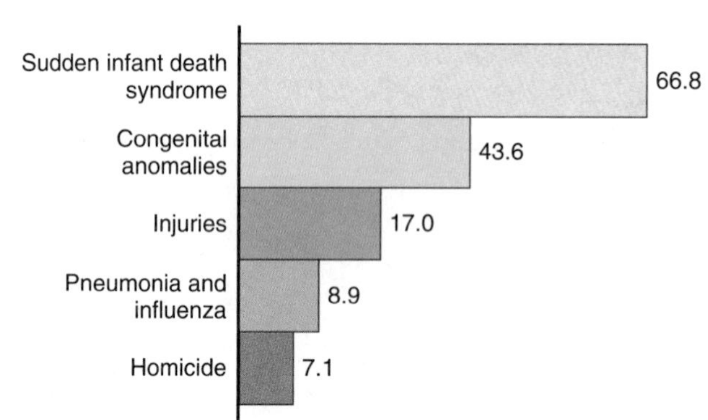

FIGURE 1-4 ◆
Leading causes of death in the United States for infants in 1998, A, Neonatal mortality (in infants up to 28 days old) and B, Postneonatal mortality (in infants between 28 days and 1 year old). In 1993 the mortality rate for Sudden Infant Death Syndrome was 109.5 per 100,000 live births. What could account for this dramatic rate reduction? (See Chap. 13 to find the answer.)
NOTE: From Murphy, S.A. (2000). *Deaths: Final data for 1998.* National Vital Statistics Reports, *48*(11). Hyattsville, MD: National Center for Health Statistics.

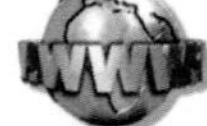

National Health Statistics

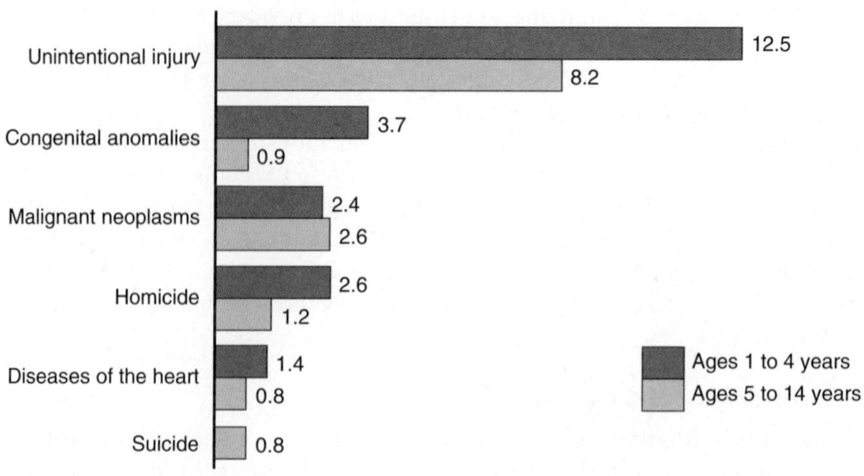

FIGURE 1-5 ◆
Age-specific death rate per 100,000 children in the United States in 1998. The leading cause of death in children between the ages of 1 and 14 years was unintentional injury. Why do you think that is? Do you think these data still apply today? Which type of injury has the highest rate of death? Drowning? Fires and Burns? Motor vehicle crashes? See Figure 1-6 for the answer.
NOTE: From Murphy, S.A. (2000). *Deaths: Final data for 1998. National Vital Statistics Reports, 48(11).* Hyattsville, MD: National Center for Health Statistics.

The most common cause of death for children between 1 and 14 years of age is unintentional injury. Congenital anomalies, cancer, diseases of the heart, homicide, and suicide are the other major causes. Figure 1-5 ◆ shows the distribution of these causes by age group. The major causes of death from unintentional injury in childhood include motor vehicle crashes (passengers and pedestrians), drowning, fires and burns, firearms, and suffocation (Figure 1-6 ◆) (Health Resources and Services Administration, 2000).

Unintentional injury continues to be the leading cause of death in adolescents 15 through 19 years. Homicide, suicide, cancer, and congenital anomalies are other major causes of death (Figure 1-7 ◆). Of all deaths from unintentional and intentional injury, motor vehicle crashes are the leading cause, followed by firearms, suffocation, drowning, and poisoning (Figure 1-8 ◆).

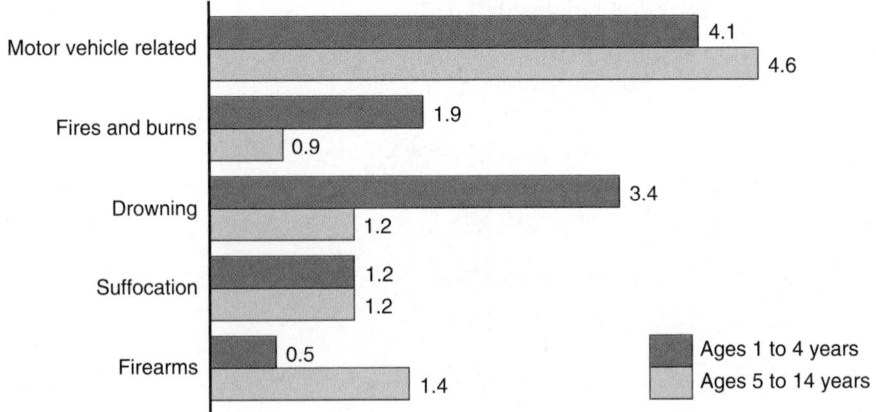

FIGURE 1-6 ◆
Death rates from unintentional and intentional injuries per 100,000 children ages 1 to 14 years in the United States in 1998. Which types of injuries are unintentional (unplanned or accidental) and intentional (violence or homicide related)?
NOTE: From Murphy, S.A. (2000). *Deaths: Final data for 1998. National Vital Statistics Reports, 48(11),* Hyattsville, MD: National Center for Health Statistics.

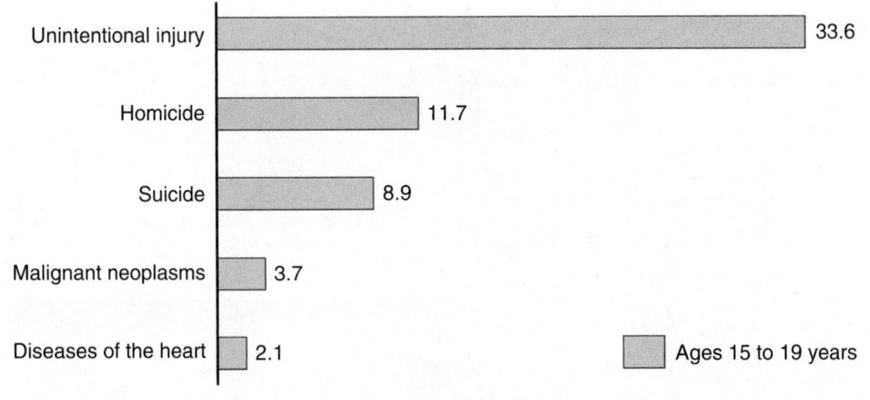

FIGURE 1-7 ◆
Death rates per 100,000 adolescents in the United States in 1998. What is the proportion of deaths that are preventable?
NOTE: From Murphy, S.A. (2000). *Deaths: Final data for 1998. National Vital Statistics Reports, 48(11).* Hyattsville, MD: National Center for Health Statistics.

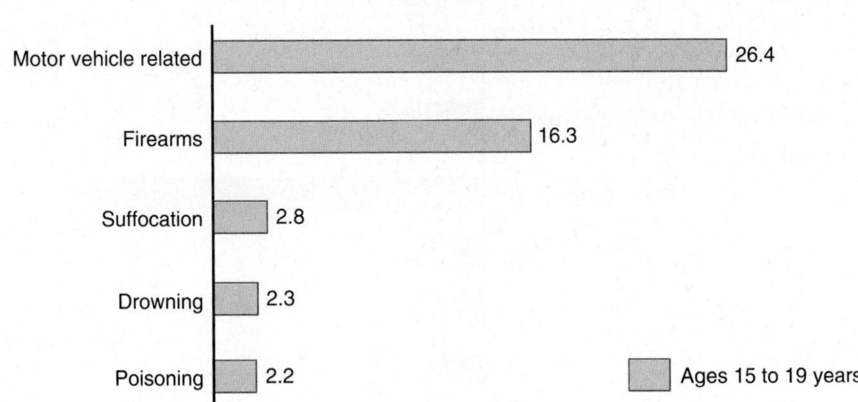

FIGURE 1-8 ◆
Death rates from all injuries per 100,000 adolescents in the United States in 1998. Of the firearm deaths, 60% are homicides and 34.2% are suicides. How many firearm deaths are thus unintentional? Can you see ways to use these data with patients and families during patient teaching and when talking with them while providing care?
NOTE: From Murphy, S.A. (2000). *Deaths: Final data for 1998. National Vital Statistics Reports, 48(11).* Hyattsville, MD: National Center for Health Statistics.

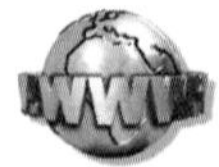

National Health Guidelines and Objectives

The U.S. government set objectives to improve the health of children and young adults in the 21st century in the report entitled *Healthy People 2010.* These objectives focus on reducing the incidence of death and disability from the major causes of death shown in Figures 1-4 through 1-8. Federal funding is available to health care organizations for the development of programs aimed at reducing the number of deaths from these factors in specific high-risk groups.

FIGURE 1-9 ◆

The leading causes of hospitalization in the United States in 1998 are much the same as those in 1993 in those 21 years of age and younger, but the number of hospital discharges [in 1000s] have changed for some causes. What do you think might account for the rise in hospital discharges for mental disorders? What do you think the current hospital discharge numbers are today?

NOTE: From *Child Health USA '95. (DHHS Publication No. HRSA-M-DSEA-96-5).* Washington, DC: Government Printing Office; and National Center for Health Statistics (1999). National Hospital Discharge Survey. Unpublished Data.

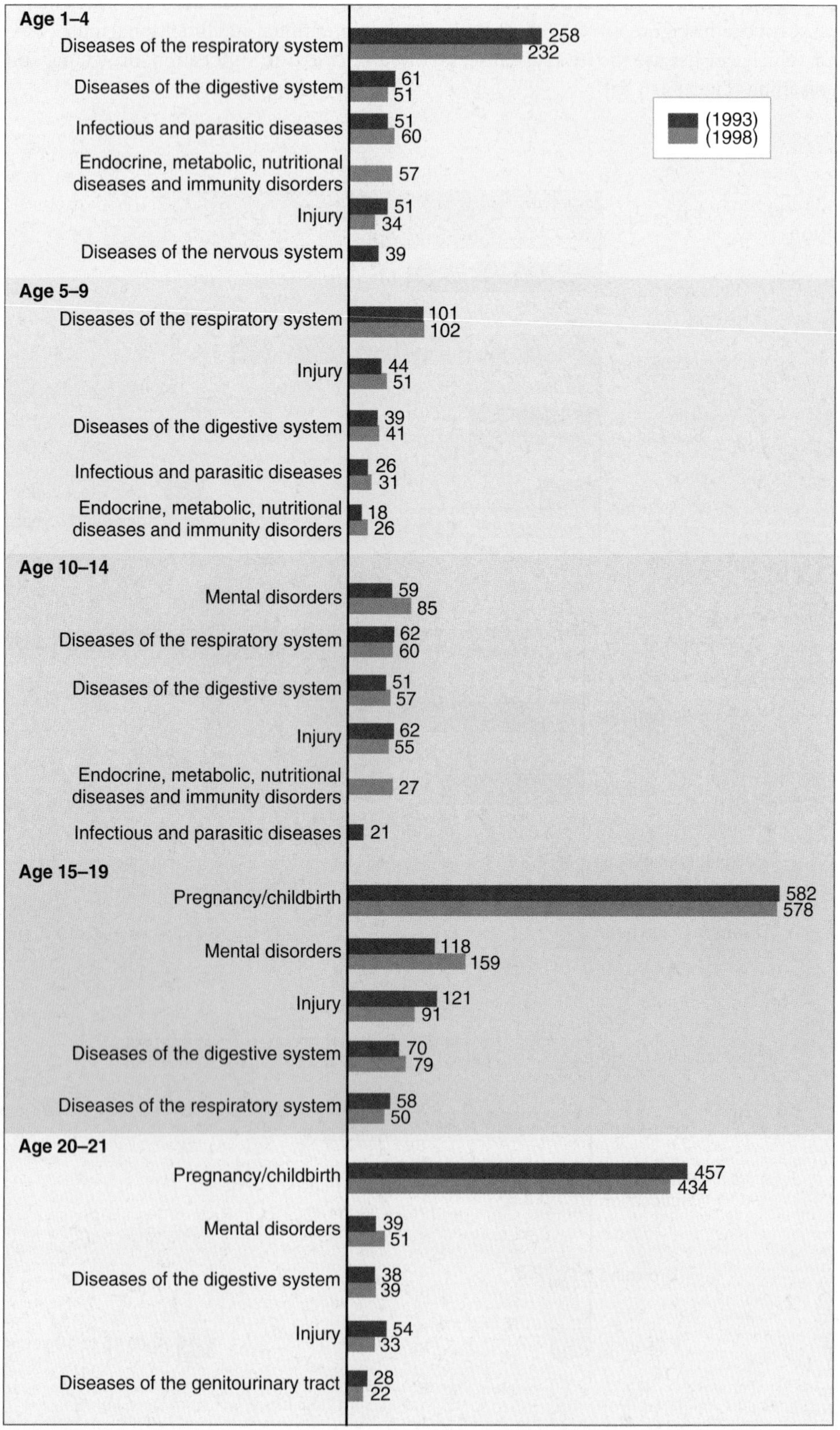

Age / Cause	(1993)	(1998)
Age 1–4		
Diseases of the respiratory system	258	232
Diseases of the digestive system	61	51
Infectious and parasitic diseases	51	60
Endocrine, metabolic, nutritional diseases and immunity disorders		57
Injury	51	34
Diseases of the nervous system	39	
Age 5–9		
Diseases of the respiratory system	101	102
Injury	44	51
Diseases of the digestive system	39	41
Infectious and parasitic diseases	26	31
Endocrine, metabolic, nutritional diseases and immunity disorders	18	26
Age 10–14		
Mental disorders	59	85
Diseases of the respiratory system	62	60
Diseases of the digestive system	51	57
Injury	62	55
Endocrine, metabolic, nutritional diseases and immunity disorders		27
Infectious and parasitic diseases	21	
Age 15–19		
Pregnancy/childbirth	582	578
Mental disorders	118	159
Injury	121	91
Diseases of the digestive system	70	79
Diseases of the respiratory system	58	50
Age 20–21		
Pregnancy/childbirth	457	434
Mental disorders	39	51
Diseases of the digestive system	38	39
Injury	54	33
Diseases of the genitourinary tract	28	22

HEALTHY PEOPLE 2010 GOALS

Goal 1: Increase Quality and Years of Healthy Life

The first goal of Healthy People 2010 is to help individuals of all ages increase life expectancy and improve their quality of life.

Goal 2: Eliminate Health Disparities

The second goal of Healthy People 2010 is to eliminate health disparities among segments of the population, including differences that occur by gender, race or ethnicity, education or income, disability, geographic location, or sexual orientation.

U.S. Department of Health and Human Services. *Healthy People* 2010. 2nd ed. With Understanding and Improving Health and Objectives for Improving Health. 2 vols. Washington, DC: U.S. Government Printing Office, November 2000.

Morbidity, an illness or injury that limits activity, requires medical attention or hospitalization, or results in a chronic condition, also varies according to the age of the child. In 1998, there were 3.4 million hospital discharges for children between 1 and 21 years of age, an average of 4.1 discharges per 100 children. Figure 1-9 ◆ compares the leading causes of hospitalization of children by age group in 1993 and 1998. Respiratory diseases are the leading cause of hospitalization in children between 1 and 14 years of age, accounting for 31% of hospital discharges in this age group. Although injury is a leading cause of death in children 1 to 14 years of age, it accounted for only 9% of hospital discharges in 1998. Respiratory diseases, injury, and digestive diseases combined accounted for 45% of discharges in children 1 to 14 years of age. Pregnancy, childbirth, and mental disorders are among the leading causes of hospitalization in adolescents between 15 and 21 years of age (Health Resources and Services Administration, 2000). What do you think could account for the increase in hospital discharges for mental disorders in children and adolescents 10 to 21 years? See Chapter 7. In 1993, chronic illnesses and impairments limited the activities of more than 4.7 million children between 1 and 19 years of age. More boys than girls had activity limitations between 1 and 19 years of age (Maternal and Child Health Bureau, 1995).

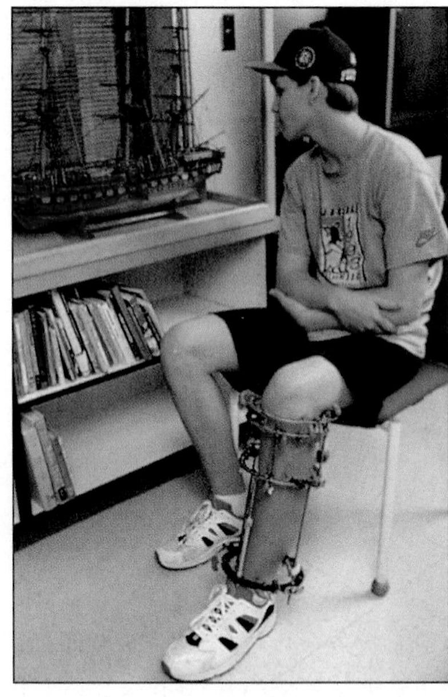

FIGURE 1-10 ◆
At the time of this photograph, Joey had been at Shriner's Hospital for over 8 months undergoing external fixation (lengthening the leg), which is a long and painful process. It is important that children undergoing long-term care continue their schooling, develop friendships with other children in the hospital, maintain contact with their friends at home, and learn self-care.

HEALTH CARE ISSUES

Health Care Technology

Research and technology have enabled many children with congenital anomalies and low birth weights to survive, with and without chronic conditions. Lifesaving technology has also created such burdens as high costs of health care and stresses on the functioning of the child's family. Many children with chronic conditions or complications of acute illnesses and injuries are managed in long-term care hospitals, rehabilitation centers, or home care programs (Figure 1-10 ◆). Approximately 400,000 children in the United States are unable to engage in normal childhood activities or depend on some form of medical technology (Klug, 1992) (Figure 1-11 ◆).

Health Care Financing

Not all children in the United States have access to health care. In 1998, 11.1 million children, 15.4% of those below 18 years of age, had no health insurance and 22.8% were covered by public insurance programs such as Medicaid. Of all children who lived in poverty in 1998, 26.4% had no health insurance and 57.7% were covered by public insurance (Health Resources and Services Administration, 2000). Most of these children had difficulty obtaining basic preventive health care, including immunizations (Figure 1-12 ◆).

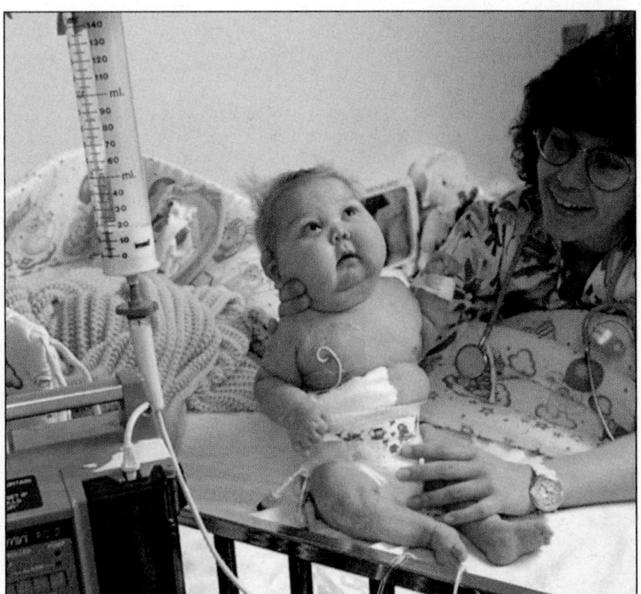

FIGURE 1-11 ◆
This child is dependent on the latest technology for necessary nutrients.

Efforts to provide universal access to health care for children continue to grow. Congress passed legislation to create the Child Health Insurance Plan in 1997 to enable more children to obtain access to essential health care services. States are allocated federal funds to encourage enrollment of children up to 200% of the federal poverty level (Smith, Wise, Chavkin, et al., 2000). Children enrolled must be provided with health benefits coverage that is substantially equal to the benefits coverage in the federal or state employee benefits plan or the plan of the largest health maintenance organization in the state. Children at 200% of poverty level are targeted by this program. More than 3 million children were enrolled in the State Children's Health Insurance Program (SCHIP) during 2000 (Health Care Finance Administration, 2000).

Managed care is an effort to coordinate and provide quality care while preventing unnecessary care and controlling costs. Significant changes in health care practices are occurring in response to these health insurance programs. Some state Medicaid programs have converted to a managed-care process.

Many children with severe chronic illnesses can be treated at home rather than by continued hospitalization. After studies in the 1980s found that home health care was

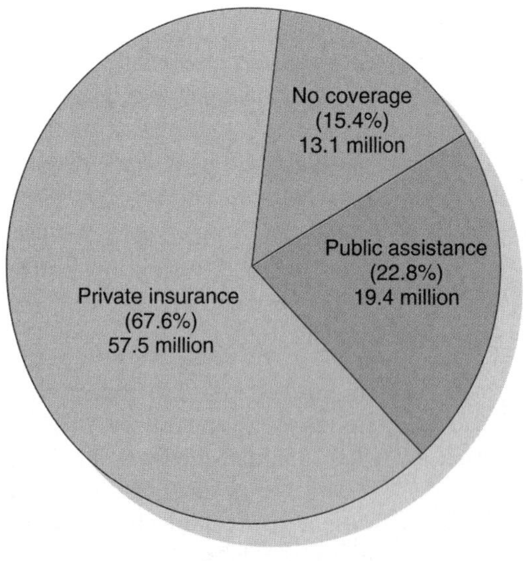

FIGURE 1-12 ◆
In the United States, how is health care of children paid for? These data from 1998 show that our taxes support 38% of the costs. What can you do to help? Something as simple as counseling parents about injury prevention and providing immunizations while a child is under care for other problems can prevent potential health problems. Part of good nursing care is supporting the well being of the child in addition to caring for the presenting problem.
NOTE: From Frontin, P., Employee Benefit Research Institute (2000). *Sources of health insurance and characteristics of the uninsured: Analysis of the March 1999 current population survey.* EBRI Issue Brief No. 217, Washington, DC: EBRI.

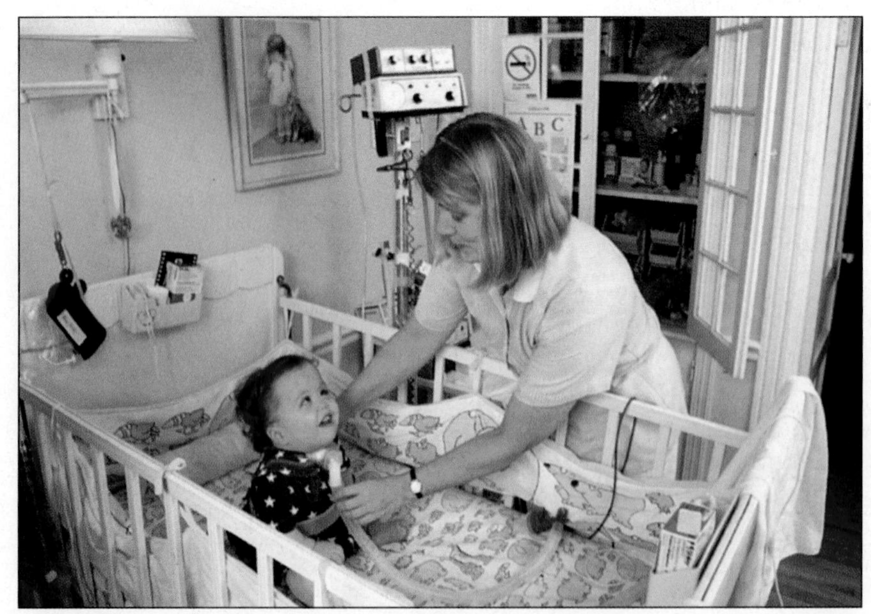

FIGURE 1-13 ◆
It is often desirable from a family and cost perspective to provide health care in the home, and technologic advances have made this possible. But is it really less costly to provide care in the home for a child with technology assistance? How does one factor in parents' out-of-pocket expenses for medical supplies that are not reimbursed? Lost time from work or the need for a parent to discontinue employment to care for the child? The emotional strain on families who care for their child 24 hours a day, 7 days a week? What support is needed by these families to continue providing this level of care at home?

substantially less expensive than hospital care, Congress amended laws to permit payment of home care services with federal funds (U.S. General Accounting Office, 1989). In 1996, nearly 600,000 children under 18 years were served by a formal home care program (National Association of Home Care, 2000). Technologic advances have resulted in the design of portable medical and infusion therapy equipment for home care. Some families have regained control over their lives by creating intensive care units in their homes (Figure 1-13 ◆). Children who 10 years ago would have died of respiratory, neurologic, or other medical conditions are thriving with home care and are participating in family, community, and school life.

LEGAL CONCEPTS AND RESPONSIBILITIES

REGULATION OF NURSING PRACTICE

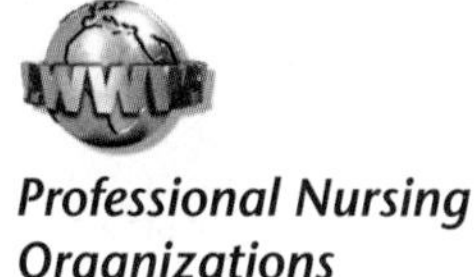

Professional Nursing Organizations

Because nurses are accountable for their professional actions, each state regulates nursing practice with a nurse practice act. In many states, nursing is defined as "the nursing diagnosis and treatment of human responses to health and to illness" (American Nurses Association, 1998). A state's nurse practice act defines the legal roles and responsibilities of nurses. Become familiar with this act in your state.

As professionals, nurses set standards for education and practice that conform to state regulations. Professional nursing organizations and state agencies that accredit nursing programs modify the standards for nursing education as the science of nursing progresses. Nurses in professional organizations develop standards of nursing practice. These standards describe the public and patient responsibilities for which nurses are accountable.

Standards of clinical nursing practice developed by the American Nurses Association in 1998 define standards for both nursing care and performance. Standards of care describe the competent level of nursing care using the nursing process and form the foundation of clinical decision making. Standards of performance describe the nurse's behavior in the professional role and include such criteria as quality of care, performance appraisal, collegiality, resource utilization, ethics, research, education, and collaboration. Specific standards have also been developed for pediatric clinical nursing practice (Table 1-2).

TABLE 1-2 Professional Practice Standards for Pediatric Clinical Nursing Practice

STANDARDS OF CARE FOR THE PEDIATRIC NURSE INCLUDE

- Collecting health data.
- Analyzing the assessment data in determining diagnoses.
- Implementing the interventions identified in the plan of care.
- Evaluating the child's and family's progress toward attainment of outcomes.

STANDARDS OF PERFORMANCE FOR THE PEDIATRIC NURSE INCLUDE

- Systematically evaluating the quality and effectiveness of pediatric nursing practice.
- Evaluating his or her own nursing practice in relation to professional practice standards and relevant statutes and regulations.
- Acquiring and maintaining current knowledge in pediatric nursing practice.
- Contributing to the professional development of peers, colleagues, and others.
- Making decisions and taking action on behalf of children and their families that are determined in an ethical manner.
- Collaborating with the child, family, and health care providers in providing patient care.
- Using research findings in practice.
- Considering factors related to safety, effectiveness, and cost in planning and delivering care.

Note: From American Nurses Association & the Society of Pediatric Nurses. (1996). *Statement on the scope and standards of pediatric clinical nursing practice.* (MCH-17). Washington, DC: American Nurses Publishing.

ACCOUNTABILITY AND RISK MANAGEMENT

Accountability

The family entrusts the child's care to the health care team. Family members expect this team to provide good medical and nursing care and to avoid mistakes that cause harm. Nurses are personally accountable for expanding their knowledge base, for recognizing important changes in the child's condition that require intervention, and for taking action as necessary to protect the child.

Risk Management

Health care institutions make every effort to promote optimal patient care and reduce liability by various activities, such as the following:

- **Risk management** is a process established by a health care institution to identify, evaluate, and reduce the risk of injury to patients, staff, and visitors, and thereby reduce the institution's liability.
- **Quality improvement** is the continuous study and improvement of the processes and outcomes of providing health care services to meet the needs of patients, by examining the systems and processes of how care and services are delivered.

CLINICAL TIP 

Policy and procedure manuals should be current and provide guidance on patient care and the use of technology specifically related to potentially serious situations.

Nurses participate in the development of institutional policies and standards of nursing practice. Hospitals and home health agencies encourage the development of diagnosis-specific nursing care plans or interdisciplinary clinical practice guidelines or critical pathways that serve as minimal institutional standards of care.

During the development of institutional standards of care, indicators of effective care by nurses and other providers are identified. These indicators may measure either the process of care, the institution's systems, or the expected outcome of care for a specific patient condition. Patient records are regularly reviewed to identify deviations from the institutional standards or clinical practice guidelines/critical pathways. When deviations from expected processes and outcomes are identified, opportunities to improve the system or processes of care provision are explored with all care providers. Recommendations for the revision of institutional standards to further improve care by nurses and other health providers in the institution often result.

LAW & ETHICS 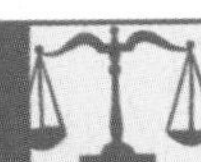

The patient's record is a legal document that is admissible evidence in court. Information in the patient's record must be legibly written in objective terms. When recording a patient's response to therapy, the nurse must include physiologic responses and exact quotes. The date, time, and nurse's signature and title are required.

Documentation of nursing care is an essential part of risk management and quality assurance. If a patient record is subpoenaed, documented care is considered the only care provided, regardless of the quality of undocumented care. The patient assessment, the nursing care plan, and the child's responses to medical therapies and nursing care, including the regularly scheduled evaluation of the patient's progress toward nursing goals, must all be documented accurately and sequentially. Nurses must also report any untoward incidents that could inhibit the patient's recovery.

LAW & ETHICS 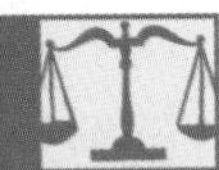

Information that the physician must provide to obtain informed consent includes an explanation of the condition, a detailed description of the treatment, possible benefits and significant risks associated with the proposed treatments, possible alternative treatments, answers to questions, and notification of a parent's or guardian's right to refuse treatment on behalf of the child.

LEGAL AND ETHICAL ISSUES IN PEDIATRIC CARE

Shanti, a 15-year-old girl with acute myelocytic leukemia, has come out of her second remission with an acute onset of fever, joint pain, and petechiae. A bone marrow transplant is one of the few remaining therapeutic options. Although Shanti has agreed to a transplant if a suitable donor is found, she does not want to be resuscitated and placed on life support equipment should she have a cardiac arrest. She has talked extensively with the hospital chaplain and social worker and feels comfortable with her decision. Her parents want an all-out effort to sustain her life until a donor is located.

Shanti's case illustrates the legal and ethical dilemmas in caring for children. At what age can children make an informed decision about whether to accept or refuse treatment? What happens when the parents and child have conflicting opinions about treatment? How are ethical decisions resolved?

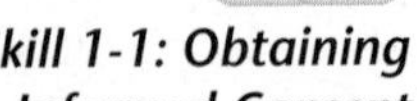

Skill 1-1: Obtaining Informed Consent

INFORMED CONSENT

Informed consent is a formal preauthorization for an invasive procedure or participation in research. Consent must be given voluntarily. Parents, as the legal custodians of minor

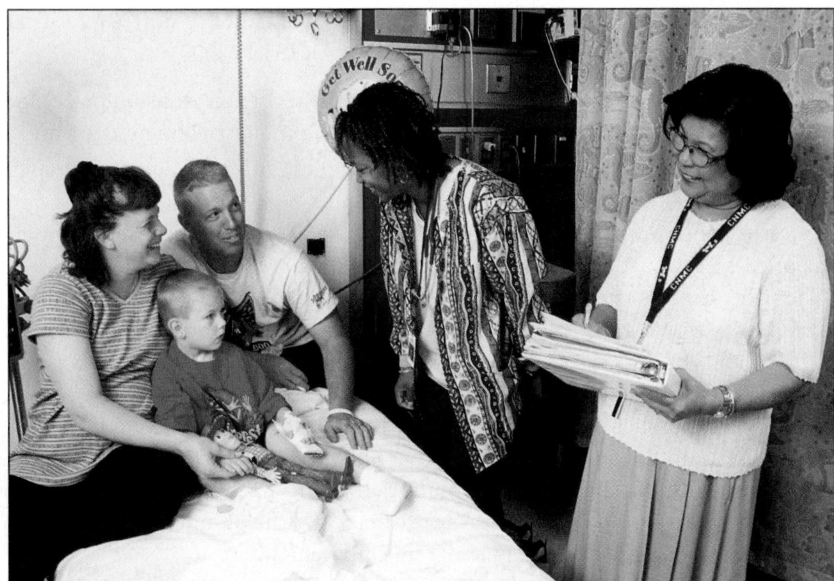

FIGURE 1-14 ◆
Children need to be actively involved in decisions regarding their care when appropriate. Here, the family and staff come together to discuss the child's care in a positive and honest manner.

children, are customarily requested to give informed consent on behalf of a child. When parents are divorced, either may give informed consent. Both children and parents must understand that they have the right to refuse treatment at any time. In an emergency, consent for treatment to preserve life or limb is not required.

Children under 18 or 21 years of age, depending on state law, can legally give informed consent in the following circumstances:

- When they are minor parents of the child patient
- When they are **emancipated minors** (self-supporting adolescents under 18 years of age, not subject to parental control)
- When they are adolescents between 16 and 18 years of age seeking birth control, mental health counseling, or substance abuse treatment (Dickey & Deatrick, 2000).

Mature minors (14- and 15-year-old adolescents who are able to understand treatment risks) can give consent for treatment or refuse treatment in some states.

Children should become more actively involved in decision making about treatment procedures as their reasoning skills develop. Children too young to give informed consent can be given age-appropriate information about their condition and asked about their care preferences. Their parents, however, make ultimate decisions regarding their care (Figure 1-14 ◆).

With regard to participation in research, federal guidelines state that children 7 years of age and older must receive information about a research project and give **assent** (the voluntary agreement to participate in a research project or to accept treatment) before they are enrolled. Children should be given adequate time to ask questions and be told that they have the right to refuse to participate in the study (U.S. Department of Health and Human Services, 1983; Lindeke, Hauck, & Tanner, 2000). The number of children asked to participate in research is expected to increase because of new Food and Drug Administration regulations requiring manufacturers to assess the safety and effectiveness of new drugs and biological products in pediatric patients (Food and Drug Administration, 1998).

CHILD'S RIGHTS VERSUS PARENTS' RIGHTS

Parents or guardians have absolute authority to make choices about their child's health care except in the following cases:

- When the child and parents do not agree on major treatment options
- When the parents' choice of treatment does not permit lifesaving treatment for the child
- When there is a potential conflict of interest between the child and parents, such as with suspected child abuse or neglect

CLINICAL TIP

The physician is legally responsible for obtaining informed consent. The nurse's role in obtaining informed consent includes the following:

- Alerting physicians to the need for informed consent
- Responding to questions asked by parents and children
- Serving as a witness when parents sign consent forms or give verbal consent by telephone

GROWTH & DEVELOPMENT

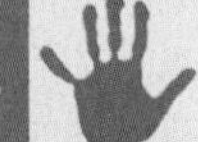

By 7 or 8 years of age, a child is able to understand concrete explanations about informed consent for research participation. By age 11, a child's abstract reasoning and logic are advanced. By age 14, an adolescent can weigh options and make decisions regarding consent as capably as an adult.

LAW & ETHICS

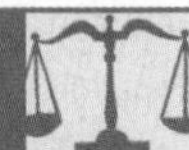

Obtain legal advice for complex family issues related to guardianship, divorced parents disagreeing over care, or a caregiver who is not the legal guardian.

- When the parents are incapacitated and cannot make a decision (e.g., critically injured in the same motor vehicle crash) (Dickey & Deatrick, 2000)

In some cases, the court may be requested to appoint a proxy decision maker for the child or to determine that the child is capable of making a major treatment decision.

CLINICAL TIP

Breaching confidentiality is a potential problem for adolescents, who are just learning whom they can trust in the health care system. Make sure you openly discuss the limits of confidentiality for such things as mandatory reporting requirements with the patient and family. Inadvertent disclosure of personal information may lead to psychologic, social, or physical harm in some patients.

CONFIDENTIALITY

Concerns about privacy and the fear of disclosure of sensitive information to parents is a major reason why adolescents do not seek health care (Ford, Bearman, & Moody, 1999). When the child is an emancipated or mature minor, many states permit health care providers to provide birth control and treatment for sexually transmitted diseases including HIV and AIDS, pregnancy, and substance abuse without informing the child's parents (Dickey, 2000). If the child has a reportable disease, confidentiality may create a public health hazard. In such cases, the health care professional is obligated to report the presence of the disease to the appropriate state or county agency (Fiesta, 1992). Suspected cases of child abuse must be reported to the appropriate agency specified by state law. In the current health care system, the complexities of treatment and the numbers of health care providers involved make it more difficult to maintain confidentiality.

PATIENT SELF-DETERMINATION ACT

The federal Patient Self-Determination Act directs health care institutions to inform hospitalized patients about their rights, which include expressing a preference for treatment options and making **advance directives** (writing a living will or authorizing a durable power of attorney for health care decisions on the patient's behalf). Nurses often discuss these issues with patients and their families. Minor children and their parents should also be informed of their rights. Adolescents with serious acute or chronic conditions with a higher risk of death should be encouraged to talk with their parents about their health care wishes and to jointly prepare advance directives (Dickey, 2000).

Do Not Resuscitate orders have become more common for children with terminal illnesses in which no further treatments are possible or desired. In many cases, these children are cared for at home or in a hospice program, but some still attend school. Implementation of Do Not Resuscitate orders for such children then becomes a community issue, to ensure that no resuscitation measures are initiated by any emergency care provider when the child has a life-threatening event. State health policies must be developed so children with these signed orders are easily identified and appropriate documentation of the orders is on file.

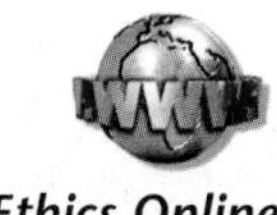

Ethics Online

ETHICAL ISSUES

Ethics is the philosophic study of morality, moral judgments, and moral problems. Ethical issues may arise from a **moral dilemma,** a conflict of social values and ethical principles that support different courses of action. Technology makes it possible to sustain the lives of children who previously would have died, thus creating many ethical issues. Problems may develop because physicians, nurses, and parents have differing opinions about treatments for an infant or child with a serious or fatal condition. Nurses often face ethical dilemmas when providing care to such a child. They witness parents struggling to decide among treatment options. Ethical issues in pediatrics are often more complex because most children lack the capacity to make or to participate in medical decisions that directly affect them.

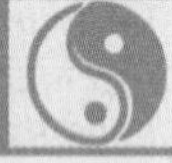

CULTURE

Jehovah's Witnesses oppose blood transfusions for themselves and their children because they believe transfusions are equivalent to the oral intake of blood, which is morally and spiritually wrong according to their interpretation of the Bible (Leviticus 17:13–14). A Jehovah's Witness who receives a transfusion believes he or she has committed a sin and may have forfeited everlasting life. Transfusions of any blood products, including plasma and the patient's own blood, are forbidden.

Ethical decision making is based on respect for persons and their ability to make decisions independently. All individuals must be treated without prejudice, regardless of race, gender, religious preference, cultural or educational background, financial status, or sexual orientation (Cassidy & Fleischman, 1996). Health care professionals may have different values from patients, based on culture and life experiences.

Certain principles guide decision making about treatment when moral dilemmas exist. A major principle is to avoid harm and provide beneficial care to the child. When making treatment decisions in pediatrics, health care professionals must determine whether their responsibility is limited to the child or includes the interests of the parents. The health care institution's ethics committee often serves the role of resolving conflicts about treatment decisions in one of the following three ways.

- By performing individual case consultations
- By serving as a forum to discuss policies about institutional ethics
- By educating health professionals and the community about ethical concepts

The committees often make treatment decisions using the process of data collection and evaluation outlined in Table 1-3. Courts should make ethical decisions only when health care professionals and parents are unable to agree about providing or withholding treatment.

Terminating Life-Sustaining Treatment

Baby Tim, at 1 day of age, has severe myelomeningocele with hydrocephalus. His physicians are seeking his parents' consent for surgical placement of a shunt to control the progression of hydrocephalus. Regardless of medical care and surgical intervention, the infant is expected to have a severe handicap. The parents, after much consideration and discussions with their family and pastor, have requested that life-sustaining treatment be withheld.

What happens when the parents' request differs from the opinion of physicians? How do federal regulations for care of infants with severe defects affect current health care practice?

Federal "Baby Doe" regulations were developed to protect the rights of infants with severe defects. Parents of such infants are usually the ultimate decision makers about the child's care. They may want to terminate treatment because of the tremendous social, emotional, and financial burden (Schrode, 2000). Physicians may believe treatment will help the child and improve the quality of life (sometimes defined as a meaningful existence or an ability to develop human relationships). Federal regulations require a formalized ethical

TABLE 1-3 Steps in Making Ethical Decisions

COLLECT INFORMATION
What decisions are needed? Who are the key persons involved? What information will help make the situation more clear? Are there any legal constraints?
IDENTIFY THE ETHICAL ISSUES OR CONCERNS OF THE SITUATION
What are their historical roots, the religious and philosophical positions? What are the current societal views of each issue?
DEFINE THE PERSONAL AND PROFESSIONAL MORAL POSITIONS ON THE ISSUES
What personal constraints are raised by the issues? What is the professional code for guidance? Are there any conflicting loyalties or obligations? What are the moral positions of the key individuals involved?
IDENTIFY ANY VALUE CONFLICTS
What is the basis for the conflict? What is the possible resolution?
DECISION MAKING
Who should make the decision? What are the possible actions and their anticipated outcome? What is the moral justification for each action? Which action fits the criteria for this situation? Decide on a course of action and carry it out.
EVALUATE THE RESULTS OF THE DECISION ACTION
Did the expected outcome occur? Is a new decision needed? Is the decision process complete?

NOTE: Adapted from Thompson, J.B., & Thompson, H.O. (1981). *Ethics in nursing.* New York: Macmillan Publishing.

decision-making process before physicians accept or reject a parent's wishes. The most common question brought before ethics committees is whether to terminate life-sustaining treatment.

Justifications for withholding, withdrawing, or limiting therapy include the following:

- The treatment in question will not work.
- The burdens of the treatment outweigh the benefits, or the quality of life is poor after treatment.
- The burdens of the disease outweigh the benefits of continued survival, or the quality of life is poor before the treatment (Cassidy, 1996).

Each of these conditions is considered according to the individual beliefs of the ethics committee members and their perceptions of the value of specific interventions for an individual child. Treatment to save the infant's life is elected if it has the potential for improving the quality of life as well. Physicians are not obligated to offer interventions that cause extreme pain and suffering when there is no or limited potential benefit. Treatments that only prolong life represent a misuse of expensive health care resources.

Organ Transplantation Issues

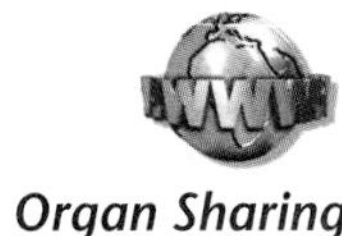

Organ Sharing

The death of a child can benefit another child through organ transplantation. The National Organ Transplant Act (Public Law 98-507) generated laws, regulations, and guidelines for organ collection and transplantation (Frader & Thompson, 1994). For example, the transplant team cannot provide care to the potential donor. The institution has specific requirements to approach family members when brain death is suspected or confirmed to request organ donation.

Regulations are important because too few organs are available for patients needing transplantation. The limited supply of organs has created numerous ethical issues. Which patients on the waiting list should receive the organs available? Should families be permitted to pay donor families for organs? Should the family's ability to pay for an organ transplant give a child higher priority for an organ? What are the brain death and nonheartbeating criteria for children that enable organ collection to proceed?

Many topics discussed in this chapter reflect the current challenges children and their families face in the health care system—access to health care, specific disease and injury risks, and ethical and legal concerns. Fortunately, pediatric nursing often involves caring for children who have episodes of acute illness or injury and who recover quickly without serious consequences. The challenge and gratification of pediatric nursing is to provide appropriate care in a supportive environment that promotes the family unit and the child's development.

Chapter Highlights

- Roles of nurses in caring for children include providing direct care, patient education, patient advocacy, and case management, and minimizing the psychologic and physical distress experienced by children and their families.
- Nurses care for children in many different settings. Within the hospital, these settings include the emergency department, observation or short-stay unit, postanesthesia unit, intensive care unit, general pediatric inpatient unit, and various outpatient clinics. Other settings include schools, child care centers, physician offices, community health centers, rehabilitation centers, and the home.
- Family-centered care is a method designed to meet the emotional, social, and developmental needs of children and families needing health care.
- Nurses must identify culturally relevant facts about their patients to provide appropriate and competent care to an increasingly diverse population.
- Unintentional injury is the leading cause of death for children between 1 and 19 years of age.
- Efforts to provide all children with access to health care include the Child Health Insurance Program currently being implemented in all states.
- Documentation of nursing care is essential for risk management and quality improvement. Documentation must include the patient assessment, the nursing care plan, the child's responses to medical therapies and nursing care, and the regular evaluation of the child's progress toward nursing goals.

- Informed consent is the formal preauthorization for an invasive procedure or participation in research. Parents typically give informed consent for children under 18 years of age unless the child is an emancipated minor, a self-supporting adolescent not subject to parental control.
- Children need to become more actively involved in decisions about their care as their decision-making abilities develop. Even though they cannot provide informed consent, federal guidelines mandate that children as young as 7 years of age receive information about treatment procedures and research project participation and give their assent.
- Because adolescents fear disclosure of confidential information, they may avoid seeking health care. When the adolescents have a reportable disease, it is important to inform them that confidentiality cannot be maintained as a report must be made to a public health agency.
- Adolescents at a higher risk of death due to a serious acute or chronic condition should be encouraged to talk with their parents and jointly prepare advance directives.
- Federal regulations require a formalized ethical decision-making process to assist health care providers and families in making important decisions about withholding, withdrawing, or limiting a child's therapy.

EXPLORE MediaLink

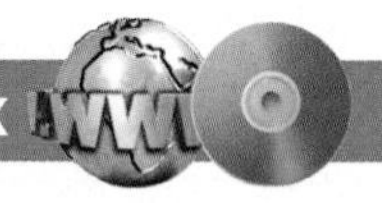

- NCLEX Review, case studies, and other interactive resources for this chapter can be found on the Companion Website at **http://www.prenhall.com/ball.** Click on Chapter 1 to select the activities for this chapter.
- For animations, more NCLEX review questions, and an audio glossary, access the accompanying CD-ROM in this book.

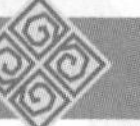

References

1. American Nurses Association. (1998). *Standards of clinical nursing practice* (2nd ed.). Washington, DC: American Nurses Publishing.
2. Cassidy, R.C., & Fleischman, A.R. (1996). *Pediatric ethics—From principles to practice.* Amsterdam, The Netherlands: Harwood Academic Publishers.
3. Dickey, S.B., & Deatrick, J. (2000). Autonomy and decision making for health promotion in adolescence. *Pediatric Nursing, 26*(5), 461–467.
4. Fiesta, J. (1992). Protecting children: A public duty to report. *Nursing Management, 23,* 14–15.
5. Food and Drug Administration. (1998, December 2). Regulations requiring manufacturers to assess the safety and effectiveness of new drugs and biological products in pediatric patients. *Federal Register, 63*(231), 66631–66672. *www.fda.gov/ohrms/dockets/98fr/120298c.txt*
6. Ford, C.A., Bearman, P.S., & Moody, J. (1999). Foregone health care among adolescents. *Journal of American Medical Association, 282*(23), 2227–2234.
7. Frader, J., & Thompson, A. (1994). Ethical issues in the pediatric intensive care unit. *Pediatric Clinics of North America, 41*(6), 1405–1421.
8. Health Care Finance Administration. (2000). The state children's health insurance program (SCHIP). *www.hcfa.gov/init/fy2000.html*
9. Health Resources and Services Administration, Maternal and Child Health Bureau. (2000). *Child health USA 2000.* Washington, DC: U.S. Government Printing Office.
10. Klug, R.M. (1992). Selecting a home care agency. *Pediatric Nursing, 8,* 504–506.
11. Lindeke, L.L., Hauck, M.R., & Tanner, M. (2000). Practical issues in obtaining child assent for research. *Journal of Pediatric Nursing, 15*(2), 99–104.
12. Maternal and Child Health Bureau. (1995). *Child health USA '94.* (DHHS Publication No. HRSA-MCH-95-1). Washington, DC: U.S. Government Printing Office.
13. Melnyk, B.M., Fineout-Overholt, E., Stone, P., & Ackerman, M. (2000). Evidence-based practice: The past, the present, and recommendations for the millennium. *Pediatric Nursing, 26*(1), 77–80.
14. Merritt, T.A., Palmer, D., Bergman, D.A., & Shiono, P.H. (1997). Clinical practice guidelines in pediatric and newborn medicine. Implications for their use in practice. *Pediatrics, 99*(1), 100–114.
15. Murray, J.E. (1999). Individuals with Disabilities Education Act (IDEA). *www.nahc.org/NAHC/Peds/News/News07021999.html*
16. National Association of Home Care. (2000). Basic statistics about home care. *www.nahc.org/Consumer/hcstats.html*
17. Population Estimates Program, Population Division, U.S. Census Bureau. (2001). Resident population estimates of the United States by age and sex: April 1, 1990, to July 1, 1999, with short-term project to November 1, 2000. *www.census.gov/population/estimates/ nation/intfile2-1.txt*
18. Schrode, K. (2000). Baby Doe and the Baby Doe regulations. *Children's National Medical Center Pediatric Ethicscope, 11*(1), 1–4.
19. Smith, L.A., Wise, P.H., Chavkin, W., Romero, D., & Zuckerman, B. (2000). Implications in welfare reform for child health: Emerging challenges for clinical practice and policy. *Pediatrics, 106*(5), 1117–1125.
20. U.S. Census (2001). Population estimates for children by age and race. *www.wonder.cdc/census*
21. U.S. Department of Health and Human Services. (1983). *Protection of human subjects: Code of federal regulations.* (45 CFR 46, Subpart D). Washington, DC: Government Printing Office.
22. U.S. Department of Health and Human Services. (2000). *Healthy People 2010,* 2nd ed. Washington, DC: U.S. Government Printing Office.
23. U.S. General Accounting Office. (1989). *Home care experiences of families with chronically ill children.* Washington, DC: Author.

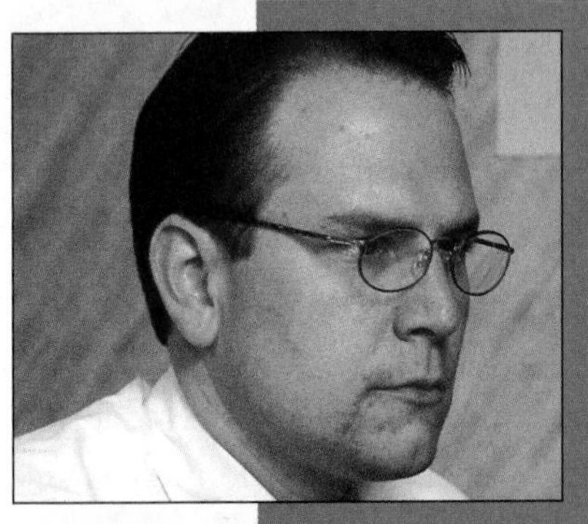

"WE WANT TO HELP IRENA GROW INTO A NORMAL AND SPECIAL CHILD. SHE HAS HAD CHALLENGES IN HER SHORT LIFE THAT WE CAN ONLY IMAGINE. WE WORRY ABOUT WHETHER SHE'LL WANT TO GO BACK TO ROMANIA WHEN SHE'S OLDER TO FIND HER FAMILY."

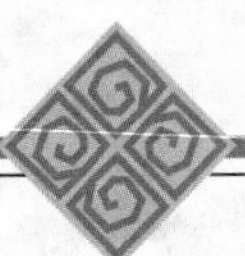

Michael and Alyssa had tried for several years to have a biologic child. After an unsuccessful in vitro fertilization, they decided to try to adopt a child. They explored opportunities with adoption agencies, and learned that international adoption was possible for them. They adopted 2-year-old Irena from Romania several months ago. Despite thorough investigation of Michael and Alyssa by the adoption agency, they received only scant information about Irena's history. She was given to an orphanage by her mother when she was about 7 months old; the mother stated that the pregnancy and delivery were normal. She was giving up the child because she had two older children to care for and her husband had left home nearly a year before and had not been heard from since. Irena appears small for her age, but is thriving in her new environment. She is learning to say a few English words and is responding appropriately to care and interactions. How can the nurse work with Michael and Alyssa to ensure special attention to Irena's growth and health care needs? What will Irena's cultural needs be as she grows older?

CHAPTER 2

GROWTH AND DEVELOPMENT

KEY TERMS

accommodation The process of changing one's cognitive structures to include data from recent experiences.

anticipatory guidance The process of understanding upcoming developmental needs and then teaching caretakers to meet those needs.

assimilation The process of incorporating new experiences into one's cognitive awareness.

associative play A type of play that emerges in preschool years when children interact with one another, engaging in similar activities and participating in groups.

autosomal chromosomes The 22 pairs of chromosomes that are responsible for characteristics other than determination of sex.

cephalocaudal development The process by which development proceeds from the head downward through the body and toward the feet.

conservation The knowledge that matter is not changed when its form is altered.

cooperative play A type of play that emerges in school years when children join into groups to achieve a goal or play a game.

defense mechanisms Techniques used by the ego to unconsciously change reality, thereby protecting itself from excessive anxiety.

development An increase in capability or function.

dramatic play A type of play in which a child acts out the drama of daily life.

ecologic theory A theory of development that emphasizes the importance of interactions between the developing child and the settings in which the child lives.

expressive jargon Use of unintelligible words with normal speech intonations as if truly communicating in words; common in toddlerhood.

growth An increase in physical size.

Human Genome Project An international effort to determine the exact DNA sequences of every human gene.

nature The genetic or hereditary capability of an individual.

nurture The effects of environment on an individual's performance.

object permanence The knowledge that an object or person continues to exist when not seen, heard, or felt.

parallel play A type of play that emerges in toddlerhood when children play side by side but demonstrate little or no social interaction.

proximodistal development The process by which development proceeds from the center of the body outward to the extremities.

puberty Period of life when the ability to reproduce sexually begins; characterized by maturation of the genital organs, development of the secondary sex characteristics, and (in females) the onset of menstruation.

sex chromosomes The pair of chromosomes that are responsible for the determination of sex; XX for females and XY for males.

MediaLink 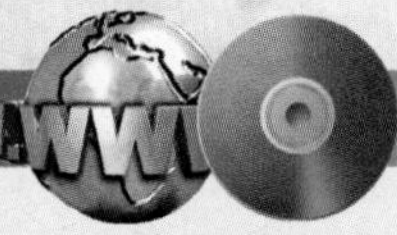

http://www.prenhall.com/ball

Resources for this chapter can be found on the CD-ROM accompanying this textbook, and on the Companion Website at http://www.prenhall.com/ball. Click on Chapter 2 to select the activities for this chapter.

CD-ROM	COMPANION WEBSITE
Audio Glossary	Web Links
NCLEX Review	NCLEX Review

GROWTH & DEVELOPMENT

Many international adoptees are small in size, due to poor nutrition of the mother during pregnancy and of the infant after birth, and to growth delay related to emotional issues. The child should be examined closely at the time of adoption for length, weight, and head circumference. Within 6 months of arrival, most children show improvement in growth patterns. If growth does not improve by this time, the child is further assessed for problems such as intestinal parasites, chronic diseases, or other medical problems (Altemeier, 2000; Miller, 2000).

Children develop as they interact with their surroundings. They learn skills at different ages, but the order in which they learn them is universal. Development is affected by factors such as nutrition and cultural practices, as well as the social situation in the country or neighborhood. While Irena will develop in a unique manner influenced by her genetic makeup, life experiences, and the interaction between these factors, certain principles of development can assist her parents and the nurse in fostering positive adaptations for her.

To highlight the important facets of development that are explored in this chapter, let us begin by examining some of Irena's characteristics (Figure 2-1 ◆).

PHYSICAL GROWTH AND DEVELOPMENT Although many international adoptees are small for their age, Irena appears well nourished. (See Chapter 3 for a discussion of nutritional needs during toddlerhood.) Her gross motor skills, including walking up steps, running, and kicking a ball, are well developed. Fine motor skills are evident in her ability to brush teeth and dress with help, scribble on paper, and build a tower of cubes.

COGNITIVE DEVELOPMENT Cognitive development relates to intellectual or thinking processes. It is hard to identify Irena's cognitive stage at this time, as she knows only a few English words and is shy during interactions with strangers. As she adapts to her new home, frequent assessments of her cognitive development will be necessary.

PLAY Irena is observed playing with toys and making sounds with her dolls. This is expected behavior, as toddlers often engage in solitary play. Toddlers also begin to enjoy the presence of other children, even though they do not yet play cooperatively with them. Irena's parents can encourage the emergence of parallel play with other toddlers by arranging to have Irena play with other children. The parents can be available at first so that Irena feels secure; once she shows comfort with other children, parents can gradually increase their absence during these playtimes.

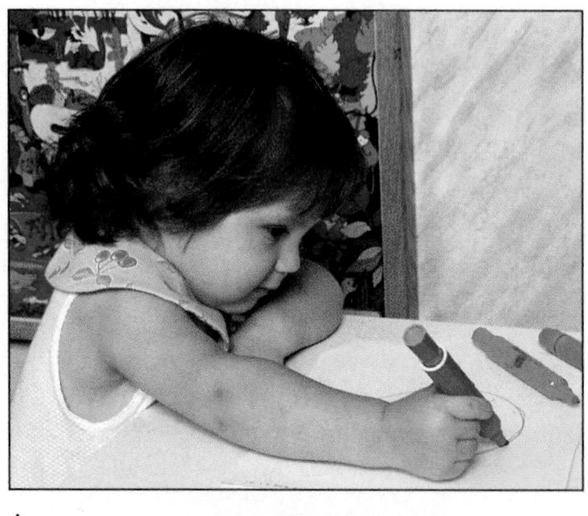

A

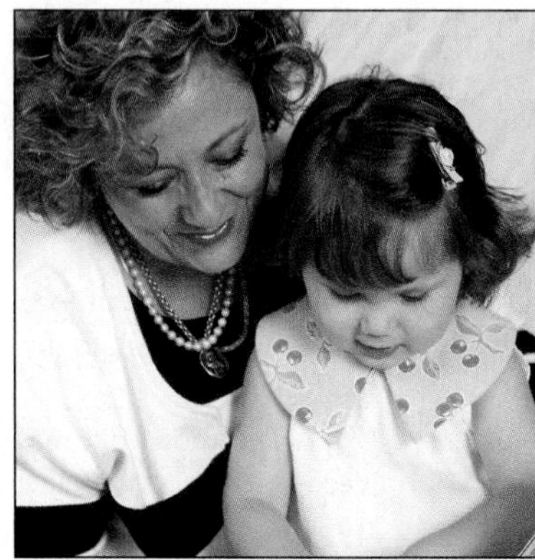

B

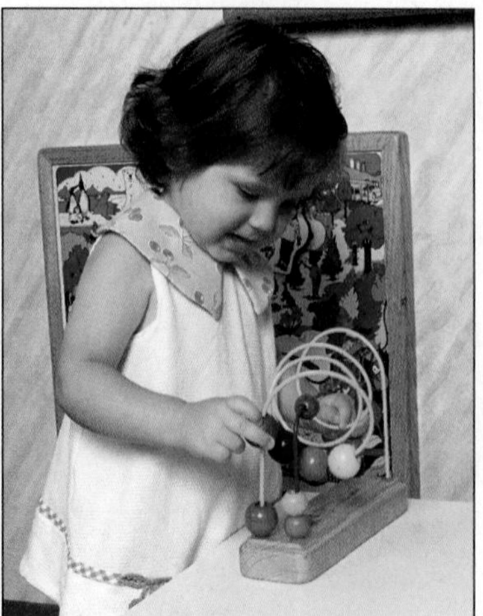

C

D

FIGURE 2-1 ◆
Observing the activities of a child provides information about developmental status.
A, Irena shows fine motor skills as she begins to scribble and color in a circle provided by a parent.
B, The parent provides positive reinforcement for activities.
C, Cognitive development is enhanced as toddlers manipulate objects.
D, Irena's parents provide comfort and a trusting environment.

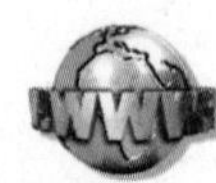

The Adoption Process

INJURY PREVENTION Cognitive and physical development mirror the changing hazards to the health and well-being of children. Irena might be injured in a car crash, particularly if not secured by a safety seat. Falls while climbing and consumption of poisons are also common injuries at her age. Injuries are a common cause of death and hospitalization during childhood. (See Chapter 1 for statistics about the relationship of injury to morbidity and mortality in childhood.) Nurses use **anticipatory guidance,** predicting the upcoming developmental tasks or needs of a child and performing appropriate teaching related to them, to discuss safety hazards and injury prevention for children of various ages with their parents.

PERSONALITY AND TEMPERAMENT Irena has been demonstrating what experts term an "easy" temperament; that is, she has readily acquired a regular schedule for eating and sleeping, her mood is generally pleasant, and she is easily comforted when upset. These temperamental characteristics will form a critical link to communication with family, teachers, and friends.

COMMUNICATION Irena has only learned a few words. This is abnormal for a toddler, since most know several hundred words. However, it is expected that Irena will learn language quickly as she adapts. Michael and Alyssa should speak with Irena often, pointing out names of people and objects. Positive reinforcement for Irena's attempts at speech can involve smiles, phrases such as "that's right," and further elaboration such as "Yes, that is a bus; it's a big, yellow bus." What else can you suggest to her parents as activities that will enhance speech development?

In this chapter, you will learn general principles of growth and development and will explore several theories related to childhood development, as well as their nursing applications. Each age group, from infancy through adolescence, is described in detail. Developmental milestones, physical and cognitive characteristics, health and safety concerns, and communication strategies are presented. This basic information will help you provide developmentally appropriate care for children in each age group. You can apply these concepts to all children, including special situations such as the one described in the opening scenario.

PRINCIPLES OF GROWTH AND DEVELOPMENT

It is essential to understand the concepts of growth and development when learning to care for children. **Growth** refers to an increase in physical size. **Development** refers to an increase in capability or function. The quantitative changes in body organ functioning, ability to communicate, and performance of motor skills unfold over time.

Each child displays a unique maturational pattern during the process of development. Although the exact age at which skills emerge differs, the sequence or order of skill performance is uniform among children. Skill development proceeds according to two processes: from the head down and from the center of the body out to the extremities. Development that proceeds from the head downward through the body and toward the feet is called **cephalocaudal development** (Figure 2-2 ◆). For example, at birth, an infant's head is much larger proportionately than the trunk or extremities. Similarly, infants learn to hold up their heads before sitting, and to sit before standing. Skills such as walking that involve the legs and feet develop last in infancy. Development that proceeds from the center of the body outward to the extremities is called **proximodistal development** (see Figure 2-2). For example, infants are first able to control the trunk, then the arms; only later are fine motor movements of the fingers possible.

During the childhood years, extraordinary changes occur in all aspects of development. Physical size, motor skills, cognitive ability, language, sensory ability, and psychosocial patterns all undergo major transformations. Nurses study normal patterns of development so they can perform thorough pediatric assessments and identify children who demonstrate slow or abnormal development. These assessments can guide the nurse in planning interventions for the child and family, such as referring the child for a diagnostic evaluation or rehabilitation, or teaching the parents how to provide adequate stimulation for the child. When development is proceeding normally, the nurse uses the knowledge of usual patterns to plan teaching approaches based on the child's cognitive and language ability, to offer appropriate toys and activities during illness, and to respond therapeutically during interactions with the child.

GROWTH & DEVELOPMENT

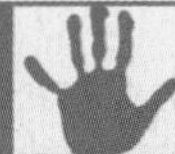

Although it is expected that international adoptees may have some developmental delays and often improve dramatically after adoption, testing of development, including verbal skills, upon arrival with their adoptive family is important. It provides a baseline upon which to measure future developmental test results and provides information needed to help parents encourage and stimulate the child appropriately (Miller, 2000). See Chapter 6 for a description of the Denver II Developmental Test.

CULTURE

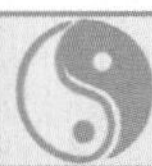

Nearly 20,000 international adoptions occur annually in the United States, up from less than half that number one decade ago. China and countries of the former Soviet Union are the major sources of adoptable children, who are an average age of 2 years (Jenista, 2000). Although these children may have an array of medical conditions such as infectious diseases, inadequate immunizations, and nutritional disorders, the effects of their early life experiences on development can also be profound. Institutionalization and multiple foster care placements can result in emotional neglect, growth and developmental delays, and behavior problems (Faber, 2000; Johnson, 2000; Miller, 2000; Aronson, 2000; Chamberlain, 2001). Nurses perform careful developmental monitoring and assist adoptive parents in fostering normal growth and development.

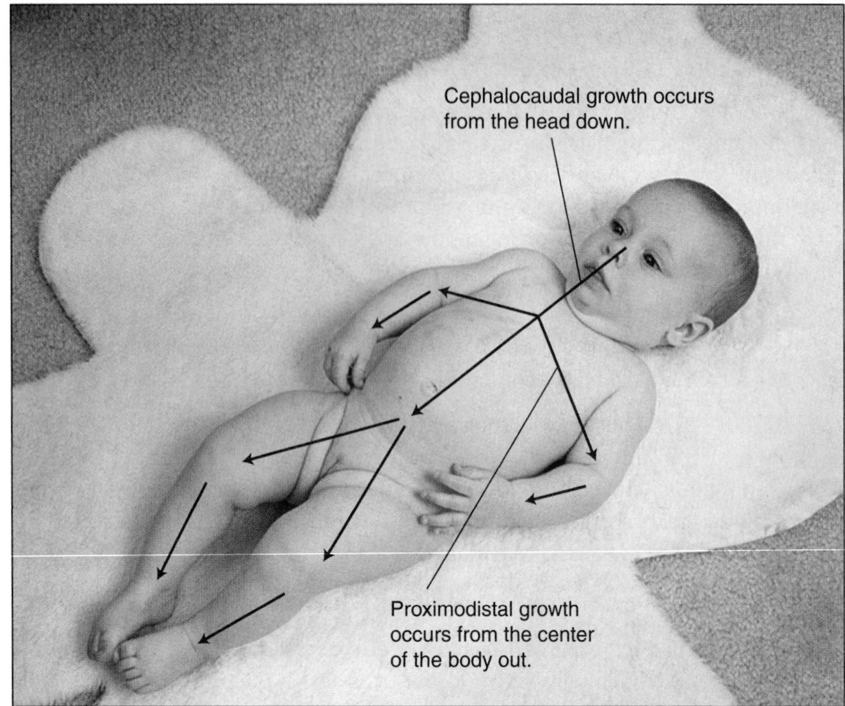

FIGURE 2-2 ◆
In normal *cephalocaudal* growth, the child gains control of the head and neck before the trunk and limbs. In normal *proximodistal* growth, the child controls arm movements before hand movements. For example, the child reaches for objects before being able to grasp them. Children gain control of their hands before their fingers; that is, they can hold things with the entire hand before they can pick something up with just their fingers.

MAJOR THEORIES OF DEVELOPMENT

Child development is a complex process. Many theorists have attempted to organize their observations of behavior into a description of principles or a set of stages. Each theory focuses on a particular facet of development. Most developmental theorists separate children into age groups by common characteristics (Table 2-1).

FREUD'S THEORY OF PSYCHOSEXUAL DEVELOPMENT

Theoretical Framework

SIGMUND FREUD (1856–1939)

Freud was a physician in Vienna, Austria. His work with adults who were experiencing a variety of nervous disorders led Freud to develop the approach called psychoanalysis, which explored the driving forces of the unconscious mind.

The psychoanalytic techniques used by Freud led him to believe that early childhood experiences form the unconscious motivation for actions in later life. He developed a theory that sexual energy is centered in specific parts of the body at certain ages. Unresolved conflict and unmet needs at a certain stage lead to a fixation of development at that stage (Gemelli, 1996).

Freud viewed the personality as a structure with three parts: the id, the basic sexual energy that is present at birth and drives the individual to seek pleasure; the ego, the realistic part of the person, which develops during infancy and searches for acceptable methods of meeting impulses; and the superego, the moral and ethical system, which develops in childhood and contains a set of values and conscience (Craig, 1999). The ego diverts impulses

TABLE 2-1 Developmental Age Groups

infancy—Birth to 12 months. Includes infants or babies up to 1 year of age who require a high level of care in daily activities.

toddlerhood—1–3 years. Characterized by increased motor ability and independent behavior.

preschool—3–6 years. The preschooler refines gross and fine motor ability and language skills and often participates in a preschool learning program.

school age—6–12 years. Begins with entry into a school system and is characterized by growing intellectual skills, physical ability, and independence.

adolescence—12–18 years. Begins with entry into the teen years. Mature cognitive thought, formation of identity, and influence of peers are important characteristics of adolescence.

TABLE 2-2 Common Defense Mechanisms Used by Children

DEFENSE MECHANISM	DEFINITION	EXAMPLE
Regression	Return to an earlier behavior	A previously toilet-trained child becomes incontinent when separated from parents during a hospitalization.
Repression	Involuntary forgetting of uncomfortable situations	An abused child cannot consciously recall episodes of abuse.
Rationalization	An attempt to make unacceptable feelings acceptable	A child explains hitting another because "he took my toy."
Fantasy	A creation of the mind to help deal with unacceptable fear	A hospitalized child who is weak pretends to be Superman.

and protects itself from excess anxiety by use of **defense mechanisms,** including regression to earlier stages and repression or forgetting of painful experiences such as child abuse (Table 2-2).

Stages

ORAL (BIRTH TO 1 YEAR) The infant derives pleasure largely from the mouth, with sucking and eating as primary desires.

ANAL (1 TO 3 YEARS) The young child's pleasure is centered in the anal area, with control over body secretions as a prime force in behavior.

PHALLIC (3 TO 6 YEARS) Sexual energy becomes centered in the genitalia as the child works out relationships with parents of the same and opposite sexes.

LATENCY (6 TO 12 YEARS) Sexual energy is at rest in the passage between earlier stages and adolescence.

GENITAL (12 YEARS TO ADULTHOOD) Mature sexuality is achieved as physical growth is completed and relationships with others occur.

Nursing Application

Freud emphasized the importance of meeting the needs of each stage in order to move successfully into future developmental stages. The crisis of illness can interfere with normal developmental processes and add challenges for the nurse who is striving to meet an ill child's needs. For example, the importance of sucking in infancy guides the nurse to provide a pacifier for the infant who cannot have oral fluids. The preschool child's concern about sexuality guides the nurse to provide privacy and clear explanations during any procedures involving the genital area. It may be necessary to teach parents that masturbation by the young child is normal and to help parents deal with it. The adolescent's focus on relationships suggests that the nurse should include questions about significant friends during history taking. Table 2-3 summarizes ways in which the nurse can apply these theoretical concepts to the care of children.

ERIKSON'S THEORY OF PSYCHOSOCIAL DEVELOPMENT

Theoretical Framework

Erikson's theory establishes psychosocial stages during eight periods of human life. For each stage, Erikson identifies a crisis, that is, a particular challenge that exists for healthy personality development to occur (Erikson, 1963, 1968). The word *crisis* in this context refers to normal maturational social needs rather than to a single critical event. Each developmental crisis has two possible outcomes: When needs are met, the consequence is healthy and the individual moves on to future stages with particular strengths. When needs are not met, an unhealthy outcome occurs that will influence future social relationships.

ERIK ERIKSON (1902–1994)

Erikson studied Freud's theory of psychoanalysis under Freud's daughter, Anna, but later established his own developmental theory emphasizing the psychosocial nature of individuals. Erikson's theory is one of the few that addresses development over the entire life span.

TABLE 2-3 Nursing Applications of Theories of Freud, Erikson, Piaget

AGE GROUP	DEVELOPMENTAL STAGES	NURSING APPLICATIONS
Infant (birth to 1 year)	Oral stage (Freud): The baby obtains pleasure and comfort through the mouth.	When a baby is NPO, offer a pacifier if not contraindicated. After painful procedures, offer a baby a bottle or pacifier or have the mother breast-feed.
	Trust versus mistrust stage (Erikson): The baby establishes a sense of trust when basic needs are met.	Hold the hospitalized baby often. **(1)** Offer comfort after painful procedures. Meet the baby's needs for food and hygiene. Encourage parents to room in. Manage pain effectively with use of pain medications and other measures.
	Sensorimotor stage (Piaget): The baby learns from movement and sensory input.	Use crib mobiles, manipulative toys, wall murals, and bright colors to provide interesting stimuli and comfort. Use toys to distract the baby during procedures and assessments.
Toddler (1–3 years)	Anal stage (Freud): The child derives gratification from control over bodily excretions.	Ask about toilet training and the child's rituals and words for elimination during admission history. Continue child's normal patterns of elimination in the hospital. Do not begin toilet training during illness or hospitalization. Accept regression in toileting during illness or hospitalization. Have potty chairs available in hospital and child care centers.
	Autonomy versus shame and doubt stage (Erikson): The child is increasingly independent in many spheres of life.	Allow self-feeding opportunities. Encourage child to remove and put on own clothes, brush teeth, or assist with hygiene. **(2)** If restraint for a procedure is necessary, proceed quickly, providing explanations and comfort.
	Sensorimotor stage (end); preoperational stage (beginning) (Piaget): The child shows increasing curiosity and explorative behavior. Language skills improve.	Ensure safe surroundings to allow opportunities to manipulate objects. Name objects and give simple explanations.
Preschooler (3–6 years)	Phallic stage (Freud): The child initially identifies with the parent of the opposite sex but by the end of this stage has identified with the same-sex parent.	Be alert for children who appear more comfortable with male or female nurses, and attempt to accommodate them. Encourage parental involvement in care. Plan for playtime and offer a variety of materials from which to choose.
	Initiative versus guilt stage (Erikson): The child likes to initiate play activities.	Offer medical equipment for play to lessen anxiety about strange objects. **(3)** Assess children's concerns as expressed through their drawings. Accept the child's choices and expressions of feelings.
	Preoperational stage (Piaget): The child is increasingly verbal but has some limitations in thought processes. Causality is often confused, so the child may feel responsible for causing an illness.	Offer explanations about all procedures and treatments. Clearly explain that the child is not responsible for causing the illness.

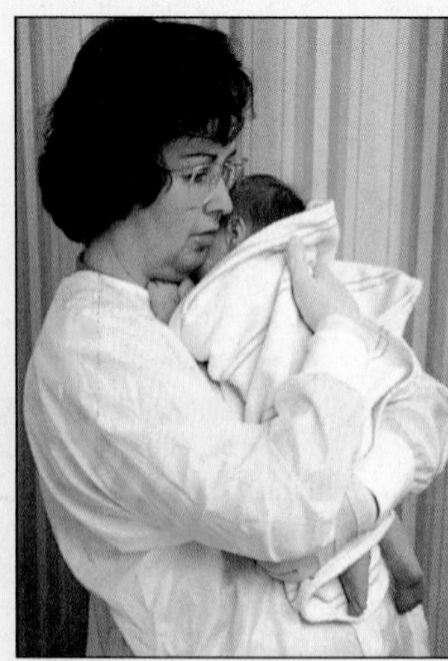

(1)

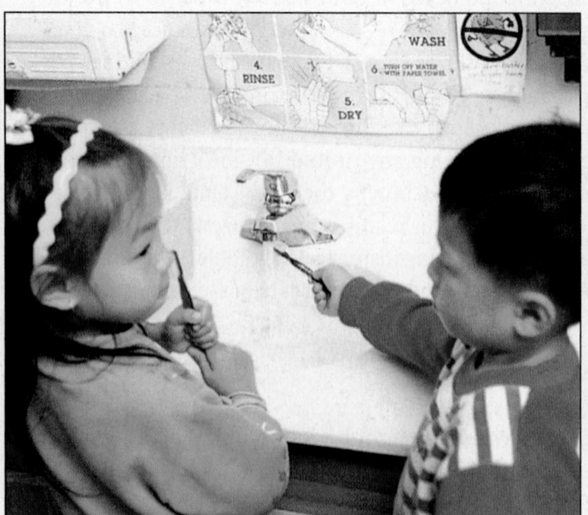

(2)

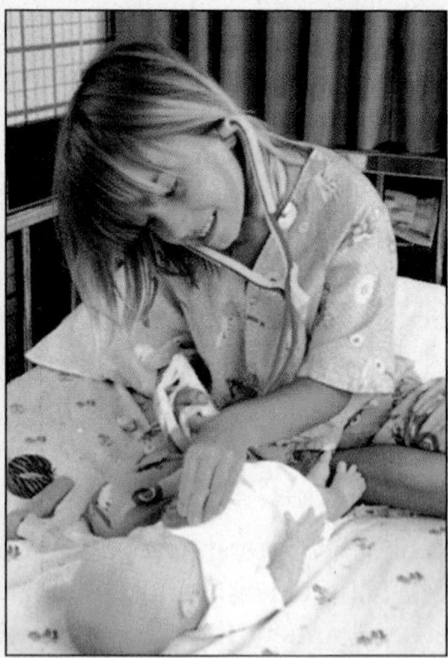

(3)

TABLE 2-3 Nursing Applications of Theories of Freud, Erikson, Piaget (continued)

AGE GROUP	DEVELOPMENTAL STAGES	NURSING APPLICATIONS
School age (6–12 years)	Latency stage (Freud): The child places importance on privacy and understanding the body.	Provide gowns, covers, and underwear. Knock on door before entering. Explain treatments and procedures.
	Industry versus inferiority stage (Erikson): The child gains a sense of self-worth from involvement in activities.	Encourage the child to continue school work while hospitalized. Encourage child to bring favorite pasttimes to the hospital. **(4)** Help child adjust to limitations on favorite activities.
	Concrete operational stage (Piaget): The child is capable of mature thought when allowed to manipulate and see objects.	Give clear instructions about details of treatment. Show the child equipment that will be used in treatment.
Adolescent (12–18 years)	Genital stage (Freud): The adolescent's focus is on genital function and relationships.	Ensure access to gynecologic care for adolescent girls. Provide information on sexuality. Ensure privacy during health care. Have brochures and videos available for teaching about sexuality.
	Identity versus role confusion stage (Erikson): The adolescent's search for self-identity leads to independence from parents and reliance on peers.	Provide a separate recreation room for teens who are hospitalized. **(5)** Take health history and perform examinations without parents present. Introduce adolescent to other teens with same health problem.
	Formal operational stage (Piaget): The adolescent is capable of mature, abstract thought.	Give clear and complete information about health care and treatments. Offer both written and verbal instructions. Continue to provide education about the disease to the adolescent with a chronic illness, as mature thought now leads to greater understanding.

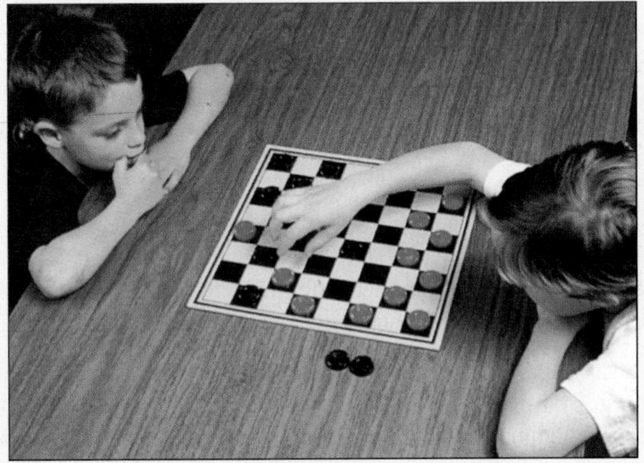

(4)

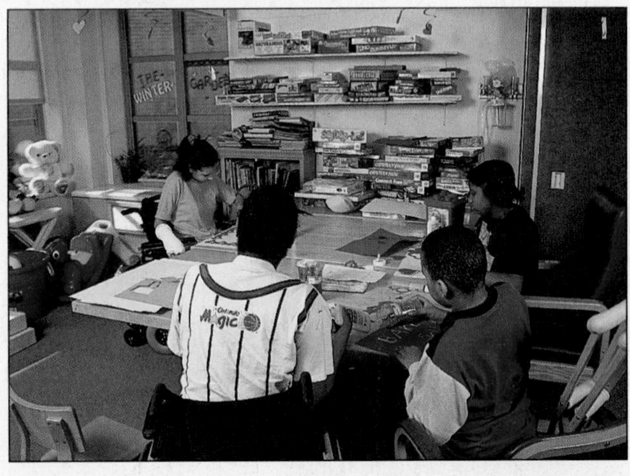

(5)

Stages

TRUST VERSUS MISTRUST (BIRTH TO 1 YEAR) The task of the first year of life is to establish trust in the people providing care. Trust is fostered by provision of food, clean clothing, touch, and comfort. If basic needs are not met, the infant will eventually learn to mistrust others.

AUTONOMY VERSUS SHAME AND DOUBT (1 TO 3 YEARS) The toddler's sense of autonomy or independence is shown by controlling body excretions, saying no when asked to do something, and directing motor activity. Children who are consistently criticized for expressions of autonomy or for lack of control—for example, during toilet training—will develop a sense of shame about themselves and doubt in their abilities.

AUTONOMY VERSUS SHAME AND DOUBT

The toddler likes to show autonomy by exerting control over toys and activities.

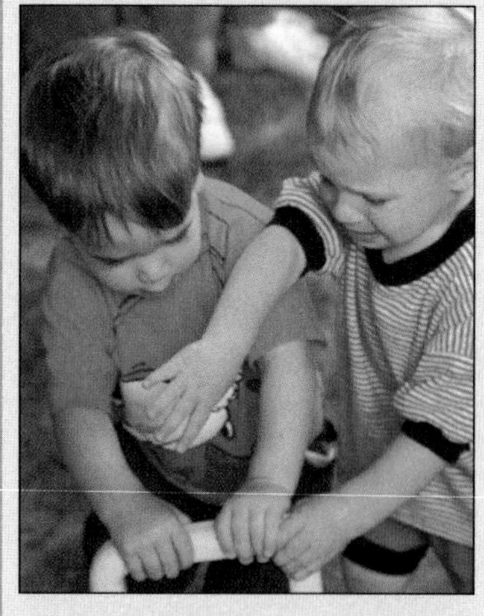

INDUSTRY VERSUS INFERIORITY

A child takes pride in accomplishments in sports.

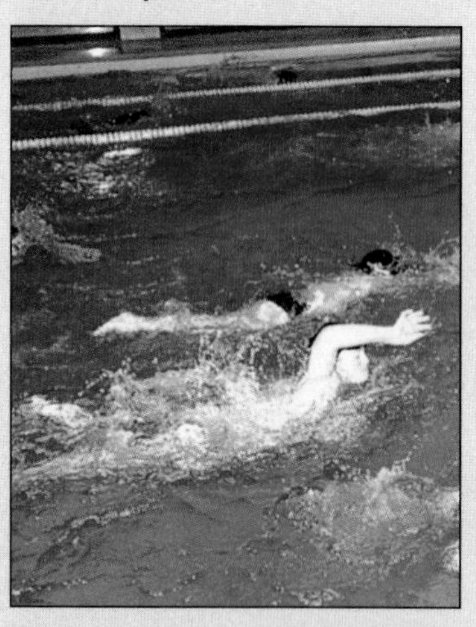

JEAN PIAGET (1896–1980)

Piaget was a 20th-century Swiss scientist who watched his own three children carefully and wrote detailed journals of their behaviors and verbalizations. He studied the intellectual abilities of children, focusing on child psychology and its application to education.

INITIATIVE VERSUS GUILT (3 TO 6 YEARS) The young child initiates new activities and considers new ideas. This interest in exploring the world creates a child who is involved and busy. Constant criticism, on the other hand, leads to feelings of guilt and a lack of purpose.

INDUSTRY VERSUS INFERIORITY (6 TO 12 YEARS) The middle years of childhood are characterized by development of new interests and by involvement in activities. The child takes pride in accomplishments in sports, school, home, and community. If the child cannot accomplish what is expected, however, the result will be a sense of inferiority.

IDENTITY VERSUS ROLE CONFUSION (12 TO 18 YEARS) In adolescence, as the body matures and thought processes become more complex, a new sense of identity or self is established. The self, family, peer group, and community are all examined and redefined. The adolescent who is unable to establish a meaningful definition of self will experience confusion in one or more roles of life.

Nursing Application

Erikson's theory is directly applicable to the nursing care of children. The social situations created by health care in the community provide opportunities for helping caregivers to meet children's needs. The child's usual support from family, peers, and others is interrupted by hospitalization. The challenge of hospitalization also adds a situational crisis to the normal developmental crisis a child is experiencing. Although the nurse may meet many of the hospitalized child's needs, continued parental involvement is necessary both during and after hospitalization to ensure progression through expected developmental stages (see Table 2-3).

PIAGET'S THEORY OF COGNITIVE DEVELOPMENT

Theoretical Framework

Based on his observations and work with children, Piaget formulated a theory of cognitive (or intellectual) development. He believed that the child's view of the world is influenced largely by age and maturational ability. Given nurturing experiences, the child's ability to think matures naturally (Ginsberg & Opper, 1988; Piaget, 1972). The child incorporates new experiences via **assimilation** and changes to deal with these experiences by the process of **accommodation.**

Stages

SENSORIMOTOR (BIRTH TO 2 YEARS) Infants learn about the world by input obtained through the senses and by their motor activity. Six substages are characteristic of this stage.

Use of Reflexes (Birth to 1 Month) The infant begins life with a set of reflexes such as sucking, rooting, and grasping. By using these reflexes, the infant receives stimulation via touch, sound, smell, and vision. The reflexes thus pave the way for the first learning to occur.

Primary Circular Reactions (1 to 4 Months) Once the infant responds reflexively, the pleasure gained from that response causes repetition of the behavior. For example, if a toy grasped reflexively makes noise and is interesting to watch, the infant will grasp it again.

Secondary Circular Reactions (4 to 8 Months) Awareness of the environment grows as the infant begins to connect cause and effect. The sounds of bottle preparation will lead to excited behavior. If an object is partially hidden, the infant will attempt to uncover and retrieve it.

Coordination of Secondary Schemes (8 to 12 Months) Intentional behavior is observed as the infant uses learned behavior to obtain objects, create sounds, or engage in other pleasurable activity. **Object permanence** (the knowledge that something continues to exist even when out of sight) begins when the infant remembers where a hidden object is likely to be found; it is no longer "out of sight, out of mind."

Tertiary Circular Reactions (12 to 18 Months) Curiosity, experimentation, and exploration predominate as the toddler tries out actions to learn results. Objects are turned in every direction, placed in the mouth, used for banging, and inserted in containers as their qualities and uses are explored.

Mental Combinations (18 to 24 Months) Language provides a new tool for the toddler to use in understanding the world. Language enables the child to think about events and objects before or after they occur. Object permanence is now fully developed as the child actively searches for objects in various locations and out of view.

PREOPERATIONAL (2 TO 7 YEARS) The young child thinks by using words as symbols, but logic is not well developed. During the preconceptual substage (2 to 4 years), vocabulary and comprehension increase greatly, but the child is egocentric (that is, unable to see things from the perspective of another). In the intuitive substage (4 to 7 years), the child relies on transductive reasoning (that is, drawing conclusions from one general fact to another). For example, when a child disobeys a parent and then falls and breaks an arm that day, the child may ascribe the broken arm to bad behavior. Cause-and-effect relationships are often unrealistic or a result of "magical thinking" (the belief that events occur because of thoughts or wishes).

CONCRETE OPERATIONAL (7 TO 11 YEARS) Transductive reasoning has given way to a more accurate understanding of cause and effect. The child can reason quite well if concrete objects are used in teaching or experimentation. The concept of conservation (that matter does not change when its form is altered) is learned at this age.

FORMAL OPERATIONAL (11 YEARS TO ADULTHOOD) Fully mature intellectual thought has now been attained. The adolescent can think abstractly about objects or concepts and consider different alternatives or outcomes.

PRIMARY CIRCULAR REACTION

A reflexive response, such as shaking a rattle, that results in pleasure and repetition is called a primary circular reaction.

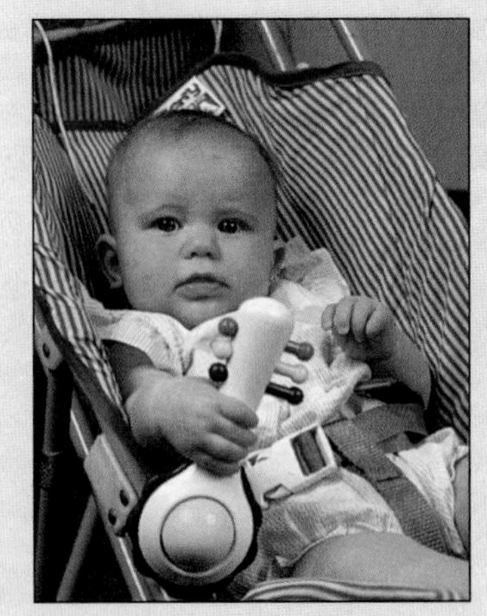

Nursing Application

Piaget's theory is essential to pediatric nursing. The nurse must understand a child's thought processes in order to design stimulating activities and meaningful, appropriate teaching plans. What activities will you plan for Irena based on her expected cognitive level? How can you encourage her cognitive development? Understanding a child's concept of time suggests to the nurse how far in advance to prepare that child for procedures. Similarly, the nurse's decision to offer manipulative toys, read stories, draw pictures, or give the child reading material to explain health care measures depends on the child's cognitive stage of development (see Table 2-3).

KOHLBERG'S THEORY OF MORAL DEVELOPMENT

Theoretical Framework

Kohlberg's work has been criticized for insensitivity to cultural differences in moral reasoning and for sexual bias; however, it remains a useful framework for some to help understand moral decision making. Kohlberg's focus is on a particular type of cognitive development concerned with moral decisions. He presented stories involving moral dilemmas to children and adults and asked them to solve the dilemmas. Kohlberg then analyzed the motives they expressed when making decisions about the best course to take. Based on the explanations given, Kohlberg established three levels of moral reasoning. Although he provided age guidelines, he stated that they are approximate and that many people never reach the highest (postconventional) stage of development (Santrock, 1999).

LAWRENCE KOHLBERG (B. 1927)

Kohlberg used Piaget's cognitive stage theory as the basis for his theory of moral development. He worked with children in his native Germany and in many other countries, including Kenya, Taiwan, and Mexico.

Stages

PRECONVENTIONAL (4 TO 7 YEARS) Decisions are based on the desire to please others and to avoid punishment.

CONVENTIONAL (7 TO 11 YEARS) Conscience or an internal set of standards becomes important. Rules are important and must be followed to please other people and "be good."

POSTCONVENTIONAL (12 YEARS AND OLDER) The individual has internalized ethical standards on which to base decisions. Social responsibility is recognized. The value in each of two differing moral approaches can be considered and a decision made.

Nursing Application

Decision making is required in many areas of health care. Children can be assisted to make decisions about health care and to consider alternatives when available. The nurse should

ALBERT BANDURA (B. 1925)

Bandura is a Canadian who has conducted psychologic research at Stanford University for many years. He believes that children learn from their social environment, particularly by modeling the observed behaviors of others.

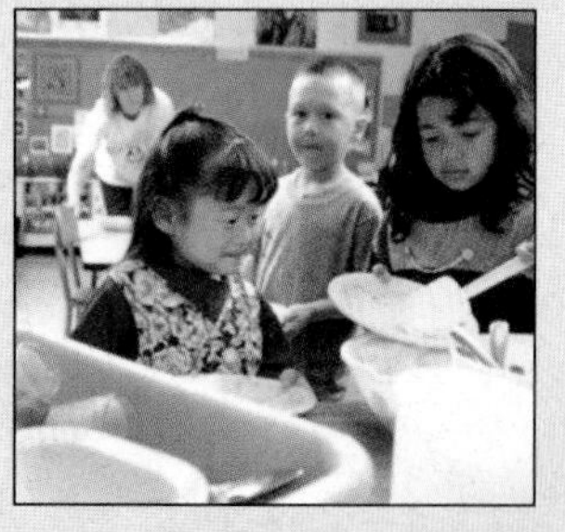

JOHN WATSON (1878–1958)

Watson was an American scientist who applied the work of animal behaviorists, such as Ivan Pavlov and B.F. Skinner, to children.

NATURE VERSUS NURTURE

Does nature or nurture have primary importance in the theories of Erikson, Kohlberg, Freud, and social learning? Think about whether each of the theories emphasizes the role of heredity (nature) or the role of the environment (nurture) in influencing the development of children.

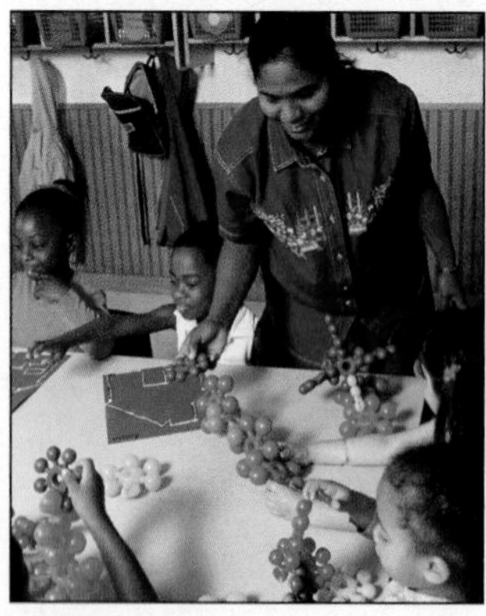

FIGURE 2-3 ◆
Children exposed to pleasant stimulation and who are supported by an adult will develop and refine their skills faster. Group activities such as these provide an environment for both motor skill and psychosocial development. Can you identify which skills are being developed?

keep in mind that young children may agree to participate in research simply because they want to comply with adults and appear cooperative. Guidelines for child participation in research are available (see Chapter 1).

SOCIAL LEARNING THEORY

Theoretical Framework

Bandura, a contemporary psychologist, believes that children learn attitudes, beliefs, customs, and values through their social contacts with adults and other children. Children imitate (or model) the behavior they see; if the behavior is positively reinforced, they tend to repeat it. The external environment and the child's internal processes are key elements in social learning theory (Bandura, 1986, 1997).

Nursing Application

The importance of modeling behavior can readily be applied in health care. Children are more likely to cooperate if they see adults or other children performing a task willingly. A frightened child may watch another child perform vision screening or have blood drawn and then decide to allow the procedure to take place. Contact with positive role models is useful when teaching children and adolescents self-care for chronic diseases such as diabetes. Positive reinforcement should be given for desired performance.

BEHAVIORISM

Theoretical Framework

Watson studied the research of Pavlov and Skinner, who demonstrated that actions are determined by responses from the environment. Pavlov and, later, Skinner worked with animals, presenting a stimulus such as food and pairing it with another stimulus such as a ringing bell. Eventually the animal being fed began to salivate when the bell rang. As Skinner and then Watson began to apply these concepts to children, they showed that behaviors can be elicited by positive reinforcement, such as a food treat, or extinguished by negative reinforcement, such as by scolding or withdrawal of attention. Watson believed that he could make of a child anyone he desired—from a professional to a thief or beggar—simply by reinforcing behavior in certain ways (Santrock, 1999).

Nursing Application

Behaviorism has been criticized for its simplicity and its denial of the inherent capability of persons to respond willfully to events in the environment. This theory does, however, have some use in health care. When particular behaviors are desired, positive reinforcement can be established to encourage these behaviors. Behavioral techniques are also used to alter behavior of children who misbehave or to teach skills to children who are physically challenged. Parents often use reinforcement in toilet training and other skills learned in childhood.

ECOLOGIC THEORY

Theoretical Framework

You may have noticed that there is controversy among theorists concerning the relative importance of heredity versus environment—or nature versus nurture—in human development. **Nature** refers to the genetic or hereditary capability of an individual. **Nurture** refers to the effects of the environment on a person's performance (Figure 2-3 ◆). Piaget believed in the importance of internal cognitive structures that unfold at their appointed times, given any environment that provides basic opportunities. He emphasized the strength of nature. The behaviorist John Watson, on the other hand, believed that behaviors are primarily shaped by environmental responses; he thus stressed the predominance of nurture. Contemporary developmental theories increasingly recognize the interaction of nature and nurture in determining the child's development.

The ecologic theory of development was formulated by Urie Bronfenbrenner to explain the unique relationship of the child in all of life's settings, from close to remote (Bronfenbrenner, 1986; Bronfenbrenner, McClelland, Ceci, Moen, Wethington, 1996). **Ecologic theory** emphasizes the presence of mutual interactions between the child and these various settings. Neither nature nor nurture is considered of more importance. Bronfenbrenner believes each child brings a unique set of genes—and specific attributes such as age, gender, health, and other characteristics—to his or her interactions with the environment. The child then interacts in many settings at different levels or systems (Figure 2-4 ◆).

URIE BRONFENBRENNER (B. 1917)

Bronfenbrenner, a professor at Cornell University, has established the ecologic theory of development. He views the child as interacting with the environment at different levels, or systems.

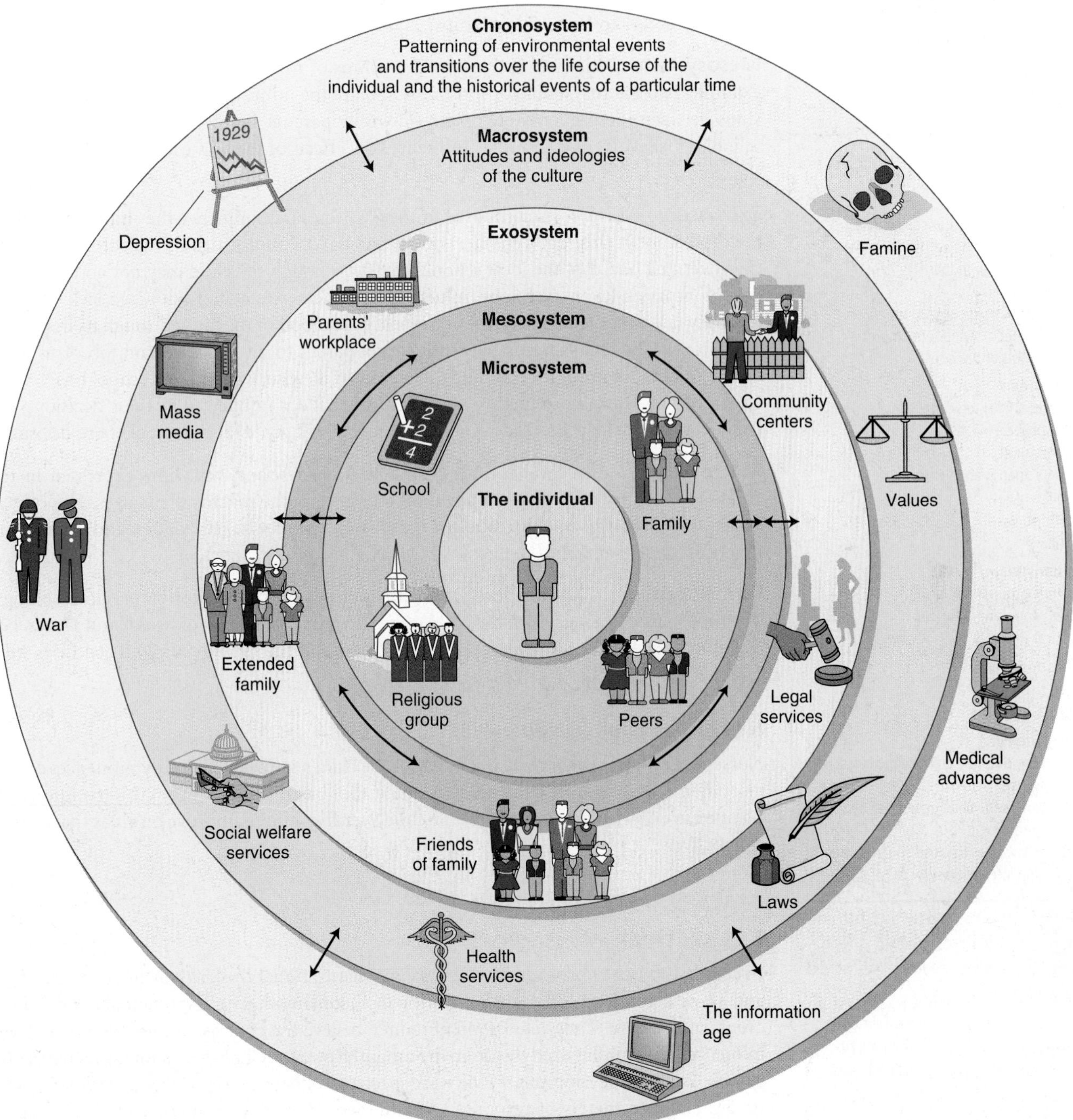

FIGURE 2-4 ◆
Bronfenbrenner's ecologic theory of development views the individual as interacting within five levels or systems. NOTE: Redrawn from Santrock, J.W. [1999]. Life Span development. Madison, WI: Brown & Benchmark. *Based on Bronenbrenner's (1979, 1986) works in Contexts of child rearing: Problems and prospects. American Psychologist, 34, 844–850; and Ecology of the family as a context for human development: Research perspectives. Developmental Psychology, 22, 723–742.*

TABLE 2-4

Assessment of Ecologic Systems in Childhood–Bronfenbrenner

Microsystems
Parents
Significant others in close contact
Child care arrangements
School
Neighborhood contacts
Clubs
Friends, peers
Religious community (e.g., churches, synagogues, mosques)

Mesosystems
Parents' involvement in child care or school
Parents' involvement in community
Parents' relationship with significant others (e.g., grandparents, care providers)
Influences of religious community (e.g., church, synagogue, mosque) on parents and school

Exosystems
Community centers
Local political influences
Parents' work
Parents' friends and activities
Social services
Health care
Libraries

Macrosystems
Cultural group membership
Beliefs and values of group
Political structure

Chronosystems
Child's age
Parents' ages

Ask yourself:
- How does the child influence each system?
- How is the child influenced by each system?
- Where does this lead you in planning interventions for the child?

STELLA CHESS AND ALEXANDER THOMAS

Chess and Thomas are psychiatrists who began the New York Longitudinal Study in 1956 with 141 children, which they expanded in 1961 with 95 additional children. Most of these individuals are still being assessed periodically as adults. Their research has identified characteristics of personality and provides a basis for the ongoing study of temperament (Chess & Thomas, 1995).

LEVELS OR SYSTEMS

Microsystem This level is defined as the daily, consistent, close relationships such as home, child care, school, friends, and neighbors. For the child with a chronic illness requiring regular care, the health care providers may even be part of the microsystem. In the ecologic model, the child influences each of these settings in addition to being influenced by them, with reciprocal interactions. Consider how Irena's microsystems have changed. Initially her mother and siblings were the important persons in her daily life, then the orphanage staff and other children, and finally Michael and Alyssa and their families and friends. How might these changes have influenced Irena? What stability is needed now to foster her ability to form relationships?

Mesosystem This level includes relationships of microsystems with one another. For example, two microsystems for most children are the home and the school. The relationships between these microsystems are shown by parents' involvement in their children's school. This involvement, in turn, influences the effects of the home and school settings on the children.

Exosystem This level is composed of those settings that influence the child even though the child is not in close daily contact with the system. Examples include the parents' jobs and the governing board of the local school district. Although the child may not go to the parents' workplaces, he or she can be influenced by policies related to health care, sick leave, inflexible work hours, overtime, travel, or even by the mood of the boss (through its impact on the parent). The child's needs may influence a parent to give up a certain job or to work harder to obtain money for the child's education. Likewise, when a local school board votes to ban certain books or to finance a field trip, the child is influenced by these decisions; the child, in turn, can help establish an atmosphere that will guide future school board decisions.

Macrosystem This level includes the beliefs, values, and behaviors expressed in the child's environment. Culture is a powerful influence in the macrosystem, as is the political system. For instance, a democratic system creates different beliefs, values, and even eating practices than an anarchic system.

Chronosystem This final level brings the perspective of time to the previous settings. The time period during which the child grows up influences views of health and illness. For example, the experiences of children with influenza in the 19th versus 20th centuries were quite different.

Nursing Application

Nurses use ecologic theory when they assess the child's settings to identify influences on development. Table 2-4 provides an assessment tool based on this theory. Interventions are planned to enhance the strengths of the child's settings and to improve on areas that are not supportive.

TEMPERAMENT THEORY

Theoretical Framework

In contrast to behaviorists such as Watson or maturational theorists such as Piaget, Chess and Thomas recognize the innate qualities of personality that each individual brings to the events of daily life. They, like Bronfenbrenner, believe the child is an individual who both influences and is influenced by the environment. However, Chess and Thomas focus on one specific aspect of development—the wide spectrum of behaviors possible in children, identifying nine parameters of response to daily events (Table 2-5). Infants generally display clusters of responses, which Chess and Thomas have classified into three major personality types (Table 2-6). Although most children do not demonstrate all behaviors described for a particular type, they usually show a grouping indicative of one personality type (Chess & Thomas, 1995, 1996).

Recent research demonstrates that personality characteristics displayed during infancy are often consistent with those seen later in life. The ability to predict future characteristics

TABLE 2-5 Nine Parameters of Personality—Chess & Thomas

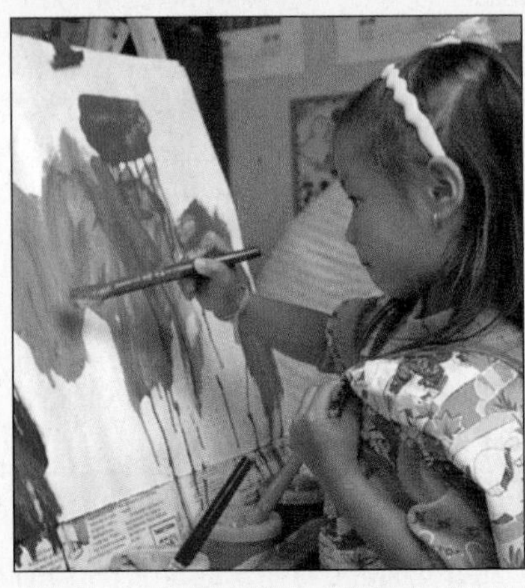

1. **Activity level.** The degree of motion during eating, playing, sleeping, bathing. Scored as high, medium, or low.
2. **Rhythmicity.** The regularity of schedule maintained for sleep, hunger, elimination. Scored as regular, variable, or irregular.
3. **Approach or withdrawal.** The response to a new stimulus such as a food, activity, or person. Scored as approachable, variable, or withdrawn.
4. **Adaptability.** The degree of adaptation to new situations. Scored as adaptive, variable, or nonadaptive.
5. **Threshold of responsiveness.** The intensity of stimulation needed to elicit a response to sensory input, objects in the environment, or people. Scored as high, medium, or low.
6. **Intensity of reaction.** The degree of response to situations. Scored as positive, variable, or negative.
7. **Quality of mood.** The predominant mood during daily activity and in response to stimuli. Scored as positive, variable, or negative.
8. **Distractibility.** The ability of environmental stimuli to interfere with the child's activity. Scored as distractible, variable, or nondistractible.
9. **Attention span and persistence.** The amount of time devoted to activities (compared with other children of the same age) and the degree of ability to stick with an activity in spite of obstacles. Scored as persistent, variable, or nonpersistent.

Note: From Chess, S., & Thomas, A. (1996). *Temperament: Theory and practice.* Philadelphia: Brunner/Mazel Publishers.

TABLE 2-6 Patterns of Temperament—Chess & Thomas

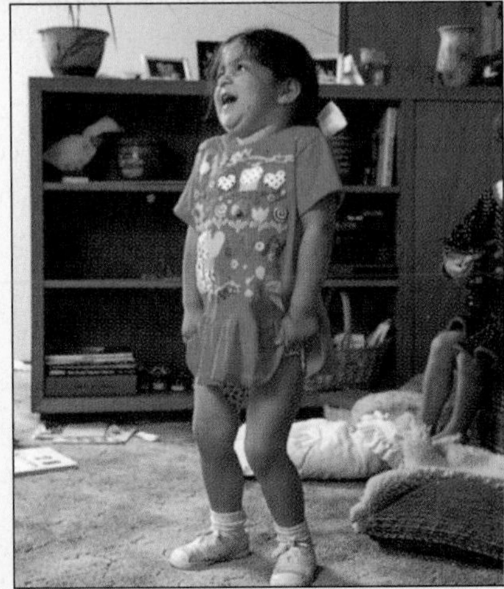

The "easy" child is generally moderate in activity; shows regularity in patterns of eating, sleeping, and elimination; and is usually positive in mood and when subjected to new stimuli. The easy child adapts to new situations and is able to accept rules and work well with others. About 40% of children in the New York Longitudinal Study displayed this personality type.

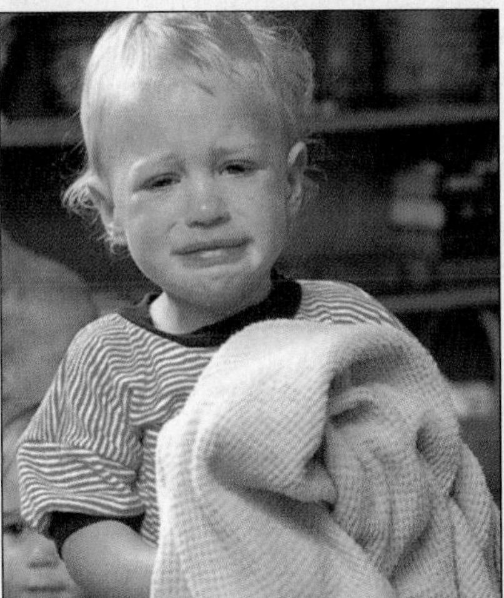

The "difficult" child displays irregular schedules for eating, sleeping, and elimination; adapts slowly to new situations and persons; and displays a predominantly negative mood. Intense reactions to the environment are common. About 10% of children in the New York Longitudinal Study displayed this personality type.

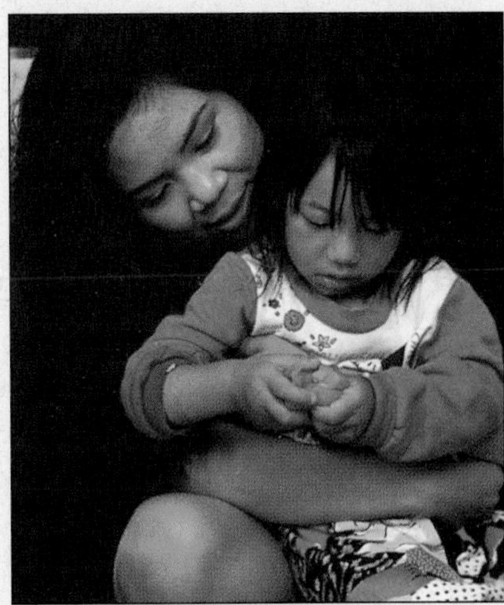

The "slow-to-warm-up" child has reactions of mild intensity and slow adaptability to new situations. The child displays initial withdrawal followed by gradual, quiet, and slow interaction with the environment. About 15% of children in the New York Longitudinal Study displayed this personality type.

The remaining 35% of children studied showed some characteristics of each personality type.

TABLE 2-7 Ways to Improve Goodness of Fit Between Parent and Child

CHILD'S BEHAVIOR	PARENT'S ACTIVITY
Extremely active	Plan periods of active play several times in day. Have restful periods before bedtime to foster sleep.
Shy	Allow time to adapt at own pace to new people and situations.
Easily stimulated	Have quiet room for sleeping as an infant. Have quiet room for homework as a school-age child.
Short attention span	Provide projects that can be completed in a short period. Gradually encourage longer periods at activities.

is not possible, however, because of the complex and dynamic interaction of personality traits and environmental reactions.

Many other researchers have expanded the work of Chess and Thomas, developing assessment tools for temperament types. The concept of "goodness of fit" is an outgrowth of this theory. Goodness of fit refers to whether parents' expectations of their child's behavior are consistent with the child's temperament type. There is a "good fit" when the properties of the environment are in accord with the child's capabilities, characteristics, and style of behavior (Chess & Thomas, 1999). As an example of lack of good fit, an active infant who reacts strongly to verbal stimuli may be unable to sleep when placed in a room with older siblings. A child who is slow to warm up may not perform well in the first few months at a new school, much to parents' disappointment. When parents understand a child's temperament characteristics, they are better able to shape the environment to meet the child's needs.

Nursing Application

The concept of personality type or temperament is a useful one for nurses (Melvin, 1995). Nurses can assess the temperament of young children and alter the environment to meet their needs. This may involve moving a hospitalized child to a single room to ensure adequate rest if the child is easily stimulated, or allowing a shy child time to become accustomed to new surroundings and equipment before beginning procedures or treatments.

Parents are often relieved to learn about temperament characteristics. They learn to appreciate their children's qualities and to adapt the environment to meet the children's needs. A burden of guilt can also be lifted from parents who feel that they are responsible for their child's actions. The nurse can teach parents ways of enhancing goodness of fit between the child's personality and the environment (Table 2-7).

INFLUENCES ON DEVELOPMENT

As we have seen, both nature and nurture are important in determining individual patterns of development. The interaction of these two forces can explain differences in time frames for acquisition of developmental skills, personality variations between identical twins, and other unique characteristics of individuals. The genetic and environmental factors that contribute to individual differences are explored in more detail next.

GENETICS

Each child inherits 23 chromosomes from the mother's egg and 23 from the father's sperm, resulting in a unique individual with 46 chromosomes. Two of these are **sex chromosomes,** and determine the child's gender; the rest are called **autosomal chromosomes,** and govern all remaining characteristics. Children can be affected by chromosomal disorders, which involve either altered numbers or structure of chromosomes. Whereas some of these mutations are incompatible with life and result in fetal death, others can lead to live births. Chromosomal disorders are caused by an array of factors such as radiation exposure, parental age, or parental

TABLE 2-8 Chromosomal Syndromes

Altered chromosome: 21 Genetic defect: trisomy 21 (Down syndrome) (secondary nondisjunction or 14/21 unbalanced translocation) Incidence: average 1 in 700 live births, incidence variable with age of mother	**Characteristics:** CNS: mental retardation: hypotonia at birth Head: flattened occiput depressed nasal bridge; mongoloid slant of eyes: epicanthal folds; white specking of the iris (Brushfield spots); protrusion of the tongue; high, arched palate; low-set ears Hands: broad, short fingers; abnormalities of finger and foot; dermal ridge patterns (dermatoglyphics); transverse palmar crease (simian line) Other: congenital heart disease and leukemia (increased incidence)
Altered chromosome: 18 Genetic defect: trisomy 18 Incidence: 1 in 3000 live births	**Characteristics:** CNS: mental retardation; severe hypotonia Head: prominent occiput: low-set ears; corneal opacities; ptosis (drooping of eyelids) Hands: third and fourth fingers overlapped by second and fifth fingers; abnormal dermatoglyphics; syndactyly (webbing of fingers) Other: congenital heart defects; renal abnormalities; single umbilical artery; gastrointestinal tract abnormalities; rocker-bottom feet; cryptorchidism; various malformations of other organs (increased incidence)
Altered chromosome: 13 Genetic defect: trisomy 13 Incidence: 1 in 5000 live births	**Characteristics:** CNS: mental retardation; severe hypotonia; seizures Head: microcephaly; microphthalmia and/or coloboma (keyhole-shaped pupil); malformed ears; aplasia of external auditory canal; micrognathia (abnormally small lower jaw); cleft lip and palate Hands: polydactly (extra digits); abnormal posturing of fingers; abnormal dermatoglyphics Other: congenital heart defects; hemangiomas; gastrointestinal tract defects; various malformations of other organs (increased incidence)
Altered chromosome: 5p Genetic defect: deletion of short arm of chromosome 5 (cri du chat, or cat cry, syndrome) Incidence: 1 in 20,000 live births	**Characteristics:** CNS: severe mental retardation; a catlike cry in infancy Head: microcephaly; hypertelorism (widely spaced eyes); epicanthal folds; low-set ears Other: failure to thrive; various organ malformations
Altered chromosome: XO (sex chromosome) Genetic defect: only one X chromosome in female (Turner syndrome) Incidence: 1 in 300–7000 live female births	**Characteristics:** CNS: no intellectual impairment; some perceptual difficulties Head: low hairline; webbed neck Trunk: short stature; dubitus valgus (increased carrying angle of arm); excessive nevi (congenital discoloration of skin due to pigmentation); broad shieldlike chest with widely spaced nipples; puffy feet; no toenails Other: fibrous streaks in ovaries; underdeveloped secondary sex characteristics; primary amenorrhea; usually infertile; renal anomalies; coarctation of the aorta (increased incidence)
Altered chromosome: XXY (sex chromosome) Genetic defect: extra X chromosome in male (Klinefelter syndrome) Incidence: 1 in 1000 live male births, approximately 1–2% of institutionalized males	**Characteristics:** CNS: mild mental retardation Trunk: occasional gynecomastia (abnormally large male breasts); eunuchoid body proportions (lack of male muscular and sexual development) Other: small, soft testes; underdeveloped secondary sex characteristics; usually sterile

Note: From Olds, S., London, M., Ladewig, P. (2000). *Maternal newborn nursing.* Upper Saddle River, NJ: Prentice Hall Health.

disease states, but their causes are often unknown. Some chromosomal disorders are outlined in Table 2-8. A disorder known as fragile X results from a different abnormality when there is a fragile site on the X chromosome that is susceptible to chromosome breakage. See Chapter 24 for a discussion of the chromosomal disorders, Down syndrome and fragile X, that result in mental retardation.

Every chromosome carries many genes that determine physical characteristics, intellectual potential, personality type, and other traits. Children are born with the potential for certain features; however, their interaction with the environment influences how and to what extent

TABLE 2-9 Laws of Mendelian Inheritance

Dominant inheritance A gene that produces a trait whenever it is present. Achondroplasia dwarfism is one example.

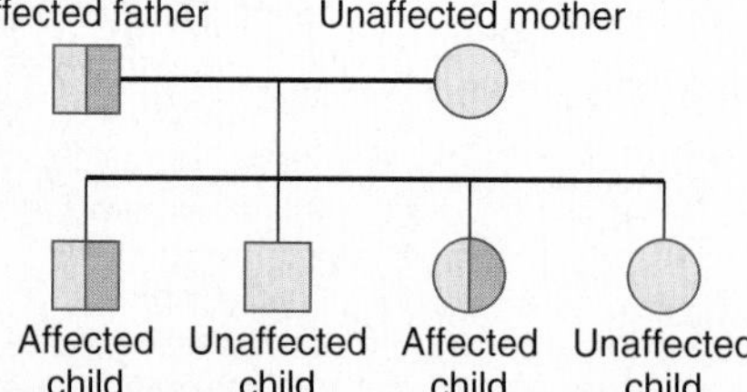

In each pregnancy there is a 50% chance that the child will have the characteristic.

Recessive inheritance A gene that produces a trait only when paired with another like gene. Examples include cystic fibrosis, Tay-Sachs disease, and phenylketonuria.

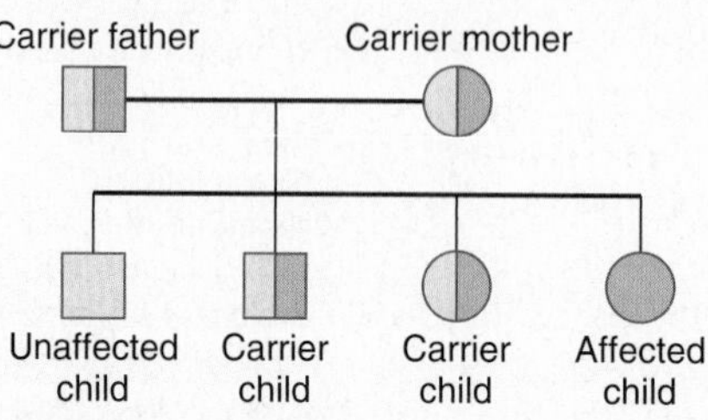

In each pregnancy, there is a 25% chance that the child will have the characteristic, a 25% chance that the child will be unaffected, and a 50% chance that the child will be a carrier of the characteristic.

X-linked inheritance A disease carried in either a dominant or recessive fashion on the X chromosome. Hemophilia is a common example of an X-linked disorder.

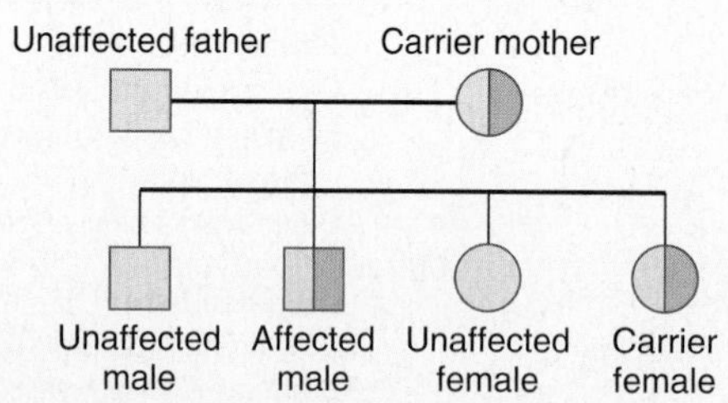

In each pregnancy with a male birth, there is a 50% chance that the child will have the characteristic and a 50% chance that the child will be unaffected. In each pregnancy with a female birth, there is a 50% chance that the child will be a carrier and a 50% chance that the child will be unaffected.

Chromosome defect Disorders caused by nondisjunction or translocation of chromosomes. Down syndrome is usually caused by a trisomy of chromosome 21.

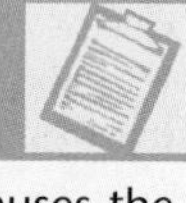

RESEARCH

In 1989, the gene that causes the inherited disease of cystic fibrosis was located on chromosome 7. This gene encodes a protein on the membrane of cells and regulates ion movement into the cells. The faulty gene leads to lung damage and gastrointestinal problems (see Chapter 13). Researchers are now attempting to insert needed DNA encoding normal ion regulation into lung tissue of cystic fibrosis patients so that lung tissue will not be damaged by the disease. Although this research is in early stages, it is an example of the potential for genetic research to revolutionize care for some inherited diseases (Jaffe, Bush, Geddes & Alton, 1999; Tolstoi & Smith, 1999).

particular traits are manifested. For example, a child may have the potential for a high level of intellectual performance, but because he or she lives in an unstimulating environment, that potential is never reached. Some children also inherit genes that lead to diseases such as cystic fibrosis (see Table 2-9 for types of genetic disease transmissions). A family history of these diseases is usually present, although they may appear without an identifiable history, because genes sometimes mutate, leading to an initial incidence of a genetic disorder.

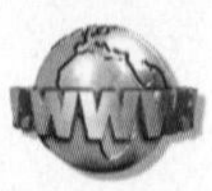

Human Genome Project/Genetics

In 1988, the U.S. Congress began funding research for mapping of all human genes, and many other nations set similar goals. The **Human Genome Project** was an international effort to determine the exact DNA sequences of every human gene. In 2000, a working draft of the human genome was achieved, several years ahead of schedule. This information about the human genetic code is freely provided to the scientific community and to the public. What does this mean for health care of children? First, it has already led to identifying the gene associated with certain abnormalities such as fragile X and cystic fibrosis (Williams, 2000). Once these genes are identified, it is possible to detect their presence in carriers and lead to better genetic counseling. New genetic material might be inserted into cells to provide important missing information, or medications can be specifically designed to target the disease on a molecular level. However, there have been concerns about ethical considerations with genetic research. What guidelines are needed to protect children and families so that genetic testing does not lead to discrimination in employment or health insurance? Who should be tested for genetic diseases, and who should have access to results? Since children cannot yet give informed consent for genetic testing (see Chapter 1 for a discussion of informed consent), it is recommended that children and adolescents should have genetic testing for a disease only when medical treatment could help if the disease is identified, or when another family member might benefit from the knowledge for their own health and the child will not be harmed by the testing (American Academy of Pediatrics Committee on Genetics, 2000). When genetic testing is performed, counseling about the results must be made available. Some nurses are choosing special educational programs to enable them to work in the growing field of genetics and health care.

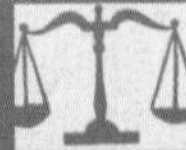

LAW & ETHICS

The explosion in knowledge and clinical therapy related to genetics will offer challenges to those in health care. Just because a genetic test for a disease can be performed, should it be done on all newborns? What might be the potential harmful uses of information obtained about someone's genetic information? What forms of disadvantage and discrimination might occur if someone was known to carry a gene for breast cancer, a neurological disease, or Alzheimer's disease? The rapidly advancing technology demands a focus on the ethical aspects of use of genetic tests and information. The Ethical, Legal, and Social Implications (ELSI) program of the National Human Genome Research Institute has been established to explore these issues (Giarelli & Jacobs, 2000; American Academy of Pediatrics, 2000).

PRENATAL INFLUENCES

Some Asian cultures calculate age from the time of conception. This practice acknowledges the profound influence of the prenatal period.

The mother's nutrition and general state of health play a part in pregnancy outcome. Poor nutrition can lead to low birth weight infants and infants with compromised neurologic performance, slow development, or impaired immune status with resultant high disease rates. Low maternal stores of iron can result in anemia in the infant (Trahms & Pipes, 1997; UNICEF, 1998). Maternal smoking is associated with low-birth-weight infants. Ingestion of alcoholic beverages, including beer and wine, during pregnancy may lead to fetal alcohol syndrome (Figure 2-5 ◆). Illicit drug use by the mother may result in neonatal addiction, convulsions, hyperirritability, poor social responsiveness, and other neurologic disturbances (Children's Defense Fund, 2000).

Even prescription drugs may adversely affect the fetus. An example is the drug thalidomide, which was commonly used in Europe to treat nausea during the 1950s. This drug resulted in the birth of infants with limb abnormalities to women who used the drug during pregnancy. Other drugs can cause bleeding, stained teeth, impaired hearing, or other defects in the infant (Briggs, Freeman, & Yaffe, 1998). Some maternal illnesses are harmful to the developing fetus. An example is rubella (German measles), which is rarely a serious disease for adults but which can cause deafness, vision defects, heart defects, and mental retardation in the fetus if it is acquired by a pregnant woman. A fetus can also acquire diseases, such as acquired immunodeficiency syndrome (AIDS) and human immunodeficiency virus (HIV) infection or hepatitis B from the mother.

Radiation, chemicals, and other environmental hazards may adversely affect a fetus when the mother is exposed to these influences during her pregnancy. The best outcomes for infants occur when mothers eat well; exercise regularly; seek early prenatal care; refrain from use of drugs, alcohol, tobacco, and excessive caffeine; and follow general principles of good health.

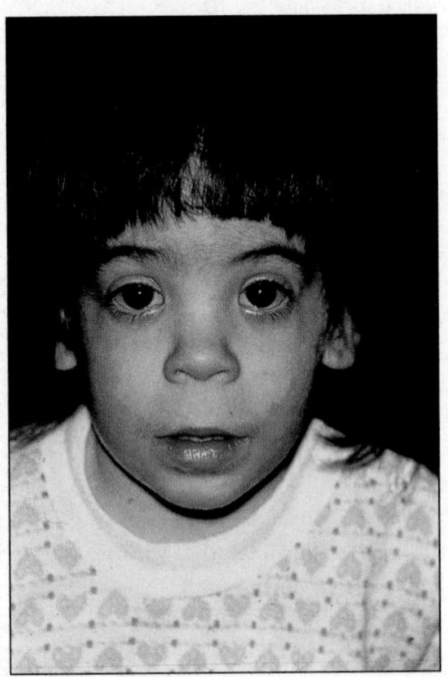

FIGURE 2-5◆
Fetal alcohol syndrome.
Courtesy of Dr. Sterling Clarren, Seattle, WA. Clarren, S.K. & Smith, D. W. (1978) The fetal alcohol syndrome. *New England Journal of Medicine, 298*, 1063–1067.

CULTURAL INFLUENCES

The traditional customs of the many cultural groups represented in North American society influence the development of the children in these groups. Foods commonly eaten vary among people with different cultural backgrounds and influence the incidence of health problems such as cardiovascular disease in these groups. The Native American practice of carrying infants on boards often delays walking when it is measured against the norm for walking on some developmental tests. Children who are carried by straddling the mother's hips or back for extended periods have a low incidence of developmental dysplasia of the hip since this keeps their hips in an abducted position. Certain groups are more prone to develop certain diseases due to genetic variations (Table 2-10).

INFANT (BIRTH TO 1 YEAR)

Can you imagine tripling your present weight in a single year? Or becoming proficient in understanding fundamental words in a new language and even speaking a few? These and many more accomplishments take place in the first year of life. Starting the year as a mainly reflexive creature, the infant can walk and communicate by the year's end. Never again in life is development so swift (Figure 2-6 ◆).

GROWTH & DEVELOPMENT

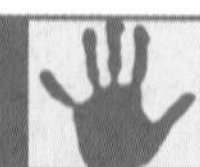

Growth charts that had been used in the United States since 1977 were not based on a wide cross section of the population. A new set of growth charts were issued in 2000 by the Centers for Disease Control and Prevention, based on national cross-sectional survey data from the second and third National Health and Nutritional Examination Survey (NHANES). In addition to previously available percentile charts for height, weight, and head circumference, charts are now available for body mass index so overweight children can more easily be identified. (See the appendix for complete copies of growth grids.)

TABLE 2-10 Diseases and Conditions More Common Among Cultural Groups

African Americans
Sickle cell disease
Hypertension
Stomach and esophageal cancer
Lactose intolerance

Asians/Pacific Islanders
Hypertension
Stomach and liver cancer
Lactose intolerance
Thalassemia

American Indians/Aleuts/Eskimos
Diabetes
Ear infections
Accidents and suicides
Cirrhosis of the liver
Overweight

Hispanic Americans
Diabetes
Overweight
Lactose intolerance

Jews
Tay-Sachs disease
Niemann-Pick disease
Werdnig-Hoffman syndrome

Mediterraneans
G6PD deficiency
β-Thalassemia
Familial Mediterranean fever

United Kingdom
Cystic fibrosis
Phenylketonuria
Hereditary amyloidosis
Hyperhomocysteinemia

Note: Adapted from Jarvis, C. (2000). *Physical examination and health assessment* (3rd ed.). Philadelphia: W.B. Saunders; and Spector, R. (2000). *Guides to heritage assessment and health traditions.* Upper Saddle River, NJ: Prentice Hall Health.

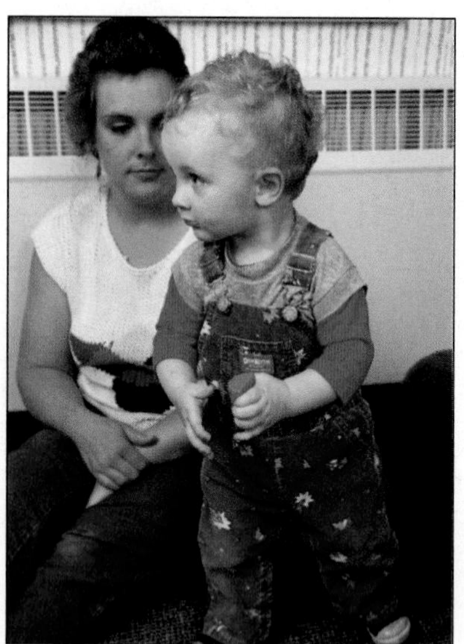

FIGURE 2-6 ◆
A 12-month-old child will have tripled his birth weight, learned to walk, and will be beginning to talk.

PHYSICAL GROWTH AND DEVELOPMENT

The first year of life is one of rapid change for the infant. The birth weight usually doubles by about 5 months and triples by the end of the first year (Figure 2-7 ◆). Height increases by approximately 1 foot during this year. Teeth begin to erupt at about 6 months, and by the end of the first year the infant has six to eight deciduous teeth (see Chapter 4). Physical growth is closely associated with type and quality of feeding. See Chapter 3 for a discussion of nutrition in infancy.

Body organs and systems, although not fully mature at 1 year of age, function differently than they did at birth. Kidney and liver maturation helps the 1-year-old excrete drugs or other toxic substances more readily than in the first weeks of life. The changing body proportions mirror changes in developing internal organs. Maturation of the nervous system is demonstrated by increased control over body movements, enabling the infant to sit, stand, and walk. Sensory function also increases as the infant begins to discriminate visual images, sounds, and tastes (Table 2-11).

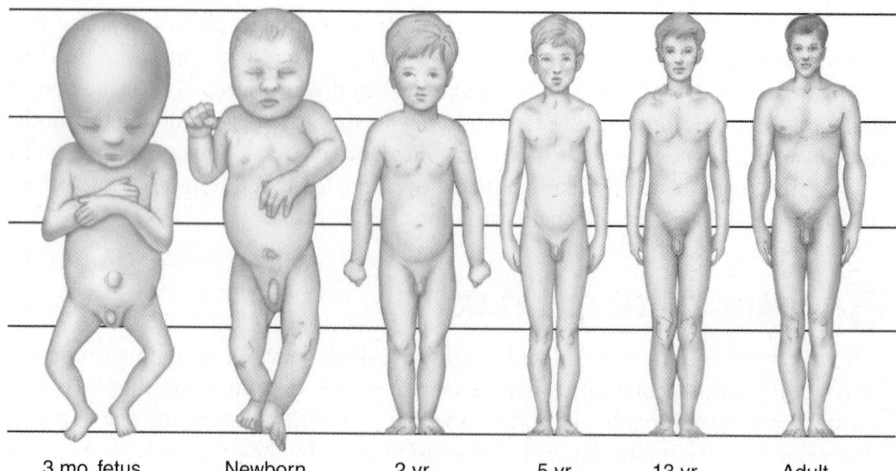

FIGURE 2-7◆
Body proportions at various ages.

TABLE 2-11 Growth and Development Milestones During Infancy

AGE	PHYSICAL GROWTH	FINE MOTOR ABILITY	GROSS MOTOR ABILITY	SENSORY ABILITY
Birth to 1 month	Gains 5–7 oz (140–200 g)/week Grows 1.5 cm (1/2 in.) in first month Head circumference increases 1.5 cm (1/2 in.)/month	Holds hand in fist **(1)** Draws arms and legs to body when crying	Inborn reflexes such as startle and rooting are predominant activity May lift head briefly if prone **(2)** Alerts to high-pitched voices Comforts with touch **(3)**	Prefers to look at faces and black-and-white geometric designs Follows objects in line of vision **(4)**

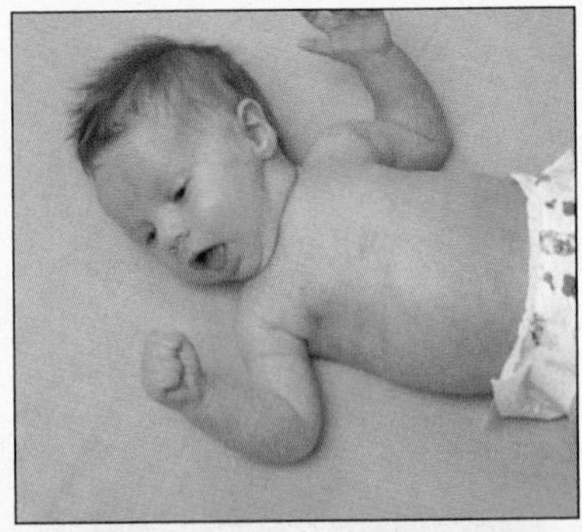

(1) Holds hand in fist

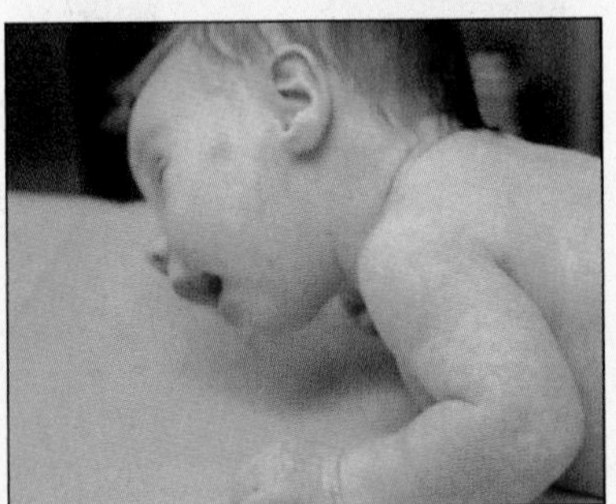

(2) May lift head

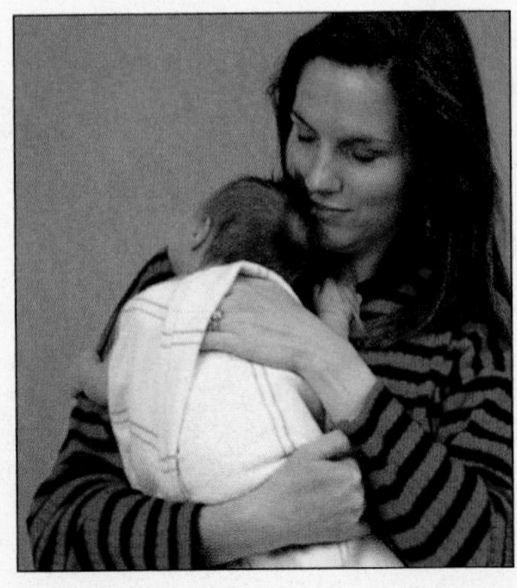

(3) Comforts with touch

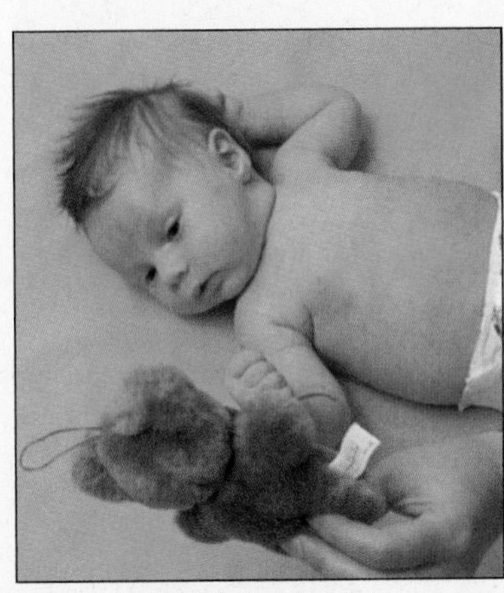

(4) Follows objects

AGE	PHYSICAL GROWTH	FINE MOTOR ABILITY	GROSS MOTOR ABILITY	SENSORY ABILITY
2–4 months	Gains 5–7 oz (140–200 g)/week Grows 1.5 cm (1/2 in.)/month Head circumference increases 1.5 cm (1/2 in.)/month Posterior fontanel closes Eats 120 mL/kg/24 hr (2 oz/lb/24 hr)	Holds rattle when placed in hand **(5)** Looks at and plays with own fingers Readily brings objects from hand to mouth	Moro reflex fading in strength Can turn from side to back and then return **(6)** Decrease in head lag when pulled to sitting; sits with head held in midline with some bobbing When prone, holds head and supports weight on forearms **(7)**	Follows objects 180° Turns head to look for voices and sounds

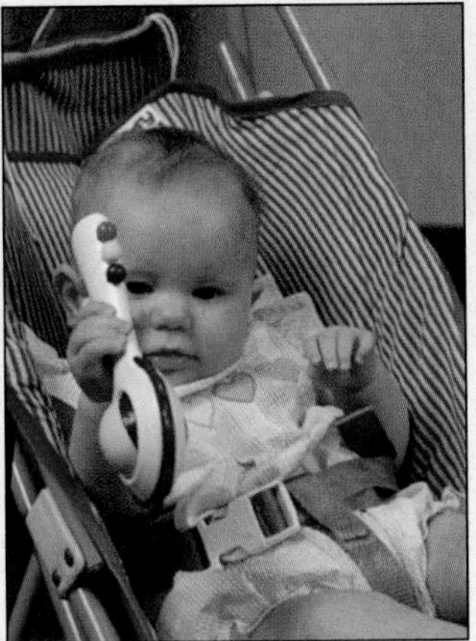

(5) Holds rattle

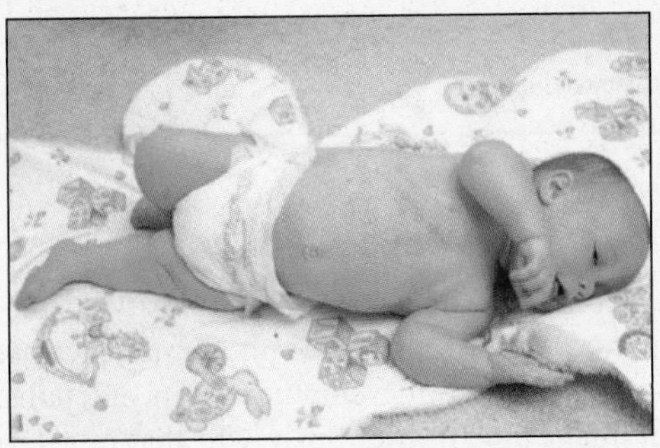

(6) Can turn from side to back

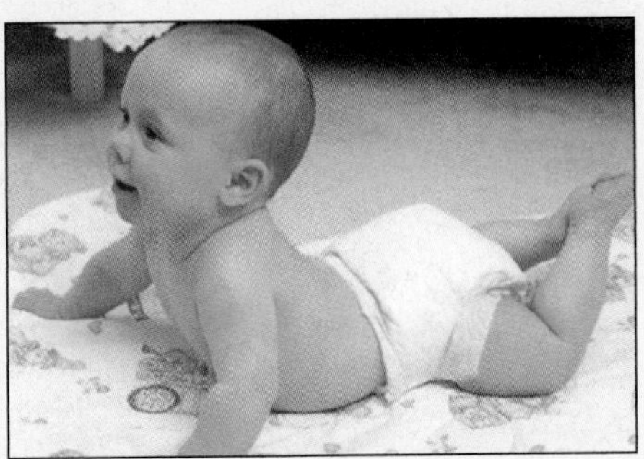

(7) Holds head up and supports weight with arms

(continued)

TABLE 2-11 Growth and Development Milestones During Infancy (continued)

AGE	PHYSICAL GROWTH	FINE MOTOR ABILITY	GROSS MOTOR ABILITY	SENSORY ABILITY
4–6 months	Gains 5–7 oz (140–200 g)/week Doubles birth weight 5–6 months Grows 1.5 cm (1/2 in.)/month Head circumference increases 1.5 cm (1/2 in.)/month Teeth may begin erupting by 6 months Eats 100 mL/kg/24 hr (1 1/2 oz/lb/24 hr)	Grasps rattles and other objects at will; drops them to pick up another offered object **(8)** Mouths objects Holds feet and pulls to mouth Holds bottle Grasps with whole hand (palmar grasp) Manipulates objects **(9)**	Head held steady when sitting No head lag when pulled to sitting Turns from abdomen to back by 4 months and then back to abdomen by 6 months When held standing supports much of own weight **(10)**	Examines complex visual images Watches the course of a falling object Responds readily to sounds
6–8 months	Gains 3–5 oz (85–140 g)/week Grows 1 cm (3/8 in.)/month Growth rate slower than first 6 months	Bangs to objects held in hands Transfers objects from one hand to the other Beginning pincer grasp at times	Most inborn reflexes extinguished Sits alone steadily without support by 8 months **(11)** Likes to bounce on legs when held in standing position	Recognizes own name and responds by looking and smiling Enjoys small and complex objects at play

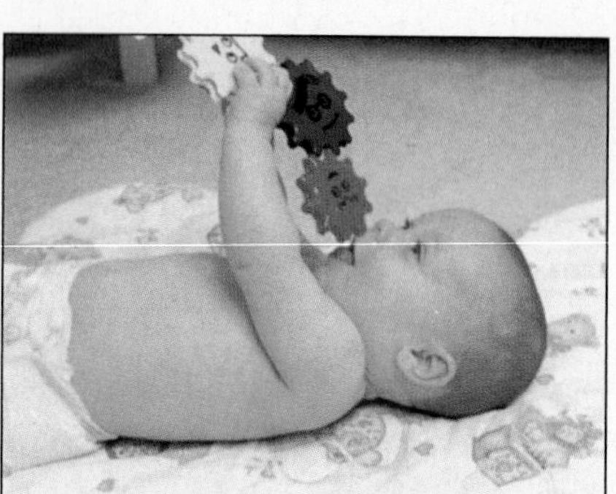

(8) Grasps objects at will

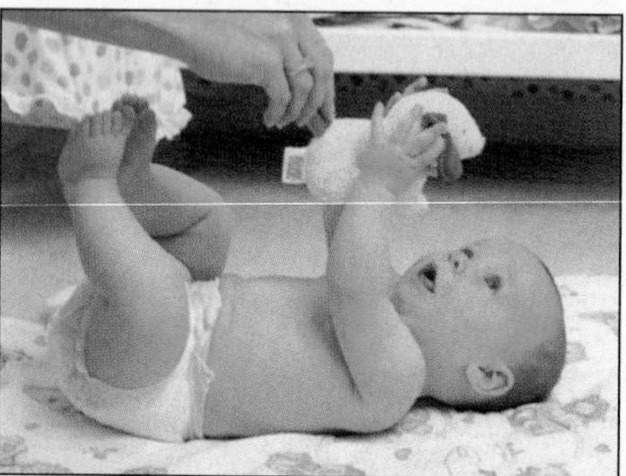

(9) Manipulates objects

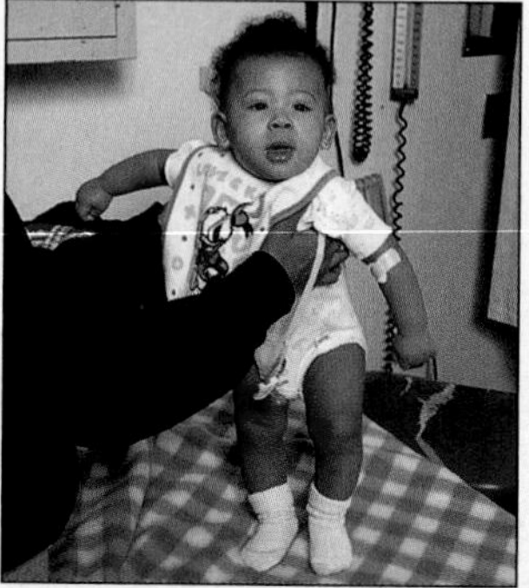

(10) Supports most of weight when held standing

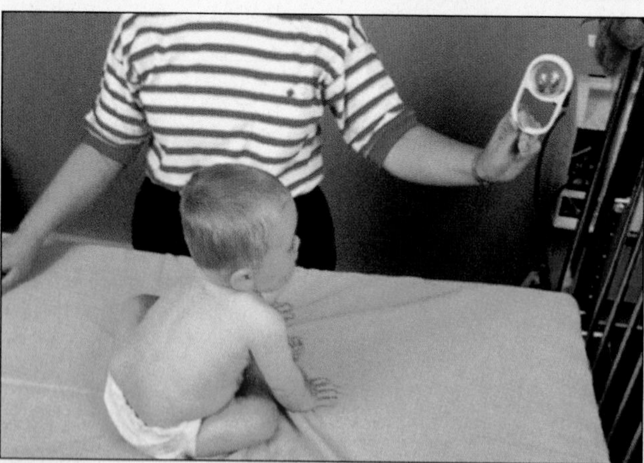

(11) Sits alone without support

COGNITIVE DEVELOPMENT

The brain continues to increase in complexity during the first year. Most of the growth involves maturation of cells, with only a small increase in cell number. This growth of the brain is accompanied by development of its functions. One has only to compare the behavior of an infant shortly after birth with that of a 1-year-old to understand the incredible maturation of brain function. The newborn's eyes widen in response to sound; the 1-year-old turns to the sound and recognizes its significance. The 2-month-old cries and coos; the

TABLE 2-11 Growth and Development Milestones During Infancy (continued)

AGE	PHYSICAL GROWTH	FINE MOTOR ABILITY	GROSS MOTOR ABILITY	SENSORY ABILITY
8–10 months	Gains 3–5 oz (85–140 g)/week Grows 1 cm (3/8 in.)/month	Picks up small objects **(12)** Uses pincer grasp well **(14)**	Crawls or pulls whole body along floor by arms **(13)** Creeps by using hands and knees to keep trunk off floor Pulls self to standing and sitting by 10 months Recovers balance when sitting	Understands words such as "no" and "cracker" May say one word in addition to "mama" and "dada" Recognizes sound without difficulty

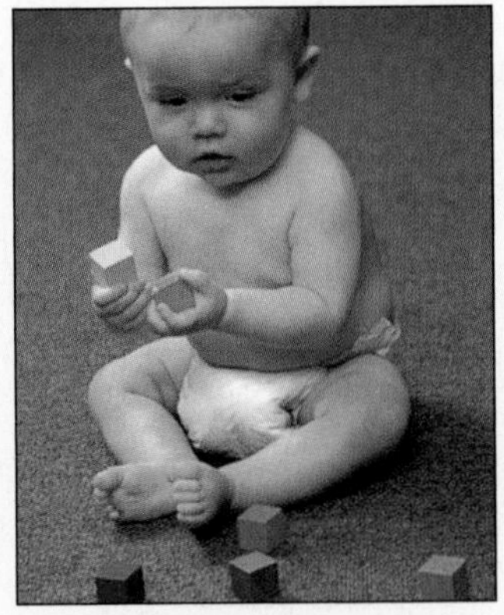

(12) Picks up small objects

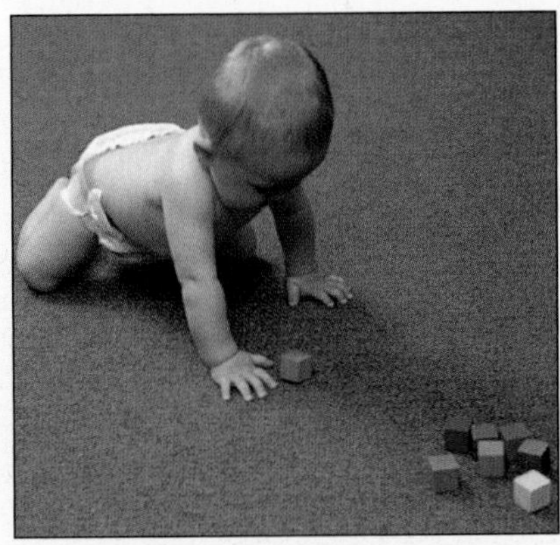

(13) Crawls or pulls body by arms

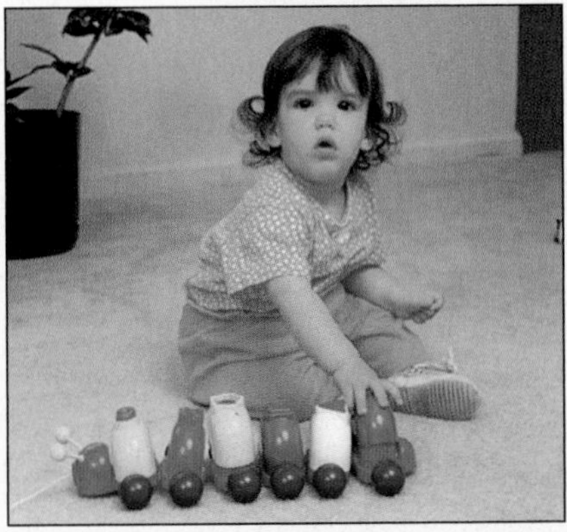

(14) Uses pincer grasp well

AGE	PHYSICAL GROWTH	FINE MOTOR ABILITY	GROSS MOTOR ABILITY	SENSORY ABILITY
10–12 months	Gains 3–5 oz (85–140 g)/week Grows 1 cm (3/8 in.)/month Head circumference equals chest circumference Triples birth weight by 1 year	May hold crayon or pencil and make mark on paper Places objects into containers through holes **(15)**	Stands alone **(16)** Walks holding onto furniture Sits down from standing **(17)**	Plays peek-a-boo and patty cake

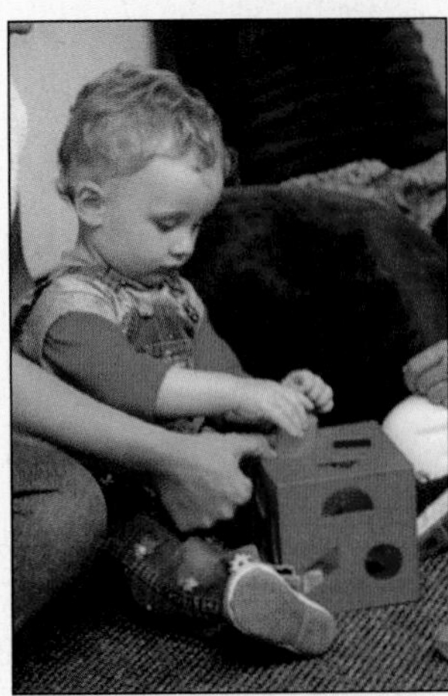

(15) Places objects in container through holes

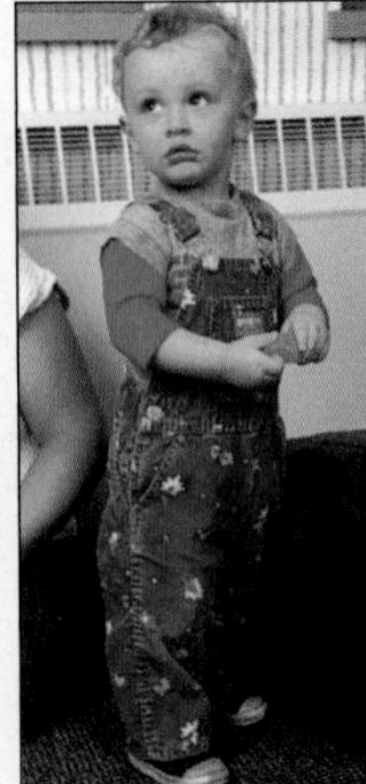

(16) Stands alone

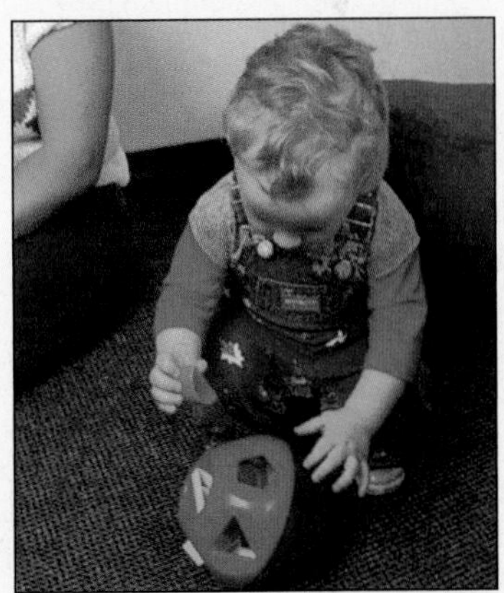

(17) Sits down from standing

1-year-old says a few words and understands many more. The 6-week-old grasps a rattle for the first time; the 1-year-old reaches for toys and self-feeds.

The infant's behaviors provide clues about thought processes. Piaget's work outlines the infant's actions in a set of rapidly progressing changes in the first year of life. The infant receives stimulation through sight, sound, and feeling, which the maturing brain interprets. This input from the environment interacts with internal cognitive abilities to enhance cognitive functioning.

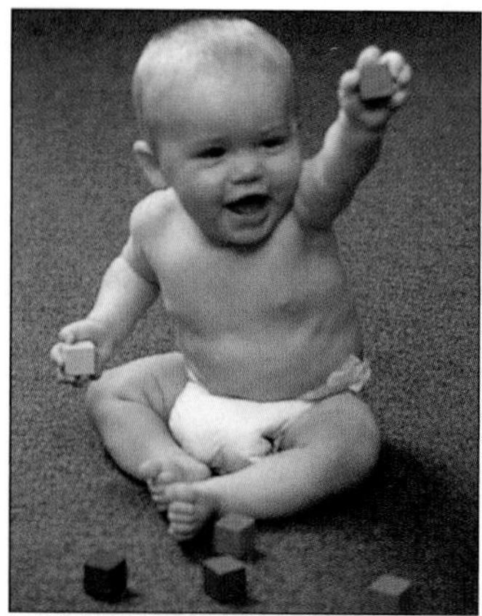

FIGURE 2-8 ◆
Garrett shows us that an 8-month-old child can play with blocks, demonstrating physical, cognitive, and social capabilities.

PLAY

An 8-month-old infant is sitting on the floor, grasping blocks and banging them on the floor. When a parent walks by, the infant laughs and waves hands and feet wildly (Figure 2-8 ◆). Physical capabilities enable the infant to move toward and reach for objects of interest. Cognitive ability is reflected in manipulation of the blocks to create different sounds. Social interaction enhances play. The presence of a parent or other person increases interest in surroundings and teaches the infant different ways to play.

The play of infants begins in a reflexive manner. When infants move extremities or grasp objects, they experience the foundations of play. They gain pleasure from the feel and sound of these activities, and gradually perform them purposefully. For example, when a parent places a rattle in the hand of a 6-week-old infant, the infant grasps it reflexively. As the hands move randomly, the rattle makes an enjoyable sound. The infant learns to move the rattle to create the sound and then finally to grasp the toy at will to play with it.

The next phase of infant play focuses on manipulative behavior. The infant examines toys closely, looking at them, touching them, and placing them in the mouth. The infant learns a great deal about texture, qualities of objects, and all aspects of the surroundings. At the same time, interaction with others becomes an important part of play. The social nature of play is obvious as the infant plays with other children and adults.

Toward the end of the first year, the infant's ability to move in space enlarges the sphere of play (Figure 2-9 ◆). Once infants crawl or walk, they can get to new places, find new toys, discover forgotten objects, or seek out other people for interaction. Play is a reflection of every aspect of development, as well as a method for enhancing learning and maturation (Table 2-12).

FOODS THAT COMMONLY CAUSE CHOKING

- Hot dogs
- Nuts
- Popcorn
- Hard candy
- Ice cubes
- Grapes
- Uncooked vegetable chunks
- Lumps of peanut butter

INJURY PREVENTION

Injuries are a major cause of death in childhood. The infant is particularly vulnerable to injuries when not adequately supervised. Increasing mobility during the second half of the first year challenges parents to childproof the home and environment. The nurse can provide anticipatory guidance to help prevent unintentional injuries (Table 2-13).

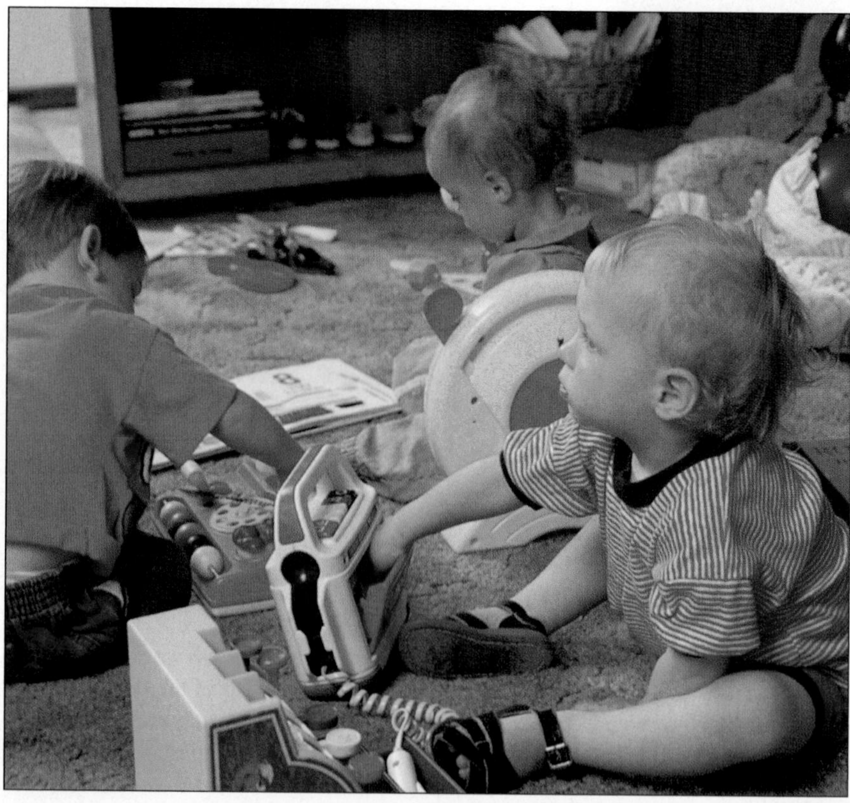

FIGURE 2-9 ◆
Mobility enlarges the sphere of play, allowing the child to seek new toys and spaces and to seek out people for interaction. Which psychosocial, cognitive, and motor skills do you see taking place in this photograph?

TABLE 2-12 Favorite Toys and Activities in Infancy

Age	Toys and activities
Birth to 2 months	Mobiles, black-and-white patterns, mirrors Music boxes, singing, tape players, soft voices Rocking and cuddling Moving legs and arms while singing and talking Varying stimuli—different rooms, sounds, visual images
3 to 6 months	Rattles Stuffed animals Soft toys with contrasting colors Noise-making objects that are easily grasped
6 to 12 months	Large blocks Teething toys Toys that pop apart and back together Nesting cups and other objects that fit into one another or stack Surprise toys such as jack-in-the-box Social interaction with adults and other children Games such as peek-a-boo Soft balls Push and pull toys

PERSONALITY AND TEMPERAMENT

Why does one infant frequently awaken at night crying while another sleeps for 8 to 10 hours undisturbed? Why does one infant smile much of the time and react positively to interactions while another is withdrawn around unfamiliar people and frequently frowns and cries? Such differences in responses to the environment are believed to be inborn characteristics of temperament. Infants are born with a tendency to react in certain ways to noise and to interact differently with people. They may display varying degrees

TABLE 2-13 Injury Prevention in Infancy

HAZARD	DEVELOPMENTAL CHARACTERISTICS	PREVENTIVE MEASURES
Falls	Mobility increases in first year of life, progressing from squirming movements to crawling, rolling, and standing	Do not leave infant unsecured in infant seat, even in newborn period. Do not place on high surfaces such as tables or beds unless holding child. **(1)** Once mobile by crawling, keep doors to stairways closed or use gates. Standing walkers have led to many injuries and are not recommended.
Burns	Infant is dependent on caretakers for environmental control. The second half of the first year is marked by crawling and increased mobility. Objects are explored by touching and placing in mouth.	Check temperature of bath water and food/liquids for drinking. Cover electrical outlets. Supervise infant so that play with electrical cords cannot occur.
Motor vehicle crashes	Infant is dependent on caretakers for placement in car. On impact with another motor vehicle, an infant held on a lap acts as a torpedo.	Use only approved restraint systems (according to Federal Motor Vehicle Safety Standards) (see Table 2-22). The seat must be used for every trip, even if very short. The seat must be properly buckled to the car's lap belt system. **(2)**
Drowning	Infant cannot swim and is unable to lift head.	Never leave infant alone in a bath of even 2.5 cm (1 in.) of water Supervise when in water even when a life preserver is worn. Flotation devices such as arm inflatabes are not certified life preservers.

(1) Never leave infant unsecured or on high surface.

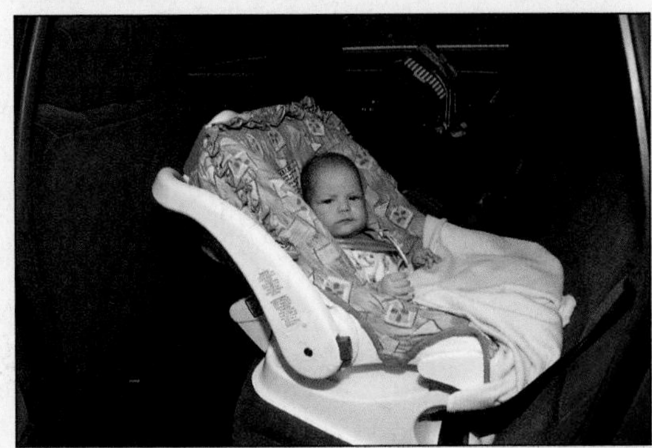

(2) Always use approved restraint system. Place infant in rear-facing seat in backseat of car

(continued)

TABLE 2-13 Injury Prevention in Infancy (continued)

HAZARD	DEVELOPMENTAL CHARACTERISTICS	PREVENTIVE MEASURES
Poisoning	Infant is dependent on caretakers to keep harmful substances out of reach.	Keep medicines out of reach. Teach proper dosage and administration of medicines to parents. Cleaning products and other harmful substances should not be stored where the infant can reach them. Remove plants from play areas. Have poison control center number by telephone.
Choking	The second half of infancy is marked by exploratory reaching and mouthing objects. Infant explores objects by placing them in the mouth. **(3)**	Avoid foods that commonly cause choking. Keep small toys away from infants, especially toys labeled "not intended for use by those under 3 years."
Suffocation	Young infant has minimal head control and may be unable to move if vomiting or having difficulty breathing.	Position infant on back for sleep. Do not place pillows, stuffed toys, or other objects near head. Do not use plastic in crib. Avoid latex balloons. **(4)**
Strangulation	Infant is able to get head into railings or crib slats but cannot remove it.	Be sure older cribs have slats spaced 6 cm (2 3/8 in.) or less apart. The mattress must fit tightly against the crib rails.

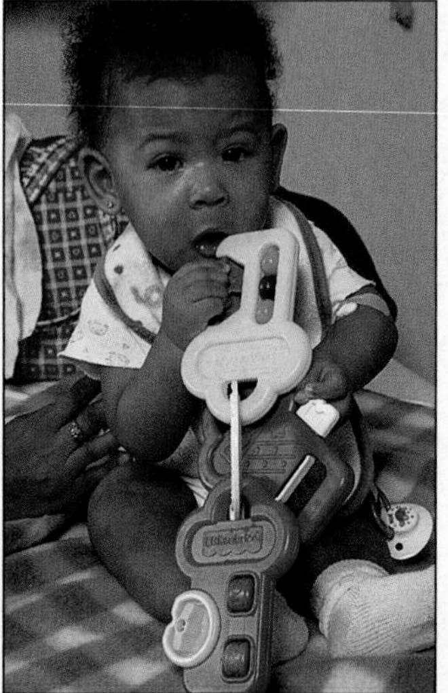

(3) Explores objects with mouth.

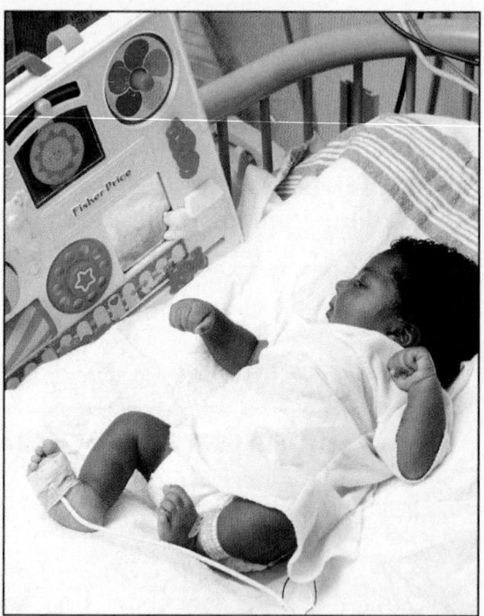

(4) Place infant on back for sleeping, keep toys clear.

of regularity in activities of eating and sleeping, and manifest a capacity for concentrating on tasks for different amounts of time (see Table 2–7).

Nursing assessment identifies personality characteristics of the infant that the nurse can share with the parents. With this information, the parents can appreciate more fully the uniqueness of their infant and design experiences to meet the infant's needs. Parents can learn to modify the environment to promote adaptation. For example, an infant who does not adapt easily to new situations may cry, withdraw, or develop another way of coping when adjusting to new people or places. Parents might be advised to use one or two babysitters rather than engaging new sitters frequently. If the infant is easily distracted when eating, parents can feed the infant in a quiet setting to encourage a focus on eating. Although the infant's temperament is unchanged, the ability to fit with the environment is enhanced.

COMMUNICATION STRATEGIES: INFANT

- Hold for feedings.
- Hold, rock, and talk to infant often.
- Talk and sing frequently during care.
- Tell names of objects.
- Use high-pitched voice with newborns.
- When the infant is upset, swaddle and hold securely.

COMMUNICATION

Even at a few weeks of age, infants communicate and engage in two-way interaction, and express comfort by soft sounds, cuddling, and eye contact. The infant displays discomfort by thrashing the extremities, arching the back, and crying vigorously. From these rudimentary skills, communication ability continues to develop until the infant speaks several words at the end of the first year of life (Table 2-14).

Nurses assess communication to identify possible abnormalities or developmental delays. Language ability may be assessed with the Denver II Developmental Test and other specialized language screening tools (see Chapter 6). Normal infants and toddlers understand

TABLE 2-14 Patterns of Infant Communication

AGE	BEHAVIOR
Birth to 2 months	Coos Babbles Comfort sounds Cries
3–6 months	Vocalizations with play and favorite people Laughs Cries less Squeals and makes pleasure sounds Multisyllabic babbling
6–9 months	Increasing vowel and consonant sounds Links syllables Speechlike rhythm when "talking" with adult
9–12 months	Understands "no" and other simple commands Says "dada" and "mama" to identify parents Learns one or two other words Receptive speech surpasses expressive speech

(receptive speech) more words than they can speak (expressive speech). Abnormalities may be caused by a hearing deficit, developmental delay, or lack of verbal stimulation from caretakers. Further assessment may be required to pinpoint the cause of the abnormality.

Nursing interventions focus on providing a stimulating environment. Parents are encouraged to speak to infants and teach words. Hospital nurses should include the infant's known words when providing care.

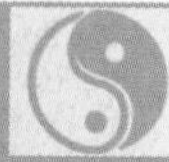

CULTURE

In traditional Native American families, children are allowed to unfold and develop naturally at their own pace. Children thus wean and toilet-train themselves with little interference or pressure from parents.

TODDLER (1 TO 3 YEARS)

Toddlerhood is sometimes called the first adolescence. An infant only months before, this child from 1 to 3 years is now displaying independence and negativism. Pride in newfound accomplishments emerges.

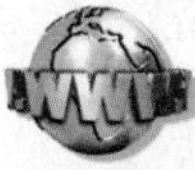

Resources for Infants, Toddlers, and Families

PHYSICAL GROWTH AND DEVELOPMENT

The rate of growth slows during the second year of life. Parents may become concerned because the child has a limited intake and need reassurance that this is normal. See Chapter 3 for further discussion of nutrition in toddlerhood. By age 2 years, the birth weight has usually quadrupled and the child is about one half of the adult height. Body proportions begin to change, with legs longer and head smaller in proportion to body size than during infancy (see Figure 2-7). The toddler has a pot-bellied appearance and stands with feet apart to provide a wide base of support. By approximately 33 months, eruption of deciduous teeth is complete, with 20 teeth present.

Gross motor activity develops rapidly (Table 2-15), as the toddler progresses from walking to running, kicking, and riding a tricycle (Figure 2-10 ◆). As physical maturation occurs, the toddler develops the ability to control elimination patterns (Table 2-16).

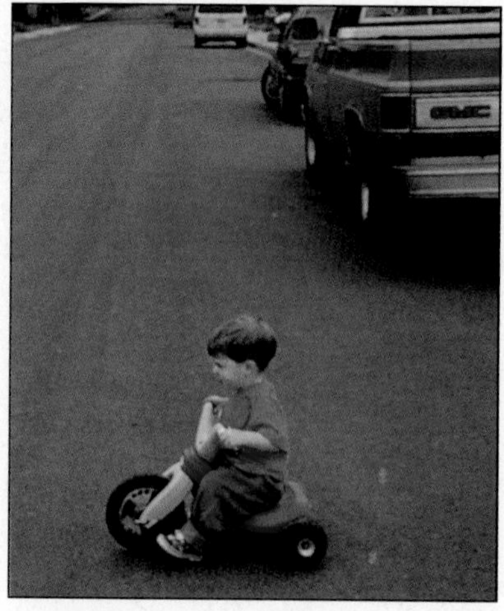

FIGURE 2-10 ◆
This toddler has learned to ride a Big Wheel, which he is doing right into the street. Toddlers must be closely watched to prevent injury.

COGNITIVE DEVELOPMENT

During the toddler years, the child moves from the sensorimotor to the preoperational stage of development. The early use of language awakens in the 1-year-old the ability to think about objects or people when they are absent. Object permanence is well developed.

At about 2 years of age, the increasing use of words as symbols enables the toddler to use preoperational thought. Rudimentary problem solving, creative thought, and an understanding of cause-and-effect relationships are now possible.

TABLE 2-15 Growth and Development Milestones During Toddlerhood

AGE	PHYSICAL GROWTH	FINE MOTOR ABILITY	GROSS MOTOR ABILITY	SENSORY ABILITY
1–2 years	Gains 8 oz (227 g) or more per month Grows 3.5–5 in. (9–12 cm) during this year Anterior fontanel closes	By end of 2nd year, builds a tower of four blocks **(1)** Scribbles on paper **(2)** Can undress self **(3)** Throws a ball	Runs Walks up and down stairs **(5)** Likes push and pull toys	Visual acuity 20/50
2–3 years	Gains 1.4–2.3 kg (3–5 lb)/year Grows 5–6.5 cm (2–2.5 in.)/year	Draws a circle and other rudimentary forms Learns to pour Learning to dress self **(4)**	Jumps Kicks ball **(6)** Throws ball overhand	

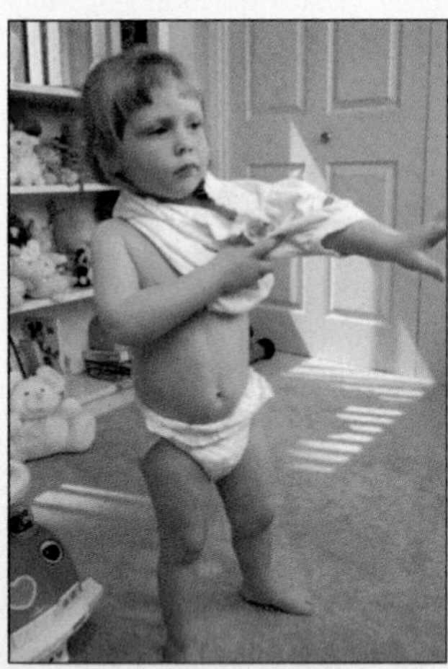

(1) Second year tower of four blocks

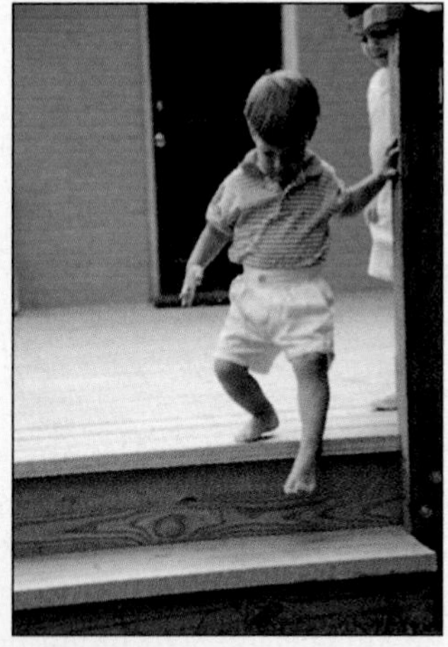

(2) Scribbles on paper

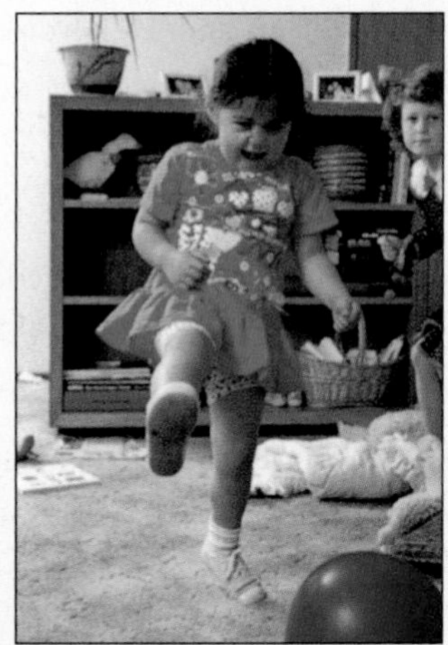

(3) Can undress self

(4) Learning to dress self

(5) Walks up and down stairs

(6) Jumps and kicks ball

PLAY

Many changes in play patterns occur between infancy and toddlerhood. The toddler's motor skills enable him or her to bang pegs into a pounding board with a hammer. The social nature of toddler play is also readily seen. Toddlers find the company of other children pleasurable, even though socially interactive play may not occur. Two toddlers tend to play with similar objects side by side, occasionally trading toys and words. This is called **parallel play.** This playtime with other children assists toddlers to develop social skills. Toddlers engage in play activities they have seen at home, such as pounding with a hammer and talking on the phone. This imitative behavior teaches them new actions and skills (Figure 2–11 ◆).

TABLE 2-16 Toilet Training

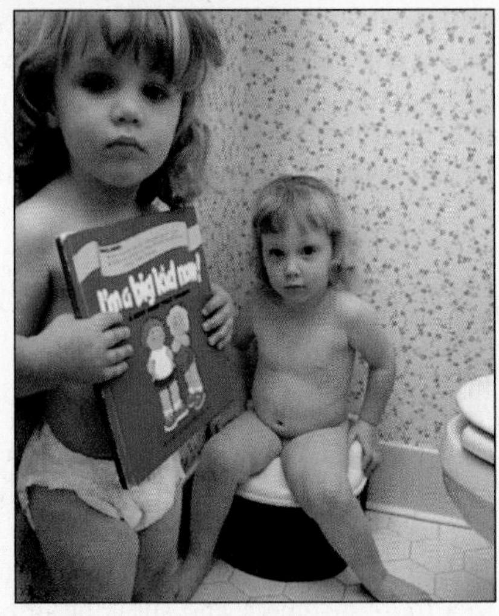

When are children ready to learn toileting? Are parents responsible for the differences in ages at which toilet training is accomplished? Does toilet training provide clues to a child's intellectual ability?

We know that children are not ready for toilet training until several developmental capabilities exist: to stand and walk well, to pull pants up and down, and to recognize the need to eliminate and then to be able to wait until in the bathroom. Once this readiness is apparent, the child can be given a small potty chair and the procedure explained.

Children often prefer their own chair on the floor to using the large toilet. The child should be placed on the chair at regular intervals for a few moments and can be given reward or praise for successes. If the child seems not to understand or does not wish to cooperate, it is best to wait a few weeks and then try again. Just as all of development is subject to individual timetables, toilet training occurs with considerable variability from one child to another. Identify for parents the developmental characteristics of their child and encourage them to appreciate without anxiety the unfolding of skills. These timetables are not predictive of future development.

The child who is ill or hospitalized or has other stress often regresses in toilet training activities. It is best to quietly reinstitute attempts at training after the trauma. Potty chairs should be available on pediatric units and toileting habits identified during initial assessment so that regular routines can be followed and the child's usual words for elimination can be used.

Physical skills are manifested in play as toddlers push and pull objects, climb in and out and up and down, run, ride a Big Wheel, turn the pages of books, and scribble with a pen. Both gross motor and fine motor abilities are enhanced during this age period.

Cognitive understanding enables the toddler to manipulate objects and learn about their qualities. Stacking blocks and placing rings on a building tower teach spatial relationships and other lessons that provide a foundation for future learning. Various kinds of play objects should be provided for the toddler to meet play needs. These play needs can easily be met whether the child is hospitalized or at home (Table 2-17).

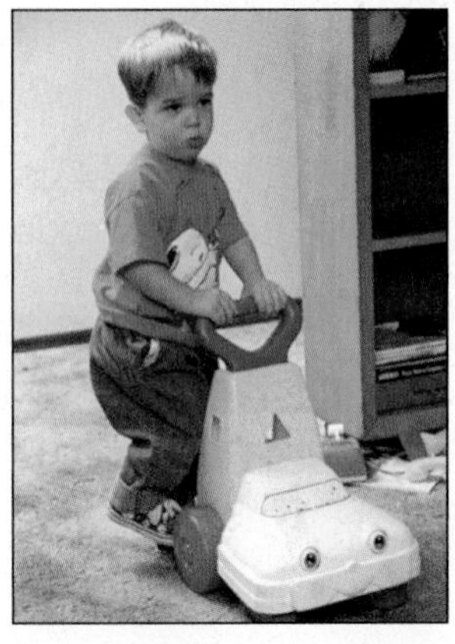

FIGURE 2-11 ◆ Imitative play such as pushing and pulling a vacuum allows the toddler to develop gross and fine motor skills.

INJURY PREVENTION

By 1 year of age, unintentional injuries are by far the leading cause of death in children (see Chapter 1). Injuries also cause disfigurement and other ongoing health problems. Nurses intervene to care for injured children in the hospital and are responsible for making sure that the hospital environment is free of safety hazards. Nurses are also instrumental in teaching parents how to make the toddler's environment safe (Table 2-18).

TABLE 2-17 Favorite Toys and Activities in Toddlerhood

PLAY NEED	TYPES OF TOYS AND ACTIVITIES
Facilitate imitative behavior	Play kitchen Grocery carts Pounding board Toy phone
Encourage gross motor activity and provide an outlet for stress	Big Wheel tricycle Soft ball and bat Water and sand Bean bag toss
Foster fine motor skills	Cloth books Large pencil and paper Wooden puzzles
Facilitate cognitive growth	Educational television shows Music Stories and books

PERSONALITY AND TEMPERAMENT

The toddler retains most of the temperamental characteristics identified during infancy, but may demonstrate some changes. The normal developmental progression of toddlerhood also plays a part in responses. For example, the infant who previously responded positively to stimuli, such as a new baby-sitter, may appear more negative in toddlerhood. The increasing independence characteristic of this age is shown by the toddler's use of the word *no.* The parent and child constantly adapt their responses to each other and learn anew how to communicate with each other.

COMMUNICATION

Because of the phenomenal growth of language skills during the toddler period, adults should communicate frequently with children in this age group. Toddlers imitate words and speech intonations, as well as the social interactions they observe.

At the beginning of toddlerhood, the child may use four to six words in addition to "mama" and "dada." Receptive speech (the ability to understand words) far outpaces expressive speech. By the end of toddlerhood, however, the 3-year-old has a vocabulary of almost 1,000 words and uses short sentences.

Communication occurs in many ways, some of which are nonverbal. Toddler communication includes pointing, pulling an adult over to a room or object, and speaking in **expressive jargon** (using unintelligible words with normal speech intonations as if truly communicating in words). Another communication method occurs when the toddler cries, pounds feet, displays a temper tantrum, or uses other means to illustrate dismay. These powerful communication methods can upset parents, who often need suggestions for handling them. It is best to verbalize the feelings shown by the toddler, for example, by saying, "You must be very upset that you cannot have that candy. When you stop crying you can come out of your room," and then to ignore further negative behavior. The toddler's search

FAMILIES WANT TO KNOW

Proper Child Safety Seat Use Chart

	INFANTS	TODDLER	YOUNG CHILDREN
WEIGHT	Birth to 1 year up to 2-22 lbs.	Over 1 year and Over 20 lbs.-40 lbs.	Over 40 lbs. Ages 4-8, unless 4'9".
TYPE OF SEAT	Infant only or rear-facing convertible	Convertible/Forward-facing	Belt positioning booster seat
SEAT POSITION	Rear-facing only	Forward-facing	Forward-facing
ALWAYS MAKE SURE:	Children to one year and at least 20 lbs. in rear-facing seats Harness straps at or below shoulder level	Harness straps should be at or above shoulders Most seats require top slot for forward-facing	Belt positioning booster seats must be used with both lap and shoulder belt. Make sure the lap belt fits low and tight across the lap/upper thigh area and the shoulder belt fits snug crossing the chest and shoulder to avoid abdominal injuries.
WARNING	All children age 12 and under should ride in the back seat	All children age 12 and under should ride in the back seat	All children age 12 and under should ride in the back seat

Note: From the National Highway Traffic Safety Administration.

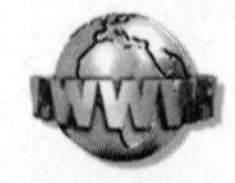

Children & Car Safety

TABLE 2-18 Injury Prevention in Toddlerhood

	HAZARD	DEVELOPMENTAL CHARACTERISTICS	PREVENTIVE MEASURES
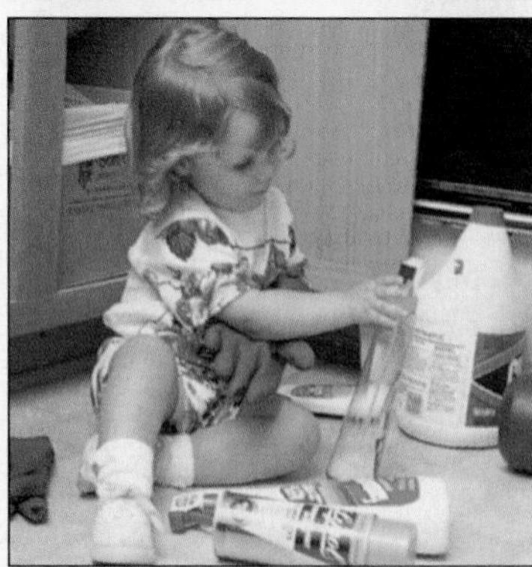	Falls	Gross motor skills improve. Toddler is able to move chairs to counters and can climb up ladders.	Supervise toddler closely. Provide safe climbing toys. Begin to teach acceptable places for climbing.
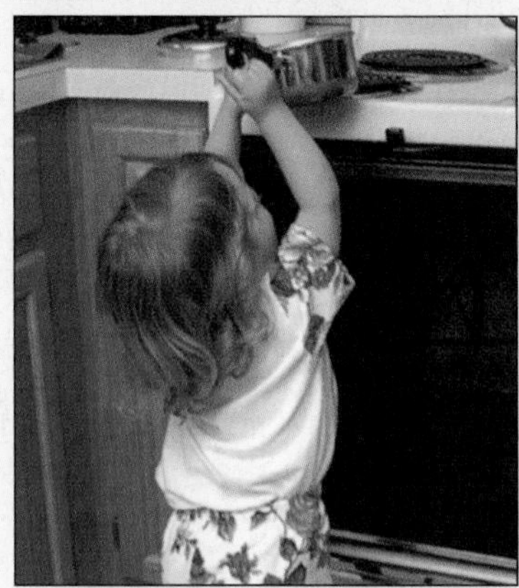	Poisoning	Gross motor skills enable toddler to climb onto chairs and then cabinets. Medicines, cosmetics, and other poisonous substances are easily reached.	Keep medicines and other poisonous materials locked away. Use child-resistant containers and cupboard closures. Have poison control center number (1-800-222-1222) by telephone. Keep syrup of ipecac in home (call Poison Control Center before using).
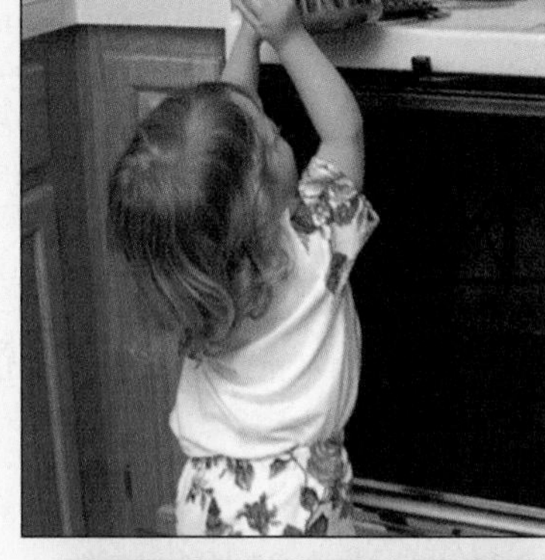	Burns	Toddler is tall enough to reach stove top. Toddler can walk to fireplace and may reach into fire.	Keep pot handles turned inward on stove. Do not burn fires without close supervision. Use a fire screen.
	Motor vehicle crashes	Toddler may be able to undo seat belt, may resist using car seat, demonstrating characteristic negativism and autonomy.	Insist on safety seat use for all trips. Use approved safety seats only, such as forward-facing convertible seat. Toddler is not large enough to use car seat belts.
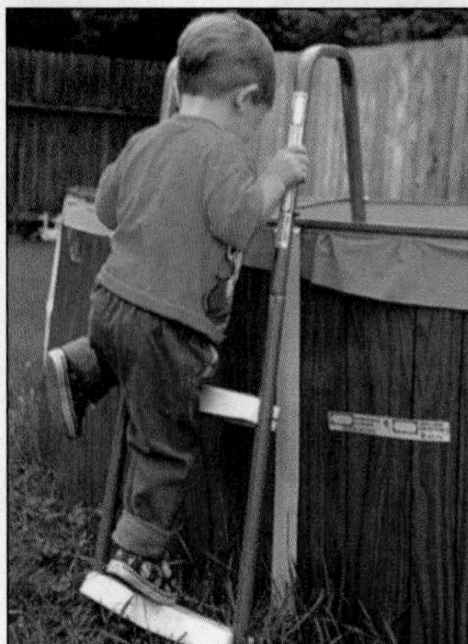	Drowning	Toddler can walk onto docks or pool decks. Toddler may stand on or climb seats on boat. Toddler may fall into buckets, toilets, and fish tanks and be unable to get top of body out.	Supervise any child near water. Swimming classes do not protect a toddler from drowning. Use child-resistant pool covers. Use approved child life jackets near water and on boats. Empty buckets when not in use.

TABLE 2-19 Communicating with a Toddler

Procedures such as drawing blood can be frightening for a toddler. Effective communication minimizes the trauma caused by such procedures:

- Avoid telling toddlers about the procedure too far in advance. They do not have an understanding of time and can become quite anxious.
- Use simple terminology: "We need to get a little blood from your arm. It will help us to find out if you are getting better." If the parent is willing, say, "Your Mom will hold your arm still so we can do it quickly."
- Allow the toddler to cry. Acknowledge that it must be frightening and that you understand.
- Perform the procedure in a treatment room so that the toddler's bed and room are a safe haven.
- Be sure the toddler is restrained, with the joints above and below the procedure immobilized.
- Use a Band-Aid to cover the site and to reassure the toddler that the body is still intact.
- Allow the toddler to choose a reward such as a sticker after the procedure.
- Praise the toddler for cooperation and acknowledge that you know this was difficult.
- Comfort the toddler by rocking, offering a favorite drink, playing music, and holding. If parents are present, they can offer the comfort needed.

COMMUNICATION STRATEGIES: TODDLER

Give short, clear instructions.
Do not give choices if none exist.
Offer a choice of two alternatives when possible.
Approach positively.
Tell toddler what you are doing, names of objects.

for autonomy and independence creates a need for such behavior. Sometimes an upset toddler responds well to holding, rocking, and stroking.

Parents and nurses can promote a toddler's communication by speaking frequently, naming objects, explaining procedures in simple terms, expressing feelings that the toddler seems to be displaying, and encouraging speech. The toddler from a bilingual home is at an optimal age to learn two languages. If the parents do not speak English, the toddler will benefit from a child care experience because both languages can then be learned.

The nurse who understands the communication skills of toddlers is able to assess expressive and receptive language and communicate effectively, thereby promoting positive health care experiences for these children (Table 2-19).

PRESCHOOL CHILD (3 TO 6 YEARS)

The preschool years are a time of new initiative and independence. Most children are in a child care center or school for part of the day and learn a great deal from this social contact. Language skills are well developed, and the child is able to understand and speak clearly. Endless projects characterize the world of busy preschoolers. They may work with play dough to form animals, then cut out and paste paper, then draw and color (Figure 2-12 ◆).

PHYSICAL GROWTH AND DEVELOPMENT

Preschoolers grow slowly and steadily, with most growth taking place in long bones of the arms and legs. The short, chubby toddler gradually gives way to a slender, long-legged preschooler (Table 2-20).

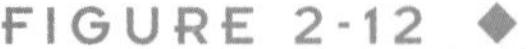

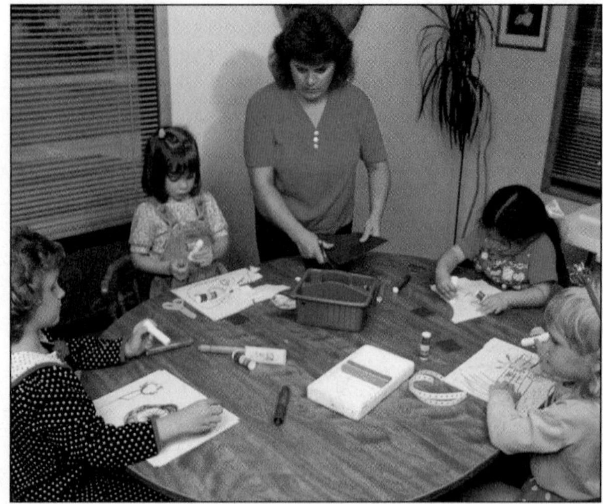

FIGURE 2-12 ◆ Preschoolers have well-developed language, motor, and social skills, and they can work creatively together on an art project, as this group is doing at an in-home child care center.

TABLE 2-20 Growth and Development Milestones During the Preschool Years

PHYSICAL GROWTH

Gains 1.5–2/5 kg (3–5 lb)/year

Grows 4–6 cm (1 1/2–2 1/2 in.)/year

FINE MOTOR ABILITY

Uses scissors **(1)**
Draws circle, square, cross **(2)**
Draws at least a six-part person
Enjoys art projects such as pasting, stringing beads, using clay
Learns to tie shoes at end of preschool years **(3)**
Buttons **(4)**
Brushes teeth **(5)**

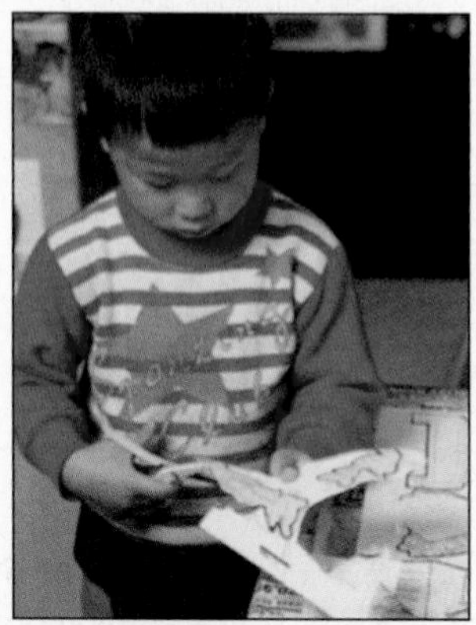

(1) Uses scissors

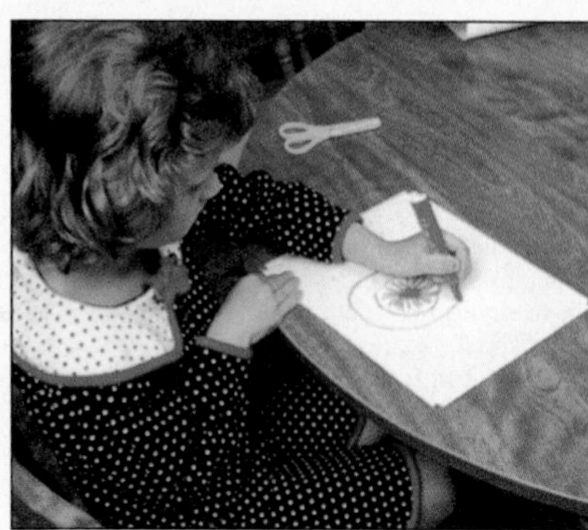

(2) Draws circle, square, cross

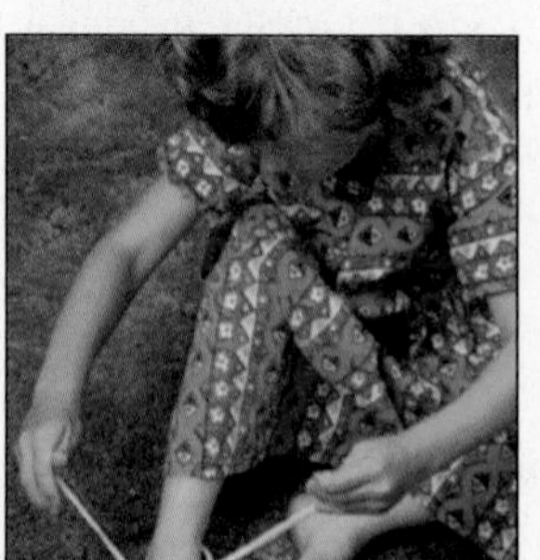

(3) Ties shoes

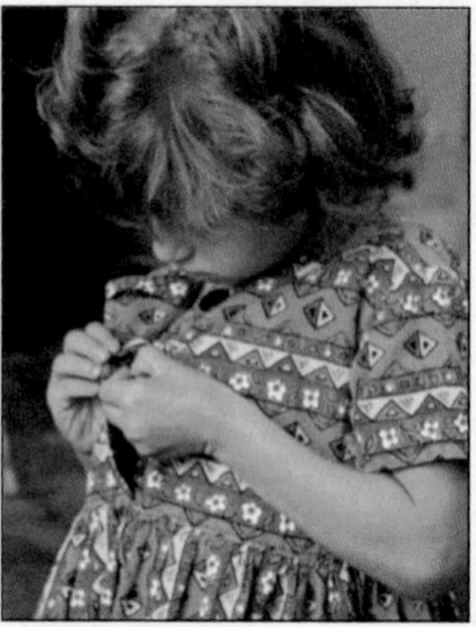

(4) Buttons clothes

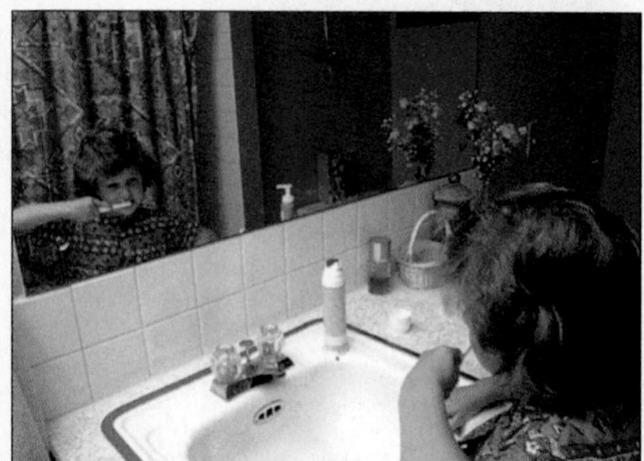

(5) Brushes teeth

GROSS MOTOR ABILITY

Throws a ball overhand
Climbs well **(6)**
Rides tricycle **(7)**

SENSORY ABILITY

Visual acuity continues to improve
Can focus on and learn letters and numbers **(8)**

FINE MOTOR ABILITY

Eats three meals with snacks
Uses spoon, fork, and knife

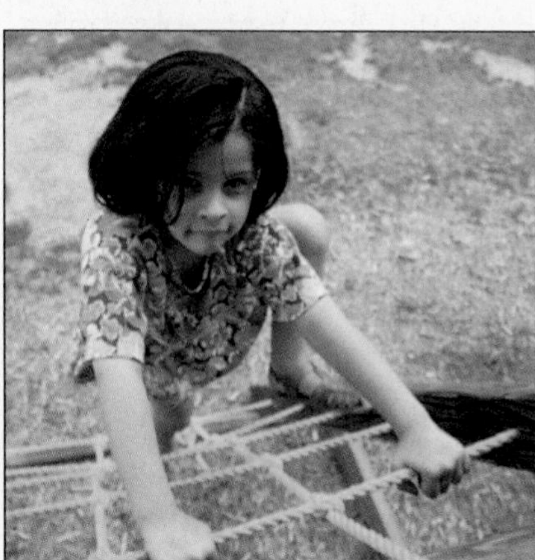

(6) Climbs well

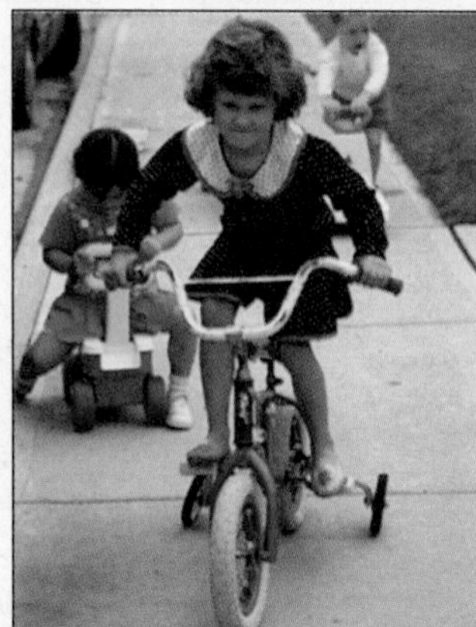

(7) Rides bicycle or bicycle with training wheels

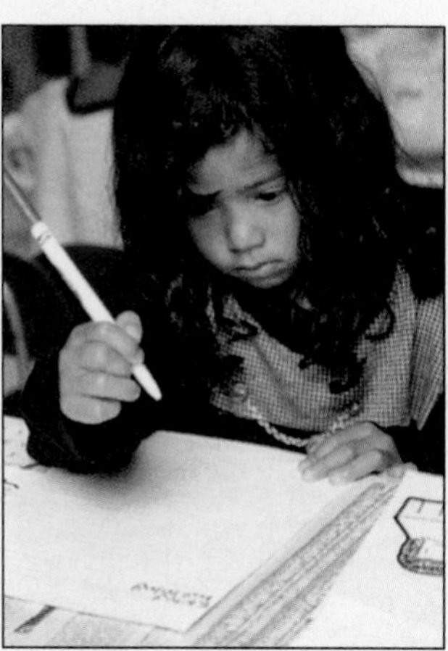

(8) Learns letters and numbers

TABLE 2-21 Recommended Daily Fluoride* Dosages

Age	AMOUNT OF FLUORIDE IN WATER SUPPLY		
	Under 0.3 ppm	*0.3–0.6 ppm*	*Above 0.6 ppm*
Under 6 months	0	0	0
6 months to 3 years	0.25 mg	0	0
3–6 years	0.50 mg	0.25 mg	0
6–16 years	1.00 mg	0.50 mg	0

ppm: parts per million
*Fluoride is available as a liquid to be mixed in a small amount of food or fluid for the infant and toddler and as a chewable tablet for the older child. It acts both systemically to promote strong teeth before they erupt and topically to strengthen tooth surfaces with which it comes in contact.
Note: From Bindler, R. M., & Howry, L. B. (1997). *Pediatric drugs and nursing implications* (2nd ed.). Stamford, CT: Appleton & Lange, 253–255.

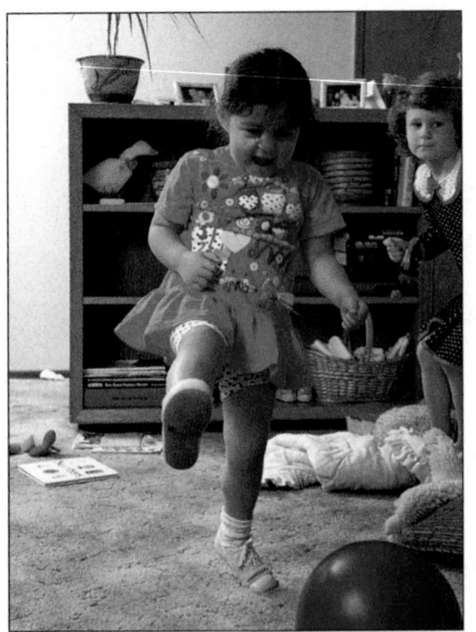

FIGURE 2-13 ◆
Preschoolers continue to develop more advanced skills, such as kicking a ball without falling down.

Physical skills continue to develop (Figure 2-13 ◆). The preschooler runs with ease, holds a bat, and throws balls of various types. Writing ability increases, and the preschooler enjoys drawing and learning to write a few letters.

The preschool period is a good time to encourage good dental habits. Children can begin to brush their own teeth with parental supervision and help to reach all tooth surfaces. Parents should floss children's teeth, give fluoride as ordered if the water supply is not fluoridated (Table 2-21), and schedule the first dental visit so the child can become accustomed to the routine of periodic dental care.

COGNITIVE DEVELOPMENT

The preschooler exhibits characteristics of preoperational thought. Symbols or words are used to represent objects and people, enabling the young child to think about them. This is a milestone in intellectual development; however, the preschooler still has some limitations in thought (Table 2-22).

PLAY

The preschooler has begun to play in a new way. Toddlers simply play side by side with friends, each engaging in his or her own activities; but preschoolers interact with others during play. One child cuts out colored paper while her friend glues it on paper in a design. This new type of interaction is called **associative play** (Figure 2-14 ◆).

TABLE 2-22 Characteristics of Preoperational Thought

CHARACTERISTIC	DEFINITION	EXAMPLE
Egocentrism	Ability to see things only from one's own point of view	The child who cannot understand why parents may need to leave the hospital for work when the child wishes them to be present
Transductive reasoning	Connecting two events in a cause–effect relationship simply because they occur together in time	A child who, awakening after surgery and feeling pain, notices the intravenous infusion and believes that it is causing the pain
Centration	Focusing on only one particular aspect of a situation	The child who is concerned about breathing through an anesthesia mask and will not listen to any other aspects of preoperative teaching
Animism	Giving lifelike qualities to nonliving things	The child who views a monitoring machine as alive because it beeps

In addition to this social dimension of play, other aspects of play also differ. The preschooler enjoys large motor activities such as swinging, riding a tricycle, and throwing a ball. Increasing manual dexterity is demonstrated in greater complexity of drawings and manipulation of blocks and modeling. These changes necessitate planning of playtime to include appropriate activities. Preschool programs and child life departments in hospitals help meet this important need.

Materials provided for play can be simple but should guide activities in which the child engages. Because fine motor activities are popular, paper, pens, scissors, glue, and a variety of other such objects should be available. The child can use them to create important images such as pictures of people, hospital beds, or friends. A collection of dolls, furniture, and clothing can be manipulated to represent parents and children, nurses and physicians, teachers, or other significant people. Because fantasy life is so powerful at this age, the preschooler readily uses props to engage in **dramatic play,** that is, the living out of the drama of human life (Figure 2-15 ◆).

The nurse can use playtime to assess the preschooler's developmental level, knowledge about health care, and emotions related to health care experiences. Observations about objects chosen for play, content of dramatic play, and pictures drawn can provide important assessment data. The nurse can also use play periods to teach the child about health care procedures and offer an outlet for expression of emotions (Table 2-23).

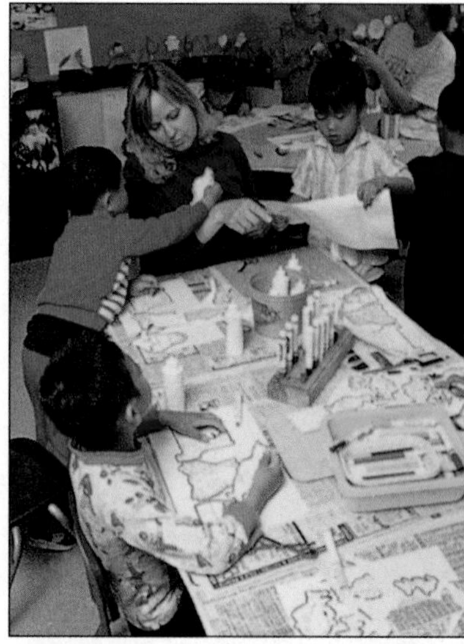

FIGURE 2-14 ◆
These preschoolers are participating in associative play, which means they can interact. One child is cutting out shapes, and the other is gluing them in place. Of course, every job needs a supervisor, who can be seen on the right.

INJURY PREVENTION

The increasing independence of preschool children puts them at risk of injury. The 3- to 7-year-old group is at high risk of injury from fire, drowning, and motor vehicle and pedestrian accidents (see Chapter 1). Nurses can teach parents preventive measures and can also begin to include preschoolers in safety teaching (Table 2-24).

PERSONALITY AND TEMPERAMENT

Characteristics of personality observed in infancy tend to persist over time. The preschooler may need assistance as these characteristics are expressed in the new situations of preschool or nursery school. An excessively active child, for example, will need gentle, consistent handling to adjust to the structure of a classroom. Encourage parents to visit preschool programs to choose the one that would best foster growth in their child. Some preschoolers enjoy the structured learning of a program that focuses on cognitive skills, whereas others are happier and more open to learning in a small group that provides much time for free play. Nurses can help parents to identify their child's personality or temperament characteristics and to find the best environment for growth.

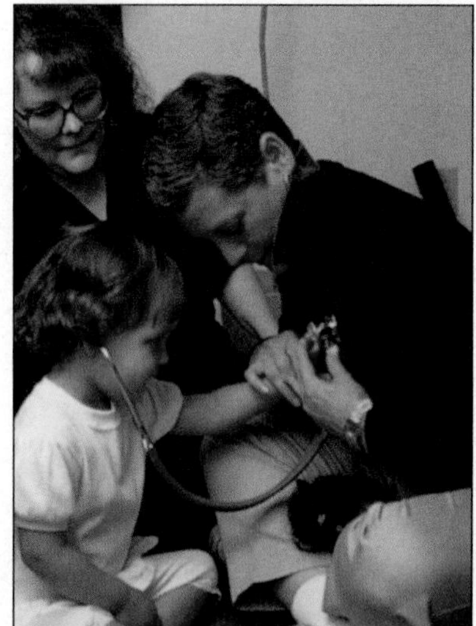

FIGURE 2-15 ◆
Jasmine is participating in dramatic play with a nurse while her mother looks on. In dramatic play, the child uses props to play out the drama of human life. It can be an excellent way for a nurse to assess the developmental level of children while talking to them. Notice that the child and the nurse are on the floor at the same level and the atmosphere is informal. Why is it important to be at the same level as the child?

TABLE 2-23 Favorite Toys and Activities in the Preschool Years

PLAY NEED	TYPES OF TOYS AND ACTIVITIES
Facilitate associative play	Simple games Puzzles Nursery rhymes, songs
Promote dramatic play	Dolls and doll clothes Play houses and hospitals Dress-up clothes Puppets
Encourage outlet for stress	Pens, paper Glue, scissors
Facilitate cognitive growth	Educational television shows Music Stories and books

TABLE 2-24 Injury Prevention in the Preschool Years

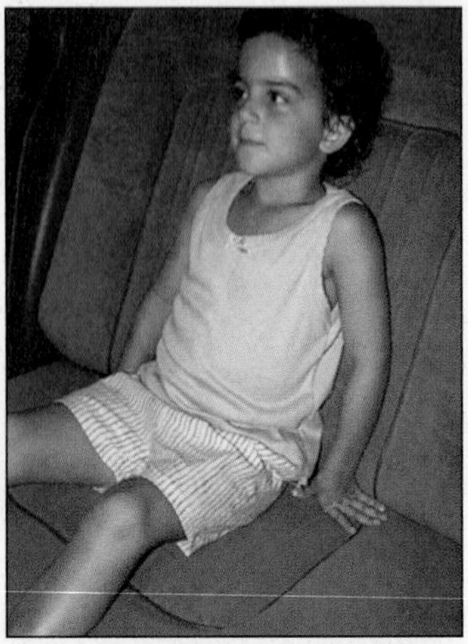

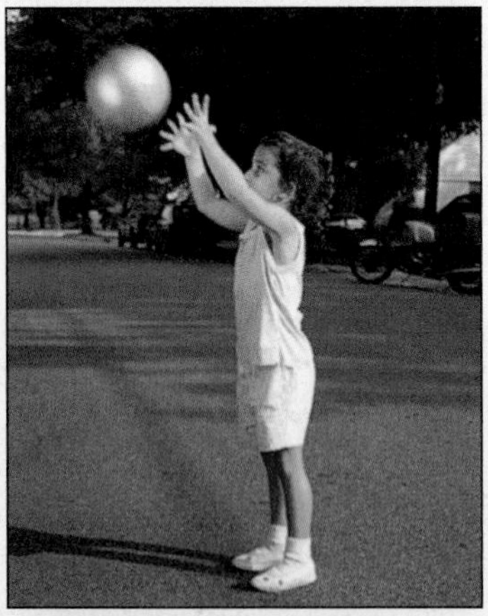

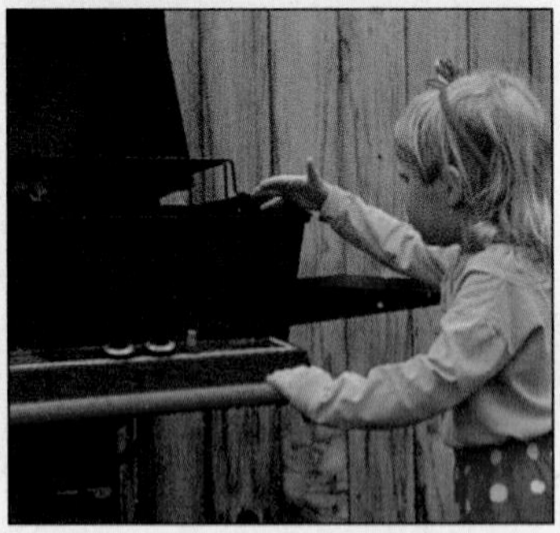

HAZARDS	DEVELOPMENTAL CHARACTERISTICS	PREVENTIVE MEASURES
Motor vehicle crashes	Older preschooler independently gets into car and puts on seat belt. Child may forget to belt up or may do so incorrectly.	Verify that child is belted in properly before starting car. Child restraint systems must be used until child weighs 18 kg (40 lb) and is 100 cm (40 in.) tall.
Motor vehicle and pedestrian accidents	Preschooler increasingly plays outside alone or with friends. Preschooler is unable to judge speed of moving car and assumes driver knows that he or she is present.	Teach child never to go into road. A safe, preferably enclosed, play yard is recommended.
Drowning	Preschooler who has had swimming lessons may choose to go into a lake or pool.	Teach child never to go into water without an adult. Provide supervision whenever child is near water.
Burns	Preschooler can understand the hazards of fire.	Teach child to stop, drop, and roll if clothes are on fire. Practice escapes from home are useful. A visit to a fire station can reinforce learning. Teach child how to call 911.
Needle sticks in hospital	Preschooler can ambulate and is interested in new objects.	Keep needles out of reach. Remove from unit immediately after use.
Electrical injury in hospital	Preschooler is mobile and may trip over cords and equipment or may choose to examine them.	Avoid use of electrical cords if possible. Keep equipment out of major traffic areas. Keep beds away from electrical outlets. Monitor child closely.

COMMUNICATION

Language skills blossom during the preschool years. The vocabulary grows to over 2,000 words, and children speak in complete sentences of several words and use all parts of speech. They practice these newfound language skills by endlessly talking and asking questions.

The sophisticated speech of preschoolers mirrors the development occurring in their minds and helps them to learn about the world around them. However, this speech can be quite deceptive. Although preschoolers use many words, their grasp of meaning is usually literal and may not match that of adults. These literal interpretations have important implications for health care providers. For example, the preschooler who is told she will be "put to sleep" for surgery may think of a pet recently euthanised; the child who is told that a dye will be injected for a diagnostic test may think he is going to die; mention of "a little stick" in the arm can cause images of tree branches rather than of a simple immunization.

The child may also have difficulty focusing on the content of a conversation. The preschooler is egocentric and may be unable to move from individual thoughts to those the nurse is proposing, as the following conversation illustrates:

Nurse: I'd like to tell you about the operation that you will have tomorrow.

Sharisse: OK. Did you know my brother just got a new squirt gun?

Nurse: That's nice. Now, first thing in the morning you will wake up early and your foot will be scrubbed with a special soap.

Sharisse: The gun can spurt for about 40 feet—you have to pump it up.

Nurse: We'll talk about that later. Let me tell you about your operation now. After your foot is scrubbed, the nurse will measure your blood pressure and temperature and feel the pulse in your arm. Do you remember my doing those things today?

Sharisse: Yes. And I got a sticker when I came into the hospital today, too. Do you know that my Mom is going to stay here tonight?

During this interchange, Sharisse engages in collective monologue, in which separate conversations occur even though each person waits for the other to speak. Though waiting for the nurse to speak, Sharisse is not generally responding to the nurse's content but is instead focusing on content from her own mind. The nurse needs to respond to Sharisse's content and then reinsert more facts about the preparations for surgery.

Concrete visual aids such as pictures of a child undergoing the same procedure or a book to read together enhance teaching by meeting the child's developmental needs. Handling medical equipment such as intravenous bags and stethoscopes increases interest and helps the child to focus. Teaching may have to be done in several short sessions rather than one long session.

COMMUNICATION STRATEGIES: PRESCHOOLER

- Allow time for child to integrate explanations.
- Verbalize frequently to the child.
- Use drawings and stories to explain care.
- Use accurate names for bodily functions.
- Allow choices.

SCHOOL-AGE CHILD (6 TO 12 YEARS)

Errol, 10 years old, arrives home from school shortly after 3 p.m. each day. He immediately calls his friends and goes to visit one of them. They are building models of cars and collecting baseball cards. Endless hours are spent on these projects and on discussions of events at school that day (Figure 2-16 ◆).

Nine-year-old Karen practices soccer two afternoons a week and plays in games each weekend. She also is learning to play the flute and spends her free time at home practicing.

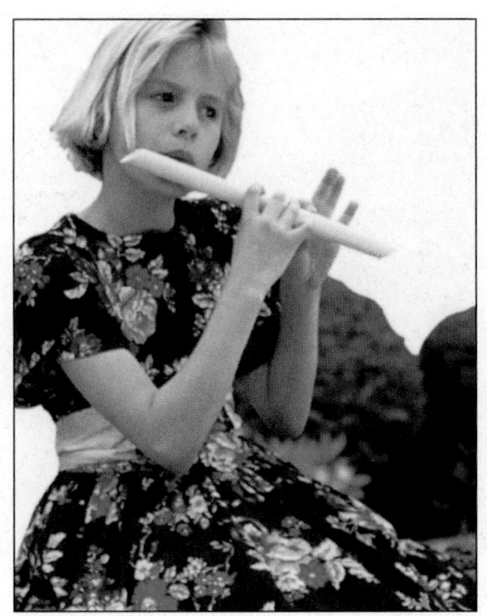

A

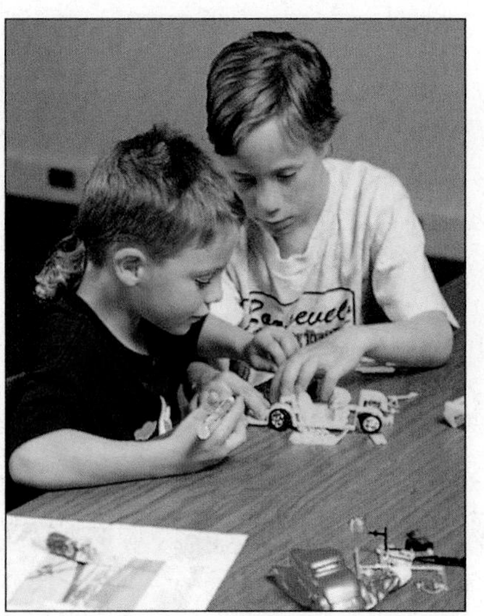

B

FIGURE 2-16 ◆ A, School-age children may take part in activities that require practice. This is a consideration when children are hospitalized and unable to practice or perform. Why? B, School-age children enjoy spending time with others the same age on projects and discussing the activities of the day. This is an important consideration when they are in an acute-care setting. When you are in the clinical setting, look for examples of this type of interaction taking place.

Although practice time is not her favorite part of music, Karen enjoys the performances and wants to play well in front of her friends and teacher. Her parents now allow her to ride her bike unaccompanied to the store or to a friend's house.

These two school-age children demonstrate common characteristics of their age group. They are in a stage of industry in which it is important to the child to perform useful work. Meaningful activities take on great importance and are usually carried out in the company of peers. A sense of achievement in these activities is important to develop self-esteem and to prevent a sense of inferiority or poor self-worth.

PHYSICAL GROWTH AND DEVELOPMENT

School age is the last period in which girls and boys are close in size and body proportions. As the long bones continue to grow, leg length increases (see Figure 2-7). Fat gives way to muscle, and the child appears leaner. Jaw proportions change as the first deciduous tooth is lost at 6 years and permanent teeth begin to erupt. Body organs and the immune system mature, resulting in fewer illnesses among school-age children. Medications are less likely to cause serious side effects, because they can be metabolized more easily. The urinary system can adjust to changes in fluid status. Physical skills are also refined as children begin to play sports, and fine motor skills are well developed through school activities (Table 2-25 and Figure 2-17 ◆).

Although it is commonly believed that the start of adolescence (age 12 years) heralds a growth spurt, the rapid increases in size commonly occur during school age. Girls may begin a growth spurt by 9 or 10 years and boys a year or so later (Figure 2-18 ◆). Nutritional needs increase dramatically with this spurt.

The loss of the first deciduous teeth and the eruption of permanent teeth usually occur at about age 6, or at the beginning of the school-age period. Of the 32 permanent teeth, 22 to 26 erupt by age 12 and the remaining molars follow during the teenage years (see Figure 2-17 inset). The school-age child should be closely monitored to ensure that brushing and flossing are adequate, that fluoride is taken if the water supply is not fluoridated, that dental care is obtained to provide for examination of teeth and alignment, and that loose teeth are identified before surgery or other events that may lead to loss of a tooth.

TABLE 2-25 Growth and Development Milestones During the School-Age Years

PHYSICAL GROWTH	FINE MOTOR ABILITY	GROSS MOTOR ABILITY	SENSORY ABILITY
Gains 1.4–2.2 kg (3–5 lb)/year Grows 4–6 cm (1 1/2–2 1/2 in.)/year	Enjoys craft projects Plays card and board games	Rides two-wheeler **(1)** Jumps rope **(2)** Roller skates or ice skates	Can read Able to concentrate for longer periods on activities by filtering out surrounding sounds **(3)**

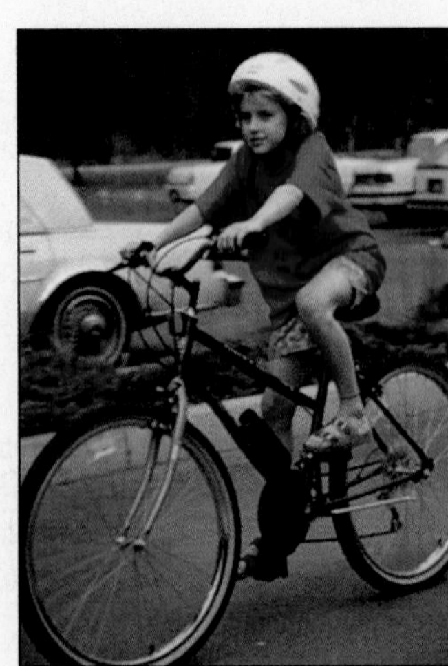

(1) Rides two-wheeler

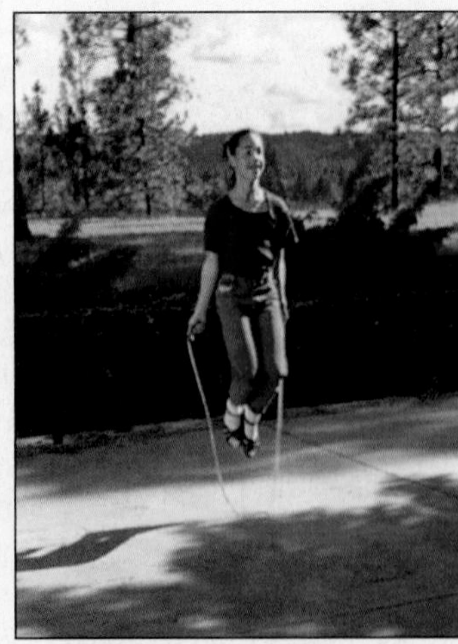

(2) Jumps rope

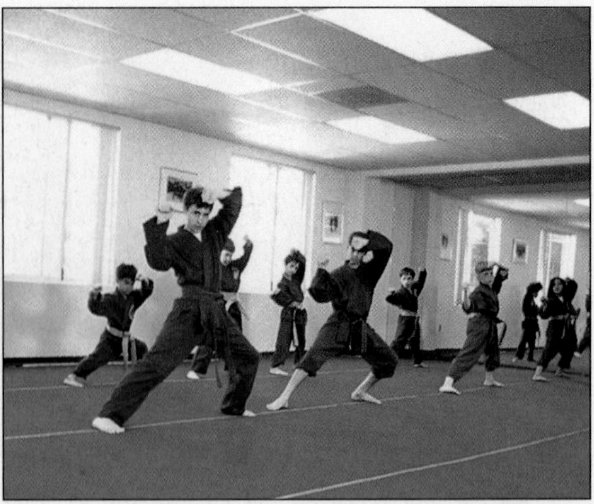

(3) Concentrates on activities for longer periods

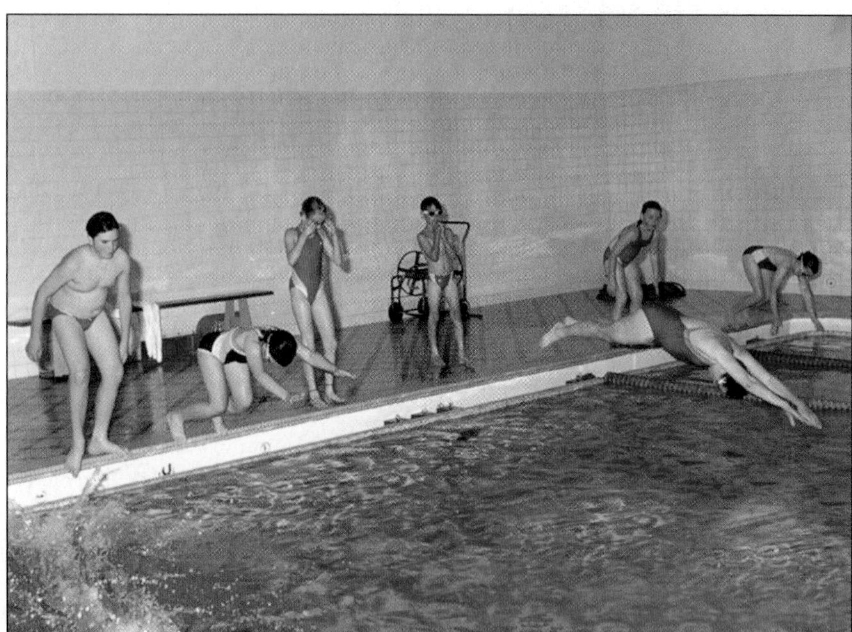

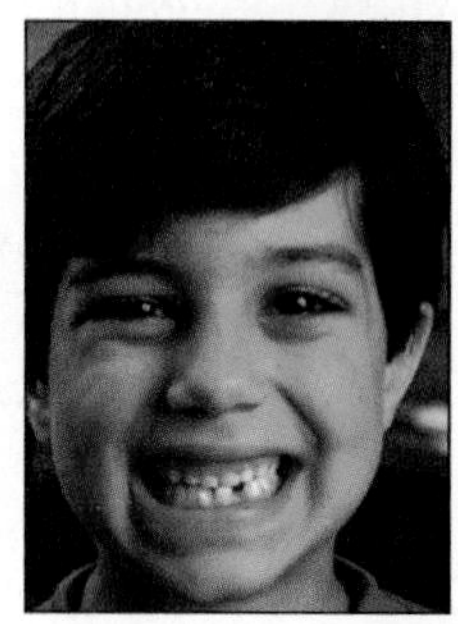

FIGURE 2-17 ◆
School-age girls and boys enjoy participating in sports. They begin to lose fat while developing their muscles, so they appear leaner than at earlier ages. *Inset,* Front teeth are lost around age 6. The family may have rituals associated with the loss of teeth that could affect the child's behavior if he loses a tooth while in the hospital.

COGNITIVE DEVELOPMENT

The child enters the stage of concrete operational thought at about 7 years. This stage enables school-age children to consider alternative solutions and solve problems. However, school-age children continue to rely on concrete experiences and materials to form their thought content.

During the school-age years, the child learns the concept of **conservation** (that matter is not changed when its form is altered). At earlier ages, a child believes that when water is poured from a short, wide glass into a tall, thin glass, there is more water in the taller glass. The school-age child recognizes that although it may look like the taller glass holds more water, the quantity is the same. The concept of conservation is helpful when the nurse explains medical treatments. The school-age child understands that an incision will heal, that a cast will be removed, and that an arm will look the same as before once the intravenous infusion is removed.

PLAY

When the preschool teacher tries to organize a game of baseball, both the teacher and the children become frustrated. Not only are the children physically unable to hold a bat and hit a ball, but they seem to have no understanding of the rules of the game and do not want to

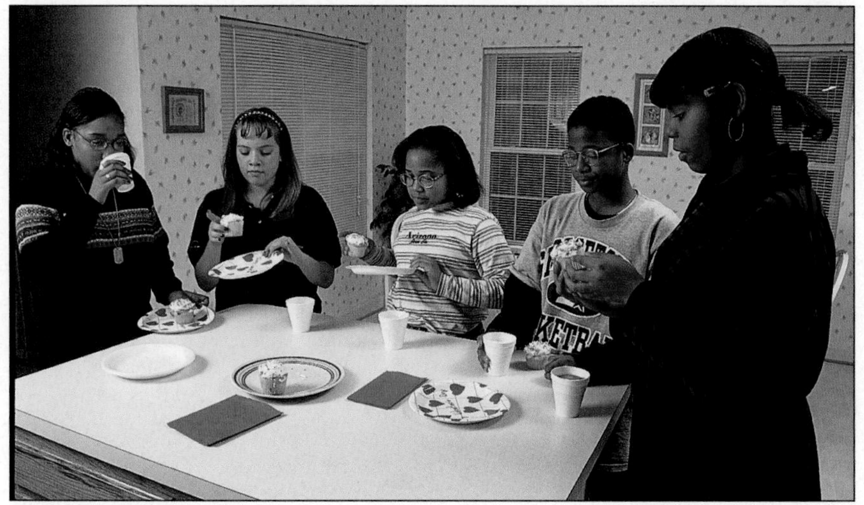

FIGURE 2-18 ◆
Because girls have a growth spurt earlier than boys, girls often are taller than boys of the same age. Remember what it was like at your first dance?

TABLE 2-26 Favorite Play Activities of School-Age Children

PLAY NEED	TYPES OF ACTIVITIES
Foster gross motor activity	Ball sports Skating Dance lessons Water and snow skiing/boarding Biking
Promote sense of industry	Musical instrument Collections (e.g., stamps, miniatures) Hobbies Board and video games
Facilitate cognitive growth	Reading Crafts Word puzzles

RESEARCH

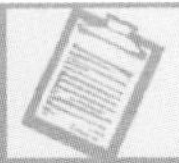

When data from food and nutrition surveys over the past three decades are analyzed, they reveal an increase in the incidence of overweight children aged 6 to 17 years from 15% to 22%. (Overweight is defined as being above the 85th percentile for weight.) This increase is attributed to such factors as availability of abundant high-energy foods (snack foods) and sedentary lifestyles (increased television watching and computer games; decreased physical activity) (Troiano, Flegel, Kuczmasski, Campbell, Johnson, 1995). The long-term risks of being overweight are well known, and children who are overweight have a greater tendency to be overweight as adults. Nurses can teach healthy snacking habits and the importance of regular daily exercise. Weigh children during each health encounter and perform a more detailed dietary history when findings suggest they are overweight.

wait for their turn at bat. By 6 years of age, however, children have acquired the physical ability to hold the bat properly and may occasionally hit the ball. School-age children also understand that everyone has a role—the pitcher, the catcher, the batter, the outfielders. They cooperate with one another to form a team, are eager to learn the rules of the game, and want to ensure that these rules are followed exactly (Table 2-26).

The characteristics of play exhibited by the school-age child are cooperation with others and the ability to play a part in order to contribute to a unified whole. This type of play is called **cooperative play.** The concrete nature of cognitive thought leads to a reliance on rules to provide structure and security. Children have an increasing desire to spend much of playtime with friends, which demonstrates the social component of play. Play is an extremely important method of learning and living for the school-age child. Active physical play has decreased in recent years as television viewing and playing of computer games have increased, leading to poor nutritional status and other health risks in children. See Chapter 3 for further discussion of nutrition and physical activity in children.

When a child is hospitalized, the separation from playmates can lead to feelings of sadness and purposelessness. School-age children often feel better when placed in multibed units with other children. Games can be devised even when children are wheelchair bound (Figure 2-19 ◆). Normal, rewarding parts of play should be integrated into care.

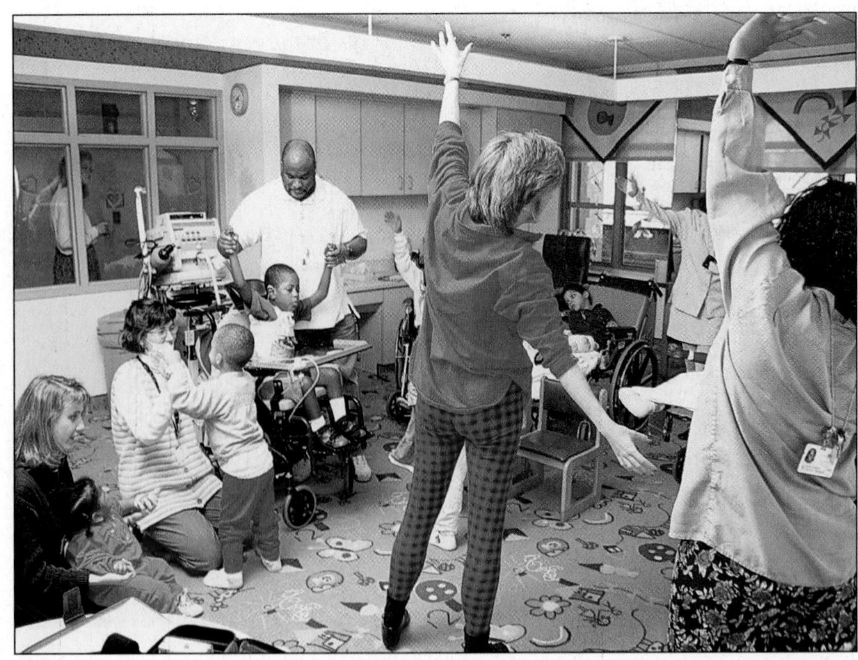

FIGURE 2-19 ◆
The nurse can help the child and family accept and adjust to new circumstances. Encouraging the child in a wheelchair to participate in group activities can help build confidence in physical skills. Good self-esteem, goal attainment, personal satisfaction, and general health are the continued benefits.

Friends should be encouraged to visit or call a hospitalized child. Discharge planning for the child who has had a cast or brace applied should address the activities in which the child can participate and those the child must avoid. Reinforce the importance of playing games with friends.

INJURY PREVENTION

Because school-age children play in unsupervised settings for longer periods, they are at risk for different types of injuries than younger children (Table 2-27). Motor vehicle crashes are still common, but firearm and burn injuries increase in incidence (see Chapter 1). Safety teaching should be an integral part of each school's curriculum. Violence anticipatory guidance can easily be integrated into health care visits, including questions for parents about how many pushing or shoving fights the child has had in the past year, how the child handles conflict, what types of discipline parents use, and which television shows are viewed by the child. The child can be asked if they have been touched in a way that makes them "feel bad," how they handle disagreements with friends, and how they spend their time (Stringham, 1998).

TABLE 2-27 Injury Prevention in the School-Age Years

	HAZARD	DEVELOPMENTAL CHARACTERISTICS	PREVENTIVE MEASURES
	Motor vehicle/ pedestrion/ biking crashes	Child plays outside; may follow ball into road; rides two-wheeler.	Teach child safe outside play, especially near streets. Reinforce use of bike helmet. Teach biking safety rules and provide safe places for riding.
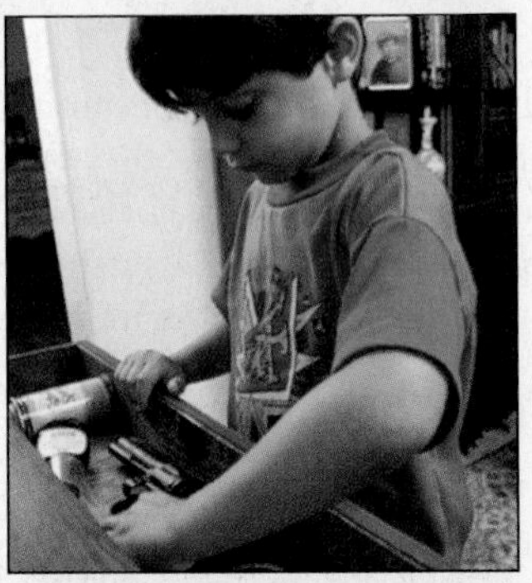	Firearms	Child may have been shown location of guns; is interested in showing them to friends.	Teach child never to touch guns without parent present. Guns should be kept unloaded and locked away. Guns and ammunition should be stored in different locations. Be sure guns have trigger locks.
	Burns	Child may perform experiments with flames or toxic substances.	Teach child what to do in case of fire or if toxic substances touch skin or eyes. Reinforce teaching about 911.
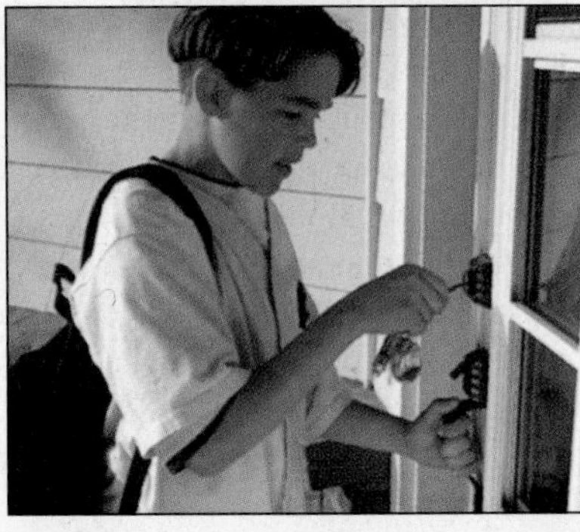	Assault	Child may be left alone after school and may walk, bike, or take public transportation alone.	Provide telephone numbers of people to contact in case of an emergency or if child feels lonely. Leave child alone for brief periods initially, and evaluate child's success in managing time. Teach child not to accept rides from or talk to or open doors to strangers. Teach child how to answer the phone.

COMMUNICATION STRATEGIES: SCHOOL-AGE CHILD

Provide concrete examples of pictures or materials to accompany verbal descriptions.
Assess knowledge before planning the instruction.
Allow child to select rewards following procedures.
Teach techniques such as counting or visualization to manage difficult situations.
Include child in discussions and history with parent.

PERSONALITY AND TEMPERAMENT

The enduring aspects of temperament continue to be manifested during the school years. The child classified as "difficult" at an earlier age may now have trouble in the classroom. Advise parents to provide a quiet setting for homework and to reward the child for concentration. For example, after homework is completed, the child may watch a television show. Creative efforts and alternative methods of learning should be valued. Encourage parents to see their children as individuals who may not all learn in the same way. The "slow-to-warm-up" child may need encouragement to try new activities and to share experiences with others, whereas the "easy" child will readily adapt to new schools, people, and experiences.

COMMUNICATION

During the school-age years, the child should learn how to correct any lingering pronunciation or grammatical errors. Vocabulary increases, and the child learns about parts of speech in school. School-age children enjoy writing and can be encouraged to keep a journal of their experiences while in the hospital as a method of dealing with anxiety. The literal translation of words characteristic of preschoolers is uncommon among school-age children.

SEXUALITY

Although children become aware of sexual differences between genders during preschool years, they deal much more consciously with sexuality during school age. As children mature physically, they need information about their bodily changes so that they can develop a healthy self-image and an understanding of the relationships between their bodies and sexuality. Children become interested in sexual issues and are often exposed to erroneous information on television shows, in magazines, or from friends and siblings. Schools and families need to use opportunities to teach school-age children factual information about sex and to foster healthy concepts of self and others. It is advisable to ask occasional questions about sexual issues to learn how much the child knows and to provide correct information when answers demonstrate confusion. Both friends and the media are common sources of erroneous ideas. Appropriate and inappropriate touch should be discussed, with lists of trusted people who can be approached (teachers, clergy, school counselors, family members, neighbors) to discuss any episodes with which the child feels uncomfortable (Finan, 1997).

ADOLESCENT (12 TO 18 YEARS)

Adolescence is a time of passage signaling the end of childhood and the beginning of adulthood. Although adolescents differ in behaviors and accomplishments, they are in a period of identity formation. If a healthy identity and sense of self-worth are not developed in this period, role confusion and purposeless struggling will ensue. The adolescents in your care will represent various degrees of identity formation, and each will offer unique challenges.

PHYSICAL GROWTH AND DEVELOPMENT

The physical changes ending in **puberty,** or sexual maturity, begin near the end of the school-age period. The prepubescent period is marked by a growth spurt at an average age of 10 years for girls and 13 years for boys (Figure 2-18). The increase in height and weight is generally remarkable and is completed in 2 to 3 years (Table 2-28). The growth spurt in girls is accompanied by an increase in breast size and growth of pubic hair. Menstruation occurs last and signals achievement of puberty. In boys, the growth spurt is accompanied by growth in size of the penis and testes and by growth of pubic hair. Deepening of the voice and growth of facial hair occur later, at the time of puberty. See Chapter 4 for a description of the pubertal stages.

During adolescence children grow stronger and more muscular and establish characteristic male and female patterns of fat distribution. The apocrine and eccrine glands mature, leading to increased sweating and a distinct odor to perspiration. All body organs are now fully mature, enabling the adolescent to take adult doses of medications.

The adolescent must adapt to a rapidly changing body for several years. These physical changes and hormonal variations offer challenges to identity formation.

TABLE 2-28 Growth and Development Milestones During Adolescence

PHYSICAL GROWTH	FINE MOTOR ABILITY	GROSS MOTOR ABILITY	SENSORY ABILITY
Variation in age of growth spurt During growth spurt, girls gain 7–25 kg (15–55 lb) and grow 2.5–20 cm (2–8 in.); boys gain approximately 7–29.5 kg (15–65 lb) and grow 11–30 cm (41/2–12 in.)	Skills are well developed **(1)**	New sports activities attempted and muscle development continues **(2)** Some lack of coordination common during growth spurt	Fully developed

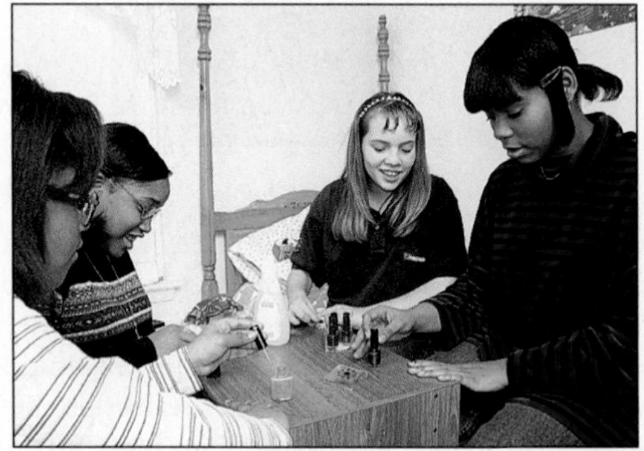

(1) Motor skills are well developed

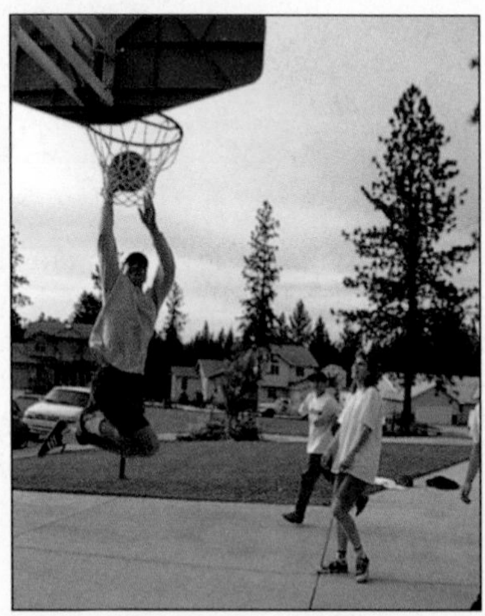

(2) New sports activities attempted

COGNITIVE DEVELOPMENT

Adolescence marks the beginning of Piaget's last stage of cognitive development, the stage of formal operational thought. The adolescent no longer depends on concrete experiences as the basis of thought but develops the ability to reason abstractly. Such concepts as justice, truth, beauty, and power can be understood. The adolescent revels in this newfound ability and spends a great deal of time thinking, reading, and talking about abstract concepts.

The ability to think and act independently leads many adolescents to rebel against parental authority. Through these actions, adolescents seek to establish their own identity and values.

ACTIVITIES

Maturity leads to new activities. Adolescents may drive, ride buses, or bike independently. They are less dependent on parents for transportation and spend more time with friends. Activities include participation in sports and extracurricular school activities, as well as "hanging out" and attending movies or concerts with friends (Table 2-29). The peer group becomes the focus of activities (Figure 2-20 ◆), regardless of the teen's interests. Peers are important in establishing identity and providing meaning. Although same-sex interactions predominate, boy–girl relationships are more common than at earlier stages. Adolescents thus participate in and learn from social interactions fundamental to adult relationships.

INJURY PREVENTION

Motor vehicle crashes, suicides, and homicides cause 75% of adolescent deaths (see Chapter 1). Teenagers have access to potentially harmful objects, such as firearms, motor vehicles, and boats and may combine them with harmful substances such as drugs and alcohol. They often believe they are immune from harm. This encourages adolescents to put themselves at high risk from dangerous behaviors (Table 2-30).

TABLE 2-29 Favorite Activities in Adolescence

Sports
Ball sports
Gymnastics
Water and snow skiing/boarding
Swimming
School team sports

School Activities
Drama
Yearbook
Class officer
Club participation

Peer Group Activities
Movies
Dances
Driving
Eating out
Attending sports events

Quiet Activities
Reading
School work
Television, computer, and video games
Music

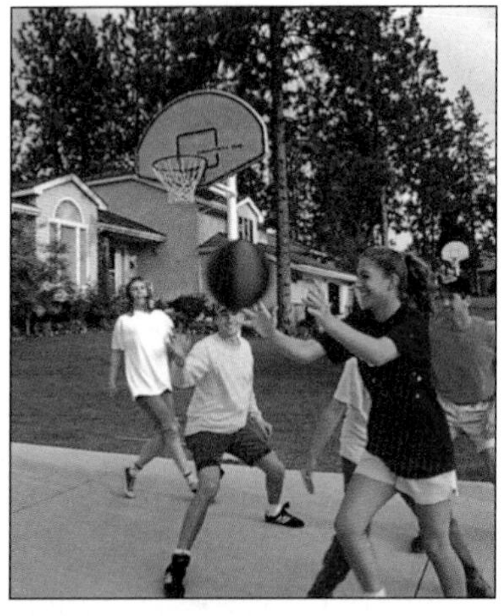

A

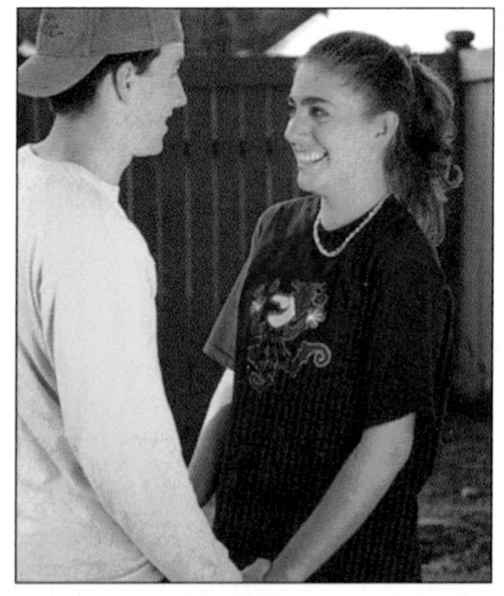

B

FIGURE 2-20 ◆
Social interaction between children of same and opposite sex is as important inside the acute care setting as it is outside. A, Teenagers enjoy playing together. B, Emotional relationships form during adolescence.

While some injuries have decreased in frequency or remained the same in recent years, others have increased. Suicide among adolescents has increased by 300% over the past four decades and is the second leading cause of death from 15 to 19 years, Morbidity Mortality Weekly Report [MMWR] 1995; Hayden & Lauer, 2000). The high rate of stress experienced by today's teenagers coupled with easy access to harmful substances and firearms promotes death by suicide. See Chater 24 for a discussion of suicide and Chapter 7 for further discussion of other violent events.

TABLE 2-30 Injury Prevention in Adolescence

HAZARD	DEVELOPMENTAL CHARACTERISTICS	PREVENTIVE MEASURES
Motor vehicle crashes	Adolescents learn to drive, enjoy new independence, and often feel invulnerable.	Insist on driver's education classes. Enforce rules about safe driving. Seat belts should be used for every trip. Discourage drug and alcohol use. Get treatment for teenagers who are known substance abusers.
Sporting injuries	Adolescents may participate in physically challenging sports such as soccer, gymnastics, or football. They may be allowed to drive motorboats.	Encourage use of protective sporting gear. Teach safe boating practices. Perform teaching related to hazards of drug and alcohol use, especially when using motorized equipment.
Drowning	Adolescents overestimate endurance when swimming. They take risks diving.	Encourage swimming only with friends. Reinforce rules and teach them about risks.

Nurses can be instrumental in assessing the potential for injury of adolescents seen in practice (see Table 2-30). Teaching about prevention is most successful when young people who have been injured share their experiences with other adolescents. National health objectives to reduce intentional and nonintentional injuries by the year 2010 have been set (Healthy People 2010, 2000).

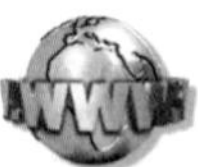

Injury Prevention

Violence is an increasingly important factor in adolescent injury. Homicide is the number one cause of death for young black males. The environment should be assessed for factors contributing to violence and adolescents at risk referred to special programs for violence prevention. Abuse in homes and schools must be reported to law enforcement agencies when nurses are aware that it may have occurred.

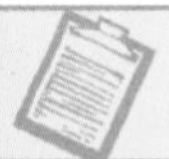

RESEARCH

The federal government administers questionnaires to a large cross section of youth annually to monitor their behaviors related to risk behavior. The Youth Risk Behavior Surveillance (YRBS) system gathers data about six high-priority areas: unintentional and intentional injury, tobacco use, alcohol and other drug use, sexual behavior, dietary behavior, and physical inactivity. How can nurses use this information to plan appropriate interventions for populations of adolescents?

PERSONALITY AND TEMPERAMENT

Characteristics of temperament manifested during childhood usually remain stable in the teenage years. For instance, the adolescent who was a calm, scheduled infant and child often demonstrates initiative to regulate study times and other routines. Similarly, the adolescent who was an easily stimulated infant may now have a messy room, a harried schedule with assignments always completed late, and an interest in many activities. It is also common for an adolescent who was an easy child to become more difficult because of the psychologic changes of adolescence and the need to assert independence.

Similar to the child's earlier ages, the nurse's role may be to inform parents of different personality types and to help them support the teen's uniqueness while providing necessary structure and feedback. Nurses can help parents to understand their teen's personality type and to work with the adolescent to meet expectations of teachers and others in authority.

COMMUNICATION

All parts of speech are used and understood by the adolescent. Colloquialisms and slang are commonly used with the peer group. The adolescent often studies a foreign language in school, having the ability to understand and analyze grammar and sentence structure.

The adolescent increasingly leaves the home base and establishes close ties with peers. These relationships become the basis for identity formation. There is generally a period of stress or crisis before a strong identity can emerge. The adolescent may try out new roles by learning a new sport or other skills, experimenting with drugs or alcohol, wearing different styles of clothing, or trying other activities. It is important to provide positive role models and a variety of experiences to help the adolescent make wise choices.

The adolescent also has a need to leave the past, to be different, and to change from former patterns to establish a self-identity. Rules that are repeated constantly and dogmatically will probably be broken in the adolescent's quest for self-awareness. This poses difficulties when the adolescent has a health problem, such as diabetes or a heart problem, that requires ongoing care. Introducing the adolescent to other teens who manage the same problem appropriately is usually more successful than telling the adolescent what to do.

Privacy should be ensured during the taking of health histories or interventions with teens. Even if a parent is present for part of a history or examination, the adolescent should be given the opportunity to relay information or ask questions alone with the health care provider. The adolescent should be given a choice of whether to have a parent present during an examination or while care is provided. Most information shared by an adolescent is confidential. Some states mandate disclosure of certain information to parents such as an adolescent's desire for an abortion. In these cases, the adolescent should be informed of what will be disclosed to the parent.

Setting up teen rooms (recreation rooms for use only by adolescents) or separate adolescent units in hospitals can provide necessary peer support during hospitalization. Most adolescents are not pleased when placed on a unit or in a room with young children. Choices should be allowed when possible, and include preference for evening or morning bathing, the type of clothes to wear while hospitalized, timing of treatments, and visitation guidelines. Use of contracts with adolescents may increase compliance. Firmness, gentleness, choices, and respect must be balanced during care of adolescent patients.

COMMUNICATION STRATEGIES: ADOLESCENT

Provide written and verbal explanations.
Direct history and explanations to teen alone; then include parent.
Allow for safe exploration of topics by suggesting that the teen is similar to other teens. ("Many teens with diabetes have questions about . . . How about you?")
Arrange meetings for discussions with other teens.

SEXUALITY

With maturation of the body and increased secretion of hormones, the adolescent achieves sexual maturity. This complex process involves growing interactions with members of the opposite sex, an interplay of the forces of society and family, and identity formation. The early adolescent progresses from dances and other social events with members of the opposite sex to the late adolescent who is mature sexually and may have regular sexual encounters. About half of all high school students in the United States have had intercourse, but only 57% used a condom at their last sexual encounter (Acquavella & Braverman, 1999).

Teenagers need information about their bodies and emerging sexuality. They should understand the interests and forces they experience. Including sex education in school classes and health care encounters is important. Information on methods to prevent sexually transmitted diseases is given, with most school districts now providing some teaching on AIDS. Far more common risks to teens, however, are diseases such as gonorrhea, herpes, and hepatitis. Health histories should include questions on sexual activity, sexually transmitted diseases, and birth control use and understanding. Most hospitals routinely perform pregnancy screening on adolescent girls before elective procedures.

Adolescents will benefit from clear information about sexuality, an opportunity to develop relationships with adolescents in various settings, an open atmosphere at home and school where problems and issues can be discussed, and previous experience in problem solving and self–decision making. Sexual issues should be among topics that adolescents can discuss openly in a variety of settings. Alternatives and support for their decisions should be available.

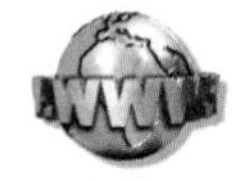

Sexual Minorities

Some adolescents identify with a sexual minority group such as lesbian, gay, bisexual, or transgendered. They are at particular risk of being stigmatized and harassed by other youth or adults. They are more likely to suffer a variety of problems such as isolation, rejection by significant others, violence, suicide, and taking sexual risks (Stevens & Morgan, 1999, 2001). Nurses are instrumental in helping these youths by providing information for them and their parents, integrating sexual minority content into sexual education curricula, and providing referrals for health and social care when needed. See Chapter 7 for further information about the health issues related to homosexuality and other sexual minority practices.

Chapter Highlights

- Development unfolds in a predictable pattern, but at different rates dependent on the particular characteristics and experiences of each child.
- Major theories of development encompass the psychosexual (Freud), psychosocial (Erikson), cognitive (Piaget), moral (Kohlberg), social learning (Bandura), and behavioral (Skinner and Watson) components of individuals.
- The ecologic theory of Bronfenbrenner and the temperament theory of Chess and Thomas emphasize the interactions of the individual within the environment.
- Influences on the developmental process include one's genetic potential and a series of environmental influences unique to each family and individual.
- Infancy spans the time from birth to 1 year, and is marked by rapid physical growth, mastery of basic fine and gross motor skills, and beginning cognitive and language skills.
- Toddlers range in age from 1 to 3 years, and become increasingly mobile and communicative. They master control over excretion and are known for exerting their own opinions and wishes to parents. Injury prevention and toilet training are specific parental teaching needs.
- Preschool years range from 3 to 6 and are marked by increasing social skills. Most preschool children attend child care programs and learn to play with other children. Continued mastery of physical coordination and language occur.
- School age spans the years from 6 to 12, when children mature in many areas. They show slow, steady growth until reaching puberty between 9 and 12 years, when a growth spurt marks increased height and weight, as well as sexual maturation. School-age children play cooperatively with other children and participate in various school and community activities.
- Adolescence occurs from about 12 years of age through the teen years. Adolescents establish their own identities distinct from parents and other adults. They are mature physically and cognitively. The peer group exerts the major influence at this age.
- The nurse is involved in assessing development at each stage, and in providing anticipatory guidance to families to foster optimal development.

EXPLORE MediaLink

- NCLEX review, case studies, and other interactive resources for this chapter can be found on the Companion Website at **http://www.prenhall.com/ball.** Click on Chapter 2 to select the activities for this chapter.
- For animations, more NCLEX review questions, and an audio glossary, access the accompanying CD-ROM in this textbook.

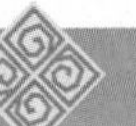

References

1. Acquavella, A., & Braverman, P. (1999). Adolescent gynecology in the office setting. *Pediatric Clinics of North America, 46,* 489–503.
2. Altemeier, W. A. (2000). Growth charts, low birth weight, and international adoption. *Pediatric Annals, 29,* 204–205.
3. American Academy of Pediatrics, Committee on Genetics. (2000). Molecular genetic testing in pediatric practice: A subject review. *Pediatrics, 106,* 1494–1497.
4. Aronson, J. (2000). Medical evaluation and infectious considerations on arrival. *Pediatric Annals, 29,* 218–223.
5. Bandura, A. (1986). *Social foundations of thought and actions: A social cognitive theory.* Englewood Cliffs, NJ: Prentice Hall.
6. Bandura, A. (1997a). *Self-efficacy: The exercise of control.* New York: W. H. Freeman.
7. Bandura, A. (1997b). *Self-efficacy in changing societies.* New York: Cambridge University Press.
8. Board on Children, Youth and Families, National Research Council and Institute of Medicine (2001). *From neurons to neighborhoods.* Washington, DC: National Academy Press.
9. Briggs, G., Freeman, R., & Yaffe, S. (1998). *Drugs in pregnancy and lactation,* (5th ed.) Baltimore: Williams & Wilkins.
10. Bronfenbrenner, U. (1986). Ecology of the family as a context for human development: Research perspectives. *Developmental Psychology, 22,* 723–742.
11. Bronfenbrenner, U., McClelland, P. D., Ceci, S. J., Moen, P., & Wethington, E. (1996). *The state of Americans.* New York: Free Press.
12. Chamberlain, L. J. (2001). Children adopted abroad could face life-long psychological problems. *Infectious Diseases in Children, 14*(1), 20.
13. Chess, S., & Thomas, A. (1995). *Temperament in clinical practice.* New York: Guilford Press.
14. Chess, S., & Thomas, A. (1996). *Temperament: theory and practice.* Philadelphia: Brunner/Mazel Publishers.
15. Chess, S., & Thomas, A. (1999). *Goodness of fit: Clinical applications from infancy through adult life.* Philadelphia: Brunner/Mazel Publishers.
16. Children's Defense Fund. (2000). *The state of America's children.* Washington, DC: Children's Defense Fund.
17. Craig, G. J. (1999). *Human development.* Upper Saddle River, NJ: Prentice Hall.
18. Erikson, E. (1963). *Childhood and society.* New York: W.W. Norton.
19. Erikson, E. (1968). *Identity: Youth and crisis.* New York: W.W. Norton.
20. Faber, S. (2000). Behavioral sequelae of orphanage life. *Pediatric Annals, 29,* 242–248.
21. Federal Interagency Forum on Child and Family Statistics. (2000). *America's children: Key national indicators of well-being.* Washington, DC: U.S. Government Printing Office.
22. Fields, J., Smith, K., Bass, L.E., & Lugaila, T. (2001). *A child's day: Home, school, and play (selected indicators of child well-being).* Washington, DC: U.S. Department of Commerce.
23. Finan, S. L. (1997). Promoting healthy sexuality: Guidelines for the school-age child and adolescent. *The Nurse Practitioner, 22,* 62–72.
24. Gemelli. R. (1996). *Normal child and adolescent development.* Washington, DC: American Psychiatric Press.
25. Giarelli, E., & Jacobs, L. A. (2000). Issues related to the use of genetic material and information. *Oncology Nursing Forum, 27,* 459–467.
26. Ginsberg, H., & Opper, S. (1988). *Piaget's theory of intellectual development* (3rd ed.). Paramus, NJ: Prentice Hall.
27. Hayden, D. C., & Lauer, P. (2000). Prevalence of suicide programs in schools and roadblocks to implementation. *Suicide and Life Threatening Behavior, 30,* 239–251.
28. Healthy People 2010. (2000). *Healthy people 2010 conference edition.* Washington, DC: United States Department of Health and Human Services.
29. Jaffe, A., Bush, A., Geddes, D. M., & Alton, E. W. F. W. (1999). Prospects for gene therapy in cystic fibrosis. *Archives of Diseases in Children, 80,* 286–289.
30. Jarvis, C. (2000). *Physical examination and health assessment* (3rd ed.). Philadelphia: W. B. Saunders.
31. Jenista, J. A. (2000). Preadoption review of medical records. *Pediatric Annals, 29,* 212–217.
32. Johnson, D. E. (2000). Long-term medical issues in international adoptees. *Pediatric Annals, 29,* 234–241.
33. Melvin, N. (1995). Children's temperament: Intervention for parents. *Journal of Pediatric Nursing, 10,* 152–159.
34. Miller, L. C. (2000). Initial assessment of growth, development, and the effects of institutionalization in internationally adopted children. *Pediatric Annals, 29,* 224–233.
35. Morbidity and Mortality Weekly Report. [MMWR]. (1995). Suicide among children, adolescents, and young adults—United States, 1980–1992. *MMWR, 44,* 289–291.
36. MMWR (2000). Youth risk behavior surveillance—United States, 1999. *MMWR, 49,* 1–99.
37. National Safety Council. (1998). *Child passenger safety.* Washington, DC: Author.
38. Piaget, J. (1972). *The child's conception of the world.* Totowa, NJ: Littlefield, Adams Co.
39. Santrock, J. (1999). *Life-span development.* Boston: McGraw-Hill.
40. Spector, R. (2000). *Guides to heritage assessment and health traditions.* Upper Saddle River, NJ: Prentice Hall Health.
41. Stevens, P., & Morgan, S. (1999). Health of lesbian, gay, bisexual, and transgender youth. *Journal of Child and Family Nursing, 2,* 237–249.
42. Stevens, P., & Morgan, S. (2001). Health of lesbian, gay, bisexual, and transgender youth. *Journal of Pediatric Health Care, 15,* 24–34.
43. Stringham, P. (1998). Violence anticipatory guidance. *Pediatric Clinics of North America, 45,* 439–448.
44. Tolstoi, L. G., & Smith, C. L. (1999). Human genome project and cystic fibrosis—a symbiotic relationship. *Journal of the American Dietetic Association, 99,* 1421–1427.
45. Trahms, C. M., & Pipes, P. L. (1997). *Nutrition in infancy and childhood* (6th ed.). New York: McGraw-Hill.
46. Troiano, R. P., Flegel, K. M., Kuczmarski, R. J., Campbell, S. M., & Johnson, C. L. (1995). Overweight prevalence and trends for children and adolescents. *Archives of Pediatric and Adolescent Medicine, 149,* 1085–1091.
47. UNICEF. (1998). The state of the world's children 1998: A UNICEF report. Malnutrition: causes, consequences, and solutions. *Nutrition Reviews, 56,* 115–123.
48. Wagner, J. D., Menke, E. M., & Ciccone, J. K. (1995). What is known about the health of rural homeless families. *Public Health Nursing, 12,* 400–408.
49. Williams, J. K. (2000). Impact of genome research on children and their families. *Journal of Pediatric Nursing, 15*(4), 207–211.
50. Worthington-Roberts, B. S., & Williams, S. R. (1997). *Nutrition in pregnancy and lactation* (6th ed.). Madison, WI: Brown & Benchmark.
51. *www.nhgri.nih.gov.* International human genome sequencing consortium announces "working draft" of human genome. Retrieved 2/8/01 www.

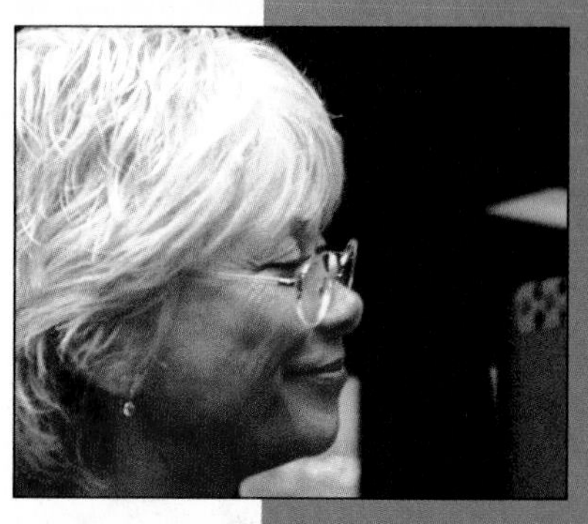

"IT IS EXCITING TO SEE JOEY PROGRESSING AFTER HIS RECENT SCOLIOSIS SURGERY. WE HAVE LEARNED TO GIVE HIM TUBE FEEDINGS SO THAT HE CAN RETURN TO THE CLASSROOM AND HAVE CONTACT WITH OTHER CHILDREN."

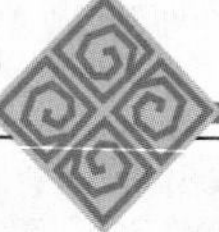

Joey was diagnosed with cerebral palsy early in life. He is now 11 years old and has returned to school after surgery for scoliosis. When evaluated prior to surgery, Joey's nutritional status showed some deficits of calories and nutrients. Joey has limited ability to swallow, related to muscle weakness of cerebral palsy, and was therefore unable to ingest enough calories by mouth to ensure his optimal growth and development. A feeding tube was inserted into his stomach to provide supplementary feedings and maximize his nutritional status prior to surgery. After several weeks of supplemental feedings, Joey was ready for surgery, and did well in his postoperative recovery.

Joey continues to have supplemental feedings throughout the day. The school nurse has met with his parents and home health nurse to learn about the amount and type of tube feedings he receives, as well as the texture of oral feedings he can manage. The nurse has planned the feeding schedule at school to facilitate adequate nutrition in that setting. In addition, careful ongoing nutritional assessment will be needed to evaluate if Joey is getting the calories and other nutrients he needs for growth and development. The school nurse is also educating the classroom teachers and other school personnel about Joey's unique nutritional requirements.

CHAPTER

3

INFANT, CHILD, AND ADOLESCENT NUTRITION

KEY TERMS

anemia A reduction in the number of red blood cells to below normal levels.

anthropometric measurement The term used to refer to growth assessment of various parts of the body.

atopy A hereditary allergic tendency.

Body Mass Index (BMI) A calculation (kilograms of weight/m^2 of height) used to determine the proportion between a child's height and weight.

Dietary Reference Intakes (DRIs) A set of nutrient values that can be used to assess and plan intake for individuals of different ages.

food insecurity An inability or uncertainty that one will be able to acquire or consume adequate quality or quantity of foods in socially acceptable ways.

food jags Eating only a few foods for several days or weeks.

food security Access at all times to enough nourishment for an active, healthy life.

nursing bottle mouth syndrome A condition that results in tooth decay when a young child is allowed to nurse or drink from a bottle for long periods, especially when sleeping.

physiologic anorexia A decrease in appetite manifested when the extremely high metabolic demands of infancy slow to keep pace with the more moderate growth rate of toddlerhood.

RAST (radioallergosorbent test) A technique in which radioimmunoassay is used to measure the presence in the blood of IgE antibodies to certain antigens.

vegan Strict vegetarian who eats no animal products.

vegetarian One who eats no poultry, meat, or fish.

MediaLink

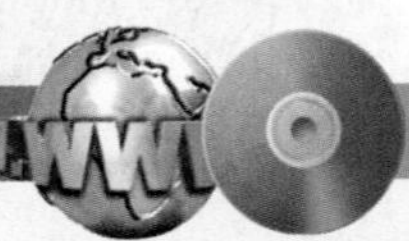

http://www.prenhall.com/ball

Resources for this chapter can be found on the CD-ROM accompanying this textbook, and on the Companion Website at http://www.prenhall.com/ball. Click on Chapter 3 to select the activities for this chapter.

CD-ROM

Audio Glossary

NCLEX Review

COMPANION WEBSITE

Web Links

NCLEX Review

MediaLink Applications

- Vegetarian Teens: Plan a 2-Day Menu
- Preschoolers: Plan a Nutrition Teaching Session
- How to Manage a Child's Peanut Allergy at School
- Analyze Your Diet

Adequate nutrition is an essential component of growth and development. The child's nutritional status begins before birth and is related to the mother's nutritional state. All children must be assessed for nutritional status, followed by teaching or other interventions to enhance health. Nurses are instrumental in giving parents information about normal nutritional needs of infants and young children. Common techniques to assess nutrition, such as measuring growth and monitoring hematocrit, provide needed information about whether intake of foods is adequate.

While all children and parents can benefit from information about nutritional needs, some children have additional issues that must be considered. The nurse recognizes the special intake requirements of children with conditions such as food allergies, cystic fibrosis, cerebral palsy, or diabetes. Nutrition monitoring is provided throughout childhood so that dietary counseling can be integrated with other teaching to promote development. How can the nurse bridge the various settings in which children's nutritional needs are met? These might include home, child care settings, schools, and hospitals. How can the nurse help the family prepare for meeting nutritional needs of a child who has special needs during travel by car or plane? If Joey's family decides to visit another state on a car trip this summer, they must plan to bring his feeding solution, tubing, and other supplies, and may need refrigeration to maintain enteral solutions.

Some children have unique nutritional needs due to their social environments. Parents may not be knowledgeable about child nutritional requirements. Perhaps the family is vegetarian and needs extra help to ensure intake of essential nutrients. If finances are limited, the family may need resources such as access to food stamps, food banks, or budget planning. The nurse considers the high rate of childhood obesity and common nutritional deficits when applying concepts of health promotion with families. Whatever the setting in which the nurse is employed, knowledge of nutrition must be integrated within nursing care.

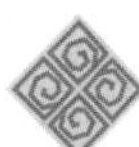

GENERAL CONCEPTS IN NUTRITION

Nutrition refers to taking in food and assimilating it metabolically for use by the body. It is an essential component of life and therefore an important topic to consider in discussions of child growth and development. The body requires a wide array of intake products, for example, carbohydrates, protein, fat, and micronutrients such as vitamins and minerals. The need for nutrients is dependent on activity level, state of health and presence of disease or other stress, and age-related needs.

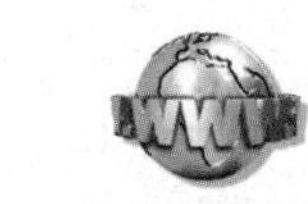

Nutrition Tools

The **Dietary Reference Intakes (DRIs)** are a set of values established by the Food and Nutrition Board of the Institute of Medicine and the National Academy of Science which can be used to assess and plan intake for individuals of different ages. They commonly include four different values that can be considered by nursing, nutrition, and other health personnel (Table 3-1). While the DRIs are the approach used in the United States, other countries have developed their own approaches to dietary standards. For example, Canada uses Adequate Intake and Reference Nutrient Intake, and the United Kingdom uses Recommended Daily Nutrient Intakes. The aim of these standards is to provide a method of evaluating individual and population diets, and of planning nutrition programs and education. DRIs are generally specific to males and females in several age categories (Table 3-2).

Although the DRIs provide useful information when evaluating diets, their use can be time consuming. What "quick check" can be performed to provide feedback about the daily diets of children? Learn the food guide pyramid and hang it in schools, clinics, and hospitals. It is a fast method of looking at children's intakes for a day and seeing if they meet most requirements. Instead of calculating amounts of nutrients ingested, the pyramid focuses on categories of foods, which readily reflects the actual intake. The numbers of servings from various categories stay constant throughout childhood while the serving sizes increase as the child gets older. See Figure 3-1 ◆ for the food guide pyramid, and consult websites for alternative pyramids for vegetarians and those from various ethnic groups, such as Hispanic and Native American.

TABLE 3-1 Daily Reference Intakes (DRIs)

Estimated Average Requirement (EAR) = daily intake needed to meet the requirements of 50% of a certain age and gender group
Use = Evaluate intake of a group; plan for intake of a group.
Example = Compare the daily intake of Vitamin C of a class of children from 24-hour recalls to this number to learn how many do not meet average requirements; plan daily menu for a child care center.

Recommended Dietary Allowance (RDA) = daily intake needed to meet the requirements of most people (97%–98%) of a certain age and gender group
Use = Set goal for daily intake.
Example = Evaluate the dietary intake of an individual for a nutrient such as vitamin C; make recommendations to an individual for a daily menu.

Adequate Intake (AI) = Used when limited information on the needs for a vitamin is available and EAR is not available, usually because studies on its metabolism in the body are hard to carry out; rather than metabolic studies, it is based on the average intake of that nutrient by a healthy group of people
Use = Evaluate intake of a group; plan intake for a group.
Example = See EAR.

Upper Intake (UI) = upper tolerable intake level; maximum level unlikely to pose a health risk
Use = Limit fortification levels of foods and provide information to limit dietary supplements.
Example = Consider intake of a fat-soluble vitamin such as vitamin A that is not readily excreted; include both food sources and supplements.

TABLE 3-2 DRI Age Groups

Pregnancy and Lactation	14–18 years
Birth to 6 months	19–30 years
6–12 months	31–50 years
1–3 years	51–70 years
4–8 years	Over 70 years
9–13 years	

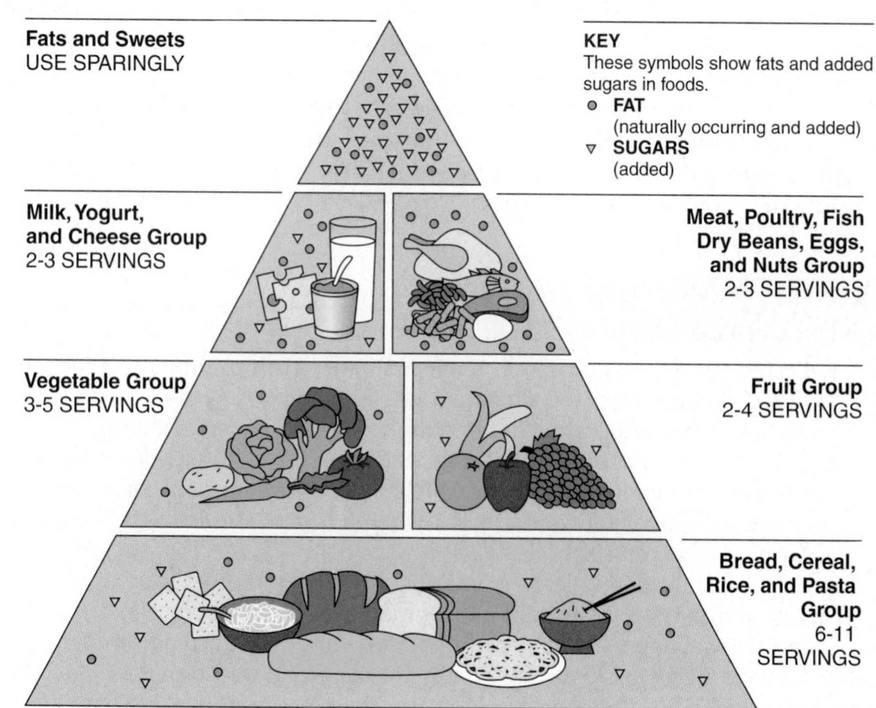

FIGURE 3-1 ◆ The Food Guide Pyramid is used to provide teaching about amounts of foods recommended for daily intake. U.S. Department of Agriculture and U.S. Department of Health and Human Services (2001). http://www.usda.gov/news/usdakids/food pyr.html.

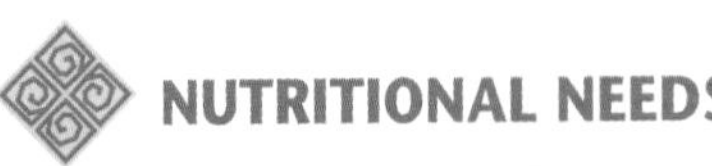

NUTRITIONAL NEEDS

INFANCY

From the first feeding of a few ounces of breast milk to a meal of soft table foods with the family at 1 year of age, the infant demonstrates an amazing growth in ability to ingest and digest a wide variety of foods. Never again will the individual have such a high metabolic rate or high intake requirements in relation to size, or such a change in the types of foods eaten. Infants have an extremely fast rate of growth, since birth weight is usually doubled by about 5 months of age, and tripled by 12 months. Meeting nutritional needs is made difficult by the small size of the infant's stomach and the immaturity of the digestive system. The great physical activity also necessitates high caloric intake. Nutrient demands for protein and vitamins must be met for the cells of the nervous system and body organs to develop properly.

Breast- and Bottle-Feeding

The natural first food is breast milk and its intake should be encouraged for all infants (Figure 3-2 ◆). It can be the only food for the first 6 months, and should continue through 12 months of age, with addition of solid foods from 6 to 12 months. Many advantages to breastfeeding are known, including excellent nutritional balance, promotion of gastrointestinal function, fostering immune defense, psychological benefits, and economic advantage. Although breast milk is the best nutritional source for infants, there may be a need for some limited supplements.

Providing breast-feeding information and instruction positively influences the number of women who decide to breast feed and increases the number of months they choose to continue breastfeeding (Kramer, 2001). Some hospitals have lactation specialists who assist breastfeeding mothers; in others, nurses provide this service. Home visits, phone calls from hospital nursing staff, early visits after the birth to obstetric and pediatric offices, and resources such as LaLeche League can provide mothers with needed breast-feeding information and problem-solving suggestions. Information is needed so that the mother gets adequate nutritional intake and sufficient rest. Support programs are especially helpful to mothers who have difficulty breastfeeding, feel unsure how it will fit into family and work life, are very young, or have an infant with problems related to feeding. The mother of a hospitalized infant will need special support to continue breastfeeding. The mother should be encouraged to come to the hospital to feed her baby on the same schedule as at home. If the infant cannot breast-feed, the hospital can provide an electric pump so the mother can maintain lactation. Often hospitals provide meals for the mother of a hospitalized baby so that she can maintain good nutrition and quality breast milk while she stays in the hospital with the baby.

Some women decide not to breast feed or are unable to do so. After several months of breastfeeding, some mothers begin to use supplemental bottles when they are away from the

AMERICAN ACADEMY OF PEDIATRICS STATEMENT ON BREASTFEEDING

The American Academy of Pediatrics states that breastfeeding is the best source of nutrition for babies at least through the first birthday and longer when possible. Mothers should receive ongoing instructions and support from medical professionals to assist them in breastfeeding.

FAMILIES WANT TO KNOW

Supplements for Breast-fed Babies

1. Each baby receives a vitamin K injection after birth to promote adequate blood clotting. After this time no further vitamin K is needed, as the baby manufactures this vitamin in the gut once he or she begins eating.
2. The need for vitamin D is not fully established, but 400 IU/day is recommended for infants who are breast fed, live in northern climates and urban settings, especially in winter or if the baby is dark skinned or is kept well covered when outside.
3. Iron is not needed unless the infant is not taking in other sources of food with iron by 4–6 months. The baby may need an iron source earlier if the mother was anemic during pregnancy or while breastfeeding.
4. Fluoride 0.25 mg is given after 6 months of age if water is not fluoridated to a level of 0.3 parts per million (ppm), or the baby is not drinking any water.

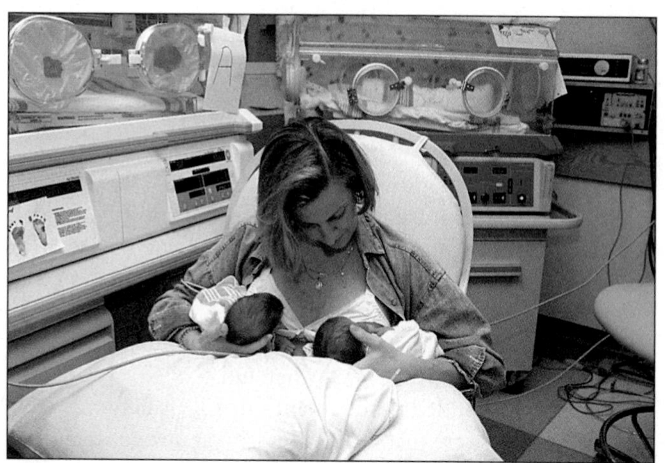

FIGURE 3-2 ◆
Breast feeding offers many physical and emotional benefits for the infant. How can nurses encourage mothers to have positive breast-feeding experiences?

infant. Nurses provide these mothers with information about formula preparation and feeding. Three types of formula are available—ready to feed, concentrate, and powder. All are nutritionally adequate for infants. The nurse can help parents decide which preparation of formula is best suited for their infant (see Table 3-3). Some infants, such as those with phenylketonuria, other metabolic disorders, or babies with cow milk allergy, require specialized formulas. Breast-or bottle-feeding is discussed at each contact with health professionals to identify potential teaching needs.

During infancy and toddlerhood, nurses should carefully examine the patterns of breast- and bottle-feeding. **Nursing bottle mouth syndrome** can occur when a young child is allowed to nurse or drink from a bottle for long periods, especially when sleeping (Figure 3-3 ◆). The milk, juice, or other fluid pools around the upper anterior teeth, salivary flow decreases, and acid buffering is decreased, resulting in tooth decay. Teach parents to avoid putting the child to bed with a bottle. Encourage pacifier use or a bottle of water instead. Mothers who breast feed should also be cautioned to limit nursing to specific times so that milk will not pool in the mouth during sleep.

Parents can be taught beginning dental care for the infant, which includes wiping the teeth off daily once they erupt with a piece of moist gauze or a small infant toothbrush.

SAFETY PRECAUTIONS

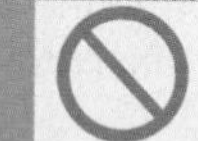

Formula can be mixed with tap water but must be refrigerated once mixed. Formula that the baby does not drink should be discarded after use and not kept for future feedings. This minimizes the chance for bacteria to grow and to cause illness in the baby. When the family lives in older housing, caution them to run tap water for about 2 minutes before using it, and to use only cold water for formula preparation. These practices will minimize the chance that lead is leached from the older pipes in the house (see Chapter 17 for further discussion of lead poisoning). If the family has a well, the water should be tested for microorganisms before being used for the baby.

TABLE 3-3 Advantages and Disadvantages of Formula Preparations

FORMULA PREPARATION	HOW PACKAGED	ADVANTAGES	DISADVANTAGES
Ready to feed	Bottles or cans	No preparation needed	Most expensive type of formula
Concentrate	Cans of concentrated liquid	Easy to add equal amounts of formula concentrate and water directly into bottle and shake	Can be incorrectly measured, leading to inadequate or unsafe nutrition for infant; requires access to clean water supply such as city tap water or bottled water; well water may have too high a mineral concentration
Powder	Cans	Least expensive type of formula	Can be incorrectly measured, leading to inadequate or unsafe nutrition for infant; requires shaking to mix thoroughly; requires access to clean water supply such as city tap water or bottled water; well water may have too high a mineral concentration

COMMON BABY FORMULAS

Milk-based Formulas
Enfamil
Similac
SMA

Soy-based Formulas
Isomil
Nursoy
Prosobee
Soyalac

Specialized Formulas
Lofenalac (low phenylketonuria)
Nutramigen (casein hydrolysate)
Pregestimil (casein hydrolysate)
Alimentum (casein hydrolysate)
Portagen (sodium caseinate)
Lactofree (lactose free)
Neocate (synthetic amino acids)

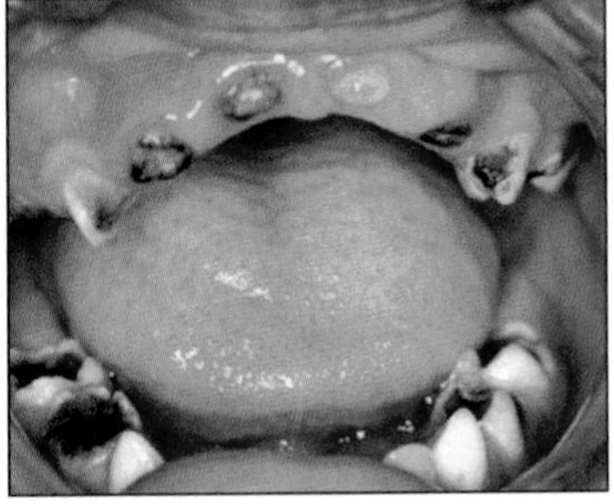

FIGURE 3-3 ◆
Nursing bottle mouth syndrome. This child has had major tooth decay related to sleeping as an infant and toddler while sucking bottles of juice and milk.
Courtesy of Dr. Lezley McIlveen, Department of Dentistry, Children's National Medical Center, Washington, DC.

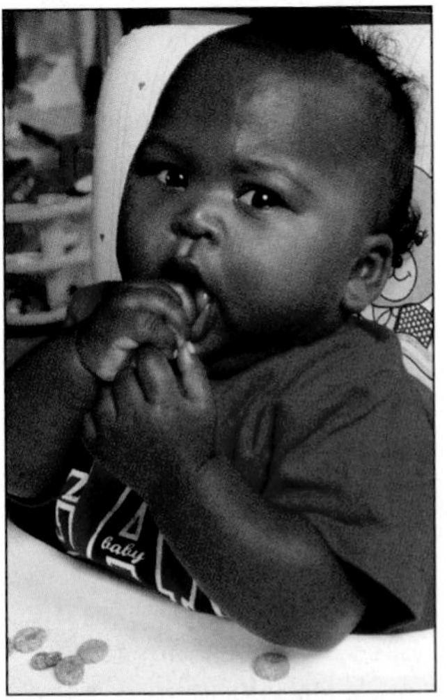

FIGURE 3-4 ◆
The baby who has developed the ability to grasp with thumb and forefinger should receive some foods that can be held in the hand.

SAFETY PRECAUTIONS

Advise parents to use caution when providing finger foods to the infant. Hard foods and some soft and malleable ones slip easily into the throat and may cause choking. Avoid hot dogs, hard vegetables, candy, whole grapes, and chunks of peanut butter. Infants and other young children should always be supervised while eating. Be sure parents are familiar with techniques for airway obstruction removal and have emergency numbers clearly listed on their phones.

Some pediatric dentists like to see the child for a first dental visit at about 1 year of age while others wait until the child is older. Have the parents select and establish contact with a dental provider when the child is nearing the end of infancy.

Introduction of Supplemental Foods

When should other foods be added to the infant's diet? Although some parents add other foods when the infant is only days or weeks old, it is best to take cues from the infant's developmental milestones. The American Academy of Pediatrics recommends introducing semisolid foods at 4 to 6 months (Committee on Nutrition, 1998). At this age the extrusion reflex (or tongue thrust) decreases and the infant can sit well with support. The infant is also developing the ability to appreciate texture and to swallow nonliquid foods, and can indicate desire for food or turn away when full.

The first food added to the infant's diet is usually rice cereal. The advantages of introducing cereal first are that it provides iron at an age when the infant's prenatal iron stores begin to decrease, it seldom causes allergy, and it is easy to digest. One to 2 tablespoons are fed to the infant once or twice daily just before formula or breastfeeding. The infant may appear to spit out food at first because of normal back-and-forth tongue movement. Parents should not interpret this early feeding behavior as indicating dislike for the food. With a little practice, the infant becomes adept at spoon-feeding.

Once the infant eats 1/4 cup of cereal twice daily, usually at 6 to 8 months of age, vegetables or fruits can be introduced (Table 3-4). By 8 to 10 months, most fruits and vegetables have been introduced and strained meats or other protein (e.g., tofu) can be added to the infant's diet. Finger foods are introduced during the second half of the first year as the infant's palmar and then finger grasps develop and as teeth begin to erupt (Figure 3-4 ◆). Infants enjoy toast, O-shaped cereal, finely sliced meats, cheese and tofu, and small pieces of cooked, softened vegetables. As food and juice intake increase, formula or breastfeedings decrease in amount and frequency (Table 3-5).

If breastfeeding is not chosen, or if supplemental feedings are given, only iron-fortified infant formula should be used during the first year of life. Cow's milk (including evaporated

TABLE 3-4 Introduction of Solid Foods in Infancy

RECOMMENDATION	RATIONALE
Introduce rice cereal at 4–6 months.	Rice cereal is easy to digest, has low allergenic potential, and contains iron.
Introduce fruits or vegetables at 6–8 months.	Fruits and vegetables provide needed vitamins.
Introduce meats at 8–10 months.	Meats are harder to digest, have high protein load, and should not be fed until close to 1 year of age.
Use single-food prepared baby foods rather than combination meals.	Combination meals usually contain more sugar, salt, and fillers.
Introduce one new food at a time, waiting at least 3 days to introduce another.	If a food allergy develops, it will be easy to identify.
Avoid carrots, beets, and spinach before 4 months of age.	Their nitrates can be converted to nitrite by young infants, causing methemoglobinemia.
Infants can be fed mashed portions of table foods such as carrots, rice, and potatoes.	This is a less expensive alternative to jars of commercially prepared baby food; it allows parents of various cultural groups to feed ethnic foods to infants.
Avoid adding sugar, salt, spices when mixing own baby foods.	Infants need not become accustomed to these flavors; they may get too much sodium from salt or develop gastric distress from some spices.
Avoid honey until at least 1 year of age.	Infants cannot detoxify *Clostridium botulinum* spores sometimes present in honey and can develop botulism.

TABLE 3-5 Infant Nutritional Pattern

Birth to 1 month
- Eats every 2–3 hours, breast or bottle
- Eats 2–3 ounces (60–90 mL) per feeding

2–4 months
- Has coordinated suck–swallow
- Eats every 3–4 hours
- Eats 3–4 ounces (90–120 mL) per feeding

4–6 months
- Begins baby food, usually rice cereal
- Eats 4 or more times daily
- Eats 4–5 ounces (100–150 mL) per feeding

6–8 months
- Eats baby food such as rice cereal, fruits, and vegetables
- Eats 4 times daily
- Eats 6–8 ounces (160–225 mL) per feeding

8–10 months
- Enjoys soft finger foods
- Eats 4 times daily
- Eats 6 ounces (160 mL) per feeding

10–12 months
- Eats most soft table foods with family
- Uses cup with lid
- Attempts to feed self with spoon though spills often
- Eats 4 times daily
- Eats 6–8 ounces (160–225 mL) per feeding

milk) can lead to bleeding and anemia (see pp. 86–87), can interfere with absorption of some nutrients, and has a high solute load which immature kidneys can have difficulty excreting. Iron-fortified formula should always be used when the infant under 12 months drinks formula. When breast-fed babies are not eating foods with iron by 4 to 6 months, supplemental iron may need to be added. Careful dietary assessment and discussion of intake by the nurse at health visits helps the practitioner decide if supplemental iron is needed.

Parents who want to make baby foods at home can be encouraged and instructed about how to do so. Some commercially prepared foods have unnecessary additives such as salt, sugar, and food starch, and they may be costly for some families. Parents can easily blend fruits and vegetables the family is eating before adding salt, sugar, or seasoning. Prepared foods should be used promptly and stored in the refrigerator between feedings. Foods can also be placed into ice cube trays and frozen; a cube or two can be defrosted at mealtime. Caution parents not to use honey in foods for infants, as it can lead to infant botulism.

SAFETY PRECAUTIONS

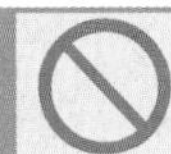

If foods or fluids are microwaved for use with infants or children, there can be "hot spots" that lead to burning. Stirring, shaking, and checking temperature before feeding are recommended to protect the child from burns to the mouth.

GROWTH & DEVELOPMENT

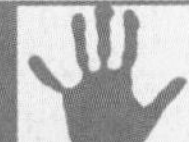

Toddlers generally eat three meals and two or three snacks daily. Toddlers can drink 2% milk starting at 2 years of age, or "follow-up" formula. Cups are recommended, with bottle use discontinued. The child is learning to use utensils but may prefer fingers and still needs small serving sizes.

TODDLERHOOD

Why do parents of toddlers frequently become concerned about the small amount of food their children eat? Why do toddlers seem to survive and even thrive with minimal food intake? The toddler often displays the phenomenon of **physiologic anorexia,** caused when the extremely high metabolic demands of infancy slow to keep pace with the more moderate growth rate of toddlerhood. Although it can appear that the toddler eats nothing at times, intake over days or a week is generally sufficient and balanced enough to meet the body's demands for nutrients and energy.

Parents often need knowledge about types of foods that constitute a healthy diet. Some easy-to-prepare foods are high in salt and other additives, and can lead to exceeding the recommendation of Healthy People 2010 for sodium intake. Provide alternatives to hot dogs, microwave meals, or fast foods with information about easy preparation of sliced meats, cheese, tofu, fruits, and vegetables. Healthy snacks for young children include yogurt, cheese, milk, slices of bread with peanut butter, thinly sliced fruits, and soft vegetables.

Advise parents to offer a variety of nutritious foods several times daily (three meals and two snacks) and let the toddler make choices from the foods offered. Offer foods only at mealtimes and have the child eat in a high chair or on a special seat at the table (Figure 3-5 ◆). Small portions are most appealing to the toddler. A general guideline for food quantity at a meal is 1 tablespoon of each food per year of age (see Table 3-6 for common serving sizes at various ages). The toddler should drink 16 to 24 ounces (1/2 to 3/4 L) of milk daily. Caution parents against giving the toddler more than 1 quart (1 L) of milk daily, since this interferes with the desire to eat other foods, leading to dietary deficiencies. Recall that the child should not be placed to bed with a bottle or allowed to carry a bottle of milk or juice around during the day, due to the risk of nursing bottle mouth syndrome (see previous discussion in chapter). In addition, parents

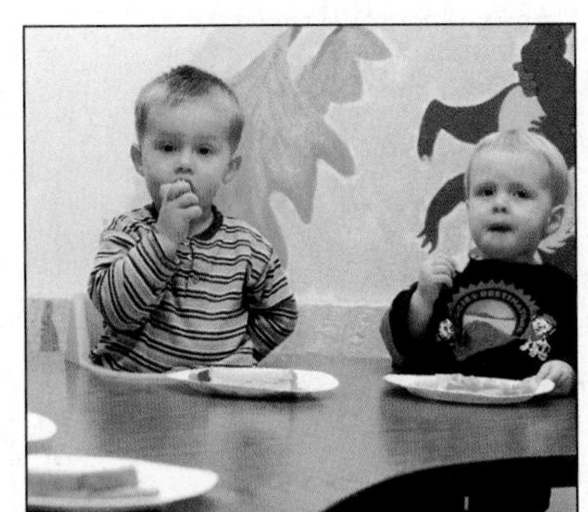

FIGURE 3-5 ◆
Toddlers should sit at a table or in a high chair to eat, to minimize chance of choking and to foster positive eating patterns.

TABLE 3-6 Typical Daily Intake at Various Ages

	BREAKFAST	SNACK	LUNCH	SNACK	DINNER	SNACK
Infant 6 months	2 T rice cereal with 2 oz (60 mL) formula	4 oz (120 mL) formula or breast milk	6 oz (180 mL) formula or breast milk	6 oz (180 mL) formula or breast milk	2 T rice cereal with 2 oz (60 mL) formula, then 6 oz (180 mL) formula or breast milk	4 oz (120 mL) formula or breast milk
12 months	1/4 to 1/2 cup (60-120 mL) apple juice 4 T rice cereal with 4 oz (120 mL) milk	3 crackers 1/2 cup (120 mL) milk	1 thin slice (1/2 oz [14 g]) of turkey 1/2 cup soft cooked carrots 1 cup (240 mL) milk	1/2 slice of cheese 1/2 cup (120 mL) milk or water	1/4 cup plain pasta 1/4 cup thin-sliced apple chunks 1/2 cup (120 mL) milk	1/2 cup yogurt
Toddler	1/4 cup (60 mL) orange juice 1/4 cup cereal with 1/2 cup (120 mL) milk 1/4 banana	5 crackers 1/2 cup (120 mL) milk	2 thin slices (1 oz [28 g]) of turkey with 1/2 slice of bread 1/2 cup cooked carrots 1 cup (240 mL) milk	1 slice cheese 1/2 cup (120 mL) juice	1/4 cup plain pasta 1/4–1/2 cup thin-sliced apple chunks 1/2 cup (120 mL) milk	1/2 cup yogurt
Preschooler	1/2 cup (120 mL) orange juice 1/3 cup cereal with 3/4 cup (180 mL) milk 1/2 banana	5 crackers 1/2 orange 1/2 cup (120 mL) milk	3 thin slices (1 1/2 oz [42 g]) of turkey with 1/2 slice bread 1/4 cup cooked carrots 3/4 cup (180 mL) milk	1 slice cheese 1/2 cup (120 mL) juice	1/4–1/2 cup plain pasta with meat sauce 1/2 cup thin-sliced apple chunks 1/2 cup (120 mL) milk	1/2 cup yogurt
School-age child	1/2 cup (120 mL) orange juice 3/4 cup cereal with 1 cup (240 mL) milk 1/2 bagel with jam		4 thin slices (2 oz [56 g]) of turkey with 1 slice bread and condiments Apple 1 cup (240 mL) milk 1 oatmeal cookie	1 1/2 cups popcorn 1 cup (240 mL) lemonade	1/2 cup pasta with meat sauce Dinner salad 1 slice garlic bread 1 cup (240 mL) milk	1 cup pudding or yogurt
Adolescent	1/2 cup (120 mL) orange juice 1 cup cereal 1 cup (240 mL) milk 1 bagel with 1 T peanut butter and jam		3 oz (84 g) meat with 2 slices of bread plus condiments Apple 1 cup (240 mL) milk 1 oatmeal cookie	3 cups popcorn 1 cup (240 mL) lemonade	1 1/2 cup pasta with meat sauce 1 slice garlic bread Salad with dressing 1 cup (240 mL) milk	1 cup pudding Fruit

should be cautioned to limit fruit juice to 4 to 6 ounces daily for children ages 1 to 6 years in order to decrease the opportunity for overweight, dental caries, and abdominal discomfort (American Academy of Pediatrics Committee on Nutrition, 2001). Using water to drink in combination with whole fruits, which provide fiber, is a healthier alternative.

Learning how to eat with others is an important task of toddlerhood. The toddler displays characteristic autonomy or independence during mealtime. Advise parents to provide opportunities for self-feeding of food with fingers and utensils, and to allow some simple choices, such as type of liquid or cup to use. Young children should eat at a table with others, not be allowed to run and play while eating, and eat at specified meal and snack times. Because social skills are developing, the hospitalized toddler may eat better if allowed to have meals with parents or other hospitalized children. See Chapter 5 for further suggestions about management of nutrition in hospitalized children.

PRESCHOOL

The diet of the preschooler is similar to that of the toddler, but mealtime is now a more social event. Preschoolers like the company of others while they eat, and they enjoy helping with food preparation and table setting (Figure 3-6 ◆). Involving them in these tasks can provide a forum for teaching about nutritious foods and principles of preparation such as the need for refrigeration, safety around stoves, and cleanliness.

Although the rate of growth is slow and steady during the preschool years, the child has periods of **food jags** (eating only a few foods for several days or weeks) and greater or lesser intake. Advise parents to assess food intake over a 1- or 2-week period rather than at each meal to obtain a more accurate impression of total intake. Food jags can be handled by providing the desired food along with other foods to foster choice. The child who chooses not to eat at snack or meal time should not be given other foods in between. Hunger will develop and the child will become accustomed to eating when food is provided. Three meals and two or three snacks daily are the norm (Table 3-6). Limit fruit juice to 8 to 12 ounces daily.

The preschool period is a good time to continue encouraging good dental habits. Children can begin to brush their own teeth with parental supervision and help to reach all tooth surfaces. See Chapter 2 for recommended doses of fluoride when the water supply is not fluoridated. If the child has not yet visited a dentist, the first dental visit should be scheduled so the child can become accustomed to the routine of dental care.

SCHOOL AGE

The school-age years are a period of gradual growth when energy requirements remain at a steady level, although sometime during these years, most children experience a preadolescent growth spurt. Girls may begin a growth spurt by 10 or 11 years, and boys a year or so later. Nutritional needs increase dramatically with this spurt, with large numbers of calories and increased amounts of other nutrients required (see Appendix B for RDAs).

School-age children are increasingly responsible for preparing snacks, lunches, and even some other meals. These years are a good time to teach children how to choose nutritious foods and how to plan a well-balanced meal. Because school-age children operate at the concrete level of cognitive thought, nutrition teaching is best presented by using pictures, samples of foods, videotapes, handouts, and hands-on experience.

School-age children often prefer the types of foods eaten at home and may be resistant to new food items. A hospitalized child may refuse to eat, slowing the recuperative process. Encourage family members to bring favorite foods from home that meet nutritional requirements. This can be especially helpful when the hospital serves food only from the dominant cultural group. A child accustomed to a diet of rice, tofu, and vegetables may not enjoy a hospital

RESEARCH

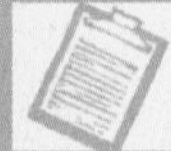

When girls experience menarche before 11 years of age, they are more frequently overweight. Early weight control and being alert for early menarche can help identify young girls in need of obesity prevention. Such prevention efforts are needed to decrease risks such as type II diabetes (Adair & Gordon-Larsen, 2001).

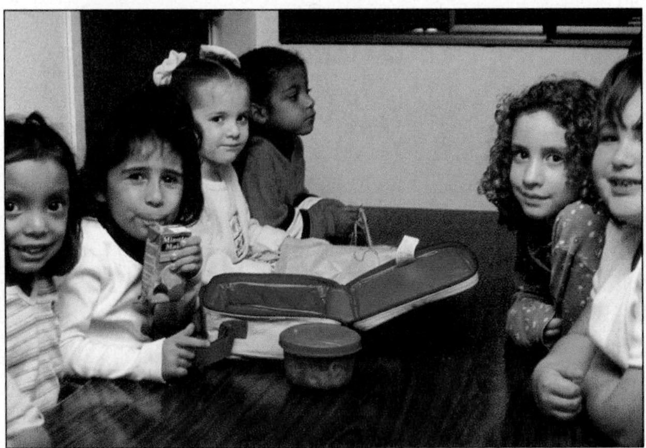

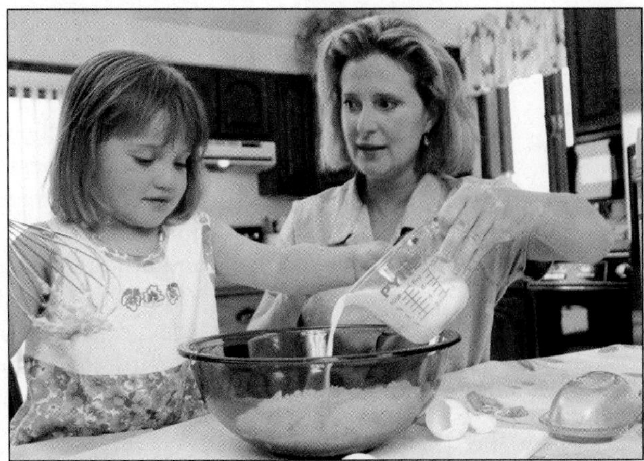

FIGURE 3-6 ◆
Preschoolers learn food habits by eating with others. Engaging them in food preparation enhances knowledge of food and promotes intake at meals.

meal of hamburger and fries. By school age, food has become strongly associated with social interaction, so it is beneficial to have children eat together or to invite family members to take the child off the unit to eat or to bring in food from home and eat with the child. Many hospitals allow children to plan a pizza night or sponsor other events to encourage eating in a social atmosphere.

Most children consume at least one meal daily in school. Although they may bring lunches to school, many children participate in the school lunch program, and perhaps the school breakfast program. Become familiar with the school district's policies in your area for providing foods, snacks, and reduced-price food to students in need. How will you plan for Joey (described in opening scenario) to be able to participate in school lunchtime with peers? What types of soft foods are commonly available at school that he might be able to enjoy?

The loss of the first deciduous teeth and the eruption of permanent teeth usually occur at about 6 years, or at the beginning of the school-age period. Of the 32 permanent teeth, 22 to 26 teeth erupt by age 12, and the remaining molars follow in the teenage years. See Chapter 4 for the typical sequence of tooth eruption. The school-age child should be closely monitored to ensure that brushing and flossing are adequate, that fluoride is taken if the water supply is not fluoridated, that dental care is obtained to provide for examination of teeth and alignment, and that loose teeth are identified before surgery or sports participation.

ADOLESCENCE

Most adolescents need well over 2,000 calories daily to support the growth spurt, and some adolescent boys require nearly 3,000 calories daily. When teenagers are active in a variety of sports, these requirements increase further. Because adolescents prepare much of their own food and often eat with friends, they need to be taught about good nutrition. Developing a diet that includes a large number of calories, meets vitamin and mineral requirements, and is acceptable to the teen may be a challenge. An adolescent who does not like the hospital lunch and reaches for a soft drink and chips may be receptive to juice and pizza, a more nutritious meal. Small improvements should be viewed positively as they may lead to further changes.

Remember that peer group influence is important, so group sessions in which adolescents eat lunch together can provide a forum for influencing food habits. What other methods can you think of to encourage positive nutritional habits among teens?

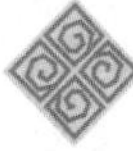

NUTRITIONAL ASSESSMENT

What is the best indication that the child's nutrition is adequate? Which data collection methods provide the most accurate information about a child's dietary intake? The nurse plays an important role in assessing the diets of children and in seeking additional evaluation from dietitians and nutritionists in complex situations.

PHYSICAL AND BEHAVIORAL MEASUREMENT

Growth Measurement

Skills 5-1 to 5-7: Growth Measurements

A common method used to evaluate the adequacy of diet is measurement of growth. **Anthropometric measurement** is the term used to refer to assessment of various parts of the body. Anthropometry of young children commonly includes weight, length, and head circumference. Standing height is substituted for length once the child can stand. Head circumference, also known as occipital-frontal circumference (OFC) is measured until the child is about 5 years. Additional measurements that may be included in special circumstances include chest circumference, mid-upper arm circumference, and skinfold measurement at sites such as triceps, abdomen, and subscapular regions. The Skills Manual presents techniques for accurate measurement of weight, length, height, chest, and head circumference.

Once the measurements are collected, plot the readings on the appropriate standardized growth curves for weight, length to height, head circumference, and body mass index (see Figure 3-7 ◆). **Body mass index (BMI)** is a calculation based on the child's weight and height, or length, and is calculated as kilograms of weight/m^2 of height. This is a useful calculation for determining if the child's height and weight are in proportion. Identify on the plots where the child falls in percentile for each measurement. Children normally fall between the 10th and 90th

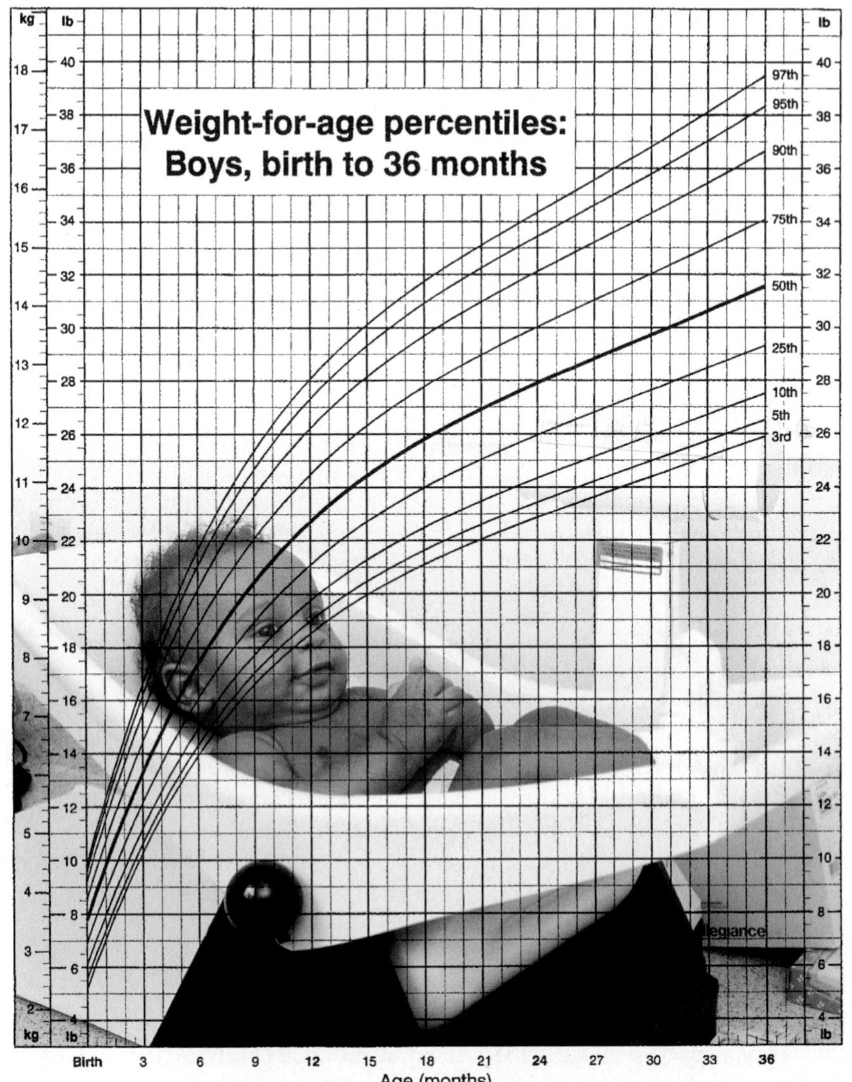

FIGURE 3-7 ◆
The nurse accurately measures the child and then places height and weight on appropriate growth grids for the child's age and gender.

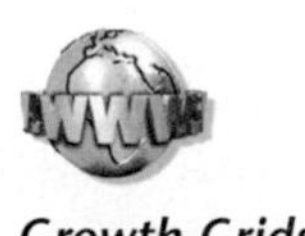

percentiles. A measurement below the 10th percentile, especially for BMI, may indicate undernutrition, whereas one over the 90th percentile can indicate overnutrition. It is important, however, to look at the differences between measurements. An infant in the 90th percentile for length, weight, and head circumference is proportional and may be a naturally large baby. On the other hand, a child who is consistently in the 10th percentile for all measurements, but is growing steadily and is at a normal development level, may simply be a small child. Much cultural and individual variation exists regarding size. See Appendix A for standardized growth curves by gender and age for infants, children, and adolescents. Visit our website to find out more about the growth curves and a course in accurate assessment techniques.

Plot your measurements on the same growth curve with earlier percentiles for the child. When measurements follow the same percentile over time, growth is generally normal for the child and nutrition is likely adequate. However, a sudden or sustained change in percentile may indicate a chronic disorder, emotional difficulty, or a nutritional intake problem. Further assessment of physical status and dietary intake will be needed.

Additional Physical Measurement

Many observations from the physical assessment provide clues to nutritional status. Every body system can be affected by dietary intake, and a combination of certain symptoms may suggest specific nutritional problems. Some of the common physical manifestations of nutritional status are outlined in Table 3-7.

Growth Grids

CLINICAL TIP

To calculate body mass index (BMI), you must:

1. Be sure that weight is in kilograms. If it is in pounds, divide that number by 2.2 to get kilograms.
2. Change height measurement to meters. Because 1 meter = 39.37 inches (or 0.0254 meters = 1 inch), you must multiply the child's height in inches by 0.0254 to obtain height in meters.
3. Now square the number of meters.
4. You are ready to calculate BMI. Put kilograms of weight/height in meters squared and divide appropriately.

If a child weighs 26.5 pounds, convert to kilograms = 12 kg. The child's height is 34.5 inches = 0.8763 m. Because m^2 = 0.7679, BMI = 15.63.

CLINICAL TIP

If you measure a child and find him or her to be either in very low or high percentiles, try the following:

1. Measure again to check for accuracy.
2. Examine if length or height, weight, and head circumference are in similar percentiles. Is the child proportional?
3. Observe if the parents are very large or very small.
4. Look at the child's chart to see if the patterns have continued over time or if they represent a sudden change.

CULTURE

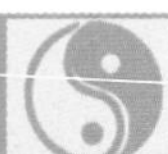

The revised growth grids now in use were standardized using a cross section of the U.S. population and are generally reflective of most children. However, children from some other countries or cultures may fall outside of these curves. For example, new immigrants or adoptees may be in lower percentiles, and "catch up" over several months or years. Children of immigrants from developing countries tend to be larger than their parents. Even when small, children should follow normal growth patterns. For example, a child may remain at the 10th or 25th percentile for height, but continue to slowly grow and not fall to a lower percentile.

RESEARCH

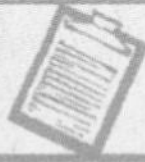

Many studies have confirmed that normal brain development requires good nutrition. Amino acids, carbohydrates, and some vitamins are precursors for neurotransmitters. Essential fatty acids are essential elements in the central nervous system. Trace elements such as zinc are found in the brain and are known to be necessary for memory. Iron is needed for central nervous system myelinization. Clearly, early nutrition plays a part in cognitive development and the importance of a good diet cannot be minimized (Wauben & Wainwright, 1999).

TABLE 3-7 Indicators of Nutritional Status

NUTRIENT DEFICIENCY	BODY SYSTEM	CLINICAL MANIFESTATIONS
Protein and Calorie	Growth	Poor growth
	Hair	Dull, scant, loss (alopecia), changed texture, depigmented
	Skin	Depigmented, poor hydration, petechiae
	Nails	Transverse ridging
Minerals	Musculoskeletal	Muscle wasting, weakness

Laboratory measurements can provide useful information when nutritional status is questionable. Some common studies include hematocrit and hemoglobin, serum glucose and fasting insulin, lipids and lipoproteins, and liver and renal function studies. Adding some further measurements such as chest circumference and skinfolds (measurement of fat at certain body sites such as triceps, scapular, and abdominal areas) may also be useful (Bessler, 1999).

DIETARY INTAKE

The mother's dietary intake during pregnancy may provide information about the child's nutritional state and it can be assessed for pertinent information. Obtain detailed information about the child's dietary intake when there is a potential for nutritional deficiency due to disease, knowledge deficit, or socioeconomic status (Hensrud, 1999). After the information is collected, compare the dietary intake with the recommended levels for a child of that age and gender (see Figure 3-1, and Appendix B for Recommended Dietary Allowances). The 24-hour recall of intake, food frequency questionnaire, and a dietary screening history provide a good overview of the infant's or child's intake and eating patterns. A food diary provides information about the child's precise food intake.

24-hour Recall of Food Intake

The 24-hour diet recall is frequently used to assess the adequacy of the diet. People can generally remember their intake in the past day, so results are fairly accurate; it is easy to gather the data and analyze results; only a few minutes are needed. Ask the parent or child to list all foods eaten during the past 24 hours (Figure 3-8 ◆). It is usually helpful to ask for a description of activities in the last day. Then start with the most recent event and move backwards, integrating food intake into the daily schedule. For example, you might begin by saying "You mentioned you got up early to come to the clinic today. What did Sam eat at home before you left? Did he have a snack as you traveled here or after you arrived?" While asking about the foods eaten, inquire specifically about the following:

- All meals and snacks
- Amounts of each food item consumed (have various-size measuring cups, bowls, and plates so accurate amounts can be indicated)
- Types of specific foods used, such as whole milk versus nonfat or 2%, brand names of cereals, specific types of margarine or butter
- Additives used, such as condiments, table salt, spices, milk to mix formula
- Food preparation methods, including adding fats to cook, removal or retention of fats on meats
- Vitamins and supplements, types, and doses
- Whether the intake is representative of the typical diet (in situations such as illness or vacation, intake may be different than usual)

Once the 24-hour recall is obtained, intake analysis is next. First, a quick check can be done to compare servings of various food types with the food guide pyramid, as described earlier. Next, a detailed analysis is done to compute calories, carbohydrate, pro-

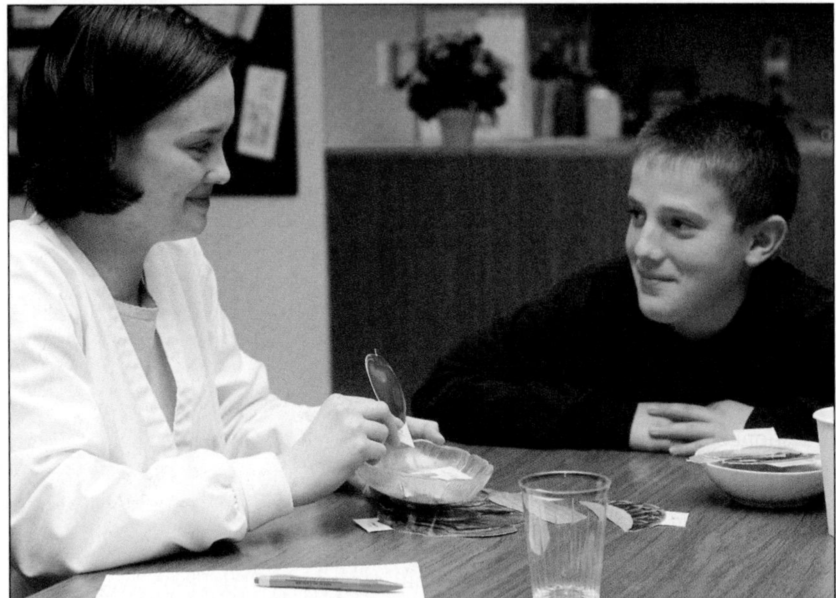

FIGURE 3-8 ◆
The nurse is interviewing a child about foods eaten in the last day. Note the models of food and dishes for accurate assessment of serving sizes.

tein, and fat intake and compare them with recommended amounts. All major vitamins and minerals are also computed and comparisons made to the DRIs. This computation may be done by hand, using a book of nutrients in common foods, or may be done on the computer. Several computer programs are available, and the federal government has a website that provides intake levels and comparisons to the RDAs—try computing your own 24-hour recall or that of a child in your clinical setting with the Healthy Eating Index.

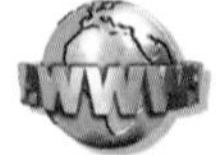

Nutrition Analysis

Food Frequency Questionnaire

Food frequency questionnaires are available that can be easily administered to parents or children. Usually they ask about how often certain types of foods are eaten in a specified period such as a week. Questionnaires can be long and evaluate a total diet, or short to focus on specific items such as fruit and vegetable intake. A short questionnaire about milk intake or fruit and vegetable intake may be helpful before the start of a teaching project on nutrition to a class of school-age children. Knowing their usual intake of a food item can provide helpful information for the project. One example of types of questions asked on a food frequency questionnaire is shown in Table 3-8.

Dietary Screening History

Ask the parent about the infant's or child's eating habits using questions in Tables 3-9 and 3-10. Responses provide information about the family's eating habits and food beliefs beyond that collected on a 24-hour dietary recall or food frequency questionnaire.

Food Diary

Parents are asked to keep a food diary when the child has a nutrition problem or disorder, such as malnutrition, obesity, or type I diabetes, that requires dietary management. All meals and snacks, with food preparation method and quantities eaten over a 1- to 7-day period, are recorded. Eating patterns change significantly for holidays or family gatherings, so ask parents to select typical days for the food diary or to record specific events affecting food intake. Food diaries can provide a great deal of helpful information, but take time and motivation to complete well (Lee & Nieman, 1996). Be sure instructions are complete and that the form has a place to record amounts, preparation, events occurring, and where food was eaten. The nurse or parent may need to obtain the school lunch menu and talk with the school lunch personnel to add accurate school intake.

The nurse completes the nutritional assessment indicated for a child, and may consult with or refer the family to a dietitian or nutritionist for additional assessment and teaching.

CULTURE

Each culture has eating practices that influence dietary intake. It is important to understand the foods commonly eaten by each cultural group and their contribution to the total nutrition of the child.

CLINICAL TIP

Parents seldom control all of the food a child eats. To help parents record an accurate food diary, remind them about all the places a child might be fed or obtain food. Older children often get snacks independently and obtain food from friends. Younger children may be fed in child care centers.

TABLE 3-8 Sample Questions – Youth Adolescent Questionnaire (YAQ)

1. Where do you usually eat breakfast?
   - Home
   - School
   - Don't eat breakfast
   - Other
2. Which cold breakfast cereal do you usually eat?
3. What type of milk do you usually drink?
   - Whole milk
   - 2% milk
   - 1% milk
   - Skim/nonfat milk
   - Don't know
   - Don't drink milk
4. How much milk (glass or with cereal) do you drink?
   - Never/less than 1 glass per month
   - 1 glass per week or less
   - 2–6 glasses per week
   - 1 glass per day
   - 2–3 glasses per day
   - 4+ glasses per day
5. How often do you eat pizza (2 slices)?
   - Never/less than once per month
   - 1–3 times per month
   - Once per week
   - 2–4 times per week
   - 5 or more times per week
6. Do you eat peanut butter sandwiches (plain or with jelly, fluff, etc.)?
   - Never/less than 1 sandwich per month
   - 1–3 sandwiches per month
   - One sandwich per week
   - 2–4 sandwiches per week
   - 5 or more sandwiches per week

From Youth/Adolescent Questionnaire (1995). Harvard Medical School. Channing Laboratory, 181 Longwood Avenue, Boston, MA 02115.

COMMON NUTRITIONAL CONCERNS

CHILDHOOD HUNGER

Although most Americans live in a "land of plenty," significant numbers of children periodically experience hunger. **Food security** is access at all times to enough nourishment for an active, healthy life (Federal Interagency Forum on Child and Family Statistics, 2000). In contrast, **food insecurity** indicates an inability to acquire or consume adequate quality or quantity of foods in socially acceptable ways, or the uncertainty that one will be able to do so (Boyle & Morris, 1999).

The major cause of hunger in children is poverty, and since one in five children is poor, their families may be unable to provide sustainable nutrition at all times (Children's Defense Fund, 2000). Many single-income families have a head of household moving into the workforce, so incomes are often not sufficient to provide for family food needs (see Chapter 1 for a description of Temporary Assistance for Needy Families [TANF]). Families may be ineligible for food assistance programs even though they are unable to purchase enough food for all their members. Children with special nutritional needs are at particular risk because it may be more costly to buy and prepare formula or foods for a child with allergies, diabetes, or an immune disorder.

TABLE 3-9 Dietary Screening History for Infants

Overview Questions
What was the infant's birth weight?
At what age did the birth weight double and triple?
Was the infant premature?
Does the infant have any feeding problems such as difficulty sucking and swallowing, spitting up, fatigue, or fussiness?

If Infant is Breast Fed
How long does the baby nurse at each breast?
What is the usual schedule for nursing?
Does the baby also take any milk or formula? Amount and frequency? What type?

If Infant Is Fed Other Foods
What formula is used? Is it iron fortified?
How is it prepared?
Do you hold or prop the bottle for feedings?
How much formula is taken at each feeding?
How many bottles are taken each day?
Does the baby take a bottle to bed for naps or nighttime? What is in the bottle?

If Infant Is Formula Fed
At what age did the baby start eating other foods?

Cereal	Finger foods
Fruit/juices	Meats
Vegetables	Other protein sources

Do you use commercial baby food or make your own?
Does the baby eat any table foods?
How often does the baby take solid foods?
How is the baby's appetite?
Do you have any concerns about the baby's feeding habits?
Does the baby take a vitamin supplement? Fluoride?
Have there been any allergic reactions to foods? Which ones?
Does the baby spit up frequently?
Have there been any rashes?
What types of stools does the baby have? Frequency? Consistency?

TABLE 3-10 Dietary Screening History for Children

What foods or beverages does the child dislike?
What types of food or beverage does the child especially like?
What is the child's typical eating schedule? Meals and snacks?
Does the child eat with the family or at separate times?
Where does the child eat each meal?
Who prepares the food for the family?
What method of cooking is used? Baking? Frying? Broiling?
What ethnic foods are commonly eaten?
Does the family eat in a restaurant frequently? What type?
What type of food does the child usually order?
Is the child on a special diet?
Does the child need to be fed, feed himself or herself, need assistance eating, or need any adaptive devices for eating?
What is the child's appetite like?
Does the child take any vitamin supplements (iron, fluoride)?
Does the child have any allergies? What types of symptoms?
What types of regular exercise does the child get?
Are there any concerns about the child's eating habits?

TABLE 3-11 Food Insecurity Screening

1. Does your household ever run out of money to buy food to make a meal?
2. Do you or members of your household ever eat less than you feel you should because there is not enough money for food?
3. Do you or members of your household ever cut the size of meals or skip meals because there is not enough money for food?
4. Do your children ever eat less than you feel they should because there is not enough money for food?
5. Do you ever cut the size of your children's meals or do they skip meals because there is not enough money for food?
6. Do your children ever say they are hungry because there is not enough food in the house?
7. Do you ever rely on a limited number of foods to feed your children because you are running out of money to buy foods for a meal?
8. Do any of your children ever go to bed hungry because there is not enough money to buy food?

Scoring: 5–8 yes = hungry; 1–4 yes = risk of hunger
From the Washington State Department of Health.

Children who have insufficient dietary intake are at risk for a wide array of health problems. They may become anemic, experience a high rate of infectious disease due to lowered immune response, have slowed developmental maturation, delayed or stunted physical growth, and learning disorders, and be at greater risk of overweight, cardiovascular disease, and diabetes in adulthood (Committee on Nutrition, 1998; Hanson, Dahlman-Hoglund, & Lundin, et al., 1997; Walter, Olivares, & Pizarro, et al., 1997). Subsequently, the national and individual cost of childhood hunger is great.

Nurses are well positioned to evaluate families for food insecurity in a variety of hospital, clinic, school, and home settings. In addition to the assessment of the individual child's nutritional status, further questions can determine families with potential problems. Administer the screening tool to identify risk in families (Table 3-11). Most parents go without food themselves in order to feed their children, so food insecurity may not necessarily have directly impacted all children. However, anxiety over providing food can be a very stressful event in families and diet quality deteriorates as insecurity increases. If families have experienced food insecurity or may be likely to at some time, be sure to provide them with access to community agencies and programs that can be of assistance. What resources are available in your community to help families with food insecurity?

OVERWEIGHT AND OBESITY

After several decades of similar statistics regarding overweight in children, the numbers are now skyrocketing. The current incidence of overweight in the United States has been called

FAMILIES WANT TO KNOW

Community Resources for Food

Food Stamp Program—Eligibility based on household size and income; refer students and those with low incomes, especially when they have young children; education services often available

Child Nutrition Programs—School lunch, breakfast, and milk programs; free and lowered cost meals in schools; assist parents to apply

Special Child Programs—Summer programs, Head Start, child care centers and homeless children programs may provide nutritional support in some communities

Women, Infants, and Children (WIC)—Supplemental foods and nutrition education to pregnant, breastfeeding, and postpartum women and to their young children; assessment of child growth often included

Nutrition Education and Training Program—Nutrition education for teachers and school food service personnel

Community Services—May include food banks, field gleaning, and other programs

Find out what services are available to provide food and nutrition education in your community. Make a list for use in clinical settings with families.

an epidemic and is associated with a wide array of health problems, such as the appearance of type II diabetes in youth (Troiano & Flegal, 1998). See Chapter 22 for a discussion of diabetes. Overweight can also influence self-image, dietary quality, and amount of physical activity. The Third National Health and Nutrition Examination Survey has found that 11% to 15% of various child and adolescent groups are now overweight (Healthy People 2010, 2000). When using the 85th percentile of BMI as indicator of overweight, from 22% to 33% of youth are affected (Troiano, Flegal, & Kuczmarski, et al., 1995). Since overweight in childhood and adolescence frequently tracks into adulthood, the implications for health care are obvious.

There are many reasons cited for the increase in overweight children. The number of calories consumed is not increasing, but children tend to exercise less, particularly on a daily basis. They infrequently walk or ride bikes, either because of the convenience of driving or due to unsafe neighborhoods. Television viewing is very high among youth and contributes to overweight both from the inactivity associated with it and the pattern of snacking during commercial time. As many as 60% of obese children view excessive television, defined as more than 5 hours daily (Gortmaker, Must, & Sobol, et al., 1996). The percentage of calories from fat consumed in the United States is among the highest in the world. Although no more than 30% of calories should come from total dietary fat, and no more than 10% from saturated fat, about 35% of calories consumed in the United States are supplied by fat and 12% by saturated fat (National Cholesterol Education Program, 1991; Krauss, Eckel, & Howard, et al. 2001). High levels of dietary fat are associated with higher cholesterol levels and decreased activity. The high rate of dietary fat is related to the large amount of fast food consumed, as fast-food restaurants are convenient and fit well into today's lifestyles. Another contributing factor to overweight is poor snacking habits, which have been on the increase in the last decade. Snacks of choice are often nutrient poor and calorie dense (Zizza, Siega-Riz, & Popkin, 2001).

Nurses can assist parents and children in building good nutritional and exercise habits throughout life, thus decreasing the incidence of overweight and its attendant health risks. Begin with an assessment of growth patterns starting early in life. Patterns of eating fast foods, meals on the run, and while watching television should be addressed in early health maintenance visits. Caution parents that television viewing should be limited to a maximum of 2 hours daily, and that television and video games should not be placed in children's bedrooms. Daily exercise routines of at least 30 minutes can be included in most families. Also, teach about the food guide pyramid and its integration into a healthy life. Healthy snacks include fruits, vegetables, grains, and nuts. "Super sizing" fast foods and eating out often should be avoided.

Risks for poor health often cluster in individuals and families, so the nurse can be alert for situations in which parents are overweight, children have elevated blood pressure, exercise infrequently, or are in upper percentiles for weight, BMI, or skinfold. Presence of risk factors necessitates further dietary and risk assessment so that a management plan can be implemented. See resources such as "Helping Your Overweight Child" and "Take Charge of Your Health: A Teenager's Guide to Better Health."

CULTURE

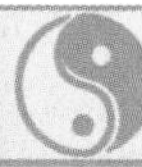

Overweight is more common among some ethnic and socioeconomic groups. Lack of knowledge about foods and physical activity, limited access to fresh produce and safe places to exercise, easy access to increasing numbers of fast foods, and ethnic differences in metabolism may constitute risk factors. Lower income and Hispanic, African American, and Native American ethnic identities are associated with higher incidence of overweight, especially among women. National goals to eliminate health disparities in income and ethnic groups have been set (Healthy People 2010, 2000).

RESEARCH

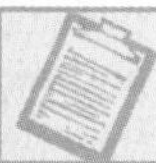

When a child has one obese parent, chances of the child being overweight are increased. In families where both parents are overweight, the incidence of obesity in children increases even more. Finally, the child who has obese parents and is overweight as an adolescent is at very high risk of becoming an obese adult (Whitaker, Wright, & Pepe, et al., 1997). Be alert for families with overweight adults and begin prevention early with the children in these families.

FOOD SAFETY

Every year in the United States, about 76 million people contract foodborne illnesses. Some are quite mild, whereas others can be severe. Children are at greater risk of severe illness and death from food and water than adults, due to their immature gastrointestinal and immune systems. The most common pathogens are *Campylobacter, Salmonella, Shigella,* and *E. coli;* infants under 1 year are at extremely high risk of *Campylobacter, Rotavirus,* and *Salmonella* illness (Morbidity and Mortality Weekly Report [MMWR], 2001a). A former common cause of food-related illness was hepatitis A. Although still prevalent in some parts of the country, effective management and prevention through immunization has decreased its incidence (see Chapter 12).

Foodborne illness is relayed by food preparation and storage practices, lack of adequate training of retail employees regarding foods and hygiene, and increasing amounts and types of foods being imported from other countries. Health personnel should integrate teaching regularly so that families can decrease risks of foodborne illness.

SAFETY PRECAUTIONS

Worldwide, over 3 million people die of illness related to unsafe drinking water each year and most of those deaths are among children. The World Health Organization is focusing on this important health problem. Children are more prone to illnesses such as diarrhea and dehydration when drinking contaminated water. Caution families with children to be sure water supplies are safe during travel and to use bottled or purified water.

FAMILIES WANT TO KNOW

Foodborne Safety Guidelines

Four Key Food Safety Practices:

1. CLEAN: Wash hands and surfaces often.
2. SEPARATE: Avoid cross contamination.
3. COOK: Cook to proper temperatures.
4. CHILL: Refrigerate promptly.

(Healthy People 2010, 2000)

____(2000). Healthy People 2010. Washington DC: U.S. Department of Health and Human Services. Retrieved April 13, 2001 from the world wide web: http://www.health.gov/ healthypeople/document.html.

CULTURE

Vitamin A deficiency is common in developing countries. The vitamin is found in liver, dairy products, and fish. Provitamin A sources are yellow and dark green vegetables. The vitamin is fat soluble and stored in the liver. When deficient, children develop night blindness, vision loss, and high rates of infection. Public health efforts have been directed at identifying children with low vitamin A status and in providing the vitamin in capsule form or in commonly ingested foods.

COMMON DIETARY DEFICIENCIES

Although there can be deficits in nearly all nutrients, certain deficiencies are more common in childhood. Either limitations in the food supply or patterns of dietary intake are the cause of most deficiencies, while children with certain disease processes, such as metabolic diseases, may have difficulty absorbing or using nutrients ingested (see Chapter 22 for a discussion of inborn errors of metabolism). The nutrient deficiencies present in a population are a result of genetic factors and characteristics of the food supply and intake patterns of particular groups.

Iron

Newborns have a store of iron obtained from their mothers in the uterus, if the maternal nutritional state was satisfactory and the baby is normal gestational age. Breast milk contains little iron, but the iron it does contain has high bioavailability. By 4 to 6 months of age, however, the baby's iron stores begin to decrease and a dietary source of iron must be added. Enriched rice cereal is commonly used to meet these initial iron needs. In babies who do not have adequate stores or do not take in enough iron, **anemia** (a reduction in the number of red blood cells) can result (Figure 3-9 ◆). Feeding cow milk during infancy can also cause anemia by irritating the gut and leading to small but consistent loss of blood from the gastrointestinal tract. When formulas are used, they should be iron fortified to help avoid iron deficiency anemia.

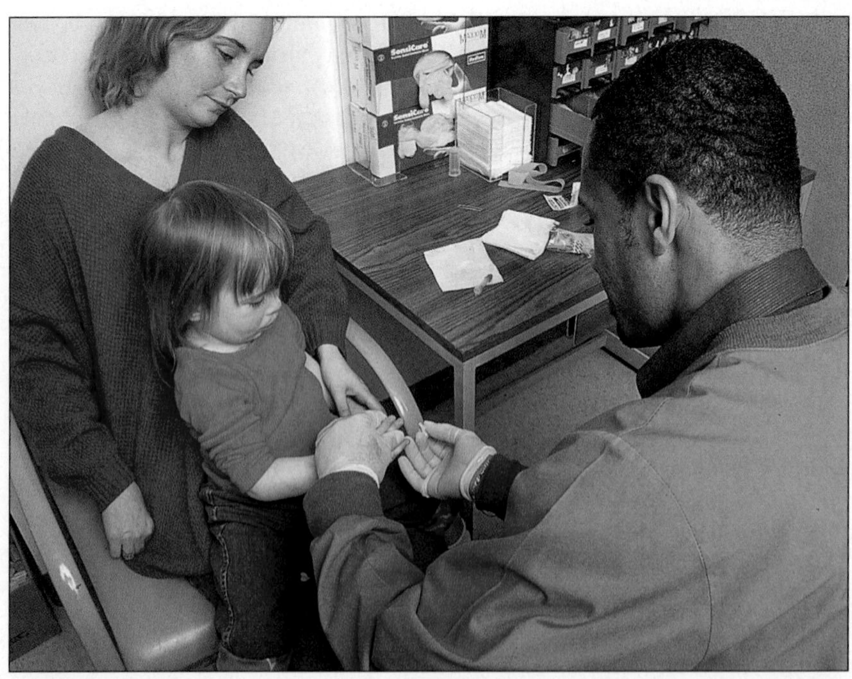

FIGURE 3-9 ◆
Most Head Start centers participate in screening programs to identify children at risk for anemia.

The other group most commonly deficient in iron is adolescent females, related to loss of blood in menses, metabolic need of the growth spurt, and poor dietary balance due to sporadic dieting. Further discussion of the symptoms and treatment of iron deficiency anemia can be found in Chapter 15.

SOURCES OF IRON

Meats
Iron-fortified formula
Iron-fortified baby cereal

Iron absorption is enhanced by vitamin C intake if taken together.
Iron is present in breast milk in a small amount, but is very well absorbed.

Calcium

Calcium is an essential nutrient for bone development during childhood and adolescence. An increased intake of soda pop and fruit juices is related to a decrease in calcium intake, especially among adolescents. During the adolescent growth spurt, almost 40% of the adult bone mass is accumulated (Trahms & Pipes, 1997). Inadequate intake puts the person at risk for osteoporosis later in life, as there is no ability to make up for earlier deficits. Although genetic variables account for some of the influence on adult bone mass, increasing calcium intake has been shown to promote bone formation. While the recommended daily intake for adolescents is 1,500 mg, the average intake for adolescent males is 1,169 mg and for females is only 753 mg—only half of the recommended level (Food and Nutrition Board, 2001).

Adolescents at highest risk for impaired bone development include female athletes and others who diet to a great degree to maintain slimness. These teens manifest the "female athlete triad" of excessive thinness, excessive exercise, and amenorrhea. A high rate of fractures and osteomalacia can result, in addition to an extreme risk of osteoporosis in adulthood. Asking about menstrual patterns, as well as exercise and diet, can be combined with physical measurements of height and weight to obtain pertinent information about the teen athlete. See Chapter 7 for a discussion of the eating disorders anorexia nervosa and bulimia nervosa.

SOURCES OF CALCIUM

Milk and milk products
Egg yolks
Grains
Legumes
Nuts
Soybeans

CLINICAL TIP

The "female athlete triad" is commonly assumed to occur only in females performing sports that emphasize thinness, but others are also affected. Anorexics often exercise excessively in an effort to lose weight. Males may diet because of anorexia or due to participation in a sport with a weight category such as wrestling or horse racing. Good history questions will help you to elicit information about factors influencing extremely thin adolescents.

Vitamin D

Vitamin D deficiencies are rare because the vitamin can be synthesized in the skin upon exposure to sunlight. However, an increased incidence in cases of vitamin D–deficient rickets has recently been observed. This vitamin is needed to enhance absorption of calcium so a lack of vitamin D can contribute to calcium deficiency as well. Human milk contains little vitamin D, and if infants are kept wrapped when outside, live in northern climates and rarely get outside in winter months, have extensive sunscreens applied, or are dark in skin color, vitamin D deficiency can result. This has led to a recommendation by the American Academy of Pediatrics that all breast-fed infants receive a 400 IU supplement of vitamin D. Formula-fed babies receive adequate amounts in commercial formulas.

Folic Acid

Epidemiologic evidence has linked increasing folic acid (folate) intake with decreased incidence of neural tube defects such as spina bifida in offspring of mothers. More recently cleft lip and palate incidence has also been found to decrease when folate intake increases. Folate levels are low among adolescents, putting them at particular risk of birth defects when they have babies. The Food and Drug Administration approved fortification of cereals and breads with folate to decrease the population risk of related congenital anomalies.

SOURCES OF FOLATE

Bread and other products with flour
Yeast
Spinach, avocado, green leafy vegetables
Beans and peas
Liver
Fruits

FEEDING DISORDER OF INFANCY AND EARLY CHILDHOOD (FAILURE TO THRIVE)

Feeding disorder of infancy and early childhood, or failure to thrive (FTT), describes a syndrome in which infants or young children fail to eat enough food to be adequately nourished. This disorder accounts for 1% to 5% of pediatric hospitalizations in children under 1 year of age, and many more children are managed in community settings (Maggioni & Lifchitz, 1995).

Etiology and Pathophysiology

The cause of FTT can be organic, as in congenital acquired immunodeficiency syndrome (AIDS) (see Chapter 11), inborn errors of metabolism (see Chapter 22), neurologic disease, and esophageal reflux (see Chapter 17). However, most cases of FTT are nonorganic in origin. FTT resulting from nonorganic causes is called feeding disorder of infancy or early childhood.

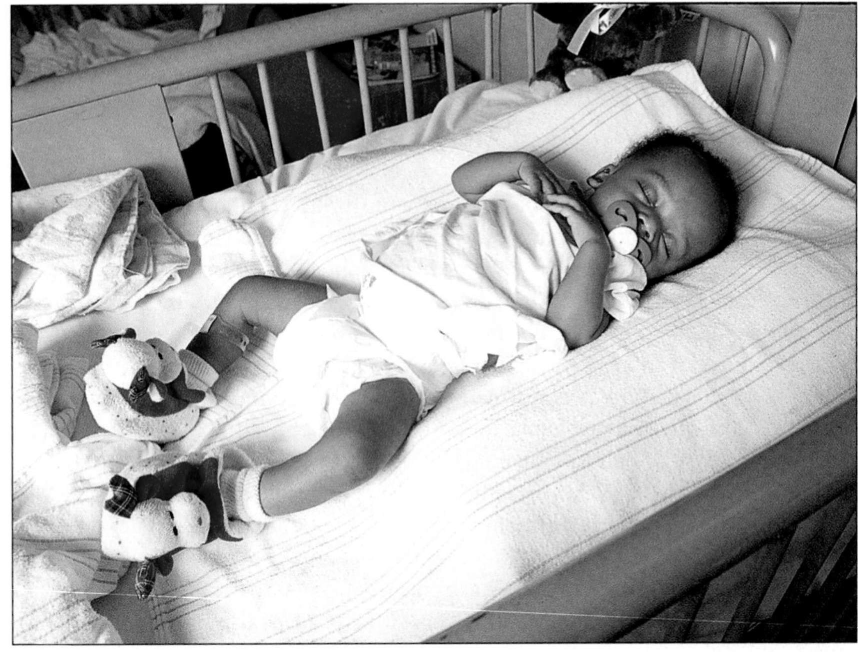

FIGURE 3-10 ◆
Infants with failure to thrive may not look severely malnourished, but they fall well below the expected weight and height norms for their age. This infant, who appears to be about 4 months old, is actually 8 months old. He has been hospitalized for failure to thrive.

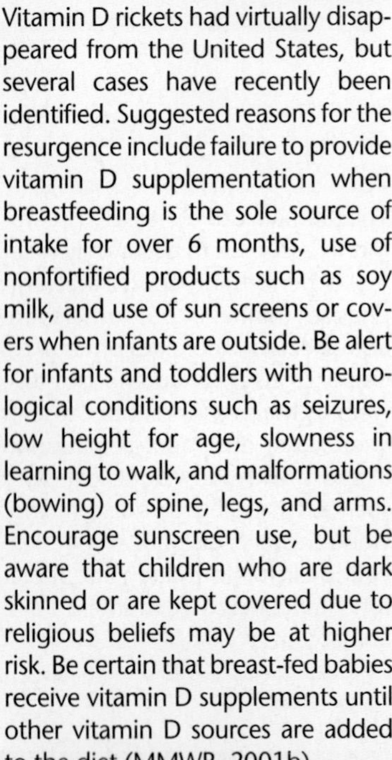

GROWTH & DEVELOPMENT

Vitamin D rickets had virtually disappeared from the United States, but several cases have recently been identified. Suggested reasons for the resurgence include failure to provide vitamin D supplementation when breastfeeding is the sole source of intake for over 6 months, use of nonfortified products such as soy milk, and use of sun screens or covers when infants are outside. Be alert for infants and toddlers with neurological conditions such as seizures, low height for age, slowness in learning to walk, and malformations (bowing) of spine, legs, and arms. Encourage sunscreen use, but be aware that children who are dark skinned or are kept covered due to religious beliefs may be at higher risk. Be certain that breast-fed babies receive vitamin D supplements until other vitamin D sources are added to the diet (MMWR, 2001b).

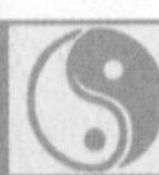

CULTURE

Each child should maintain a height and weight growth pattern similar to the population standard. Asian-American children may normally be below the 5th percentile on growth charts and not have an eating disorder. Suspect an eating disorder when the infant or child falls one standard deviation below his or her own curve and either fails to gain weight or loses weight over several months.

Infants and children whose parents or caretakers suffer from depression, substance abuse, mental retardation, or psychosis are at risk for this disorder. Parents may be socially and emotionally isolated, or may lack knowledge of infant nutritional and nurturing needs. A reciprocal interaction pattern may exist whereby the parent does not offer enough food or is not responsive to the infant's hunger cues, and the infant is irritable, not soothed, and does not give clear cues about hunger (Corrales & Utter, 1999).

Clinical Manifestations

The characteristics of this feeding disorder are persistent failure to eat adequately with no weight gain or with weight loss in a child under 6 years of age, which is not associated with other medical conditions or mental disorders, and is not caused by lack of or unavailability of food (American Psychiatric Association Working Group on Eating Disorders, 2000). Infants with feeding disorders refuse food, may have erratic sleep patterns, are irritable and difficult to soothe, and are often developmentally delayed (Figure 3-10 ◆).

Clinical Therapy

A thorough history and physical examination are needed to rule out any chronic physical illness. The infant or child may be hospitalized so that health care providers can establish a routine for feeding and sleeping. The goals of treatment are to provide adequate caloric and nutritional intake, promote normal growth and development, and assist parents in developing feeding routines and responding to the infant's cues of physical and psychologic hunger.

NURSING MANAGEMENT

Nursing Assessment and Diagnosis

Assessment of the child by the nurse is essential for establishing the best intervention plan. Accurate measurement of weight and height each time any child is seen for health care provides an important record of growth patterns over time. This helps in identification of the child with an eating disorder. The child's activity level, developmental milestones, and interaction patterns provide important information. When feeding the child, the nurse observes how the child indicates hunger or satiety, the ability of the child to be soothed, and general interaction patterns such as eye contact, touch, and cuddliness.

Parents are questioned about stresses in their lives; these may prevent appropriate interaction with the child. Asking about the pregnancy and delivery can elicit information about early disturbances in the child–parent relationship. Are there other children in the family and have eating problems occurred with them? Observe the child and parent behaviors while they feed the child; cues given by each person and interactional modes such as rocking, singing, talking, and body postures are important.

Following are nursing diagnoses pertinent for the young child with an eating disorder:

- *Altered nutrition: Less than body requirements,* related to inability to ingest proper amounts of food
- *Altered growth and development,* related to inadequate intake
- *Altered parenting,* related to lack of knowledge about nutritional needs
- *Fatigue,* related to malnutrition

Planning and Implementation

Nursing care centers on performing a thorough history and physical assessment, observing parent–child interactions during feeding times, and providing necessary teaching to enable parents to respond appropriately to their child's needs. The child is often hospitalized initially and evaluated for physical growth while staff members feed the child. Accurate weights, nutritional assessments, and developmental evaluation should be done to see if the child grows more normally. Additional diagnostic tests may be carried out at this time to rule out organic causes of the poor growth.

Once a diagnosis of nonorganic failure to thrive is confirmed, parents become involved in feeding the child. Observations of feeding and continued careful physical assessments are needed. The child's intake is carefully recorded at each meal or feeding. Parents are taught how to understand and respond to the child's cues of hunger and satiety. They are taught to hold, rock, and touch the infant during feedings, and to establish eye contact with infants and older children.

Upon discharge, referral to an agency that can continue monitoring of the home situation is needed. This provides an opportunity to observe feeding during a home visit and evaluate stresses and behavior patterns among family members. Frequent growth measurement and development must be ensured so the child is adequately nourished. Parents may need referral to community resources to help them manage stressful situations in their lives and to enhance their parenting skills.

Evaluation

Expected outcomes of nursing care include the following:

- Adequate growth and normal development of the infant is achieved.
- An improved parent–child relationship is established.

FOOD REACTIONS

Food reaction encompasses any adverse reaction to foods or substances ingested in foods. The foods that most commonly cause a reaction are fish, shellfish, nuts, eggs, soy, wheat, corn, strawberries, and cow milk products. Chemical additives, antibiotics, preservatives, and food colorings also can cause food sensitivity reactions.

Allergic reactions are a common cause of reaction. These IgE-mediated reactions are potentially systemic, characteristically rapid in onset, and may be manifest as swelling of the lips, mouth, uvula, or glottis, generalized urticaria, and, in severe reactions, anaphylaxis. Food allergies are the most common cause of anaphylaxis and are most prevalent in children with a family history of allergic reactions to various substances and foods (**atopy**). Children with allergies may experience urticaria of the lips, mouth, and throat upon eating certain foods (Pongracic, 2000). Allergic individuals need to be aware of "hidden" substances in prepared foods. For example, the child who is allergic to nuts will experience a reaction to a food if nut extracts are used in its preparation.

Delayed hypersensitivity reactions are attributed to digestive products of food and require a thorough diet history over several days to identify the offending food. These reactions are more difficult to diagnose, because the reaction can occur up to 24 hours after

CULTURE

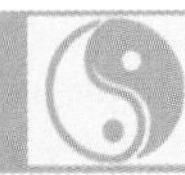

Some ethnic groups have a high incidence of lactose intolerance due to low amounts of the enzyme lactase in the gut. Although most members of the group have adequate amounts of lactase in childhood to drink milk products, by adulthood 70%–100% of some groups are lactose intolerant. African Americans, Native Americans, and Asians often have lactase deficiency which may begin to emerge during childhood. When intolerance to milk products develops, suggest alternative sources of calcium and other nutrients found in milk.

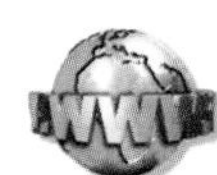

Food Allergy

COMMUNITY CARE

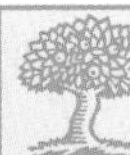

Children with food allergies should wear an alert tag and carry an emergency medication such as Epipen®. Nurses in schools and offices must instruct families, school teachers, and others about the child's allergy and what to do in case of accidental ingestion of the food product.

ingestion of the food. There may also be biphasic reactions that occur 1 to 30 hours after an initial anaphylaxis. Such reactions can be severe and life threatening.

Food intolerance refers to an abnormal physiologic response to a food and is not IgE-mediated. Examples include indigestion or flatulence upon eating certain foods, or a sweating reaction to some spices (Burks, 2000).

Cow milk may cause an allergy or food intolerance. An allergy leads to an IgE-mediated systemic reaction. An intolerance leads to a gastrointestinal response to milk proteins (diarrhea, vomiting, abdominal pain) as a result of lack of the enzyme lactase in the gastrointestinal tract. Infants have difficulty absorbing cow milk and, when ingesting it, may have vomiting and watery, blood-streaked, mucoid diarrhea. Even without such overt signs, they may have anemia induced by blood loss not noted by care providers.

Diagnostic tests to identify suspected food allergies include measurement of serum IgE levels, scratch tests, and the **radioallergosorbent test (RAST),** in which radioimmunoassay is used to measure IgE antibodies to specific allergens (see Chapter 11). A diet diary helps to track the date, types of foods eaten, and reaction(s), if any. Foods should be eaten singly for several days to determine whether they cause a reaction.

Treatment consists of eliminating the offending foods from the child's diet.

Nursing Management

Prevention is the first step. Instruct parents of infants to introduce new foods at a rate of not more than one new food every 3 to 5 days. If a sensitivity is noted, the causative food can be easily identified. Discuss any changes in diet or preparation of formula. Reassure parents that the child's symptoms will disappear when the offending foods are removed from the diet.

Be alert for skin, respiratory, and other characteristic manifestations of sensitivity or allergy. Many nurses are involved in administering and measuring skin prick tests for possible allergies.

Nursing care of a child with food allergies is primarily supportive. Help the family identify the offending foods. Explain to parents all tests, use of a food diary, and care of the child should a reaction occur. The child and school may need an Epipen® or other fast treatment of the allergic child. Emphasize the importance of reading food labels for hidden foods that can trigger an allergic reaction (Bock, Munoz-Furlong, & Sampson, 2001). The child with a true food allergy should wear a medical alert tag. Be sure that school personnel know about the allergy and to avoid giving the child the food product. Refer the family to the Food Allergy Network. Recognize that food allergies can be life threatening and plan carefully with the family, child care facilities, schools, and other community contacts to ensure avoidance of food and fast treatment if needed.

NUTRITIONAL SUPPORT

SPORTS NUTRITION

Regular physical activity should be encouraged for all children, with at least 30 minutes of activity recommended daily. However, during vigorous or prolonged exercise, or during hot weather, there may be special nutritional needs of child and adolescent athletes. A well-balanced diet, reflective of the food pyramid, is needed. A wide variety of fresh fruits and vegetables, grains, and complex carbohydrates usually provides for adequate caloric intake. When the child is hungry, extra calories should come from the food groups listed here, rather than from increased intake of fat. When the child or teen is very active, sports bars or drinks can provide the additional needed calories in a nutritionally balanced manner. As always, the height, weight, and BMI percentiles are the best assurance that the individual is growing adequately over time. Adequate energy to perform the sport as well as be attentive and productive at school and for other activities should also be considered.

Water should be increased during activity both to minimize chance of dehydration and to maximize performance. About 1 hour before vigorous exercise, the child should drink one or two glasses (8 to 16 ounces) of water, and should repeat the same amount of fluid just before the exercise begins. Young children may not feel thirsty, and should be encouraged to drink 4 to 6 ounces of fluid every 15 minutes during exercise (Trahms & Pipes,

1997). Water is usually the best replacement, but during extended exercise, sports drinks may be a good alternative for some of the fluid intake. Additional water is needed after activity. Weight loss of 1 pound indicates a loss of about 0.5 quart of fluid. Be sure the child takes in fluid to replace all losses.

Some common nutrients that may be deficient in all teens, but even more often in the athlete, are calcium and iron. The increased blood volume common in the well-conditioned person necessitates greater intake. Calcium foods such as milk products and dark green vegetables, and iron foods such as adequate meats and grains, can guard against deficiencies. Many adolescents believe that they need extra protein during athletic seasons; however, most Americans ingest adequate protein to meet even the increased needs of sports, although the vegetarian child or adolescent may need assistance to plan a diet with adequate protein.

Many teens ingest a wide variety of dietary supplements, believing that they enhance performance during sports. Most of the claims of these products are unproven, and their safety has not usually been investigated, especially in the young. Offer guidance and help the family and teen to investigate claims before choosing to use a product. Be sure they know doses, desired effects, and potential side effects of supplements. Be aware that some sports and coaches may encourage small size and dieting. Consider that children and adolescents in activities such as ballet, wrestling, track or running, and horse racing may have health risks associated with inconsistent or poor intake.

Some common amino acid nutritional supplements include creatine, carnitine, and glutamine. Although side effects to these substances are minimal, their possible enhancement of performance is temporary and outcomes of long-term use are unknown. Increasing overall intake to meet needs during high activity is a better alternative. Creatine has been studied more than most supplements; it is made by the body and is present in many protein sources. Supplemental creatine increases the creatine level in muscle and may help to increase performance in short bursts of activity, while not affecting endurance sports. The increase in muscle mass that can occur is actually due to water and will be lost quickly when the supplement is discontinued (Johnson, 2001). Some athletes obtain steroids, which can cause serious side effects, lead to endocrine disturbance, and interfere with growth; their use is also illegal in sports. Minerals such as chromium, iron, and calcium are used by some youths. The nurse can ask careful and sensitive questions, such as "Many athletes take supplements to aid in performance in sports. What supplements do you take or are you considering?" Information can then be provided to enhance the youth's understanding of nutrition and sports performance. Generally, intake of a balanced diet with adequate carbohydrate, protein, and fat will meet the needs of most athletes and lead to maximal sport performance.

HEALTH-RELATED CONDITIONS

Many health conditions influence the nutritional state of the child. Conversely, the child's nutritional state can influence the state of health. Figure 3-11 ◆ shows some common conditions that influence nutritional needs. These conditions are discussed in various chapters throughout the text. When you read about them, discuss with classmates how you will adjust normal nutritional assessment and teaching due to the presence of a health care concern. Which conditions influence absorption of nutrients? Which cause changes in nutritional intake requirements? Some children benefit from special dietary aids, such as eating utensils and cups that are easy to grasp. Therapists can evaluate and make recommendation about devices that can assist the child at meals.

GROWTH & DEVELOPMENT

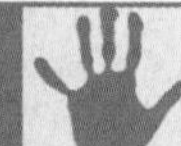

When a pregnant teen follows a vegetarian diet, additional help will be needed to encourage adequate nutrition (Rudys-Shapard, 2001). A 24-hour or 2-day diet record will help identify nutritional needs. Consider additional pregnancy needs for protein, iron, and calcium, and note that vitamin B_{12} is recommended as a supplement. Use the vegetarian food guide pyramid available through the American Dietetic Association.

VEGETARIANISM

Some families choose to eat vegetarian diets and can be helped and encouraged in their endeavors. Several variations of intake occur. **Vegetarians** eat no poultry, meat, or fish. Lacto-ovovegetarians eat eggs and dairy products, while lacto-vegetarians eat dairy products. In contrast, **vegans** are strict vegetarians and eat no animal products. When someone says they are vegetarian, it is best to ask specific questions about what they will and will not eat.

The vegetarian can be very healthy, but may need some additional help to ensure nutritional adequacy. Some common deficiencies are listed in Table 3-12. Completing a 24-hour

PATHOPHYSIOLOGY ILLUSTRATED

FIGURE 3-11 ◆
Conditions That Influence Nutritional Needs

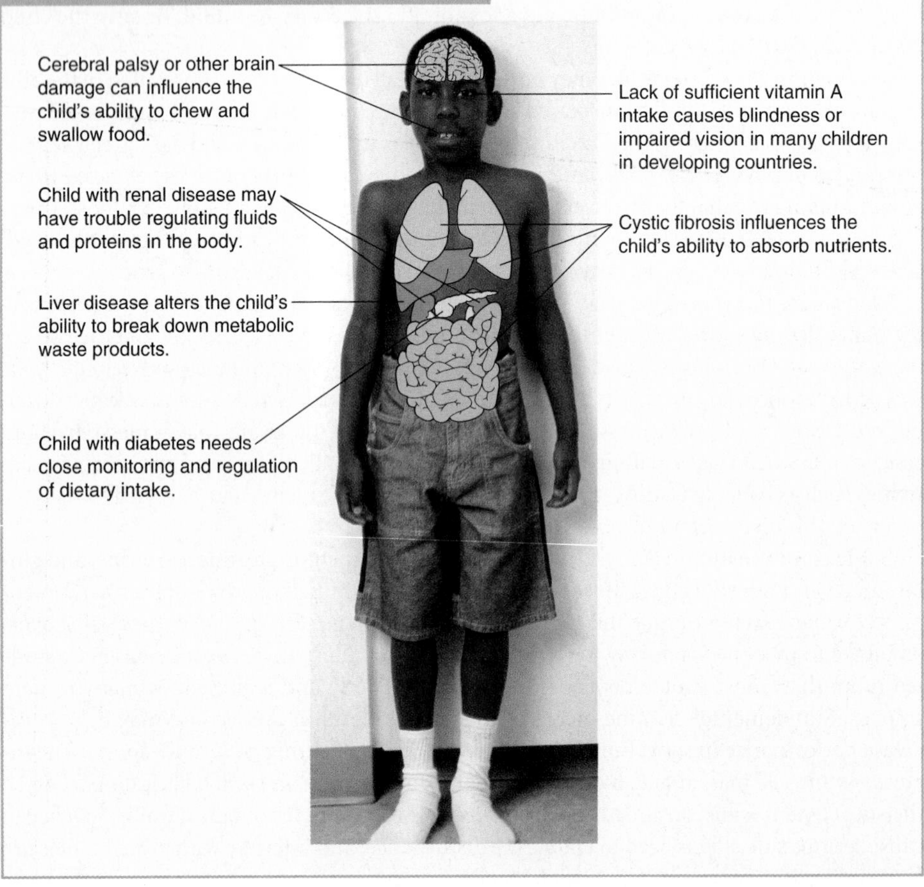

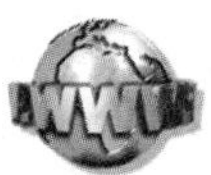
Alternative Food Pyramids

diet recall for the pregnant or lactating woman, and for vegetarian children, with analysis for RDAs, can be helpful. Be sure to routinely assess growth and other nutritional measures as well. Provide ideas of various foods to meet nutritional needs and perform other general nutritional teaching. When a vegetarian child is hospitalized, plan with the nutrition department and the child's family to meet intake needs.

ENTERAL THERAPY

Skill 11-3: Administering a Gavage Feeding

Enteral nutrition is a form of nutritional support provided when a child cannot take in enough food orally to sustain health. Since it is the closest form of nutritional support to the natural method of eating, it has the least untoward effects and greatest rate of success. Some of the children who use enteral therapy are those with cerebral palsy or other neurological conditions which lead to weakness of the throat and mouth, children with neoplasm or immune dysfunction, and those in acute states of recovery from accidents or illness. A tube can be inserted into the nasal opening and placed through the esophagus into the stomach; however, a tube that is surgically placed into the stomach through an abdominal opening, a jejunal or gastric tube, is preferred for long-term use. As long as the child can absorb and use

TABLE 3-12 Common Nutritional Deficiencies of Vegans

Vitamin D and calcium	Fiber	Protein
Vitamin B_{12}	Calories	Fat
Minerals: zinc, iron		

nutrients, enteral therapy can be successful in providing calories and essential nutrients. Commercially prepared formulas are available and specially formulated solutions can be adapted for children with specific dietary needs. The tube and entry site are cared for to prevent infection and skin breakdown. See Chapter 17 for suggestions on management of nursing care during tube feedings.

As Joey, from the opening scenario, continues to recover from his surgery, physical therapy will focus on increasing motor control of the head, neck, and hands. This will enable him to receive more feedings by mouth and less by the tube-feeding route. What information do Joey's family, teachers, and classmates need to provide safe feedings, effective intake, and adequate growth?

TOTAL PARENTERAL NUTRITION

Parenteral nutrition has made it possible to provide intravenous nutritional support for individuals who cannot eat or are unable to absorb nutrients from the intestinal tract in a normal manner and are at risk of severe malnutrition (Matarese & Gottschlich, 1998). Examples of children who benefit from this method of nutrition are those with congenital malformation of the gastrointestinal tract, head injury, severe burns, or for support after bone marrow transplant, sepsis, or other critical conditions. A catheter is inserted so that a sterile nutrition solution is infused directly into the bloodstream. A central venous catheter is inserted to promote safe infusion. Fluids usually contain glucose; electrolytes such as sodium, potassium, calcium, magnesium, phosphate, and chloride; vitamins; and proteins. Lipid emulsions are another type of TPN used in some children. Meticulous care is needed, whether in the hospital or at home, to ensure safe TPN infusion and treatment. The nurse performs initial assessment and ongoing evaluation and monitoring of treatment, and administers the solutions in hospital or other settings (Skipper, 1998). See the protocols for TPN management in the Skills Manual.

LAW & ETHICS

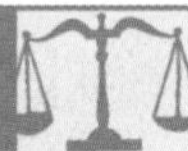

Total parenteral nutrition (TPN) is expensive, complicated to administer, and can have adverse side effects. How are decisions made about when to institute this type of nutritional support? Should it be used in all situations? If someone is unconscious or dying, is this method of nutrition started? These ethical issues are often difficult and have no easy answers. Nurses usually administer TPN in the home and hospital and may feel stressed if families, the patient, and other health professionals do not agree on its use (Breier, 2000). Guidelines are available to help health care professionals make decisions about treatments, and nurses should seek the guidance of ethics professionals in their agencies when needed.

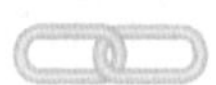

Skill 8-7: Administering Total Parenteral Nutrition

Chapter Highlights

- Adequate nutritional intake is necessary for the normal growth and development of children.
- Children with medical or psychosocial conditions require additional nutritional support.
- Dietary intake patterns vary throughout childhood as the child grows, is able to metabolize different types of food, and gains greater gross and fine motor control.
- Nutritional assessment is an essential part of nursing care and may involve approaches such as growth measurement and intake records.
- Common nutritional concerns in childhood include hunger, overweight, foodborne illness, and dietary deficiencies.
- The child with feeding disorder of infancy and childhood requires comprehensive assessment and ongoing management to foster parent–child interaction and adequate nutritional intake.
- Children engaging in sports and those who eat vegetarian diets may need guidance to meet nutritional needs.
- Alternative feeding methods such as enteral and parenteral feedings are required by some children.

EXPLORE MediaLink

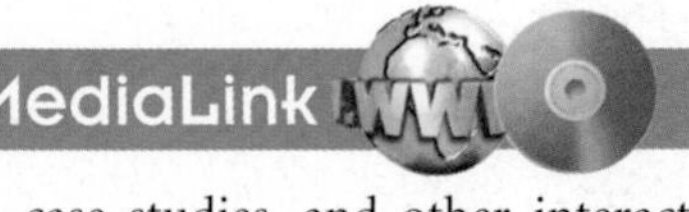

- NCLEX review, case studies, and other interactive resources for this chapter can be found on the Companion Website at **http://www.prenhall.com/ball.** Click on Chapter 3 to select the activities for this chapter.
- For animations, more NCLEX review questions, and an audio glossary, access the accompanying CD-ROM in this textbook.

References

1. Adair, L. S., & Gordon-Larsen, P. (2001). Maturational timing and overweight prevalence in U.S. adolescent girls. *American Journal of Public Health, 91,* 642–644.
2. American Academy of Pediatrics Committee on Nutrition. (2001). The use and misuse of fruit juice in pediatrics. *Pediatrics, 107,* 1210–1213.
3. American Psychiatric Association Working Group on Eating Disorders. (2000). Practice guidelines for the treatment of patients with eating disorders. *American Journal of Psychiatry, 157,* 1–39.
4. Bessler, S. (1999). Nutritional assessment. In P. Q. Samour, K. K. Helm, & C. E. Lang, *Handbook of pediatric nutrition* (2nd ed., pp. 17–42). Gaithersburg, MD: Aspen.
5. Bock, S. A., Munoz-Furlong, A., & Sampson, H. A. (2001). Fatalities due to anaphylactic reactions to foods. *Journal of Allergy and Clinical Immunology, 107,* 191–193.
6. Boyle, M. A., & Morris, D. H. (1999). *Community nutrition in action,* (2nd ed.). Belmont, CA: West/Wadsworth.
7. Breier, S. J. (2000). Ethics and total parenteral nutrition. *Journal of Intravenous Nursing, 23,* 52–57.
8. Burks, W. (2000). Diagnosis of allergic reactions to food. *Pediatric Annals, 29,* 744–752.
9. Children's Defense Fund. (2000). *The state of America's children.* Washington, DC: Author.
10. Committee on Nutrition. (1998). *Pediatric nutrition handbook* (4th ed.). Elk Grove Village, IL: American Academy of Pediatrics.
11. Corrales, K. M., & Utter, S. L. (1999). Failure to thrive. In P. Q. Samour, K. K. Helm, & C. E. Lang, *Handbook of pediatric nutrition* (2nd ed., pp. 395–412). Gaithersburg, MD: Aspen.
12. Federal Interagency Forum on Child and Family Statistics. (2000). *America's children: Key national indicators of well-being, 2000.* Washington, DC: Author.
13. Food and Nutrition Board. (2001). *Dietary reference intakes.* Washington DC: National Academy Press.
14. Gortmaker, S. L., Must, A., Sobol, A. M., Peterson, K., Colditz, G. A., & Dietz, W. H. (1996). Television viewing as a cause of increasing obesity among children in the United States. *Archives of Pediatric and Adolescent Medicine, 150,* 356–362.
15. Hanson, L. A., Dahlman-Hoglund, A., Lundin, S., Karllson, M., Dahlgren, U., Ahlstedt, S., & Telemo, E. (1997). Early determinants of immunocompetence. *Nutrition Reviews, 55,* S12–S17.
16. Healthy People 2010. (2000). *Healthy people 2010.* Washington, DC: U.S. Department of Health and Human Services. Retrieved at April 13, 2001 *http://www.health.gov/healthypeople/document.html.*
17. Hensrud, D. D. (1999). Nutrition screening and assessment. *Medical Clinics of North America, 83,* 1525–1546.
18. Johnson, W. A. (2001). Nutritional supplements: What you need to know. *Contemporary Pediatrics, 18*(7), 63–74.
19. Kramer, M. S. (2001). Promotion of breastfeeding intervention trial (PROBIT). *Journal of the American Medical Association, 285,* 413–420.
20. Krauss, R. M., Eckel, R. H., Howard, G., Appel, L. J., Daniels, S. R., Deckelbaum, R. J., Erdman, J. W., Kris-Etherton, P., Boldberg, I. J., Kotchen, T. A., Lichtenstein, A. H., Mitch, W. E., Mullis, R., Robinson, K., Wylie-Rosett, J., St. Jeor, S., Suttie, J., Tribble, D. L., & Bazzarre, T. L. (2001). AHA scientific statement: AHA dietary guideline. *Journal of Nutrition, 131,* 132–146.
21. Lee, R. D., & Nieman, D. C. (1996). *Nutrition assessment* (2nd ed.). Boston: McGraw-Hill.
22. Maggioni, A., & Lifchitz, F. (1995). Nutritional management of failure to thrive. *Pediatric Clinics of North America, 42,* 791–810.
23. Matarese, L. E., & Gottschlich, M. M. (1998). *Contemporary nutrition support practice.* Philadelphia: W. B. Saunders.
24. MMWR. (2001a). Preliminary FoodNet data on the incidence of foodborne illnesses. *Morbidity and Mortality Weekly Report, 50,* 241–246.
25. MMWR. (2001b). Severe malnutrition among young children—Georgia, January 1997 to June 1999. *Morbidity and Mortality Weekly Report, 50,* 224–227.
26. National Cholesterol Education Program. (1991). *Report of the expert panel on blood cholesterol levels in children and adolescents.* Washington, DC: U.S. Department of Health and Human Services.
27. Pongracic, J. A. (2000). Is it food allergy? *Contemporary Pediatrics, 17,* 101–112, 117–121.
28. Rudys-Shapard, R. (2001). Adolescent, pregnant, and vegetarian: A turbulent time for a teen. *Journal of Pediatric Health Care, 15,* 35–40.
29. Skipper, A. (1998). *Dietitian's handbook of enteral and parenteral nutrition (2nd ed.).* Gaithersburg, MD: Aspen.
30. Trahms, C. M., & Pipes, P. L. (1997). *Nutrition in infancy and childhood (6th ed.).* New York: WCB/McGraw-Hill.
31. Troiano, R. P., & Flegal, K. M. (1998). Overweight children and adolescents: Description, epidemiology, and demographics. *Pediatrics, 101* (Suppl. 3), 497–504.
32. Troiano, R. P., Flegal, K. M., Kuczmarski, R. J., Campbell, S. M., & Johnson, C. L. (1995). Overweight prevalence and trends for children and adolescents. *Archives of Pediatric and Adolescent Medicine, 149,* 1085–1091.
33. Walter, T., Olivares, M., Pizarro, F., & Munoz, C. (1997). Iron, anemia, and infection. *Nutrition Reviews, 55,* 111–124.
34. Wauben, I. P., & Wainwright, P. E. (1999). The influence of neonatal nutrition on behavioral development: A critical appraisal. *Nutrition Reviews, 57,* 35–44.
35. Whitaker, R., Wright, J. A., Pepe, M. S., Seidel, K. D., & Dietz, W. H. (1997). Predicting obesity in young adulthood from childhood and parental obesity. *New England Journal of Medicine, 337,* 869–873.
36. Zizza, C., Siega-Riz, A. M., & Popkin, B. M. (2001). Significant increase in young children's snacking between 1977–1978 and 1994–1996 represents a cause for concern! *Preventive Medicine, 32,* 303–310.

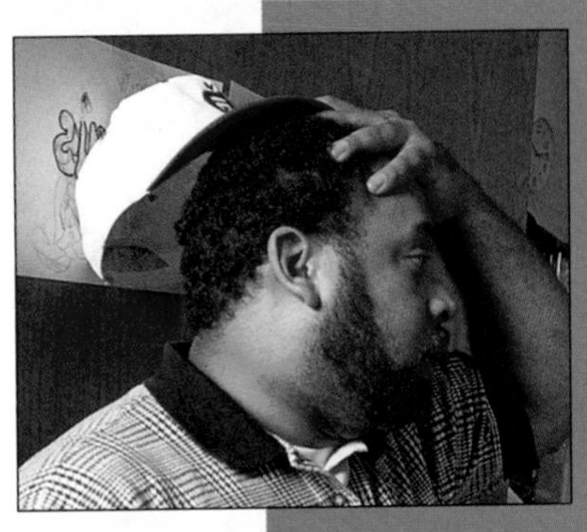

"I WAS SCARED WHEN WE BROUGHT LATOYA TO THE HOSPITAL. SHE LOOKED HELPLESS, AFRAID, AND SICK. THE NURSES AND DOCTORS TOOK OVER WHEN WE GOT TO THE HOSPITAL, AND I FELT BETTER BECAUSE THEY SEEMED TO KNOW WHAT TO DO."

Latoya, 6 months old, is brought by her mother and father to the emergency room. She is an emergency admission from the local pediatrician's office with a diagnosis of bronchiolitis. As Latoya's nurse, you are responsible for assessing her condition after she arrives on the pediatric nursing unit.

What information do you look for, and in what order do you gather this information? What techniques can you use to obtain information about Latoya's condition? How do you organize your findings to make sense of them?

The patient history and physical examination provide a structure and a sequence for collecting and analyzing relevant **assessment** data. The initial physical examination findings provide the baseline for monitoring Latoya's response to treatment. Analysis of the assessment data also enables you to form nursing diagnoses and to develop a nursing care plan to direct the nursing care that Latoya will receive.

CHAPTER

4

PEDIATRIC ASSESSMENT

KEY TERMS

assessment The process of collecting information about a child and family to develop the nursing diagnoses. The assessment process includes the patient history, physical examination, and analysis of the collected data to identify relevant information.

auscultation The technique of listening to sounds produced by the airway, lungs, stomach, heart, and blood vessels to identify their characteristics. Auscultation is usually performed with the stethoscope to enhance the sounds heard.

clinical judgment Analyzing and synthesizing data from the patient history, physical examination, screening tests, and laboratory studies to make decisions about the child's health problems. This is also called diagnostic reasoning.

effective communication Information exchanged among the nurse, parent, and child that is clearly understood by all persons involved in the conversation.

inspection The technique of purposeful observation by carefully looking at the characteristics of the child's physical features and behaviors. Physical feature characteristics include size, shape, color, movement, position, and location.

nonverbal behavior The use of facial expression, eye contact, touch, posture, gestures, and body movements that communicate feelings during a conversation.

palpation The technique of touch to identify characteristics of the skin, internal organs, and masses. Characteristics include texture, moistness, tenderness, temperature, position, shape, consistency, and mobility of masses and organs.

percussion The technique of striking the surface of the body, either directly or indirectly, to set up vibrations that reveal the density of underlying tissues and borders of internal organs.

range of motion The direction and extent to which a particular joint is capable of moving, either independently or with assistance.

review of systems A comprehensive interview to identify and record the parent's or child's health concerns and health problems by body system; provides an overview of the child's health status.

MediaLink

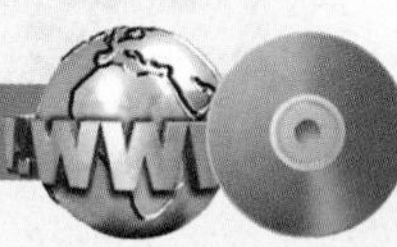

http://www.prenhall.com/ball

Resources for this chapter can be found on the CD-ROM accompanying this textbook, and on the Companion Website at http://www.prenhall.com/ball. Click on Chapter 4 to select the activities for this chapter.

CD-ROM

Animation
- Otoscope Examination
- Mouth and Throat Examination

Audio Glossary

NCLEX Review

COMPANION WEBSITE

Web Links

NCLEX Review

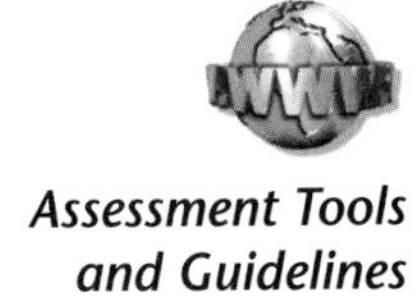

Assessment Tools and Guidelines

Do examination techniques need to vary for children of different ages? How does the nurse gain cooperation for the examination from infants and toddlers? This chapter answers these questions and provides an overview of pediatric assessment, including history taking and examination techniques geared to the unique needs of pediatric patients. Strategies for obtaining the child's history are presented first. The remainder of the chapter then outlines a systematic process for physical examination of the child.

ANATOMIC AND PHYSIOLOGIC CHARACTERISTICS OF CHILDREN

It is readily apparent that infants and children are smaller than adults. Significant differences in physiology also normally exist between children and adults. Knowledge of pediatric anatomic and physiologic differences will aid in recognizing normal variations found during the physical examination. It also assists with understanding the different physiologic responses children have to illness and injury. Figure 4-1 ◆ provides an overview of important anatomic and physiologic differences between children and adults.

AS THEY GROW

Anatomic & Physiologic Characteristics of Children

FIGURE 4-1 ◆

Children are not just small adults. There are important anatomic and physiologic differences between children and adults that will change based on a child's growth and development. Can you identify which of these differences are of greatest concern for the hospitalized child and why?

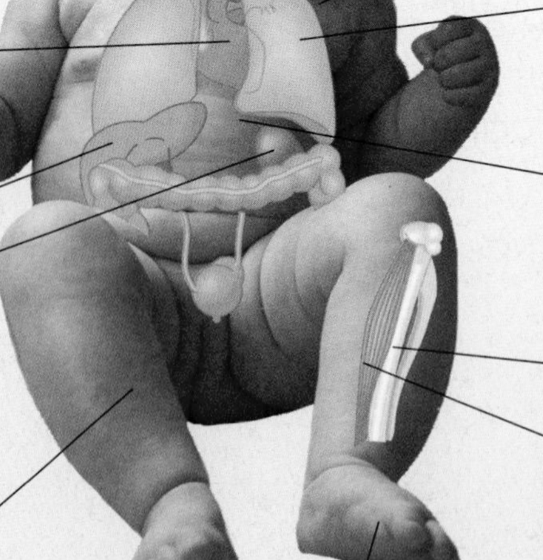

OBTAINING THE CHILD'S HISTORY

COMMUNICATION STRATEGIES

What makes communication effective? What does it mean when a parent or caretaker will not look you in the eye when speaking with you? What types of cues indicate that a parent may be withholding historical information?

The health history interview is a personal conversation with a parent, caretaker, or adolescent during which private concerns and feelings are shared. Try to ensure that this exchange of information with the parent or the child is clearly understood by both parties, that it is an **effective communication.** Effective communication is difficult to accomplish because parents and children often do not correctly interpret what the nurse says, just as you may not understand completely what the parent or child says. People's interpretation of information is based on their life experiences, culture, and education.

Strategies to Build a Rapport with the Family and Child

As you begin the history, make sure the parents understand the purpose of the interview and that the information will be used appropriately. To develop rapport, demonstrate your interest in and concern for the child and family during the interview. This rapport forms the foundation for the collaborative relationship between the nurse and parent that will provide the best nursing care for the child. The following strategies help to establish rapport with the child's family during the nursing history.

- *Introduce yourself* (your name, title or position, and your role in caring for the child). To demonstrate respect, ask all family members present what name they prefer you to use when talking with them.
- *Explain the purpose of the interview* and why the nursing history is different from the information collected from other health professionals. For example, "The nurses will use this information to plan nursing care best suited for your child."
- *Provide privacy* and remove as many distractions as possible during the interview. If the patient's room does not offer privacy, attempt to find a vacant patient room or lounge.
- *Direct the focus of the interview* with open-ended questions. Use close-ended questions or directing statements to clarify information. Open-ended questions are useful to initiate the interview, develop a rapport, and understand the parent's perceptions of the child's problem; for example, "Tell me what problems led to Roberto's admission to the hospital." Close-ended questions are used to obtain detailed information; for example, "How high was Tommy's fever this morning?"
- *Ask one question at a time* so that the parent or child understands what piece of information you want and so that you know which question the parent is answering. "Does any member of your family have diabetes, heart disease, or sickle-cell anemia?" is a multiple question. Ask about each disease separately to ensure the most accurate response.
- *Involve the child in the interview* by asking age-appropriate questions. Young children can be asked, "What is your doll's name?" or "Where does it hurt?" Demonstrating an interest in the child initiates development of rapport with both child and parents. Ask older children and teens questions about their illness or injury. Offer them an opportunity to privately discuss their major concerns when their parents are not present.
- *Be honest* with the child when answering questions or when giving information about what will happen. Children need to learn that they can trust you.
- *Choose the language style* that is best understood by the parent and child. Commonly used phrases can have different meanings to persons in various regions of the country or to different ethnic groups. To improve communication, request frequent feedback from the parents or child to ensure that their interpretation of phrases is accurate.
- *Use an interpreter to improve communication* when you are not fluent in the family's primary language (Figure 4-2 ◆).

> **CULTURE** 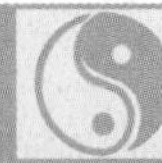
>
> Some cultural groups, particularly Asians, try to anticipate the answers you want to hear, or they say yes even if they do not understand the question. This practice is done in an effort to please you or as an expression of politeness. Remember to phrase your questions in a neutral manner.

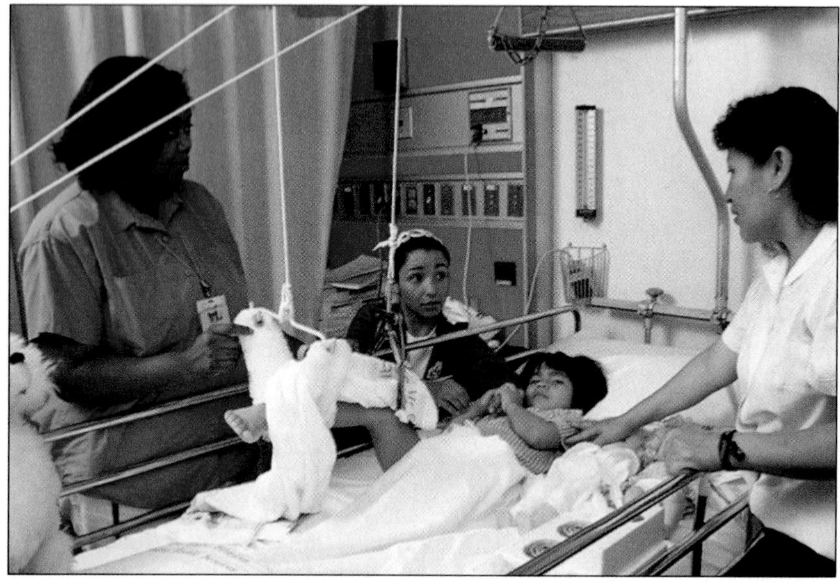

FIGURE 4-2 ◆
Most hospitals have designated interpreters that you should use. If not, find a professional interpreter whom you have identified beforehand and who knows medical terms and the cultural norms of the family. The interpreter (*center*) should be positioned to improve communication. Maintain eye contact with the parent or patient, not the interpreter. To ensure confidentiality of information for parents, avoid using a family member for history taking.

Careful Listening

Complete attention is necessary to "hear" and accurately interpret information the parents and child give during the nursing history. Carefully *listen* to the information provided by the parent, as well as how it is expressed, and *observe behavior* during the interaction.

- Does the parent hesitate or avoid answering certain questions?
- Pay attention to the parent's attitude or tone of voice when the child's problems are discussed. Determine if it is consistent with the seriousness of the child's problem. The tone of voice can reveal anxiety, anger, or lack of concern.
- Be alert to any underlying themes. For example, the parent who talks about the child's diagnosis, but repeatedly refers to the impact of the illness on the family's finances or on meeting the needs of other family members, is requesting that these issues be addressed.
- Observe the parent's **nonverbal behavior** (posture, gestures, body movements, eye contact, and facial expression) for consistency with the words and tone of voice used. Is the parent interested in and appropriately concerned about the child's condition? Behaviors such as sitting up straight, making eye contact, and appearing apprehensive reflect appropriate concern for the child. Physical withdrawal, failure to make eye contact, or a happy expression could be inconsistent with the child's serious condition.

CULTURE 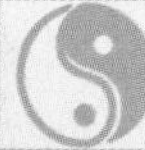

Eye contact with the interviewer may be avoided by many cultural groups (Asian, Native American, and Middle Eastern patients) because it is considered impolite, aggressive, or a sign of disrespect (Spector, 2000).

Subtle nonverbal and verbal cues often indicate that the parent has not provided complete information about the child's problem. Observe for behaviors such as avoiding eye contact, change in voice pitch, or hesitation when responding to a question. Being supportive and asking clarifying questions encourage further description or the expression of information that is difficult for the parent or child to share; for example, "It sounds like that was a very difficult experience. How did Latasha react?"

Encourage parents to share information, even if it is private or sensitive, especially when it influences nursing care planning. Often parents avoid sharing some information because they want to make a good impression, or they do not understand the value of the missing information. If a hesitation to share information is detected, briefly explain why the question was asked, for example, to make their child's hospital experience more pleasant or to begin planning for the child's discharge and home care.

In some cases, the parent becomes too agitated, upset, or angry to continue responding to questions. When the information is not needed immediately, move on to another portion of the history to determine whether the parent is able to respond to other questions. Depending on the emotional status of the parent, it may be more appropriate to collect the remaining historical data at a later time.

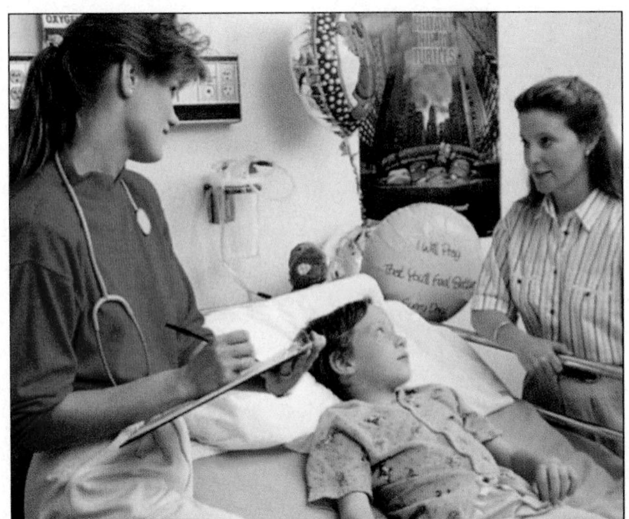

FIGURE 4-3 ◆
While you are collecting physiologic data you should be observing patient behavior.

DATA TO BE COLLECTED

The child's health, medical, and personal-social history is collected and organized to plan the child's nursing care. A modification of the Burns Classification System is the data-collection framework selected for this text (Burns, 1992; Byrnes, 1996). Physiologic, psychosocial, and developmental data are organized to help develop the nursing diagnoses and the nursing care plan. Be alert for nonverbal cues (Figure 4-3 ◆).

Patient Information

Obtain the child's name and nickname, age, sex, and ethnic origin. The child's birth date, race, religion, address, and phone number can be obtained from the admission form. Ask the parent for an emergency contact address and phone number, as well as a work phone number. The person providing the patient history and that person's relationship to the patient are recorded.

Physiologic Data

Information about the child's health problems and diseases is collected chronologically in a format similar to the traditional medical history.

- The *chief complaint* is the child's primary problem or reason for hospital admission or visit to a health care setting, stated in the parent's or child's exact words.
- The *history of the present illness or injury* is a detailed description of the current health problem. This includes the onset and sequence of events, characteristics of and changes in symptoms over time, influencing factors, and the current status of the problem. Each problem is described separately. Table 4-1 lists the specific data to be collected about each illness and injury.
- The *past history* is a more detailed description of the child's prior health problems. It includes the birth history and all major past illnesses and injuries. A detailed and complete birth history is obtained when the child's present problem may be related to the birth history (Table 4-2). Record the child's age at the time of each illness, injury, related surgery, or hospitalization. Obtain information about each specific diagnosis, treatment, outcome, complication or residual problem, and the child's reaction to the event (Table 4-3).
- The *current health status* is a detailed description of the child's typical health status. Obtain information about allergies, current medications, immunization status, activities and exercise, sleep patterns, nutrition, safety measures used, and health maintenance care (Table 4-4).
- The ***review of systems*** provides a comprehensive overview of the child's health. This is an opportunity to identify additional signs and symptoms associated with the child's admission problem or to identify other problems that have no direct relationship to

TABLE 4-1 History of Present Illness or Injury

CHARACTERISTIC	DEFINING VARIABLES
Onset	Sudden or gradual, previous episodes, date and time began
Type of symptom	Pain, itching, cough, vomiting, runny nose, diarrhea, rash, etc.
Location	Generalized or localized—anatomically precise
Duration	Continuous or episodic, length of episodes
Severity	Effect on daily activities, e.g., interrupted sleep, decreased appetite, incapacitation
Influencing factors	What relieves or aggravates symptoms, what precipitated the problem, recent exposure to infection or allergen
Past evaluation for the problem	Laboratory studies, physician's office or hospital where done, results of past examinations
Previous and current treatment	Prescribed and over-the-counter drugs used, other measures tried (heat, ice, rest), response to treatments

TABLE 4-2 Birth History

PRENATAL
Mother's age, health during pregnancy, prenatal care, weight gained, special diet, expected date of delivery Details of illnesses, x-ray findings, hospitalizations, medications, complications, and timing during pregnancy Prior obstetric history
ANTENATAL—DESCRIPTION OF DELIVERY
Site of delivery (hospital, home, birthing center) Labor induced or spontaneous Vaginal or cesarean section, forceps or suction used, vertex or breech position Single or multiple birth
CONDITION OF BABY AT BIRTH
Weight, Apgar score, cried immediately Need for incubator, oxygen, suctioning, ventilator Any abnormalities detected, meconium staining
POSTNATAL
Difficulties in the nursery—feeding, respiratory difficulties, jaundice, cyanosis, rashes Length of hospital stay, special nursery, home with mother Breast or bottle fed, weight gained in hospital Medical care needed in first week—admission to hospital

TABLE 4-3 Past Illnesses and Injuries

Illnesses	Major illnesses including common communicable diseases
Injuries	Major injuries, their mechanism (cause) and severity
Surgeries	Specific types, day surgery or hospitalized
Hospitalizations	Reasons and length of hospitalizations
Transfusions	Circumstances, reactions

the child's significant health problem but could be factors complicating nursing care or home care. For example, asking about any urinary problems may reveal that a child still wets the bed at 7 years of age, although the admission is for a femur fracture. The nurse would then need to consider how bedwetting might cause problems with the spica cast. For each problem, obtain the treatment, outcomes, residual problems, and age at time of onset. Data-collection guidelines are given in Table 4-5.

- The *familial and hereditary diseases* summarize the major familial and hereditary diseases in three generations of family members, including the parents, grandparents, aunts, uncles, cousins, child, and siblings. Collect information about the health status of each parent. Record information in either a pedigree or a narrative format. Specific diseases the nurse inquires about are listed in Table 4-6.

Psychosocial Data

Obtain information about family composition to establish a socioeconomic and sociologic context within which to plan the child's care in the hospital and at home.

- Family composition, including family members living in the home, their relationship to the child, marital status of parents or other family structure, and persons participating in the care of the child

TABLE 4-4 Current Health Status

HEALTH MAINTENANCE
Name of primary health care provider; last visit Name of dentist; last visit Other health care providers
ALLERGIES
To food, medication, animals, insect bites, environment, etc. Type of reaction
IMMUNIZATIONS
Types, dates received, unexpected reactions
SAFETY MEASURES USED
Car restraint system Window guards Medication storage Sports protective gear Smoke detectors Bicycle helmet Firearm storage Other
SOCIOCULTURAL FACTORS
Environment Family financial status Health insurance
ACTIVITIES AND EXERCISE
Physical mobility Play and/or sports activities Limitations and adaptive equipment
NUTRITION
Formula or breast fed When solid foods introduced Eating and snacking habits Variety of foods consumed, junk foods eaten Appetite
SLEEP
Length and timing of naps and nighttime sleep Nightmares or night terrors Other sleep disturbances Where the child sleeps Bedtime rituals

TABLE 4-5 Review of Systems

BODY SYSTEMS	EXAMPLES OF PROBLEMS TO IDENTIFY
General	General growth pattern, overall health status, ability to keep up with other children or tires easily with feeding or activity, fever, sleep patterns Allergies, type of reaction (hives, rash, respiratory difficulty, swelling, nausea), seasonal or with each exposure
Skin and lymph	Rashes, dry skin, itching, changes in skin color or texture, tendency for bruising, swollen or tender lymph glands
Hair and nails	Hair loss, changes in color or texture, use of dye or chemicals on hair Abnormalities of nail growth or color
Head	Headaches, head injuries
Eyes	Vision problems, squinting, crossed eyes, lazy eye, wears glasses, eye infections, redness, tearing, burning, rubbing, swelling eyelids
Ears	Ear infections, frequent discharge from ears, or tubes in ears Hearing loss (no response to loud noises or questions, inattentiveness, was hearing test ever done?)
Nose and sinuses	Nosebleeds, nasal congestion, colds with runny nose, sinus pain or infections Nasal obstruction, difficulty breathing, snoring at night
Mouth and throat	Mouth breathing, difficulty swallowing, sore throats, strep infections Tooth eruption, cavities, braces Voice change, hoarseness, speech problems
Cardiac and hematologic	Heart murmur, anemia, hypertension, cyanosis, edema, rheumatic fever, chest pain
Chest and respiratory	Trouble breathing, choking episodes, cough, wheezing, cyanosis, exposure to tuberculosis, other infections
Gastrointestinal	Bowel movements, frequency, color, regularity, consistency, discomfort, constipation or diarrhea, abdominal pain, bleeding from rectum, flatulence Nausea or vomiting, appetite
Urinary	Frequency, urgency, dysuria, dribbling, enuresis, strength of urinary stream Toilet trained—age when day and night dryness attained
Reproductive	For pubescent children
Female	Menses onset, amount, duration, frequency, discomfort, problems; vaginal discharge, breast development
Male	Puberty onset, emissions, erections, pain or discharge from penis, swelling or pain in testicles
Both	Sexual activity, use of contraception, sexually transmitted diseases
Musculoskeletal	Weakness, clumsiness, poor coordination, balance, tremors, abnormal gait, painful muscles or joints, swelling or redness of joints, fractures
Neurologic	Seizures, fainting spells, dizziness, numbness, learning problems, attention span, hyperactivity, memory problems

- Household members employed, family income, and financial resources or agencies used such as health insurance, food stamps, or Temporary Assistance for Needy Families
- Description of the housing and home environment (atmosphere, emotional stresses, family activities); safe play area; use of city or well water; and availability of electricity, heat, and refrigeration

TABLE 4-6 Familial or Hereditary Diseases

Infectious diseases	Tuberculosis, HIV, or hepatitis
Heart disease	Heart defects, myocardial infarctions, hypertension, hyperlipidemia
Allergic disorders	Eczema, hay fever, or asthma
Eye disorders	Glaucoma, cataracts, vision loss
Ear disorders	Hearing loss
Hematologic disorders	Sickle-cell anemia, thalassemia, G6PD deficiency, leukemia
Lung disorders	Cystic fibrosis
Cancer	Type, early age of onset
Endocrine disorders	Diabetes mellitus
Mental disorders	Mental retardation, epilepsy, Huntington chorea, psychiatric disorders
Musculoskeletal disorders	Arthritis, muscular dystrophy
Gastrointestinal disorders	Ulcers, colitis, kidney disease
Repeated miscarriages, stillbirths, or sudden childhood deaths	
Learning problems	

TABLE 4-7 Daily Living Patterns

ROLE RELATIONSHIPS
Family relationships/alterations in family process Peer relationships Social interactions: e.g., childcare, preschool, school, neighborhood Communication
SELF-PERCEPTION/SELF-CONCEPT
Personal identity and role identity Self-esteem Body image/nonvisible disorder
COPING/STRESS TOLERANCE
Temperament Coping behaviors Discipline Any substance abuse
VALUES AND BELIEFS
Religion Personal values/beliefs
HOME CARE PROVIDED FOR CHILD'S CONDITION
Resources needed/available Knowledge and skills of parents, other family members Respite care available
SENSORY/PERCEPTUAL PROBLEMS
Adaptations to daily living for any sensory loss (vision, hearing, cognitive, or motor)

Note: Adapted from Burns, C. (1992). A new assessment model and tool for pediatric nurse practitioners. *Journal of Pediatric Health Care, 6*, 73–81.

- School or childcare arrangements; description of the neighborhood, including playgrounds, transportation, and proximity to stores
- Changes in family or lifestyle since last seen; number of times the family has moved; how the child and family members have coped with the changes

Information about daily routines, psychosocial data, and other living patterns forms the basis for many nursing diagnoses and development of an individualized nursing care plan. Collection of information should focus on issues that have an impact on the quality of daily living, even if some data seem to overlap with disease data (Table 4-7). The psychosocial history for adolescents should focus on critical areas in their lives (home environment, employment and education, activities, drugs, sexual activity/sexuality, suicide and depression, and safety) that may contribute to a less-than-optimal environment for normal growth and development (Goldenring & Cohen, 1988). Possible screening questions can be found in Table 4-8.

EXAMINATION TECHNIQUES

- **inspection** Purposeful observation of the child's physical features and behaviors. Physical feature characteristics include size, shape, color, movement, position, and location.
- **palpation** Use of touch to identify characteristics of the skin, internal organs, and masses. Characteristics include texture, moistness, tenderness, temperature, position, shape, consistency, and mobility of masses and organs.
- **auscultation** Listening to sounds produced by the airway, lungs, stomach, heart, and blood vessels to identify their characteristics. Auscultation is usually performed with a stethoscope to enhance the sounds heard.
- **percussion** Striking the surface of the body, either directly or indirectly, to set up vibrations that reveal the density of underlying tissues and borders of internal organs.

TABLE 4-8 Adolescent Psychosocial Assessment Using the HEADSSS Screening Tool

HOME ENVIRONMENT

- With whom do you live?
- Have there been any recent changes in your living situation?
- How are things between your parents (or parent and significant other adult) at home?
- Are your parents employed?

EMPLOYMENT AND EDUCATION

- Are you currently in school?
- What are your favorite subjects?
- How are your school grades?
- Have you ever been expelled from school or missed many days?
- Do your friends attend school?
- What are your future education or employment plans?

ACTIVITIES

- What do you do in your spare time?
- What do you do for fun?
- With whom do you spend time?

DRUGS

- Have you ever tried street drugs? Alcohol? Steroids? Have you ever smoked or chewed tobacco?
- Are you still using these drugs? Are any of your friends using or selling drugs?

SEXUAL ACTIVITY/SEXUALITY

- What is your sexual orientation?
- Are you sexually active?
  At what age did you start having sex?
  How many sexual partners do you have?
  Do you (or your partner) use condoms?
  Do you (or your partner) use contraceptives?
- Have you ever been abused, either physically or sexually?

SUICIDE/DEPRESSION

- Are you ever sad or tearful? Tired or unmotivated?
- Have you ever felt that life is not worth living? Have you ever thought about or tried to hurt yourself? Do you have a suicide plan?

SAFETY

- Do you use a seat belt or bicycle helmet?
- Do you ever get into dangerous situations where you could be hurt?
- Is there a gun in your home? Have you ever learned about gun safety?

Note: Adapted from Goldenring, J. M., & Cohen, E. (1988). Getting into adolescent heads. *Contemporary Pediatrics, 5*, 75–90.

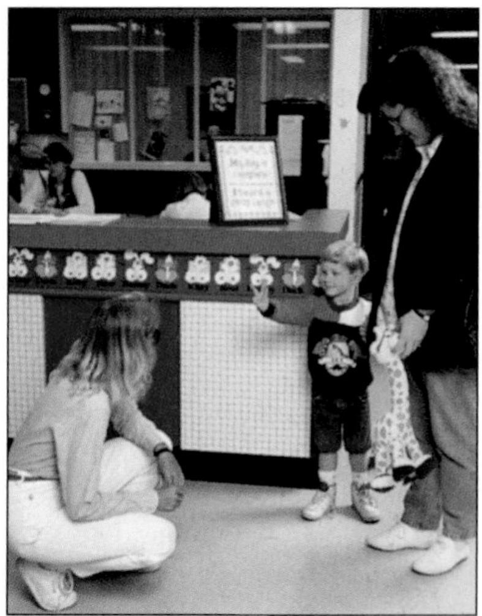

FIGURE 4-4 ◆
Examination of the child begins from the first contact. You should be observing the behavior of the child and parent by using visual cues to make a proper assessment. Does the child appear well nourished? Does the child appear secure with the parent?

Developmental Data

Information about the child's motor, cognitive, language, and social development is recorded. Ask the parent about the child's milestones and current fine and gross motor skills. Obtain the age at which the child first used words appropriately and the current words used or language ability. For children in school, ask about academic performance to assess cognitive development. Ask the parent about the child's manner of interaction with other children, family members, and strangers.

The developmental data will help the nurse plan nursing care that is appropriate for the child. Guidelines for a nursing assessment of development can be found in Chapter 2.

GENERAL APPRAISAL

The examination begins when you first meet the child, either when admitting the child to the nursing unit or in the patient's room (Figure 4-4 ◆). Measure the infant's weight, length, and head circumference. If the child can stand, a standing height measurement is substituted for length (Figure 4-5 ◆). Take the child's temperature, heart rate, respiratory rate, and blood pressure.

Observe the child's general appearance and behavior. The child should appear well nourished and well developed. Infants and young children are often fearful and seek reassurance from their parents. The child may resist interacting with you until rapport is established.

Observe the behavior and tone of voice used by the parent when he or she is talking to the child. Is the child encouraged to speak? Is the child appropriately reassured or supported by the parent? The child should feel secure with the parent and perceive permission to interact with the nurse.

ASSESSING SKIN AND HAIR CHARACTERISTICS AND INTEGRITY

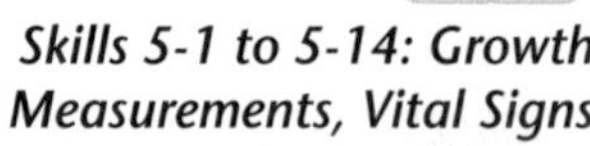

Skills 5-1 to 5-14: Growth Measurements, Vital Signs

What is indicated when the child's skin is not uniform in color or when it feels spongy to the touch? What are each of the primary skin lesions called, and what characteristics are used to describe each of them? How can cyanosis and jaundice be detected in children of darker skin? Why is skin turgor assessed? How is the presence of head lice identified in a child?

Examination of the skin requires good lighting to detect variations in skin color and to identify lesions. Daylight is preferred when available. Rather than inspecting the entire skin surface of the child at one time, examine the skin simultaneously with other body systems as each region of the body is exposed.

INSPECTION OF THE SKIN

The child's skin is inspected for color and the presence of imperfections, elevations, or other lesions.

Skin Color

The color of the child's skin usually has an even distribution. The skin is inspected for color variations—such as increased or decreased pigmentation, pallor, mottling, bruises, erythema, cyanosis, or jaundice—that may be associated with local or generalized conditions. Some variations in skin color are common and normal, such as freckles found in the white population and Mongolian spots found on infants of dark skin (Figure 4-6 ◆). Bruises are common on the knees, shins, and lower arms as children stumble and fall. Bruises on other parts of the body, especially in various stages of healing, should raise a suspicion of child abuse.

When a skin color abnormality is suspected, the buccal mucosa and tongue should be inspected to confirm the color change. This is especially important in children of darker skin because the mucous membranes are usually pink, regardless of skin color. The gums are pressed lightly for 1 to 2 seconds. Any residual color, such as jaundice or cyanosis, is more easily detected in blanched skin. Jaundice may also be noticed in the sclerae of the eyes. Generalized cyanosis is associated with respiratory and cardiac disorders. Jaundice is associated with liver disorders.

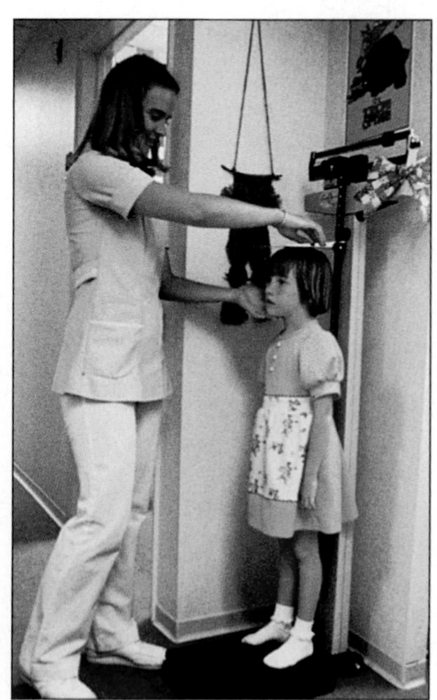

FIGURE 4-5 ◆
Standing height measurements are taken routinely at each well-child visit to assess the child's rate of growth.

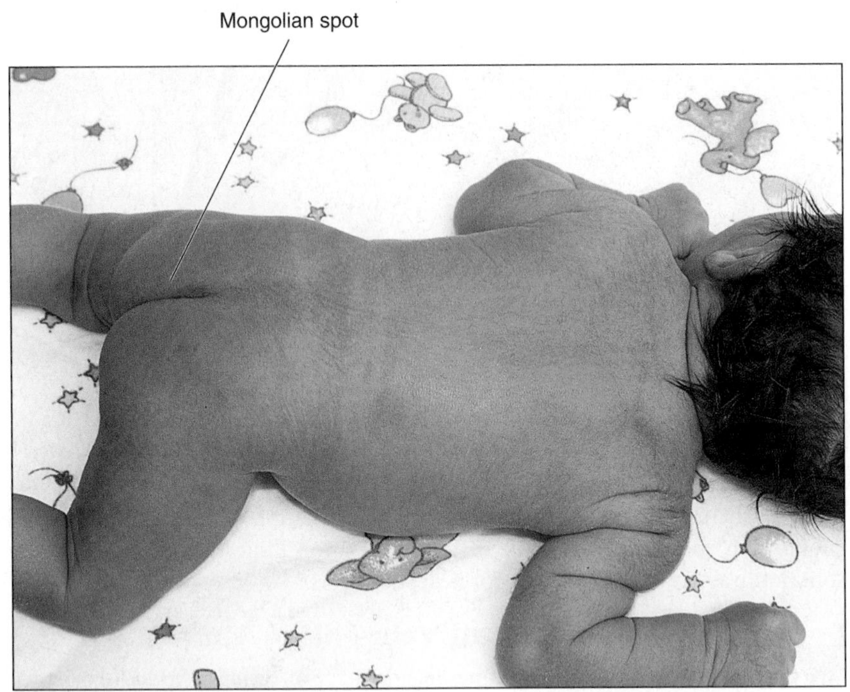

FIGURE 4-6 ◆
Mongolian spots are large patches of bluish-colored skin often seen on the buttocks. They are a normal occurrence in dark-skinned infants, but are sometimes incorrectly thought to be bruises.

CLINICAL TIP

The palms of the hands and soles of the feet are often lighter than the rest of the skin surface in children of darker skin. In addition, their lips may appear slightly bluish.

CLINICAL TIP

The color of the bruise provides clues to its age (Wilson, 1977).

Color	*Age of Bruise*
Reddish blue	Up to 48 hours
Brownish blue	2–3 days
Brownish green	4–7 days
Greenish yellow	7–10 days
Yellow-brown	More than 8 days
Normal skin color	2–4 weeks

EQUIPMENT NEEDED

Gloves

PALPATION OF THE SKIN

Palpation of the skin provides a sense of its characteristics: temperature, texture, moistness, and resilience or turgor. To evaluate these characteristics, the nurse lightly touches or strokes the skin surface. The nurse follows standard precautions by wearing gloves when palpating mucous membranes, open wounds, and lesions.

Temperature

The child's skin normally feels cool to the touch. A general evaluation of skin temperature can be obtained by placing the wrist or dorsum of the hand against the child's skin. Excessively warm skin may indicate the presence of fever or inflammation, whereas abnormally cool skin may be a sign of shock or cold exposure.

Texture

Children have soft, smooth skin over the entire body. Any areas of roughness, thickening, or induration (area of extra firmness with a distinct border) should be identified. Abnormalities in texture are associated with endocrine disorders, chronic irritation, and inflammation.

Moistness

The child's skin is normally dry to the touch. The skin may feel slightly damp when the child has been exercising or crying. Excessive sweating without exertion is associated with a fever or with an uncorrected congenital heart defect.

Resilience (Turgor)

The child's skin is taut, elastic, and mobile because of the balanced distribution of intracellular and extracellular fluids. To evaluate skin turgor, the examiner pinches a small amount of skin on the abdomen between the thumb and forefinger, releases the skin, and watches the speed of recoil (Figure 4-7 ◆). If the skin rapidly returns to its previous contour, good skin turgor is indicated. When poor skin turgor is present, the skin tents or stands up rather than resuming its previous contour. Poor skin turgor is commonly associated with dehydration.

If *edema,* an accumulation of excess fluid in the interstitial spaces, is present, the skin feels doughy or boggy. To test for the degree of edema present, the examiner presses for 5 seconds against a bone beneath the area of puffy skin, releases the pressure, and observes

CLINICAL TIP

The degree of dehydration, or weight loss caused by dehydration, can be estimated from the time it takes tented skin to return to its natural contour (Seidel, Ball, Dains, & Benedict, 2003).

Weight Loss from Dehydration	*Time to Return to Normal*
<5%	<2 sec
5–8%	2–3 sec
9–10%	3–4 sec
>10%	>4 sec

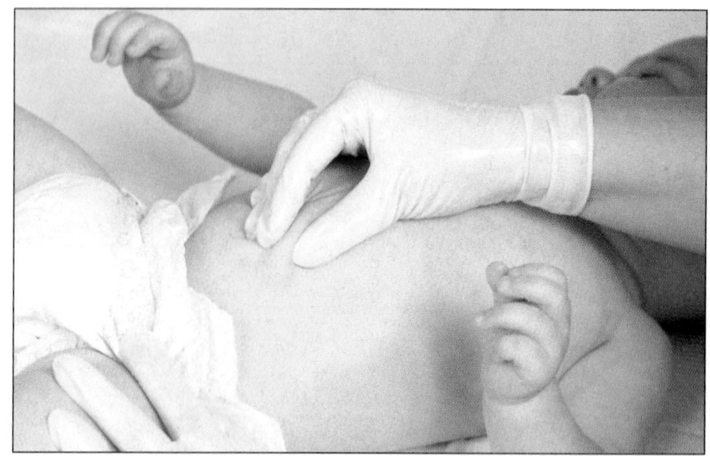

FIGURE 4-7 ◆
Tenting of the skin is associated with poor skin turgor. Skin with normal turgor will quickly return to a flat position.

how rapidly the indentation disappears. If the indentation disappears rapidly, the edema is "nonpitting." Slow disappearance of the indentation indicates "pitting" edema, which is commonly associated with kidney or heart disorders.

Capillary Refill and Small-Vein Filling Times

Two techniques are used to determine the adequacy of *tissue perfusion* (oxygen circulating to the tissues). When tissue perfusion is inadequate, immediately assess the child for shock or a physical constriction such as a cast or bandage that is too tight. The capillary refill time is normally less than 2 seconds (Figures 4–8A and B ◆). The small-vein filling time is normally less than 4 seconds (Figures 4–8C and D ◆).

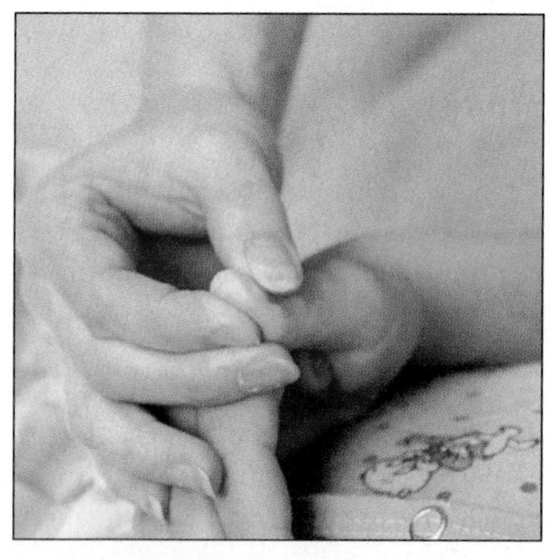

A

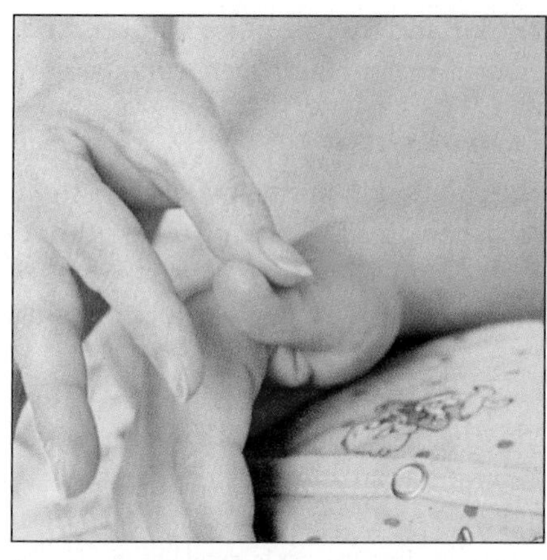

B

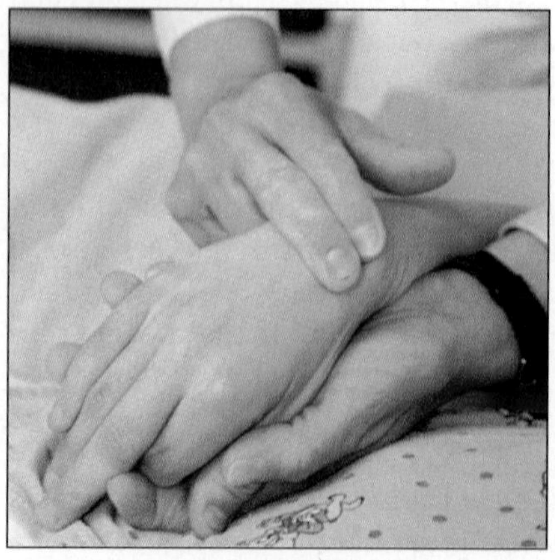

C

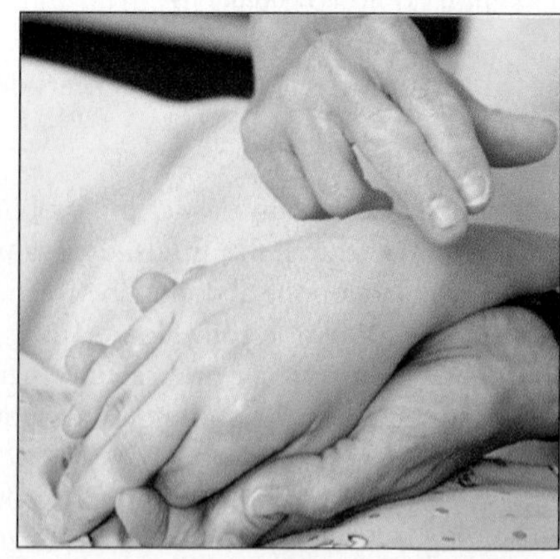

D

FIGURE 4-8 A-D ◆
Capillary refill technique: A, Pinch the end of a finger until the skin is blanched. B, Quickly release the finger and watch the blood return to the veins. Count the seconds it takes for the color to return or veins to fill. Slow color return or vein filling time could be related to shock or constriction due to a tight bandage or cast. Small vein filling time technique: C, Using the index finger, milk a vein on the dorsum of the hand or foot from proximal to distal. D, Release your pressure and color should return promptly.

SKIN LESIONS

Skin lesions are usually an indication of an abnormal skin condition. Characteristics of these lesions—location, size, type of lesion, pattern, and discharge, if present—provide clues about the cause of the condition. Inspect and palpate the isolated or generalized skin color abnormalities, elevations, lesions, or injuries to describe all characteristics present.

Primary lesions (such as macules, papules, and vesicles) are often the skin's initial response to injury or infection. Mongolian spots and freckles are normal findings also classified as primary lesions. Secondary lesions (such as scars, ulcers, fissures) are the result of irritation, infection, and delayed healing of primary lesions. Figure 4-9 ◆ describes common primary lesions.

PATHOPHYSIOLOGY ILLUSTRATED

FIGURE 4-9 ◆
Common Primary Skin Lesions and Associated Condition

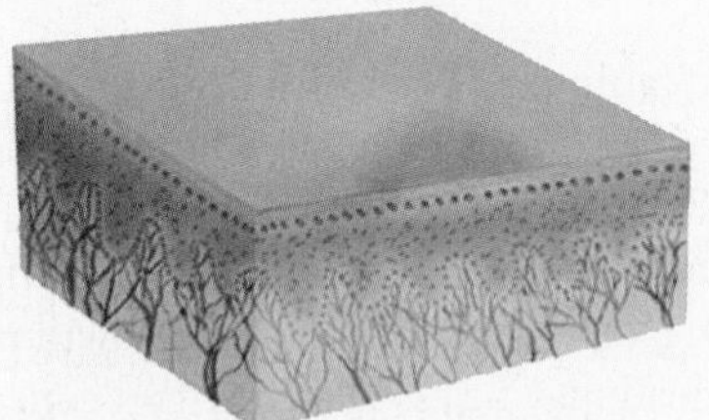

Lesion Name: Macule
Description:
Flat, nonpalpable, diameter <1 cm (1/2 in.)
Example: Freckle, rubella, rubeola, petechiae

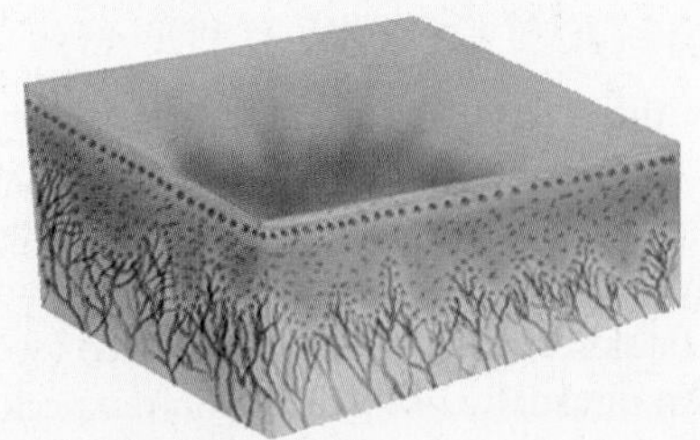

Lesion Name: Patch
Description:
Macule diameter >1 cm (1/2 in.)
Example: Vitiligo, Mongolian spot

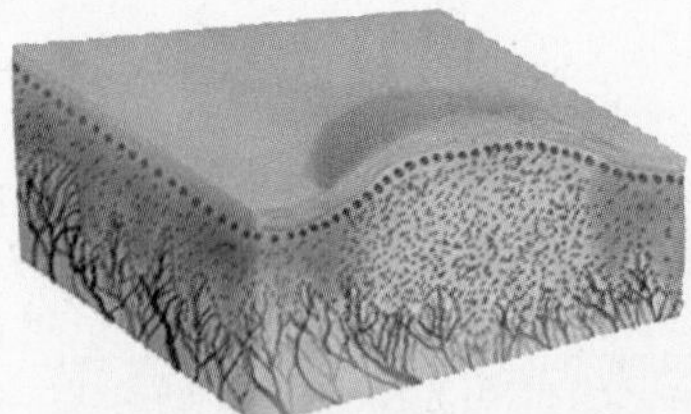

Lesion Name: Papule
Description:
Elevated, firm, diameter <1 cm (1/2 in.)
Example: Warts, pigmented nevi

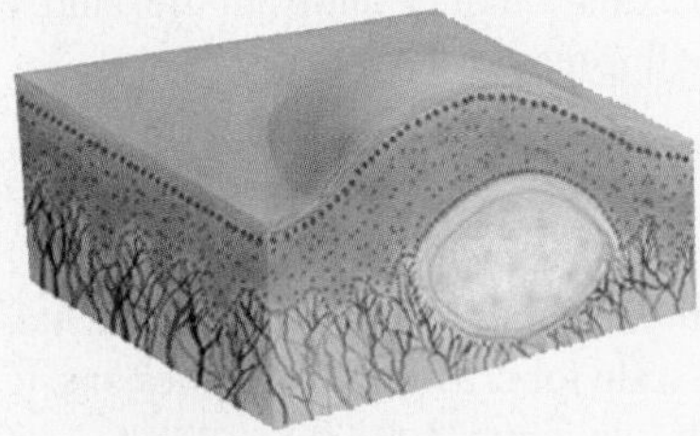

Lesion Name: Nodule
Description:
Elevated, firm, deeper in dermis than papule, diameter 1-2 cm (1/2 in.-1 in.)
Example: Erythema nodosum

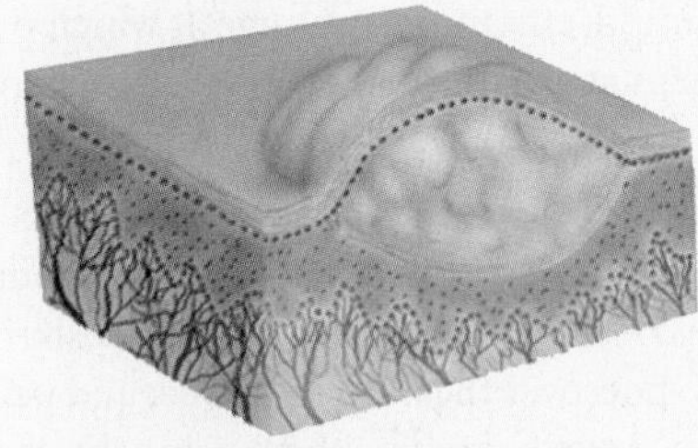

Lesion Name: Tumor
Description:
Elevated, solid, diameter >2 cm (1 in.)
Example: Neoplasm, hemangioma

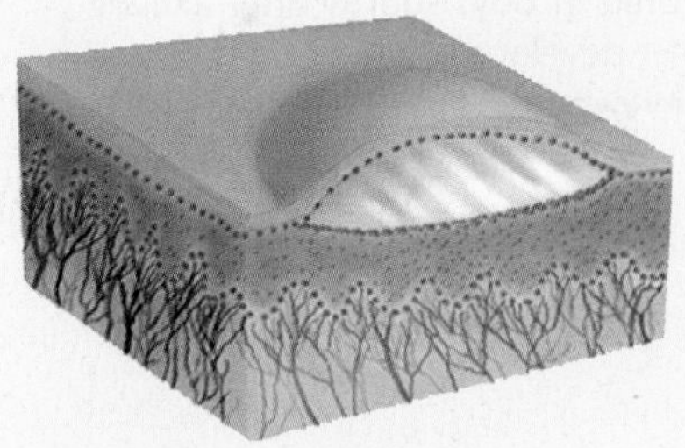

Lesion Name: Vesicle
Description:
Elevated, filled with fluid, diameter <1 cm (1/2 in.)
Example: Early chicken pox, herpes simplex

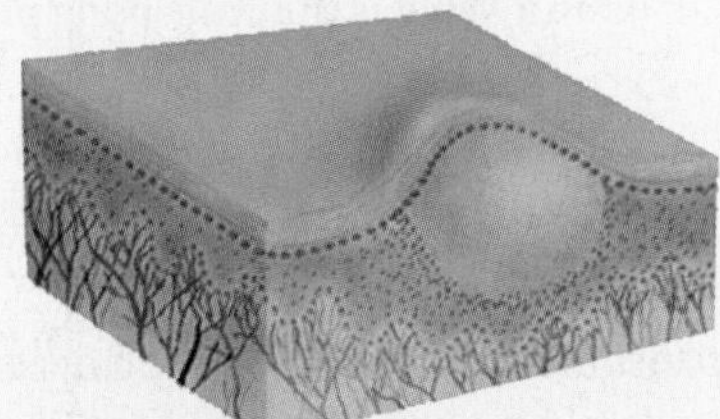

Lesion Name: Pustule
Description:
Vesicle filled with purulent fluid
Example: Impetigo, acne

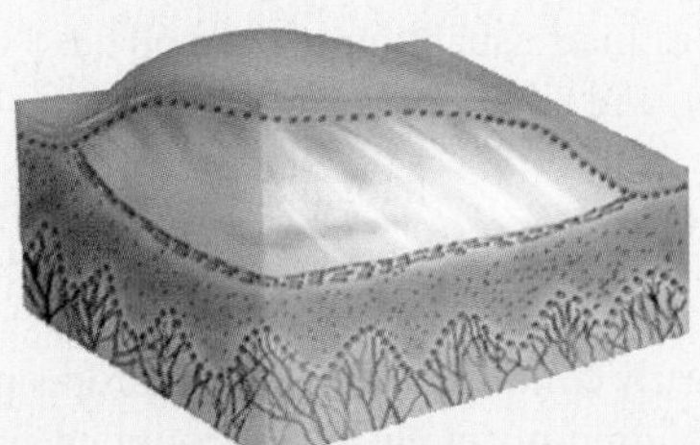

Lesion Name: Bulla
Description:
Vesicle diameter >1 cm (1/2 in.)
Example: Burn blister

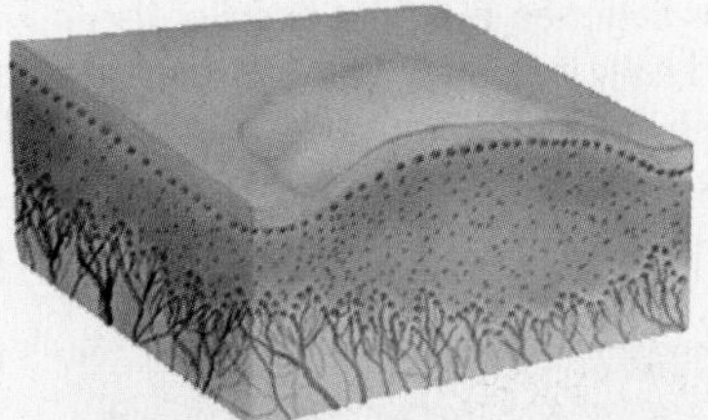

Lesion Name: Wheal
Description:
Irregular elevated solid area of edematous skin
Example: Urticaria, insect bite

COMMON PATTERNS OF SKIN LESIONS

Annular:	Circular, begins in center and spreads to periphery
Polycyclic:	Annular lesions running together
Linear:	In a row or stripe
Groups:	Clustered
Gyrate:	Twisted, spiral, coiled

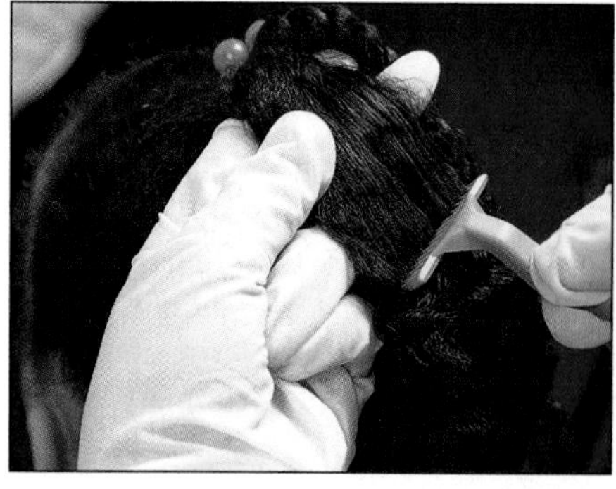

A

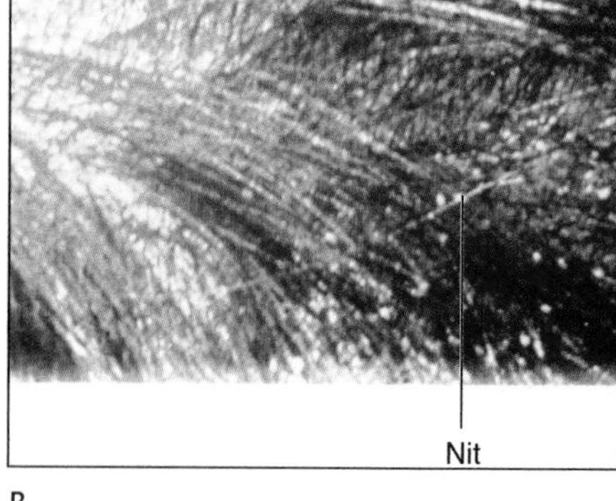

B

FIGURE 4-10 ◆

A, Inspecting for head lice with a fine-tooth comb. B, Nits in the hair.
Courtesy of Centers for Disease Control

INSPECTION OF THE HAIR

Inspect the scalp hair for color, distribution, and cleanliness. The hair shafts should be evenly colored, shiny, and either curly or straight. Variation in hair color not caused by bleaching can be associated with a nutritional deficiency. Normally, hair is distributed evenly over the scalp. Investigate areas of hair loss. Hair loss in a child may result from tight braids or skin lesions such as ringworm (see p. 891). Notice any unusual hair growth patterns. An unusually low hairline on the neck or forehead may be associated with a congenital disorder such as hypothyroidism.

Children are frequently exposed to head lice. Inspect the individual hair shafts for small nits (lice eggs) that adhere to the hair (Figure 4-10 ◆). None should be present.

Observe the distribution of body hair as other skin surfaces are exposed during examination. Fine hair covers most areas of the body. The presence of body hair in unexpected places should be noted. For example, a tuft of hair at the base of the spine often indicates a spinal defect.

It is important to note the age at which pubic and axillary hair develops in the child. Development at an unusually young age is associated with precocious puberty.

GROWTH & DEVELOPMENT

Pubic hair begins to develop in children between 8 and 12 years of age, and axillary hair develops about 6 months later. Facial hair is noted in boys shortly after axillary hair develops.

PALPATION OF THE HAIR

Palpate the hair shafts for texture. Hair should feel soft or silky with fine or thick shafts. Endocrine conditions such as hypothyroidism may result in coarse, brittle hair. Part the hair in various spots over the head to inspect and palpate the scalp for crusting or other lesions. If lesions are present, describe them using the characteristics in Figure 4–9.

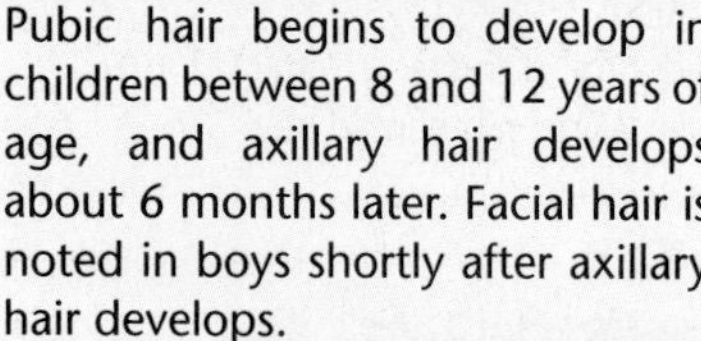

CLINICAL TIP

Children who were low-birth-weight infants often have a flat, elongated skull because the soft skull bones were flattened by the weight of the head early in infancy. Head flattening is also associated with the side- and back-lying sleep positions of infants.

ASSESSING THE HEAD FOR SKULL CHARACTERISTICS AND FACIAL FEATURES

What can cause a child's head or face to be asymmetric? How does a normal fontanel feel? What does an unusually large or small head suggest in an infant? What is the ping-pong phenomenon and what does it indicate?

INSPECTION OF THE HEAD AND FACE

Head

During early childhood, the skull's sutures permit expansion for brain growth. Infants and young children normally have a rounded skull with a prominent occipital area. The shape of the head changes during childhood, and the occipital area becomes less prominent. An abnormal skull shape can result from premature closure of the sutures.

The head circumference of infants and young children is routinely measured until 5 years of age to ensure that adequate growth for brain development has occurred. The Skills Manual describes proper technique. A larger than normal head is associated with hydrocephalus, and a smaller than normal head suggests microcephaly.

EQUIPMENT NEEDED

Tape measure

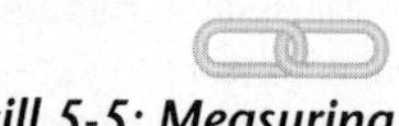

Skill 5-5: Measuring Head Circumference

Face

Inspect the child's face for symmetry during several facial expressions such as resting, smiling, talking, and crying (Figure 4-11 ◆). Significant asymmetry may result from paralysis of trigeminal or facial nerves (cranial nerves V or VII), in utero positioning, and swelling from infection, allergy, or trauma.

Next inspect the face for unusual facial features such as coarseness, wide eye spacing, or disproportionate size. Tremors, tics, and twitching of facial muscles are often associated with seizures.

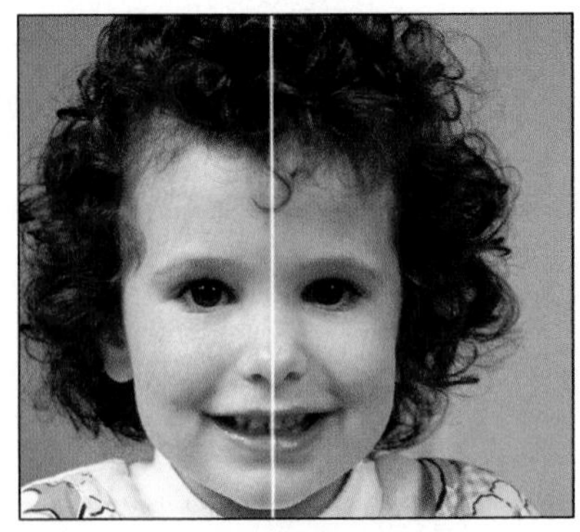

FIGURE 4-11 ◆ Draw an imaginary line down the middle of the face over the nose and compare the features on each side. Significant asymmetry may be caused by paralysis of cranial nerve V or VII, in utero positioning, or swelling from infection, allergy, or trauma.

PALPATION OF THE SKULL

Palpate the skull in infants and young children to assess the sutures and fontanels and to detect soft bones (Figure 4-12 ◆).

Sutures

Use your fingerpads to palpate each suture line. The edge of each bone in the suture line is felt, but normally there is no separation of the two bones. If additional bone edges are felt, it may indicate a skull fracture.

Fontanels

At the intersection of the sutures, palpate the anterior and posterior fontanels. The fontanel should feel flat and firm inside the bony edges. The anterior fontanel is normally smaller than 5 cm (2 in.) in diameter at 6 months of age and then becomes progressively smaller. It

AS THEY GROW 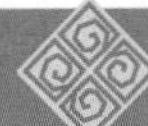 Sutures and Fontanels of the Skull

FIGURE 4-12 ◆

The sutures are separations between the bones of the skull that have not yet joined. The fontanels are formed at the intersection of these sutures where bone has not yet formed. Fontanels are covered by tough membranous tissue that protects the brain. The posterior fontanel closes between 2 and 3 months. The anterior fontanel and sutures are palpable up to the age of 18 months. The suture lines of the skull are seldom palpated after 2 years of age. After that time, the sutures rarely separate.

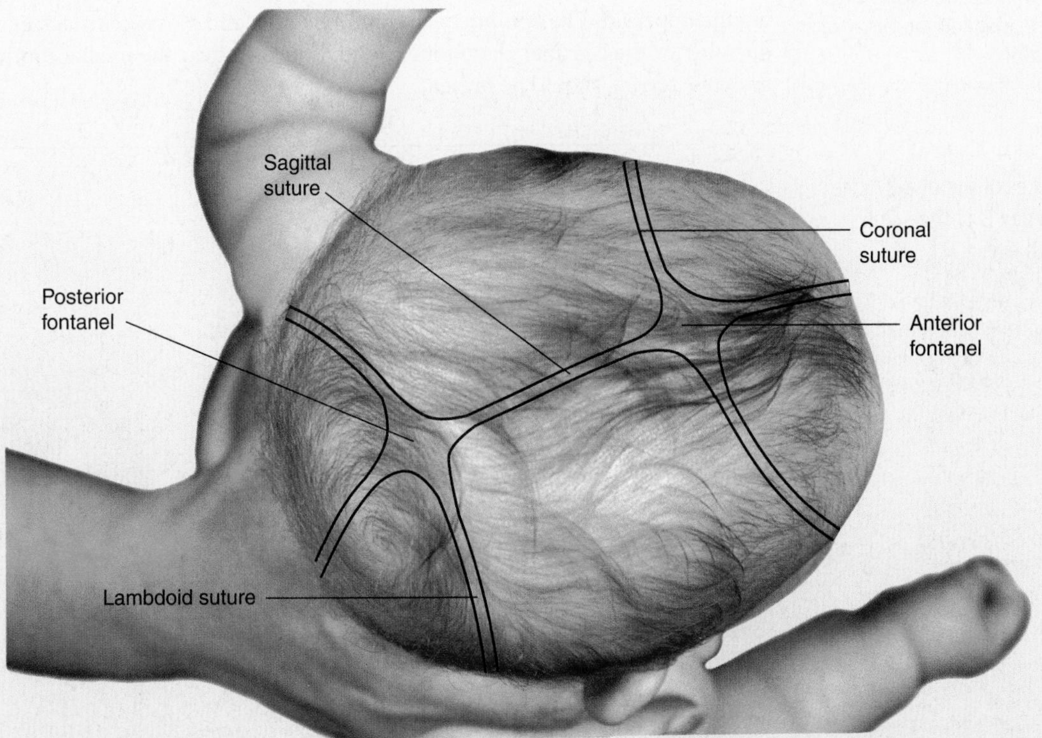

closes between 12 and 18 months of age. The posterior fontanel closes between 2 and 3 months of age.

A tense fontanel, bulging above the margin of the skull, is an indication of increased intracranial pressure. A soft fontanel, sunken below the margin of the skull, is associated with dehydration.

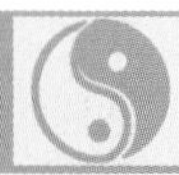

CULTURE

The head is a sacred part of the body to Southeast Asians. Ask for permission before touching the infant's head to palpate the sutures and fontanels (Spector, 2000). When a Hispanic child is examined, however, not touching the head is considered bad luck.

ASSESSING EYE STRUCTURES, FUNCTION, AND VISION

What is one of the most common eye problems that occurs during childhood? What do bulging or sunken eyeballs look like? What is the red reflex and what does it indicate? How is eye muscle balance tested? Is it normal for a child's visual acuity to be different at certain ages?

INSPECTION OF THE EXTERNAL EYE STRUCTURES

The function of the external and internal eye structures and related cranial nerves makes vision possible. The external eye structures, including the eyeballs, eyelids, and eye muscles, are inspected. The function of cranial nerves II, III, IV, and VI, which innervate the eye structures, is also tested (Figure 4-13 ◆).

EQUIPMENT NEEDED

Ophthalmoscope
Vision chart
Penlight
Small toy
Index card or paper cup

Eye Size and Spacing

Inspect the eyes and surrounding tissues simultaneously when examining facial features. The eyes should be the same size but not unusually large or small. Observe for eye bulging, which can be identified by retracted eyelids or a sunken appearance. Bulging may be associated with a tumor, and a sunken appearance may reflect dehydration.

Next inspect the eyes to see if they are appropriately distanced from each other. *Hypertelorism,* or widely spaced eyes, can be a normal variation in children.

Eyelids

Inspect the eyelids for color, size, position, mobility, and condition of the eyelashes. Eyelids should be the same color as surrounding facial skin and free of swelling or inflammation along the edges. Sebaceous glands that look like yellow striations are often present near the hair follicles. Eyelashes curl away from the eye to prevent irritation of the conjunctivae.

Inspect the conjunctivae lining the eyelids by pulling down the lower lid and then everting the upper lid. The conjunctivae should be pink and glossy. The lacrimal punctum, the opening for the lacrimal gland on each lid, is located near the medial canthus. No redness or excess tearing should be present.

CLINICAL TIP

The eyelids of newborns are often swollen and difficult to open after antibiotics are instilled at birth to prevent infection.

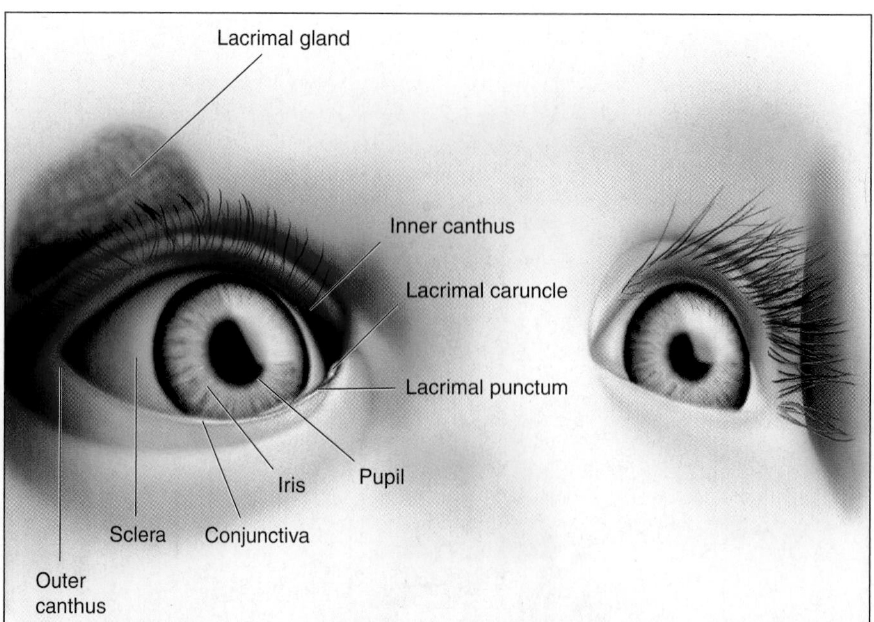

FIGURE 4-13 ◆
External structures of the eye. Notice that the light reflex is at the same location on each eye.

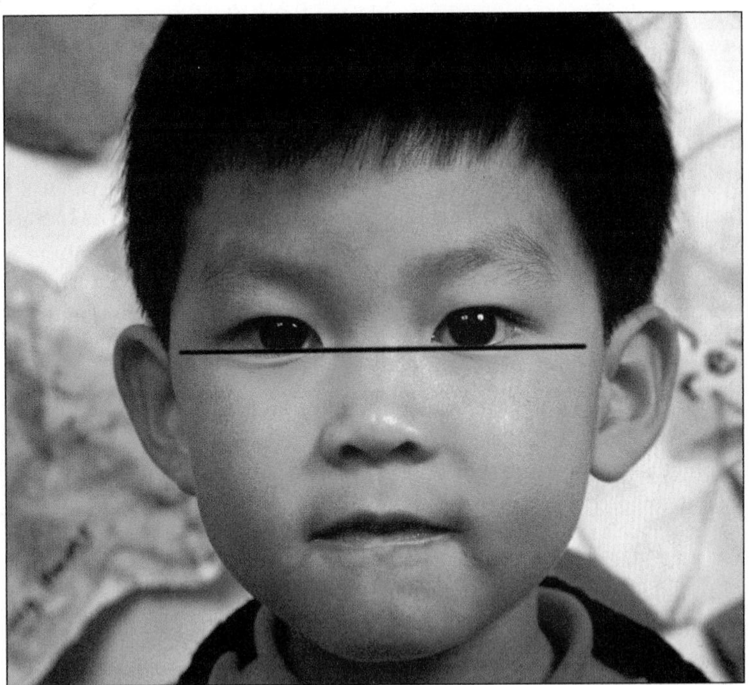

FIGURE 4-14 ◆
Draw an imaginary line across the medial canthi and extend it to each side of the face to identify the slant of the palpebral fissures. When the line crosses the lateral canthi, the palpebral fissures are horizontal and no slant is present. When the lateral canthi fall above the imaginary line, the eyes have an upward or Mongolian slant. A downward or anti-Mongolian slant is present when the lateral canthi fall below the imaginary line. Epicanthal folds are present when an extra fold of skin partially or completely covers the caruncles in the medial canthi. What type of slant does this child have?

When the eyes are open, inspect the level at which the upper and lower lids cross the eye. Each lid normally covers part of the iris but not any portion of the pupil. The lids should also close completely over the iris and cornea. Ptosis, drooping of the lid over the pupil, is often associated with injury to the oculomotor nerve, cranial nerve III. Sunset sign, in which the sclera is seen between the upper lid and the iris, may indicate retracted eyelids or hydrocephalus.

Inspect the eyes for the palpebral slant (Figure 4-14 ◆). The eyelids of most people open horizontally. An upward or Mongolian slant is a normal finding in Asian children; however, children with Down syndrome also often have a Mongolian slant (Figure 4-15 ◆). A downward or anti-Mongolian slant is seen in some children as a normal variation.

CLINICAL TIP

Children of Asian descent often have an extra fold of skin, known as the epicanthal fold, covering all or part of the medial canthus of the eye.

Eye Color

Inspect the color of each sclera, iris, and bulbar conjunctiva. The sclera is normally white or ivory in children of darker skin. Sclerae of another color suggest the presence of an underlying disease. For example, yellow sclerae indicate jaundice. Typically the iris is blue or light colored at birth and becomes pigmented within 6 months. Inspect the iris for the presence of Brushfield spots, white specks in a linear pattern around the iris circumference, which are often associated with Down syndrome. The bulbar conjunctivae, which cover the sclera to the edge of the cornea, are normally clear. Redness can indicate eyestrain, allergies, or irritation.

Pupils

Inspect the pupils for size and shape. Normally the pupils are round, clear, and equal in size. Some children have a coloboma, a keyhole-shaped pupil caused by a notch in the iris. The presence of this sign can indicate that the child has other congenital anomalies.

To test the pupillary response to light, shine a bright light into one eye. A brisk constriction of both the pupil exposed to direct light and the other pupil is a normal finding.

To test pupillary response to accommodation, ask the child to look first at a near object (for example, a toy) and then at a distant object (for example, a picture on the wall). The expected response is pupil constriction with near objects and pupil dilation with distant objects. This procedure tests the optic nerve, cranial nerve II.

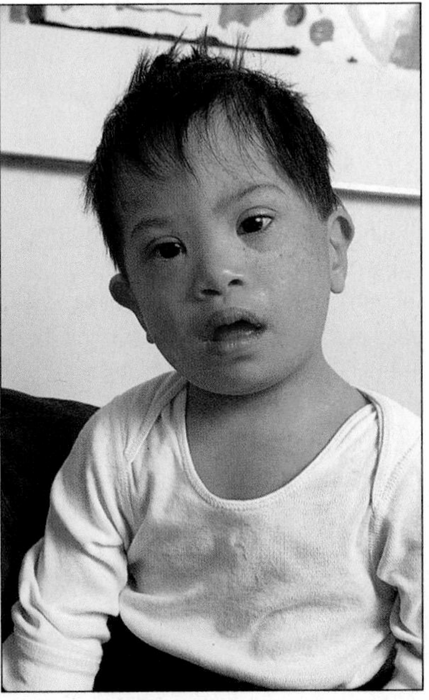

FIGURE 4-15 ◆
The eyes of this boy with Down syndrome show a Mongolian slant.

INSPECTION OF THE EYE MUSCLES

A common pediatric eye disorder is strabismus, or crossed eyes. This condition is important to detect because, if uncorrected, it can cause vision impairment. Several tests are used to detect the presence of a muscle imbalance that can result in strabismus. These tests include the evaluation of extraocular movements, the corneal light reflex, and the cover–uncover test.

Extraocular Movements

Seat the child at your eye level to evaluate the extraocular movements. Hold a toy or penlight 30 cm (12 in.) from the child's eyes and move it through the six cardinal fields of gaze. The child's head may need to be held still until fine motor eye movement develops. Both eyes should move together, tracking the object. This procedure tests the oculomotor, trochlear, and abducens nerves (cranial nerves III, IV, and VI) (Figure 4-16 ◆).

Corneal Light Reflex

To test the corneal light reflex, shine a light on the child's nose, midway between the eyes. Identify the location where the light is reflected on each eye. The light reflection is normally symmetric, at the same spot on each cornea. An asymmetric corneal light reflex indicates strabismus (see Figure 4-13 ◆).

Cover–Uncover Test

The cover–uncover test can be used only for older, cooperative children. While standing slightly to one side, but in a position from which you are still able to see the child's eyes, ask the child to look at a picture on the wall. Cover one of the child's eyes with an index card and simultaneously inspect the uncovered eye for movement as it focuses on the picture. Then remove the card from the covered eye and inspect it for movement as it focuses on the picture. Repeat the procedure with the child's other eye covered. Because the eyes work together, no obvious movement of either eye is expected. Eye movement indicates a muscle imbalance.

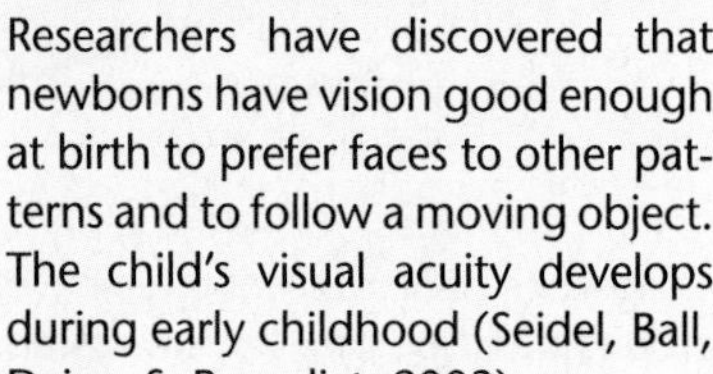

Researchers have discovered that newborns have vision good enough at birth to prefer faces to other patterns and to follow a moving object. The child's visual acuity develops during early childhood (Seidel, Ball, Dains, & Benedict, 2003).

Age	*Visual Acuity*
3 years	20/50
4 years	20/40
5 years	20/30
6 years	20/20

VISION ASSESSMENT

Because vision is such an important sense for learning, assessment is essential to detect any serious problems. Vision is evaluated using an age-appropriate vision test, but no simple method exists. It is possible to assess the presence of vision in infants and children by observing their behavior in response to certain maneuvers and during play.

Infants and Toddlers

When the infant's eyes are open, test the blink reflex by moving your hand quickly toward the infant's eyes. A quick blink is the normal response. Absence of the blink reflex can indicate that the infant is blind.

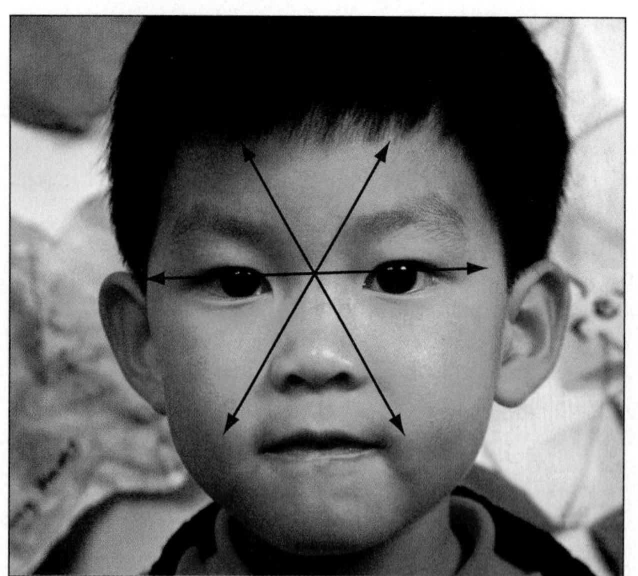

FIGURE 4-16 ◆
Begin the eye muscle examination with inspection of the extraocular movements. Have the child sit at your eye level. Hold a toy or penlight about 30 cm (12 in.) from the child's eyes and move it through the six cardinal fields of gaze. Both eyes should move together, tracking the object. This procedure tests cranial nerves III, IV, and VI.

To test an infant's ability to visually track an object, hold a light or toy about 15 cm (6 in.) from the infant's eyes. When the infant has fixated on or is staring at the object, move it slowly to each side. The infant should follow the object with the eyes and by moving the head.

Once an infant has developed skills to reach for and then pick up objects, observe play behavior to evaluate vision. The ability to easily find and pick up small toys is a good indicator of vision in children under 3 years of age.

Skills 5-17 to 5-19: Visual Acuity Screening

Standardized Vision Charts

Standardized vision charts cannot be used to test vision until the child can understand directions and cooperate, usually at about 3 or 4 years of age. The Snellen E chart or Picture chart can be used to test visual acuity of preschool-age children just as the Snellen Letter chart is used for school-age children and adolescents. The Skills Manual describes the use of these charts.

CLINICAL TIP

A difference of two lines or more between the eyes is an indication for further evaluation.

INSPECTION OF THE INTERNAL EYE STRUCTURES

The funduscopic examination allows you to inspect the structures of the internal eye—the retina, optic disc, arteries and veins, and macula (Figure 4-17 ◆). This examination takes extensive practice because the ophthalmoscope is a complex instrument to master and because the examination is difficult to perform on uncooperative children. Most often it is performed by experienced examiners.

Darkening the room will cause the child's pupils to dilate. Explain the procedure to the child to gain full cooperation. Have a picture on the wall or have the parent or assistant hold a toy for the child to stare at so that the child's eye will not have to be held open forcibly.

Using the Ophthalmoscope

The ophthalmoscope has a lens-and-mirror system and a bright light for inspecting the structures of the internal eye (Figure 4-18 ◆). Different lens powers are arranged on the rotating disk of the ophthalmic head. This system permits compensation for vision difference between the child and the examiner. The black-numbered plus lenses magnify images, and the red-numbered minus lenses reduce them in a range of powers. The lenses can be changed by turning the disk with the forefinger.

Turn the ophthalmoscope on and set the lens power at zero. Keep your forefinger on the disk to change the lens power as needed. Hold the ophthalmoscope so you can see through the lens. Rest the top against your eyebrow and the handle against your cheek to keep the instrument stabilized. The right eye is used to examine the child's right eye and the left eye to examine the child's left eye. This position is best for visualizing the eye, and it reduces direct exposure to infection. Place a hand on the child's head for stabilization.

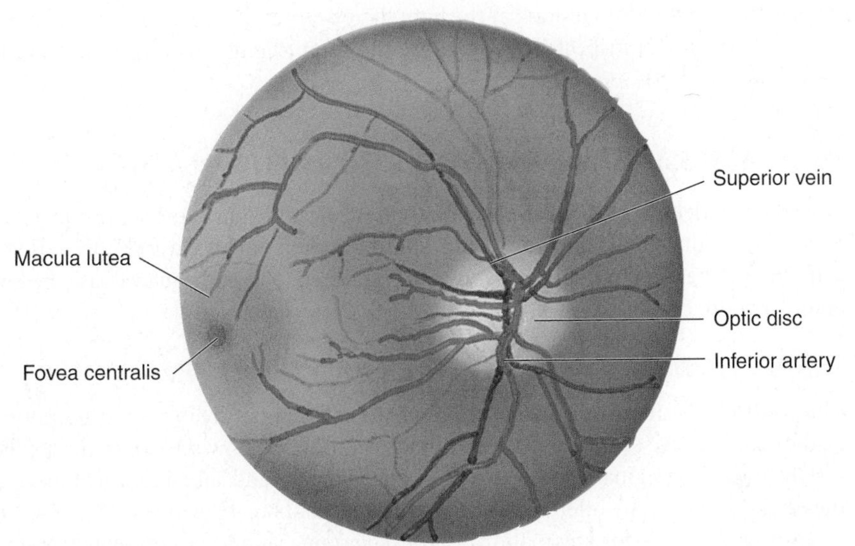

FIGURE 4-17 ◆ Normal fundus.

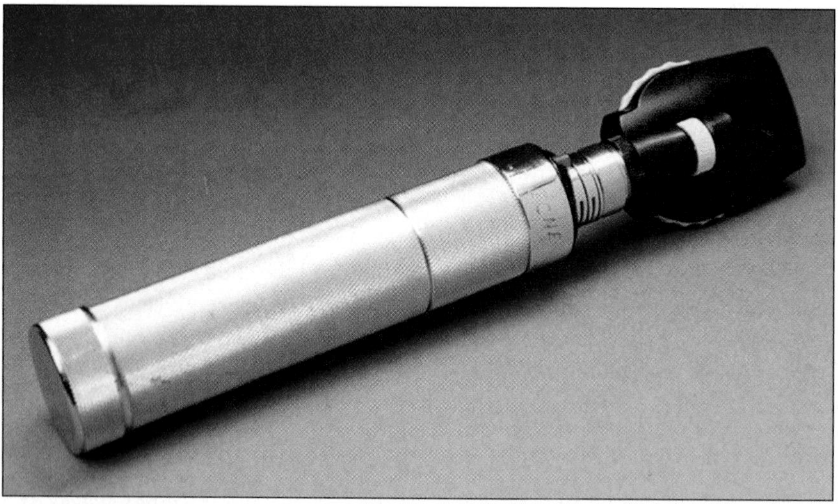

FIGURE 4-18 ◆
Ophthalmoscope.

RED REFLEX Shine the ophthalmoscope light at the child's eye from a distance of 30 cm (12 in.). The first image seen is the red reflex, the red glow of the vascular retina. When you see the red reflex, know that you are using the ophthalmoscope correctly and that the child's lens is clear. Black spots or opacities within the red reflex are abnormal and may indicate congenital cataracts. If a white reflex is seen rather than a red reflex, a retinoblastoma may be present. The red reflex can also be tested by shining a small flashlight into the eye.

CLINICAL TIP

Keep the red reflex in view to make sure your head and the ophthalmoscope move as one unit. If you lose the red reflex when moving closer to the child, move back, find the red reflex, and start again.

VISUALIZING THE INTERNAL EYE STRUCTURES Slowly move closer to the child. Deeper levels of the vitreous humor are inspected before the pink retina comes into view. The retina is a deeper pink in children of darker skin. A blood vessel is the first retinal structure usually seen. Continue moving closer to the child's eye and adjust the plus or minus lenses to focus on this blood vessel. Retinal arteries appear smaller and brighter red than veins. The blood vessels branch to spread and cover the retina.

Inspect and follow the branching of the blood vessels toward the nose until they merge into the optic disc. Dark areas along the blood vessels may indicate retinal hemorrhages. Carefully inspect sites where arteries and veins cross. Notches and indentations at these sites are associated with hypertension.

The optic disc margin is normally sharply defined, round, and yellow to creamy pink. Blurring of the disc margins or bulging of the optic disc is a sign of increased intracranial pressure. The diameter of the optic disc is used to identify the location of other landmarks on the retina.

The macula is located approximately two disc diameters lateral to the optic disc. To see the macula, ask the child to look at the light. It appears as a yellow dot surrounded by deep pink. The macula is inspected last because the bright light causes the child to blink and look away.

ASSESSING THE EAR STRUCTURES AND HEARING

How do you identify proper ear placement on the head? What is the significance of low-set ears? Why is otitis media the most common ear problem during early childhood? What play activities can be used to test hearing in young children? How do you evaluate the hearing of an older child?

INSPECTION OF THE EXTERNAL EAR STRUCTURES

EQUIPMENT NEEDED

Otoscope
Noisemakers (bell, rattle, tissue paper)
Tuning fork, 500–1,000 Hz

The position and characteristics of the pinna, the external ear, are inspected as a continuation of the head and eye examination. The pinna is considered "low set" when the top lies completely below an imaginary line drawn through the medial and lateral canthi of the eye toward the ear. Low-set ears are often associated with congenital renal disorders (Figure 4-19 ◆).

Inspect the pinna for any malformation. The pinna should be completely formed, with an open auditory canal. Next, inspect the tissue around the pinna for abnormalities. A pit

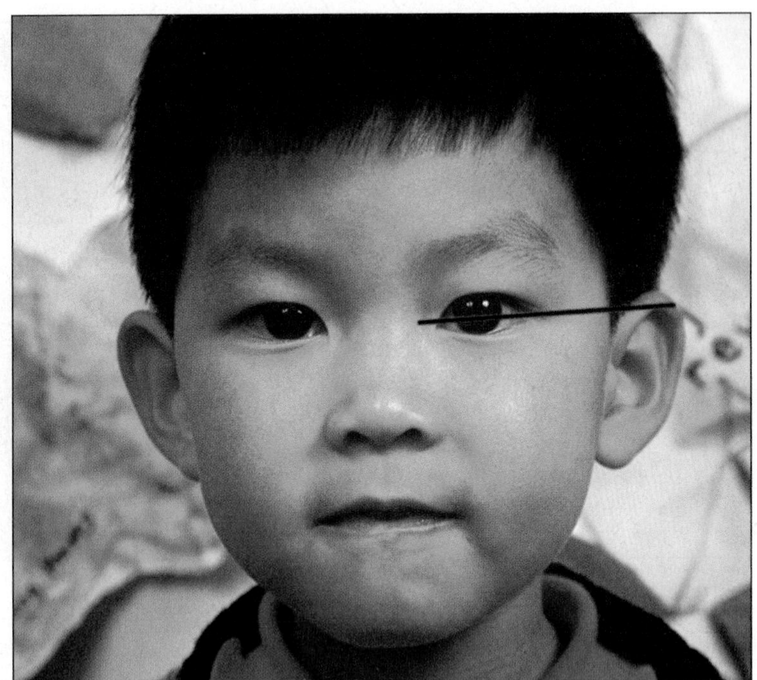

FIGURE 4-19 ◆
To detect the correct placement of the external ears, draw an imaginary line through the medial and lateral canthi of the eye toward the ear. This line normally passes through the upper portion of the pinna. The pinna is considered "low set" when the top lies completely below the imaginary line. Low-set ears are often associated with renal disorders. Is this a normal ear placement? Yes, it is.

or hole in front of the auditory canal may indicate the presence of a sinus. If the pinna protrudes outward, there may be swelling behind the ear, a sign of mastoiditis.

Inspect the external auditory canal for any discharge. A foul-smelling, purulent discharge may indicate the presence of a foreign body or an infection in the external canal. Clear fluid or a blood-tinged discharge may indicate a cerebrospinal fluid leak caused by a basilar skull fracture.

INSPECTION OF THE TYMPANIC MEMBRANE

Examination of the tympanic membrane is important in infants and young children because they are prone to otitis media, a middle ear infection. The eustachian tubes are shorter, wider, and more horizontally positioned in infants and young children than in older children and adults. This positioning enables bacteria to move up the eustachian tube from the pharynx, causing an infection.

The otoscope, an instrument with a magnifying lens, bright light, and speculum, is used to examine the internal auditory canal and tympanic membrane. Infants and young children often resist having their ears inspected with the otoscope because of past painful experiences. The otoscopic examination is often delayed until portions of the assessment requiring cooperation are completed. Use simple explanations to prepare the child. Let the child play with the otoscope or demonstrate how it is used on the parent or a doll. Figure 4-20 ◆ illustrates one method that can be used to restrain an uncooperative child.

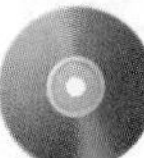

Otoscopic Exam

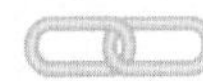

Skill 2-3: Positioning a Child for an Otoscopic Exam

Using the Otoscope

To begin the otoscopic examination, hold the handle of the otoscope in the palm of your hand with your thumb pointed toward the base of the handle. If a pneumatic squeeze bulb is used, hold it between the index finger and the handle. Choose the largest ear speculum that fits into the auditory canal to form a seal for testing the movement of the tympanic membrane. A large speculum is also less likely to injure the auditory canal if the child moves suddenly.

Hold the otoscope in the hand closest to the child's face and when the child is cooperative rest the back of your hand against the child's head to stabilize it. Use your other hand to pull the pinna toward the back of the head and either up or down. Pulling the pinna straightens the auditory canal and improves inspection of the tympanic membrane (Figure 4-21 ◆).

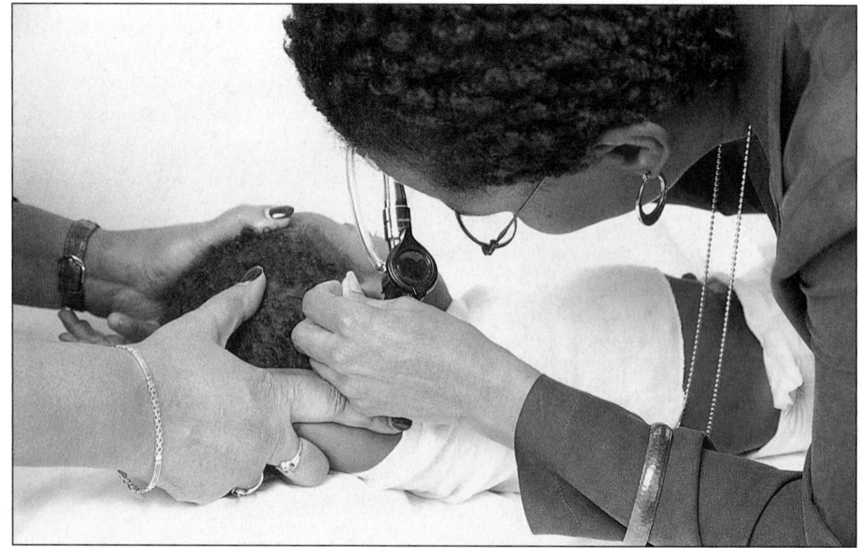

FIGURE 4-20 ◆
To restrain an uncooperative child, place the child prone on the examining table. Have an assistant hold the child's arms next to the head to restrain the child's head movements. Restrain the child's body movements by lying across the child's body. Keep your hands free to hold the otoscope and position the external ear.

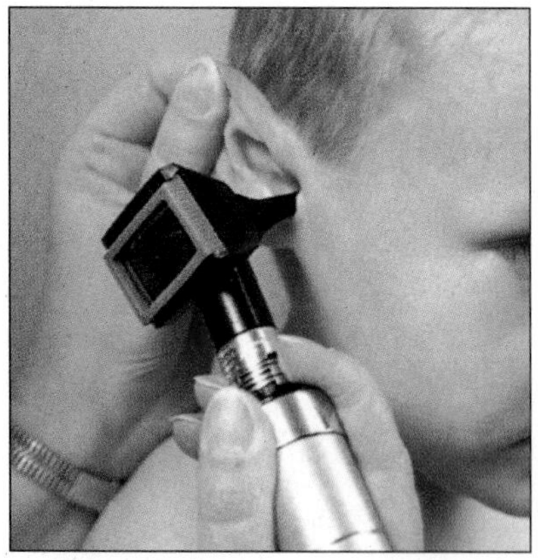

FIGURE 4-21 ◆
To straighten the auditory canal: pull the pinna back and up for children over 3 years of age; pull the pinna down and back for children under 3 years of age.

TABLE 4-9 Unexpected Findings on Examination of the Tympanic Membrane and Their Associated Conditions

CHARACTERISTICS OF TYMPANIC MEMBRANE	UNEXPECTED FINDINGS	ASSOCIATED CONDITIONS
Color	Redness Slight redness Amber Deep red or blue	Infection in middle ear Prolonged crying Serous fluid in middle ear Blood in middle ear
Light reflex	Absent Distorted, loss of triangular shape	Bulging tympanic membrane, infection in middle ear Retracted tympanic membrane, serous fluid in middle ear
Bony landmarks	Extra prominent	Retracted tympanic membrane, serous fluid in middle ear
Movement	No motility Excess motility	Infection or fluid in middle ear Healed perforation

SAFETY PRECAUTIONS

Never irrigate the ear canal if any discharge is present. Cold water should never be used for irrigation.

Slowly insert the speculum into the auditory canal, inspecting the walls for signs of irritation, discharge, or a foreign body. The walls of the auditory canal are normally pink, and some cerumen is present. Children often put beads, peas, or other small objects into their ears. If the auditory canal is obstructed by cerumen or a foreign body, irrigation can be used to clean the canal.

The tympanic membrane, which separates the outer ear from the middle ear, is usually pearly gray and translucent. It reflects light, and the bones (ossicles) in the middle ear are normally visible. When the pneumatic attachment is squeezed, the tympanic membrane normally moves in and out in response to the positive and negative pressure applied (Figure 4-22 ◆). Table 4-9 lists the abnormal findings of a tympanic membrane examination and their associated conditions.

HEARING ASSESSMENT

Hearing evaluation is important in children of all ages because hearing is essential for normal speech development and learning. With new technology, even newborns can have their hearing screened, and many states require such screening prior to hospital discharge. Often

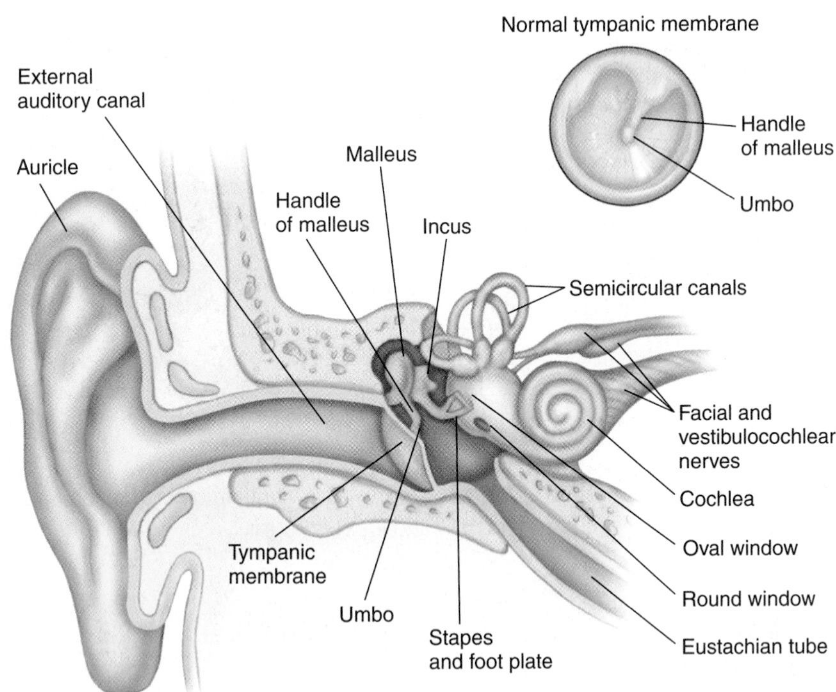

FIGURE 4-22 ◆
Cross section of the ear. The tympanic membrane normally has a triangular light reflex with the base on the nasal side pointing toward the center. The bony landmarks, the umbo and handle of malleus, are seen through the tympanic membrane.

Skills 5-20, 5-21: Hearing Acuity Screening

hearing must be evaluated by inspection of the child's responses to various auditory stimuli. Hearing loss may occur at any time during early childhood as the result of birth trauma, frequent otitis media, meningitis, or antibiotics that damage cranial nerve VIII.

Use hearing and speech articulation milestones as an initial hearing screen. Select an age-appropriate method to screen hearing. When a hearing deficiency is suspected as a result of screening, the child is referred for audiometry, tympanometry, or evoked response to obtain the most accurate evaluation of hearing.

Infants and Toddlers

Select noisemakers with different frequencies, such as a rattle, bell, and tissue paper, that will attract the young child's attention. Ask the parent or an assistant to entertain the infant with a quiet toy, such as a teddy bear. Stand behind the infant, about 60 cm (2 feet) away from the infant's ear but outside the infant's field of vision, and make a soft sound with the noisemaker. Have the parent or your assistant observe the child for any of the following responses when the noisemaker is used: widening the eyes, briefly stopping all activity to listen, or turning the head toward the sound. Repeat the test in the other ear and with the other noisemakers.

Preschool and Older Children

Whispered words are used to evaluate the hearing of children over 3 years of age. Position your head about 30 cm (12 in.) away from the child's ear, but out of the range of vision so the child cannot read your lips. Use words easily recognized by the child, such as Mickey Mouse, hot dog, and Popsicle, and ask the child to repeat the words. Repeat the test with different words in the opposite ear. The child should correctly repeat the whispered words.

Bone and Air Conduction of Sound

A tuning fork is used to evaluate the hearing of school-age children who can follow directions. Stroke the tines of the tuning fork to begin the vibration. Avoid touching the vibrating tines, which will dampen the sound. Bone conduction is tested when the handle of the tuning fork is placed on the child's skull. Air conduction is tested when the vibrating tines are held close to the child's ear (Figure 4-23 ◆).

To perform the Weber test, place the vibrating tuning fork on top of the child's skull in the midline. Ask the child to tell you where the sound is heard the best, either in both ears equally or in one ear. The sound should be heard equally in both ears.

GROWTH & DEVELOPMENT

Indicators of hearing loss in an infant:

- No startle reaction to loud noises
- Does not turn toward sounds by 4 months of age
- Babbles as a young infant but does not keep babbling or develop speech sounds after 6 months of age

Indicators of hearing loss in a young child:

- No speech by 2 years of age
- Speech sounds are not distinct at appropriate ages

CLINICAL TIP

An alternative procedure is used to assess hearing when the child will not cooperate by repeating the whispered words. In a whisper, direct the child to point to different parts of the body or objects, for example, "Show me your eyes" and "Point to your mouth." Children should point to the correct body part each time.

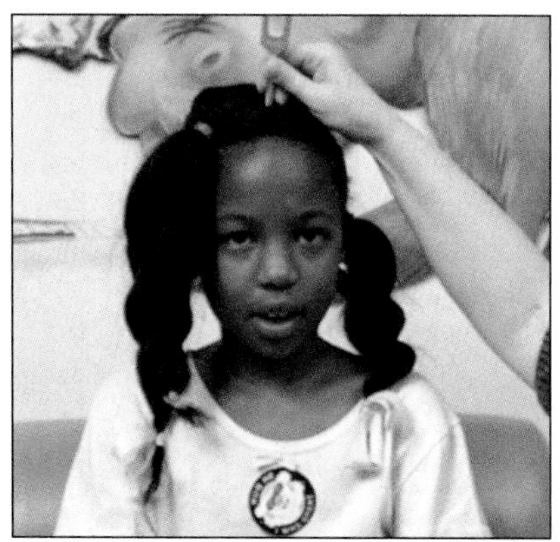
A

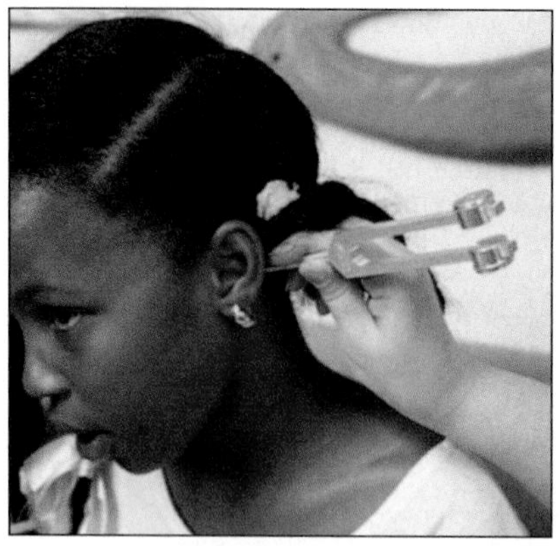
B

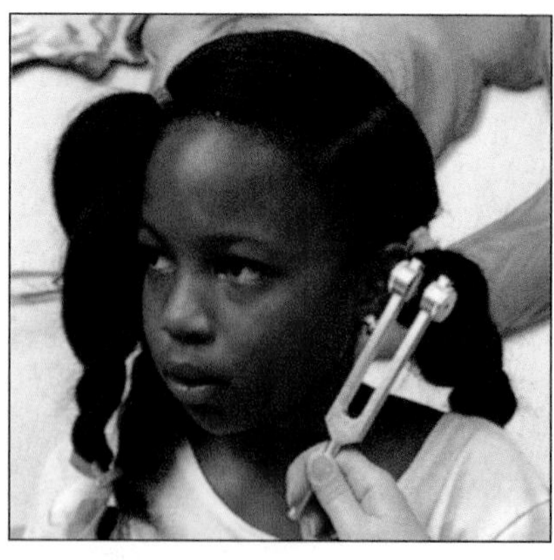
C

FIGURE 4-23 ◆
A, Weber test. Place vibrating tuning fork on midline of the child's head. B, Rinne test, step 1. Place vibrating tuning fork on mastoid process. C, Rinne test, step 2. Reposition still vibrating tines between 2.5 and 5 cm (1 and 2 in.) from ear.

TABLE 4-10 Interpretation of the Weber and Rinne Tests of Hearing

TEST AND RESULT	ASSOCIATED CONDITION
Weber Test	
Sound heard equally in both ears	No hearing loss
Sound heard better in one ear (lateralized)	Conductive hearing loss if sound lateralized to deaf ear
Rinne Test	
Sound heard by air conduction twice as long as bone conduction	No hearing loss
Sound heard longer by bone conduction than air conduction	Conductive hearing loss in affected ear
Sound heard longer by air conduction than bone conduction, but less than twice as long	Sensorineural hearing loss in affected ear

To perform the Rinne test, place the vibrating tuning fork handle on the mastoid process behind an ear. Ask the child to tell you when the sound is no longer heard. Immediately move the tuning fork, holding the vibrating tines about 2.5 to 5 cm (1 to 2 in.) from the same ear. Again, ask the child to indicate when the sound is no longer heard. The child normally hears the air-conducted sound twice as long as the bone-conducted sound. Repeat the Rinne test on the other ear. Table 4-10 provides an interpretation of the Weber and Rinne tests.

ASSESSING THE NOSE AND SINUSES FOR AIRWAY PATENCY AND DISCHARGE

What is the most common cause of a nasal obstruction in children? What does nasal flaring indicate? What signs indicate that a foreign body might be lodged in the nose? What does it mean if the child frequently wipes the nose upward with a hand?

INSPECTION OF THE EXTERNAL NOSE

The external nose characteristics and placement on the face are examined simultaneously with the facial features. Inspect the external nose for size, shape, symmetry, and midline placement on the face. The nose should be proportional in size to other facial features and positioned in the middle of the face. A flattened nasal bridge is the expected finding in Asian and black children.

The nasolabial folds are normally symmetric. Asymmetry of these folds may be associated with injury to the facial nerve (cranial nerve VII). A saddle-shaped nose is associated with congenital defects such as cleft palate.

Inspect the external nose for the presence of unusual characteristics. For example, a crease across the nose between the cartilage and bone is often caused by the allergic child's wiping an itchy nose upward with a hand.

PALPATION OF THE EXTERNAL NOSE

When a deformity is noted, gently palpate the nose to detect any pain or break in contour. No tenderness or masses are expected. Pain and a contour deviation are usually the result of trauma.

Nasal Patency

The child's airway must be patent to ensure adequate oxygenation. To test for nasal patency, occlude one nostril and observe the child's effort to breathe through the open nostril with the mouth closed. Repeat the procedure with the other nostril. Breathing should be noiseless and effortless. *Nasal flaring,* an effort the child makes to widen the airway, is a sign of respiratory distress and should not be present.

If the child struggles to breathe, a nasal obstruction may be present. Nasal obstruction may be caused by a foreign body, congenital defect, dry mucus, discharge, polyp, or trauma. Newborns may have respiratory distress because of *choanal atresia,* a congenital membranous or bony obstruction between the nose and the nasopharynx. Young children commonly place objects up their nose, and unilateral nasal flaring is a sign of such an obstruction.

GROWTH & DEVELOPMENT

Infants under 6 months of age will not automatically open their mouths to breathe when their nose is occluded, such as by mucus.

ASSESSMENT OF SMELL

The olfactory nerve (cranial nerve I) is rarely tested in preschool children, but it can be tested in school-age children and adolescents. When testing smell, choose scents the child will easily recognize such as orange, chocolate, and mint. When the child's eyes are closed, occlude one nostril and hold the scent under the nose. Ask the child to take a deep sniff and identify the scent. Alternate odors between the nares. The child can normally identify common scents.

INSPECTION OF THE INTERNAL NOSE

Inspect the internal nose for color of the mucous membranes and the presence of any discharge, swelling, lesions, or other abnormalities. Use a bright light, such as an otoscope light or penlight. For infants and young children, push the tip of the nose upward and shine the light at the end of the nose (Figure 4-24 ◆). The nasal speculum for the otoscope can be used in older children. Avoid touching the septum of the nose with the speculum. Injury to the septum can cause a nosebleed.

EQUIPMENT NEEDED

Otoscope with nasal speculum
Penlight

Mucous Membranes

The mucous membranes should be dark pink and glistening. A film of clear discharge may also be present. Turbinates, if visible, should be the same color as the mucous membranes and have a firm consistency. When the turbinates are pale or bluish gray, the child may have allergies. A *polyp,* a rounded mass projecting from the turbinate, is also associated with allergies.

Nasal Septum

Inspect the nasal septum for alignment, perforations, bleeding, or crusting. The septum should be straight. Crusting will be noted over the site of a nosebleed.

Discharge

Observe for the presence of nasal discharge, noting if the drainage is from one or both nares. Nasal discharge is not a normal finding unless the child is crying. Discharge may be watery, mucoid, purulent, or bloody. The character of the discharge depends on the condition present. A foul-smelling discharge in only one nostril is often associated with a foreign body. Table 4-11 lists conditions associated with nasal discharge.

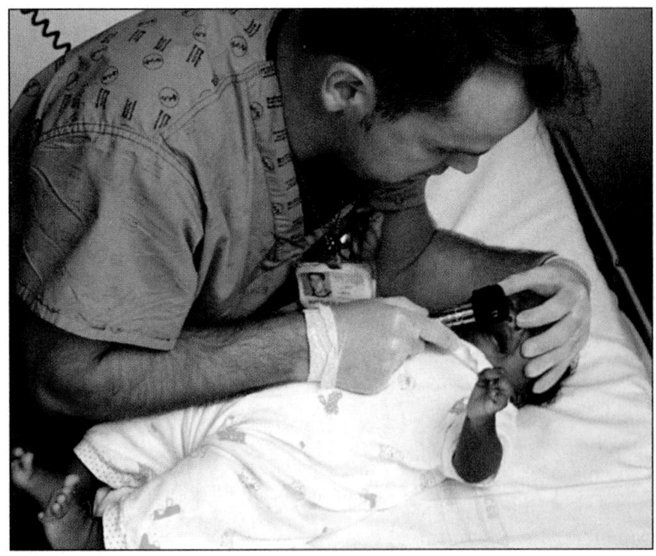

A

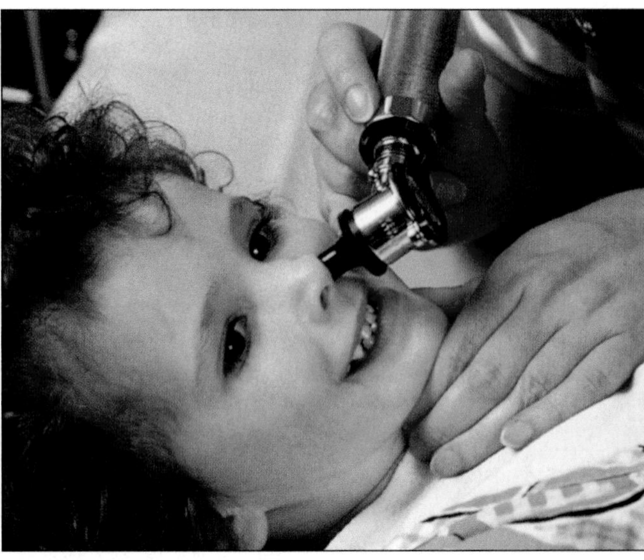

B

FIGURE 4-24 ◆
Techniques for examining nose. A, Technique for infant or small child. B, Technique for older child.

TABLE 4-11 Nasal Discharge Characteristics and Associated Conditions

DISCHARGE DESCRIPTION	ASSOCIATED CONDITION
Watery	
Clear, bilateral	Allergy
Serous, unilateral	Spinal fluid from fracture of cribriform plate
Mucoid or purulent	
Bilateral	Upper respiratory infection
Unilateral	Foreign body
Bloody	Nose bleed, trauma

INSPECTION OF THE SINUSES

The maxillary and ethmoid sinuses develop during early childhood (Figure 4-25 ◆). Sinus infections can occasionally occur in young children. Suspect a sinus problem when the child has a headache or pain and swelling around one or both eyes.

Inspect the face for any puffiness around one or both eyes. Puffiness and swelling are not normally present. To palpate over the maxillary sinuses, press up under both zygomatic arches with the thumbs. To palpate the ethmoid sinuses, press up against the bone above both eyes with the thumbs. No swelling or tenderness is expected. Tenderness may be an indication of sinusitis.

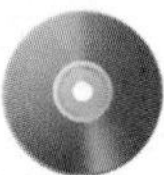

Mouth and Throat Examination

EQUIPMENT NEEDED

Tongue blade
Penlight
Gloves

ASSESSING THE MOUTH AND THROAT FOR COLOR, FUNCTION, AND SIGNS OF ABNORMAL CONDITIONS

What is the best site to evaluate cyanosis in children? What is the expected sequence of tooth eruption? How is it determined that the tongue has adequate movement for all speech sounds? How can the throat be inspected without causing the child to gag?

INSPECTION OF THE MOUTH

Young children often need coaxing and simple explanations before they will cooperate with the mouth and throat examination. Most children readily show their teeth. If the child re-

AS THEY GROW ◈ Sinus Development

FIGURE 4-25 ◆

Sinuses grow and develop during childhood. Maxillary sinuses can be identified in 1-year-old children. Ethmoid sinuses have developed in children by 6 years of age. Sinus problems under 7 years occur infrequently.

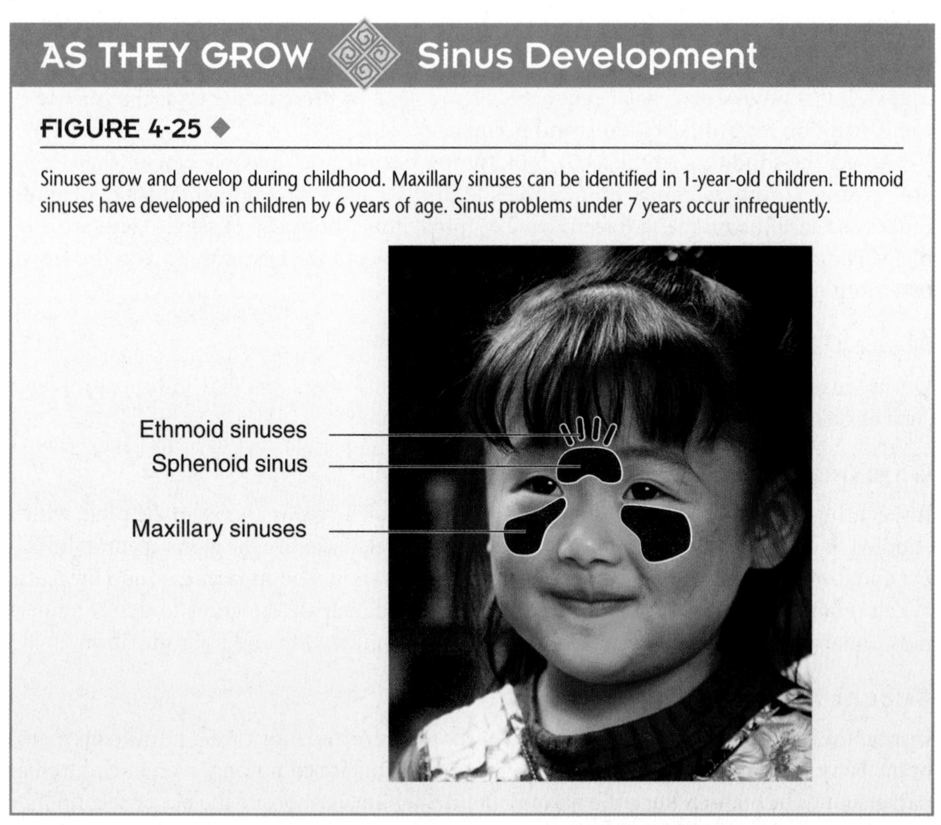

sists by clenching the teeth, they can be gently separated with a tongue blade. Wear gloves when examining the mouth because of contact with mucous membranes (Figure 4-26 ◆).

Lips

Inspect the lips for color, shape, symmetry, moisture, and lesions. The lips are normally symmetric without drying, cracking, or other lesions. Lip color is normally pink in white children and more bluish in children of darker skin. Pale, cyanotic, or cherry red lips are indicators of poor tissue perfusion caused by various conditions.

SAFETY PRECAUTIONS 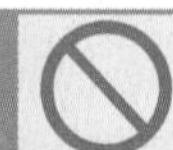

Avoid examining the mouth if there are signs of respiratory distress, high fever, drooling, and intense apprehension. These may be signs of epiglottitis. Inspecting the mouth may trigger a total airway obstruction. See Chapter 13 for more information.

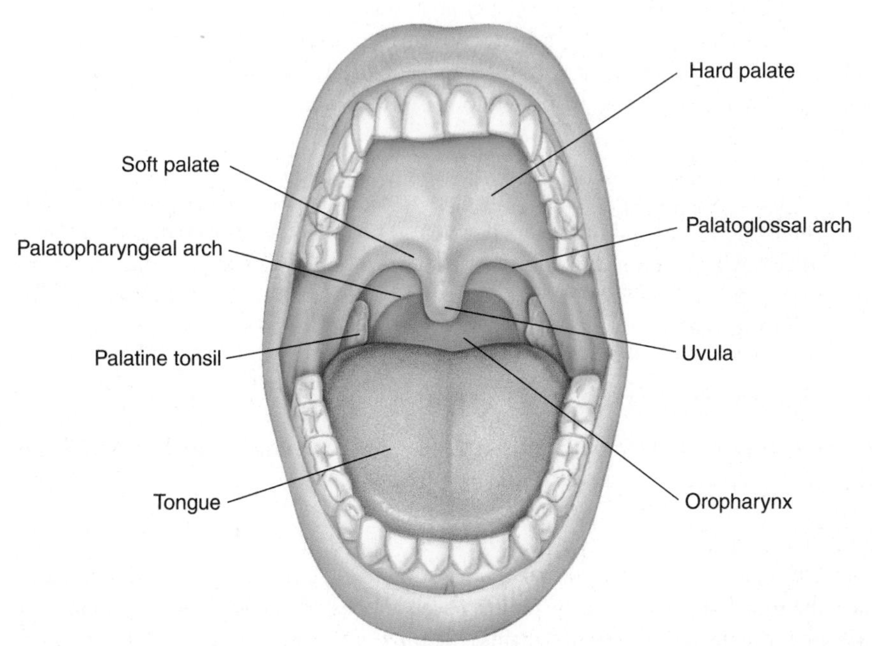

FIGURE 4-26 ◆
The structures of the mouth.

Teeth

Inspect and count the child's teeth. The timing of tooth eruption is often genetically determined, but it involves a regular sequence. Figure 4-27 ◆ presents the typical sequence of tooth eruption for both deciduous and permanent teeth.

Inspect the condition of the teeth, look for loose teeth, and note any spaces where teeth are missing. Compare empty tooth spaces with the child's developmental stage of tooth eruption. Once the permanent teeth have erupted, none should be missing. Teeth are normally white, without a flattened, mottled, or pitted appearance. Discoloration on the crown of a tooth may indicate caries.

Mouth Odors

During inspection of the teeth, be alert to any abnormal odors that may indicate problems such as diabetic ketoacidosis, infection, or poor hygiene.

Gums

Inspect the gums for color and adherence to the teeth. The gums are normally pink, with a stippled or dotted appearance. Use a tongue blade to help visualize the gums around the upper and lower molars. No raised or receding gum areas should be apparent around the teeth. When inflammation, swelling, or bleeding is observed, palpate the gums to detect tenderness. Inflammation and tenderness are associated with infection and poor nutrition.

Buccal Mucosa

Inspect the mucous membrane lining the cheeks for color and moisture. The mucous membrane is usually pink, but patches of hyperpigmentation are commonly seen in children of darker skin. The Stensen duct, the parotid gland opening, is opposite the upper second molar bilaterally. Normally pink, the duct opening becomes red when the child is infected with mumps. Small pink sucking pads can be present in infants. No areas of redness, swelling, or ulcerative lesions should be present.

Tongue

Inspect the tongue for color, moistness, size, tremors, and lesions. The child's tongue is normally pink and moist, without a coating. The tongue's size permits it to fit easily into the mouth. A pattern of gray, irregular borders that form a design (geographic tongue) is often normal, but it may be associated with fever, allergies, or drug reactions. Tremors are abnormal. A white adherent coating on an infant's tongue may be caused by thrush, a *Candida* infection.

Observe the mobility of the tongue. The child should be able to touch the gums above the upper teeth with the tongue. This tongue movement is adequate to enunciate all speech sounds clearly. Ask the child to stick out the tongue and lift it so the underside of the tongue and the floor of the mouth can be inspected for distended veins.

Palate

Inspect the hard and soft palate to detect any clefts, masses, or an unusually high arch. The palate is normally pink, with a dome-shaped arch and no cleft. The uvula hangs freely from the soft palate. Newborns often have Epstein pearls, white papules in the midline of the palate that disappear in a few weeks. A high-arched palate can be associated with sucking difficulties in young infants.

PALPATION OF THE MOUTH STRUCTURES

Palpate any masses seen in the mouth to determine their characteristics, such as size, shape, firmness, and tenderness. No masses should be found.

Tongue

To assess the tongue's strength, simultaneously testing the hypoglossal nerve (cranial nerve XII), place the index finger against the child's cheek and ask the child to push against your finger with the tongue. Some pressure against the finger is normally felt.

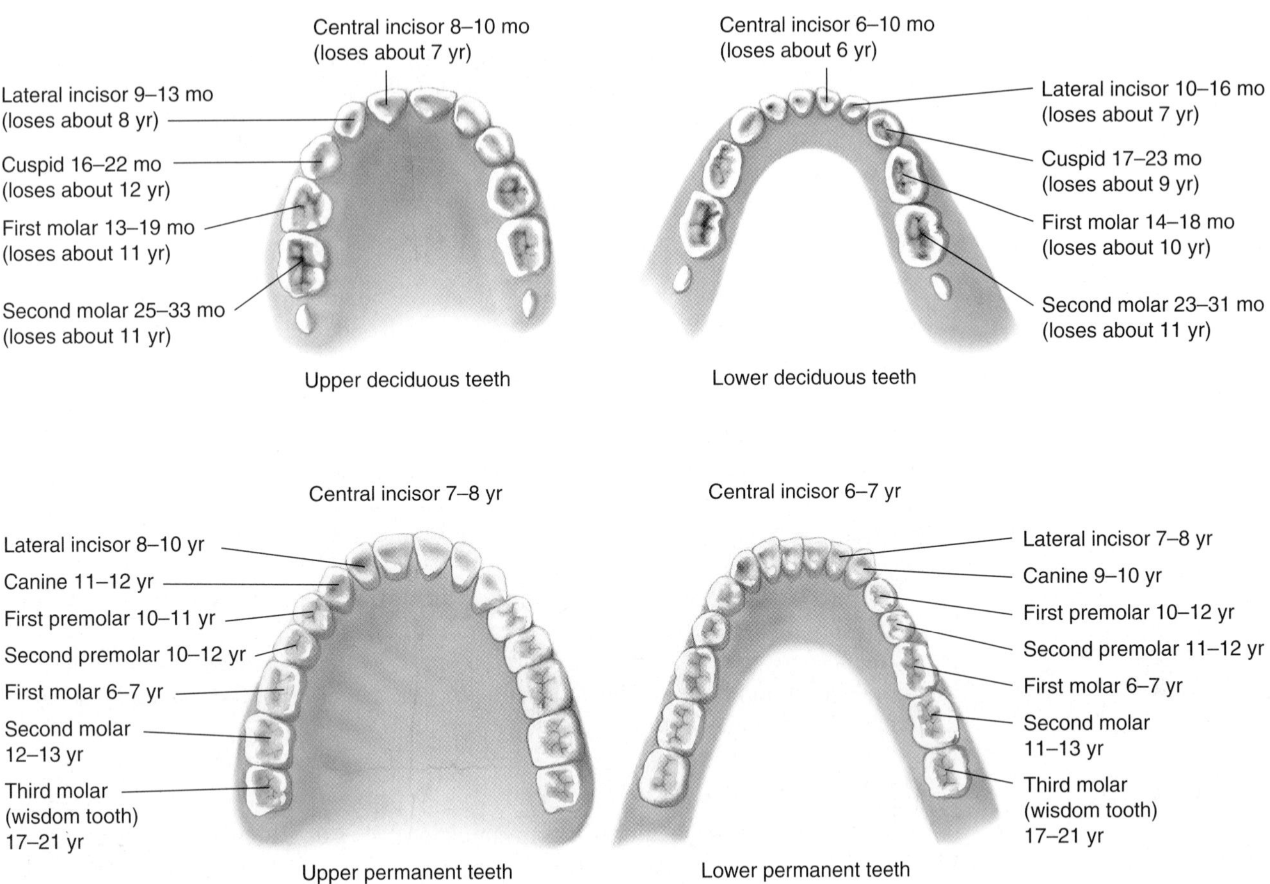

FIGURE 4-27 ◆
Typical sequence of tooth eruption for both deciduous and permanent teeth. Notice that bottom teeth come in first for each kind of tooth, incisors, cuspids, and molars. They are lost in the same pattern.

Palate

To palpate the palate, insert the little finger, with the fingerpad upward, into the mouth. While the infant sucks against your finger, palpate the entire palate. This procedure also tests the strength of the sucking reflex, innervated by the hypoglossal nerve (cranial nerve XII). No clefts should be palpated.

INSPECTION OF THE THROAT

Inspect the throat for color, swelling, lesions, and the condition of the tonsils. Ask the child to open the mouth wide and stick out the tongue. A flashlight is used to illuminate the throat. A tongue blade can be used, if needed, to visualize the posterior pharynx. Moistening the tongue blade may decrease the child's tendency to gag. The throat is normally pink without lesions, drainage, or swelling. Swelling or bulging in the posterior pharynx may be associated with a peritonsillar abscess.

Tonsils

During childhood the tonsils are large in proportion to the size of the pharynx because lymphoid tissue grows fastest in early childhood. The tonsils should be pink without exudate, but *crypts* (fissures) may be present as a result of prior infections.

Gag Reflex

Use a tongue blade when you are unable to see the posterior pharynx or need to test the gag reflex. The gag reflex is tested at the end of the examination because children dislike the gagging sensation. Prepare the child for what will happen. Ask the child to say "Ah" and watch for the symmetric rising movement of the uvula. This reflex tests the glossopharyngeal and vagal nerves (cranial nerves IX and X). If the uvula does not rise or rises to one side, cranial nerves IX and X may be paralyzed. The epiglottis lies behind the tongue and is normally pink like the rest of the buccal mucosa.

ASSESSING THE NECK FOR CHARACTERISTICS, RANGE OF MOTION, AND LYMPH NODES

What does it mean when a child's head is tilting to one side? By what age should an infant be able to control his or her head? What does a lymph node feel like? What does an enlarged lymph node feel like?

INSPECTION OF THE NECK

Inspect the neck for size, symmetry, swelling, and any abnormalities. A short neck with skin folds is normal for infants. The neck is normally symmetric. No swelling should be present. Swelling may be caused by local infections such as mumps or a congenital defect. The neck lengthens between 3 and 4 years of age.

Inspect the child's neck for any *webbing*, an extra skin fold on each side of the neck. Webbing is commonly associated with Turner syndrome.

Infants develop head control by 2 months of age. By this age, an infant can lift the head up and look around when lying on the stomach. A lack of head control can result from neurologic injury, such as an anoxic episode.

PALPATION OF THE NECK

Face the child and use the fingerpads to simultaneously palpate both sides of the neck for lymph nodes, as well as the trachea and thyroid.

Lymph Nodes

To palpate the lymph nodes, slide the fingerpads gently over the lymph node chains in the head and neck. The sequence for lymph node palpation is as follows: around the ears, under the jaw, in the occipital area, and in the cervical chain of the neck (Figure 4-28 ◆). Firm,

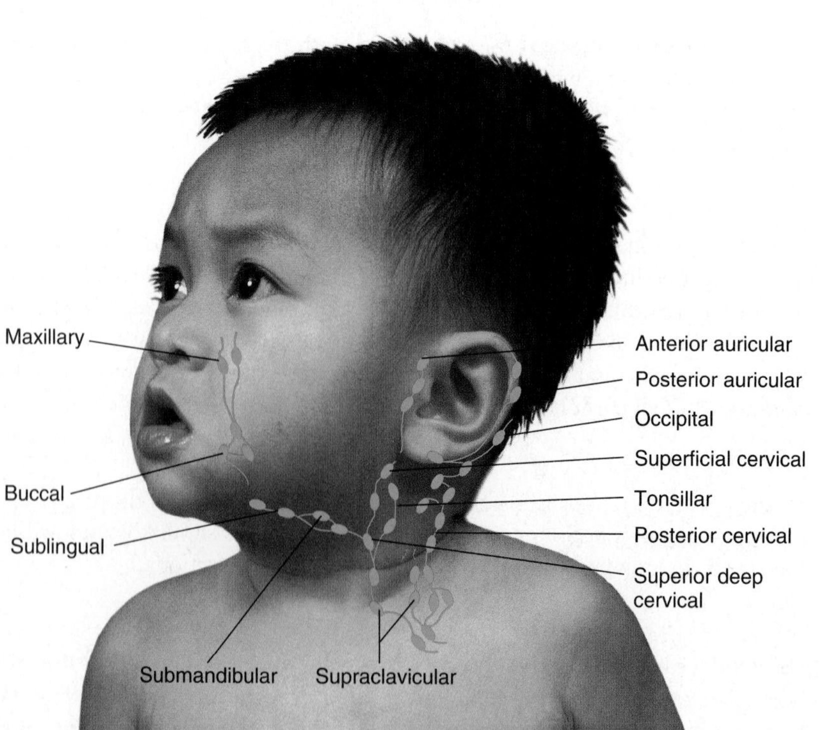

FIGURE 4-28 ◆
The neck is palpated for enlarged lymph nodes around the ears, under the jaw, in the occipital area, and in the cervical chain of the neck.

clearly defined, nontender, movable lymph nodes up to 1 cm (1/2 in.) in diameter are common in young children. Enlarged, firm, warm, tender lymph nodes indicate the presence of local infection.

Trachea

Palpate the trachea to determine its position and to detect the presence of any masses. The trachea is normally in the midline of the neck. It is difficult to palpate in children less than 3 years of age because of their short necks. To palpate the trachea, place the thumb and forefinger on each side of the trachea near the chin and slowly slide them down the trachea. Any shift to the right or left of midline may indicate a tumor or a collapsed lung.

Thyroid

As the fingers slide over the trachea in the lower neck, attempt to feel the isthmus of the thyroid, a band of glandular tissue crossing over the trachea. The lobes of the thyroid wrap behind the trachea and are normally covered by the sternocleidomastoid muscle. Because of the anatomic position of the thyroid, the lobes of the thyroid are not usually palpable in the child unless they are enlarged.

RANGE OF MOTION ASSESSMENT

To test the neck's **range of motion,** ask the child to touch the chin to each shoulder and to the chest and then to look at the ceiling. Move a light or toy in all four directions when assessing infants. Children should freely move the neck and head in all four directions without pain.

When the child is unable to move the head voluntarily in all directions, passively move the child's neck through the expected range of motion. Limited horizontal range of motion may be a sign of *torticollis,* persistent head tilting. Torticollis results from a birth injury to the sternocleidomastoid muscle or from unilateral vision or hearing impairment. Pain with flexion of the neck toward the chest (Brudzinski sign) may indicate meningitis.

ASSESSING THE CHEST FOR SHAPE, MOVEMENT, RESPIRATORY EFFORT, AND LUNG FUNCTION

What terms are used to describe the location of specific sounds heard when auscultating the chest? What does it mean when a child's chest is rounded in shape? What are retractions and what do they indicate? How can normal and adventitious breath sounds be distinguished when auscultating the lungs?

Examination of the chest includes the following procedures: inspecting the size and shape of the chest, palpating chest movement that occurs during respiration, observing the effort of breathing, and auscultating breath sounds.

TOPOGRAPHIC LANDMARKS OF THE CHEST

The chest skeleton provides most of the landmarks used to describe the location of findings during examination of the chest, lungs, and heart. The intercostal spaces are the horizontal markers. The sternum and spine are the vertical landmarks. When both a horizontal and a vertical landmark are used, the location of findings can be precisely described (Figures 4–29 and 4–30 ◆). Be sure to indicate whether the finding is on the right or left side of the patient's chest (Table 4-12).

INSPECTION OF THE CHEST

Position the child on the parent's lap or on the examining table with all clothing above the waist removed to inspect the chest. The thoracic muscles and subcutaneous tissue are less developed in children than in adults, so the chest wall is thinner. As a result, the rib cage is more prominent.

EQUIPMENT NEEDED
Stethoscope

Size and Shape of the Chest

Inspect the chest for any irregularities in shape. A rounded chest is present when the anteroposterior diameter is approximately equal to the lateral diameter. If a rounded chest is

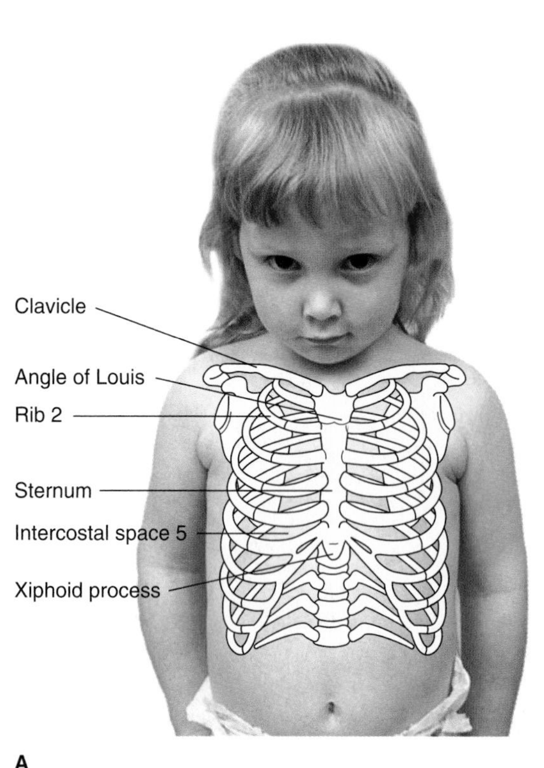

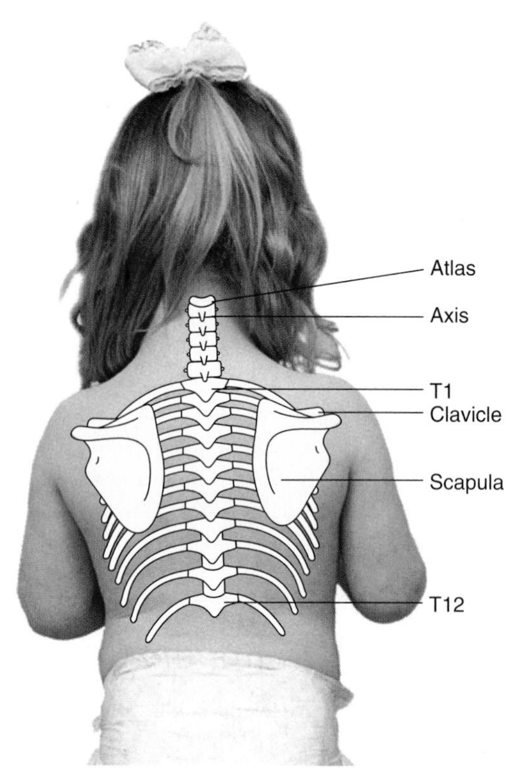

FIGURE 4-29 ◆

Intercostal spaces and ribs are numbered to describe the location of findings. A, To determine the rib number on the anterior chest, palpate down from the top of the sternum until a horizontal ridge, the Angle of Louis, is felt. Directly to the right and left of that ridge is the second rib. The second intercostal space is immediately below the second rib. Ribs 3–12 and the corresponding intercostal spaces can be counted as the fingers move toward the abdomen. B, To determine the rib number on the posterior chest, find the protruding spinal process of the seventh cervical vertebra at the shoulder level. The next spinal process belongs to the first thoracic vertebra, which attaches to the first rib.

TABLE 4-12 Vertical Landmarks of the Chest

VERTICAL LINES FOR EXAMINING THE CHEST	LOCATION OF VERTICAL LINES
Midsternal	Through the middle of the sternum
Midclavicular	From the middle of the clavicle
Anterior axillary	From the anterior axillary fold
Midaxillary	From the middle of the axilla
Posterior axillary	From the posterior axillary fold
Spinal	Through the spinous processes of the vertebrae

found in a child over 2 years of age, a chronic obstructive lung condition such as asthma or cystic fibrosis may be present.

An abnormal chest shape results from two different structural deformities (Figure 4-31 ◆). If the sternum protrudes, increasing the anteroposterior diameter, pigeon chest (pectus carinatum) may be present. If the lower portion of the sternum is depressed, decreasing the anteroposterior diameter, funnel chest (pectus excavatum) may be present. *Scoliosis,* curvature of the spine, causes a lateral deviation of the chest (see Chapter 21).

GROWTH & DEVELOPMENT

In infants the chest is rounded with the anteroposterior diameter approximately equal to the lateral diameter. The chest becomes more oval with growth and by 2 years of age the lateral diameter is greater than the anteroposterior diameter.

Chest Movement and Respiratory Effort

Inspect for simultaneous chest expansion and abdominal rise. Chest movement is normally symmetric bilaterally, rising with inspiration and falling with expiration. The chest move-

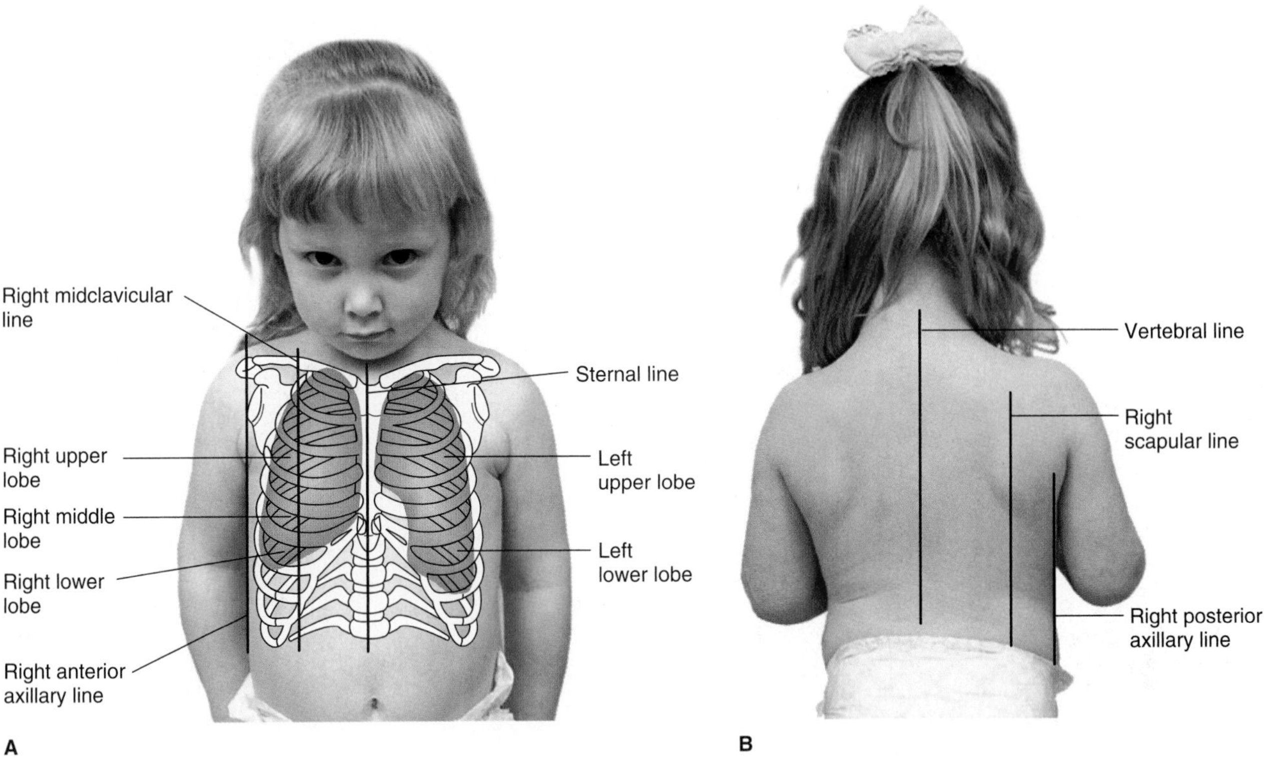

FIGURE 4-30 ◆
The sternum and spine are the vertical landmarks used to describe the anatomic location of findings. The distance between the finding and the center of the sternum (midsternal line) or the spinal line can be measured with a ruler. Imaginary vertical lines, parallel to the midsternal and spinal lines, are used to further describe the location of the findings.

ment of infants and young children is less pronounced than the abdominal movement. The diaphragm is the primary breathing muscle in infants and children under 6 years old. The thoracic muscles are less developed and serve as accessory muscles in cases of respiratory distress. As the thoracic muscles develop, they become primarily responsible for ventilation. On inspiration the chest and abdomen should rise simultaneously. Asymmetric chest rise is associated with a collapsed lung. Retractions, depression of sections of the chest wall with each inspiration, are seen when the accessory muscles are used for breathing in cases of respiratory distress.

GROWTH & DEVELOPMENT

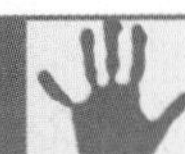

Infants and children have a faster respiratory rate than adults because of a higher metabolic rate and need for oxygen. Young children are also unable to increase the depth of respirations because not all the alveoli are developed (Hazinski, 1999).

Respiratory Rate

Because young children use the diaphragm as the primary breathing muscle, observe or feel the rise and fall of the abdomen to count the respiratory rate in children under age 6 years. Table 4-13 gives the normal respiratory rates for each age group. Make every effort to count the respiratory rate when the child is quiet. The respiratory rate rises in response to excitement, fear, respiratory distress, fever, and other conditions that increase oxygen needs.

A sustained respiratory rate greater than 60 breaths per minute is an important sign of respiratory distress. At that rate, children develop hypoxemia if treatment is not started. The child's airway is very narrow, resulting in higher airway resistance than occurs in adults. When the respiratory rate exceeds 60 breaths per minute, inspired oxygen does not reach the alveoli for gas exchange because air moves no farther than the upper airway (Eichelberger, Ball, Pratsch, Clark, 1998).

CLINICAL TIP

To get the most accurate reading of a newborn's respiratory rate, wait until the baby is sleeping or resting quietly. Use the stethoscope to auscultate the rate or place your hand on the abdomen. Count the number of breaths for an entire minute, because newborns often have irregular respirations.

PALPATION OF THE CHEST

Palpation is used to evaluate chest movement, respiratory effort, deformities of the chest wall, and tactile fremitus.

FIGURE 4-31 ◆
Two types of abnormal chest shape. A, Funnel chest. B, Pigeon chest.

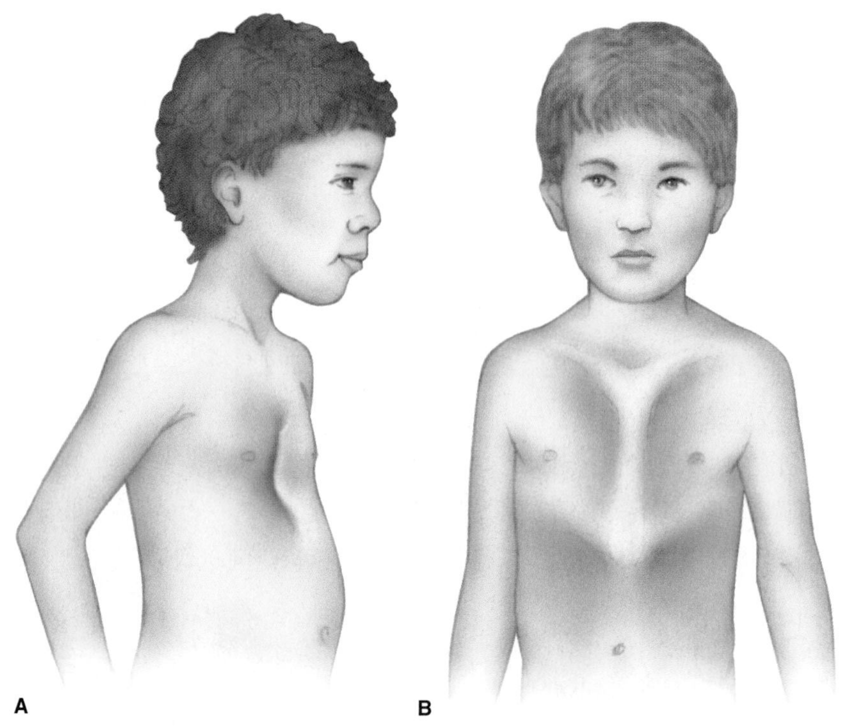

TABLE 4-13 Normal Respiratory Rate Ranges for Each Age Group

AGE	RESPIRATORY RATE PER MINUTE
Newborn	30–80
1 year	20–40
3 years	20–30
6 years	16–22
10 years	16–20
17 years	12–20

Chest Wall

To palpate the chest motion with respiration, place the palms of your hands with fingers spread on each side of the child's chest. Confirm the bilateral symmetry of chest motion. Use your fingerpads to palpate any depressions, bulges, or unusual chest wall shape that might indicate abnormal findings such as tenderness, cysts, other growths, crepitus, or fractures. None should be found. *Crepitus,* a crinkly sensation palpated on the chest surface, is caused by air escaping into the subcutaneous tissues. It often indicates a serious injury to the upper or lower airway. Crepitus may also be felt near a fracture.

Tactile Fremitus

Crying and talking produce vibrations, known as *tactile fremitus,* that can be palpated on the chest. Place the palms of your hands on each side of the chest to evaluate the quality and distribution of these vibrations. Ask the child to repeat a series of words or numbers, such as Mickey Mouse or ice cream. As the child repeats the words, move your hands systematically over the anterior and posterior chest, comparing the quality of findings side to side. The vibration or tingling sensation is normally palpated over the entire chest. Decreased sensations indicate that air is trapped in the lungs, as occurs with asthma. Increased sensations indicate lung consolidation, as occurs with pneumonia.

AUSCULTATION OF THE CHEST

Auscultate the chest with a stethoscope to assess the quality and characteristics of breath sounds, to identify abnormal breath sounds, and to evaluate vocal resonance. Use an infant or pediatric stethoscope when available to help you localize any unexpected breath sounds. Use the stethoscope diaphragm because it transmits the high-pitched breath sounds better.

Breath Sounds

Evaluate the quality and characteristics of breath sounds over the entire chest, comparing sounds between the sides. Select a routine sequence for auscultating the entire chest so you will consistently assess all lobes of the lungs. Figure 4-32 ◆ shows one suggested chest auscultation sequence. Listen to an entire inspiratory and expiratory phase at each spot on the chest before you move to the next site.

Three types of normal breath sounds are usually heard when the chest is auscultated. *Vesicular* breath sounds are low-pitched, swishing, soft, short expiratory sounds. They are usually heard in older children but not in infants and young children. *Bronchovesicular* breath sounds are medium-pitched, hollow, blowing sounds heard equally on inspiration and expiration in all age groups. The location of these sounds on the chest is related to the child's developmental status. *Bronchial/tracheal* breath sounds are hollow and higher pitched than vesicular breath sounds.

Breath sounds normally have equal intensity, pitch, and rhythm bilaterally. Absent or diminished breath sounds generally indicate a partial or total obstruction, such as from a foreign body or mucus, that does not permit airflow.

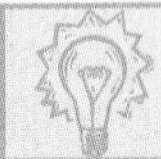

CLINICAL TIP

Auscultation of breath sounds is difficult when an infant is crying. First, try to quiet the infant with a pacifier, bottle, or toy. If the infant continues to cry, all is not lost. At the end of each cry the infant takes a deep breath, which you can use to assess breath sounds, vocal resonance, and tactile fremitus. Encourage toddlers and preschoolers to take deep breaths by providing a pinwheel or mobile to blow.

Vocal Resonance

Auscultate the chest to evaluate how well voice sounds are transmitted. Have the child repeat a series of words, either the same as or different from those used for evaluating tactile fremitus. Use the stethoscope to auscultate the chest, comparing the quality of sounds from

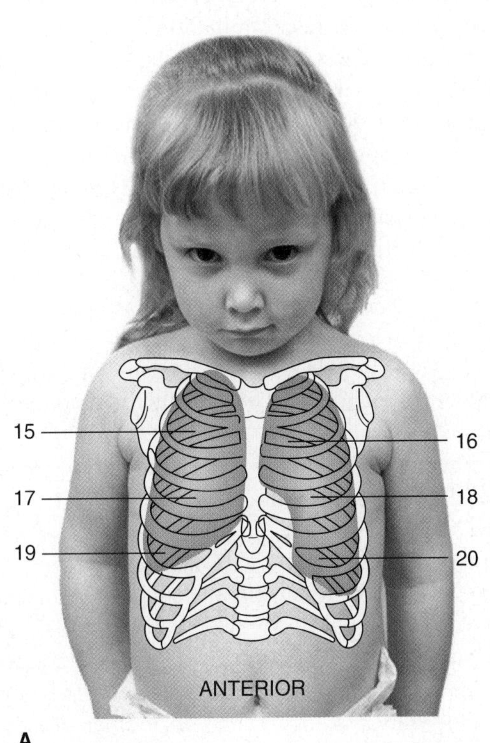

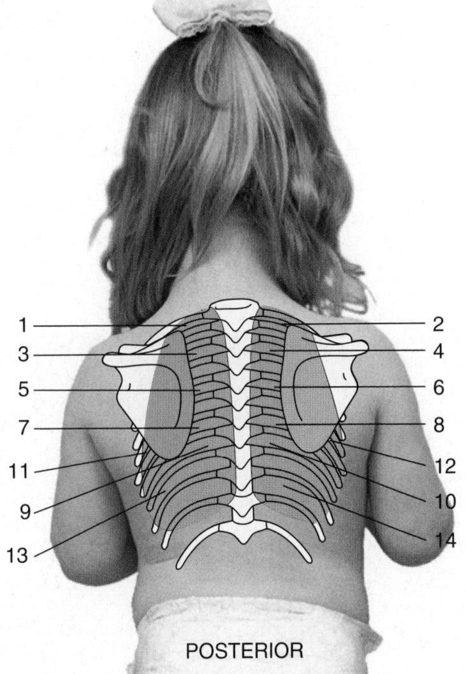

FIGURE 4-32 ◆
One example of a sequence for auscultation of the chest.

GROWTH & DEVELOPMENT

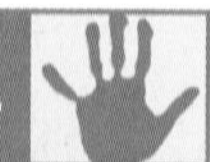

Infants and young children have a thin chest wall because of immature muscle development. The breath sounds of one lung are heard over the entire chest. It takes practice to accurately identify absent or diminished breath sounds in infants and young children. Because the distance between the lungs is greatest at the apices and midaxillary areas in young children, these sites are best for identifying absent or diminished breath sounds. Carefully auscultate, comparing the quality of breath sounds heard bilaterally.

CLINICAL TIP

When trying to get the child to breathe normally while auscultating the chest, use suggestive language to increase cooperation: "You certainly are good at breathing slowly. Have you been practicing?" The child will often deepen and slow the breathing pattern as you give praise and draw attention to it.

side to side and over the entire chest. Voice sounds, with words and syllables muffled and indistinct, are normally heard throughout the chest.

If voice sounds are absent or more muffled than usual, an airway obstruction condition such as asthma may be present. When a lung consolidation condition such as pneumonia is present, the vocal resonance quality changes in characteristic ways. These abnormal characteristics are called whispered pectoriloquy, bronchophony, and egophony. *Whispered pectoriloquy* is present when syllables are heard distinctly in a whisper. *Bronchophony* is the increased intensity and clarity of sounds while the words remain indistinct. *Egophony* is the transmission of the "eee" sound as a nasal "ay" sound.

Abnormal Breath Sounds

Abnormal breath sounds, also called adventitious sounds, generally indicate the presence of a disease process. Examples of abnormal breath sounds are crackles, rhonchi, and friction rubs. To further assess abnormal breath sounds, determine their location, the respiratory phase in which they are present, and whether they change or disappear when the child coughs or shifts position. To routinely identify these adventitious sounds takes practice. Table 4-14 describes adventitious sounds.

Abnormal Voice Sounds

Observing the quality of the voice and other audible sounds is also important during an examination of the lungs. Examples of these sounds are hoarseness, wheezing, stridor, and cough. *Stridor* is a noise resulting from air moving through a narrowed trachea and larynx; it is associated with croup. *Wheezing* is a noise resulting from the passage of air through mucus or fluids in a narrowed lower airway; it is associated with asthma. A *cough* is a reflexive clearing of the airway associated with a respiratory infection. *Hoarseness* is associated with inflammation of the larynx.

PERCUSSION OF THE CHEST

Percussion is a method sometimes used to assess the resonance of the lungs and the density of underlying organs, such as the heart and liver. Today there is less reliance on percussion to evaluate the lungs because of the frequent use of x-ray examination.

When percussing the anterior and posterior chest, choose a sequence that covers the entire chest and permits comparison bilaterally. The same sequence as that used for auscultation is effective. To perform *indirect percussion,* lay the middle finger of your nondominant hand on the child's chest at an intercostal space. Keep the other fingers off the chest. With a springlike motion, use the fingertip of your other hand to tap the finger in contact with the chest (Figure 4-33A ◆). *Direct percussion* is a technique effective for infants. Tap the chest at an intercostal space with a fingertip to elicit the quality of resonance (Figure 4-33B ◆).

TABLE 4-14 Description of Selected Adventitious Sounds and Their Cause

TYPE	DESCRIPTION	CAUSE
Fine crackles	High-pitched, discrete, noncontinuous sound heard at end of inspiration *(Rub pieces of hair together beside your ear to duplicate the sound.)*	Air passing through watery secretions in the smaller airways (alveoli and bronchioles)
Sibilant rhonchi	Musical, squeaking, or hissing noise heard during inspiration or expiration, but generally louder on expiration	Bronchospasm or an anatomic narrowing of the trachea, bronchi, or bronchioles
Sonorous rhonchi	Coarse, low-pitched sound like a snore, heard during inspiration or expiration; may clear with coughing	Air passing through thick secretions that partially obstruct the larger bronchi and trachea

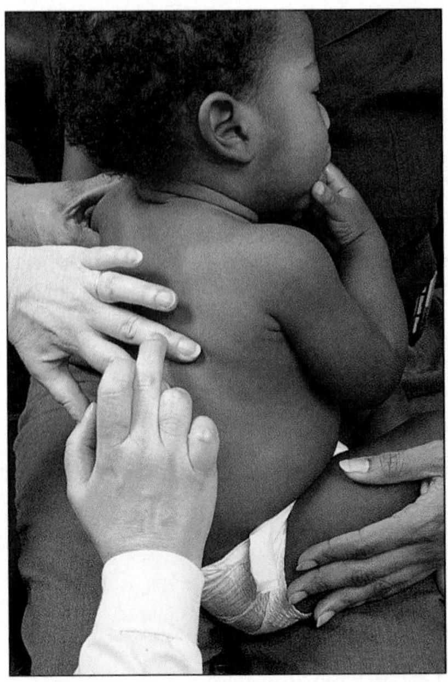
A

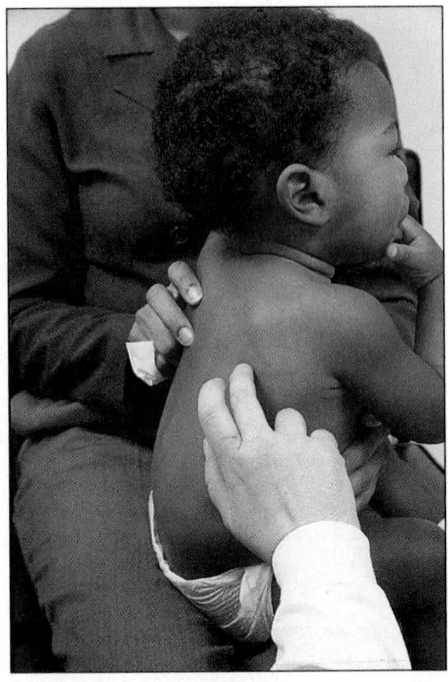
B

FIGURE 4-33 ◆
A, Indirect percussion. Place the middle finger on the child's chest at an intercostal space with the other fingers off of the chest. Tap the finger with a springlike motion with the fingertip of the other hand. B, Direct percussion. Tap the infant's chest with the fingertip directly at an intercostal space.

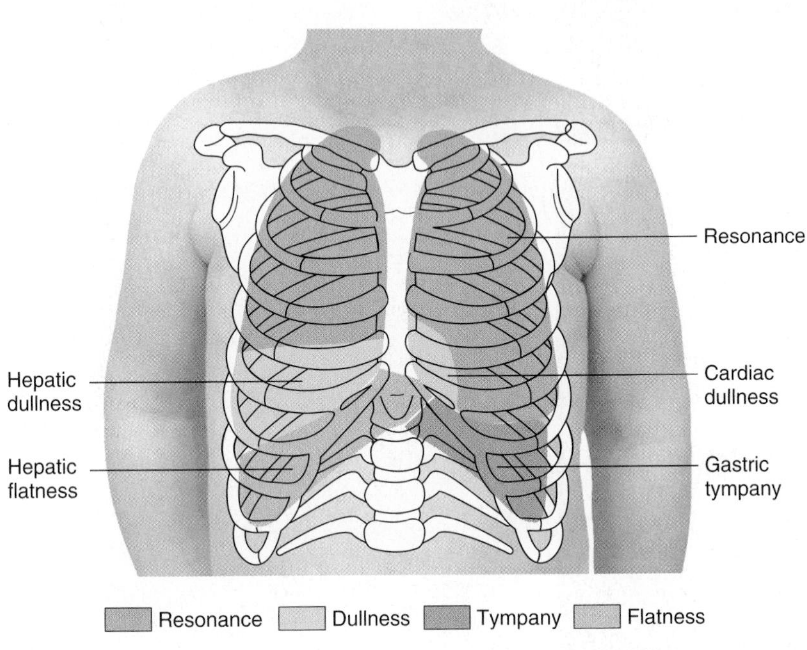

FIGURE 4-34 ◆
Normal resonance patterns expected over the chest. *Tympany* is a loud, high-pitched sound, like a drum. It is usually heard over an air-filled stomach. *Flatness* is a soft, dull sound, like the sound made when percussing your thigh. It is heard over dense muscle and bone. *Dullness* is a moderately loud, thudlike sound. It is heard when percussing over the liver and heart, and at the base of the lungs (at the level of the diaphragm). *Resonance* is a loud, low-pitched, hollow sound, like the sound made when percussing a table. It is heard over the lungs. *Hyperresonance* is a loud, very low-pitched, booming sound. It is usually heard over superinflated lungs. However, because of the thin chest wall in young children, hyperresonance may be a normal finding.

Characteristic patterns of percussion resonance are expected (Figure 4-34 ◆). Characteristic descriptions of sounds heard with percussion of the chest include tympany, flatness, dullness, resonance, and hyperresonance.

 ASSESSING THE BREASTS FOR DEVELOPMENT AND MASSES

What is the first stage of breast development in girls? Do boys have breast development during puberty? What does breast tissue feel like?

INSPECTION OF THE BREASTS

Stages of Development

Inspect the breasts for current stage of development. Breast development in girls precedes other pubertal changes. Breast budding, the first stage of pubertal development in girls, normally occurs between 9 and 14 years of age. Breast development before 6 years of age in

CULTURE 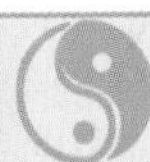

The age of onset of pubertal changes can vary with race and ethnicity, environmental conditions, geographic location, and nutrition. The mean age for breast development in black girls is 8.87 years and for white girls is 9.96 years (Herman-Giddens, et al., 1997).

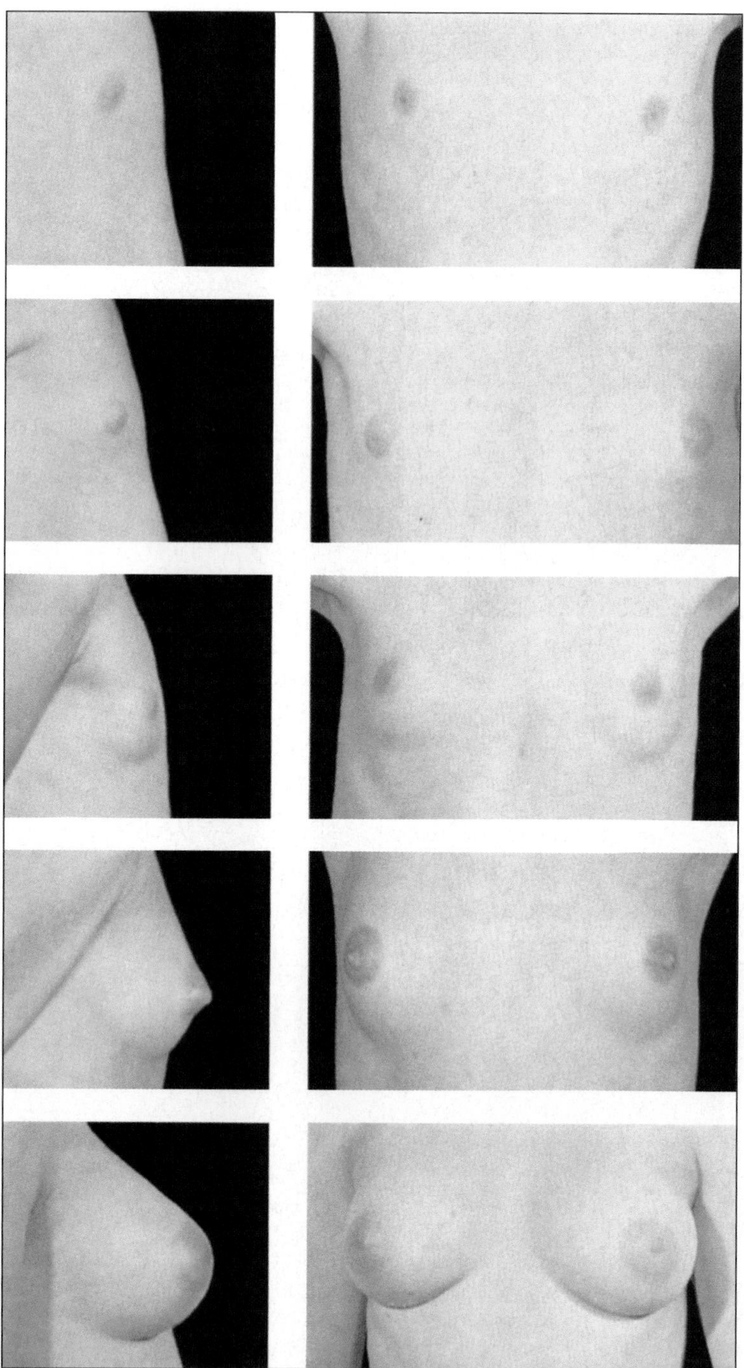

FIGURE 4-35 ◆
Normal stages of breast development.

black girls and 7 years of age in white girls is abnormal (Herman-Giddens, Slora, Wasserman, et al., 1997; Kaplowitz, Oberfield, & the Drug and Therapeutics and Executive Committees of the Lawson Wilkins Pediatric Endocrine Society, 1999). Figure 4-35 ◆ shows normal breast development. A girl's breasts may develop at different rates and appear asymmetric. Boys often have unilateral or bilateral breast enlargement during adolescence. This enlargement can occur as breast buds or actual breast tissue (gynecomastia). It generally disappears without treatment, usually within a year.

Nipples

The nipples of prepubertal boys and girls are symmetrically located near the midclavicular line at the fourth to sixth ribs. The areola is normally round and more darkly pigmented than the surrounding skin. Inspect the anterior chest for other dark spots that may be *su-*

pernumerary nipples, which are small, undeveloped nipples and areola that may be mistaken for moles. Their presence may be associated with congenital renal or cardiac anomalies.

PALPATION OF THE BREASTS

The developing breasts of adolescent females are palpated for abnormal masses or hard nodules. Breast tissue normally feels dense, firm, and elastic.

ASSESSING THE HEART FOR HEART SOUNDS AND FUNCTION

What is the point of maximum intensity and where is it located? Where are the pulse points to assess pulse quality? What heart sounds are associated with systole and diastole? What is the normal heart rate of infants and children? What is the difference between heart sounds and murmurs?

EQUIPMENT NEEDED

Stethoscope
Sphygmomanometer

INSPECTION OF THE PRECORDIUM

Begin the heart examination by inspecting the *precordium,* or anterior chest. Place the child in a reclining or semi-Fowler's position, either on the parent's lap or on the examining table. Inspect the shape and symmetry of the anterior chest from the front and side views. The rib cage is normally symmetric. Bulging of the left side of the chest wall may indicate an enlarged heart.

Observe for any chest movement associated with the heart's contraction. The *apical impulse,* sometimes called the point of maximum intensity, is located where the left ventricle taps the chest wall during contraction. The apical impulse can normally be seen in thin children. A *heave,* an obvious lifting of the chest wall during contraction, may indicate an enlarged heart.

PALPATION OF THE PRECORDIUM

Place the entire palmar surface of the fingers together on the chest wall to palpate the precordium. Systematically palpate the entire precordium to detect any pulsations, heaves, or vibrations. Palpating with minimal pressure increases the chance of detecting abnormal findings.

GROWTH & DEVELOPMENT

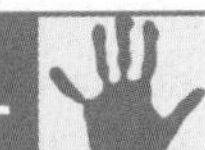

The location of the apical impulse changes as the child's rib cage grows. In children under 7 years, it is located in the fourth intercostal space just lateral to the left midclavicular line. In children over 7 years, it is located in the fifth intercostal space at the left midclavicular line.

Apical Impulse

The apical impulse is normally felt as a slight tap against one fingertip. Use the topographic landmarks of the chest to describe its location (see Figures 4–29 and 4–30). Any other sensation palpated is usually abnormal.

Abnormal Sensations

A *lift* is the sensation of the heart lifting up against the chest wall. It may be associated with an enlarged heart or a heart contracting with extra force. A *thrill* is a rushing vibration that feels like a cat's purr. It is caused by turbulent blood flow from a defective heart valve and a heart murmur. If present, the thrill is palpated in the right or left second intercostal space. To describe a thrill's location, use the topographic landmarks of the chest (see Figures 4–29 and 4–30) and estimate the diameter of the thrill palpated.

PERCUSSION OF THE HEART BORDERS

Percussion of the heart borders is rarely performed during physical examination. The borders of the heart are better identified by x-ray examination. Percussion of the heart should be performed only by an experienced examiner.

AUSCULTATION OF THE HEART

Auscultation is used to count the apical pulse, to assess the characteristics of the heart sounds, and to detect abnormal heart sounds. Use the bell of the stethoscope to detect lower pitched sounds.

To assess heart sounds completely, auscultate the heart with the child in both sitting and reclining positions. Differences in heart sounds caused by a change in the child's position or by a change in the position of the heart near the chest wall can then be detected. If differences in heart sounds are detected with a position change, then place the child in the left lateral recumbent position and auscultate again.

TABLE 4-15 Normal Heart Rates for Children of Different Ages

AGE	HEART RATE RANGE (BEATS/MIN)	AVERAGE HEART RATE (BEATS/MIN)
Newborns	100–170	120
Infants to 2 years	80–130	110
2–6 years	70–120	100
6–10 years	70–110	90
10–16 years	60–100	85

GROWTH & DEVELOPMENT

The child's heart rate varies with age, decreasing as the child grows older. The heart rate also increases in response to exercise, excitement, anxiety, and fever. Such stresses increase the child's metabolic rate, creating a simultaneous need for more oxygen. Children respond to the need for more oxygen by increasing their heart rate, a response called sinus tachycardia. They cannot increase their cardiac stroke volume to deliver more oxygen to the tissues as adults do.

Heart Rate and Rhythm

The apical heart rate can be counted at the site of the apical impulse, either by palpation or by auscultation. Count the apical rate for 1 minute in infants and in children who have an irregular rhythm. The brachial or radial pulse rate should be the same as the auscultated apical heart rate. Table 4-15 gives normal heart rates in children of different ages.

Listen carefully to the heart rate rhythm. Children often have a normal cycle of irregular rhythm associated with respiration called sinus arrhythmia. With *sinus dysrhythmia,* the child's heart rate is faster on inspiration and slower on expiration. When any rhythm irregularity is detected, ask the child to take a breath and hold it while you listen to the heart rate. The rhythm should become regular during inspiration and expiration. Other rhythm irregularities are abnormal.

Differentiation of Heart Sounds

Heart sounds are due to the closure of the valves and vibration or turbulence of blood produced by that valve closure. Two primary sounds, S_1 and S_2, are heard when the chest is auscultated.

S_1, the first heart sound, is produced by closure of the tricuspid and mitral valves when the ventricular contraction begins. The two valves close almost simultaneously, so only one sound is normally heard.

S_2, the second heart sound, is produced by the closure of the aortic and pulmonic valves. Once blood has reached the pulmonic and aortic arteries, the valves close to prevent leakage back into the ventricles during diastole. The timing of the valve closure varies with respirations. Sometimes S_2 is heard as a single sound and at other times as a *split sound,* that is, two sounds heard a fraction of a second apart.

Sound is easily transmitted in liquid, and it travels best in the direction of blood flow. Auscultate heart sounds at specific areas on the chest wall in the direction of blood flow, just beyond the valve (Figure 4-36 ◆). The sounds produced by the heart valves or blood tur-

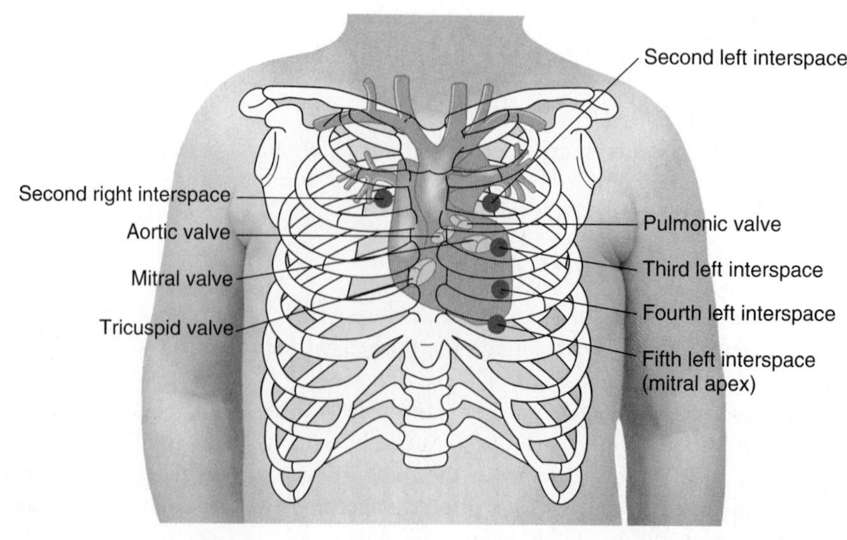

FIGURE 4-36 ◆
Sound travels in the direction of blood flow. Rather than listen for heart sounds over each heart valve, auscultate heart sounds at specific areas on the chest wall away from the valve itself. These areas are named for the valve producing the sound. *Aortic:* Second intercostal space near the sternum. *Pulmonic:* Second left intercostal space near the sternum. *Tricuspid:* Fifth right or left intercostal space near the sternum. *Mitral (apical):* In infants—third or fourth intercostal space, just left of the left midclavicular line. In children—fifth intercostal space at the left midclavicular line.

TABLE 4-16 Identification of the Listening Sites for Auscultation of the Quality and Intensity of Heart Sounds

HEART SOUND	LOCATIONS BEST HEARD	WHERE HEARD SOFTLY
S_1	Apex of the heart Tricuspid area Mitral area	Base of the heart Aortic area Pulmonic area
S_2	Base of the heart Aortic area Pulmonic area	Apex of the heart Tricuspid area Mitral area
Physiologic splitting	Pulmonic area	
S_3	Mitral area	

bulence are heard throughout the chest in thin infants and children. Both S_1 and S_2 can be heard in all listening areas.

Auscultate heart sounds for quality (distinct versus muffled) and intensity (loud versus weak). First, distinguish between S_1 and S_2 in each listening area. Heart sounds are usually distinct and crisp in children because of their thin chest wall. Muffling or indistinct sounds may indicate a heart defect or congestive heart failure. Document the area where heart sounds are heard the best. Table 4-16 and Figure 4-36 review the location where each sound is normally best heard for assessment of quality and intensity.

CLINICAL TIP

Palpate the carotid pulse when auscultating the heart to distinguish between the two heart sounds. The heart sound heard simultaneously with the pulsation is S_1.

Splitting of the Heart Sounds

After the first and second heart sounds are successfully distinguished, try to detect *physiologic splitting.* The split second heart sound is more apparent during inspiration when the child takes a deep breath. More blood returns to the right ventricle, causing the pulmonic valve to close a fraction of a second later than the aortic valve. To detect physiologic splitting, auscultate over the pulmonic area while the child breathes normally and then while the child takes a deep breath. Splitting is normally more easily detected after a deep breath. The splitting returns to a single sound with regular breathing. If splitting does not vary with respiration, then it is called fixed splitting, which is an abnormal finding associated with an atrial septal defect.

Third Heart Sound

A third heart sound, S_3, is occasionally heard in children as a normal finding. S_3 occurs when blood rushes through the mitral valve and splashes into the left ventricle. It is heard in diastole, just after S_2. It is distinguished from a split S_2 because it is louder in the mitral area than in the pulmonic area.

Murmurs

Occasionally abnormal heart sounds are auscultated. These sounds are produced by blood passing through a defective valve, great vessel, or other heart structure.

To hear murmurs in children takes practice. Often murmurs must be very loud to be detected. For softer murmurs, normal heart sounds must be distinguished before an extra sound is recognized. Once a murmur is detected, define the characteristics of the extra sound.

Murmurs are classified by the following characteristics:

- *Intensity.* How loud is it? Can a thrill also be palpated?
- *Location.* Where is the murmur the loudest? Identify the listening area and precise topographic landmarks. Is the child sitting or lying down?
- *Radiation.* Is the sound transmitted over a larger area of the chest, to the axilla, or to the back?
- *Timing.* Is the murmur heard best after S_1 or S_2? Is it heard during the entire phase between S_1 and S_2?
- *Quality.* What does the murmur sound like? For example, is it machinelike, musical, or blowing?

GUIDELINES FOR GRADING THE INTENSITY OF A MURMUR

Intensity	*Description*
Grade I	Barely heard in a quiet room
Grade II	Quiet, but clearly heard
Grade III	Moderately loud, no thrill palpated
Grade IV	Loud, a thrill is usually palpated
Grade V	Very loud, a thrill is easily palpated
Grade VI	Heard without the stethoscope in direct contact with the chest wall

COMPLETING THE HEART EXAMINATION

A complete assessment of cardiac function also includes measuring the blood pressure, palpating the pulses, and evaluating signs from other systems.

Blood Pressure

Skill 5-10: Assessing the Blood Pressure

Assessment of blood pressure is important to detect conditions of hypertension or hypovolemic shock. The technique for obtaining the blood pressure in children can be found in the Skills Manual. Table 4-17 gives upper limits (95th percentile) of blood pressure readings

GROWTH & DEVELOPMENT

Infants have a low systolic blood pressure, and detecting the distal pulses is often difficult. Use the brachial artery in the arms and the popliteal or femoral artery in the legs to evaluate the pulses. The radial and distal tibial pulses are normally palpated easily in older children.

TABLE 4-17 Upper Limits (95th Percentile) of Systolic and Diastolic Blood Pressure Values for Children of Different Ages by Selected Height Percentiles

BOYS

	Systolic BP (mm Hg) by Height Percentile			*Diastolic BP (mm Hg) by Height Percentile*		
Age in Years	**10th**	**50th**	**90th**	**10th**	**50th**	**90th**
1	99	103	106	54	56	58
2	103	107	110	59	61	63
3	106	109	112	63	65	67
4	108	111	114	68	69	71
5	109	113	116	71	73	75
6	110	114	117	75	76	78
7	111	115	118	77	79	81
8	113	116	119	79	81	83
9	114	118	121	81	82	84
10	116	119	123	82	83	85
11	118	121	125	82	84	86
12	120	124	127	83	85	87
13	122	126	129	83	85	87
14	125	129	132	84	86	87
15	128	132	135	85	86	88
16	131	134	138	86	88	90
17	133	137	140	88	90	92

GIRLS

	Systolic BP (mm Hg) by Height Percentile			*Diastolic BP (mm Hg) by Height Percentile*		
Age in Years	**10th**	**50th**	**90th**	**10th**	**50th**	**90th**
1	102	104	107	56	58	59
2	103	106	108	61	62	64
3	104	107	109	65	66	68
4	106	108	111	68	69	71
5	107	110	112	71	72	74
6	109	111	114	73	74	76
7	111	113	115	75	76	78
8	113	115	117	77	78	79
9	115	117	119	78	79	81
10	117	119	122	79	81	82
11	119	121	124	81	82	83
12	121	123	126	82	83	85
13	123	125	128	83	84	86
14	125	127	129	84	85	87
15	126	128	131	85	86	88
16	127	129	132	85	87	88
17	127	130	132	86	87	88

Note: Data from Rosner, B., Prineas, R. J., Loggie, J. M. H., and Daniels, S. R. (1993). Blood pressure nomograms for children and adolescents, by height, sex, and age, in the United States. *Journal of Pediatrics, 123:* 871–886.

of children at different ages by selected height percentiles. Persistent readings at or above this level are associated with hypertension.

Palpation of the Pulses

Palpate the characteristics of the pulses in the extremities to assess the circulation. The technique and sites for palpating the pulse are the same as those used for adults (Figure 4-37 ◆). Evaluate the pulsation for rate, regularity of rhythm, and strength in each extremity and compare your findings bilaterally. The femoral and brachial pulses are the most important pulses to evaluate.

Palpate the femoral arteries and compare their strength with the strength of the brachial pulse. The femoral pulsations are usually stronger than or as strong as the brachial pulsations. A weaker femoral pulse is associated with coarctation of the aorta.

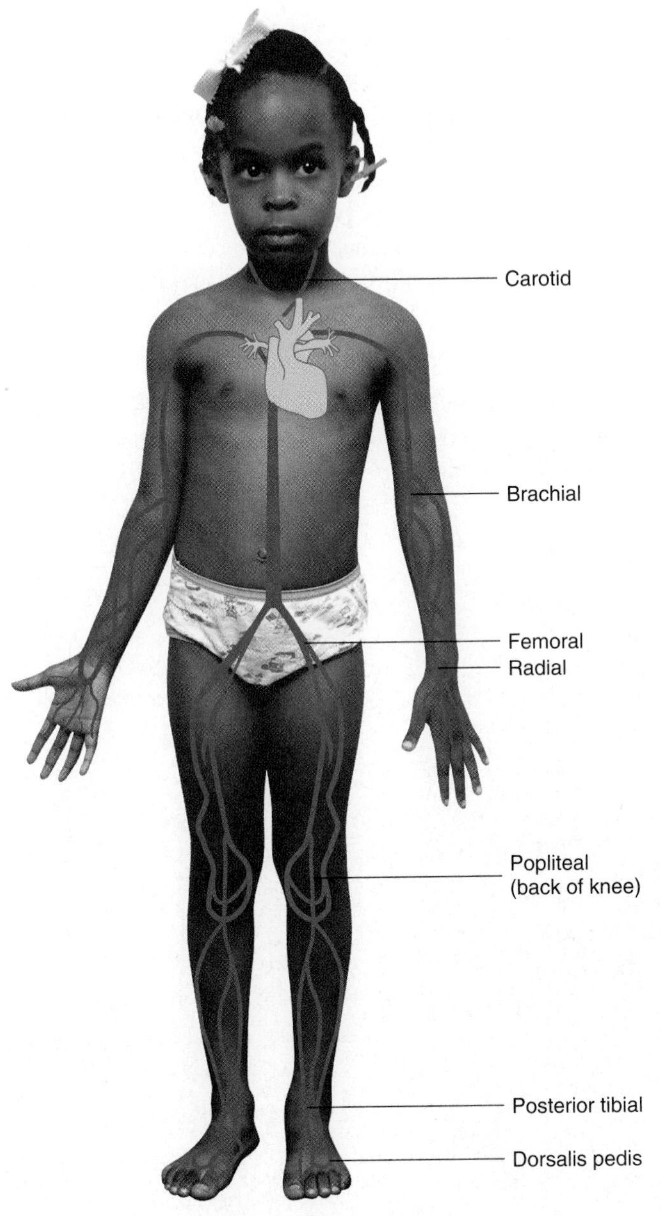

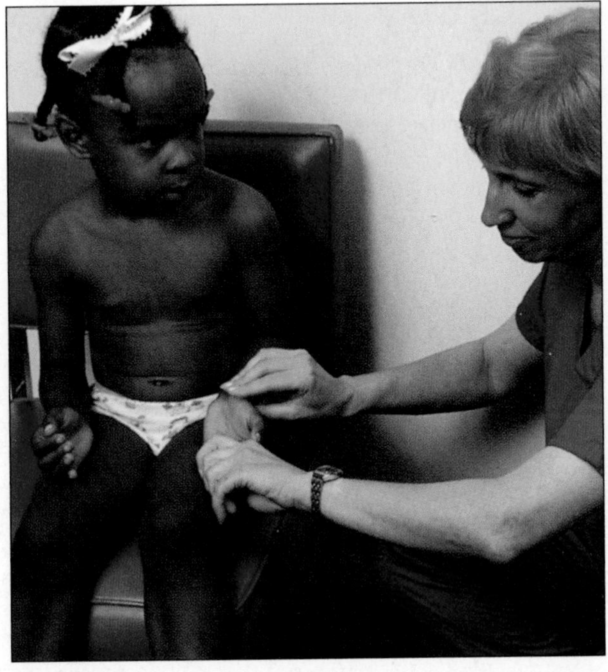

FIGURE 4-37 ◆

A, The sites used to assess pulses in children. B, Place your fingerpads firmly over each pulse point to evaluate the pulsation.

Other Signs

To assess the heart and tissue perfusion, other signs should be considered. These signs include skin color, capillary refill, and respiratory distress. The mucous membranes are usually pink. Cyanosis is most commonly associated with a congenital heart defect in children. Capillary refill is normally less than 2 seconds, indicating good circulation and perfusion of the tissues. Signs of respiratory distress, such as tachypnea, flaring, and retractions, may be associated with the child's attempts to compensate for hypoxemia caused by a congenital heart defect.

ASSESSING THE ABDOMEN FOR SHAPE, BOWEL SOUNDS, AND UNDERLYING ORGANS

What does a sunken abdomen indicate? What do bowel sounds normally sound like? How frequently should bowel sounds be heard in children? What do the various percussion tones indicate? What does a rigid abdomen indicate?

TOPOGRAPHIC LANDMARKS OF THE ABDOMEN

The location of underlying organs and structures of the abdomen must be considered upon examination. The abdomen is commonly divided by imaginary lines into quadrants for the purpose of identifying underlying structures (Figure 4-38 ◆).

INSPECTION OF THE ABDOMEN

Begin the examination of the abdomen by inspecting the shape and contour, condition of the umbilicus and rectus muscle, and abdominal movement. Inspect the child's abdomen from the front and side with good lighting.

EQUIPMENT NEEDED
Stethoscope

Shape

Inspect the shape of the abdomen to identify an abnormal contour. The child's abdomen is normally symmetric and rounded or flat when the child is supine. A scaphoid or sunken abdomen is abnormal and may indicate dehydration.

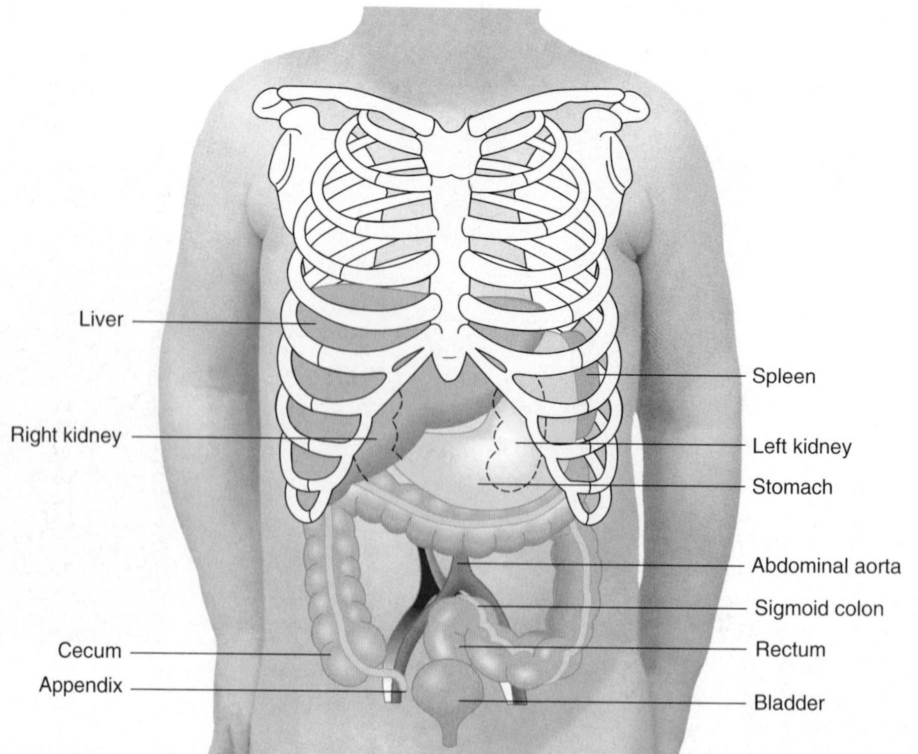

FIGURE 4-38 ◆
Topographic landmarks of the abdomen. The abdomen is commonly divided by imaginary lines into quadrants for the purpose of identifying underlying structures.

Umbilicus

Observe the newborn's umbilical stump for color, bleeding, odor, and drainage. The stump becomes black, dry, and hard within a couple of days after birth. It normally falls off between 7 and 14 days after birth. After the stump falls off, inspect the umbilicus for complete healing. Continued drainage may indicate an infection or a granuloma.

Inspect the umbilicus in older infants and toddlers. Children in these age groups often have an umbilical hernia, a protrusion of abdominal contents through an open umbilical muscle ring.

Rectus Muscle

Inspect the abdominal wall for any depression or bulging at midline above or below the umbilicus, indicating separation of the rectus abdominis muscles. The depression may be up to 5 cm (2 in.) wide. Measure the width of the separation to monitor change over time. As abdominal muscle strength develops, the separation usually becomes less prominent. However, the splitting may persist if congenital muscle weakness is present.

Abdominal Movement

Infants and children up to 6 years of age breathe with the diaphragm. The abdomen rises with inspiration and falls with expiration, simultaneously with the chest rise and fall. When the abdomen does not rise as expected, peritonitis may be present.

Other abdominal movements such as peristaltic waves are abnormal. *Peristaltic waves* are visible rhythmic contractions of the intestinal wall smooth muscle, which move food through the digestive tract. Their presence generally indicates an intestinal obstruction, such as pyloric stenosis.

CLINICAL TIP 

Inspection and auscultation are performed before palpation and percussion because touching the abdomen may change the characteristics of bowel sounds.

AUSCULTATION OF THE ABDOMEN

To evaluate bowel sounds, auscultate the abdomen with the diaphragm of the stethoscope. Bowel sounds normally occur every 10 to 30 seconds. They have a high-pitched, tinkling, metallic quality. Loud gurglings (*borborygmi*) are heard when the child is hungry. Listen in each quadrant long enough to hear at least one bowel sound. Before determining that bowel sounds are absent, auscultate at least 5 minutes. Absence of bowel sounds may indicate peritonitis or a paralytic ileus. Hyperactive bowel sounds may indicate gastroenteritis or a bowel obstruction.

Next auscultate over the abdominal aorta and the renal arteries for a vascular hum or murmur. No murmur should be heard. A murmur may indicate a narrowed or defective artery.

CLINICAL TIP 

Expected pattern of percussion tones over the abdomen: Dullness is found over organs such as the liver, spleen, and full bladder. Tympany is found over the stomach or the intestines when an obstruction is present. Tympany may be found over areas beyond the stomach in infants because of air swallowing. A resonant tone may be heard over other areas.

PERCUSSION OF THE ABDOMEN

Use indirect percussion to evaluate borders and sizes of abdominal organs and masses. Percussion is performed with the child supine. Choose a sequence that permits you to systematically percuss the entire abdomen (Figure 4-39 ◆).

Different tones are expected when the abdomen is percussed, depending on the underlying structures. Organ size can be identified by listening for a percussion tone change at the border of an organ. For example, when you percuss down the chest, the upper edge of the liver is usually detected by a tone change from resonant to dull near the fifth intercostal space at the right midclavicular line. The lower liver edge is usually detected 2 to 3 cm (about 1 in.) below the right costal margin in infants and toddlers, but closer to the costal margin in older children.

CLINICAL TIP 

Use suggestive words to help the child relax so you can palpate the abdomen. "How soft will your tummy get when my hand feels it? Does it get softer than this? Yes. See, it softens as you breathe out. Will it also be softer here?" In this way, the child learns to relax the abdomen and is challenged to do it better.

PALPATION OF THE ABDOMEN

Both light and deep palpation are used to examine the abdomen's organs and to detect any masses. *Light palpation* is used to evaluate the tenseness of the abdomen (how soft or hard it is), the liver, the presence of any tenderness or masses, and any defects in the abdominal wall. *Deep palpation* is used to detect masses, define their shape and consistency, and identify tenderness in the abdomen.

To make the most accurate interpretation, perform the abdominal examination when the child is calm and cooperative. Organs and other masses are more easily palpated when the abdominal wall is relaxed. Infants and toddlers often feel more secure lying supine across

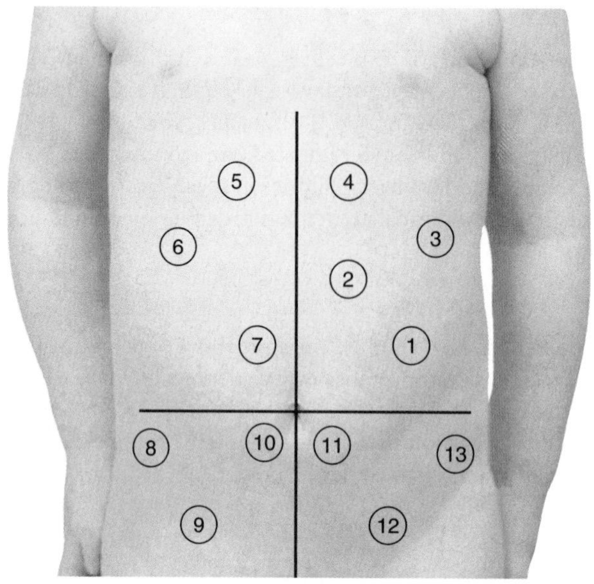

FIGURE 4-39 ◆
Sequence for indirect percussion of the abdomen.

both the parent's and the examiner's laps. A bottle, pacifier, or toy may distract the child and improve cooperation for the examination.

To begin palpation, position the child supine with knees flexed. Stand beside the child and place your warmed fingertips across the child's abdomen. Palpate with the edge of your fingers, not just your fingerpads, and palpate in a sequence to examine the entire abdomen. Watch the child's face as you palpate for a grimace or constriction of the pupils, which indicates the presence of pain.

CLINICAL TIP

When children are ticklish, some special approaches are needed to gain their cooperation. Use a firm touch and do not pretend to tickle the child at any point in the examination. Alternatively, put the child's hand on the abdomen and place your hand over the child's. Let your fingertips slide over to touch the abdomen. The child has a sense of being in control, and you may be able to palpate directly.

Light Palpation

For light palpation, use a superficial, gentle touch that slightly depresses the abdomen. Usually the abdomen feels soft and no tenderness is detected. Palpate any bulging along the abdominal wall, especially along the rectus muscle and umbilical ring, which could indicate the presence of a hernia. Measure the diameter of the muscle ring, rather than the protrusion, to monitor change over time. The muscle ring normally becomes smaller and closes by 4 years of age. An umbilical hernia that persists beyond this age may need surgical repair.

LIVER Locate and lightly palpate the lower liver edge. Place the fingers in the right midclavicular line at the level of the umbilicus and gently move them toward the costal margin during expiration. As the liver edge descends with inspiration, a flat, narrow ridge is usually felt by your finger. Measure the distance of the liver edge from the right costal margin at the right midclavicular line. The liver edge is normally palpated 2 to 3 cm (approximately 1 in.) below the right costal margin in infants and toddlers. It may not be palpable in older children. The liver is enlarged when the edge is more than 3 cm (1.25 in.) below the right costal margin. An enlarged liver may be associated with congestive heart failure or hepatic disease.

CLINICAL TIP

Older children often need distraction, especially when there is a question of abdominal tenderness and guarding or when the child is ticklish. Have the child perform a task that requires some concentration, such as pressing the hands together or pulling locked hands apart.

Deep Palpation

To perform deep palpation, press the fingers of one hand (for small children) or two hands (for older children) more deeply into the abdomen. Because the abdominal muscles are most relaxed when the child takes a deep breath, ask the child to take regular deep breaths when each area of the abdomen is palpated.

SPLEEN Palpate for the spleen at the left costal margin in the midclavicular line. The spleen tip may be felt when the child takes a deep breath. The spleen is enlarged when it can be easily palpated below the left costal margin.

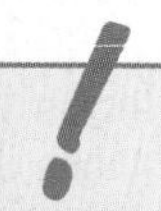

NURSING ALERT

If an enlarged kidney or mass is detected, do not continue to palpate the kidney. Pressure on the mass may release cancerous cells.

KIDNEYS Palpate for the kidneys deep in the abdomen along each side of the spinal column. The kidneys are difficult to palpate in all children, except newborns, because of the deep layer of abdominal muscles and intestines. If a kidney is actually palpated, an abnormal mass may be present.

OTHER MASSES Occasionally other masses, both normal and abnormal, can be palpated in the abdomen. A tubular mass commonly palpated in the lower left or right quadrant is often an intestine filled with feces. A distended bladder is often palpated as a firm, central, dome-shaped mass above the symphysis pubis in young children. Any fixed mass that moves laterally, pulsates, or is located along the vertebral column may be a neoplasm.

ASSESSMENT OF THE INGUINAL AREA

The inguinal area is inspected and palpated during the abdominal examination to detect enlarged lymph nodes or masses. The femoral pulse, a part of the heart examination, may be assessed simultaneously with the abdominal examination.

Inspection

Inspect the inguinal area for any change in contour, comparing sides. A small bulging noted over the femoral canal in girls may be associated with a femoral hernia. A bulging in the inguinal area in boys may be associated with an inguinal hernia.

Palpation

Palpate the inguinal area for lymph nodes and other masses. Small lymph nodes, less than 1 cm (0.5 in.) in diameter, are often present in the inguinal area because of minor injuries on the legs. Any tenderness, heat, or inflammation in these palpated lymph nodes could be associated with a local infection.

EQUIPMENT NEEDED

Gloves
Lubricant
Penlight

ASSESSING THE GENITAL AND PERINEAL AREAS FOR PUBERTAL DEVELOPMENT AND EXTERNAL STRUCTURAL ABNORMALITIES

How is the stage of pubertal development determined in girls and boys? What can a vaginal discharge indicate in a preadolescent girl? Is swelling in a newborn's scrotum normal? Where is the proper location of the urethral meatus on the penis?

PREPARATION OF CHILDREN FOR THE EXAMINATION

Examination of the genitalia and perineal area can cause stress in children because they sense their privacy has been invaded. To make young children feel more secure, position them on the parent's lap with their legs spread apart. Children can also be positioned on the examining table with their knees flexed and the legs spread apart like a frog.

In younger children the genital and perineal examination is performed immediately after assessment of the abdomen. The genitals and perineum may be examined last in older children and adolescents.

GROWTH & DEVELOPMENT

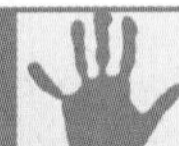

Preschool-age children are often taught that strangers are not permitted to touch their "private parts." When a child this age actively resists examination of the genital area, ask the parent to tell the child you have permission to look at and touch these parts of the body. Some children develop modesty during the preschool period. Briefly explain what you need to examine and why. Then calmly and efficiently examine the child.

INSPECTION OF THE FEMALE GENITALIA

The external genitalia of girls are inspected for color, size, and symmetry of the mons pubis, labia, urethra, and vaginal opening (Figure 4-40 ◆). The stage of pubertal maturation is also determined. Simultaneously look for any abnormal findings such as swelling, inflammation, masses, lacerations, or discharge.

Mons Pubis

Inspect the mons pubis for pubic hair. The presence, amount, and distribution of pubic hair indicates the sexual maturation stage in the girl. Preadolescent girls have no pubic hair. Initial pubic hair is lightly pigmented, sparse, and straight. Pubic hair develops in consistent stages for all girls, but the timing of pubic hair stages is individually determined (Tanner, 1962). Figure 4-41◆ illustrates the normal stages of female pubic hair development. Breast development usually precedes pubic hair development. The presence of pubic hair before 8 years of age is unusual.

Labia

The labia minora are usually thin and pale in preadolescent girls but become dark pink and moist after puberty. In young infants, the labia minora may be fused and cover the structures in the vestibule. These adhesions may need to be separated.

GROWTH & DEVELOPMENT

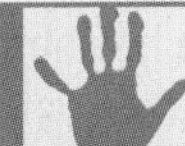

The newborn's external genital structures are strongly influenced by maternal hormones. The labia majora are swollen and the labia minora may be more prominent. The clitoris is relatively large. A white mucoid vaginal discharge can also be seen. As the hormonal influence decreases over a few weeks, these structures attain normal size.

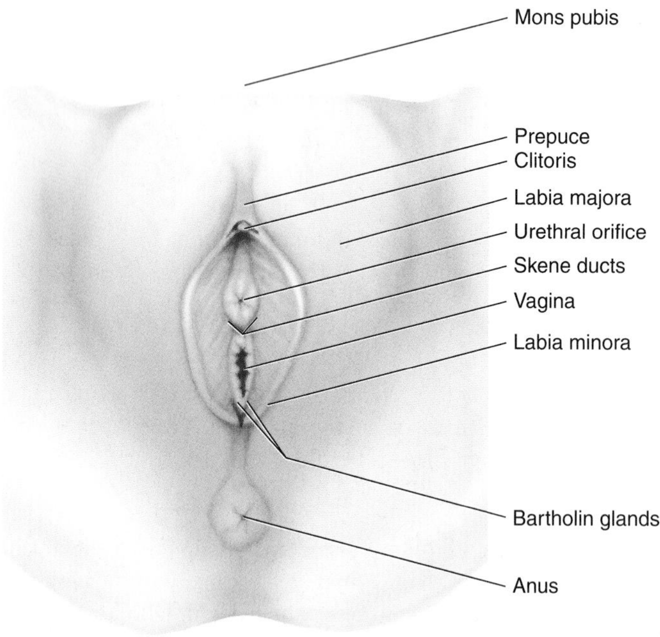

FIGURE 4-40 ◆
Anatomic structures of the female genital and perineal area.

Hymen

Use the thumb and forefinger of one hand to separate the labia minora for viewing structures in the vestibule. The hymen is just inside the vaginal opening. In preadolescents it is usually a thin membrane with a crescent-shaped opening. The vaginal opening is usually about 1 cm (0.5 in.) in adolescents when the hymen is intact. Sexually active adolescents may have a vaginal opening with irregular edges.

NURSING ALERT

Signs of sexual abuse in young children include bruising or swelling of the vulva, foul-smelling vaginal discharge, enlarged opening of the vagina, and rash or sores in the perineal area.

Urethral and Vaginal Openings

Inspect the vestibule for lesions. No lesions or signs of inflammation are expected around the urethral or vaginal opening. Redness and excoriation are often associated with an irritant such as bubble bath.

Vaginal Discharge

Preadolescent girls do not normally have a vaginal discharge. Adolescents often have a clear discharge without a foul odor. Menses generally begin approximately 2 years after breast

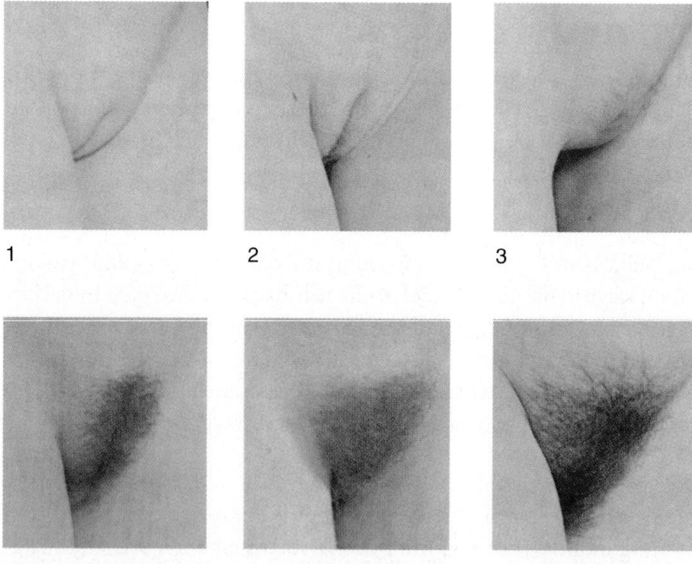

FIGURE 4-41 ◆
The stages of female pubic hair development with sexual maturation. Soft downy hair along the labia majora is an indication that sexual maturation is beginning. Hair grows progressively coarse and curly as development proceeds.
From Van Wieringen et al. (1971), *Growth diagrams 1965 Netherlands.* Groningen: Walters-Noardhof.

bud development. A foul-smelling discharge in preschool-age children may be associated with a foreign body. Various organisms may cause a vaginal infection in older children.

An internal vaginal examination is indicated when abnormal findings such as a vaginal discharge or trauma to the external structures is noted. The vaginal examination of the child should be performed only by an experienced examiner.

PALPATION OF THE FEMALE GENITALIA

Palpate the vaginal opening with a finger of your free hand. The Bartholin and Skene glands are not usually palpable. Palpation of these glands in preadolescent children indicates enlargement because of an infection such as gonorrhea.

INSPECTION OF THE MALE GENITALIA

The male genitalia are inspected for the structural and pubertal development of the penis, scrotum, and testicles. Boys are placed in tailor position, seated with their legs crossed in front of them. This position puts pressure on the abdominal wall to push the testicles into the scrotum.

Penis

The penis is inspected for size, foreskin, hygiene, and position of the urethral meatus. The length of the nonerect penis in the newborn is normally 2 to 3 cm (1 in.). The penis enlarges in length and breadth during puberty. The penis is normally straight. A downward bowing of the penis may be caused by a *chordee*, a fibrous band of tissue associated with hypospadias.

When the penis is circumcised, the glans penis is exposed. To inspect the glans penis of an uncircumcised boy, ask the child or parent to pull the foreskin back. Alternatively, the examiner may retract the foreskin. The foreskin of children over 6 years of age normally retracts easily. If the foreskin is tight and cannot be retracted, phimosis is present.

The glans penis is normally clean and smooth without inflammation or ulceration. The urethral meatus is a slit-shaped opening near the tip of the glans. No discharge should be present. A round, pinpoint urethral meatus may indicate meatal stenosis. Location of the urethral meatus at another site on the penis is abnormal, indicating hypospadias or epispadias. Inspect the urinary stream. The stream is normally strong without dribbling.

Scrotum

Inspect the scrotum for size, symmetry, presence of the testicles, and any abnormalities. The scrotum is normally loose and pendulous with rugae, or wrinkles. The scrotum of infants often appears large in comparison to the penis. A small, undeveloped scrotum that has no rugae indicates that the testicles are undescended. Enlargement or swelling of the scrotum is abnormal. It may indicate an inguinal hernia, hydrocele, torsion of the spermatic cord, or testicular inflammation. A deep cleft in the scrotum may indicate ambiguous genitalia.

Pubic Hair

Inspect the presence, amount, and distribution of pubic hair. Straight, downy pubic hair first develops at the base of the penis. The hair becomes darker, dense, and curly, extending over the pubic area in a diamond pattern by the completion of puberty. The presence of pubic hair before 9 years of age is uncommon. Stages of pubic hair development follow a standard pattern, as illustrated in Figure 4-42 ◆.

GROWTH & DEVELOPMENT

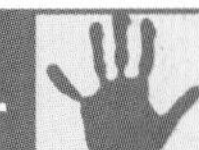

The foreskin is usually not completely separated from the glans at birth. Separation is normally completed by 3 to 6 years of age. A foreskin opening large enough for a good urinary stream is normal, even when the foreskin does not fully retract.

SAFETY PRECAUTIONS

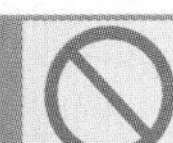

When the boy's foreskin does not easily retract, do not forcefully pull it back. Force may result in torn tissues that heal with adhesions between the foreskin and the glans.

GROWTH & DEVELOPMENT

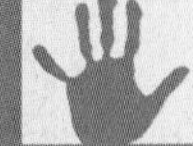

The stage of pubertal maturation is determined by inspecting the amount of pubic hair, size of the penis, and development of the testicles and scrotum. Pubic hair usually appears after the scrotum and testicles start to grow but before the penis begins enlarging (Tanner, 1962).

PALPATION OF THE MALE GENITALIA

Penis

Palpate the shaft of the penis for nodules and masses. None should be present.

Testicles

Palpate the scrotum for the presence of the testicles. Make sure your hands are warm to avoid stimulating the cremasteric reflex that causes the testicles to retract. Place your index finger and thumb over both inguinal canals on each side of the penis. This keeps the testicles from retracting into the abdomen (Figure 4-43 ◆).

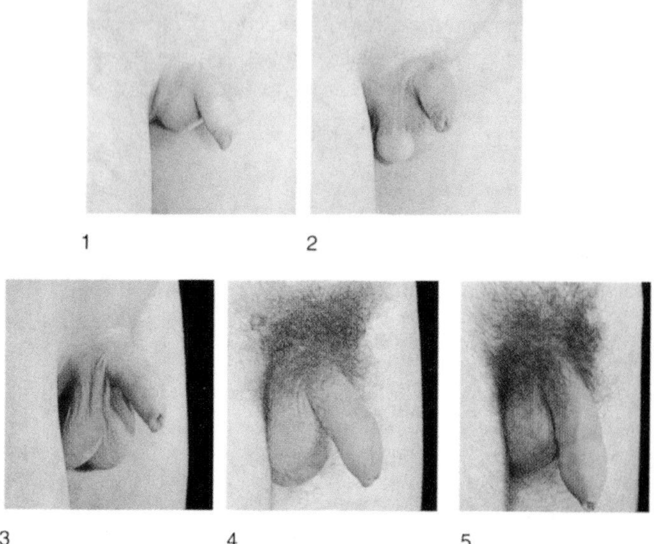

FIGURE 4-42 ◆
The stages of male pubic hair and external genital development with sexual maturation.
From Van Wieringen et al. (1971) *Growth diagrams 1965 Netherlands.* Groningen: Walters-Noardhof.

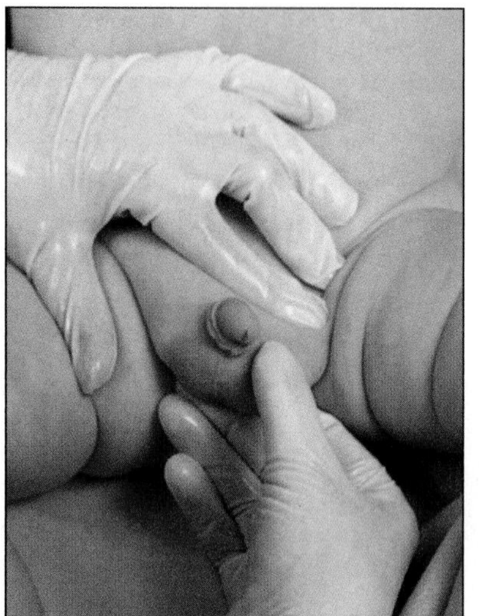

FIGURE 4-43 ◆
Palpating the scrotum for descended testicles and spermatic cords.

Gently palpate each testicle with only enough pressure to identify the shape and size. The testicles are normally smooth and equal in size. They are approximately 1 to 1.5 cm (0.5 in.) in diameter until puberty, when they increase in size. A hard, enlarged, painless testicle may indicate a tumor.

If a testicle is not palpated in the scrotum, the examiner palpates the inguinal canal for a soft mass. When the testicle is found in the inguinal canal, try to move it to the scrotum to palpate the size and shape. The testicle is descendable when it can be moved into the scrotum. An undescended testicle is one that does not descend into the scrotum or cannot be palpated in the inguinal canal.

Spermatic Cord

Palpate the length of the spermatic cord between the thumb and forefinger from the testicle to the inguinal canal. It normally feels solid and smooth. No tenderness is expected.

Enlarged Scrotum

When bulging or swelling of the scrotum is present, palpate the scrotum to identify the characteristics of the mass. Try to determine whether the mass is unilateral or bilateral and attempt to reduce the mass by pushing it back through the external inguinal ring. A mass that decreases may indicate an inguinal hernia. A mass that does not decrease may indicate a hydrocele or an incarcerated hernia.

CLINICAL TIP

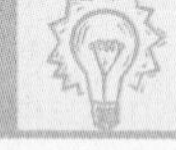

To distinguish between a hydrocele and an incarcerated hernia, place a bright penlight under the scrotum and look for a red glow or transillumination through the scrotum. A hydrocele transilluminates; a hernia does not.

Inguinal Canal

Attempt to insert your little finger into the external inguinal canal to determine whether the external inguinal ring is dilated. The inguinal ring is normally too small for the finger to pass into the canal. If the finger passes into the inguinal canal, ask the child to cough. A sensation of abdominal contents coming down to touch the fingertip may indicate an inguinal hernia.

Cremasteric Reflex

Stroke the inner thigh of each leg to stimulate the cremasteric reflex. The testicle and scrotum normally rise on the stroked side. This response indicates intact function of the spinal cord at the T12, L1, and L2 levels.

INSPECTION OF THE ANUS AND RECTUM

Inspect the anus for sphincter control and any abnormal findings such as inflammation, fissures, or lesions. The external sphincter is usually closed. Inflammation and scratch marks around the anus may be associated with pinworms. A protrusion from the rectum may be associated with a rectal wall prolapse or a hemorrhoid.

PALPATION OF THE ANUS AND RECTUM

Lightly touching the anal opening should stimulate an anal contraction or "wink." Absence of a contraction may indicate the presence of a lower spinal cord lesion.

Patency of the Anus

Passage of meconium by newborns indicates a patent anus. When passage of meconium is delayed, a lubricated catheter can be inserted 1 cm (0.5 in.) into the anus. Resistance in passage of the catheter may indicate an obstruction.

Rectal Examination

A rectal examination is not routinely performed on children. It is indicated for symptoms of intraabdominal, rectal, bowel, or stool abnormalities. The rectal examination should be performed only by an experienced examiner.

ASSESSING THE MUSCULOSKELETAL SYSTEM FOR BONE AND JOINT STRUCTURE, MOVEMENT, AND MUSCLE STRENGTH

What do extra skin folds on an arm or leg indicate? What causes poor muscle tone? What condition does a rib hump indicate? At what age is it normal for children to be knock-kneed and bowlegged?

INSPECTION OF THE BONES, MUSCLES, AND JOINTS

Bones and Muscles

Inspect and compare the arms and then the legs for differences in alignment, contour, skin folds, length, and deformities. The extremities normally have equal length, circumference, and numbers of skin folds bilaterally. Extra skin folds and a larger circumference may indicate a shorter extremity.

Joints

Inspect and compare the joints bilaterally for size, discoloration, and ease of voluntary movement. Joints are normally the same color as surrounding skin, with no sign of swelling. Children should voluntarily flex and extend joints during normal activities without pain. Redness, swelling, and pain with movement may indicate injury or infection.

PALPATION OF THE BONES, MUSCLES, AND JOINTS

Bones and Muscles

Palpate the bones and muscles in each extremity for muscle tone, masses, or tenderness. Muscles normally feel firm, and bony masses are not normally present. Doughy muscles may indicate poor muscle tone. Rigid muscles, or *hypertonia,* may be associated with an active seizure or cerebral palsy. A mass over a long bone may indicate a recent fracture or a bone tumor.

Joints

Palpate each joint and surrounding muscles to detect any swelling, masses, heat, or tenderness. None is expected when the joint is palpated. Tenderness, heat, swelling, and redness can result from injury or a chronic joint inflammation such as juvenile rheumatoid arthritis.

RANGE OF MOTION AND MUSCLE STRENGTH ASSESSMENT

Active Range of Motion

Observe the child during typical play activities, such as reaching for objects, climbing, and walking, to assess range of motion of all major joints. Children spontaneously move their joints through the full normal range of motion with play activities when no pain is present. Limited range of motion may indicate injury, inflammation of a joint, or a muscle abnormality.

GROWTH & DEVELOPMENT

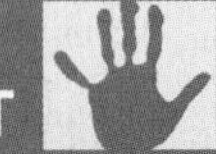

Palpate the clavicles of the newborn from the sternum to the shoulder. These bones are often fractured during delivery. A mass and crepitus may indicate a fracture.

GROWTH & DEVELOPMENT

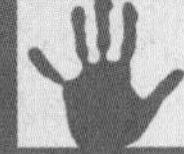

Newborns typically have a limited extension of the hips, knees, and elbows, resulting from their flexed fetal position. When the newborn's arms and legs are extended and released, the extremities rapidly return to their flexed fetal position.

TABLE 4-18 Selected Gross Motor Milestones for Age

GROSS MOTOR MILESTONES	AGE ATTAINED
Rolls over from prone to supine position	4 months
Sits without support	8 months
Pulls self to standing position	10 months
Walks around room holding onto objects	11 months
Walks alone well	15 months
Kicks ball	24 months
Jumps in place	30 months
Throws ball overhand	36 months

Note: From Frankenburg, W. K., Dodds, J., Archer, P., Shapiro, H., & Bresnick, B. (1992). The Denver II: A major revision and restandardization of the Denver Developmental Screening Test. *Pediatrics, 89,* 91–97.

CLINICAL TIP

To check the muscle strength in a newborn, hold the infant upright with your hands under the infant's arms. An infant who is held lightly will normally not slip through the hands. Muscle weakness is present when the infant slides through the hands.

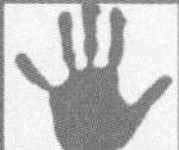

GROWTH & DEVELOPMENT

After beginning to walk, young children often have a pot-bellied stance because of a lumbar lordosis. This posture generally disappears by 5 years of age.

Passive Range of Motion

When a joint is suspected of having limited active range of motion, perform passive range of motion. Flex and extend, abduct and adduct, or rotate the affected joint cautiously to avoid causing extra pain. Full range of motion without pain is normal. Limitations in movement may indicate injury, inflammation, or malformation. Increased passive range of motion may indicate muscle weakness.

Muscle Strength

Observe the child's ability to climb onto an examining table, throw a ball, clap the hands, or move around on the bed. The child's ability to perform age-appropriate play activities indicates good muscle tone and strength. Attainment of age-appropriate motor development is another indicator of good muscle strength (Table 4-18).

To assess the strength of specific muscles in the extremities, engage the child in some games. Muscle strength is compared bilaterally to identify muscle weakness. For example, ask the child to squeeze your fingers tightly with each hand; push against and pull your hands with his or her hands, lower legs, and feet; and resist extension of a flexed elbow or knee. Children normally have good muscle strength bilaterally. Unilateral muscle weakness

TABLE 4-19 Normal Development of Posture and Spinal Curves

Infant

2–3 months

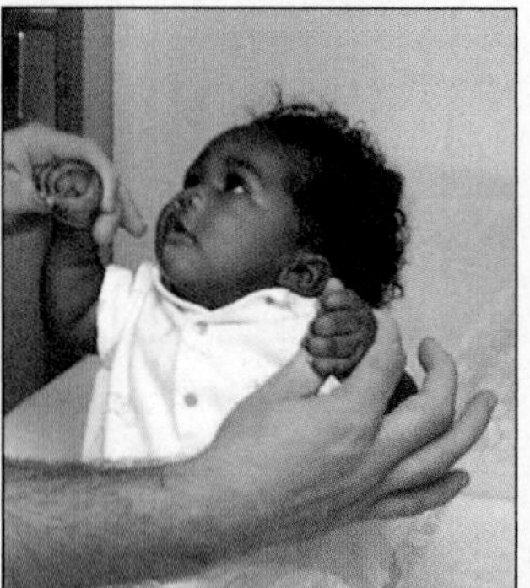

Holds head erect when held upright; thoracic kyphosis when sitting.

6–8 months

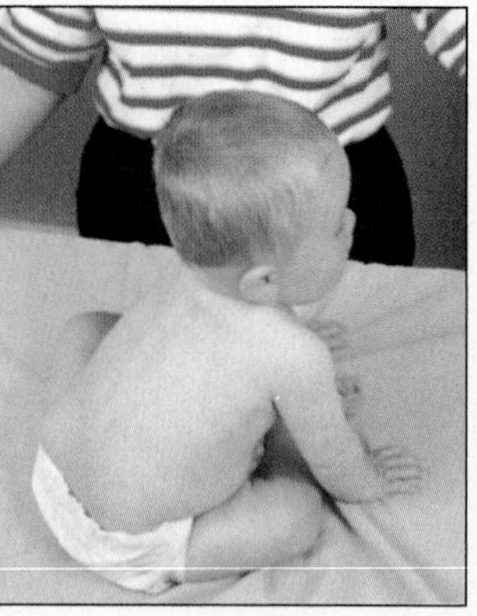

Sits without support; spine is straight.

10–15 months

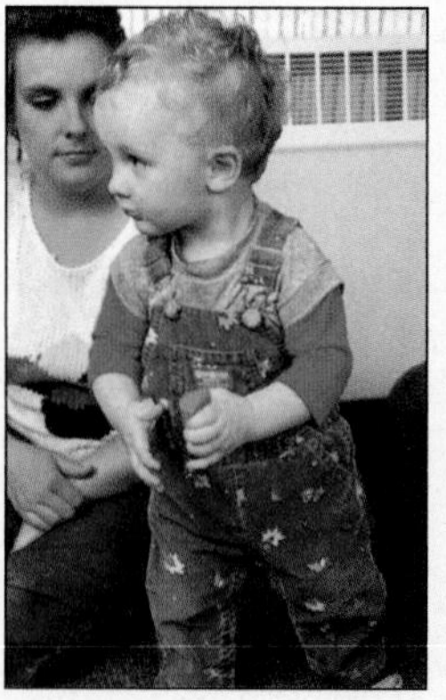

Walks independently; straight spine.

Toddler

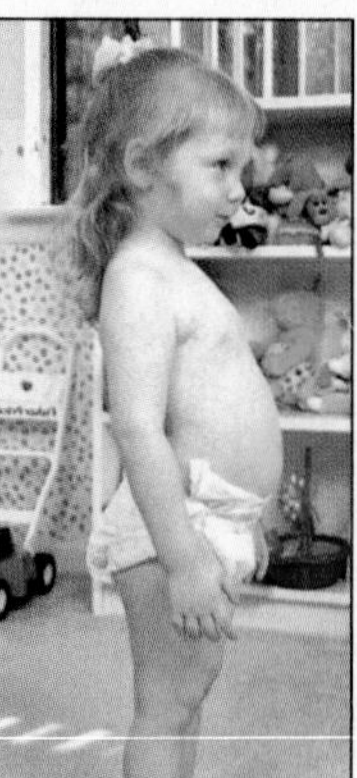

Protruding abdomen; lumbar lordosis.

School-age child

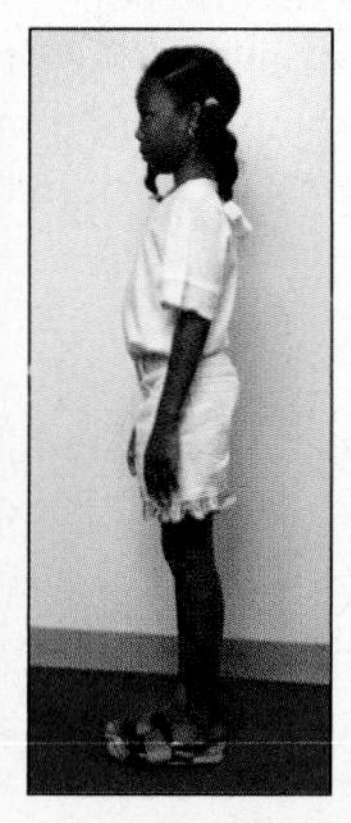

Height of shoulders and hips is level; balanced thoracic convex and lumbar concave curves.

may be associated with a nerve injury. Bilateral muscle weakness may result from hypoxemia or a congenital disorder such as Down syndrome.

When generalized muscle weakness is suspected in a preschool- or school-age child, ask the child to stand up from the supine position. Children are normally able to rise to a standing position without using their arms as levers. Children who push their body upright using the arms and hands may have generalized muscle weakness, known as a *positive Gower sign*. This may indicate muscular dystrophy (see Figure 21–16.)

POSTURE AND SPINAL ALIGNMENT

Posture

Inspect the child's posture when standing from a front, side, and back view. The shoulders and hips are normally level. The head is held erect without a tilt, and the shoulder contour is symmetric. The spine has normal thoracic convex and lumbar concave curves after 6 years of age. Table 4-19 shows normal posture and spinal curvature development.

Spinal Alignment

Assess the school-age child and adolescent for *scoliosis,* a lateral spine curvature. Stand behind the child, observing the height of the shoulders and hips (Figure 4-44 ◆). Ask the child to bend forward slowly at the waist, with arms extended toward the floor. No lateral curve should be present in either position. The ribs normally stay flat bilaterally. The lumbar concave curve should flatten with forward flexion (Figure 4-45 ◆). A lateral curve to the spine or a one-sided rib hump is an indication of scoliosis (see also Chapter 21).

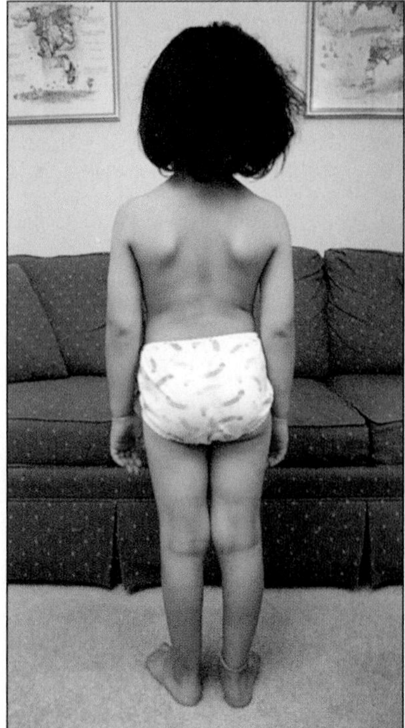

FIGURE 4-44 ◆
Does this child have legs of different lengths or scoliosis? Look at the level of the iliac crests and shoulders to see if they are level. See the more prominent crease at the waist on the right side? This child could have scoliosis.

INSPECTION OF THE UPPER EXTREMITIES

Arms

The alignment of the arms is normally straight, with a minimal angle at the elbows, where the bones articulate.

Hands

Count the fingers. Extra finger digits (*polydactyly*) or webbed fingers (*syndactyly*) are abnormal. Inspect the creases on the palmar surface of each hand. Multiple creases across the palm are normal. A single crease that crosses the entire palm of the hand, a simian crease, is associated with Down syndrome (Figure 4-46 ◆).

Nails

Inspect the nails for size, shape, and color. Nails are normally convex, smooth, and pink. *Clubbing,* widening of the nailbed with an increased angle between the proximal nail fold and nail, is abnormal (see Figure 14–7). Clubbing is associated with chronic respiratory and cardiac conditions.

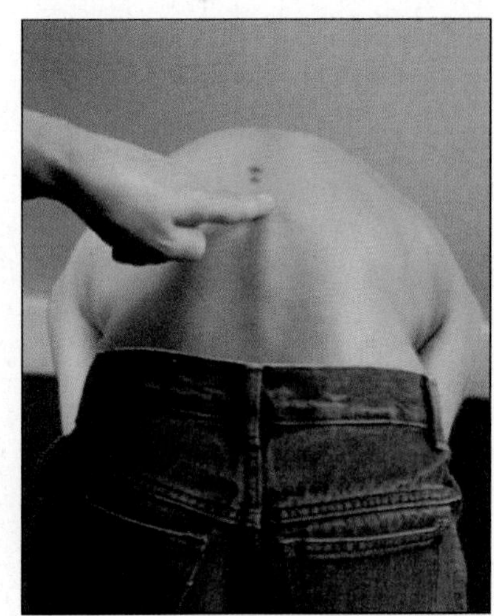

FIGURE 4-45 ◆
Inspection of the spine for scoliosis. Ask the child to slowly bend forward at the waist, with arms extended toward the floor. Run your forefinger down the spinal processes, palpating each vertebra for a change in alignment. A lateral curve to the spine or a one-sided rib hump is an indication of scoliosis.

INSPECTION OF THE LOWER EXTREMITIES

Hips

Assess the hips of newborns and young infants for dislocation or subluxation. The skin folds on the upper legs are inspected first. The same number of skin folds should be present on each leg. Uneven skin folds may indicate a hip dislocation or difference in leg length (Allis sign). Then check for a difference in knee height symmetry (Figure 4-47 ◆). The Ortolani–Barlow maneuver is used to assess an infant's hips for dislocation or subluxation (Figure 4-48 ◆).

The child is asked to stand on one leg and then the other. The iliac crests should stay level. If the iliac crest opposite the weight-bearing leg appears lower, the hip that is bearing weight may be dislocated.

Legs

Inspect the alignment of the legs. After a child is 4 years of age, the alignment of the long bones is straight, with minimal angle at the knees and feet where the bones articulate. Alignment of the lower extremities in infants and toddlers is assessed to ensure that normal

FIGURE 4-46 ◆

A, Normal palmar creases. B, Simian crease associated with Down Syndrome.

Photo B from Zitelli, B. J., & Davis, H. W. (Eds.). (1997). *Atlas of pediatric physical diagnosis* (3rd ed.). St. Louis: Mosby-Year Book.

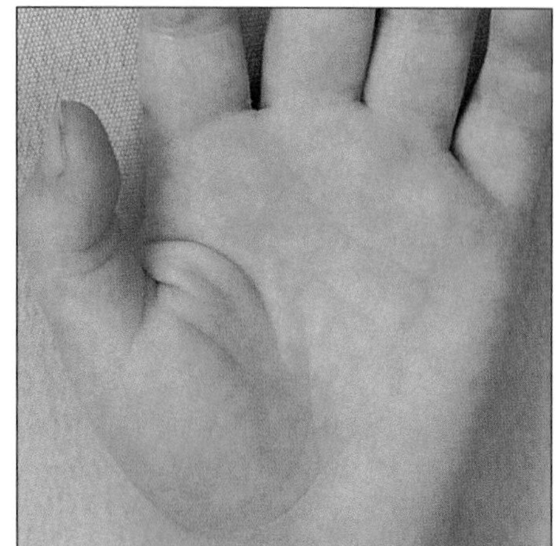

A

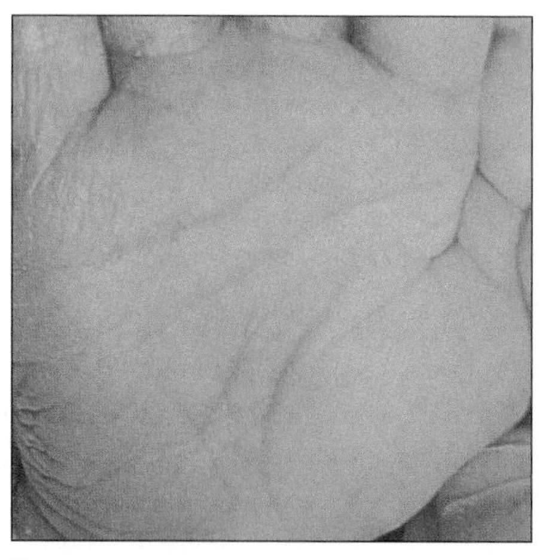

B

FIGURE 4-47 ◆

Flex the infant's hips and knees so the heels are as close to the buttocks as possible. Place the feet flat on the examining table. The knees are usually the same height. A difference in knee height (Allis sign) is an indicator of hip dislocation (see also Chap. 21).

Courtesy of Dee Corbett, RN, Children's National Medical Center, Washington, DC.

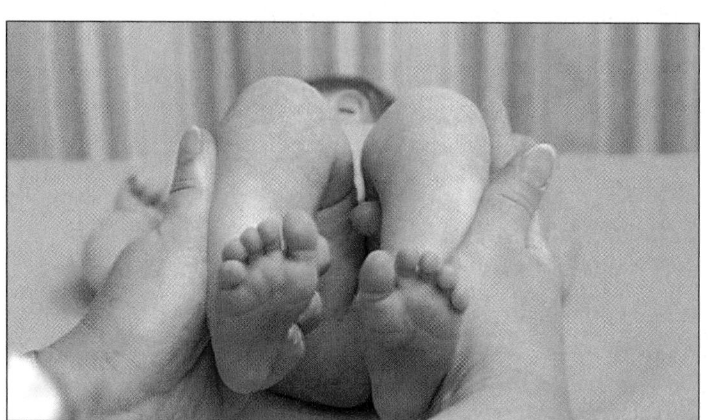

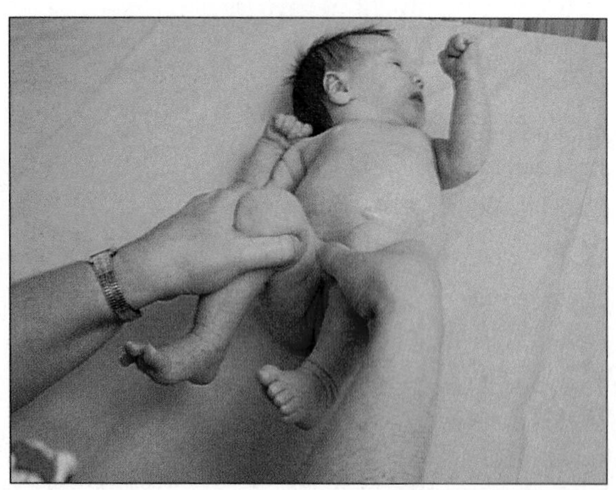

A

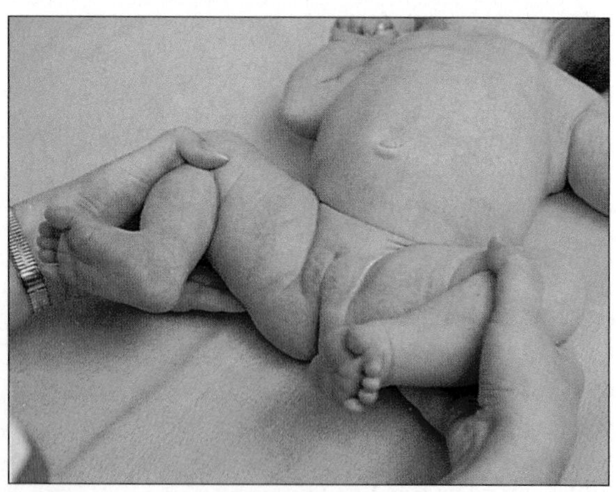

B

FIGURE 4-48 ◆

Ortolani-Barlow maneuver. A, Place the infant on his or her back and flex the hips and knees at a 90 degree angle. Place a hand over each knee with the thumb over the inner thigh, and the first two fingers over the upper margin of the femur. Move the infant's knees together until they touch, and then put downward pressure on one femur at a time to see if the hips easily slip out of their joints or dislocate. B, Slowly abduct the hips, moving each knee toward the examining table. Keep pressure on the hip joints with the fingers in a lever-type motion. Equal hip abduction, with the knees nearly touching the examining table, is normal. Any resistance to abduction or a clunk felt on palpation can be an indication of a congenital hip dislocation.

changes are occurring. To evaluate the toddler with bowlegs, have the child stand on a firm surface. Measure the distance between the knees when the child's ankles are together. No more than 3.5 cm (1.5 in.) between the knees is normal. See Figure 4-49 ◆ for assessment of knock-knees.

Feet

Inspect the feet for alignment, the presence of all toes, and any deformities. The weight-bearing line of the feet is usually in alignment with the legs. Many newborns have a flexible forefoot inversion (metatarsus adductus) that results from uterine positioning. Any fixed deformity is abnormal.

Inspect the feet for the presence of an arch when the child is standing. Children up to 3 years of age normally have a fat pad over the arch, giving the appearance of flat feet. Older children normally have a longitudinal arch. The arch is usually seen when the child stands on tiptoe or is sitting.

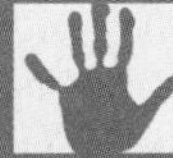

GROWTH & DEVELOPMENT

Infants are often born with a twisting of the tibia caused by positioning in utero (tibial torsion). The infant's toes turn in as a result of the tibial torsion. Toddlers go through a skeletal alignment sequence of bowlegs (genu varum) and knock-knees (genu valgum) before the legs assume a straight alignment.

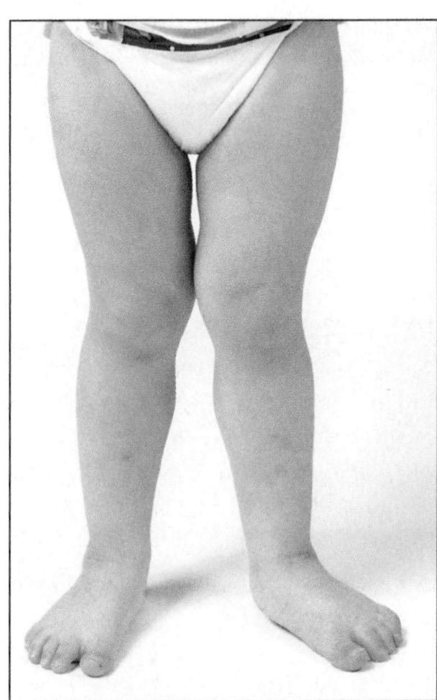

FIGURE 4-49 ◆
To evaluate the child with knock-knees, have the child stand on a firm surface. Measure the distance between the ankles when the child stands with the knees together. The normal distance is not more than 2 in. (5 cm) between the ankles.

ASSESSING THE NERVOUS SYSTEM FOR COGNITIVE FUNCTION, BALANCE, COORDINATION, CRANIAL NERVE FUNCTION, SENSATION, AND REFLEXES

What aspects of developmental information are useful for assessment of cognitive function? How are the infant's and child's levels of consciousness evaluated? How are cranial nerves assessed in infants? A scissoring gait is associated with what condition? At what age does a Babinski response become abnormal? What response is expected when a deep tendon reflex is stimulated?

COGNITIVE FUNCTION

Observe the child's behavior, facial expressions, gestures, communication skills, activity level, and level of consciousness to assess cognitive functioning. Match the neurologic examination to the child's stage of development. For example, cognitive function is evaluated much differently in infants than in older children because infants cannot use words to communicate.

Behavior

The alertness of infants and children is indicated by their behavior during the assessment. Infants and toddlers are curious but seek the security of the parent, either by clinging or by making frequent eye contact. Older children are often anxious and watch all of the examiner's actions. Lack of interest in assessment or treatment procedures may indicate a serious illness. Excessive activity or an unusually short attention span may be associated with an attention deficit hyperactivity disorder.

Communication Skills

Speech, language development, and social skills provide good clues to cognitive functioning. Listen to speech articulation and words used, comparing the child's performance with standards of social development and speech articulation for the child's age (Table 4-20). Toddlers can normally follow simple directions such as "Show me your mouth." By 3 years of age, the child's speech should be easily understood. Delay in language and social skill development may be associated with mental retardation.

Memory

Immediate, recent, and remote memory can be tested in children starting at approximately 4 years of age. To evaluate recent memory, ask the child to remember a special name or object. Then 5 to 10 minutes later during the examination, have the child recall the name or object. To evaluate remote memory, ask the child to repeat his or her address or birth date or a nursery rhyme. By 5 or 6 years of age, children are normally able to recall this information without difficulty.

CLINICAL TIP

The neurologic examination provides an opportunity to develop rapport with the child. Many of the procedures can be presented as games that young children enjoy. Cognitive function can be assessed by how well the child follows directions for the game. As the assessment proceeds, the child develops trust and is more likely to cooperate with examination of other systems.

GROWTH & DEVELOPMENT

Immediate memory can be tested by asking the child to repeat a series of words or numbers, such as the names of Disney or Sesame Street characters. Children can remember more words or numbers with age.

Age	*Recall Ability*
4 years	3 words or numbers
5 years	4 words or numbers
6 years	5 words or numbers

TABLE 4-20 Expected Language Development for Age

LANGUAGE MILESTONES	AGE ATTAINED
Understands Mama and Dada	10 months
Says Mama, Dada, 2 other words; imitates animal sounds	12 months
4–6 word vocabulary, points to desired objects	13–15 months
7–20 word vocabulary, points to 5 body parts	18 months
2-word combinations	20 months
3-word sentences, plurals	36 months

Note: From Capute, A. J., Shapiro, B. K., & Palmer, R. B. (1987). Marking the milestones of language development. *Contemporary Pediatrics, 4,* 24–4.

Level of Consciousness

When approaching the infant or child, observe his or her level of consciousness and activity, including facial expressions, gestures, and interaction. Children are normally alert, and sleeping children arouse easily. The child who cannot be awakened is unconscious. A lowered level of consciousness may be associated with a number of neurologic conditions such as a brain injury, seizure, infection, or brain tumor.

CEREBELLAR FUNCTION

EQUIPMENT NEEDED

Reflex hammer
Cotton balls
Penlight
Tongue blades

Observe the young child at play to assess coordination and balance. Development of fine motor skills in infants and preschool children provides clues to cerebellar function.

Balance

Observe the child's balance during play activities such as walking, standing on one foot, and hopping (Table 4-21). The Romberg procedure can also be used to test balance in children over 3 years of age (Figure 4-50 ◆). Once balance and other motor skills are attained, chil-

TABLE 4-21 Expected Balance Development for Age

BALANCE MILESTONES	AGE ATTAINED
Stands without support briefly	12 months
Walks alone well	15 months
Walks backwards	2 years
Balances on 1 foot for 5 seconds	4 years
Hops on 1 foot, heel-toe walking	5 years
Heel-toe walking backwards	6 years

TABLE 4-22 Expected Fine Motor Development for Age

FINE MOTOR MILESTONES	AGE ATTAINED
Transfers objects between hands	7 months
Picks up small objects	10 months
Feeds self with cup and spoon	12 months
Scribbles with crayon or pencil	18 months
Builds 2-block tower	24 months
Builds 4-block tower	30 months
Unfastens front buttons	36 months

Note: From Frankenburg, W.K., Dodds, J., Archer, P., Shapiro, H., & Bresnick, B. (1992). The Denver II: A major revision and restandardization of the Denver Developmental Screening Test. *Pediatrics, 89,* 91–97.

dren do not normally stumble or fall when tested. Poor balance may indicate cerebellar dysfunction or an inner ear disturbance.

Coordination

Tests of coordination assess the smoothness and accuracy of movement. Development of fine motor skills can be used to assess coordination in young children (Table 4-22). After 6 years of age, the tests for adults (finger-to-nose, finger-to-finger, heel-to-shin, and alternating motion) can be used (Figure 4-51 ◆). The child usually responds enthusiastically when these tests are presented as games. Jerky movements or inaccurate pointing (*past pointing*) indicates poor coordination, which can be associated with delayed development or a cerebellar lesion.

Gait

A normal gait requires intact bones and joints, muscle strength, coordination, and balance. Inspect the child when walking from both a front and a rear view. The iliac crests are normally level during walking, and no limp is expected. A limp may indicate injury or joint disease. Staggering or falling may indicate cerebellar ataxia. *Scissoring,* in which the thighs tend

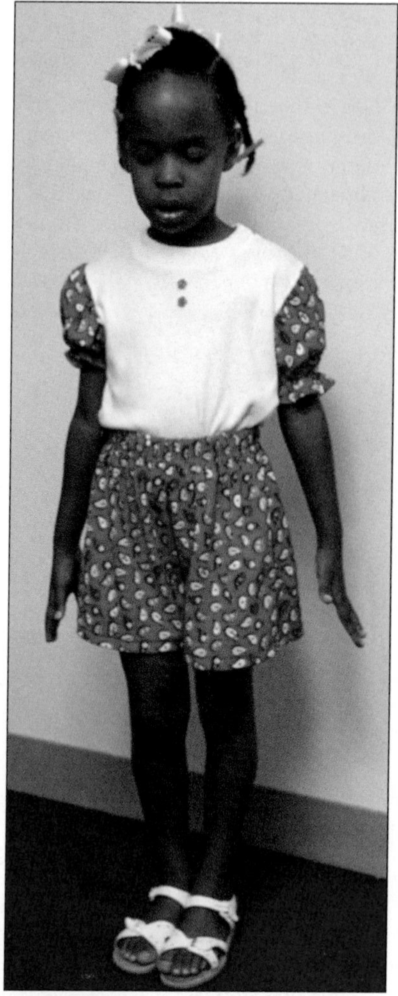

FIGURE 4-50 ◆
Romberg procedure. Ask the child to stand with feet together and eyes closed. Protect the child from falling by standing close. Preschool-age children may extend their arms to maintain balance, but older children can normally stand with their arms at their sides. Leaning or falling to one side is abnormal and indicates poor balance.

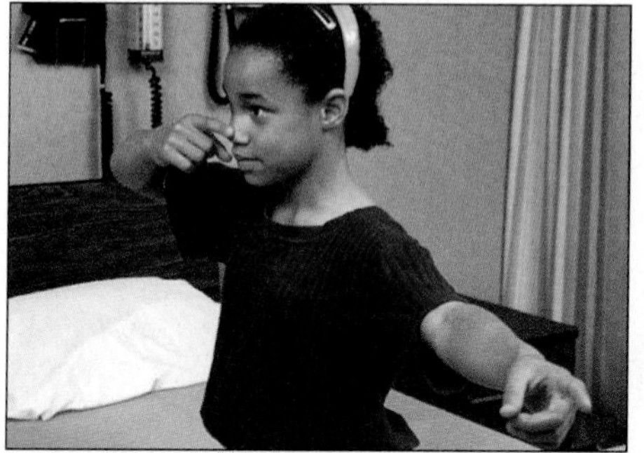

A

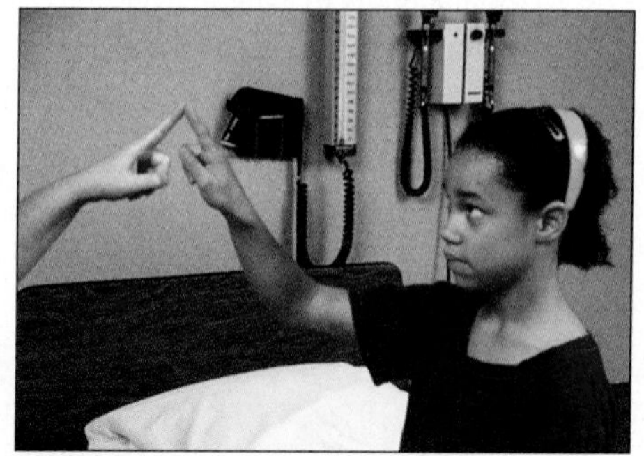

B

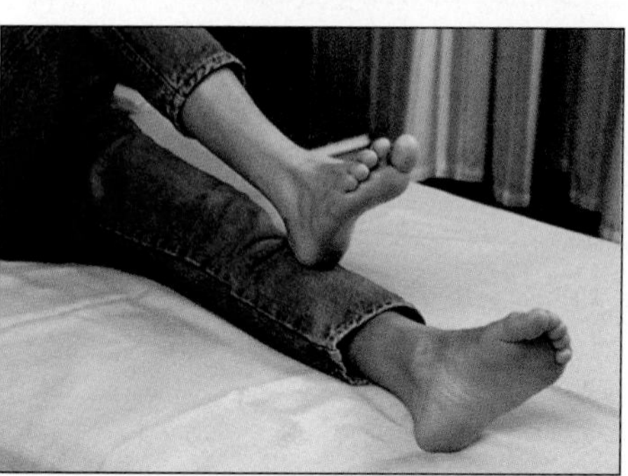

C

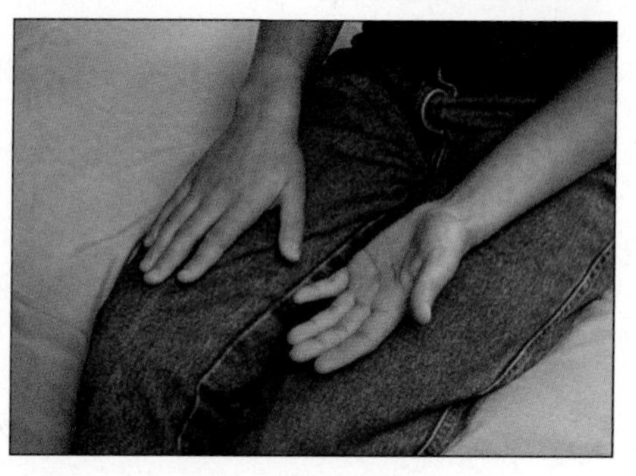

D

FIGURE 4-51 A-D ◆
Tests of coordination. A, *Finger-to-nose test.* Ask the child to close the eyes and touch his or her nose, alternating the index fingers of the hands. B, *Finger-to-finger test.* Ask the child to alternately touch his or her nose and your index finger with his or her index finger. Move your hand to several positions within the child's reach to test pointing accuracy. Repeat the test with the child's other hand. C, *Heel-to-shin test.* Ask the child to rub his or her leg from the knee to the ankle with the heel of the other foot. Repeat the test with the other foot. This test is normally performed without hesitation or inappropriate placement of the foot. D, *Rapid alternating motion test.* Ask the child to rapidly rotate his or her wrist so the palm and dorsum of the hand alternately pat the thigh. Repeat the test with the other hand. Hesitating movements are abnormal. Mirroring movements of the hand not being tested indicates a delay in coordination skill refinement.

GROWTH & DEVELOPMENT

Gait stance is related to the motor development of the child. Toddlers beginning to walk have a wide-based gait and limited balance. With practice, the toddler's balance improves and the gait develops a narrower base.

to cross forward over each other with each step, may be associated with cerebral palsy or other spastic conditions.

CRANIAL NERVE FUNCTION

To assess the cranial nerves in infants and young children, modifications can be made to the procedures used to assess school-age children and adults (Table 4-23). Abnormalities of cranial nerves may be associated with compression of an individual nerve, brain injury, or infections.

SENSORY FUNCTION

To assess sensory function, compare the responses of both sides of the body to various types of stimulation. Equal responses bilaterally are normal. Loss of sensation may indicate a brain or spinal cord lesion.

CLINICAL TIP

An infant's sensory function is not routinely assessed. Withdrawal responses to painful procedures indicate normal sensory function.

Superficial Tactile Sensation

Stroke the skin on the lower leg or arm with a cotton ball or a finger while the child's eyes are closed. Cooperative children over 2 years of age can normally point to the location touched.

Superficial Pain Sensation

Break a tongue blade to get a sharp point. After asking the child to close the eyes, touch the child in various places on each arm and leg, alternating the sharp and dull ends of the tongue blade. Children over 4 years of age can normally distinguish between a sharp and dull sen-

TABLE 4-23 Age-Specific Procedures for Assessment of Cranial Nerves in Infants and Children

CRANIAL NERVE[a]	ASSESSMENT PROCEDURE AND NORMAL FINDINGS[b]
I Olfactory	Infant: Not tested. Child: Not routinely tested. Give familiar odors to child to smell, one naris at a time. *Identifies odors such as orange, peanut butter, and chocolate.*
II Optic	Infant: Shine a bright light in eyes. *A quick blink reflex and dorsal head flexion indicate light perception.* Child: Test vision and visual fields if cooperative. *Visual acuity appropriate for age.*
III Oculomotor IV Trochlear VI Abducens	Infant: Shine a penlight at the eyes and move it side to side. *Focuses on and tracks the light to each side.* Child: Move an object through the six cardinal points of gaze. *Tracks object through all fields of gaze.* All ages: Inspect eyelids for drooping. Inspect pupillary response to light. *Eyelids do not droop and pupils are equal sized and briskly respond to light.*
V Trigeminal	Infant: Stimulate the rooting and sucking reflex. *Turns head toward stimulation at side of mouth and sucking has good strength and pattern.* Child: Observe the child chewing a cracker. Touch forehead and cheeks with cotton ball when eyes are closed. *Bilateral jaw strength is good. Child pushes cotton ball away.*
VII Facial	All ages: Observe facial expressions when crying, smiling, frowning, etc. *Facial features stay symmetric bilaterally.*
VIII Acoustic	Infant: Produce a loud sound near the head. *Blinks in response to sound, moves head toward sound, or freezes position.* Child: Use a noisemaker near each ear or whisper words to be repeated. *Turns head toward sound and repeats words correctly.*
IX Glossopharyngeal X Vagus	Infant: Observe swallowing during feeding. *Good swallowing pattern.* All ages: Elicit gag reflex. *Gags with stimulation.*
XI Spinal accessory	Infant: Not tested. Child: Ask child to raise the shoulders and turn the head side to side against resistance. *Good strength in neck and shoulders.*
XII Hypoglossal	Infant: Observe feeding. *Sucking and swallowing are coordinated.* Child: Tell the child to stick out the tongue. Listen to speech. *Tongue is midline with no tremors. Words are clearly articulated.*

[a]Brocketed nerves are tested together.
[b]Italic indicates normal findings.

sation each time. To improve the child's accuracy with the test, let the child practice telling you the difference between the sharp and dull stimulation.

An inability to identify superficial touch and pain sensation may indicate sensory loss. Identify the extent of sensory loss, such as all areas below the knee. Other sensory function tests (temperature, vibratory, deep pressure pain, and position sense) are performed when sensory loss is found. Refer to other texts for description of these procedures.

INFANT PRIMITIVE REFLEXES

Evaluate the movement and posture of newborns and young infants by the Moro, palmar grasp, plantar grasp, placing, stepping, and tonic neck primitive reflexes (Table 4-24). These reflexes appear and disappear at expected intervals in the first few months of life as the central nervous system develops. Movements are normally equal bilaterally. An asymmetric response may indicate a serious neurologic problem on the less responsive side.

SUPERFICIAL AND DEEP TENDON REFLEXES

Evaluate the superficial and deep tendon reflexes to assess the function of specific segments of the spine.

Superficial Reflexes

Assess superficial reflexes by stroking a specific area of the body. The plantar reflex, testing spine levels L4 through S2, is routinely evaluated in children (Figure 4-52 ◆). Assess the cremasteric reflex in boys (see p. 146).

Deep Tendon Reflexes

To assess the deep tendon reflexes, tap a tendon near specific joints with a reflex hammer (or with the index finger for infants), comparing responses bilaterally. The biceps, triceps, brachioradialis, patellar, and Achilles tendons are usually evaluated in children. Inspect for movement in the associated joint and palpate the strength of the expected muscle contraction (Table 4-25). Table 4-26 outlines the numeric scoring of deep tendon reflexes. Responses are normally symmetric bilaterally. The absence of a response is associated with decreased muscle tone and strength. Hyperactive responses are associated with muscle spasticity.

CLINICAL TIP

The best response to deep tendon reflex testing is achieved when the child is relaxed or distracted. Children often anticipate the knee jerk and either tighten up or exaggerate the response. Making the child focus on another set of muscles may provide a more accurate response. When testing the reflexes on the lower legs, have the child press his or her hands together or try to pull them apart when gripped together.

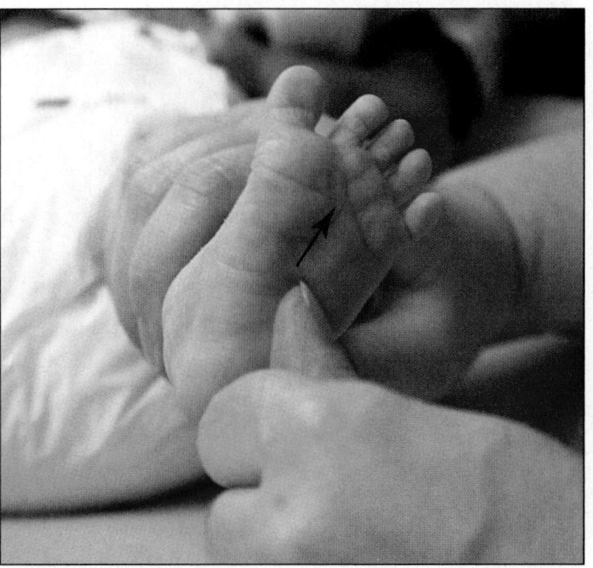

FIGURE 4-52 ◆
To assess the plantar reflex, stroke the bottom of the infant's or child's foot in the direction of the arrow. Watch the toes for plantar flexion or the Babinski response, fanning and dorsiflexion of the big toe. The Babinski response is normal in children under 2 years of age. Plantar flexion of the toes is the normal response in older children. A Babinski response in children over 2 years of age can indicate neurologic disease.

TABLE 4-24 Techniques for Assessing Selected Primitive Reflexes, With Normal Findings and Their Expected Age of Occurrence

PRIMITIVE REFLEX	TECHNIQUE AND NORMAL FINDINGS[a]	NORMAL APPEARANCE AND DISAPPEARANCE
Moro 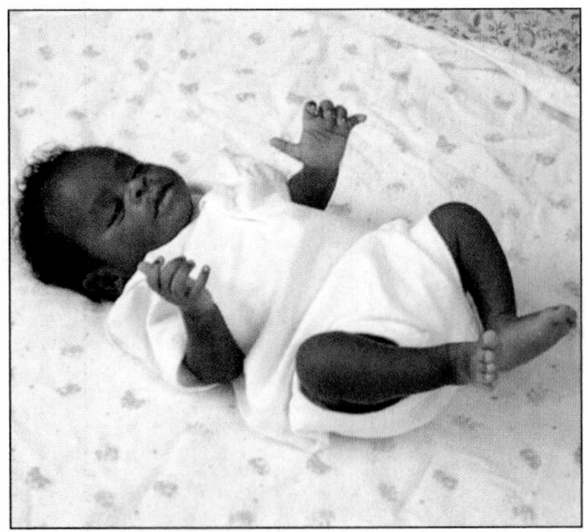	Startle the infant with a sudden noise or change in position. *The arms extend and the fingers form a C as they spread. The arms slowly move together as in a hug. The legs may make a similar motion.*	Present at birth. Decreases in strength by 4 months of age. Disappears by 6 months of age.
Palmar grasp 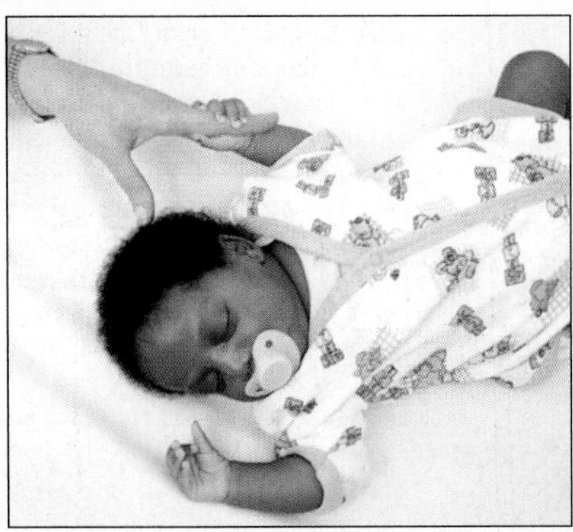	Place finger across the infant's palm and avoid touching the thumb. *A strong grip around the finger is normal.*	Present at birth. Disappears by 3 months of age.
Plantar grasp 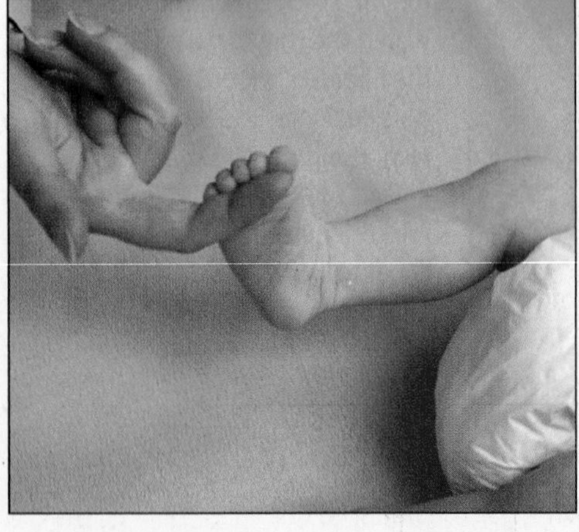	Place finger across the foot at the base of the toes. *The toes normally curl as if gripping the finger.*	Present at birth. Disappears at about 8 months of age.

[a]Italics indicate normal findings.

(continued)

TABLE 4-24 Techniques for Assessing Selected Primitive Reflexes, With Normal Findings and Their Expected Age of Occurrence (continued)

PRIMITIVE REFLEX	TECHNIQUE AND NORMAL FINDINGS[a]	NORMAL APPEARANCE AND DISAPPEARANCE
Placing 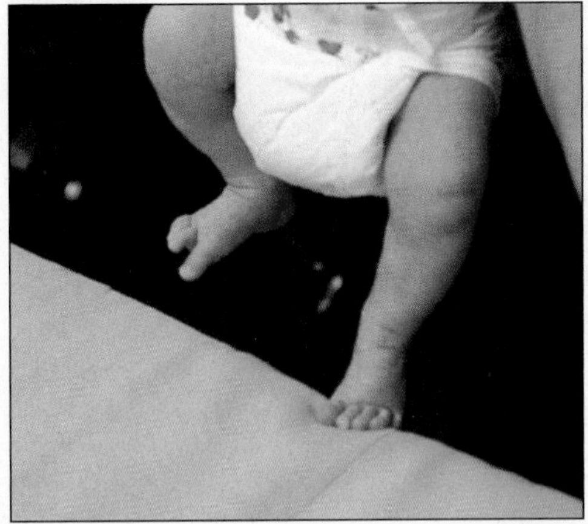	Hold the infant erect and touch the top of one foot with the edge of a table or chair. *The infant normally lifts the foot, as if to step up onto the surface.*	Present within days of birth. Disappears at various times.
Stepping 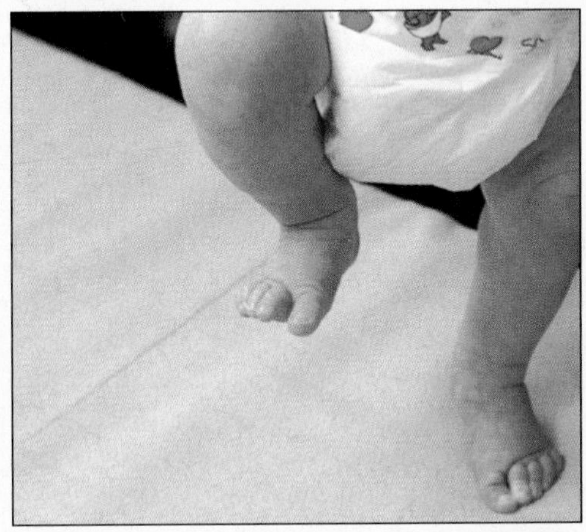	Hold the infant erect and touch the bottom of one foot on the surface of a table or chair. *The feet lift in an alternating pattern as if to walk.*	Present at birth. Disappears between 4 and 8 weeks of age.
Tonic neck 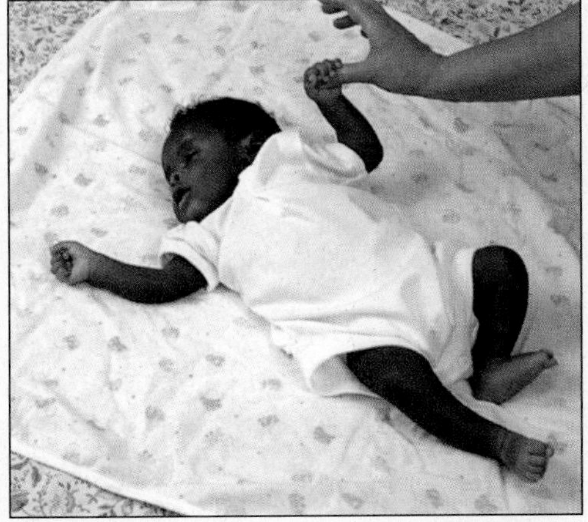	Place the infant in a supine position and, when relaxed, turn the head to one side. Repeat by turning the head to the opposite side. *The arm and leg on the face side normally extend and the opposite arm and leg flex, as if to assume a fencing position.*	Appears about 2 months of age. Decreases by 4 months of age. Disappears no later than 6 months of age. This reflex must disappear before the infant can turn over.

[a] Italics indicate normal findings.

TABLE 4-25 Assessment of Deep Tendon Reflexes and the Spinal Segment Tested With Each

DEEP TENDON REFLEX	TECHNIQUE AND NORMAL FINDINGS[a]	SPINE SEGMENT TESTED
Biceps 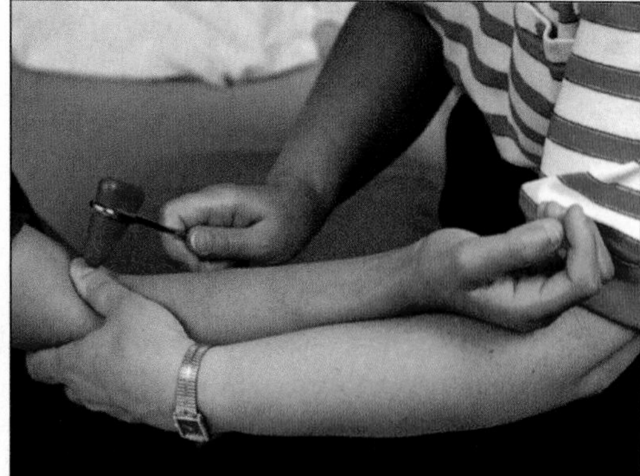	Flex the child's arm at the elbow, and place your thumb over the biceps tendon in the antecubital fossa. Tap your thumb. *Elbow flexes as the biceps muscle contracts.*	C5 and C6
Triceps 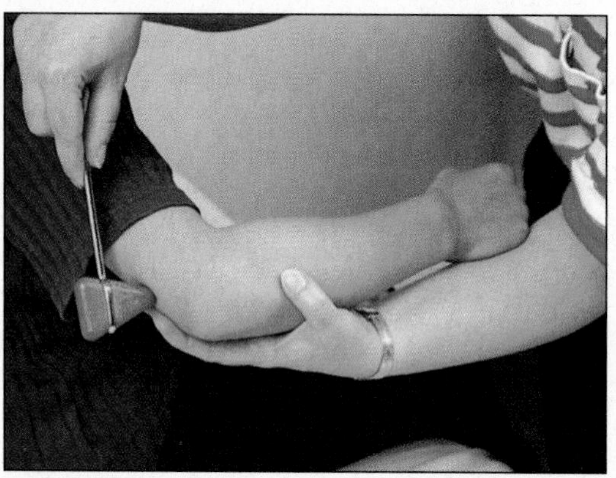	With the child's arm flexed, tap the triceps tendon above the elbow. *Elbow extends as the triceps muscle contracts.*	C6, C7, and C8
Brachioradialis 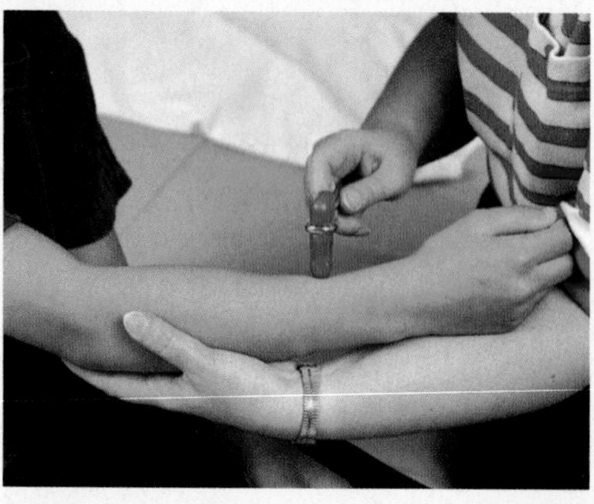	Lay the child's arm with the thumb upright over your arm. Tap the brachioradial tendon 2.5 cm (1 in.) above the wrist. *Forearm pronates (palm facing downward) and elbow flexes.*	C5 and C6

[a] Italics indicate normal findings.

(continued)

TABLE 4-25 Assessment of Deep Tendon Reflexes and the Spinal Segment Tested With Each (continued)

DEEP TENDON REFLEX	TECHNIQUE AND NORMAL FINDINGS[a]	SPINE SEGMENT TESTED
Patellar 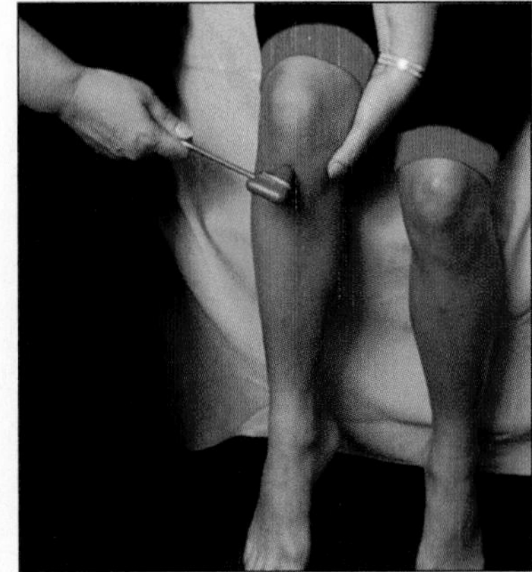	Flex the child's knees, and when the legs are relaxed, tap the patellar tendon just below the knee. *Knee extends (knee jerk) as the quadriceps muscle contracts.*	L2, L3, and L4
Achilles 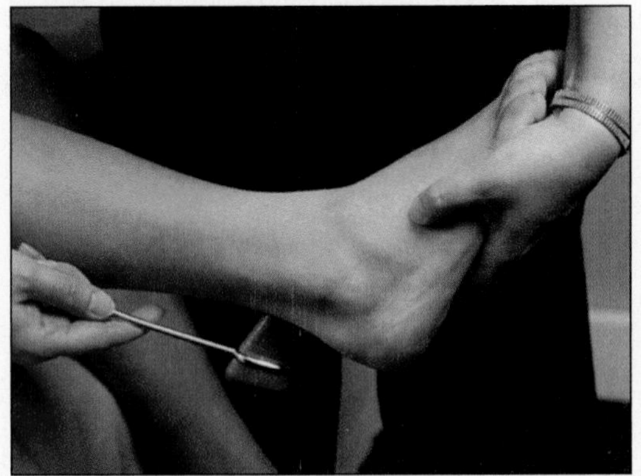	While the child's legs are flexed, support the foot and tap the Achilles tendon. *Plantar flexion (ankle jerk) as the gastrocnemius muscle contracts.*	S1 and S2

[a] Italics indicate normal findings.

TABLE 4-26 Numeric Scoring of Deep Tendon Reflex Responses

GRADE	RESPONSE INTERPRETATION
0	No response
1+	Slow, minimal response
2+	Expected response, active
3+	More active or pronounced than expected
4+	Hyperactive, clonus may be present

ANALYZING DATA FROM THE PHYSICAL EXAMINATION

Once the physical examination has been completed, any abnormal findings for each system should be grouped with those of other systems. **Clinical judgment** is used to identify common patterns of physiologic responses associated with medical conditions. Individual abnormal physiologic responses are also the basis of many nursing diagnoses.

LAW & ETHICS 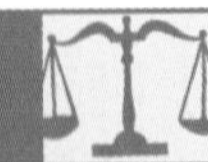

Be sure to record all findings from the physical assessment legibly, in detail, and in the format approved by your institution.

Let us return to the vignette at the beginning of the chapter. Your thorough physical assessment of Latoya has revealed signs of respiratory distress and inadequate tissue perfusion from several body systems. These signs include mottled skin color, an increased resting respiratory rate, retractions, increased respiratory effort, nasal flaring, tachycardia, and lethargy. These signs represent the integumentary, respiratory, cardiac, and neurologic systems. Based on these findings, you would be able to select nursing diagnoses appropriate for an infant with bronchiolitis, for example, Ineffective Breathing Pattern, use of accessory muscles to breathe related to respiratory muscle fatigue; and Caregiver Role Strain related to unpredictability of the care situation. These diagnoses, in turn, would direct your nursing care of this child.

Chapter Highlights

- Establish a rapport with the family and use careful listening techniques to collect historical information about the child's health status.
- Historical data to collect include the chief complaint, history of the present illness or injury, past history, current health status, review of systems, and family history. In addition, psychosocial and developmental data are collected.
- The physical examination sequence includes assessment of the following:
  - Skin and hair
  - Head, eyes, ears, nose, and mouth structures and function
  - Neck
  - Chest and lungs
  - Breasts
  - Heart and pulses
  - Abdomen
  - Inguinal area
  - Genitalia and perineal areas
  - Musculoskeletal system
  - Nervous system
- Clinical judgment is used to identify common patterns of physiologic responses associated with medical conditions.
- The physiologic responses and family and child responses to their health conditions become the basis for many nursing diagnoses.

EXPLORE MediaLink

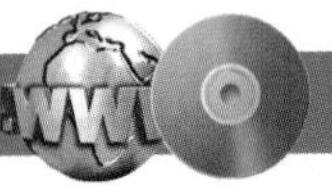

- NCLEX review, case studies, and other interactive resources for this chapter can be found on the Companion Website at **http://www.prenhall.com/ball.** Click on Chapter 4 to select the activities for this chapter.
- For animations, more NCLEX review questions, and an audio glossary, access the accompanying CD-ROM in this textbook.

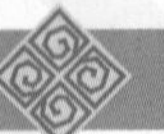

References

1. Burns, C. (1992). A new assessment model and tool for pediatric nurse practitioners. *Journal of Pediatric Health Care, 6,* 73–81.
2. Byrnes, K. (1996). Conducting the pediatric health history: A guide. *Pediatric Nursing, 22,* 135–137.
3. Eichelberger, M. R., Ball, J. W., Pratsch, G. S., & Clark, J. R. (1998). *Pediatric emergencies: A manual for prehospital care providers* (2nd ed.). Upper Saddle River, NJ: Brady, Prentice Hall.
4. Goldenring, J. M., & Cohen, E. (1988). Getting into adolescent heads. *Contemporary Pediatrics, 5,* 75–90.
5. Hazinski, M. F. (1999). *Manual of pediatric critical care* (pp. 289–293). St. Louis: Mosby.
6. Herman-Giddens, M. E., Slora, E. J., Wasserman, R. C., Bourdony, C. J., Bhapkar, M. V., et al. (1997). Secondary sexual characteristics and menses in young girls seen in office practice: A study from the pediatric research in office setting network. *Pediatrics, 99*(4), 505–512.
7. Kaplowitz, P. B., Oberfield, S. E., and the Drug and Therapeutics and Executive Committees of the Lawson Wilkins Pediatric Endocrine Society. (1999). Reexamination of the age limit for defining when puberty is precocious in girls in the United States: Implications for evaluation and treatment. *Pediatrics, 104*(4), 936–941.
8. Seidel, H. M., Ball, J. W., Dains, J., & Benedict, G. W. (2003). *Mosby's guide to physical examination* (5th ed.). St. Louis: Mosby.
9. Spector, R. E. (2000). *Cultural diversity in health and illness* (5th ed.). Upper Saddle River, NJ: Prentice Hall Health.
10. Tanner, J. M. (1962). *Growth at adolescence* (2nd ed.). Oxford: Blackwell Scientific Publications, Inc.
11. Wilson, E. F. (1977). Estimation of the age of cutaneous contusions in child abuse. *Pediatrics, 60,* 750.

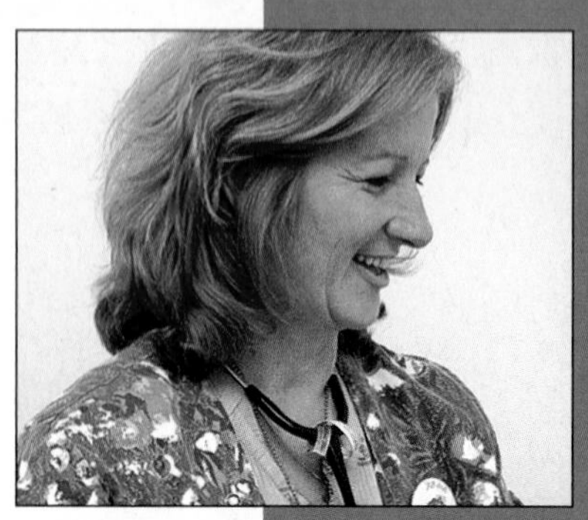

"USING A DOLL TO DEMONSTRATE PROCEDURES IS A HELPFUL TECHNIQUE IN PREPARING A CHILD OF SABRINA'S AGE FOR SURGERY. ALTHOUGH SHE IS ANXIOUS AT FIRST, PLAYING WITH THE DOLL HELPS HER TO FEEL MORE CONTROL OVER WHAT WILL HAPPEN."

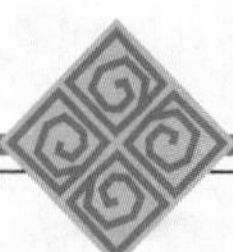

Four-year-old Sabrina has had several nosebleeds and fainting spells recently. After examination by her physician and a number of diagnostic studies such as chest x-ray examination, echocardiography, and electrocardiography, coarctation of the aorta is diagnosed. Sabrina will come in this week for a cardiac catheterization. In 2 weeks, she is scheduled to have open heart surgery.

Sabrina and her family live about 50 miles from the medical center. Her parents have three other children, ages 9, 7, and 2. The parents are both employed, but Sabrina's mother plans to take several days off at the time of surgery. Sabrina attends preschool, and she is used to spending time with other children.

Sabrina has had few health problems, and her experiences with health care professionals are limited. Her parents, who are anxious about the heart surgery, are concerned about how their daughter will adapt to hospitalization.

How should you prepare Sabrina for the cardiac catheterization and for the surgery? How far in advance should teaching take place? What teaching aids are helpful? How can Sabrina's parents be involved in and reinforce the teaching? What kind of support do her parents, siblings, and friends need during hospitalization?

CHAPTER

5

NURSING CONSIDERATIONS FOR THE HOSPITALIZED CHILD

KEY TERMS

case manager Person who coordinates health care to prevent gaps or overlaps.

child life specialist Trained professional who plans therapeutic activities for hospitalized children.

Individualized Education Plan Formulation of a specific learning approach for a child with a physical or mental disability, following thorough assessment of the child's capabilities and areas of need.

Individualized Transition Plan A plan that focuses on assisting the individual in moving successfully from school and home into other community settings.

rehabilitation Assisting a child with physical or mental challenges to reach his or her fullest potential through therapy and education that considers the physiologic, psychologic, and environmental strengths and limitations of the child.

rooming in Practice in which parents stay in the child's hospital room and care for the child.

separation anxiety Distress behaviors observed in young children separated from familiar caregivers.

therapeutic play Planned play techniques that provide an opportunity for children to deal with their fears and concerns related to illness or hospitalization.

MediaLink 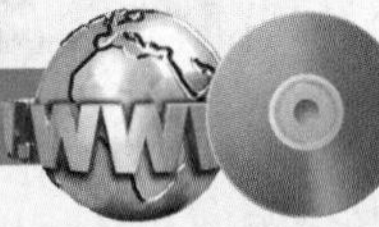

http://www.prenhall.com/ball

Resources for this chapter can be found on the CD-ROM accompanying this textbook, and on the Companion Website at http://www.prenhall.com/ball. Click on Chapter 5 and select the activities for this chapter.

CD-ROM

Audio Glossary

NCLEX Review

COMPANION WEBSITE

Web Links

NCLEX Review

MediaLink Applications

Communication Strategy: Preparing a Toddler for Venipuncture

Hospitalization, whether it is elective, planned in advance, or the result of an emergency or trauma, is stressful for children of all ages and their families. Today, children are infrequently hospitalized, because most pediatric conditions can be managed within the community. Hospitalized children are usually very ill. They are in an unknown environment, surrounded by strange people, equipment, and frightening sights and sounds. These children are subjected to unfamiliar procedures, some of which are invasive, and may even have surgery or be in an intensive care unit. For both children and families, routines are disrupted and normal coping strategies are tested.

To minimize the stress of hospitalization, nurses need to provide support to children and their families before, during, and after hospitalization. Through preadmission preparation, children and their families are introduced to the acute care setting. During hospitalization, nurses work collaboratively with parents to use various strategies that promote coping and adaptation, or prepare children for procedures and surgery. Nurses are instrumental in ensuring that the developmental and educational needs of children are met, especially when hospitalization is prolonged. Nurses also work with families to help prepare for discharge or transfer to a long-term care or rehabilitation facility.

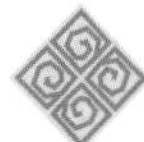

EFFECTS OF ILLNESS AND HOSPITALIZATION ON CHILDREN AND FAMILIES

CHILDREN'S UNDERSTANDING OF HEALTH AND ILLNESS

Can you remember as a child thinking that yelling at your mother caused your strep throat? Perhaps as an adolescent you believed that you would never become ill or have an accident. Maybe you feared being in a car crash like that of a friend. Children have limited knowledge about the body and its relation to health and illness. Their understanding is based primarily on their cognitive ability at various developmental stages and on previous experiences with health care professionals.

Infant

By about 6 months of age, infants have developed an awareness of themselves as separate from their mother or father. They are able to identify primary caretakers and to feel anxious when in contact with strangers. Hospitalization can be a traumatic time for an infant, particularly if the parents are not staying with the child.

Three phases of **separation anxiety** were first identified in young children who were separated from their parents for long periods or permanently and lacked a close relationship with one caretaker after separation (Bowlby, 1960). Characteristic behaviors of children in the three phases of separation anxiety are listed in Table 5-1. Infants and young children who are hospitalized often display some of these behaviors, particularly if parents are unable to remain with the child.

Before the 1970s, health care professionals assumed that the despair and denial manifested by infants and young children after prolonged separation were signs of positive adaptation, since the child in these stages seemed calm and quiet. Infants sometimes protested when their parents visited, and parents were therefore advised not to visit often. However, the protest phase is now viewed as a healthy response to separation from loved ones and as an indication that the infant has meaningful, close relationships. Parents should be encouraged to remain with and provide care to the hospitalized infant, and to visit as often as possible if they cannot remain with the young child.

Toddler and Preschooler

Toddlers and preschoolers are beginning to understand illness but not its cause. Two unrelated events may appear to have a cause-and-effect relationship for young children, who may consider the sun, an animal, bad behavior, or even magic to be the cause of their illness. These children may blame other people, events, or themselves for an illness (Bibace & Walsh, 1981), especially if the other event occurs shortly before the illness.

The child's concept of the body usually is limited to names and locations of some body parts. Although toddlers and preschoolers are not likely to understand how lungs, the heart,

TABLE 5-1 Stages of Separation Anxiety in Young Children

PROTEST
Screaming, crying Clinging to parents Withdrawal from other adults
DESPAIR
Sadness, depression Withdrawal or compliant behavior Crying when parents appear
DENIAL
Lack of protest when parents leave Appearance of being happy and content with everyone Close relationships not established Developmental delay possible

Note: From Separation Anxiety by J. Bowlby, 1960. *International Journal of Psychoanalysis, 41,* 89–113. Adapted.

bones, or other body parts function, they are learning concepts of safety and other health-related issues (Mobley, 1996).

Separation from parents remains the major stressor for the child. When a parent cannot be present, reminders can be left with the child. These might include a piece of cloth saturated with the mother's favorite perfume or father's cologne, an object belonging to the parent, or an audiotape with messages from the parents. Toddlers and preschoolers fear bodily mutilation and change. If, like Sabrina, the child is undergoing an operation, the nurse should explain to the child that surgery will fix the body. The nurse should encourage the parents to be present as much as possible for important rituals such as toileting, carrying out bedtime routines, and singing favorite nursery rhymes.

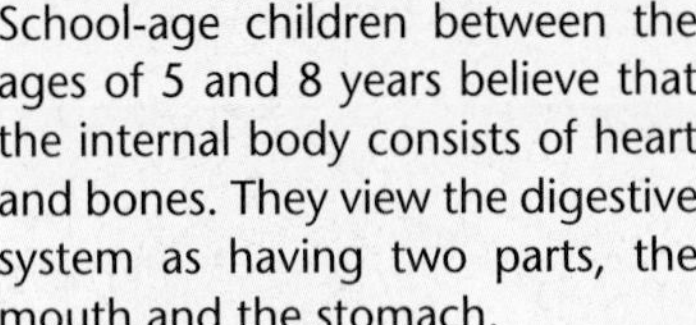

School-age children between the ages of 5 and 8 years believe that the internal body consists of heart and bones. They view the digestive system as having two parts, the mouth and the stomach.

School-Age Child

Older children have a more realistic understanding of the reasons for illness and are able to comprehend explanations. The child's concept of body parts and function is maturing. Concepts of time are well formed, and parents should be encouraged to tell the child when they will return. Parents should also be available for telephone calls to provide support and comfort. Stressful procedures can lead to regression or other behavioral changes. The child relies on parents and others for support and understanding during these events.

Adolescent

After 11 years of age, adolescents become increasingly aware of the physiologic, psychologic, and behavioral causes of illness and injury. Adolescents are concerned with appearance and perceive an illness or injury in terms of its effect on their body image. Allowing choices in clothing, hair, and music acknowledges the importance of their self-identity (Rosenbaum & Carty, 1996). Privacy and modesty are major concerns of adolescents because their physical characteristics are rapidly changing. Nurses should respect their feelings.

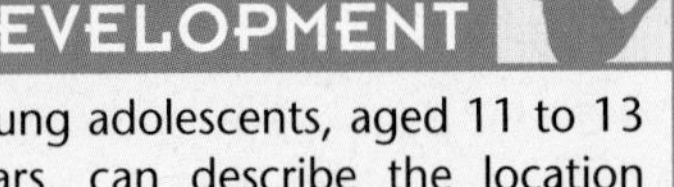

Young adolescents, aged 11 to 13 years, can describe the location and function of major organs such as the brain, nose, eyes, heart, and stomach.

Adolescents are in the process of becoming independent of their parents' influence, so control over aspects of their care is important. The peer group is a major influence in their lives, and having recreation and teen lounge facilities available during hospitalization is recommended. Separation from peers, home, and school are cited as major stressors of hospitalization by adolescents (Gusella & Ward, 1998).

FAMILY RESPONSES TO HOSPITALIZATION

The illness and hospitalization of a child disrupt a family's usual routines. Sometimes roles are altered as one parent stays at the hospital while the other parent or siblings take on additional tasks at home. Family members may be anxious and fearful, especially when the outcome is unknown or potentially serious. Watching a child in pain is difficult for a parent. Adjustment is made more difficult by a serious emergency, lengthy illness, chronic condition, poor prognosis, lack of family support, and lack of financial or community services. (See Chapter 8 for a description of nursing support for the child with life-threatening illness or injury.)

Parents report greater satisfaction with their children's care when nurses tailor actions to the family needs and preferences. Maintaining positive communication with medical personnel and viewing care as a partnership between parents (as well as other key family members) and clinicians are considered predictive of parental satisfaction with their child's hospital care (Marino & Marino, 2000; Conner & Nelson, 1999). Nurses need to see the families as the people who know and understand the child best, ask for their participation and partnership in care, and carefully explain all aspects of treatment. Parents need support to lessen their anxiety, because those with many fears may not be able to parent children effectively and perform protective, nurturing, and decision-making roles (Melnyk, 2000).

The siblings of an ill child often receive little attention from the parents. Parents are preoccupied and may not think to take the siblings to visit the child in the hospital. The siblings may fantasize about the illness or injury and the appearance of their brother or sister. Siblings who are not adequately informed about the hospitalized child's condition may fear that the child will be disabled or die, even when this is unlikely. They may feel guilty about fighting with or being mean to their brother or sister in the past and believe that they played a role in causing his or her illness.

As family roles and routines change, siblings may feel insecure and anxious. Behavioral problems may develop, or school performance may deteriorate. Siblings may feel jealous because the ill brother or sister seems to monopolize the parents' attention. Given support, however, the siblings of an ill child manage well. Chapter 8 describes strategies for working with the siblings of a hospitalized child.

CULTURE 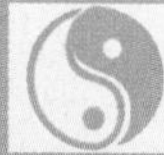

For Mexican Americans, family is a strong support. Extended family and godparents (compadres) may want to be with a hospitalized child. Although the father of the child is often the spokesperson, mothers commonly are influential in decisions regarding child health care (Lipson, Dibble, & Minarik, 1996). The nurse should be inclusive of all people the family wishes to have present in the hospital and for explanations about health care.

 PREPARATION FOR HOSPITALIZATION

Hospitalization may be planned or unexpected. A child may be hospitalized for one of the following reasons:

- The child who has been ill at home gradually or suddenly becomes worse.
- The child needs diagnostic or treatment procedures or requires elective surgery.
- The child who was previously healthy suffers an injury, necessitating unexpected hospitalization.

When hospitalization is planned, children and their parents have time to prepare for the experience. Assess the family's knowledge and expectations and then provide information about what is likely to happen. A variety of approaches can be used to provide information and allay fears:

- Tours of the hospital unit or surgical area are helpful. During tours, preschoolers and school-age children should be allowed to see and touch items with which they will come in contact. The surgical team's attire is less frightening if the child has had a chance to try it on (Figure 5–1 ◆). Medical equipment is not as scary when the child learns what it does and sees how it is used, for example, through demonstration on a doll (Figure 5–2 ◆).
- If a tour is not possible, photographs or a videotape can be used to show the medical setting and procedures.
- Many hospitals offer health fairs to explain health procedures to children. During a tour, while hospitalized, or at home, the child can be exposed to books or films that explain in age-appropriate terms what to expect during various procedures (Table 5-2). Use coloring books or other methods to reinforce teaching.

Parents can be instrumental in preparing a child for hospitalization by reviewing material presented, being available to answer questions, and being truthful and supportive (see p. 168; Figure 5-3 ◆).

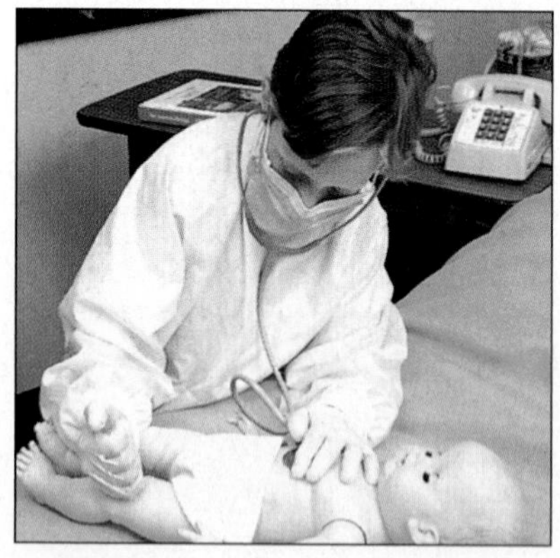

FIGURE 5-1 ◆
Allowing the child to dress up as a doctor or a nurse helps prepare the child for hospitalization. This helps the child adjust to treatment, care, and the recovery process. Why? What might the child's concerns be? Can you think of any concerns that might be related to cultural background?

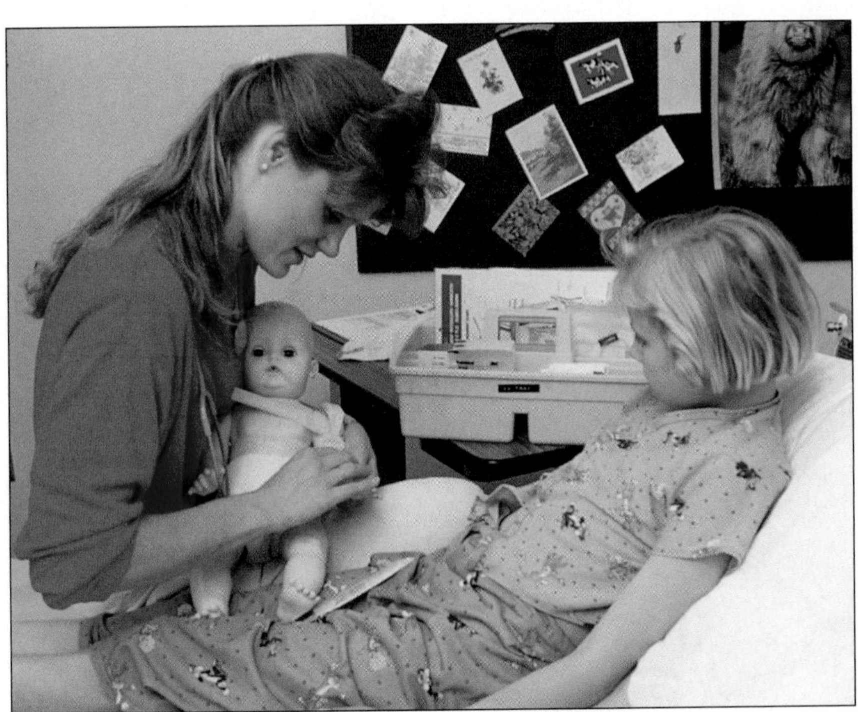

FIGURE 5-2 ◆
The child's anxiety and fear often will be reduced if the nurse explains what is going to happen and demonstrates how the procedure will be done by using a doll. Based on your experience, can you list five things you can do to prepare a school-age child for hospitalization?

TABLE 5-2 Sample Teaching Materials for Children Regarding Hospitalization and Health Care

VIDEOTAPES	PUBLISHER
Clean Intermittent Catheterization	Learner Managed Designs, Inc.
I Have Epilepsy Too	Epilepsy Foundation
What Do I Tell My Children? How to Help a Child Cope with the Death of a Loved One	Life Cycle Productions
BOOKS	
Barney Is Best, by N. W. Carlstrom	HarperCollins
Barney and Baby Bop Go to the Doctor, by M. Larsen	Lyrick Publishers
The Berenstain Bears Go to the Doctor, by S. Berenstain & B. Berenstain	Random House
Chris Gets Ear Tubes, by B. Pace & K. Hutton	Kendall Green Publishers
Curious George Goes to the Hospital, by M. Rey & H. A. Rey	Houghton Mifflin Company
Cut, by P. McCormick & P. McCormick (Mental health hospitalization of a teen.)	Front Street Publishers
David's Story: A Book About Surgery, by B. Brink	Lerner Publications
Doctors and Nurses: What Do They Do? C. Green	HarperCollins
The Fall of Freddie the Leaf, by L. Buscaglia	Henry Holt & Co.
Going to the Hospital, by F. Rogers & J. Judkis	Penguin Putnam Books
The Hospital Book, by J. Howe	Crown Publishers
Let's Talk About Going to the Hospital, by M. Johnston	Rosen Publishers
A Night Without Stars, by J. Howe	Avon
No Measles, No Mumps for Me, by P. Showers	Thomas Y. Crowell
Corduroy Goes to the Doctor, by D. Freeman & L. McCue	A Golden Book
Rita Goes to the Hospital, by M. Davison	Random Books
Tubes in My Ears: My Trip to the Hospital, by V. Dooley & M. Katon	Mondo Publishers
A Visit to the Sesame Street Hospital, by D. Hautzig	Random Books
When Molly Was in the Hospital: A Book for Brothers and Sisters of Hospitalized Children, by D. Duncan	Rayve Productions
Why Am I Going to the Hospital? by C. Cilliota & C. Livingston	Lyle Stuart

RESEARCH

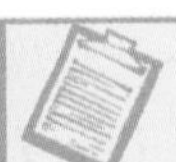

Children who focus on the concrete details of a health care procedure are better able to cope emotionally and recover faster than those who worry about vague aspects of their condition or treatment. Researchers suggest that nurses communicate clearly and tell children about the concrete aspects of their treatment (LaMontagne, 2000).

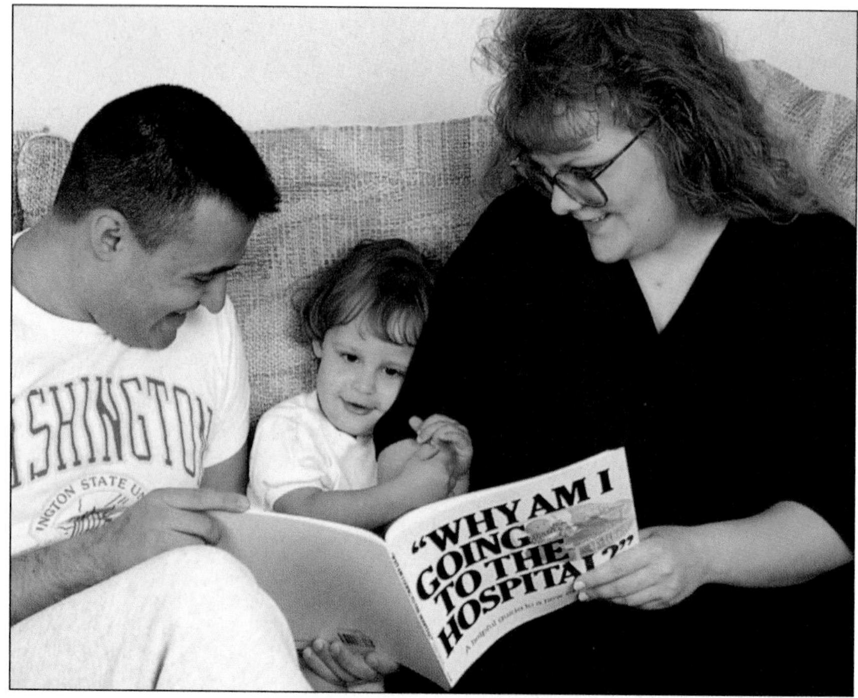

FIGURE 5-3 ◆
Jasmine's parents are taking the time to prepare her for hospitalization by reading a book recommended by the nurse. Such material should be appropriate to the child's age and culture. Why do you think that having the parents read this material is valuable?

FAMILIES WANT TO KNOW

Parental Preparation of Children for Hospitalization

- Read stories to the child about the experience.
- Talk about going to the hospital, what it will be like. Talk about coming home.
- Encourage the child to ask questions.
- Encourage the child to draw pictures of what the hospital will be like.
- Visit the hospital unit if possible.
- Let the child touch or see equipment if possible.
- Plan for support via parents' presence, telephone calls, special items of the parents that child can keep during the stay.
- Be honest.

Different approaches are useful when adolescents are being prepared for hospitalization. They learn not only from written materials, models, and videotapes, but also from talking with peers who have had similar experiences. An opportunity for asking questions without parents present should be provided.

ADAPTATION TO HOSPITALIZATION

SPECIAL UNITS AND TYPES OF CARE

Children who are admitted to a hospital may be cared for in one or more of the following units: emergency department, intensive care unit, or short-stay unit. They may require surgical treatment involving preoperative and postoperative care. Children with infectious diseases may require isolation precautions. Other children may need rehabilitative care to achieve or restore maximum potential.

Emergency Care

When a child is brought to an emergency department, the parents are usually frightened and insecure and may even be in a state of shock. The fast pace and critical nature of the unit create an atmosphere in which parents are hesitant to ask questions and are anxious about the outcome. Keep both the child and the family informed about what is being done and when more news may be available. The parents and child should remain together as much as possible. It is recommended that parents who wish to remain with a child during even invasive procedures or resuscitation efforts should be allowed to do so. However, further research needs to be performed to study the impact of such presence on family, patients, and health care personnel (Emergency Nurses Association, 1998). Nurses need to ask family members about their desired presence in critical situations and keep them informed about the health care provided.

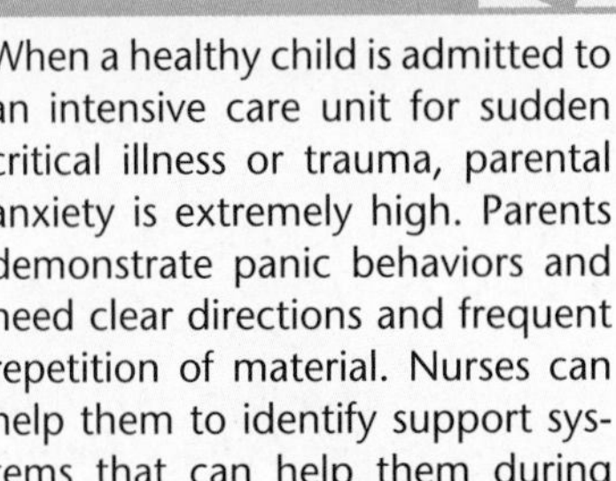

RESEARCH

When a healthy child is admitted to an intensive care unit for sudden critical illness or trauma, parental anxiety is extremely high. Parents demonstrate panic behaviors and need clear directions and frequent repetition of material. Nurses can help them to identify support systems that can help them during this very stressful time (Huckabay & Tilem-Kessler, 1999).

Intensive Care

Parents of a child in an intensive care unit are also likely to be anxious, particularly since the child's illness may be severe and the prognosis may be guarded. The unfamiliar equipment may create an atmosphere of fear. Numerous health care professionals come and go, and parents may not know whom to question or even what questions to ask. Provide emotional support, explain the purpose of treatments and machines, help parents to hold or touch their child, and provide support and referral to other services if appropriate. (See Chapter 8 for a discussion of stressors in parents and children in an intensive care unit and the nursing strategies intended to address these stressors.)

Preoperative and Postoperative Areas

Many hospitals now allow parents to be with their child right up until surgery begins and again in the postanesthesia recovery area. Parents often want to support their child before and immediately after a surgical procedure, and their presence may offer reassurance and comfort to the child.

Prepare family members for what will happen and what is expected of them. In some hospitals, only one or two close family members are allowed to see the child. They may need to wear special gowns, shoes, or hats, and they may be restricted to certain areas. Special equipment such as intravenous setups and monitoring devices should be explained.

Short-Stay Units

Hospitalizations have generally become short, with minor surgery, diagnostic tests such as radiology studies, and treatments such as chemotherapy performed in 1 day. The child may be admitted in the morning and go home in the afternoon. In addition, children who have potentially serious illnesses may be placed on a short-stay or 23-hour unit for monitoring or limited treatment, after which a decision is made to either hospitalize the child for additional treatment or send the child home if improvement occurs (Figure 5-4 ◆). These short

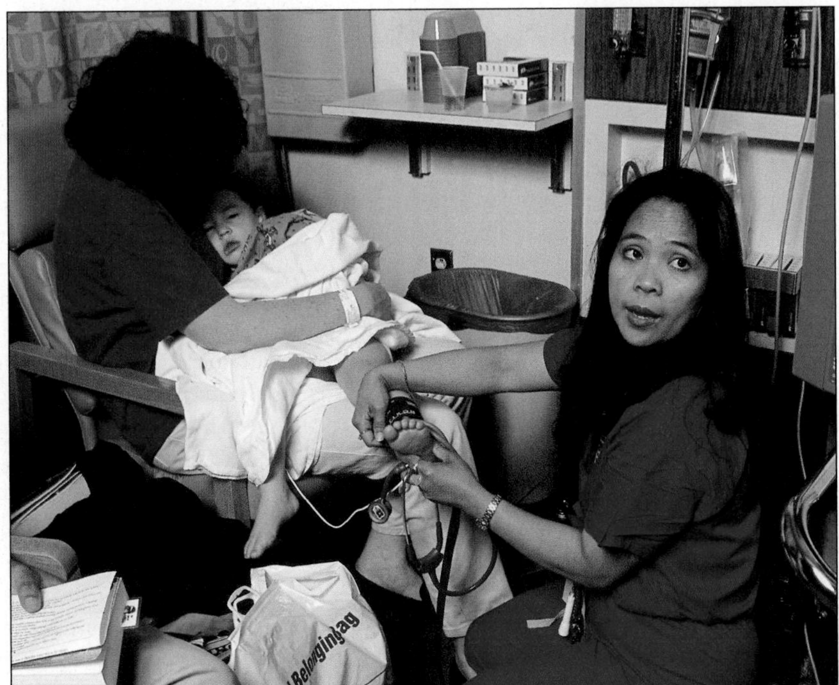

FIGURE 5-4 ◆
The nurse is monitoring a young child who is in a short-stay unit for treatment of dehydration and fever. What support does the mother need?

TABLE 5-3 Nursing Considerations in Preparing Parents and Child for Planned Short-Stay Admission

- Are there special requirements, such as not being permitted food or drink or needing extra fluid intake?
- What time and where must the child appear?
- Are any special forms, insurance numbers, or previous records needed?
- How long will the child stay in the hospital?
- Are parents expected or encouraged to be with the child or stay in the health facility?
- Is there a chance the child may need to remain longer than expected?
- What will the child's condition be for transfer home?
- Will special equipment or care be needed?
- What symptoms can indicate problems?
- Where can the family go or whom can they call in case of problems or questions?

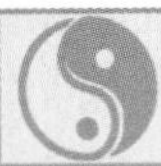

Chapter 4: Infection Control Methods

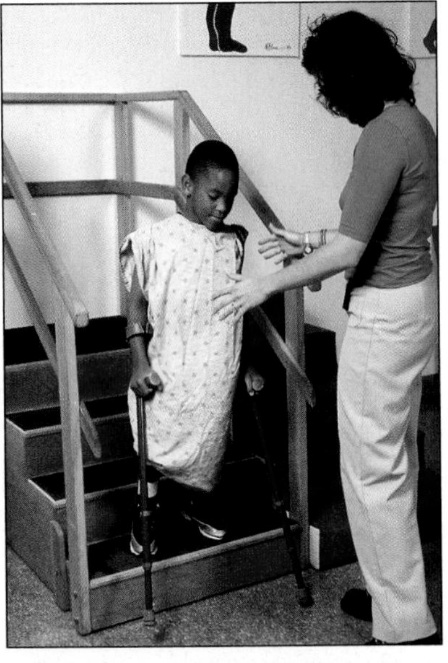

FIGURE 5-5 ◆
Rehabilitation units provide an opportunity for the child to relearn tasks like walking and climbing stairs. They provide an important transition from hospital to home and community.

stays are beneficial because they cause minimal disruption of family patterns and are cost effective. Nurses can help parents prepare the child properly for planned admissions, monitor the child during the procedures, encourage family participation in care, and keep families well informed (Table 5-3).

Isolation

Children who are placed in isolation may suffer lack of stimulation due to limited contact with other children. Frequent family visits are important and should be encouraged. Family members may be reluctant to wear protective garments either out of fear of using them incorrectly or a belief that they are unnecessary. Be sure the family understands the reason for isolation and any special procedures. Having contact with and holding the child should be encouraged when possible. (Standard precautions are described in the Skills Manual.)

Rehabilitation

Rehabilitation units provide children with ongoing care and support to continue recovery beyond the initial period of illness or injury (Figure 5-5 ◆). These may be separate units within a hospital or independent centers. The objective of **rehabilitation** is to help the child with physical or mental challenges reach his or her fullest potential and to promote achievement of developmentally appropriate skills. Parental involvement is essential.

FAMILY ASSESSMENT

To develop a plan of care that involves all family members, assess the impact of the child's illness or hospitalization on the family (Table 5-4). Teaching the child and family, providing support, and referring them to community resources are key elements of the plan.

The family's resources should be assessed frequently. These resources include the coping strategies of family members, financial resources, access to health care, and availability of community services. One family may manage quite well with limited financial support because they have good coping strategies, but another family with greater financial resources may have difficulty caring for an ill child. Staying with a hospitalized child can be a financial drain for parents if they must miss work, and perhaps travel to another location and stay away from home.

It is important to assess the family dynamics. Evaluate the quality of communication, methods of handling problems, and sources of strength. Examine how the family has been dealing with the health needs of the child if the child has been hospitalized or required home care in the past. Ask about the roles they want to play in the child's treatment and the roles they would like the nurse to fulfill. Referrals to family service agencies or other community organizations may be needed. Support groups in the community or agencies that provide medical equipment can also be helpful.

CULTURE

Many ethnic groups, such as Chinese Americans and Mexican Americans, use a combination of Western medicine and traditional therapies such as home treatments or a traditional healer (*curandismo* for Mexican Americans). This information may not be shared with nurses or physicians, both out of respect and in fear that they will be told not to use these methods. Recognizing and supporting use of both Western and traditional practices can promote health and provide comfort for children and families.

CHILD AND FAMILY TEACHING

Teaching is an essential part of the nurse's role in care of hospitalized children and their parents. Teaching may be informal, as when the nurse provides an explanation during routine

TABLE 5-4 Family Assessment

FAMILY ROLES
■ What changes will the child's illness create in the family? ■ Will household tasks need to be reallocated? ■ Will a burden be placed on certain family members? ■ Will one parent room in or spend a great deal of time in the hospital?
KNOWLEDGE
■ What knowledge does the family have about the child's condition and treatment? Do they need further information? ■ Is there a need to start discharge planning and teaching early?
SUPPORT SYSTEMS
■ Does the family have medical insurance? What percentage of costs will it cover? Will other financial support be needed? ■ Are close friends or family available to provide child care for other children, assist with family tasks, or help in other ways? ■ Are there community services such as support groups, camps for children with disabilities, education sessions, or equipment and financial resources to which the nurses can refer the family?
SIBLINGS
■ Have siblings been informed of the ill child's condition and the expected outcome? ■ Have they been reassured that they did not cause the illness? ■ Do they understand the change in roles and family routines? ■ Are they able to visit the ill child? ■ Have their teachers been informed of the family stress? ■ If the hospitalized child's life is threatened, are the siblings involved in a therapy plan to assist them in dealing with that stress?

care, or structured, as when the nurse plans and implements a formal teaching program. Be sure that explanations or reading materials are at a level the parent can understand. If translators are needed to facilitate understanding, be sure they are arranged for and available for teaching sessions. Teaching about the behaviors seen in hospitalized children and the strategies to deal with these behaviors is helpful for parents. For instance, it has been shown that providing information for parents of hospitalized toddlers on the typical behaviors of hospitalized children, and on the strategies to assist children, leads to less anxiety on the part of the parents and to greater parental involvement and support of the child during the hospitalization (Melnyk, 1995). How can you plan to provide such information for parents?

Teaching directed at children must take into account their developmental level and cognitive abilities. Learning is easier when teaching involves more than one sense (such as hearing, vision, and touch). Teaching directed at parents must be geared to their level of understanding. If English is not spoken or is the parents' second language, then a translator may be necessary.

Timing is a critical factor in teaching. Parents and children are less receptive to teaching when they are preoccupied with other thoughts or activities. Scheduling specific times for teaching sessions may be helpful.

Depending on the information to be presented, teaching may use the cognitive, psychomotor, or affective domains of learning. Teaching that includes all three domains is more effective.

Teaching Plans

A teaching plan is a written plan that includes goals and expected outcomes, interventions needed to achieve the specified goals, and a method and time for evaluation of the expected outcomes. The teaching plan may also specify teaching methods and types of materials to be used. Developing a teaching plan helps to ensure that all the necessary information is included and makes teaching more efficient.

The child's primary caretaker should participate in the development of the teaching plan as well as the implementation. The primary caretaker is most often a parent but may be a

LAW & ETHICS

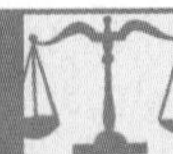

The American Nurses Association's 1996 Statement on the Scope and Standards of Pediatric Clinical Nursing Practice mandates teaching as a component of pediatric nursing care.

LAW & ETHICS

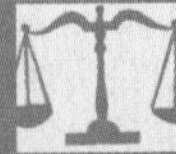

When children are hospitalized for illness or injury, they are in a vulnerable position. Whereas adults are able to refuse or question treatment, children are often not given those rights. This may be in conflict with the United Nations Convention on the Rights of the Child, which gives children the right to be heard in all matters affecting them. Nurses can carefully examine each situation, being careful not to take for granted that hospitalized children should be unhappy and in pain. We can seek to allow them to speak their wishes and to provide strategies that will best help them during health care (Bricher, 2000).

GROWTH & DEVELOPMENT

For children who can hear, touch, see a model or equipment, read, look at pictures, or even smell such things as alcohol swabs, learning is more complete. This basis is particularly important for the school-age child in the stage of concrete operational thought, who must be able to manipulate materials in order to learn.

close family member (uncle, aunt, grandparent). The first step in establishing a teaching plan is to assess the child's or parent's knowledge, skills, and feelings by asking the following questions:

- What does the parent or child know about the health issue?
- What is the cognitive level or ability to learn?
- Is there a desire to learn?
- What previous experiences affect the learning experience, either positively or negatively?
- What resources are available to the parents, child, and nurse that enhance understanding of the health condition?
- Are there feelings or beliefs that might interfere with the learning process?
- What complimentary care does the family use, and how does this relate to the teaching plan?

The second step involves deciding what knowledge, skill, or change in attitude is desired. Outcome criteria or objectives are established with the parent and child.

- A learning objective for a parent might be: The parent states the importance of checking the child's toes in the casted leg twice daily for temperature, movement, sensations, color, and edema (cognitive domain).
- An objective for a child might be: The child self-catheterizes using correct technique and records the amount of urine in a log (psychomotor domain).
- An objective for an adolescent might be: The adolescent explores methods of managing feelings of loss of control related to diabetes management (affective domain).

Possible teaching methods and approaches should be explored. A variety of sources, including written materials (books, pamphlets, handouts, and stories), computer software, audiovisual presentations, and others, are available (see Table 5-2). In some settings, audiovisual and computer resources may be limited. Small-group teaching sessions (e.g., for children with recently diagnosed diabetes or cystic fibrosis) may be another option. Gathering two or three parents or children together on a unit to learn and share experiences may be helpful.

For some conditions, standardized teaching plans are available in books and from health care agencies (see p. 173 for an example). These plans can serve as a guide in developing an individualized teaching plan.

Children Who Have Special Health Care Needs

Children who have disabilities may have special learning needs. If they have visual impairment or perceptual difficulty, then material must be presented in auditory and tactile ways. Children who have hearing deficits need visual and tactile presentations. Children who have learning disabilities may need more frequent reinforcement and shorter teaching sessions. They should be evaluated for comprehension often so teaching can be adjusted as necessary. When psychomotor skill performance is needed, special aids may be necessary so the child can hold a syringe, draw up a liquid, or perform other tasks. Adequate assessment of the child's strengths and disabilities, along with consultation with parents and the child's teachers, can help the nurse to plan teaching methods.

Children who have chronic illnesses may have been hospitalized numerous times and have received other health care at home and in the community. They usually have adapted coping mechanisms that help them deal with the chronic illness. Nurses can talk with them to see what has helped in the past, provide information about what to expect during this hospitalization, assign staff members who are familiar when possible, and follow each child's lead in assisting his or her coping (Boyd & Hunsberger, 1998).

STRATEGIES TO PROMOTE COPING AND NORMAL DEVELOPMENT

During hospitalization, care of the child focuses not only on meeting physiologic needs, but also on meeting psychosocial and developmental needs. Several strategies may be used to help children adapt to the hospital environment, promote effective coping, and provide de-

FAMILIES WANT TO KNOW

Standardized Teaching Plan: Care During a Seizure

Seizures are characterized as periods of involuntary muscle contractions and relaxations that the child has no control over. Seizures may be caused by high fever, head trauma, birth defects, and other neurological problems. It is very hard to predict when a seizure is going to occur. Some safety measures can help to prevent injuries to your child during a seizure.

WHAT TO DO DURING A SEIZURE

Seizure activity often means that the child is at risk for injury. Here are some safety guidelines to remember when your child has a seizure.

- Remain calm and stay with your child.
- Protect your child from any injury.
    - Place your child on the floor when the seizure occurs.
    - Remove any dangerous objects from your child's reach, such as furniture, glass, or objects that can fall on the floor. Do not restrain or hold down your child during a seizure.
    - If the floor is hard (tile, cement, uncarpeted), place a small pillow, sweater, or your hand under your child's head.
    - Loosen your child's clothing if it is too tight.
    - Turn your child's head to one side to prevent choking. Do not put anything into your child's mouth during a seizure.
- Provide time for your child to recover after the seizure stops. Reassure your child that he or she is okay. Speak softly. Explain what happened. Do not give food or drink until your child has fully recovered from the seizure.

WHEN TO CALL FOR EMERGENCY HELP

- If your child's seizure continues for more than 5 minutes
- If your child has trouble breathing or does not breathe after the seizure
- If your child has one seizure after the other without waking up between each

EVERYDAY SAFETY GUIDELINES

- Have your child wear a safety helmet while riding a bike or skating to reduce the chances of a head injury.
- Keep bathroom and bedroom doors unlocked. It will be easier for you or other family members to get into a room to help.
- If the child prefers a bath rather than a shower, use just a few inches of water in the tub. Supervise the young child during the bath. Be sure someone is at home when a teenager is bathing.
- Your child should always swim with a buddy. If a seizure occurs, it is easier to rescue a child in a pool than a child in a pond or lake.
- Teach your child to hold onto the handrails when using stairs.
- Move glass, furniture, and extra pillows away from the child's bed to reduce the chance of injury during a seizure. Think about placing your child's mattress on the floor. This would keep the child from falling out of bed during a seizure.
- Give antiseizure medicines as prescribed to decrease the number of times your child has a seizure.
- Have your child wear a medical identification bracelet at all times.
- Inform relatives, baby-sitters, and teachers that your child has seizures. Tell them about any special care to be given during a seizure.

Note: From *Pediatric Patient Teaching Guides* by J. Ball, 1998, Mosby–Year Book, p. I–4.

velopmentally appropriate activities (Figure 5-6 ◆). These strategies include child life programs, rooming in, therapeutic play, and therapeutic recreation.

Child Life Programs

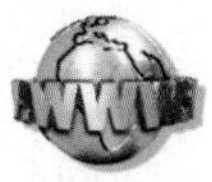

Child Life Programs

Many hospitals have child life programs that focus on the psychosocial needs of hospitalized children. Professional child life specialists, paraprofessionals, and volunteers staff these departments. A **child life specialist** plans activities to provide age-appropriate playtime for children either in the child's room or in a playroom. Some of the planned activities are designed

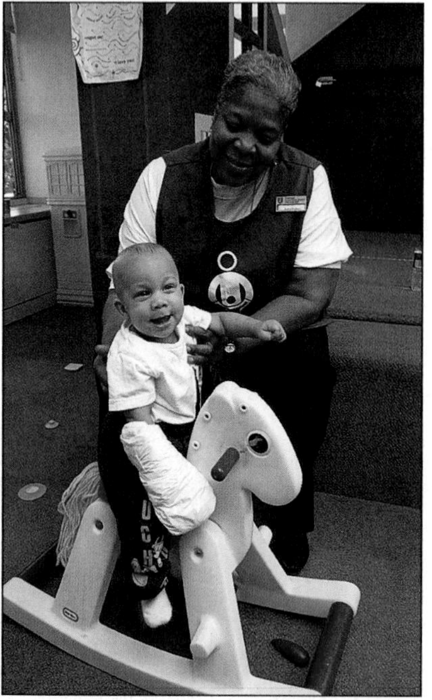

A

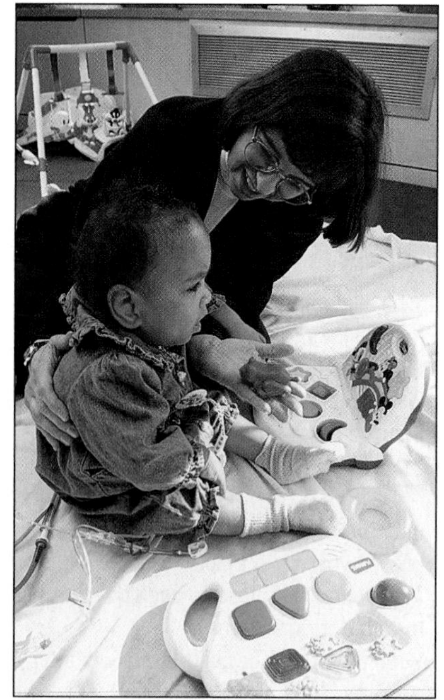

B

FIGURE 5-6 ◆
A, Volunteers such as this foster grandmother can provide stimulation and nurturing to help young children adapt to lengthy hospitalizations.
B, Child life specialists plan activities for young children in the hospital to facilitate play and stress reduction.

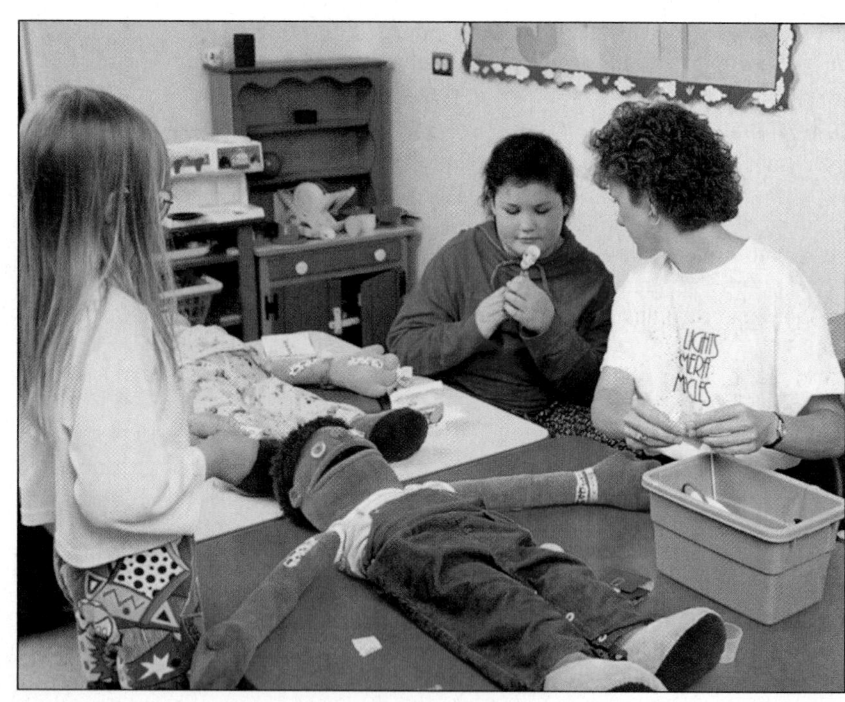

FIGURE 5-7 ◆
A child life specialist works with children being treated for cancer. Special dolls are used to familiarize children with the procedures they undergo.

CHANGING HEALTH CARE SYSTEM

Due to changes in the health care system, more children today are receiving care in outpatient centers, day surgery units, and other community centers. Pediatric inpatient units are consequently small, and play therapy programs are being curtailed. It is important for nurses to plan for provision of play in care, whatever the unit may be. Play therapists can become involved in the wide variety of units in which children receive health care (De Pasquale, 1999).

to assist children in working through feelings about illness. Examples include playing with medical equipment or drawing pictures about hospital treatments (Figure 5-7 ◆). A trusted child life specialist may stay with a child during a particularly frightening procedure such as a venipuncture or bone marrow aspiration.

Both the child life department and the nursing staff focus on the emotional needs of hospitalized children. Child life specialists and nurses may formulate a plan together to assist children with particular needs.

Rooming In

The practice of **rooming in** involves having a parent stay in the child's hospital room and care for the hospitalized child. Some hospitals provide cots, others have special built-in beds on pediatric wards, and in some institutions a parent stays in a separate room on the unit. A parent who is rooming in may want to perform all of the child's basic care or help with some of the medical care. Communication between nurse and parent is important so that the parent's desire for involvement is supported.

Therapeutic Play

Play is an important part of childhood. The stress of illness and hospitalization increases the value of play. Not only is normal development facilitated by play, but play sessions can provide a means for the child to learn about health care, to express anxieties, to work through feelings, and to achieve a sense of mastery or control over frightening or little-understood situations. In the present era of cost containment, play programs may be minimized in hospitals, so nurses should document the need for and benefits of play. Play that presents an opportunity to deal with the fears and concerns of health experiences is called **therapeutic play.**

Through therapeutic play, the child's knowledge of his or her illness or injury can be assessed. A common technique involves using an outline drawing of the body (Figure 5-8 ◆) or stories and asking the child to draw in or talk about what the illness or injury means to him or her (Ramsey, 2000). Alternatively, the child may be asked to draw a picture or make up a story, enabling the nurse to assess fears and other emotions. The Goodenough Draw-A-Person test helps to assess the cognitive level of children between 3 and 13 years of age (Table 5-5). The Gellert Index is another tool that helps to assess the child's knowledge of the body (Table 5-6). In addition to assessment, drawing can be used as a nursing intervention. Show to the child on a drawing what will happen during surgery or a treatment. The child's drawings of health care experiences allow him or her to express fears and gain mastery over the situation.

A variety of techniques may be used to promote therapeutic play (Table 5-7). Specific techniques are chosen to reflect the child's developmental stage.

TODDLER Play is important for toddlers. Through play they explore the environment and learn to identify with significant people in their lives. Play is also an acceptable way for toddlers to release tensions caused by stress or aggressive impulses.

Toddlers should be approached slowly, and the initial approach should be made in their parents' presence, if possible, to decrease feelings of stranger anxiety (wariness of strangers). Playing a variation of peek-a-boo or hide-and-seek using the curtain surrounding the toddler's crib or bed helps promote the realization that objects out of sight, such as parents, do return. The use of transitional objects, such as a familiar blanket or

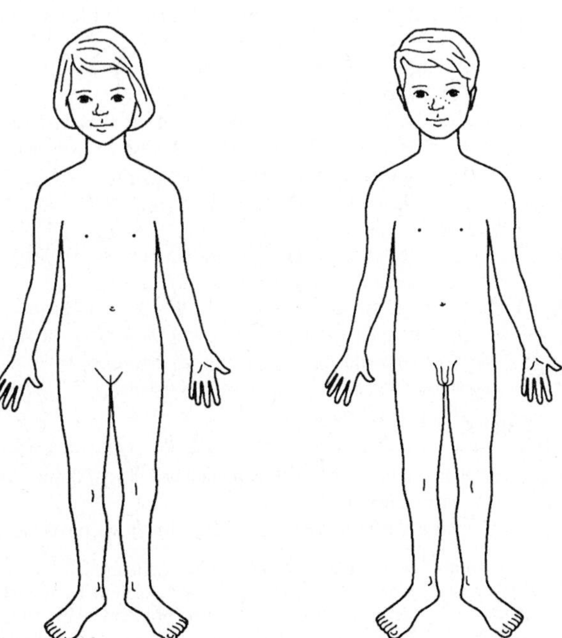

FIGURE 5-8 ◆
The nurse can use a simple gender-specific outline drawing of a child's body to encourage children to draw what they think about their medical problem. Such drawings reveal a child's interpretation, which the nurse can work with to provide appropriate care.

stuffed animal, can temporarily substitute for the security of parents. The toddler who is restrained can be read familiar stories. Repetition of stories promotes a sense of stability in the unfamiliar hospital environment.

A doll is a familiar toy that can be used to recreate a stressful environment, thereby providing an opportunity for the child to express and work through feelings. Other developmentally appropriate toys for toddlers include familiar objects from home such as measuring cups or spoons, wooden puzzles, building blocks, and push-and-pull toys. Playing with safe hospital equipment (bandages, syringes without needles, and stethoscopes) helps tod-

TABLE 5-5 Goodenough Draw-A-Person Test

- The child is asked to draw a picture of a person and to do so carefully and completely, taking his or her time. It is preferable to have the child take the test alone, away from parents.
- Points are assigned for specific details included in the drawing, for example, 1 point each for the presence of head, legs, arms, trunk, and eyes. Additional points are assigned depending on the complexity of details.
- For every 4 points assigned, another year is added to a baseline age of 3 years. For example, a child who scores 24 points (by including 24 details) would have a total score of 9 years (6 plus 3 baseline years). This number is compared to the child's chronologic age to determine his or her cognitive level.

The Goodenough Test may be obtained from the Psychological Corporation, 555 Academic Court, San Antonio, TX 78204; 1–800–872–1726; *www.psychcorp.com.*

TABLE 5-6 Gellert Index of Body Knowledge

PART A

What do you have inside you? Tell me as many things as you can think of that are inside you.

PART B

1. Show me the head. What is in the head? (Tell me all the things that are in the head.)
2. Make a circle showing where and about how big the heart is. What does the heart do? (What is it for?) What would happen if we didn't have a heart?
3. Show me some places where you have bones. (Try for a minimum of five locations.) What do we have bones for? What would happen if we didn't have bones?
4. Make a circle showing where and about how big the stomach is. What does the stomach do? Show me where the food goes after you swallow it. (Sketch in diagram.) And then? (If excretion is not mentioned spontaneously, ask: Does it ever come out anywhere? If the answer is affirmative, ask: Show me where it comes out.)
5. Make a circle showing about where and about how big the ribs are. Why do we have ribs? (What for?) What would happen if we didn't have ribs?
6. Make a circle showing about where and about how big the liver is. What does the liver do? What would happen if we didn't have a liver?
7. What do you think we have a skin for? What would happen if we didn't have a skin?
8. Make a circle showing where and about how big the lungs are. How many lungs are there? What do we have lungs for? What would happen if we didn't have lungs?
9. Do you have any nerves? (If no, ask: Does anybody else? If so, who?) What would happen if we didn't have any nerves?
10. Make a circle showing where and about how big the bladder is. What do we have a bladder for? What would happen if we didn't have a bladder?
11. How come we have bowel movements? (What for?) Where do bowel movements come from? (Probe for derivation from food, stomach, intestines.) Show me on the diagram. What would happen if we didn't have bowel movements? About how often (how many times) should people have bowel movements? About how often do you have bowel movements?

PART C

1. What do you think is the most important part of you? (If you picked one part of you as the most important, which one would you pick?)
2. Are there any parts of you that you could live (get along) without? Which ones?

Note: From "Children's conceptions of the content and functions of the human body," by E. Gellert, 1962, Genetic Psychology Monographs 65, 293–405. Reprinted with permission of the Helen Dwight Reid Education Foundation. Published by Heldref Publications, 1319 18th St NW, Washington DC 20036-1802.

TABLE 5-7 Therapeutic Play Techniques

TECHNIQUE	ASSESSMENT	INTERVENTION
Stories	Have the child make up a story about a picture. Analyze content and emotional clues in the story. Have children tell a story about an important experience in a group of other children.	Read or make up stories to explain illness, hospitalization, or other specific aspects of health care. Emotions such as fear can be included.
Drawings	Administer Goodenough Draw-A-Person test (see Table 5-5) to evaluate cognitive level. Consider subject matter, size and placement of items in drawings, colors used, presence or absence of physical barriers, and general emotional feeling. Administer Gellert Index (Table 5-6) to learn about the child's knowledge of the body and its functioning before planning teaching.	Use the child's drawings or outlines of the body to explain care, procedures, or conditions. Provide an opportunity for the child to draw pictures of his or her choice or directed topics such as a picture of the child's family or health care encounter. Ask the child: "Tell me about your picture." Be alert to the child's emotions: "This child must be frightened by the big x-ray machine."
Music	Observe types of music chosen and effects of played music on behavior.	Encourage parents and children to bring favorite tapes to the hospital for stress relief. Have tapes playing during tests and procedures. Parents can tape their voices to play for infants and young children during separations. During longer hospitalizations children can tape messages for siblings or classmates, who are then encouraged to retape their responses. Playtime can include the opportunity to play instruments and sing.
Puppets	The puppets can ask questions of young children, who are often more likely to answer the puppet than a person.	Perform short skits to teach children necessary health care information. Include emotional content when appropriate.
Dramatic play	Provide dolls and medical equipment, and analyze the roles assigned to dolls by the child, the behavior demonstrated by the dolls in the child's play, and the apparent emotions. Dolls with handicaps like those of the child are especially helpful (see Figure 5-9B).	Provide dolls and equipment for play sessions. To ensure safety, supervise closely when actual equipment is used. Respond to emotions and behavior shown. Use dolls and equipment such as casts, nebulizer, intravenous apparatus, and stehoscope to explain care. Use dolls with problems or handicaps similar to those of the child when available. Provide toys that foster expression of emotion, such as a pounding board and indoor darts.
Pets	Provide pet therapy. Watch the interaction between child & animal. (See Figure 5-10)	Respond to emotions the child shows. Facilitate touch and stroking of animals.

Additional techniques, such as sand or water play or pet therapy, may be appropriate in specific situations.

dlers to overcome the anxiety associated with these items. Supervise these play sessions and remove hospital equipment when you leave.

PRESCHOOLER The nurse can intervene to reduce the stress produced by preschoolers' fears through the use of some kinds of play. A simple outline of the body or a doll can be used to address the child's fantasies and fears of bodily harm. Playing with safe hospital equipment may help preschoolers to work through feelings such as aggression (Figure 5-9 ◆).

Preschoolers like crayons and coloring books, puppets, felt and magnetic boards, play dough, books, and recorded stories. Preschoolers and older children often enjoy pet therapy. Children's hospitals and units can have visits from pets, most commonly dogs, that provide diversion and physical contact (Figure 5-10 ◆). Both preschool and school-age children may enjoy playing with a toy hospital.

SCHOOL-AGE CHILD Although play begins to lose its importance in the school-age years, the nurse can still use some techniques of therapeutic play to help the hospitalized child deal with stress. School-age children often regress developmentally during hospitalization, demonstrating behaviors characteristic of an earlier state, such as separation anxiety and fear of bodily injury. Outlines of the body and, occasionally, dolls can be used to illustrate the cause and treatment of the child's illness. Terms for body parts that are suitable for older children should be used. Drawings provide an outlet for expression of fears and anger.

School-age children enjoy collecting and organizing objects and often ask to keep disposable equipment that has been used in their care. They may use these items later to relive the experience with their friends. Games, books, schoolwork, crafts, tape recordings, and computers provide an outlet for aggression and increase self-esteem in the school-age child. The type of play used should promote a sense of mastery and achievement.

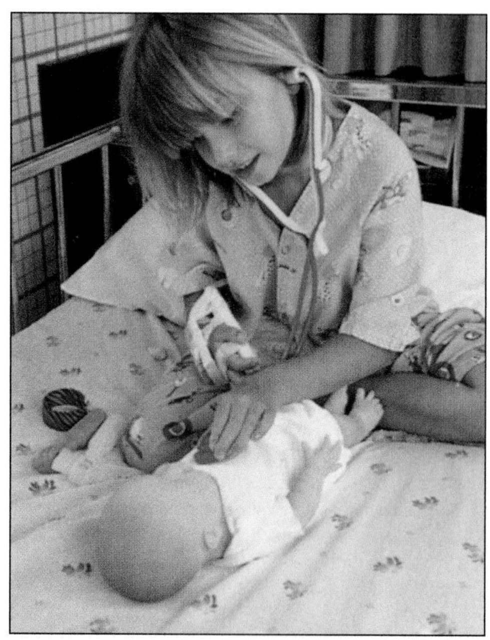

A

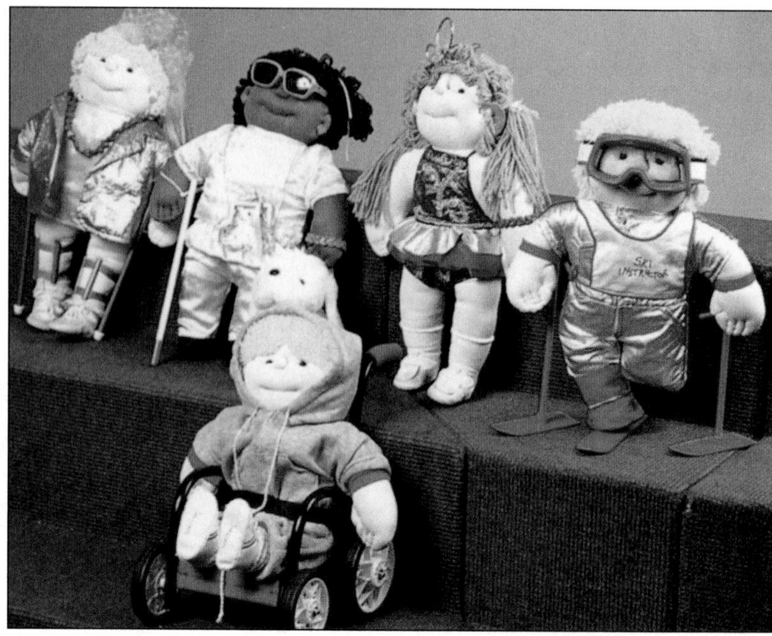

B

FIGURE 5-9 ◆
A, Age-appropriate play will help the child to adjust to hospitalization and care. B, Having the child play with dolls that have "disabilities" similar to his or her own will help the child adjust. Such play helps the child realize what activities are possible.

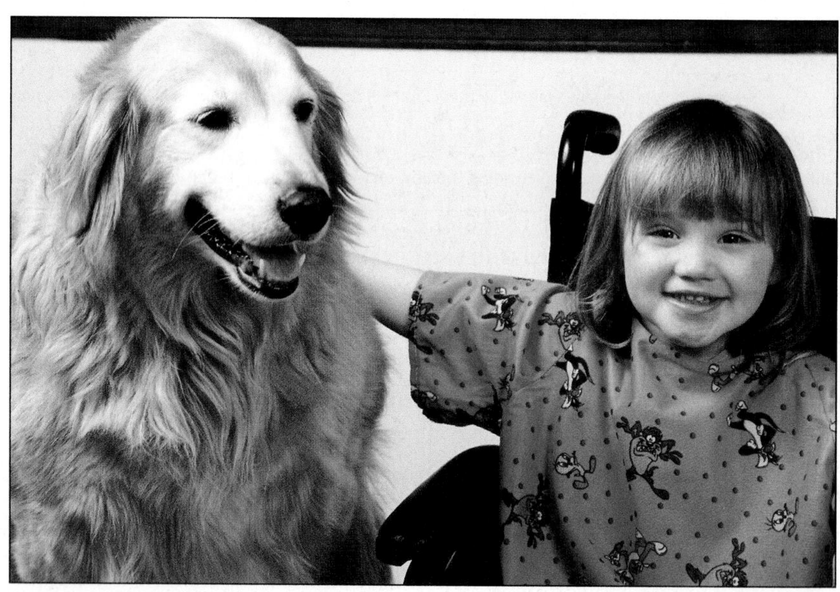

FIGURE 5-10 ◆
Hospitals may have pet therapy from specially trained animals to provide comfort and distraction during health care. Both the child and the dog seem to be smiling!

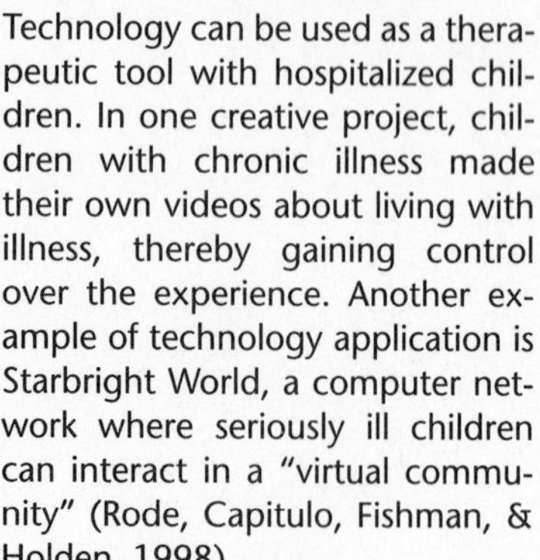

CLINICAL TIP

Technology can be used as a therapeutic tool with hospitalized children. In one creative project, children with chronic illness made their own videos about living with illness, thereby gaining control over the experience. Another example of technology application is Starbright World, a computer network where seriously ill children can interact in a "virtual community" (Rode, Capitulo, Fishman, & Holden, 1998).

Therapeutic Recreation

Many of the special play techniques used with younger children are not suitable for adolescents. However, adolescents do need a planned recreation program to assist them in meeting developmental needs during hospitalization. Peers are important, and the isolation of hospitalization can be difficult. Telephone contact with other teenagers and visits from friends should be encouraged. Interactions with other teenagers at a pizza party, video game, or movie night or during other activities can help adolescents feel normal (Figure 5-11 ◆). Physical activities that provide an outlet for stress are recommended. Even adolescents on bed rest or in wheelchairs can play a modified form of basketball.

The independence of adolescence is interrupted by illness. Nurses can provide choices for teenagers to assist them in regaining control. Giving them options and letting them

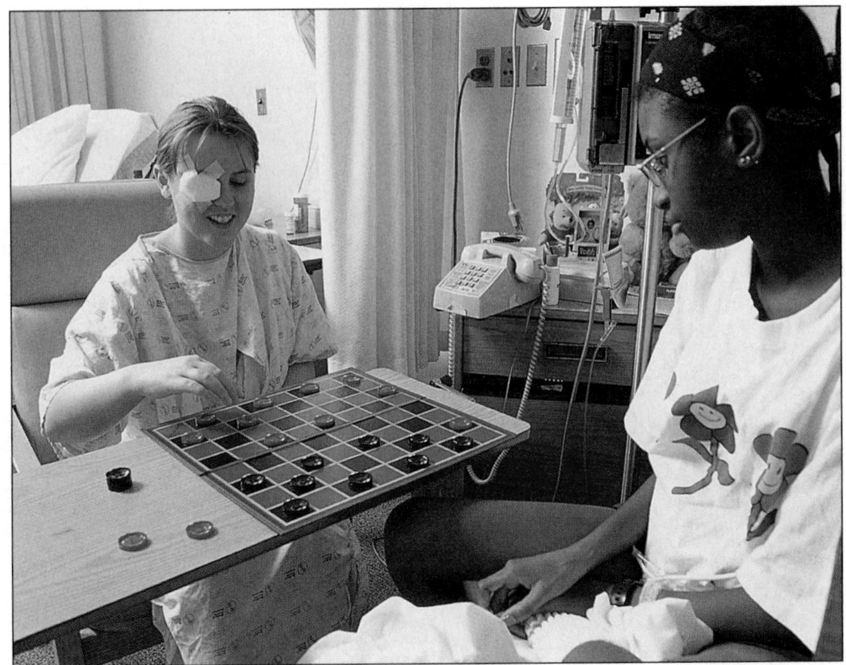

FIGURE 5-11 ◆
Having interaction with other hospitalized adolescents and maintaining contact with friends outside the hospital are very important so that the teenager does not feel alone. A friendly yet competitive checkers game helps to stimulate these teenagers and allows for self-expression. What are the other benefits?

choose an evening recreational activity can promote their feelings of independence. Passes to leave the hospital for special activities may be possible.

STRATEGIES TO MEET EDUCATIONAL NEEDS

Some hospitalizations are so short that the absence of the child or adolescent from school and peers is of minimal concern. However, if hospitalization is expected to last longer than a few days or if the child's condition will change, necessitating special school arrangements, the nurse should assess the effects of hospitalization on the child's education.

When an elective procedure occurs, families should be encouraged to arrange the extended school absence with teachers. The child can then be provided with schoolwork to do in the hospital or at home when well enough. This minimizes educational deficits and future problems for the child. Pencils, paper, comfortable work areas, computers, and quiet work times should be provided (Figure 5-12 ◆). Telephone calls or Internet connections with teachers can be arranged as needed.

The social aspects of school and peers should also be considered. Peers can be encouraged to visit a hospitalized classmate, send cards and letters, call on the phone, or communicate via the Internet. When the child returns to school, the nurse can visit the classroom to provide classmates with information about the child's medical condition.

The hospital nurse may contact the child's school nurse when special arrangements are necessary. For example, the child who is wearing a large cast or who needs medications or other treatments may offer challenges in a traditional school setting.

The child with chronic health problems or requiring long-term hospitalization has other needs with regard to school. Hospitals or rehabilitation units may have classrooms, teachers, and facilities to promote learning (Figure 5-13 ◆). Many school districts provide tutors or computer connections for students who are hospitalized or receiving home care for long periods. Teachers can visit children at the hospital or at home. Parents are often pivotal in making arrangements to meet the child's educational needs, since they interact with the child, the school, and the health care team.

LAW & ETHICS

The Joint Commission on Accreditation of Healthcare Organizations (1992) mandates provision for schooling of the child in a health care facility for an extended period.

PREPARATION FOR PROCEDURES

A number of procedures take place during hospitalization, from collection of urine or blood specimens to spinal taps and surgery. Special techniques can help the child to understand and cope with feelings about these procedures. Nurses should never assume that a procedure will not be traumatic for the child. Even providing urine in a specimen cup or undergoing x-ray

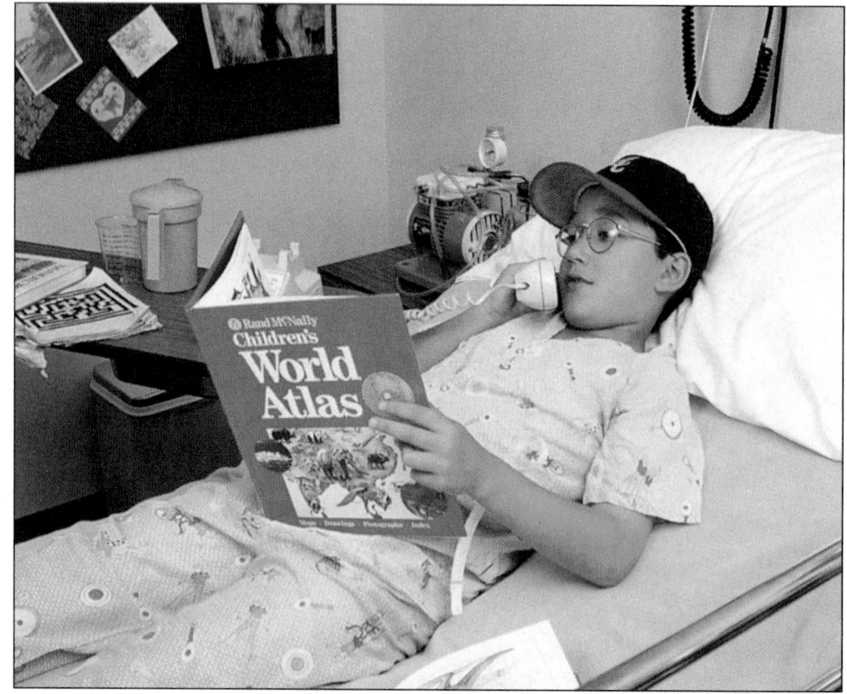

FIGURE 5-12 ◆
It is important that the hospitalized child not fall behind in schoolwork. As soon as the child is able, schoolwork should be resumed. If the child is unable to get out of bed, all necessary study materials should be brought to the child. The child can consult with teachers on the phone or via computer.

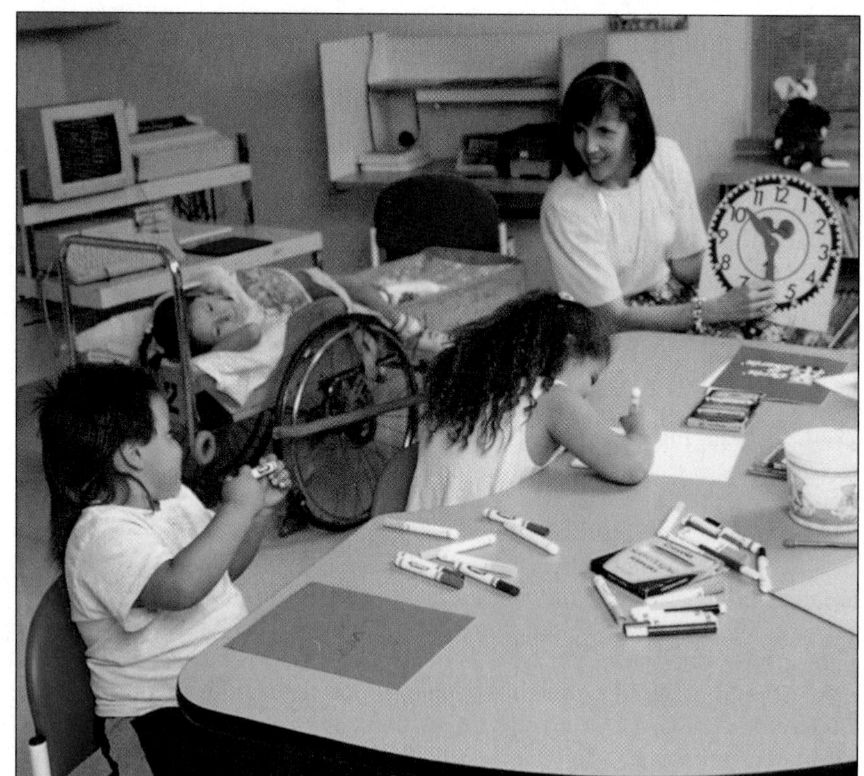

FIGURE 5-13 ◆
Shriner's Hospital in Spokane, Washington, has a special classroom and teacher for children undergoing a lengthy hospital stay, enabling them to remain current with their schoolwork. The child who falls behind other students might not fit in when he or she returns to school or might be required to repeat a grade. What are the potential consequences of these situations?

Skills 7-1 to 7-13: Administration of Medication

examination can be frightening if the child does not understand the reason for the procedure or what to expect. Administration of medication can also be frustrating for the child. The nurse should prepare the child for medication administration and adapt techniques used with adults so the correct medication is safely given (Table 5-8).

To assess the child's feelings about the procedure, ask the following questions:

- Does the child know the purpose of the procedure?
- Has the child experienced this procedure before? Was the experience painful, frightening, or reassuring?

TABLE 5-8 Variations in Medication Administration to Children

ROUTE	DEVELOPMENTAL CONSIDERATIONS	TECHNIQUES
Oral	Children under 5 years cannot generally swallow pills and capsules.	■ Medications are usually given in liquid form (elixir, syrup, or suspension) ■ Sometimes tablets are crushed or capsules are opened and mixed with one spoon of food. Check with pharmacy to be sure this does not inactivate the drug. Never crush enteric-coated or timed-release medicine. ■ When choosing a vehicle for crushed tablets, use only one spoonful of applesauce, pudding, jelly, or similar food. ■ Use TB syringe for amounts less that 1 mL to increase accuracy.
	Children may not want to take medicine.	■ Position young children upright to avoid choking and aspiration. ■ Give liquid medicines slowly by oral syringe (for infants) aimed at the inside of the cheek or by medicine cup (for toddler and preschooler) for drinking. ■ Have the expectation that the medicine will be taken. Let children choose the type of fluid to drink after, but do not ask if they will take their medicine now.
Rectal	Colon is small in size.	■ For children under 3 years, the nurse's gloved fifth finger is used for insertion. After this age, the index finger can usually be used. ■ Lubricate the tip of the suppository.
Ophthalmic and Otic	Young children may be fearful of medicines placed in the eyes or ears.	■ Adequate restraint is needed to avoid injury. ■ The nurse's hand can be stabilized by resting the wrist on the child's head. ■ Explanations and therapeutic play can be used with children old enough to explain the process of administration. ■ Have medication at room temperature.
Topical	Skin of infants is thin and fragile.	■ Only prescribed doses and medicines appropriate for young children should be used on the skin. ■ Covering the area or keeping the child's hands occupied may be necessary to ensure adequate contact of medication with the skin.
Intramuscular	Anatomy and physiology of children differ from that of adults.	■ Gluteus maximus muscle (dorsal gluteal site) must not be used until the child has been walking for at least 1 year. ■ Vastus lateralis site is preferred for young children. ■ Amounts to be administered should be limited to no more than 1–2 mL for ventrogluteal site depending on muscle size. ■ The deltoid muscle is rarely used in young children except for the small amounts injected in some vaccines.
Intravenous	Veins are small and fragile. Fluid balance is critical.	■ Careful maintenance of sites is needed. ■ Common infusion sites include hands and feet, although scalp veins are sometimes used in infants. ■ Infusion pumps require frequent monitoring. ■ Syringe pumps are often used when minimal fluid is to be given over an extended period of time. ■ Central lines are commonly used for long-term intravenous medication therapy.

See Skills Manual for further medication administration techniques.

- What does the child think will happen? Are the child's beliefs accurate?
- Is the procedure painful?
- What techniques does the child use to gain control in challenging situations?
- Will the parents or adult friends be present to provide support?

Preparation may begin a few moments to several days before the procedure, depending on the child's age. Use words that the child understands to describe the procedure and its purpose (see Chapter 2). Older children need explanations geared to their cognitive level

CLINICAL TIP

When a potentially painful procedure will be occurring, an anesthetic cream or disk, such as EMLA, should be applied to the skin 1 to 2 hours before the planned procedure. This can lessen discomfort and, therefore, fear in the child.

and previous experiences (Figure 5-14 ◆). They will want to know what is happening, why, and what they can do to cope during the procedure (Table 5-9).

Provide written information for adolescents, and schedule time for questions and discussions. Adolescents can make many choices about their own health care. They can be asked such questions as, "Do you want a local or general anesthetic?" or "Do you want your hand numbed for the intravenous start?" Some adolescents want their parents involved in their care, while others prefer to minimize the parents' role.

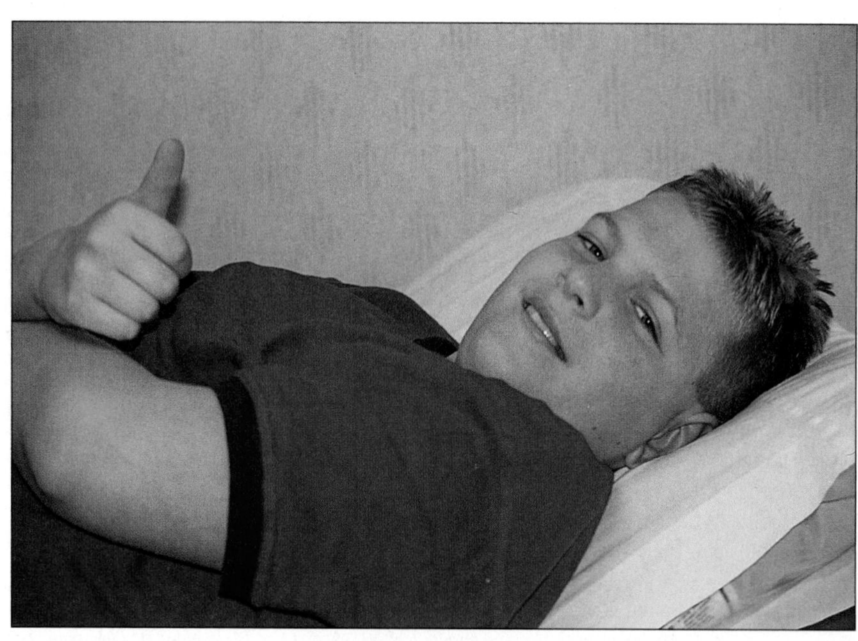

FIGURE 5-14 ◆
This boy was formerly afraid of blood draws but with the aid of health professionals has overcome his fear and can now have the procedure done calmly. He shows us his mastery over the situation. What can you do to help children afraid of procedures to develop coping mechanisms to assist them?

TABLE 5-9 Assisting Children Through Procedures

DEVELOPMENTAL STAGE	BEFORE PROCEDURE	DURING PROCEDURE
Infant	None for infant. Explain to parents the procedure, the reason for it, and their role.	Restrain infant securely and gently. Perform procedure quickly. Use touch, voice, pacifier, and bottle as distractions. Have parent hold, rock, and sing to infant after procedure.
Toddler	Give explanation just before procedure, since toddler's concept of time is limited. Explain that child did nothing wrong; the procedure is simply necessary.	Perform in treatment room. Give short explanations and directions in a positive manner. Avoid giving choices when none are available. For example, "We are going to do this now" is better than "Is it okay to do this now?" Allow child to cry or scream. Comfort child after procedure. Give child a choice of favorite drink or special sticker.
Preschool child	Give simple explanations of procedure. Basic drawings may be useful. While providing supervision, allow the child to touch and play with equipment to be used if possible. Since any entry into the body is viewed as a threat, state that the child's body will remain the same, and use adhesive bandages to reassure the child that the body is intact and parts will not "fall out."	Perform in treatment room. Restrain securely. Give short explanations and directions in a positive manner. Encourage control by having the child count to 10 or spell name. Allow child to cry. Give positive feedback for cooperation and getting through procedure. Encourage the child to draw afterward to explore the experience.
School-age child	Clear, thorough explanations are helpful. Use drawings, pictures, books, and contact with equipment. Teach stress-reduction techniques such as deep breathing, and visualization. Offer a choice of reward after procedure is completed.	Be ready to restrain child if needed. Allow child to remain in position by self if child is able to be still. Explain throughout procedure what is happening. Facilitate use of stress-control techniques. Praise cooperative efforts.
Adolescent	Give clear explanations orally and in writing. Teach stress-reduction techniques. Explore fear of certain procedures, such as staple removal or venipuncture.	Assist adolescent in self-control. Avoid using restraints. Assist with use of stress-control techniques. Explain expected outcome and tell when results of test will be completed.

The procedure should be performed as quickly and efficiently as possible. Parents may wish to be involved or may prefer to be available afterward to comfort the child. The parents or nurse can be designated to support the child by way of a gentle touch, talking, singing, reassurance, or a stress-reduction technique.

Procedures on young children are generally performed in a treatment room so the child's own room is viewed as a "safe" and relatively pain-free site. After the procedure, the child can be taken back to his or her room for comfort and reassurance. A choice of reward often soothes the young child. A common procedure for which children need support is venipuncture.

Preparation for Surgery

A child's surgical experience can be elective, planned in advance, or a result of an emergency or trauma. How a child responds to the experience depends on the psychologic and physical preparation he or she receives. The accompanying Nursing Care Plan for the Child Undergoing Surgery summarizes key elements of preoperative and postoperative care.

Preoperative Care

Preoperative care of the child includes both psychosocial and physical preparation for surgery.

PSYCHOSOCIAL PREPARATION The goal of preoperative teaching is to reduce the fear associated with the unknown and decrease stress and anxiety associated with surgery. Teaching should be geared to the child's developmental level. If child life teachers are available, they can play an important role in preparing the child for surgery.

If the child will be in an intensive care unit or recovery room after surgery, a visit there before surgery can reduce the fear and anxiety associated with waking up in a strange environment filled with frightening sights, sounds, and smells. The use of tapes, anatomically correct puppets and dolls, drawings, and models is encouraged to teach the child about the surgical procedure. For example, a doll was used as a teaching aid in preparing Sabrina, the preschooler described in the opening vignette, for surgery. Playing with stethoscopes, gowns, masks, and syringes without needles also helps the child feel more in control. Children should be reassured that their parents can accompany them to the operating room floor and will be waiting when they awaken from surgery.

PHYSICAL PREPARATION Preoperative procedures and guidelines vary among hospitals and outpatient surgical centers. Preoperative checklists are used in ambulatory and acute care settings to ensure proper physical preparation of patients for surgery. A sample checklist is provided in Table 5-10.

TABLE 5-10 Preoperative Checklist

____Check that consent forms are witnessed and signed and in the patient's chart.
____Be sure the child's name band is in place.
____Be sure any allergies are prominently noted in the child's chart.
____Remove any prosthetic devices, including orthodontic appliances.
____Check the child's mouth for loose teeth and tonque piercings.
____Remove eyeglasses and jewelry.
____Bathe and cleanse the operative site if ordered.
____Put the child in an operating room gown, allowing the child to wear underwear.
____Check that all special tests have been completed and the results are in the child's chart.
____Have the child void before surgery.
____Keep the child NPO before surgery.
____Give the child prescribed medications.
____Transport the child safely to the operating room.

NURSING CARE PLAN The Child Undergoing Surgery

GOAL	INTERVENTION	RATIONALE	EXPECTED OUTCOME
Preoperative Care			
1. Knowledge deficit related to preoperative and postoperative events			
	NIC Priority Intervention: **Teaching, Preoperative:** Assisting a patient to understand and mentally prepare for surgery and postoperative recovery		NOC Suggested Outcome. **Knowledge:** Extent of understanding conveyed about treatment regimen
The child and family will acquire knowledge related to the operation.	■ Ask questions of the parent and child about surgery. ■ Teach about preoperative and postoperative events using appropriate developmental methods such as dolls, drawings, stories, and tours. ■ Reinforce information the family has received about the purpose of surgery. ■ Have the child demonstrate postoperative events that pertain to his or her case such as deep breathing, putting bandage on doll, taping intravenous line on doll, and pressing patient-controlled analgesia button. ■ Allow the parents and child to ask questions.	■ Prior knowledge and understanding can be reinforced and used to guide your presentation. ■ Developmental level determines the cognitive approach that works best for teaching. ■ The physician may have explained operation. ■ Concrete experience promotes learning. ■ Learners must have opportunity to ask questions.	The child and family are able to verbalize details about expected preoperative and postoperative events. They ask questions that demonstrate understanding. The child demonstrates skills needed in the postoperative period.
2. Anxiety related to change in health status			
	NIC Priority Intervention: **Anxiety Reduction:** Minimizing apprehension, dread, foreboding, or uneasiness related to an unidentified source of anticipated danger.		NOC Suggested Outcome: **Coping:** Actions to manage stressors that tax an individual's resources.
The child and family will show decreased behavior indicating anxiety.	■ Question the child about expectations of hospitalization and previous experiences. ■ Orient the child to the hospital setting, routines, staff, and other patients. ■ Institute age-appropriate play and interactions with the child. ■ Explain procedures and prepare for those that might cause trauma. Encourage parents to support the child. ■ Allow the parents and child to ask questions.	■ Previous experiences can influence present anxiety level. ■ Familiarity with the setting and people can decrease anxiety by removing unknown factors. ■ Play can increase trust level and decrease anxiety. ■ The child is more likely to trust caregivers if they are truthful and if parents are present. ■ Questioning provides an opportunity to explain the unknown, which decreases anxiety.	The child and family demonstrate less anxiety. They verbalize understanding and comfort in hospital routines. Parents support the child for traumatic procedures.

(continued)

NURSING CARE PLAN The Child Undergoing Surgery (continued)

GOAL	INTERVENTION	RATIONALE	EXPECTED OUTCOME
3. Risk for infection and injury related to exposure to nosocomial infection and use of preoperative medication			
	NIC Priority Intervention: **Infection Control and Fall Prevention:** Minimizing the acquisition and transmission of infectious agents, and instituting special precautions with patient at risk of falling.		NOC Suggested Outcome: Actions to eliminate or reduce actual, personal, and modifiable health risks.
The child will show no signs of infection.	■ Monitor vital signs at least every 4 hours. Inspect skin and respiratory status each shift.	■ Increase in vital sign levels, skin lesions, nasal drainage, or adventitious breath sounds can indicate signs of infection in the child.	The child's vital signs and assessment are within normal limits.
The child will remain free of injury.	■ Report any variations from expected vital signs. ■ Keep side rails up after preoperative medication is given. Maintain NPO status when ordered. Transport the child to the operating room safely secured.	■ Symptoms are reported so surgery can be canceled if necessary. ■ Preoperative medication can alter level of consciousness. NPO status prevents aspiration.	The child is transported safely to the operating room.
Postoperative Care			
4. Impaired skin integrity related to disruption of skin surface			
	NIC Priority Intervention: **Wound Care:** Prevention of wound complications and promotion of wound healing.		NOC Suggested Outcome: **Wound Healing:** The extent to which cells and tissues have regenerated following intentional closure.
The child will be free of infection.	■ Monitor vital signs per hospital routine. Record and report changes from baseline. ■ Monitor surgical dressing and drains every hour. ■ Change or reinforce dressings when wet. ■ Check the intravenous site every 2 hours for redness, swelling, pain, or pallor. ■ Teach parents signs of infection before discharge. Teach parents aseptic technique for dressing change and wound care.	■ Changes in vital signs, especially increased temperature and pulse, can indicate infection. ■ Excess drainage may indicate infection. ■ Wet dressing can allow organisms to come into contact with surgical wound. ■ Intravenous lines may become infiltrated or cause thrombophlebitis. ■ Parents report signs of infection and perform home care as needed.	The child shows no signs of infection. The surgical wound heals without infection. The intravenous line remains patent without signs of infection. The child continues to demonstrate no signs of infection at home.
5. Risk for constipation related to surgical procedure and anesthetics			
	NIC Priority Intervention: **Constipation Management:** Establishment and maintenance of regular bowel elimination		NOC Suggested Outcome: **Bowel Elimination:** Ability of the gastrointestinal tract to form and evacuate stool effectively.
The child will achieve and maintain normal bowel functioning by the fourth postoperative day.	■ Auscultate bowel sounds every 4 hours. Offer liquids only when bowel sounds are present. Assess the abdomen for distention. ■ Document the character and frequency of bowel movements. ■ Advance the diet as tolerated. ■ Increase activity as ordered and tolerated.	■ Restricting fluids avoids distention if peristalsis is not normal. ■ Knowledge of bowel status ensures early identification of constipation. ■ Fluids and roughage promote normal bowel functioning. ■ Physical activity promotes peristalsis.	The child has bowel movement within 2 to 3 days after surgery with normal pattern by the fourth post-operative day.

(continued)

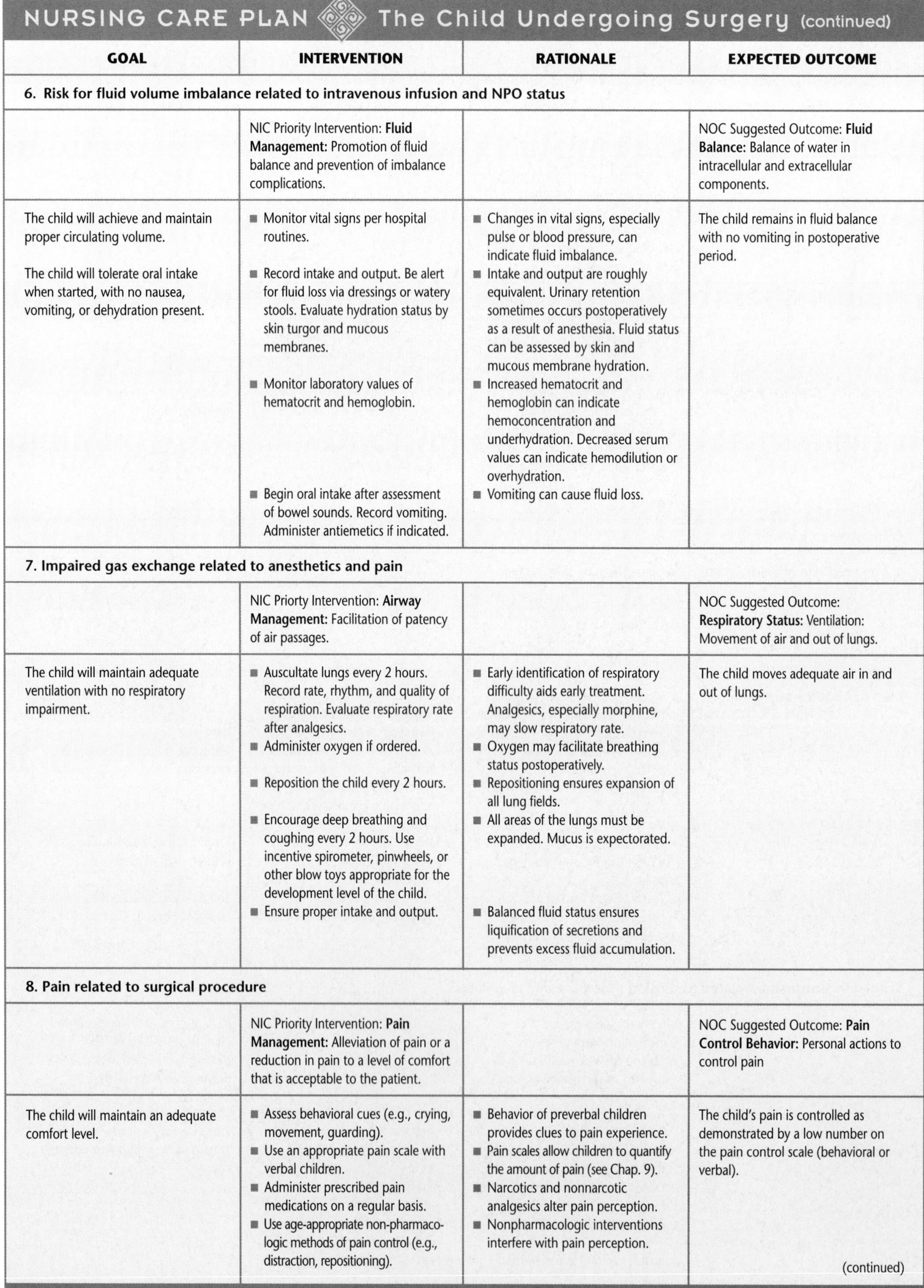

NURSING CARE PLAN The Child Undergoing Surgery (continued)

GOAL	INTERVENTION	RATIONALE	EXPECTED OUTCOME
6. Risk for fluid volume imbalance related to intravenous infusion and NPO status			
	NIC Priority Intervention: **Fluid Management:** Promotion of fluid balance and prevention of imbalance complications.		NOC Suggested Outcome: **Fluid Balance:** Balance of water in intracellular and extracellular components.
The child will achieve and maintain proper circulating volume. The child will tolerate oral intake when started, with no nausea, vomiting, or dehydration present.	■ Monitor vital signs per hospital routines. ■ Record intake and output. Be alert for fluid loss via dressings or watery stools. Evaluate hydration status by skin turgor and mucous membranes. ■ Monitor laboratory values of hematocrit and hemoglobin. ■ Begin oral intake after assessment of bowel sounds. Record vomiting. Administer antiemetics if indicated.	■ Changes in vital signs, especially pulse or blood pressure, can indicate fluid imbalance. ■ Intake and output are roughly equivalent. Urinary retention sometimes occurs postoperatively as a result of anesthesia. Fluid status can be assessed by skin and mucous membrane hydration. ■ Increased hematocrit and hemoglobin can indicate hemoconcentration and underhydration. Decreased serum values can indicate hemodilution or overhydration. ■ Vomiting can cause fluid loss.	The child remains in fluid balance with no vomiting in postoperative period.
7. Impaired gas exchange related to anesthetics and pain			
	NIC Priorty Intervention: **Airway Management:** Facilitation of patency of air passages.		NOC Suggested Outcome: **Respiratory Status:** Ventilation: Movement of air and out of lungs.
The child will maintain adequate ventilation with no respiratory impairment.	■ Auscultate lungs every 2 hours. Record rate, rhythm, and quality of respiration. Evaluate respiratory rate after analgesics. ■ Administer oxygen if ordered. ■ Reposition the child every 2 hours. ■ Encourage deep breathing and coughing every 2 hours. Use incentive spirometer, pinwheels, or other blow toys appropriate for the development level of the child. ■ Ensure proper intake and output.	■ Early identification of respiratory difficulty aids early treatment. Analgesics, especially morphine, may slow respiratory rate. ■ Oxygen may facilitate breathing status postoperatively. ■ Repositioning ensures expansion of all lung fields. ■ All areas of the lungs must be expanded. Mucus is expectorated. ■ Balanced fluid status ensures liquification of secretions and prevents excess fluid accumulation.	The child moves adequate air in and out of lungs.
8. Pain related to surgical procedure			
	NIC Priority Intervention: **Pain Management:** Alleviation of pain or a reduction in pain to a level of comfort that is acceptable to the patient.		NOC Suggested Outcome: **Pain Control Behavior:** Personal actions to control pain
The child will maintain an adequate comfort level.	■ Assess behavioral cues (e.g., crying, movement, guarding). ■ Use an appropriate pain scale with verbal children. ■ Administer prescribed pain medications on a regular basis. ■ Use age-appropriate non-pharmacologic methods of pain control (e.g., distraction, repositioning).	■ Behavior of preverbal children provides clues to pain experience. ■ Pain scales allow children to quantify the amount of pain (see Chap. 9). ■ Narcotics and nonnarcotic analgesics alter pain perception. ■ Nonpharmacologic interventions interfere with pain perception.	The child's pain is controlled as demonstrated by a low number on the pain control scale (behavioral or verbal).

(continued)

NURSING CARE PLAN The Child Undergoing Surgery (continued)

GOAL	INTERVENTION	RATIONALE	EXPECTED OUTCOME
9. Risk for impaired skin integrity related to limited mobility after surgery			
	NIC Priority Intervention: **Skin Surveillance and Pressure Management:** Collection and analysis of patient data to maintain skin integrity and minimizing pressure to body parts.		NOC Suggested Outcome: **Risk Control:** Actions to eliminate or reduce actual personal and modifiable health threats.
The child's skin will remain intact.	■ Turn and reposition the child every 2 hours. ■ Keep linens clean and dry. ■ Check pressure areas when turning and rub erythematous areas with lotion. ■ Get the child up and ambulating when ordered. ■ Check the incision for drainage, redness, and intactness of staples or stitches every 4–8 hours.	■ Repositioning takes pressure off the skin and allows increased circulation. ■ Clean linen decreases the chance of skin break-down. ■ Rubbing increases circulation. ■ Movement decreases pressure on skin. ■ Early identification of infection or problems with wound healing can ensure fast treatment.	The child develops no pressure areas. The wound heals without complication.
10. Anxiety (child and family) related to equipment and surgical outcome			
	NIC Priority Intervention: **Anxiety Reduction:** Minimizing apprehension, dread, foreboding, or uneasiness related to an unidentified source of danger.		NOC Suggested Outcome: **Coping:** Actions to manage stressors that tax an individuals' resources.
The child and family will verbalize comfort with postoperative care and outcome.	■ Explain monitors, drainage dressings, intravenous lines, and procedures. ■ Reassure the child and family that anxiety is a normal response to the stressful event of surgery. ■ Encourage parental presence and care of the child. ■ Use touch and other nonverbal and verbal communication with the child and family	■ Knowledge of purpose decreases anxiety. ■ Knowledge of what is expected decreases anxiety. ■ The child's anxiety decreases with parental presence. ■ Effective communication reassures child and family.	The child and family demonstrate coping skills to deal with hospitalization.
11. Knowledge deficit (child and family) related to needed home care			
	NIC Priority Intervention: **Teaching, Postoperative:** Health System Guidance: Facilitating a patient's location and use of appropriate health services.		NOC Suggested Outcome: **Knowledge:** Home Care Extent of understanding conveyed about home care.
The child and family will verbalize self-care required at home.	■ Provide oral and written home care instructions regarding surgical wound care, medications, activities, and diet. ■ Provide a number to call for questions or concerns. Instruct on follow-up visits.	■ Teaching regarding home care is necessary early in hospitalization. ■ Parents need to know emergency information and that follow-up care is required.	The child and family demonstrate skills needed for home care following discharge. They verbalize plans for future care.

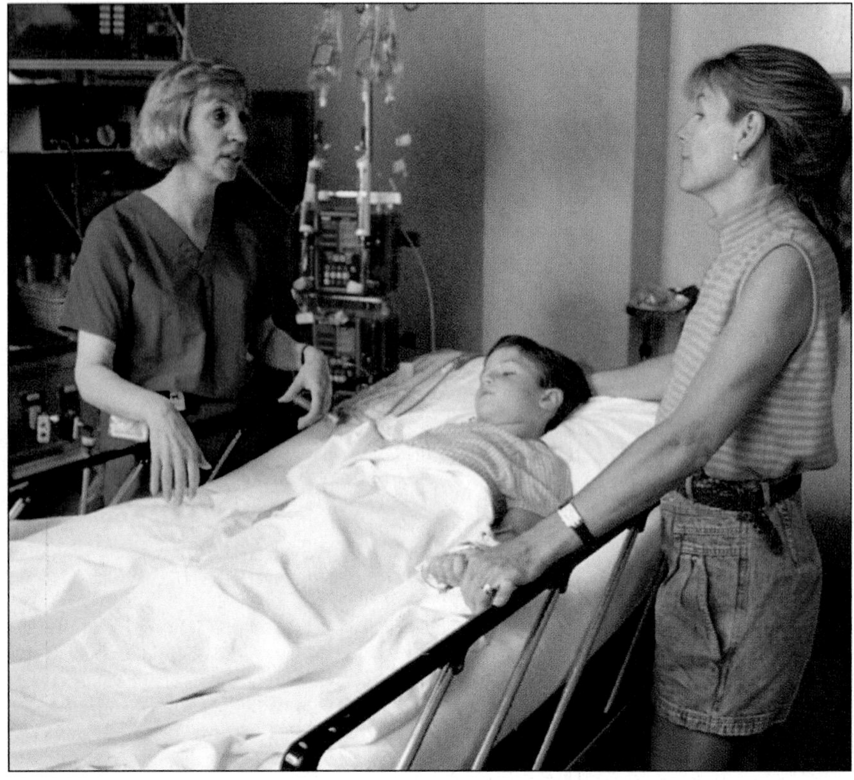

FIGURE 5-15 ◆
This child has just undergone surgery and is in the PICU. Although the child's physical care is immediate and important, remember that both the child and the family have strong psychosocial needs that must be addressed concurrently. It is important to reunite the family as soon as possible after surgery.

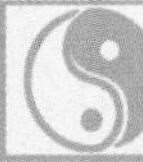

CULTURE

Many American Indian tribes use "smudging" or burning of native plants as a blessing and purifying of the spirit. This practice is thought to enhance healing and protect the child. The nurse can provide a safe, facilitative environment for this important ceremony in the hospital.

Postoperative Care

Postoperative care of the child includes both physical and psychologic care. The child's level of consciousness is evaluated, and vital signs are taken frequently. The surgical site is observed for drainage, and dressings are checked. The nurse monitors the child's intake and output and provides comfort and pain relief. (See Chapter 9 for details concerning pain management.) Parents are allowed to visit with the child as soon after surgery as possible and culturally competent care is implemented (Figure 5-15 ◆). Refer to the Nursing Care Plan for the Child Undergoing Surgery.

PREPARATION FOR LONG-TERM CARE

When ill or injured children require long-term care, they are often transferred from an acute care hospital to a rehabilitation center or other long-term care facility. The rehabilitation phase of the treatment does not begin at the time of discharge from the acute care hospital but, instead, early in the hospitalization phase. The plan of care is instituted in the hospital, interventions and therapies are begun, and plans are made for continued care.

When it becomes apparent that a child will need long-term care, the health care team explores with the family the options and resources available to provide such care:

- Home care with support services such as visiting nurses and physical therapists
- A long-term care facility
- A specialized rehabilitation center that can provide care for an extended period

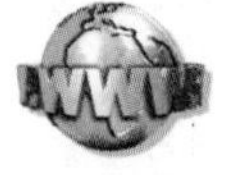

Brain Injury Resources

The family should make the decision about which option will work best, considering the needs of the child, the financial implications, the roles and supports available to the family unit, and the resources available in the community. Guidelines to assist parents in evaluating rehabilitation centers are available from the Brain Injury Association.

Nurses in acute care hospitals frequently coordinate services when transfer to another facility occurs. This involves giving information about the child's history, plan of care, and treatment to the new facility. Forms are available to assist the person responsible for coordinating the transfer. Families will need support and assistance in dealing with the transfer from the acute care setting to another facility.

PREPARATION FOR HOME CARE

Nurses play an important role in preparing the child and family for discharge home; this preparation starts early during the hospitalization. The nurse works with the social service department, home care agencies, and the family to plan for equipment, procedures, and other home care needs. Home care nurses then take over the child's care and assist families to meet the child's health care needs.

ASSESSING THE CHILD IN PREPARATION FOR DISCHARGE

Discharge plans should begin early in the child's hospitalization. A health care team, including the physician, nurse, social worker, discharge planner, and family, works together to ensure a smooth transition home. An assessment of the family's ability to manage the child's care and of the appropriateness of the home for providing care should be made (Votroubek & Townsend, 1997).

Children with multisystem problems may require home care involving specialized equipment and personnel. Early planning gives the family time to investigate health insurance benefits, support services in the community, and other needs before discharge.

When a child is to be discharged home, the school district should be contacted and plans for education made. This involves an assessment of the child by the school district and formulation of an **Individualized Education Plan (IEP)**. The IEP may include home tutors, specialized services from persons such as physical or speech therapists, or arrangements for transport of the child with a disability to the school and provisions for special medical care as needed. For each child with a chronic disability who is 14 years or older, an **Individualized Transition Plan** focuses on assisting the individual in moving successfully from school or home into other community settings as they grow older (Jackson & Vessey, 2000).

Some common problems that interfere with successful discharge planning include financial concerns, the family's unavailability for teaching and planning, and poor communication and lack of teamwork among involved health care disciplines. Nurses should be alert to these potential problems from the initial contact with the child and family and should take precautions to solve them as soon as possible (Proctor, Morrow-Howell, Kitchen, & Wang, 1995).

PREPARING THE FAMILY FOR HOME CARE

The family may need to learn physical and rehabilitative procedures for the child's care. Short-term care may be necessary until the child regains full function. In other situations, care may be required throughout the child's life. This may involve measuring vital signs or determining blood glucose levels. For the child requiring complex long-term care, parents may need to learn about intravenous lines, medications, oxygen administration, or ventilators (Figure 5-16 ◆). Parents need to be taught how to use the equipment needed for the child's care and must show that they can use it correctly. They must be able to identify symptoms of distress and report them immediately to the health care provider. The education provided and the parents' ability to perform care are discussed with a visiting nurse or individual who manages the home care program. Parents should be encouraged to learn cardiopulmonary resuscitation (refer to Chapter 6). Some families need help to become providers of end-of-life care.

Help parents explore options for respite. If they cannot provide daily care or need a break, they should be able to rely on others for a short period. Some agencies are available to provide respite care. Ongoing assistance may be needed to help families deal with financial, time, and other challenges. Families with the greatest burdens in caring for their children will require the most interventions.

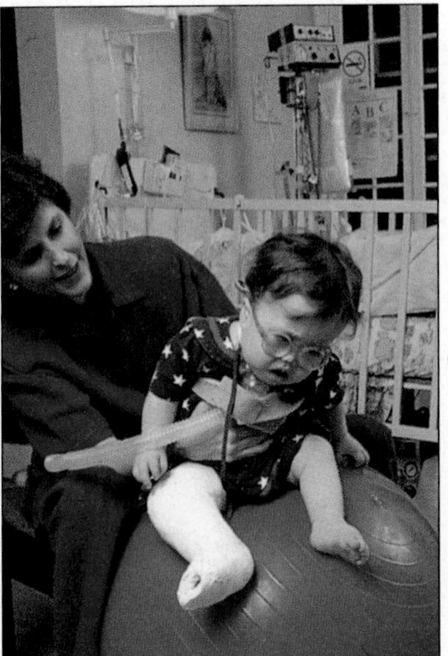

FIGURE 5-16 ◆
This child with chronic medical problems is being cared for at home. Are there any legal implications for the hospital and the nurse associated with the preparation of the child and family for home care?

PREPARING PARENTS TO ACT AS CASE MANAGERS

The family is an integral part of the plan of care for an ill or hospitalized child. The child with a chronic illness or an injury requiring long-term care will probably require the services of numerous health care personnel or health care agencies. One person needs to be identified as a **case manager,** to coordinate health care and to prevent gaps and overlaps. In some hospitals, nurses act as case managers. They may organize a patient care conference while the child with a chronic condition is hospitalized. Management goals are set and decisions are made about which health care provider or agency is responsible for helping the child meet each goal.

Parents can also act as case managers. The parent as case manager coordinates medical care, hospital stays, and visits to specialists; meets with school district representatives to plan the IEP for the child; finds equipment, personnel, and other services for home care; and manages the child's overall care.

Nurses should strongly encourage parents who want to take over case management to do so. They can be assisted in learning the management skills required. Many communities have workshops for parents who are managing the complex care of their children.

Chapter Highlights

- Hospitalization is a stressful event for all children and their families, especially when the hospitalization was unplanned and sudden.
- The understanding of children about their illnesses and hospitalizations is based on cognitive abilities at each developmental stage, and upon previous health care experiences.
- Nurses assess the impact of the child's illness or hospitalization on the family unit.
- Families are always disrupted by a child's hospitalization, and various approaches can help them to understand the process and cope more successfully with this challenge.
- When hospitalization is planned, both the child and parents can prepare for the experience. Nurses assist this process by teaching about what to expect.
- A teaching plan includes goals and expected outcomes, interventions needed to achieve the specified goals, and a method and time for evaluation of the expected outcomes.
- Strategies such as child life programs, rooming in, therapeutic play, and therapeutic recreation help meet the psychosocial needs of the hospitalized child.
- The nurse assists the family to plan for the child's long-term health care needs and home care issues. Culturally competent care is integrated throughout all provisions of care. Parents may be trained to act as case managers for the child with long-term needs, or the task is delegated to a health care provider.

EXPLORE MediaLink

- NCLEX review, case studies, and other interactive resources for this chapter can be found on the Companion Website at **http://www.prenhall. com/ball**. Click on Chapter 5 to select the activities for this chapter.
- For animations, more NCLEX review questions, and an audio glossary, access the accompanying CD-ROM in this textbook.

References

1. Bibace, R., & Walsh, M. (1981). Children's conception of illness. In R. Bibace & M. Walsh (Eds.), *Children's conceptions of health, illness and bodily function.* San Francisco: Jossey-Bass.
2. Bowlby, J. (1960). Separation anxiety. *International Journal of Psychoanalysis, 41*(2/3), 89–113.
3. Boyd, J. R., & Hunsberger, M. (1998). Chronically ill children coping with repeated hospitalizations: Their perceptions and suggested interventions. *Journal of Pediatric Nursing, 13,* 330–342.
4. Bricher, G. (2000). Children in the hospital: Issues of power and vulnerability. *Pediatric Nursing, 26,* 277–282.
5. Conner, J. M., & Nelson, E. C. (1999). Neonatal intensive care: Satisfaction measured from a parent's perspective. *Pediatrics, 103,* 336–349.
6. De Pasquale, S. (1999, November). Serious play. *Johns Hopkins Magazine,* 30–36.
7. Emergency Nurses Association. (1998). *Family presence at the bedside during invasive procedures and/or resuscitation.* Des Plains, IL: Author.
8. Gusella, J. L., Ward, A. M., & Butler, G. S. (1998). The experience of hospitalized adolescent: How well do we meet their developmental needs? *Children's Health Care, 27,* 131–145.
9. Huckabay, L. M. D., & Tilem-Kessler, D. (1999). Patterns of parental stress in PICU admission. *Dimensions of Critical Care Nursing, 18*(2), 36–42.
10. Jackson, P. L., & Vessey, J. A. (2000). *Primary care of the child with a chronic condition* (3rd ed.). St. Louis: Mosby, Inc.
11. LaMontagne, L. L. (2000). Effects of surgery type and attention focus on children's coping. *Nursing Research, 49,* 245–252.
12. Lipson, J. G., Dibble, S. L., & Minarik, P. A. (1996). *Culture and nursing care: A pocket guide.* San Francisco: UCSF Nursing Press.
13. Marino, B. L., & Marino, E. K. (2000). Practice applications of research. Parents' report of children's hospital care: What it means for your practice. *Pediatric Nursing, 26,* 195–198.
14. Melnyk, B. M. (1995). Parental coping with childhood hospitalization: A theoretical framework to guide research and clinical interventions. *Maternal-Child Nursing Journal, 23,* 123–131.
15. Melnyk, B. M. (2000). Intervention studies involving parents of hospitalized young children: An analysis of the past and future recommendations. *Journal of Pediatric Nursing, 15,* 4–13.
16. Mobley, C. E. (1996). Assessment of health knowledge in preschoolers. *Children's Health Care, 25,* 11–18.
17. Proctor, E. K., Morrow-Howell, N., Kitchen, A., & Wang, Y. T. (1995). Pediatric discharge planning: Complications, efficiency, and adequacy. *Social Work in Health Care, 22,* 1–18.
18. Ramsey, C. A. (2000). Storytelling can be a valuable teaching aid. *Association of Operating Room Nurses Journal, 72,* 497–499.
19. Rode, D., Capitulo, K. L., Fishman, M., & Holden, G. (1998). The therapeutic use of technology. *American Journal of Nursing, 98*(12), 32–35.
20. Rosenbaum, J. N., & Carty, L. (1996). The subculture of adolescence: Beliefs about care, health and individuation within Leininger's theory. *Journal of Advanced Nursing, 23,* 741–746.
21. Votroubek, W., & Townsend, J. L. (1997). *Pediatric home care.* Gaithersburg, MD: Aspen Publishers.

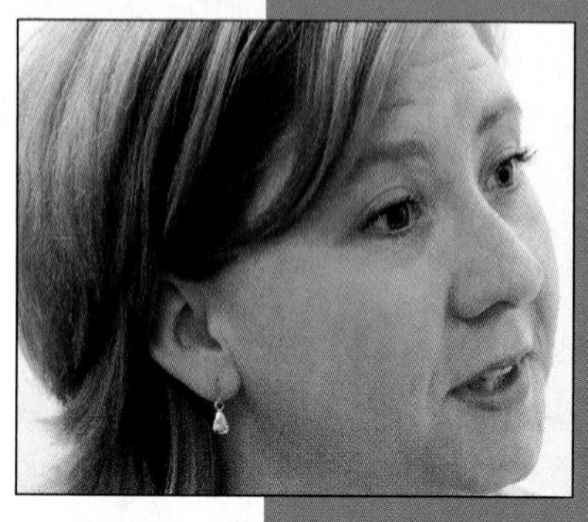

"SOMETIMES JESSICA'S ASTHMA ATTACKS REALLY FRIGHTEN ME BECAUSE SHE STRUGGLES SO HARD TO BREATHE. I DON'T LIKE TO SEND HER OUT OF CLASS TOO SOON, BUT I DON'T WANT TO MAKE HER CONDITION WORSE. I WISH I KNEW WHAT TO DO!"

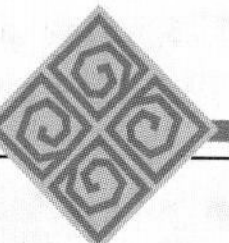
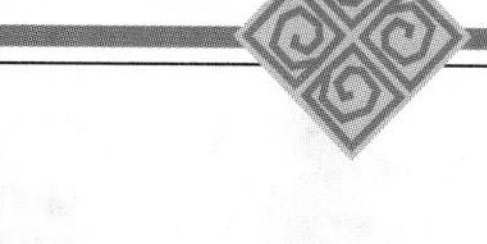

Jessica, 8 years old, is anxious because her asthma attack is getting worse. Her teacher sees that she is having trouble breathing, so she sends her to the school health office for treatment. Jessica has such severe asthma that a nebulizer is kept at school for her to use. This treatment will often relieve Jessica's symptoms and permit her to return to classes. However, in this case, the asthma attack does not respond to the treatment, and the school nurse contacts her mother to come pick her up from school. This means another visit to the emergency department for treatment.

Jessica has had asthma since she was 2 years old and has needed to stay in the hospital for severe asthma attacks twice over the past 2 years. Fortunately, her asthma attack improves with the medications provided in the emergency department, and she can go home after a couple of hours. Jessica does not like to miss school or to worry her mother. Her mother wishes there were some way to reduce the number and severity of her asthma attacks.

What are some possible triggers of Jessica's asthma attacks at school? What measures can be taken to control her asthma on a daily basis and reduce the number of attacks? What special arrangements are needed to permit a child to receive care for asthma or another chronic condition while at school?

CHAPTER 6

NURSING CONSIDERATIONS FOR THE CHILD IN THE COMMUNITY

KEY TERMS

chronic condition A health condition that lasts or is expected to last 3 months or more.

developmental surveillance A continuous process of skilled observations of a child's fine and gross motor, language, and psychosocial behavior milestones at health visits during childhood.

disability Impairment in one or more of five categories of function—cognition, communication, motor abilities, social abilities, or patterns of interactions.

health supervision The process of health promotion services, growth and development monitoring, and disease and injury prevention throughout the child's life.

medical home A primary care provider or regular source of health care.

medically fragile Children who need skilled nursing care with or without medical equipment to support vital functions.

screening tests Procedures used to detect the presence of a health condition before symptoms are apparent.

sensitivity Screening test value stated as the percentage of children testing positive for a condition who truly have that condition.

specificity Screening test value stated as the percentage of children testing negative for a condition who do not have that condition.

MediaLink 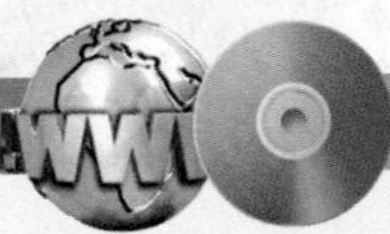

http://www.prenhall.com/ball

Resources for this chapter can be found on the CD-ROM accompanying this textbook, and on the Companion Website at http://www.prenhall.com/ball. Click on Chapter 6 to select the activities for this chapter.

CD-ROM

Audio Glossary

NCLEX Review

COMPANION WEBSITE

Web Links

NCLEX Review

MediaLink Applications

- Plan a Health Supervision Visit
- Provide Health Education in the Schools
- Identify Health Issues in Child Care Settings
- Develop an Individual School Health Plan (ISHP)
- Complete an Emergency Information Form (EIF)

Nurses care for children in a wide variety of community settings. Some of these settings include child care centers, schools, camps, physician offices, hospital or public health clinics, homeless shelters, and the home. The range of nursing care varies from monitoring the health and safety of children in child care centers and schools to providing acute care to a child at home. Falling within this range are the provision of health supervision or well-child care, care for episodic illnesses and injuries, and assisting families to learn optimal management of their child's chronic conditions. Each of these nursing roles is important in promoting the health of children in the community.

Children receive most of their health care (health supervision and episodic health care for acute illnesses and injuries) in community settings. Depending on the community, health care resources, and age of the child, this care may be provided in any of the settings previously described.

During the past decade, the United States has begun to place a greater emphasis on health promotion and disease and injury prevention (health protection). The purpose is not only to promote optimal well-being and to reduce the pain and suffering of children and families, but also to reduce health care costs. Other patterns of health care delivery are also changing to reduce the costs of health care. Examples of these changes include day surgery in ambulatory surgical centers, newborn discharge after 24 to 48 hours, home care for long-term intravenous antibiotics, and short-stay units associated with emergency departments. Health plans and other health care providers continue to explore options to provide safe, high-quality care with fewer hospitalizations or shorter stays when hospitalization is needed. Home care services have developed to support families who now care for more acutely ill children.

LAW & ETHICS

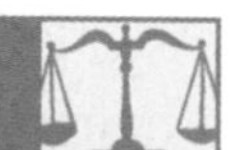

The 1975 Education for All Handicapped Children Act, Public Law 94–142, and the Education of the Handicapped Amendments of 1986, Public Law 99–457, guarantee a free and appropriate education for all children with disabilities between 3 and 21 years of age. This legislation was renamed the Individuals with Disabilities Education Act (IDEA) in 1991 and reauthorized by Congress in 1997. As a result of these laws, children with complex health conditions must be managed in school settings in the least restrictive educational environment.

This trend in out-of-hospital care is also seen among children with chronic health conditions and advanced disease states. Technologic advances, such as portable medical equipment, now make it possible to provide complex health care services in the home and other community settings (Figure 6-1 ◆). Strategies to support families who provide care to their children in the home have developed. Additionally, federal law mandates that education be provided to all children with disabilities, regardless of health care status. As a result, schools are now obligated to provide complex health care to children.

Care of children continues to shift from the hospital to community settings at a rapid rate. The nurse working with families in a community setting must use the knowledge of how the larger environment influences the child's health and development and the family's activities. To work effectively in the community, the nurse's role includes:

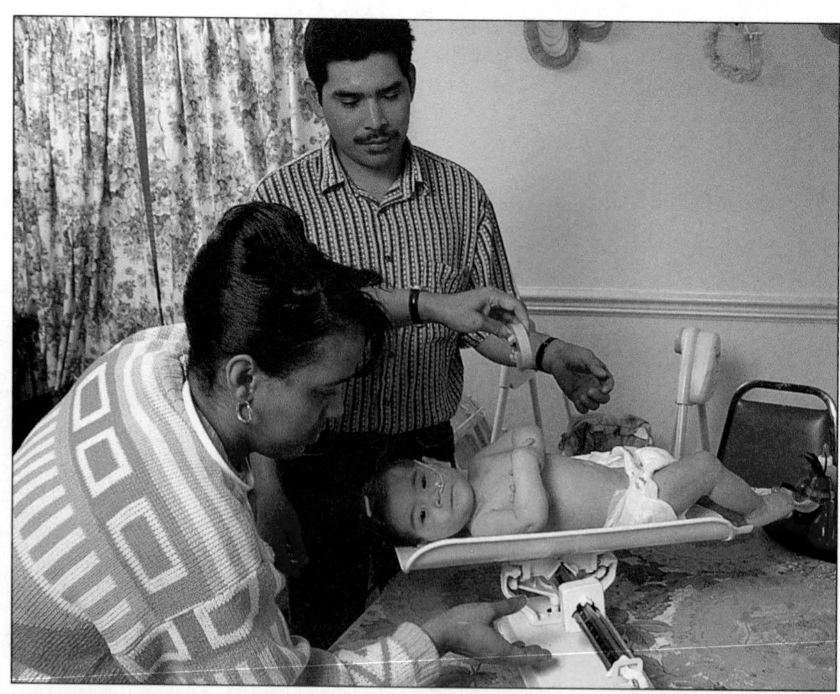

FIGURE 6-1 ◆
Nurses provide both short-term and long-term services to families in the home setting. In some cases, families need support for a short time after the child is discharged from the hospital following an acute illness. In other cases, families need assistance with complex nursing care for the child dependent on technology for survival.

- Making assessments, planning strategies, and implementing and evaluating approaches to care that match the family's economic and social situation, and available resources.
- Working with others in the community (schools, churches, and other community-based resources) to make assessments, plan strategies, and implement and evaluate approaches addressed to the health care needs of the community's children (Pridham, Broome, & Woodring, 1996).

HEALTH SUPERVISION

How often do children need health supervision visits? What are the elements of a health supervision visit? Why are children screened for health conditions at certain times?

All children need a regular source of health care, a primary care provider or **medical home** that supports the family and child during the important developmental years. When a family has an established relationship with a primary care provider, comprehensive, family-centered health services can be provided based on the provider's knowledge of the family's strengths and weaknesses.

Health supervision is the provision of services that focus on disease and injury prevention, growth and developmental surveillance, and health promotion at key intervals during the child's life (Figure 6-2 ◆). It is not just a periodic visit for health care services. National guidelines for preventive health services have been developed for infants, children, and adolescents by the U.S. Department of Health and Human Services (DHHS) and the American Medical Association. Settings for health supervision visits vary widely within a community and include physician offices, community health centers, the home, schools or child care centers, or shelters.

The health supervision visit must be individualized to the family and child. Every health visit, including an episodic illness visit or maintenance care for a chronic condition, is a potential health promotion visit. A tracking system in the primary care setting helps to identify appropriate health supervision activities for each child at every visit. For example, needed immunizations may sometimes be given during a visit for an acute condition if the child has missed a prior health supervision visit. Refer to Chapter 12 for immunization guidelines.

Nurses play an important role in managing these health supervision visits. Depending on the setting, the nurse may provide all services or support the physician by obtaining an updated health history, screening for diseases and other conditions, conducting a developmental assessment, and providing immunizations, anticipatory guidance, and health education.

COMMUNITY CARE

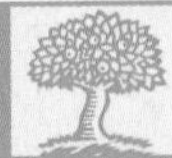

A medical home includes:

1. Provision of preventive services
2. Assurance of ambulatory and inpatient care 24 hours a day
3. Continuity of care from infancy to adolescence
4. Appropriate use of subspecialty consultation and referrals
5. Interaction with school and community agencies
6. A central record and database containing all pertinent information (Green & Palfrey, 2000).

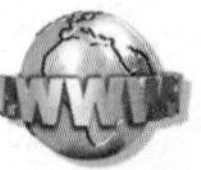

Guidelines for Health Promotion & Supervision

NATIONAL GUIDELINES FOR HEALTH PROMOTION

- *Bright Futures*, Maternal and Child Health Bureau, Health Resources and Services Administration, DHHS
- *Put Prevention into Practice*, Office of Disease Prevention and Health Promotion, Public Health Service, DHHS
- *Guidelines for Adolescent Preventive Services*, American Medical Association

Health supervision

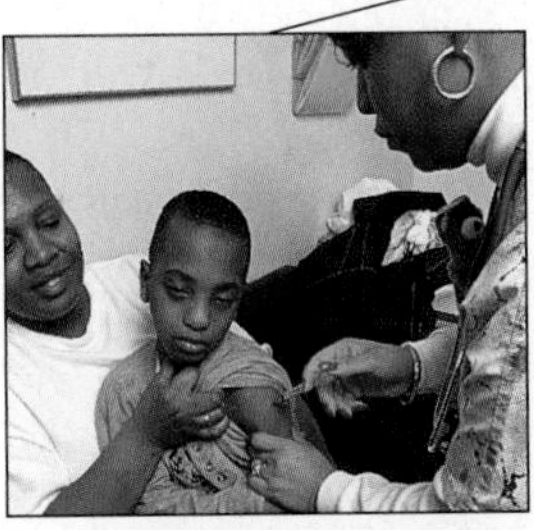

Disease and injury prevention
Screening tests
Immunizations
Safety teaching
Anticipatory guidance

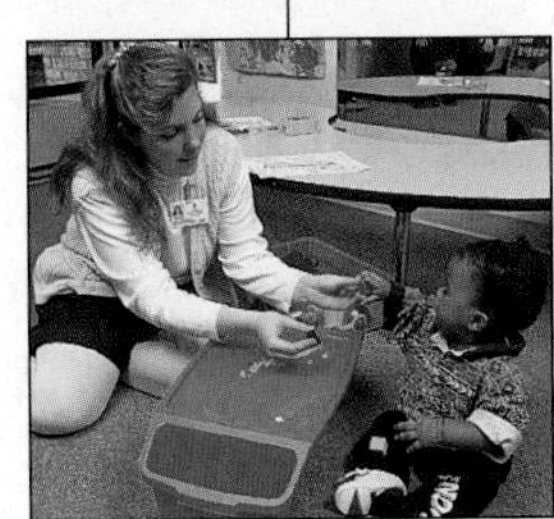

Developmental surveillance
Observation of progress in areas of fine motor, gross motor, language, adaptive skills, and cognition.

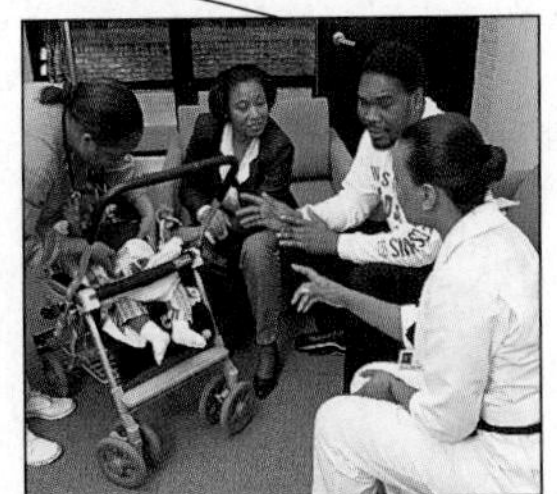

Health promotion
Child and family guidance to promote family strengths in areas of healthy life styles, social development, coping, and family interactions.

FIGURE 6-2 ◆
Model of pediatric health supervision visits.

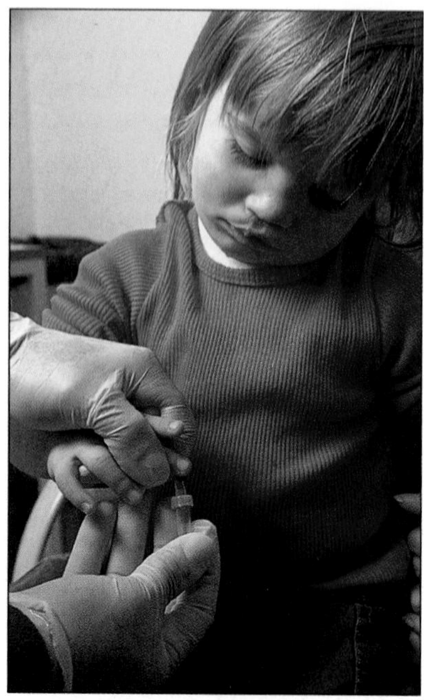

FIGURE 6-3 ◆
This 18-month-old toddler is having a blood screening test to detect iron deficiency anemia. Children are often screened for adequate levels of iron in the latter stages of infancy and during toddlerhood.

NURSING MANAGEMENT

Nursing Assessment and Diagnosis

Nursing assessment of the child and family at each visit for health supervision focuses on the following:

- Interviewing the family and child to update the health history, assessing the child's developmental or educational progress, identifying nutritional status and dietary habits, and discussing any concerns of the parent or child (see Chapters 3 and 4)
- Observing the family–child relationships
- Conducting developmental surveillance assessments
- Performing age-appropriate screening tests (Figure 6-3 ◆)
- Performing a physical assessment

DISEASE AND INJURY PREVENTION **Screening tests** are procedures used to detect the presence of a health condition before symptoms are apparent. Once a screening test identifies the existence of a health condition, early intervention can begin, with the goal of reducing the severity or complications of the condition. For example, all newborns are screened within 1 week of birth for at least two genetic diseases, congenital hypothyroidism and phenylketonuria. Appropriate interventions (medication or diet therapy) reduce the chances or severity of mental retardation if either of these conditions is present. (See Chapter 22 for more information about newborn screening.)

Screening tests are administered at times when children are most likely to develop a condition or to identify the greatest number of children at highest risk for the condition. Screening tests are also expected to correctly identify children who truly have the condition. Some children are at greater risk of contracting certain conditions because of their envi-

SCREENING TEST INTERPRETATION

Sensitivity is the proportion of children with a condition who test positive for that condition. Some children who test positive do not have the condition; they are false positives.

Specificity is the proportion of children who do not have a condition who test negative for that condition. Some children who test negative actually have the condition; they are false negatives.

The best screening tests have both a high sensitivity and high specificity. If a child tests positive on a screening test, then additional tests are usually performed to confirm the presence of the condition (Curry & Duby, 1994).

TABLE 6-1 Clinical Preventive Services for Normal-Risk Children, birth to 18 years of age*

SCREENING TEST	AGE	FREQUENCY
Newborn screening (PKU, sickle-cell hemoglobinopathies, hypothyroidism)	Newborn	Once
Hearing	Newborn, 3 to 8 years, 10 years, 12 years, 15 years, 18 years	Once in each age interval
Head circumference	Birth to 2 years	Periodically
Height and weight	Birth to 18 years	Periodically
Lead	1 year, 2 years	Once at each age
Eye screening	Birth, 3 to 4 years	Once
	5 to 18 years	Periodically
Blood pressure	6 to 12 months	Once
	3 to 18 years	Periodically
Dental	1 to 18 years	Periodically
Alcohol use	11 to 18 years	Periodically
COUNSELING	**AGE**	**FREQUENCY**
Development, nutrition, physical activity, safety, unintentional injuries and poisoning, violent behaviors, firearms, sexually transmitted diseases and HIV, family planning, tobacco use, drug use	Birth to 18 years	As appropriate for age

*For recommended immunization schedule, see Chapter 12.
Note: From Office of Public Health and Science and Office of Disease Prevention and Promotion (1998). *Put prevention into practice: Clinician's handbook of preventive services* (2nd ed.). Washington, DC: U.S. Department of Health and Human Services, Public Health Services, Fig. A.2(a).

ronment (Figure 6-4 ◆). For example, young children living in housing built before 1960 are screened more frequently for lead poisoning than children who live in newer houses where only lead-free paints have been used. Table 6-1 outlines the recommended screening tests by age for infants, children, and adolescents.

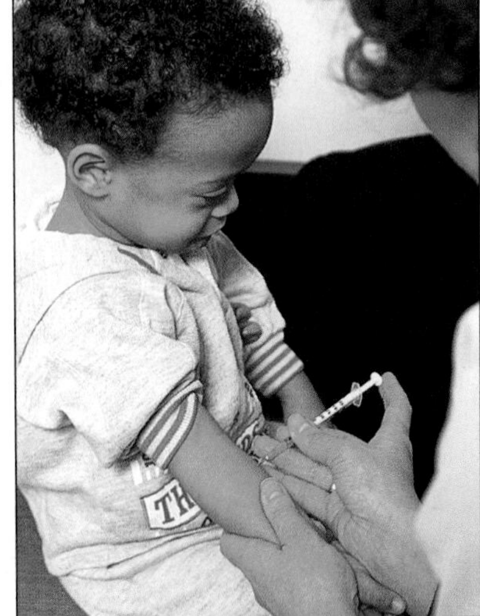

FIGURE 6-4 ◆
Children who live in an area where active tuberculosis has been detected or is epidemic need tuberculosis screening more frequently.

DEVELOPMENTAL SURVEILLANCE **Developmental surveillance** is a flexible, continuous process of skilled observations of children's fine and gross motor skills, language, and psychosocial behavior milestones throughout encounters during child health visits. Information may be collected from several sources; for instance, a questionnaire that the parent completes, trigger questions asked during the interview, or observation of the child during the visit. Parents can also be interviewed to identify any developmental concerns they may have about the child. To initiate general health supervision and developmental surveillance, questions such as the following may be used (Deloian, 1997):

- Do you have any concerns about Sam's vision and hearing?
- What changes have you seen in Hannah's development?
- What kind of baby is Jamal?
- What do you and Brianna enjoy doing together?
- What are Brandon's favorite play activities?

Standardized developmental questionnaires are effective for developmental surveillance of most children, especially when time for health supervision visits is limited. These questionnaires are easy to administer, do not require the child's cooperation, and can be completed by parents in the waiting area. Children in need of more extensive developmental surveillance can be identified. See Table 6-2 for a list of commonly used developmental screening questionnaires that have been tested for validity and reliability.

When talking with parents, review physical, social, and communication milestones for infants and young children. Be aware that parents' recall of past developmental milestones is often faulty. The child is often reported to have achieved milestones at ages earlier than actually occurred. When accuracy of developmental milestones is critical, ask to see the

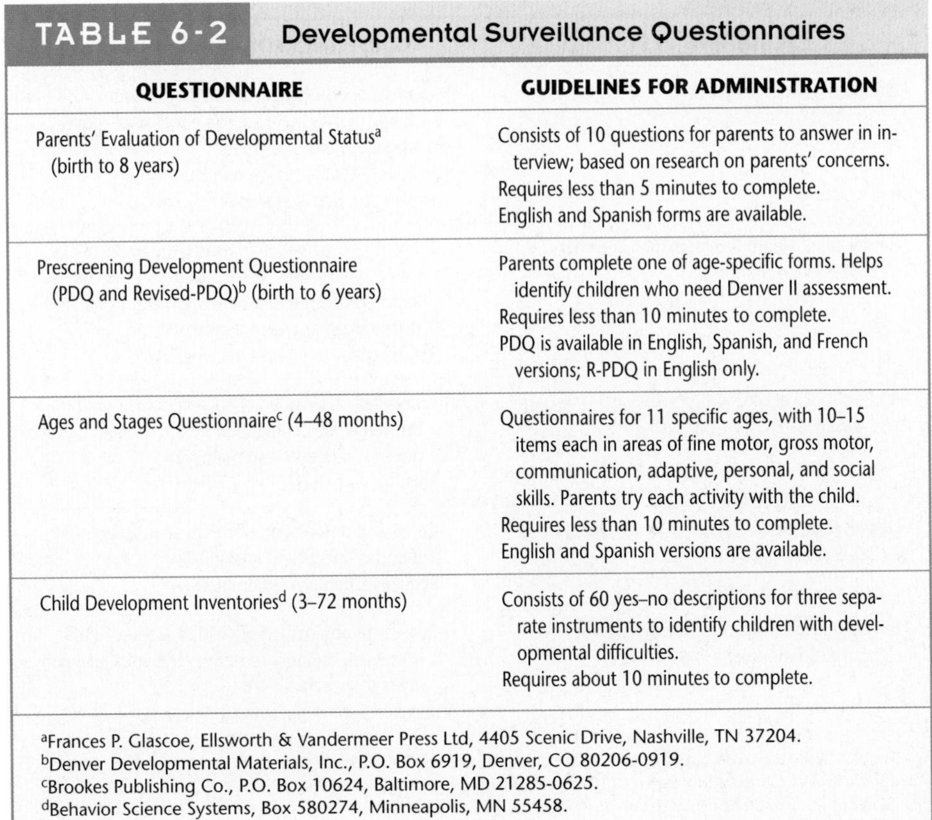

TABLE 6-2 Developmental Surveillance Questionnaires

QUESTIONNAIRE	GUIDELINES FOR ADMINISTRATION
Parents' Evaluation of Developmental Status[a] (birth to 8 years)	Consists of 10 questions for parents to answer in interview; based on research on parents' concerns. Requires less than 5 minutes to complete. English and Spanish forms are available.
Prescreening Development Questionnaire (PDQ and Revised-PDQ)[b] (birth to 6 years)	Parents complete one of age-specific forms. Helps identify children who need Denver II assessment. Requires less than 10 minutes to complete. PDQ is available in English, Spanish, and French versions; R-PDQ in English only.
Ages and Stages Questionnaire[c] (4–48 months)	Questionnaires for 11 specific ages, with 10–15 items each in areas of fine motor, gross motor, communication, adaptive, personal, and social skills. Parents try each activity with the child. Requires less than 10 minutes to complete. English and Spanish versions are available.
Child Development Inventories[d] (3–72 months)	Consists of 60 yes–no descriptions for three separate instruments to identify children with developmental difficulties. Requires about 10 minutes to complete.

[a]Frances P. Glascoe, Ellsworth & Vandermeer Press Ltd, 4405 Scenic Drive, Nashville, TN 37204.
[b]Denver Developmental Materials, Inc., P.O. Box 6919, Denver, CO 80206-0919.
[c]Brookes Publishing Co., P.O. Box 10624, Baltimore, MD 21285-0625.
[d]Behavior Science Systems, Box 580274, Minneapolis, MN 55458.

child's baby diary or review the past health history at ages closer to the milestone achievement. The parents' report of current skills and achievements is usually accurate.

Review school performance for older children and adolescents. Review report cards, school achievement records, and any performance on psychoeducational tests when indicated. Inquire about the child's participation in sports and other activities, as well as noted abilities.

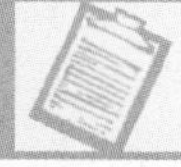

RESEARCH

Past research has indicated that carefully eliciting parents' concerns about their child's development can be as accurate as screening tests in identifying true developmental problems (Glascoe, 1999).

If a developmental delay or abnormality is suspected, a specific developmental screening test is needed to document developmental progress. See Table 6-3 for a list of commonly used developmental screening tests. Some health care providers actually use the Denver II as a developmental chart, like a growth curve, to monitor the child's developmental progress (see Figures 6–5 ◆ and 6–6 ◆). Remember that developmental screening tests are not diagnostic tests. They simply help to confirm that most children are progressing along an age-appropriate norm, and they help document suspicions or patterns of developmental problems.

To perform developmental screening with any of the standardized screening tools, make sure all directions are followed:

- Read directions thoroughly or utilize specific training tools available.
- Calculate the infant's age correctly, especially if premature.
- Attempt to develop rapport with the infant or child to get the best performance.
- In some cases, parents can be asked if a child demonstrates specific skills at home, especially if the child is not cooperative.
- Note the behavior and cooperativeness of the child during the screening process.
- Analyze the findings to make the correct interpretation.

Failure to perform a single item in a single domain does not mean the child has failed the test. The child should be reevaluated at a future visit. Provide parents with guidance on specific methods for stimulating the child. Failure of multiple items within one domain or

TABLE 6-3 Developmental Screening Test for Infants and Young Children

SCREENING TEST	GUIDELINES FOR ADMINISTRATION
Denver II[a] (birth to 6 years)	Consists of observation of the child in four domains: personal-social, fine motor–adaptive, language, and gross motor. Requires 30 minutes to complete. A training video is available.
Bayley Infant Neurodevelopmental Screener (BINS)[b] (3–24 months)	Consists of observation of child with 10–13 items for each of six age-specific scales to assess neurological processes, neurodevelopmental skills, and developmental accomplishments. Requires 10–15 minutes to complete.
McCarthy Scales of Children's Abilities[b] (2.5–8.5 years)	Consists of observation of child in domains of motor, verbal, perceptual-performance, quantitative, general cognition, and memory. Requires 45 minutes to complete.
Denver Articulation Screening Exam (DASE)[a] (2.5–6 years)	Consists of observation of child's articulation of 30 sound elements and intelligibility. Requires 5 minutes to complete.
Early Language Milestone Scale—2 (ELM)[c] (birth to 36 months)	Consists of observation of child to assess auditory expressive, auditory receptive, and visual components of speech. Requires 5–10 minutes to complete.

[a]Denver Development Materials, Inc., P.O. Box 6919, Denver, CO 80206-0919
[b]Psychological Corporation, 304 E. 45th Street, New York, NY 10017-3425
[c]PRO-ED, Inc., 8700 Shoal Creek Blvd., Austin, TX 78758-6897

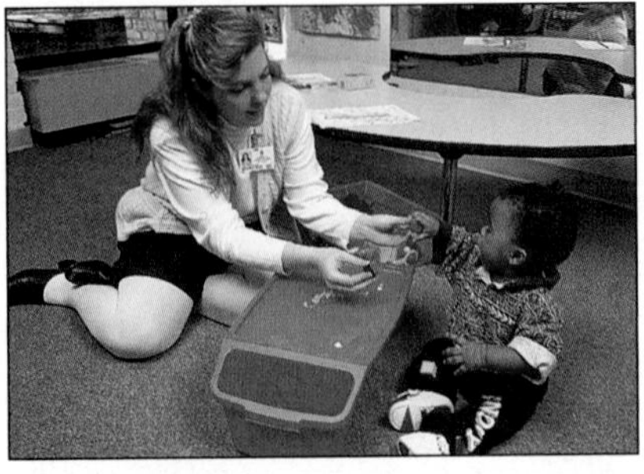
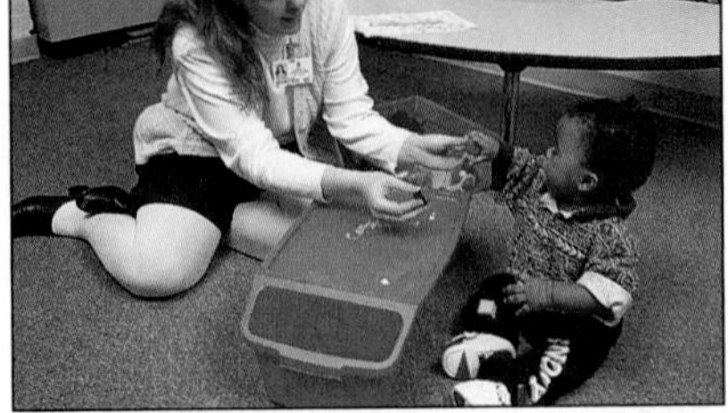

A

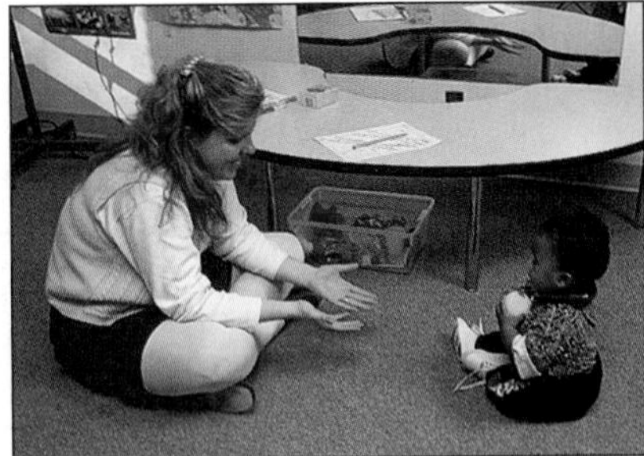

B

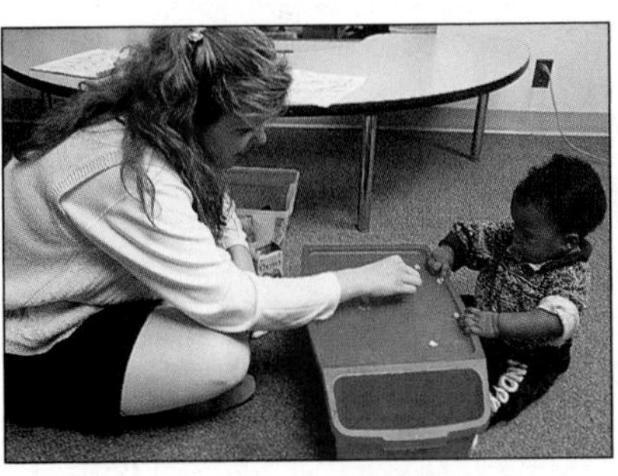

C

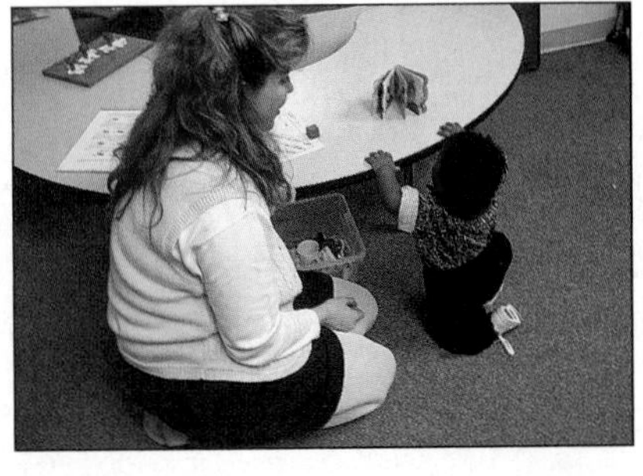

D

FIGURE 6-5 ◆
Follow all directions for performing the Denver II assessment and for interpreting responses. Develop rapport with the child and approach the assessment as fun. This often helps the child participate more actively during the entire Denver II assessment. The 9-month-old boy in this sequence is able to perform the following age-appropriate behaviors: Banging two cubes, A; playing ball with the examiner, B; using a thumb-finger grasp, C; and pulling to stand, D.

across multiple domains is of greatest concern. When poor development patterns in one or more domains are revealed, referral for diagnostic developmental assessment is needed.

Examples of nursing diagnoses for an 18-month-old child who is brought by parents for regular health supervision and immunizations may include the following:

- *Altered nutrition: more than body requirements* related to lack of basic nutritional knowledge
- *Risk for poisoning* related to lack of proper precautions with increased mobility to reach and climb
- *Health-seeking behaviors* related to needed immunizations
- *Risk for altered parenting* related to mother's plans to return to full-time work

Planning and Implementation

Nursing management for health supervision visits includes providing immunizations, offering anticipatory guidance, educating parents and children about healthy behaviors, carrying out collaborative nurse–family planning for health promotion, and providing referrals for follow-up care. For more information about the recommended schedule for immunizations and the nurse's role in ensuring full immunization status for children, refer to Chapter 12.

Most parents want to know how to contribute to their child's growth and development. Discussions at the conclusion of the health supervision assessments should focus on building family strengths by promoting the development of competence, confidence, and self-esteem in the growing child.

Although some specific interventions are most likely to take place only in a health care facility or physician's office, most of the nursing management for health supervision can occur in any setting.

PROVIDE ANTICIPATORY GUIDANCE Anticipatory guidance provides the family with information on what to expect during the child's current and next stage of development. Topics for each visit should include age-appropriate information about healthy habits, prevention of illness and injury, prevention of poisoning, nutrition, oral health, and sexuality. Health promotion guidance also helps the child and family to develop strategies to support and enhance social development, family relationships, parental health, community interactions, self-responsibility, and school or vocational achievement.

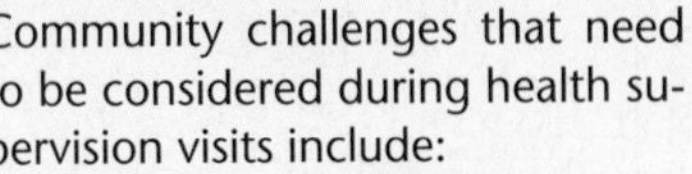

Community challenges that need to be considered during health supervision visits include:

- Poverty; inadequate housing; limited opportunities for employment; lack of affordable, high-quality child care
- Environmental hazards; unsafe neighborhood; community violence
- Isolation in a rural community; lack of programs for families with special needs; lack of social support; inadequate public services
- Lack of educational programs and social services for adolescent parents; lack of social, educational, cultural, and recreational opportunities
- Lack of access to medical or dental services; inadequate fluoride levels in community water

Parents who are experiencing more than two of these problems in their community may need extra assistance or guidance to provide a supportive environment for their child that fosters growth and development.

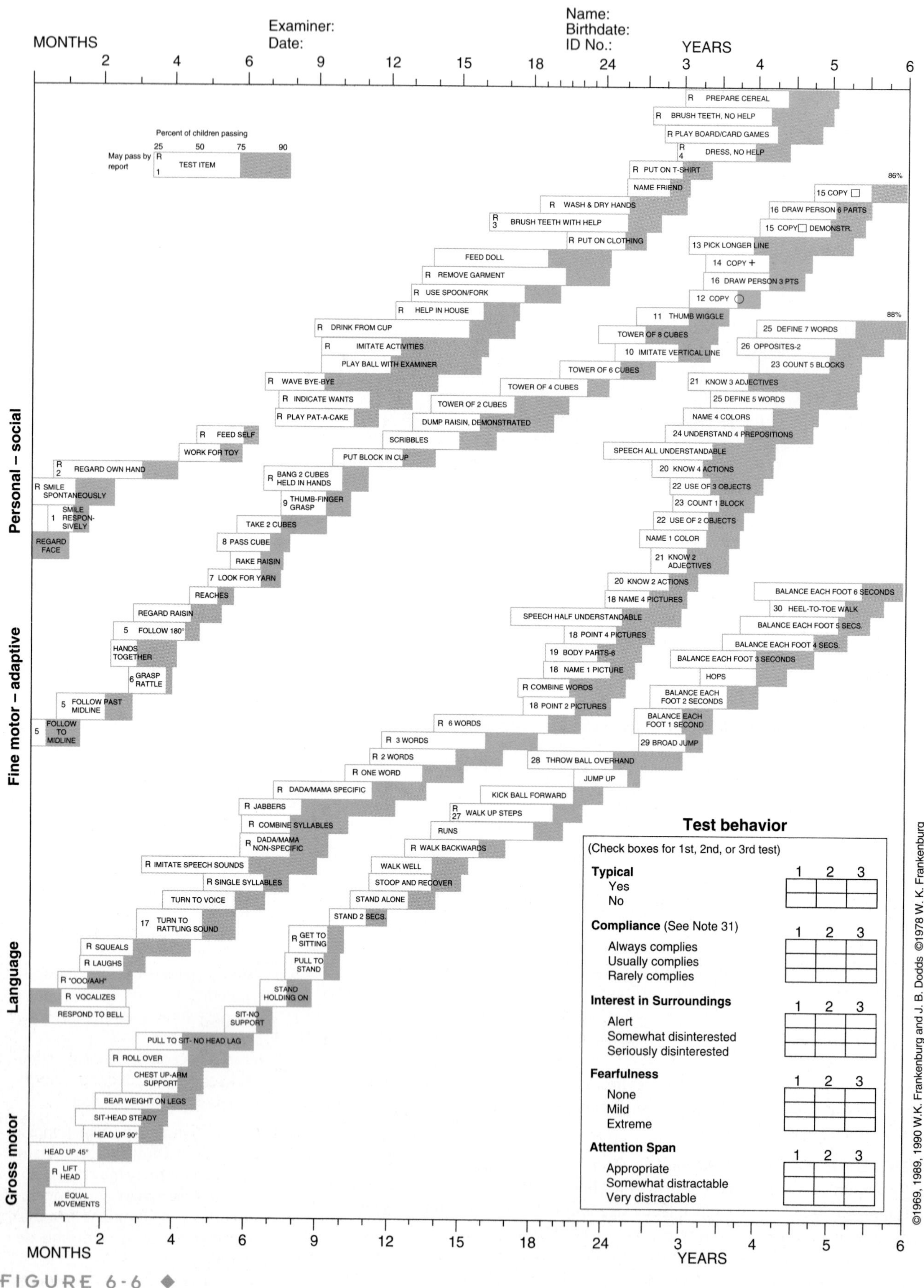

FIGURE 6-6 ◆

Denver II. *From W. K. Frankenburg, Denver, CO.*

DIRECTIONS FOR ADMINISTRATION

1. Try to get child to smile by smiling, talking or waving. Do not touch him/her.
2. Child must stare at hand several seconds.
3. Parent may help guide toothbrush and put toothpaste on brush.
4. Child does not have to be able to tie shoes or button/zip in the back.
5. Move yarn slowly in an arc from one side to the other, about 8" above child's face.
6. Pass if child grasps rattle when it is touched to the backs or tips of fingers.
7. Pass if child tries to see where yarn went. Yarn should be dropped quickly from sight from tester's hand without arm movement.
8. Child must transfer cube from hand to hand without help of body, mouth, or table.
9. Pass if child picks up raisin with any part of thumb and finger.
10. Line can vary only 30 degrees or less from tester's line.
11. Make a fist with thumb pointing upward and wiggle only the thumb. Pass if child imitates and does not move any fingers other than the thumb.

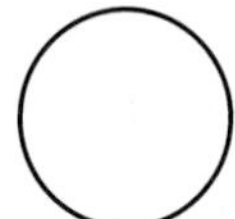

12. Pass any enclosed form. Fail continuous round motions.

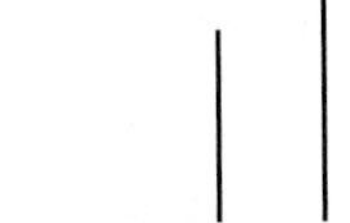

13. Which line is longer? (Not bigger.) Turn paper upside down and repeat. (pass 3 of 3 or 5 of 6).

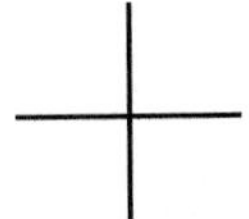

14. Pass any lines crossing near midpoint.

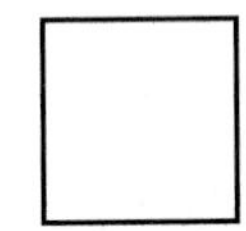

15. Have child copy first. If failed, demonstrate.

When giving items 12, 14, and 15, do not name the forms. Do not demonstrate 12 and 14.

16. When scoring, each pair (2 arms, 2 legs, etc.) counts as one part.
17. Place one cube in cup and shake gently near child's ear, but out of sight. Repeat for other ear.
18. Point to picture and have child name it. (No credit is given for sounds only.) If less than 4 pictures are named correctly, have child point to picture as each is named by tester.

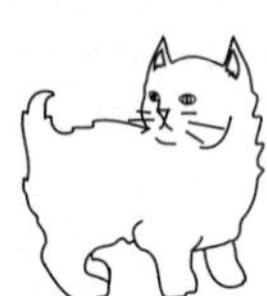
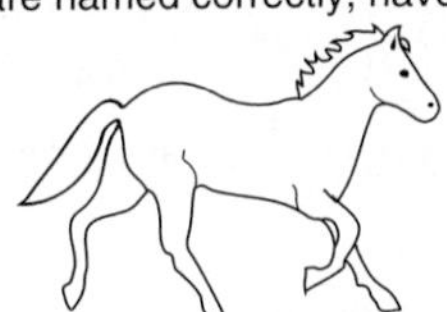
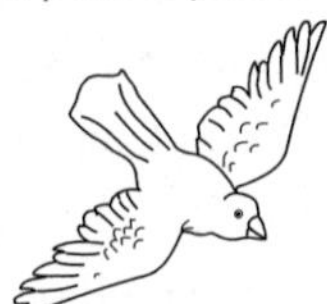
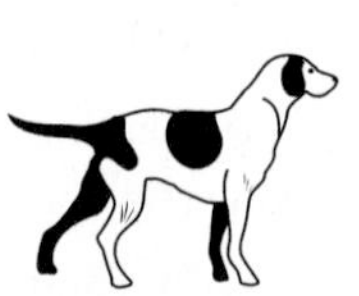
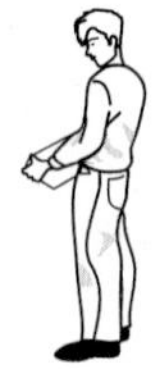

19. Using doll, tell child: Show me the nose, eyes, ears, mouth, hands, feet, tummy, hair. Pass 6 of 8.
20. Using pictures, ask child: Which one flies?... says meow?... talks?... barks?... gallops? Pass 2 of 5, 4 of 5.
21. Ask child: What do you do when you are cold?... tired?... hungry? Pass 2 of 3, 3 of 3.
22. Ask child: What do you do with a cup? What is a chair used for? What is a pencil used for? Action words must be included in answers.
23. Pass if child correctly places <u>and</u> says how many blocks are on paper. (1, 5).
24. Tell child: Put block **on** table; **under** table: **in front of** me, **behind** me. Pass 4 of 4. (Do not help child by pointing, moving head or eyes.)
25. Ask child: What is a ball?... lake?... desk?... house?... banana?... curtain?... fence?... ceiling? Pass if defined in terms of use, shape, what it is made of, or general category (such as banana is fruit, not just yellow). Pass 5 of 8, 7 of 8.
26. Ask child: If a horse is big, a mouse is_____? If fire is hot, ice is_____? If sun shines during the day, the moon shines during the ____? Pass 2 of 3.
27. Child may use wall or rail only, not person. May not crawl.
28. Child must throw ball overhand 3 feet to within arm's reach of tester.
29. Child must perform standing broad jump over width of test sheet (8 1/2 inches).
30. Tell child to walk forward, ⊂⊃⊂⊃⊂⊃⊂⊃ → heel within 1 inch of toe. Tester may demonstrate. Child must walk 4 consecutive steps.
31. In the second year, half of normal children are non-compliant.

OBSERVATIONS:

FIGURE 6-6 ◆ **(continued)**
Directions for admistration of Denver II. *From W. K. Frankenburg, Denver, CO.*

Because the time for each visit is limited, build upon the parents' current knowledge and care practices. Time can be used to focus on anticipatory guidance to introduce new information, to reinforce what the family is doing well, and to clear up any poorly understood concepts.

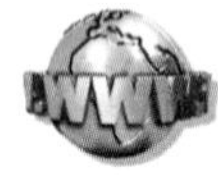

Injury and Violence Prevention

Take advantage of other sources of information in the community to enhance the guidance provided. For example, state and local SAFE KIDS Coalitions help inform families about injury-prevention strategies. School health programs such as the National Fire Prevention Association's "Risk Watch" may educate children about injury prevention, and other school programs may educate students about smoking and drug avoidance. Keep informed about the types of health education provided in different community settings so it is easier to reinforce the concepts already being taught. See Chapter 7 for more information on health promotion in the community.

ENCOURAGE HEALTH PROMOTION ACTIVITIES Often families need health education and counseling to promote healthy behaviors in their own child. Examples of focused health education and counseling may be information about environmental control to reduce lead exposure, dietary changes to increase iron-rich foods, and reduction of milk intake for weight control or loss strategies. Counseling in the case of the 18-month-old toddler for whom nursing diagnoses were previously stated could focus on child care arrangements and the anticipation and management of potential behavior problems.

Patient education and counseling are most effective when the family understands the relationship between the behavior change needed and the health outcome. The parents and child then work in partnership with the nurse or health care provider and make a commitment to the change or changes needed. Steps in promoting patient education and counseling include:

- Working with families to assess barriers to behavior change.
- Involving patients in selecting a risk factor to change and the outcome goal.
- Gaining commitment from the parents and child to change.
- Using a combination of strategies.
- Designing a behavior modification program.
- Monitoring progress through follow-up contact (Curry & Duby, 1994).

PERFORM HEALTH SUPERVISION INTERVENTIONS After all of the information from the interviews, physical assessment, and screening tests is collected and analyzed, specific health and developmental achievements should be summarized for the parents and child. Immunizations are provided as appropriate. (See Chapter 12 for the recommended immunization schedule.) Anticipatory guidance may be offered at various points during the health supervision visit.

When a child is found to be at risk for a health condition or an actual health problem is detected, follow-up care must be arranged. The child may need to return for another visit to the primary care provider for further evaluation, or referral to another provider may be needed. The nurse needs to learn about all of the available community resources to make appropriate referrals. The range of such services may include the following:

- Hospital and community-based health care specialists from many disciplines (dentists, physicians, physical therapists, speech therapists, nutritionists, social workers)
- Community-based programs (child care centers, developmental stimulation programs, home visitor programs, early intervention programs, mental health centers, diagnostic and evaluation centers, schools, family support centers, food and nutrition referral centers, public health clinics, churches, and other organizations that support families and children)

Expected outcomes of nursing care include the following:

- The child and family collaborate with the health care provider in joint problem solving and decision making regarding the management of the child's condition after appropriate education and counseling.
- The child and family prepare for future health supervision visits by identifying questions or concerns they want to discuss.

HEALTH SUPERVISION BY AGE GROUP

Infancy (Birth to 1 Year)

Health supervision visits occur frequently during the first year of life because growth and developmental changes are so rapid. Examples of developmental surveillance questions to use during infancy include the following:

- Do you have any specific concerns about Colin's development or behavior?
- How does Taneka communicate what she wants?
- How does Bruce move?
- What do you think Joshua understands?
- How does Tasha act around family members? Around other people?
- Tell me about Emily's typical play.

Anticipatory guidance should focus on the infant's stages of rapid growth and development, injury prevention, and nutrition (e.g., adequate amounts of formula or breast milk, when to start solid foods, and avoidance of honey) (see Chapters 2 and 3). Make sure the parents recognize their strengths in caring for the infant and other family members.

Health education focuses on issues such as colic, normal sleep patterns, sleep positions, dental hygiene, hand washing, bowel movements, skin and hair care, appropriate dress for weather, safe car transport, and prevention of sunburn. Teach parents how to recognize signs of early illness in their children, including fever, failure to eat, vomiting, diarrhea, dehydration, unusual irritability or sleepiness, and skin rash.

RECOMMENDED SCHEDULE FOR HEALTH SUPERVISION VISITS DURING INFANCY

Prenatal
Newborn
First week
1 month
2 months
4 months
6 months
9 months

Note: From Green & Palfrey (2000).

Early Childhood (1 to 5 Years)

Health supervision visits are needed frequently during early childhood for developmental surveillance, screening for health problems, and immunizations. Examples of developmental surveillance questions to ask during these visits include the following:

- Do you have any specific concerns about Jawan's development or behavior?
- How does Nicki communicate what she wants?
- What do you think Jerry understands?
- How does Penny get from one place to another?
- How does Kevin act around family members? Around other children?
- How does Lataye react to strangers?
- To what extent does Chris eat independently?
- Tell me about Jodie's typical play.

Anticipatory guidance should focus on promoting growth and development, nutrition, setting limits and discipline, toilet training, injury prevention, family activities, conflict with siblings, child care or play groups, and showing interest in the child's achievements (see Chapters 2 and 3).

Health education should focus on good nutrition; feeding and mealtime strategies; tooth brushing, fluoride supplements (as needed), and dental visits; the child's natural curiosity about genital differences and masturbation; safety approaching dogs; safe car transport; and management of common minor illnesses.

RECOMMENDED SCHEDULE FOR HEALTH SUPERVISION VISITS DURING EARLY CHILDHOOD

1 year
15 months
18 months
2 years
3 years
4 years

Note: From Green & Palfrey (2000).

Middle Childhood (5 to 10 Years)

Health supervision visits occur less frequently during middle childhood as the health of most children is stable, growth has slowed, and screening for health conditions is needed less frequently. Examples of developmental surveillance questions to ask of both the parent and child during visits with children in this age range include the following:

- Do you have any specific concerns about Shanelle's development or behavior?
- How do you think Ben is performing in school? How is his attendance? Do you have any concerns about his grades?

RECOMMENDED SCHEDULE FOR HEALTH SUPERVISION VISITS DURING MIDDLE CHILDHOOD

5 years
6 years
8 years
10 years

Note: From Green & Palfrey (2000).

- Does Shawn seem able to follow the rules at school?
- When Richie plays with other children, can he keep up with them?
- Is Marta proud of her achievements at school? Does she talk with you about what goes on at school? How do you acknowledge or praise these achievements? Is she in any special classes?
- Have you visited Jorge's classroom? Do you participate in activities at his school? What does the teacher say about him during your parent–teacher conference?

Anticipatory guidance should focus on issues such as growth and development, school entry and educational progress, the growing influence of peers, injury prevention, sports safety, setting reasonable expectations, recognition of achievements, setting limits and discipline, respecting authority, promoting independence, and beginning to have responsibility for chores.

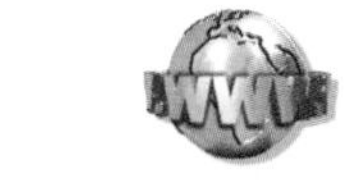

Health Education

Health education should focus on oral health, nutrition, need for regular physical activity, and teaching the child about personal care and hygiene, preparation for puberty and sexual development, dangers of smoking and smokeless tobacco, and managing anger and resolving conflict.

Adolescence (11 to 18 Years)

Health supervision visits should occur annually during adolescence because of the dramatic changes occurring in physical, social, and emotional development. Adolescents need comprehensive clinical preventive services to deter them from participating in behaviors that jeopardize their health; to detect physical, emotional, and behavioral problems early; and to encourage behaviors that will promote healthy lifestyles (Department of Adolescent Health, 1996). See Table 6-4 for recommended health supervision activities by age.

Developmental surveillance questions should focus on physical, social, and emotional development (Figure 6-7 ◆). The assessment of health behaviors and developmental surveillance become more closely related as the adolescent becomes more heavily influenced by peers.

Examples of questions to ask include the following:

- What do you do for fun? What is your favorite activity?
- Who is your best friend? What do you do together? About how many friends do you have? How old are your friends? What do you and your friends do outside of school?
- What are some of the things that worry you? Make you sad? Make you angry? What do you do about these things? Whom do you talk to about them? What do you do when

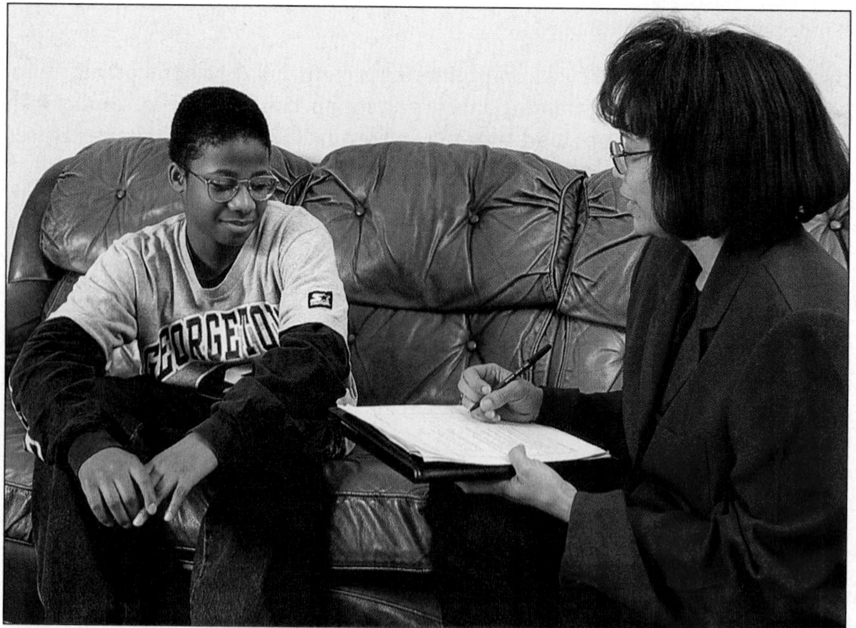

FIGURE 6-7 ◆
With adolescents, in contrast to earlier developmental stages, developmental surveillance questions should be directed to the child rather than the parent.

TABLE 6-4 Recommended Adolescent Preventive Health Services by Age and Procedure

<table>
<tr><th rowspan="3">Procedure</th><th colspan="11">AGE OF ADOLESCENT</th></tr>
<tr><th colspan="4">Early</th><th colspan="3">Middle</th><th colspan="4">Late</th></tr>
<tr><th>11</th><th>12</th><th>13</th><th>14</th><th>15</th><th>16</th><th>17</th><th>18</th><th>19</th><th>20</th><th>21</th></tr>
<tr><td>Health guidance</td><td colspan="11"></td></tr>
<tr><td>Parenting[a]</td><td colspan="4">■</td><td colspan="3">■</td><td colspan="4"></td></tr>
<tr><td>Development</td><td>■</td><td>■</td><td>■</td><td>■</td><td>■</td><td>■</td><td>■</td><td>■</td><td>■</td><td>■</td><td>■</td></tr>
<tr><td>Diet and physical activity</td><td>■</td><td>■</td><td>■</td><td>■</td><td>■</td><td>■</td><td>■</td><td>■</td><td>■</td><td>■</td><td>■</td></tr>
<tr><td>Healthy lifestyles[b]</td><td>■</td><td>■</td><td>■</td><td>■</td><td>■</td><td>■</td><td>■</td><td>■</td><td>■</td><td>■</td><td>■</td></tr>
<tr><td>Injury prevention</td><td>■</td><td>■</td><td>■</td><td>■</td><td>■</td><td>■</td><td>■</td><td>■</td><td>■</td><td>■</td><td>■</td></tr>
<tr><td>Screening history</td><td colspan="11"></td></tr>
<tr><td>Eating disorders</td><td>■</td><td>■</td><td>■</td><td>■</td><td>■</td><td>■</td><td>■</td><td>■</td><td>■</td><td>■</td><td>■</td></tr>
<tr><td>Sexual activity[c]</td><td>■</td><td>■</td><td>■</td><td>■</td><td>■</td><td>■</td><td>■</td><td>■</td><td>■</td><td>■</td><td>■</td></tr>
<tr><td>Alcohol and other drug use</td><td>■</td><td>■</td><td>■</td><td>■</td><td>■</td><td>■</td><td>■</td><td>■</td><td>■</td><td>■</td><td>■</td></tr>
<tr><td>Tobacco use</td><td>■</td><td>■</td><td>■</td><td>■</td><td>■</td><td>■</td><td>■</td><td>■</td><td>■</td><td>■</td><td>■</td></tr>
<tr><td>Abuse</td><td>■</td><td>■</td><td>■</td><td>■</td><td>■</td><td>■</td><td>■</td><td>■</td><td>■</td><td>■</td><td>■</td></tr>
<tr><td>School performance</td><td>■</td><td>■</td><td>■</td><td>■</td><td>■</td><td>■</td><td>■</td><td>■</td><td>■</td><td>■</td><td>■</td></tr>
<tr><td>Depression</td><td>■</td><td>■</td><td>■</td><td>■</td><td>■</td><td>■</td><td>■</td><td>■</td><td>■</td><td>■</td><td>■</td></tr>
<tr><td>Risk for suicide</td><td>■</td><td>■</td><td>■</td><td>■</td><td>■</td><td>■</td><td>■</td><td>■</td><td>■</td><td>■</td><td>■</td></tr>
<tr><td>Physical assessment</td><td colspan="11"></td></tr>
<tr><td>Blood pressure</td><td>■</td><td>■</td><td>■</td><td>■</td><td>■</td><td>■</td><td>■</td><td>■</td><td>■</td><td>■</td><td>■</td></tr>
<tr><td>Body Mass Index</td><td>■</td><td>■</td><td>■</td><td>■</td><td>■</td><td>■</td><td>■</td><td>■</td><td>■</td><td>■</td><td>■</td></tr>
<tr><td>Comprehensive examination</td><td colspan="4">■</td><td colspan="3">■</td><td colspan="4">■</td></tr>
<tr><td>Tests</td><td colspan="11"></td></tr>
<tr><td>Cholesterol</td><td colspan="4">1</td><td colspan="3">1</td><td colspan="4">1</td></tr>
<tr><td>TB</td><td colspan="4">2</td><td colspan="3">2</td><td colspan="4">2</td></tr>
<tr><td>GC, chlamydia, syphilis, and HPV</td><td colspan="4">3</td><td colspan="3">3</td><td colspan="4">3</td></tr>
<tr><td>HIV</td><td colspan="4">4</td><td colspan="3">4</td><td colspan="4">4</td></tr>
<tr><td>Pap smear</td><td colspan="4">5</td><td colspan="3">5</td><td colspan="4">5</td></tr>
<tr><td>Immunizations</td><td colspan="11"></td></tr>
<tr><td>MMR</td><td colspan="2">■</td><td></td><td></td><td colspan="3"></td><td colspan="4"></td></tr>
<tr><td>Td</td><td colspan="2">■</td><td></td><td></td><td colspan="3">O</td><td colspan="4"></td></tr>
<tr><td>Hepatitis B</td><td colspan="2">■</td><td></td><td></td><td colspan="3">6</td><td colspan="4">6</td></tr>
<tr><td>Hepatitis A</td><td colspan="4">7</td><td colspan="3">7</td><td colspan="4">7</td></tr>
<tr><td>Varicella</td><td colspan="4">8</td><td colspan="3">8</td><td colspan="4">8</td></tr>
</table>

[a]A parent health guidance visit is recommended during early and middle adolescence.
[b]Includes counseling regarding sexual behavior and avoidance of tobacco, alcohol, and other drug use.
[c]Includes history of unintended pregnancy and STD.
1. Screening test performed once if family history is positive for early cardiovascular disease or hyperlipidemia.
2. Screen if positive for exposure to active TB or lives/works in high-risk situation, e.g., homeless shelter, health care facility.
3. Screen at least annually if sexually active.
4. Screen if high risk for infection.
5. Screen annually if sexually active or if 18 years or older.
6. Vaccinate if high risk for hepatitis B infection.
7. Vaccinate if at risk for hepatitis A infection.
8. Vaccinate if no reliable history of chicken pox.

O Do not give if administered in last 5 years.

Note: *From Department of Adolescent Health. (1996).* Guidelines for adolescent preventive services (GAPS). Chicago, IL: American Medical Association.

you are really down or depressed? Do these feelings sometimes last more than a week? Have you ever been in trouble at school or with the law? Have you thought about running away? Have you ever thought about hurting yourself or killing yourself?

- What kind of changes have you noticed in your body over the past 6 months? Do you think you are developing pretty much like the rest of your friends? How do you feel about these changes? Has anyone talked with you about what to expect as your body develops?
- How do you feel about your weight? Are you trying to change your weight? Do you ever fast, vomit, or take laxatives or diet pills to control your weight?

- How are you doing in school?
- What type of responsibilities do you have at home?
- Did you drink alcohol in the last month? How much? What is the most you have ever had to drink? Have you ever tried other drugs? How often have you taken them in the past month? Do you ever drink and drive? Are you worried about any friends or family members and how much they drink and drive?
- Have you smoked any cigarettes in the last month? Chewed tobacco?
- Do your friends pressure you to do things you don't want to do? How do you handle that?
- Have you started dating? Do you date one person or go out as a group? Do you have a steady partner? Are you happy with dating or with this relationship?
- Have you ever been frightened by violent or sexual things someone has said to you? Has anyone ever tried to harm you physically? Has anyone ever touched you in a way you don't like? Forced you to have sex?
- How do you get along with members of your family? What would you like to change about your family if you could?
- Do you own a gun or have access to one?

Anticipatory guidance should focus on future healthy behaviors such as the following: school achievement, identification of talents and interests to pursue, stress-reduction techniques, use of protective sports gear, use of car safety belts, violence prevention, and use of sunscreen to prevent skin cancer (see Chapters 2, 7, and 23).

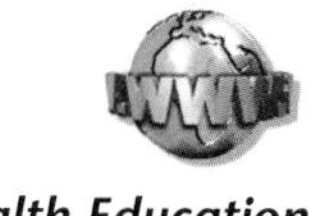
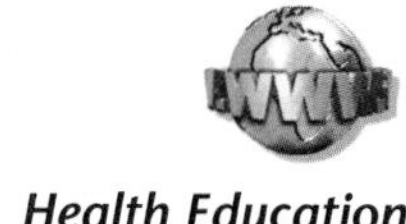

Health Education

Health education should focus on the avoidance of tobacco products, drugs and alcohol; sexuality, sexual activity options (abstinence, contraception, and safe sex); and good health behaviors including nutrition, oral health, exercise, and sleep. See Chapter 7 for more information on health education.

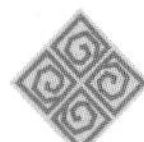

HEALTH PROMOTION FOR CHILDREN IN COMMUNITY SETTINGS

What nursing care does the child with a chronic illness need in different community health care settings? How can you ease the transition back to school for the child with a chronic condition? How do you identify families that need extra support to care for their child at home? Nursing care in all community health care settings (home, school, specialty clinic, primary care office) is focused on minimizing the impact of the health condition on the child's physical and emotional development and functioning.

EPISODIC CARE FOR ILLNESSES AND INJURIES

During childhood, most children have several episodes of illnesses and injuries that require health care. In most cases, care is provided by the primary health care provider. At other times, the urgency of the condition requires that the child go to an urgent care center or emergency department. The nurse's role in the cases of these episodic health care visits includes the following:

- Collecting health information about the condition
- Performing an assessment
- Assisting the primary care provider with any diagnostic or therapeutic procedures
- Educating the child and family about care of the child at home and how to identify any signs that the health problem is getting more serious

CARE OF THE CHILD WITH SPECIAL HEALTH CARE NEEDS

Children with a **chronic condition,** one that lasts or is expected to last 3 months or more, are also defined as children with special health care needs. Many of these children have a **disability,** an impairment in one or more of five categories of function (cognition, communication, motor abilities, social abilities, or patterns of interactions). Most children with chronic conditions are cared for in the home without home nursing or other health care services. Children with chronic health conditions need regular health supervision, as well as additional health services to help the child and family manage the condition.

Health promotion, disease prevention, and anticipatory guidance have greater significance for the child with special health care needs. This child already has a condition that places him or her at higher risk for other problems, such as infectious diseases, injury, or developmental delay. The goal is to permit the child, such as Jessica in the opening scenario, to have as normal a childhood as possible.

The provider of care for children with chronic conditions varies by the type of condition, type of health insurance coverage, preferences of the family, and availability of pediatric specialty resources. Most children with chronic conditions, such as asthma, have a primary care provider. The primary care provider is usually the most knowledgeable about local community resources that may help the child and family. The child is often referred to pediatric specialists, as needed, for a review of the management of the child's health condition, and to make new recommendations according to the child's health status.

A pediatric specialist and advanced practice nurses may collaborate with the primary care provider to coordinate care of the child with chronic conditions, such as spina bifida, cystic fibrosis, or diabetes mellitus. In this manner, the child benefits from the most current health care guidelines and expertise in care for the specific condition. The child and family usually retain a primary care provider, who provides health supervision care and episodic illness care while serving as the child's advocate in the larger health care system. Sometimes a pediatric specialist serves as the child's primary care provider, but it is important to make sure regular health supervision services are not forgotten during the care of acute exacerbations of the chronic condition. Some children with chronic conditions may even require additional health supervision visits for added immunizations, such as the meningococcal and influenza vaccines.

Nurses working in hospital specialty clinics and other community settings can help ensure that these children receive the appropriate health supervision services. The nurse in a tertiary care facility needs to identify appropriate resources and to help the family establish linkages with those existing in the child's community. This is a greater challenge if the child and family have traveled a distance to obtain the specialty services. It is often best to make sure the child has a primary care provider in the home community to provide regular care and to help with the coordination of local community resources.

The role of the nurse in caring for the chronically ill child in a community setting includes providing health supervision, teaching the parents to manage the child's care at home, providing guidelines to promote the child's growth and development, monitoring the child's health status, and referring the family to appropriate community services. Nurses providing care to children with specific chronic conditions need the following knowledge and skills (Jackson, 2000):

- Knowledge of the pathophysiology of the chronic condition and anticipated disease trajectory
- Knowledge of child and family reactions to the stress of the chronic condition
- The ability to work with family members in their efforts to manage the child's normal growth and development
- The ability to provide culturally sensitive care to the child and family experiencing a chronic health condition
- Assessment skills to identify any changes in the child's condition requiring referral or consultation
- The ability to communicate effectively with appropriate health professionals regarding any changes in the child's physical or psychosocial health
- The ability to work collaboratively with other health professionals
- Knowledge of resources (community agencies, tertiary care centers, specialty professionals) appropriate for the child and family with a chronic condition
- The ability to identify a dysfunctional family needing intervention

GROWTH & DEVELOPMENT

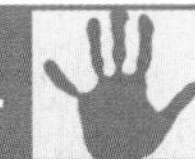

"Children with special health care needs are those who have or are at risk for a chronic physical, developmental, behavioral, or emotional condition and who also require health and related services of a type or amount beyond that required by children generally" (McPherson et al., 1998). Of the 12.6 million U.S. children less than 18 years, 18% match the definition for children with special health care needs (Newacheck, McManus, Fox, et al., 2000).

RESEARCH

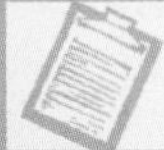

The overall incidence of children with chronic conditions has not changed much in the last 20 years. The number of years of survival of these children has changed with technology, surgical techniques, and other health care advances (Jackson, 2000).

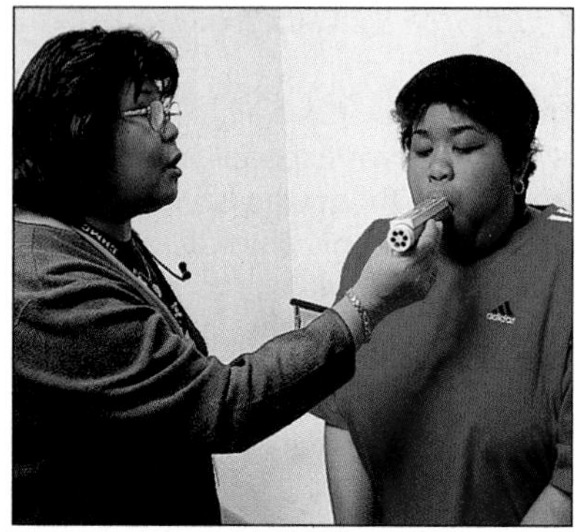

FIGURE 6-8 ◆
Nurses provide patient education to help families learn to recognize the early stages of an asthma attack by using a peak flow meter. The child learns the proper method for taking a deep breath and blowing into the peak flow meter so the best reading is obtained.

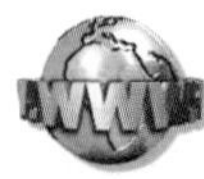

School Health

NURSING PRACTICE

Healthy People 2010 includes a specific national objective for the health education of children in school settings to prevent health problems such as unintentional injury, violence, suicide, tobacco use and addiction, alcohol and other drug use, unintended pregnancy, HIV/AIDS and STD infections, unhealthy dietary patterns, inadequate physical activity, and environmental health.

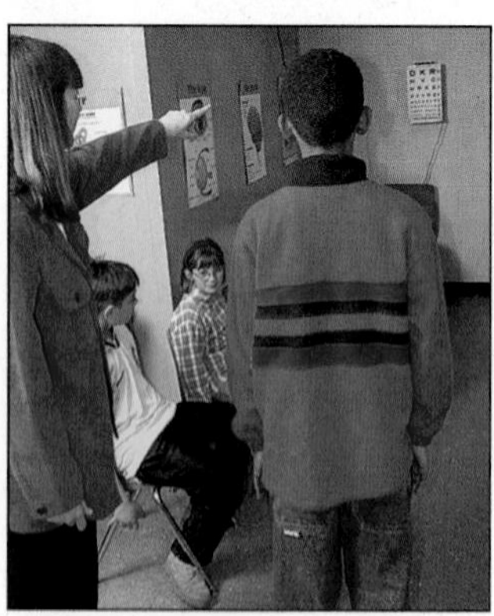

FIGURE 6-9 ◆
The school is often the setting for screening tests of large groups of students at risk for a problem. Screening tests are often organized so all children in a particular grade are assessed, as in this test to detect vision problems.

In Jessica's case, a nurse with some of the above knowledge and skills could collaborate with the primary care provider to help Jessica improve her asthma control. The recommended care of children with asthma has changed from episodic care for acute asthma attacks with minimal daily management to guidelines for aggressive daily management by the child and family (Figure 6-8 ◆). Recognition of early warning signs of an asthma attack can lead to the initiation of extra medications in an effort to avert a severe attack. (See Chapter 13 for a discussion of asthma management.) The accompanying Nursing Care Plan outlines community-based strategies that can be used when working with a child such as Jessica and her family to improve asthma management.

NURSING IN A SCHOOL SETTING

School nurses work to remove or minimize the health barriers to learning so students can perform academically. Nursing actions for all children focus on the following strategies:

- Reducing infectious disease transmission so school attendance is improved
- Promoting healthy behaviors through health education for many different and diverse audiences
- Providing safe school facilities by inspecting the school environment for hazards
- Assessing health status and screening children for health conditions that are common among school-age children (such as vision and hearing impairments, and scoliosis) (Figure 6-9 ◆)
- Referring and managing acute and chronic health conditions
- Participating as the health specialist on the team developing a child's individualized education plan (IEP) and individualized school health plan (ISHP)
- Building effective support systems between student, family, school, and community

Table 6-5 presents standards of school nursing care.

Emergency preparedness is important and a plan of managing the emergency care of all students should be developed. Injuries and acute illnesses occur frequently during school hours. School personnel (administrators, secretaries, and health aides in the absence of the school nurse) need to be trained to distinguish between an emergency and an

TABLE 6-5 Standards of Professional School Nursing Practice

1. The school nurse collects client data.
2. The school nurse analyzes the assessment data in determining nursing diagnoses.
3. The school nurse identifies expected outcomes individualized to the client.
4. The school nurse develops a plan of care/action that specifies interventions to attain expected outcomes.
5. The school nurse implements the interventions identified in the plan of care/action.
6. The school nurse evaluates the client's progress toward attainment of outcomes.
7. The school nurse systematically evaluates the quality and effectiveness of school nursing practice.
8. The school nurse evaluates one's own nursing practice in relation to professional practice standards and relevant statutes, regulations, and policies.
9. The school nurse acquires and maintains current knowledge and competency in school nursing practice.
10. The school nurse interacts with and contributes to the professional development of peers and school personnel as colleagues.
11. The school nurse's decisions and actions on behalf of clients are determined in an ethical manner.
12. The school nurse collaborates with the student, family, school staff, community, and other providers in providing student care.
13. The school nurse promotes use of research findings in school nursing practice.
14. The school nurse considers factors related to safety, effectiveness, and cost when planning and delivering care.
15. The school nurse uses effective written, verbal, and nonverbal communication skills.
16. The school nurse manages school health services.
17. The school nurse assists students, families, school staff, and community to achieve optimal levels of wellness through appropriately designed and delivered health education.

Note: From the National Association of School Nurses. (1999). *Standard of Professional School Nursing Practice*. Scarborough, ME: Author.

NURSING CARE PLAN The Child with Asthma in the Community Setting

GOAL	INTERVENTION	RATIONALE	EXPECTED OUTCOME
1. Family Coping: Potential for growth related to increased control of asthma with daily therapeutic care			
	NIC Priority Intervention: **Family Support:** Promotion of family interests and goals.		NOC Suggested Outcome: None developed for this nursing diagnosis.
The child and parents will work in partnership with the nurse to improve the child's asthma management.	■ Listen to the family's concerns about asthma management and respond with information to correct any misconceptions. ■ Teach the family skills (assessment, use of equipment, and giving medications) for managing the child's asthma attacks. ■ Provide telephone consultation to the parents during management of the first few asthma attacks. ■ Educate the parents about when to call for future medical advice or to seek emergency treatment.	■ The parents' concerns may not be the same as the nurse's. If the parents' concerns are not addressed, the parents may not comply with recommended care. ■ Proper use of equipment and appropriate medication dosage will help alleviate asthma symptoms. ■ Support and reinforcement of learning during an asthma attack will increase the parents' confidence in managing future attacks. ■ Parents need guidelines for judging the severity of asthma attacks.	The parents express greater confidence in averting and managing their child's asthma attacks.
2. Management of Therapeutic Regimen, Family Ineffective related to knowledge deficit			
	NIC Priority Intervention: **Family Involvement:** Facilitating family participation in the emotional and physical care of the patient.		NOC Suggested Outcome: None developed for this nursing diagnosis.
The child and parents will recognize early signs of an asthma attack and begin taking medications.	■ Teach the child and parents to use a peak flow meter. ■ Help the child recognize his or her personal best peak flow and range indicating development of asthma symptoms. ■ Teach the family and child to give medications when the peak flow falls to the yellow range. ■ Teach the child and family to monitor the child's response to medications with peak flow meter.	■ The peak flow meter helps quantify changes in respiratory status before symptoms are detected. ■ Identifying a personal best peak flow helps establish the ranges to be used for future symptom identification. ■ Giving medications before an asthma attack becomes established may help avert the actual attack. ■ Monitoring the response gives the family information to determine when home care is inadequate and medical intervention is needed.	The number of asthma attacks requiring medical intervention is reduced.
3. Health Maintenance Altered, related to lack of school asthma management plan			
	NIC Priority Intervention: **Health System Guidance:** Facilitating a patient's location and use of appropriate health services.		NOC Suggested Outcome: **Health Promoting Behavior:** Actions to sustain or promote optimal wellness, recovery, and rehabilitation.
An individual school health plan (ISHP) will be developed to help control and manage the child's asthma symptoms.	■ Provide the family with educational materials to give to the school nurse and school administrators. ■ Advocate for all children to have an asthma management plan developed.	■ School personnel need the latest information about effective asthma management in school settings. ■ Establishing a school policy will help all children with asthma receive appropriate care.	Implementation of the school health plan reduces the number of school absences for asthma attacks that occur during school hours and increases participation in school activities.

(continued)

NURSING CARE PLAN — The Child with Asthma in the Community Setting (continued)

GOAL	INTERVENTION	RATIONALE	EXPECTED OUTCOME
3. Health Maintenance Altered, related to lack of school asthma management plan (continued)			
	■ Support the family to have a school health plan that includes the physician's written orders customized for the child. ■ Include in the ISHP participation in regular school/class activities such as field trips and physical education, and what to do if asthma symptoms occur at school. ■ Help the family to obtain extra equipment and medications that can be provided to the school. ■ Work with the parents and school nurse to teach the specific asthma interventions to a designated person in the school nurse's absence.	■ The child with severe asthma needs a personalized care plan to be most successful in controlling asthma attacks. ■ Participation, even with modification or premedication, prior to activities promotes self-esteem and peer relationships. ■ Schools will provide care, but the families must provide all supplies, equipment, and medications. ■ School nurses often travel between several schools. The school administrator or secretary often serves as the backup care provider.	
4. Self-Esteem Disturbance (child), related to need to seek special care during school hours			
	NIC Priority Intervention: **Self-Esteem Enhancement:** Assisting a patient to increase his or her personal judgment of self-worth.		NOC Suggested Outcome: **Child Development, Middle Childhood:** Milestones of physical, cognitive, and psychosocial progression by 8 years of age.
The child's improved control over asthma will increase his or her self-esteem and peer relationships.	■ Assess the child's peer relationships and opportunities for age-appropriate interactions. ■ Motivate the child and family to gain increased control of asthma so the child can participate in normal childhood activities. ■ Identify types of conflict and teasing the child experiences with peers, and teach the child defense tactics to deal with them.	■ Assessment is important to identify the best strategies to support the child and family. ■ Motivation may increase compliance with recommended daily asthma control interventions. ■ If the child is able to gain some control over these situations, his or her self-esteem will be improved.	The child establishes friendships and engages in activities with peers.

urgent problem that parents should be called to manage. Guidelines for activation of the community's emergency medical services (EMS) should be developed in collaboration with the local EMS agency.

Children with chronic conditions may have special challenges when attending school. An individual school health plan (ISHP), developed collaboratively by the parent, child, school nurse, school administrator, and teachers, is a formal mechanism to ensure that the child's health needs are managed in the school setting (Figure 6-10 ◆). The nursing process is the format used for development of the ISHP. In some cases the health plan is integrated into the child's individualized education plan or individual family service plan. The information in this plan is treated confidentially, but stored in an easily accessible area for personnel who may have to provide care. The parent provides medications, supplies, and equipment along with the physician's written instructions for care. In some cases, school personnel must be trained to care for the child who needs medications or has special equipment, including special precautions when providing care. The school nurse often provides the training to school personnel who will be responsible for providing care.

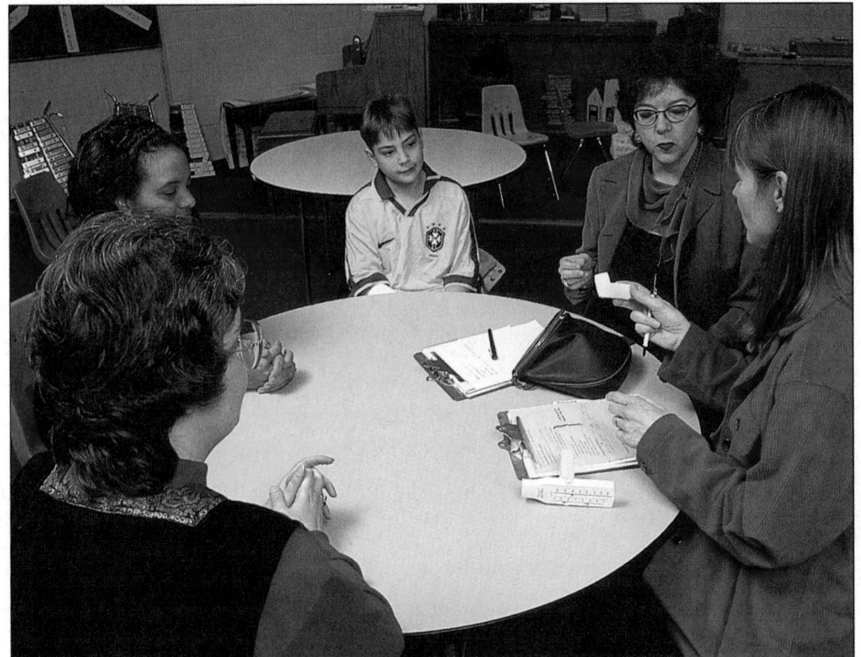

FIGURE 6-10 ◆
Because some children need medications or other therapies during school hours, the parents and child, school nurse, teacher, and school administrators develop a plan to manage the child's condition during school hours. This document is the child's Individual School Health Plan.

When a child returns to school following the diagnosis of a chronic condition or a significant change in condition, the child's nurse (in either the hospital or community setting) can help with the transition of the child back to the classroom. Contact the school administrators and school nurse. Work with the family to begin preparing teachers and school administrators for the child's special needs. Send educational materials about the child's condition to the school. Often an ISHP must be developed or modified. In Jessica's case, the school nurse should educate her teacher to recognize the signs of an asthma attack and the importance of having Jessica get her medication before the symptoms worsen. Work with the child's family and teachers to prepare classmates for the visible changes they will see in the child. Help them understand more about the child's condition.

CLINICAL TIP

Make sure the individual school health plan (ISHP) includes directions for care of the child on the bus, on field trips, and during extracurricular activities.

NURSE'S ROLE IN OTHER COMMUNITY SETTINGS

In several other settings in the community, the nurse's role may parallel that in a school setting. Promoting health and preventing disease and injury are equally important in child care centers, camps, health department clinics, and disaster or homeless shelters. For example, nurses work with child care center administrators to address infection control issues and to assess the safety of the children's environment. Nurses in camps assess the safety of the children's environment, but also provide nursing care to children with acute illnesses and injuries and plan activities to promote health. Some special camps for children with chronic conditions must have trained personnel to provide needed medical and nursing care while children are participating in recreational activities. Children in health department clinics and shelters need health supervision services as well as linkage with other community resources to promote health.

FAMILY ASSESSMENT

The strength, resilience, coping skills, and resources of a child's family plays a major role in fostering the child's growth and development, as well as managing the child's health problems. When providing care to children in all settings, taking time to assess the family will help you to plan and provide nursing care that corresponds to the family's values, resources, and abilities. Information about the family's structure, home and community environments, occupation and education, and cultural characteristics should be collected. Information about the way the family functions in nurturing its members, problem solving, and communicating may help identify strategies that are potentially more effective for management of the child's health care. Tables 4–4 and 4–7 provide suggestions for information that should be collected for the family assessment.

The presence of a chronic illness or disability adds a dimension of developmental risk for an infant, child, or youth. The child and family members can respond with either psychologic or behavioral problems. Families need support to increase their resources and coping behaviors so they can successfully manage the multiple stressors, strains, and hassles of daily living along with the child's chronic condition.

Resilient families are able to bounce back from the stresses and challenges while adapting to successfully manage the child's chronic illness or disability. These families have effective coping behaviors and the ability to acquire and maintain needed resources for managing the demands of the child's condition. Following are characteristics of a resilient family (Patterson, 1991):

- Balancing the child's illness with other family needs
- Forming collaborative relationships with health care professionals
- Maintaining a professional relationship rather than a friendship relationship with providers
- Developing competence in communication skills
- Maintaining family flexibility and adapting to changing circumstances
- Maintaining a commitment to the family as a unit
- Attributing positive meaning to the situation
- Maintaining supportive relationships outside the family
- Engaging in active coping efforts with effective and efficient problem-solving abilities

NURSING MANAGEMENT

Most families do not naturally develop resilience. Often nursing support is needed to help family members learn new skills, make adaptations, and gain confidence in their abilities to manage the challenges they face. Nurses can help families identify their strengths and areas for improvement that will lead to increased resiliency.

Nursing Assessment and Diagnosis

FAMILY ASSESSMENT TOOLS Several family assessment tools have been developed that help measure family coping and functioning. Identification of family strengths and deficits gives nurses information that can be used to support family development—to reinforce family functioning, for family education, for intervention directed to meet special needs, and for referrals to community resources for long-term follow-up.

The Family APGAR is a good initial screening tool that focuses on the family's adaptation, partnership, growth, affection, and resolve (Table 6-6). The five-item questionnaire can be administered quickly. All family members are asked to complete the questionnaire, so the nurse gains a picture of the family's perspective on family functioning. Be more concerned if the majority of responses fall in the "hardly ever" category or responses vary greatly among family members. This variation may indicate a family that needs much more support to cope with the demands of daily life and management of the child's condition. Discuss the findings with the family members.

The Family Profile (Table 6-7) is another family assessment tool that will be of help when parents are caring for a child with special health care needs in the home. The parents complete this survey of their resources and current use of community services. This assessment may set the stage for the family to become a fully collaborative partner in caring for the child with a serious chronic condition.

HOME ASSESSMENT TOOLS Assess the home environment to determine factors that promote the child's growth and development. Both assessments will help the nurse plan care that will promote safety for the child and strategies to promote the child's development.

TABLE 6-6 The Family APGAR Questionnaire

PART I

The following questions have been designed to help us better understand you and your family. You should feel free to ask questions about any item in the questionnaire.

The space for comments should be used when you wish to give additional information or if you wish to discuss the way the question is applied to your family. Please try to answer all questions.

Family is defined as the individual(s) with whom you usually live. If you live alone, your "family" consists of persons with whom you now have the strongest emotional ties.[a]

	For each question, check only one box		
	Almost Always	**Some of the time**	**Hardly ever**
I am satisfied that I can turn to my family for help when something is troubling me. Comments:	☐	☐	☐
I am satisfied with the way my family talks over things with me and shares problems with me. Comments:	☐	☐	☐
I am satisfied that my family accepts and supports my wishes to take on new activities or directions. Comments:	☐	☐	☐
I am satisfied with the way my family expresses affection and responds to my emotions, such as anger, sorrow, and love. Comments:	☐	☐	☐
I am satisfied with the way my family and I share time together. Comments:	☐	☐	☐

[a]According to which member of the family is being interviewed, the interviewer may substitute for the word *family* either *spouse, significant other, parents,* or *children.*

Note: From Smilkstein, G. (1978). The family APGAR: A proposal for a family function test and its use by physicians. *Journal of Family Practice, 6(6),* 1231–1239.

The Home Observation for Measurement of the Environment (HOME) is an assessment tool developed to measure the quality and quantity of stimulation and support available to the child in the home environment (Caldwell & Bradley, 1984) (Figure 6-11 ◆). Four age-specific scales are available (birth to 3 years, 3 to 6 years, 6 to 10 years, and 10 to 15 years). Examples of subscales within each age-specific scale include parental responsivity, acceptance of child, the physical environment, learning materials, variety in experience, and parental involvement. Data are collected during an informal, low-stress interview and observation over approximately 1 hour. The child must be awake during the majority of the interview. Observation of the parent–child interaction is an essential part of the assessment. The intent is to allow family members to act normally.

Several nursing diagnoses may result from the family and home assessment, for example:

- *Risk for caregiver role strain* related to child with a newly diagnosed chronic condition and its financial burden
- *Impaired social interaction (parents and child)* related to lack of family or respite support for community interaction
- *Risk for altered parent/child attachment* related to child's dependence on technology

TABLE 6-7 Questions from the Family Profile

FAMILY STRUCTURE/ROLES

Do you want to care for your child at home?
Are you aware of any alternatives to home care?
Who are your child's primary caregivers?
Who are the other members of your household?
Can you identify another person to act as backup caregiver for your child?
Are there others (friends/family members) who can assist you with your child with special needs, with your other children, or with your family obligations?

MEDICAL MANAGEMENT

Have you completed the hospital training in your child's care? If no, what is left to learn?
Has your child's backup caregiver completed training? If no, what is left to learn?
Do you or your backup caregiver need refresher training for anything?
Do you have transportation to medical appointments?
Do you need help in selecting a nursing provider?
Do you need help in selecting a vendor?

NUTRITION

How is your child fed? If formula, will you need help to buy/locate the formula?
Have you applied for WIC?
Does your child have a special need for diapers that is greater than the norm?

EDUCATION

Will your child be going out to school?
Do you know which school your child will attend?
Has your child been referred for the infant and toddler program?
Do you have an IEP for your child?
Do you have a contact person in the school program?
Will your child need adaptive equipment at home?

PARENTING/CHILD CARE

What hours/shifts do you think you will need nursing for your child?
In the event you need to leave home quickly or if you become incapacitated, who will watch your child with special needs? Your other children?
What is your plan for child care in the event of the nurse's absence?
Will you need help in finding child care for your other children?
Do you work outside the home? Any plans for the future?
Do you go to school? Any plans for the future?

FINANCIAL RESOURCES

Does your child have medical insurance? Are your other children covered under a family insurance plan?
Do you need more information about or referrals to WIC, SSI, TANF, food stamps, housing, respite care?
Do you need help in obtaining everyday supplies for your child?
Do you need a referral for help in obtaining other items for your child, such as furniture, clothing, toys?
Do you need help with budgeting?

COMMUNITY RESOURCES

Are you involved with any other helping agencies or persons, especially those you would like to include in this planning process?
Do you or other family members belong to a church? Social groups? Clubs? Associations?
Would you like to talk with another parent who has a child with special needs?
Would you like a referral to a support group?
Do you want a referral for counseling? Individual? Marital? Family? Child? Sibling?

FAMILY LIFE

Do you see your child's homecoming as making a significant change in your lifestyle, and if so, how?
Do you have concerns about your other children?
Can you describe how you see your child in a few months? What are your short-term goals for your child?
Can you describe how you see your child in a few years? What are your long-term goals for your child?
How would you describe your family strengths?
What are your family's needs at this time?

Note: From McCord, B. (1993). *Family profile.* Millersville, MD: Coordinating Center for Home and Community Care.

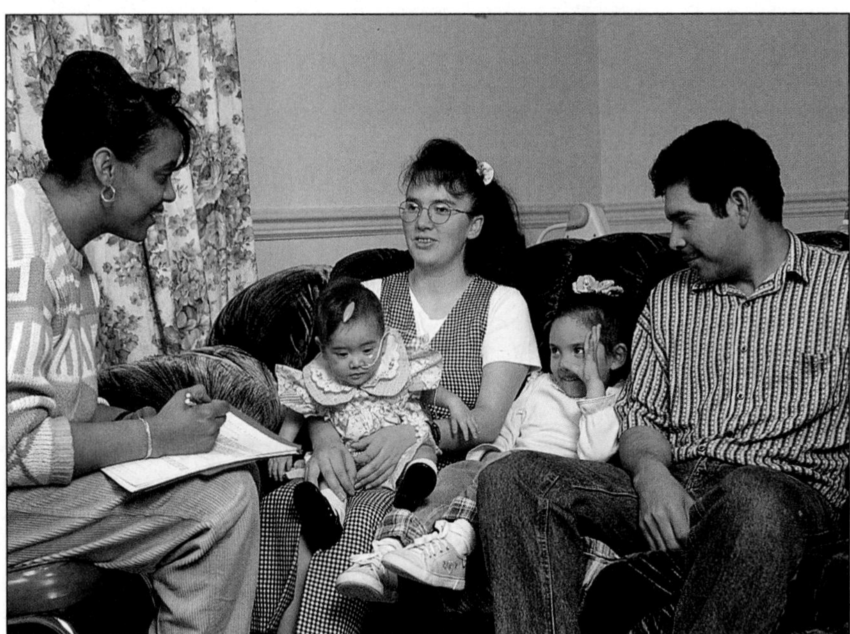

FIGURE 6-11 ◆
A visit to the home when all family members are present provides the best information for completion of an assessment tool such as the Home Observation for Measurement of the Environment (HOME).

Planning and Implementation

Work to establish a therapeutic relationship with the family, characterized by empathy and trust, as well as the development of mutually identified goals for the child's care. To help families develop resiliency, focus on family competence and strengths. Acknowledge and validate their emotions. Provide information in a clear, timely, and sensitive manner. Ask questions that help direct the family's thinking rather than providing them with all of the answers. Work with families to create solutions until they are able to solve problems independently (Patterson, 1995). Linkage with other families who have faced similar situations may be helpful.

Refer families with moderate or severe dysfunctioning to community resources for social support and counseling as appropriate. Make sure the family has a coordinator of care, especially when a family member seems to be unable to assume the case management role initially. When families seem unable to use referrals and recommendations for identifying and obtaining community assistance, the nurse can help in some additional ways (Taylor & Edwards, 1995):

- Call and act as the family's advocate.
- Help with role rehearsal.
- Provide instructions and support.
- Connect the family with a volunteer who can accompany the family to services.
- Perform or refer the family for case management services.

Expected outcomes of nursing care include the following:

- The family assumes the role of case manager, or works effectively with an assigned case manager, with effective interventions by nurses and the health care team.
- The care needed by the child with a chronic condition is provided by the family according to recommended guidelines.

 HOME HEALTH CARE NURSING

Home health care is a component of the continuum of comprehensive health care provided to individuals and families in the home. Many of the children needing home health care are **medically fragile,** and thus require skilled nursing care with or without medical equipment to support vital functions. Only 2% to 5% of these children have chronic conditions serious enough to need regular home health care services (Ahmann, 1996). Home health care services may also be provided for short intervals to help families during the child's acute recovery, such as a child with a osteomyelitis receiving home antibiotic infusion therapy. Following are two major goals of working with families in the home care setting:

- Promoting or restoring health while attempting to minimize the effects of the disability and illness, including terminal illness
- Promoting child or family self-care capacity in the home

CLASSIFICATIONS OF MEDICALLY FRAGILE CHILDREN

- Children with prolonged dependence on a medical device that is required to sustain life (mechanical ventilators, intravenous nutrition or drugs, tracheostomy, suctioning, oxygen, or tube feedings)
- Children with prolonged dependence on other medical devices that compensate for vital body functions who require daily or near daily nursing care (apnea monitors, renal dialysis, urinary catheters, and colostomies)

Note: From Office of Technology Assessment (1987).

Home care nursing is focused on assisting a family to gain a greater ability to manage the care of a child with a chronic condition more independently. The home is also seen as a much better environment to promote the child's growth and development.

Parents and other care providers without backgrounds in health care are given tremendous responsibilities to provide technology-assisted health care to their child. Technology assistance includes any of the following: ventilators; tracheostomies; suctioning; nasogastric, gastrostomy, or parenteral feeding with feeding pumps; intravenous fluids and medications with intravenous pumps. In some cases, families have created mini intensive care units in their home. Examples of some serious chronic conditions cared for by families in the home include children with congenital heart defects before corrective surgery, bronchopulmonary dysplasia, and cancer in its terminal stage.

Health care systems (health care providers and insurers) are challenged to simultaneously address the child's illness and developmental needs while providing the support needed by these families so that children do well in their environments. The family also needs help to support the growing child in the school and other peer settings.

To work in the home care setting, nurses need a variety of skills:

- Knowledge and experience in acute care practice with various medical technologies to work with these children (These skills enable nurses to provide direct care, teach the family and child self-care practices, and monitor the child's progress. This may involve collaboration with other health care team members.)
- Community assessment skills; an understanding of community resources, financing mechanisms, and multiagency collaboration; and good communication skills (Taylor & Edwards, 1995)
- An understanding of these resources to better assist families to find the most supportive services to match the child's and family's needs
- Skill in educating family members to assume care of the child

SAFETY PRECAUTIONS

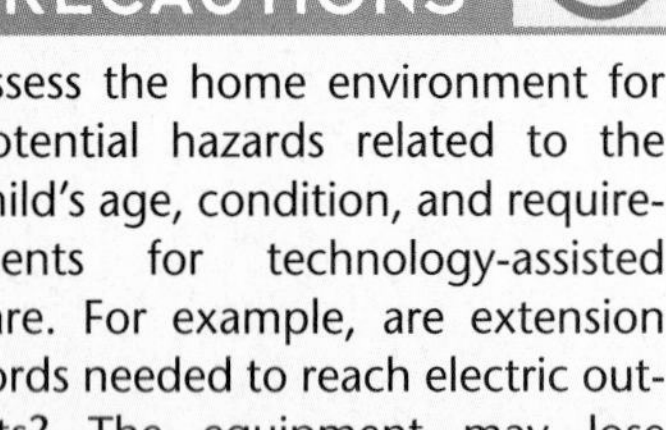

Assess the home environment for potential hazards related to the child's age, condition, and requirements for technology-assisted care. For example, are extension cords needed to reach electric outlets? The equipment may lose power if someone trips over the cord and disconnects it by mistake.

NURSING MANAGEMENT

Nursing Assessment and Diagnosis

Assessment in the home is focused on the child being cared for, the family's strengths and coping, and utilization of community resources.

TRANSITION FROM THE HOSPITAL For most children, home health care is initiated after an acute hospitalization. The hospital or home care nurse can be responsible for coordinating and linking the transition steps. Clinical care guidelines or case management are methods for promoting a smooth transition. Expected outcomes for the child are documented. The home care nurse works in collaboration with hospital nurses by assessing the following:

- Caregiver readiness
- Home readiness (safe sleeping arrangements, adequate supplies, ability to meet nutritional and fluid needs, telephone access, heat, electricity, refrigeration, and lack of any communicable diseases in the home)

SAFETY PRECAUTIONS

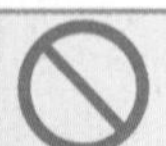

Consider any features of the child's home environment that could cause an acute illness. For example, use of a woodstove or fireplace for heating could cause respiratory distress; renovation of a house built before 1960 could expose the child to lead dust.

Nursing diagnoses that could apply as the child transitions from the hospital to home setting include the following:

- *Ineffective management of therapeutic regimen: family* related to complexity of therapeutic regiment and excessive demands made on the family
- *Knowledge deficit* related to information misinterpretation

Planning and Implementation

Nurses help families in the home setting in the following ways (Ahmann, 1996):

- Assuring competent care to the child
- Providing information about the child's condition and community resources
- Assisting families in time management skills and patient care management
- Advocating for increased insurance coverage or locating other sources of financial assistance
- Identifying appropriate programs in the community such as respite care, therapeutic recreation, or educational opportunities

Recognize that control belongs to the family in the home care setting. The parents are the employer with the ability to hire and fire. Every interaction is negotiated with the family, or between the family and child if there are differences in what they want. The nurse must be flexible and able to set aside power. House rules for such things as parking, private areas in the home, routines, and discipline of the child must all be followed. Role expectations of the nurse must be clearly understood to reduce stress in the family. The success of home care is also based upon effective cultural communication.

The range of nursing care activities that may be included in a child's care plan in the home setting include sensory stimulation, routines of daily living, positioning and skin care with gentle handling, respiratory care, nutrition and elimination, medications, and other supportive therapies. A plan for safe evacuation of the home is needed in case of fire. An emergency care plan should be developed for the child that includes an emergency medical history readily available to emergency care providers. The emergency health care provider needs enough information to understand the basics of the child's problem, to prevent delays in disease-specific treatment, and to minimize unnecessary interventions until the child's personal physician can be consulted. The family also needs to notify the emergency medical services agency and the power company about the presence of a technology-assisted child in the home. Backup generators may be needed if electrical power for life-sustaining equipment is essential. Meeting the child and family before an emergency will help emergency medical technicians to be better prepared to care for the child with special health care needs.

Expected outcomes of nursing care include the following:

- Care of the child's medical needs are integrated into the family's routines when possible.
- The family has an emergency care plan for the child in the event of a disaster or weather emergency, or the child's condition suddenly worsens.

CULTURE 

When providing care in the home, recognize potential conflicts between "mainstream" medical care and the family's cultural preferences after carefully listening to the parents' perspectives. Learn and use the family's perspectives of health and disease in discussions and in development of the plan of care (Ahmann, 1996).

LAW & ETHICS 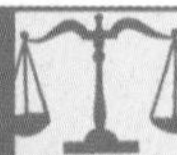

Home care assumes the presence of the child's primary caregiver. Invasive treatments and decisions for provision of emergency care to avoid serious risk to life and limb require informed consent. When the caregiver is not present and the home care nurse provides such care, the home health care agency and the nurse are at significant liability risk (Hogue, 1993).

EMERGENCY MEDICAL DATA

Special medical emergencies can develop quickly in a child with severe and complex medical problems. An Emergency Information Form should provide a summary of the child's medical history, baseline physical findings, and important and unique management requirements (American Academy of Pediatics, Committee on Pediatric Emergency Medicine, 1999).

Chapter Highlights

- Care in the community involves health supervision, care for episodic illnesses or injuries, and assisting families to manage their child's chronic health condition.
- Working with the child and family in the community setting requires an understanding of how the larger environment influences the child's health and development and integration of that knowledge into the nursing care plan.
- Health supervision is the provision of services that focus on disease and injury prevention, growth and developmental surveillance, and health promotion at key intervals during the child's life.
- Anticipatory guidance provides the family with information about what to expect during the child's current and future stage of development on topics such as healthy habits; prevention of illness, injury, and poisoning; nutrition; oral health; and sexuality.
- During episodic care for illnesses and injuries, the nurse collects health information, assesses the child, assists the primary care provider with diagnostic or therapeutic procedures, and educates the child and family about care of the child at home.
- Caring for the chronically ill child in the community includes health supervision and monitoring the child's health status, teaching the family to manage the child's condition and promote the child's growth and development, and making referrals to community resources.

- An individualized school health plan describes the school-based care of the child with a chronic condition for optimal participation in school and class activities.
- Family assessment tools help nurses identify the family strengths and deficits to support family development and coping.
- Home care nursing is focused on helping the family to gain the ability to manage the child with a chronic condition more independently.

EXPLORE MediaLink

- NCLEX review, case studies, and other interactive resources for this chapter can be found on the Companion Website at **http://www.prenhall.com/ball.** Click on Chapter 6 to select the activities for this chapter.
- For animations, more NCLEX review questions, and an audio glossary, access the accompanying CD-ROM in this textbook.

References

1. Ahmann, E. (1996). *Home care for the high risk infant: A family centered approach* (2nd ed.). Gaithersburg, MD: Aspen Publishers.
2. American Academy of Pediatrics, Committee on Pediatric Emergency Medicine. (1999). Emergency preparedness of children with special health care needs. *Pediatrics, 104*(4), e53.
3. Caldwell, B. M., & Bradley, R. H. (1984). *The home observation for measurement of the environment.* Little Rock, AR: University of Arkansas.
4. Curry, D. M., & Duby, J. C. (1994). Developmental surveillance by pediatric nurses. *Pediatric Nursing, 20*(1), 40–44.
5. Deloian, B. J. (1997). Screening tests. In J. A. Fox (Ed.), *Primary health care of children* (pp. 148–157). St. Louis: Mosby.
6. Department of Adolescent Health. (1996). *Guidelines for adolescent preventive services (GAPS).* Chicago: American Medical Association.
7. Glascoe, F. P. (1999). Using parents' concerns to detect and address developmental and behavioral problems. *Journal of the Society of Pediatric Nurses, 4*(1), 24–35.
8. Green, M., & Palfrey, J. S. (2000). *Bright futures: Guidelines for health supervision of infants, children, and adolescents* (2nd ed.). Arlington, VA: National Center for Education in Maternal and Child Health.
9. Hogue, E. (1993). Care in the absence of primary caregivers. *Pediatric Nursing, 19*(1), 49–50.
10. Jackson, P. L. (2000). The primary care provider and chidren with chronic conditions. In P. L. Jackson & J. A. Vessey (Eds.), *Primary care of the child with a chronic condition* (3rd ed., pp. 3–19). St. Louis: Mosby.
11. McPherson, M., Arango, P., Fox, H., Lauver, C., McManus, M., et al. (1998). A new definition of children with special health care needs. *Pediatrics, 102*(1), 137–140.
12. National Association of School Nurses. (1999). *Standards of professional school nursing practice.* Scarborough, ME: Author.
13. Newacheck, P. A., McManus, M., Fox, H. B., Hung, Y. Y., & Halfon, N. (2000). Access to health care for children with special health care needs. *Pediatrics, 105*(4), 760–766.
14. Office of Public Health and Science and Office of Disease Prevention and Promotion. (1998). *Put prevention into practice: Clinician's handbook of preventive services* (2nd ed.). Washington, DC: U.S. Department of Health and Human Services, Public Health Services.
15. Office of Technology Assessment. (1987). *Technology-dependent children: Hospital vs. home care. A technical memorandum.* Washington, DC: Congress of the United States.
16. Patterson, J. M. (1991). Family resilience to the challenge of a child's disability. *Pediatric Annals, 20*(9), 491–499.
17. Patterson, J. M. (1995). Promoting resilience in families experiencing stress. *Pediatric Clinics of North America, 42*(1), 47–63.
18. Pridham, K. F., Broome, M., & Woodring, B. (1996). Education for the nursing of children and their families: Standards and guidelines for prelicensure and early professional education. *Journal of Pediatric Nursing, 11*(5), 273–280.
19. Taylor, E. H., & Edwards, R. L. (1995). When community resources fail: Assisting the frightened and angry parent. *Pediatric Clinics of North America, 42*(1), 209–216.

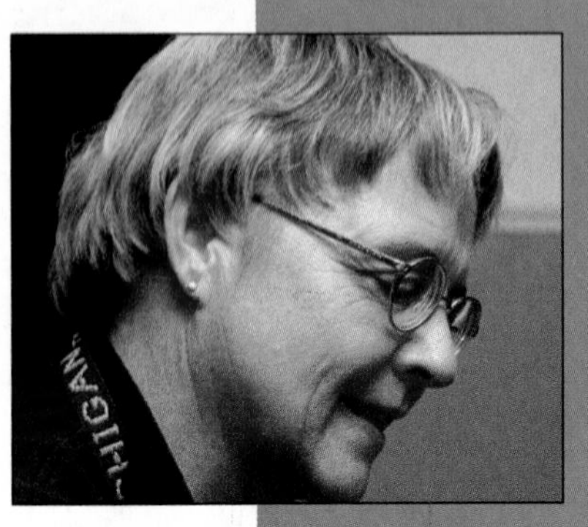

"It is important to make the right compromises for a teen like Amy. She needs love, a nurturing environment, and clear guidelines about behavior. Most of all she needs to value herself as a person so she can make the right decisions in the years ahead."

Amy is 15 years old and attends an alternative high school. She recently had an ear piercing and it is sore. She comes to the health room to ask the advice of the school nurse. Upon examination, the area around the piercing is inflamed and mildly edematous. After asking some questions, the nurse learns that Amy's ear was pierced by a friend, using a needle that had been "sterilized" by passing it through a match flame. She has had a slight fever, but otherwise feels fine.

In her home state, adolescents under 18 years of age must have the signature of a parent for body piercings and tattoos, so Amy chose to have the procedure done by a friend. She believes this is safe since her friend has done many piercings on others. She admits that her parents are not very pleased with her body art, but that they allow her to do it as long as she agrees to stay in high school. She had previously run away and spent several weeks living on the streets.

What health care and social needs does Amy have? How can you support both her and her parents? What signs of resilience does Amy show? This chapter examines the complex social contexts in which children live, learn, and grow, and explores the role of nurses in supporting them to reach their potentials. The challenges of providing comprehensive health care for all children and adolescents, no matter their lifestyles, are discussed.

CHAPTER

7

SOCIAL AND ENVIRONMENTAL INFLUENCES ON THE CHILD

KEY TERMS

adaptation phase Period during a crisis when the child and family meet the challenge and use resources effectively.

adjustment phase Period just after a family is confronted by a crisis, characterized by disorganization and unsuccessful attempts to deal with the problem.

child sexual abuse The exploitation of a child for the sexual gratification of an adult.

emotional abuse Shaming, ridiculing, embarrassing, or insulting a child.

emotional neglect A caretaker's inability to meet the psychosocial needs of a child.

physical abuse The deliberate maltreatment of another individual that inflicts pain or injury and may result in permanent or temporary disfigurement or even death.

physical neglect The deliberate withholding of or failure to provide the necessary and available resources to a child.

protective factors Characteristics of a child and family that provide strength and assistance in dealing with a crisis.

resilience The ability to function with healthy responses, even with significant stress and adversity.

risk factors Characteristics of a child and family that promote or contribute to health system challenges.

violence Threatened or actual use of physical force that leads to potential or actual physical or emotional trauma.

MediaLink 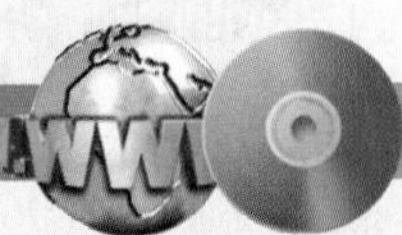 http://www.prenhall.com/ball

Resources for this chapter can be found on the CD-ROM accompanying this textbook, and on the Companion Website at http://www.prenhall.com/ball. Click on Chapter 7 to select the activities for this chapter.

CD-ROM

Audio Glossary

NCLEX Review

COMPANION WEBSITE

Web Links

NCLEX Review

MediaLink Applications

Plan a Smoking Cessation Program for Teens

Plan for the Aftereffects of Violence

Many of the major causes of mortality and morbidity in children are closely linked with social influences in the child's environment. The social contexts for young children growing up today are different from those of even a decade ago. Examining the social contexts in which children live and grow can provide insights into the behavior of children and adults, and present opportunities for nursing interventions. All nurses must examine the social influences and apply the knowledge gained to plan health care that will benefit youth as they grow into adulthood.

What are the challenges of today's society that children must often face at a very young age? How can nurses help children to face these challenges and to emerge as healthy and contributing members of society? What roles do nurses play in identifying and using the protective factors and in minimizing the risk factors of youth? This chapter will help you to examine and apply these concepts in a variety of nursing settings.

Examine again the major causes of death for children from 1 year of age through adolescence that are presented in Chapter 1 (Figures 1-5, 1-6, 1-7, and 1-8). Did you notice that most morbidity is related to preventable causes linked to present-day lifestyles? Car crashes, fires, drownings, and homicides are a few examples of common causes of death in children.

Now examine the major reasons for hospitalization (Figure 1-9). By the time children are 5 years of age, injuries rank as the second cause, and by 10 years, mental disorders are the major cause of hospitalization. By the teen years, pregnancy and mental disorders are the most common admitting diagnoses to hospitals. These conditions are related, at least in part, to the environmental settings in which we live. These settings and their influences must be examined in order to understand how to best intervene with children.

BASIC CONCEPTS

In this chapter, two main theories will be used to provide a framework in which to examine societal influences on children. The ecological model is discussed in Chapter 2, and should be reviewed now to assist in evaluating the environmental settings that influence children (see Figure 2-4). This theory views the child and the environment as interacting forces, with children influencing systems around them, even while they are influenced by these systems (Lackey & Walker, 1998). Close systems providing daily contact are microsystems, but other systems such as parental work and political or cultural environments are also important. Understanding these systems, or the forces in which children function, can provide information that guides care providers. For example, if the parents' employment agencies do not provide health care insurance, their children may not obtain necessary health care such as immunizations, treatment for diseases, and growth monitoring.

Another model that provides a useful framework for understanding the societal influences on child health is the resiliency model. **Resilience** is the ability to function with healthy responses, even with significant stress and adversity (Stewart, Reid, & Mangham, 1997). In this model, the individual or family members experience a crisis that provides a source of stress, and the family interprets or deals with the crisis based on the family's resources. (See Chapter 6 for family assessment tools.) Families may have **protective factors** that provide strength and assistance in dealing with crises, and **risk factors** that promote or contribute to health system challenges. Risk and protective factors can be identified in children, in their families, and in their communities. The combination and interplay of these factors determine adaptation to a crisis.

Once confronted by a crisis, the child and family first experience the **adjustment phase,** characterized by disorganization and unsuccessful attempts at meeting the crisis. In the **adaptation phase,** the child and family meet the challenge and use resources to deal with the crisis (Malone, 1998). The model and examples are described in Table 7-1. Table 7-2 lists questions that can be helpful as the nurse gathers information from the youth or family members which can be used to maximize resilience in individuals and families. These concepts can be applied to Amy's family in the opening scenario. She experienced disruption in family stability. The risk and protective factors interacted with her own personality in ways that resulted in her desire to appear as an independent person, establishing her identity by body decorations.

TABLE 7-1	Components of Resiliency Model	
COMPONENT	**MEANING**	**EXAMPLE**
A = Crisis Event or Health Challenge	Nature of health care challenge	Parent leaving home
V = Vulnerability; risk factors	Stresses and risks related to dealing with the health challenge	Prior abandonment; financial instability; child's developmental understanding of abandonment
T = Typology	Family methods of functioning	Reliance on extended family; parent alcoholism
B = Protective factors	Strengths for dealing with challenge	Child's desire to succeed in school; positive role modeling of maternal grandparents
C = Appraisal	Family's interpretation of crisis event	Abandonment by loved one; inability to trust others
PS = Problem-solving or coping techniques	Skills that help family work toward solution	Use of community resources; acceptance of school and community counselors; child's involvement in classroom activities
X = Response	Positive or negative response to tension created by the health challenge	Remaining parent using counseling available; child identifying with a teacher in school; establishment of sense of mutual interdependence among remaining family members

Note: From Malone, J.A. (1998). The resiliency model of family stress, adjustment, and adaptation. In B. Vaughan-Cole, M.A. Johnson, J.A. Malone & B.L. Walker, *Family Nursing Practice.* Philadelphia: WB Saunders, pg 42. Adapted.

TABLE 7-2 Assessment Questions to Determine Resilience Capability

QUESTIONS TO DETERMINE RISK FACTORS

- Describe the event that occurred and what it has been like for your family.
- What other stressors do you have in your family right now?
- Are there financial worries?
- Are there things you think and worry about late at night?
- Describe your job, your friends.
- Describe your typical day.
- Describe your neighborhood.
- Do you have friends, people to call in emergencies?

QUESTIONS TO DETERMINE PROTECTIVE FACTORS

- What gives you strength?
- How do you deal with this stress?
- What do you think you do well in your family?
- Who do you call when you need help?
- Do you have a computer? Internet access?
- Are you religious? Spiritual?
- Do you exercise regularly?
- How do you spend free time?

Nurses use concepts of resiliency theory in planning interventions for children and families. Nursing strategies can target risk factors, such as encouraging family behaviors to ensure gun safety by teaching use of gun locks and locked gun cabinets in families with firearms. In addition, protective factors can be emphasized, such as when regular exercise is suggested to help maintain normal weight and cardiovascular function.

RESEARCH

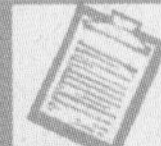

The ADD Health Study (National Longitudinal Study of Adolescent Health) was conducted with over 100,000 adolescents and helped to determine the family, school, and individual characteristics associated with risk factors. Parent–family connectedness, school connectedness, a belief in a higher being, and academic success were predictive of youth having the lowest health risks.

EXTERNAL INFLUENCES ON CHILD HEALTH

POVERTY

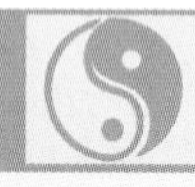

CULTURE

Ethnic disparities are apparent in poverty with 10% of white children classified as poor, 34% of Hispanic children, and 36% of black children (Federal Interagency Forum on Child and Family Statistics, 2000).

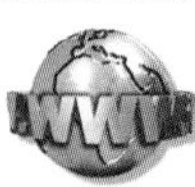

National Health Guidelines and Statistics

An important risk factor that influences the health of children is poverty. Conversely, basic financial stability is a protective factor that contributes to the general health and well-being of children. Children who are poor are overrepresented in nearly every health indicator. One in 5 children is poor, or earning less than $9,000 annually for a family of three persons (Children's Defense Fund, 2000). Children who are poor are more likely to have unmet health needs, to have difficulty in school, to become teen parents, and to experience multiple health problems. Children are the poorest group in this country and more children are poor now than at any time in our past (Board on Children, Youth, and Families, 2001). Children comprise about 38% of the poor in this country and the proportion of poor children in all ethnic groups is increasing (Stein, 1997).

Poverty leads to homelessness for some children. Children comprise one-third and women represent 20% of the homeless population. Families are the fastest growing group of homeless people. On any night, about 100,000 children are homeless in the United States (Menke, 1998; Crook, 1998). The reasons for homelessness are also common risks for a number of the other challenges to health discussed in this chapter. Homeless people often have poor finances, may have been abused or victims of other violence, and have mental instability.

Children who experience homelessness often have multiple physical and mental health problems, and lack health insurance to provide care for these problems. Teens who have been homeless are more likely to engage in other risky behavior, such as unprotected sex with multiple partners and substance abuse. They are more likely to need emergency care, to be depressed, and to become pregnant than other teens (Ensign & Santelli, 1998).

Health problems related to homelessness and other family characteristics continue even after finding a place to live (Vostanis, Grattan, & Cumella, 1998). Complex ongoing care is needed. This may begin in a shelter for the homeless, but should continue while the family obtains a place to live, accesses other community services, gets the children safely enrolled in school, and attains financial and mental stability.

Nursing management for families with children that are poor or homeless focuses on identification of poverty, careful assessment of health risks, and linking the family to resources that can assist with stability and health. There is often no way to identify a poor child from appearance and they may hide their status when in school or at a health care facility. Addresses given may not be accurate, or the address of a shelter might be used. Children living at shelters or in cars and on the street usually do not take the school bus but prefer to walk to avoid stigma. Be alert for children who have multiple health problems and repeated infectious diseases. They are often hungry, and have varying degrees of personal hygiene depending on access to laundry and bathing facilities. See Table 7-3 for examples of nursing care needs for homeless children and families.

STRESS

The adverse effect of stress on adults is well documented. More recently the impact of stress on children has been recognized. Children manifest stress in a variety of ways, including regressive behavior, interrupted sleep, hyperactive behavior, gastrointestinal symptoms, crying, and withdrawal from normal events. Common stressful events for children include moving to a new home or school, marital difficulties in the family, abuse, and being expected to achieve at an extremely high level in school or sports. The busy pace of today's lifestyles and the impact of the media in encouraging early development of children may put undue stress upon some children (Elkind, 1998). For poor families, commonly reported stressors are related to food provision, shelter, transportation, medical care, and personal-time needs.

The child experiencing stress has more frequent respiratory and gastrointestinal illnesses and is more likely to be the victim of an injury. The negative long-term effects of stress on body organs and systems suggest that children under stress are more likely to develop illnesses such as strokes, hypertension, and heart attacks later in life.

TABLE 7-3 Common Health Problems and Nursing Management of Poor and Homeless Children

COMMON HEALTH PROBLEMS	NURSING MANAGEMENT
Lack of immunizations	Check immunization records. Provide immunizations at schools and in homeless shelters.
Common infectious diseases	Facilitate free clinics in shelters, schools, and community settings. Teach hygiene measures. Provide resources for disease management. Arrange for medications when needed. Provide information about resources for bathing, hygiene.
Sleep deficits	Inform parents about respite facilities. Arrange for children to have quiet sleep time in school if possible.
Vision and hearing deficits	Perform screening for deficits. Provide resources for eye glasses, hearing aids, care for ear infections (e.g., service organizations such as Lion's Club).
Nutritional deficits	Perform height and weight checks and nutritional assessment. Evaluate family for food security (see Chapter 3). Be sure child is registered for school breakfast and lunch programs if available. Ensure that children are linked to summer food programs at end of academic year. Link to Women, Infants and Children (WIC) Nutrition Program. Inform about resources for meals and field gleaning in the community.
Dental care problems	Teach oral hygiene. Provide tooth brushes and toothpaste. Provide bottled water for use if child lives in a car or on the street. Perform oral assessment. Refer to dental programs for people with low incomes.
Injuries	Teach basic safety precautions. Visit the living situation if possible to assess for safety hazards. Teach "street safe" skills. Provide helmets, car seats, or other gear needed.
Adolescent pregnancy and sexually transmitted diseases	Provide sexuality teaching. Inform about access to family planning services. Assess for child abuse and prostitution.
Mental illness	Assess for depression. Evaluate for suicide potential. Provide links to services. Plan programs to foster self-esteem. Arrange for a Big Brother or Big Sister. Refer to extracurricular activities in the school and community. Arrange for a school bus stop away from a shelter so other students do not stigmatize the homeless child.

Nurses help children to manage stress by encouraging good coping strategies. Healthy lifestyles including good nutrition, exercise, and plenty of sleep can be emphasized with all children. The National Heart, Lung, and Blood Institute has launched a 5-year program to encourage children to get at least 9 hours of sleep nightly. Parents can be encouraged to provide youth with activities that foster self-esteem and to avoid unrealistic expectations about performance in sports and other activities. Resources to assist with food acquisition, shelter, transportation, and medical care should be provided for families needing the assistance.

GROWTH & DEVELOPMENT

First-born children tend to be concerned with achievement and grades, often become leaders, and more commonly obtain advanced degrees. Last-born children more often demonstrate a relaxed approach to school and achievements (Santrock, 1999).

FAMILY STRUCTURE

The families into which children are born influence them profoundly. Children are supported in different ways and acquire different worldviews depending on such factors as whether one or both parents work, how many siblings are present, and whether an extended family is nearby. Note should be made of variations in family structure such as single parent, homosexual parents, extended family, and stepparents. Societal changes have impacted family life and the needs of children immensely. Working parents often raise children with little time for quality relationships and without the financial resources needed for optimum development (Board on Children, Youth, and Families, 2001). All factors influence the physical and mental health of children and can determine their needs for nursing intervention.

About half of all marriages in the United States end in divorce. Divorce has a profound effect on children, varying with the child's age and cognitive stage. Young children who have limited ability to understand divorce may show such behavioral manifestations as crying, sleep disturbance, regression, and aggressive behavior (Wallerstein, Corbin, & Lewis, 1988; Wallerstein & Kelly, 1996; Wallerstein, Lewis, & Blakeslee, 2000) (see Table 7-4). Older children and adolescents more commonly show inadequate social skills related to cooperation and negotiation, increased aggression, and substance abuse (Thompson, 1998). After divorce, children most often live (about 80% of the time) in a single-parent household with the mother (Friedman, 1998). This can lead to financial strain, decreased health insurance coverage, parental role strain, and other stresses that impact the children. Remarriage, stepparenting, and joint custody arrangements create additional challenges for families. Nurses can help them recognize the challenges the children are experiencing, cope with their particular needs, and provide resources such as family mediation sessions, financial assistance, and support groups (Melnyk & Alpert-Gillis, 1997).

Nurses can complete family diagrams during home visits and in other settings to evaluate the people who are important in a child's life. Both the risk factors of the family (e.g., recent separation, parental stress, and limited health care coverage) and the strengths manifested (e.g., loving relationships, influential grandparents or other extended family members, and general good health) should be identified and used in planning care. Nurses can help family members who are experiencing divorce to recognize the challenges the children are experiencing, cope with their particular needs, and provide resources such as mediation sessions, financial assistance, and support groups (Melnyk & Alpert-Gillis, 1997).

TABLE 7-4 Effects of Divorce

AGE (YEARS)	BEHAVIOR
3–5	Fear, anxiety, and dread in daily life events Regression Searching and questioning Self-blame Increased aggression
6–8	Extreme sadness Fantasies and panic Worries about lack of food, money, caretaking
9–12	Intense anger Somatic complaints Confused self-identity
13–18	Withdrawal from family Concern about sex and marriage Sense of loss Anger

Note: From Wallerstein, J., & Kelly, J. (2000). *Surviving the breakup.* New York: Harper Collins. Adapted.

SCHOOL AND CHILD CARE

Once a child is 5 or 6 years of age, several hours daily are spent in a school setting. Physical skills are developed through participation in education and sports. Psychosocial stages are met as the child interacts with children and adults and achieves social interaction patterns and pride in accomplishments. The presentation of concepts that challenge thought processes enhances cognitive development.

Although the primary role of schools is educational, they also perform several health-related functions. School health screening programs play an important role in identifying children with such health problems as hearing loss, visual impairment, and scoliosis. Nurses provide assessment, teaching, and clinical management related to some health problems. Consider the case of Amy in the opening scenario. She went to the school nurse when her body piercing was potentially infected; the nurse examined the site and made suggestions for cleaning and taught the symptoms Amy needed to be aware of what could indicate serious infections. Some schools have clinics that examine and provide even more complete health care for children. Many schools teach good nutrition, healthful living, safe sexual practices, and other health-related subjects. A school nurse may be present, at least part time, to plan these classes or to work with teachers. Nurses assist school districts in providing plans for emergency health care when needed. With the increase in mainstreaming, school staff now have the responsibility for administering medications, maintaining urinary catheters, and providing respiratory care and other treatments to ensure the child's proper growth and development. See Chapter 6 for a further discussion of school nurse activities.

Some children spend part or nearly all of their days in child care settings (Figure 7-1 ◆). Nearly half of all children are in regular child care by their first birthday (Fields, Smith, & Bass, et al., 2001). While there has been debate about whether child care has a positive or negative impact on children, it appears now that the closeness of the parent–child relationship, the quality of care, and the length of the child care day are important in determining child care effects on children (National Institute of Child Health and Human Development, 1997).

Nursing management involves helping parents to explore types of child care options available and to evaluate programs in their communities (Table 7-5). Care options for young school-age children, either before or after school, can also be shared with parents. Early intervention programs with at-risk children, such as the Zero to Three Project and Head Start, have been influential in contributing to the health and welfare of children and should be recommended when available. Nurses frequently manage the health programs in early intervention, providing for screening and health evaluations and establishing early intervention education plans.

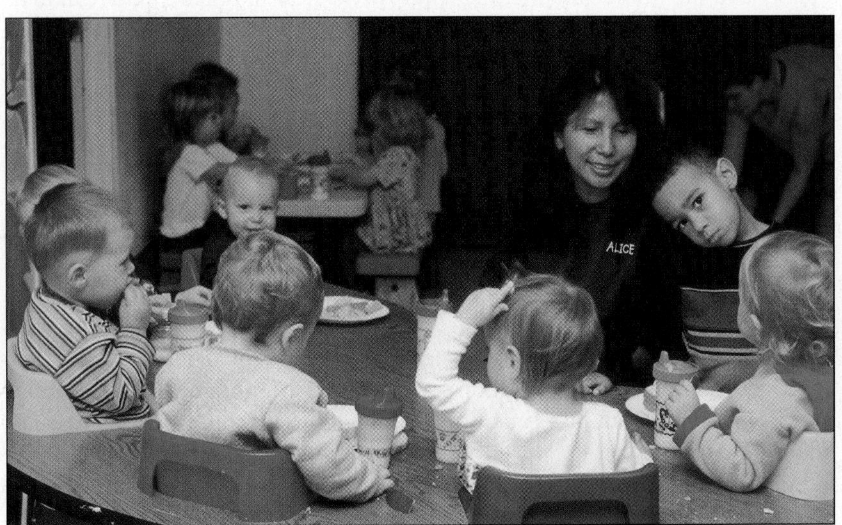

FIGURE 7-1 ◆
Most children will spend time in child care settings. It is important to explore options and find the best fit for the child's needs.

TABLE 7-5 Types of Child Care

TYPE OF CARE	DESCRIPTION	ADVANTAGE/DISADVANTAGE
In home	Caretaker comes to home of the child	Child can remain at home Little exposure to infectious diseases No need for alternative care when child is ill Limited contact with other children to encourage development Most costly
Family child care	Parent brings child to home of a caretaker	Limited number of children Some exposure to other children and encouragement of development Family-type atmosphere Little governmental regulation or examination
Center care *a. Private, nonprofit (e.g., church, YMCA)* *b. Public (e.g., Head Start)* *c. Private proprietary*	Parent brings child to a center where many children receive care	A learning curriculum plan is in place Contact with other children can enhance development Exposure to multiple children increases infectious disease risk

COMMUNITY

The community in which a child lives may support the child's development or, conversely, expose the child to hazards. Social programs such as Head Start preschools, sports activities, after-school programs, and child abuse treatment centers offer valuable services that improve the experience of growing children. On the other hand, an economically depressed community with scant services and a high homicide rate is unsupportive and hazardous for growing children.

The physical environment is supportive when the child is provided with sidewalks on which to walk to school, open spaces in which to learn and play, and clean air to breathe. Children who must walk to school on unsafe roads, have access to contaminated drinking supplies, or live near polluting manufacturing companies or in crowded housing or old structures are at risk for injuries and health problems such as lead poisoning (see Chapter 17).

Nurses should be aware of the types of neighborhoods in the community. Learn about local resources and hazards. Assessment of every child involves information about the community and the health care that the family needs help to obtain. Refer children when appropriate for lead poisoning and safe programs after school, and teach them about injury prevention specific to their communities.

CULTURE

The child's cultural group may influence the use of traditional and contemporary health care practices. If the parents or children are recent immigrants, they may still be learning the English language and finding out about health care resources. Even in families that have been in this country for some time, a combination of approaches to health care is common.

Recent immigrants may experience culture shock, a state of crisis related to the difference in values and lifestyle. This can lead to stress-related symptoms, and create a need for health care intervention. Children whose parents immigrated from another country may feel different than peers and develop conflict with their parents, particularly during adolescence.

All cultural groups have rules regarding patterns of social interaction. Schedules of language acquisition are determined by the number of languages spoken and the amount of speech in the home. The particular social roles assumed by men and women in the culture

FAMILIES WANT TO KNOW

Evaluation of Child Care

The nurse can help parents to evaluate child care options and make decisions about placement for their children. Parents should always be welcomed to visit an agency or home child care—this is essential so they can see the routines in action. Following are suggested questions for them to ask.

ADMINISTRATION

Is the facility licensed?
Who are the administrators? What is their training and experience?
How many staff are employed? What is their training?
Is there a parent board? What part do they play in administering the center?

PHYSICAL ENVIRONMENT, HEALTH, AND SAFETY

What is the neighborhood like? Is transportation to the center convenient?
What is the condition of lighting, heat, cooling, ventilation system, play spaces (inside and out), and the building's general condition?
Is playground equipment safe?
Is there a soft material such as bark, sand, or rubber tiles under climbing equipment?
Is there always supervision for the children?
Are there emergency medical forms and signed forms for field trips?
Who may pick up children? How are they signed in and out?
What is the immunization policy and how are records examined and maintained?
Are criminal background checks of staff done for potential child abuse and other problems?
What is the policy for children with infectious diseases and other illness?
How are foods prepared? Are staff licensed in food handling?
What is the state of general cleanliness?
Who changes diapers? Are recommendations for standard precautions to prevent pathogen transfer followed?
What arrangements and routines are made for naps and quiet times?

DEVELOPMENTAL APPROACHES

Is the curriculum appropriate for different age groups?
Are there materials and plans for gross motor, fine motor, language, and social development?
How much time do children spend in structured time? Free time?
How is discipline handled?
Do the children appear occupied and happy?
What reading materials are available?
What type and quantity of field trips are planned?
What is the educational level and longevity of the child care workers?
Is there a diversity among the children's backgrounds and experiences?

affect school activities and ultimately career choices. Attitudes toward touching and other methods of encouraging developmental skills vary among cultures.

Nurses must become aware of common characteristics of the cultural groups they are serving in order to establish culturally competent nursing care. Arrange for translators when needed. Be aware that traditional and westernized health care are often both accepted and used; remain nonjudgmental about traditional healing practices. Provide ethnic foods in health care facilities. Evaluate youth in immigrant families for conflict between family and societal expectations.

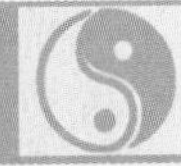

CULTURE

Cultural differences in child rearing influence personality. For example, Japanese children are taught to respect parents and elders. Gender distinctions are the basis for social behaviors. Girls are praised for maintaining poise, grace, and control; boys for showing determination and strength of will in overcoming obstacles.

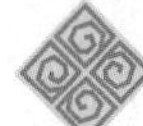

LIFESTYLE ACTIVITIES AND THEIR INFLUENCE ON CHILD HEALTH

Many of the patterns of daily life play a part in determining the length and quality of one's life. The child's use of tobacco products and controlled substances influences both physical and mental health. Patterns of exercise and use of protective gear help to avoid early disabilities. Tattoos that can introduce pathogens are an example of a lifestyle pattern that influences mental and physical health, and body image.

COMMUNITY CARE

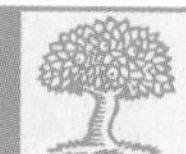

Forms of tobacco other than cigarettes may be popular among certain groups or in specific parts of the country. Chewing tobacco may be used by adolescents in school without staff being aware of the behavior. Bidis are small, brown, hand-rolled cigarettes that are popular among some youths. Try to learn what types of tobacco are most common in the local community and plan to integrate history questions during health exams to learn about cigarette and other tobacco use.

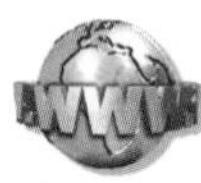

Smoking Prevention

RESEARCH

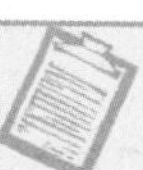

The Youth Risk Behavior Surveillance System is conducted on large representative numbers of youth by the Centers for Disease Control and Prevention. The categories of priority health-risk behaviors investigated in each survey are:

- Tobacco use
- Alcohol and other drug use
- Behaviors contributing to unintentional and intentional injury
- Sexual behaviors contributing to unintended pregnancy and sexually transmitted diseases
- Physical inactivity
- Unhealthy dietary behaviors

TOBACCO USE

Tobacco use is the most preventable cause of adult death in the United States. It leads to 430,000 deaths annually, and will be responsible for the premature death of 5 million of today's youth as they reach adult years (Healthy People 2010, 2000). Major health problems linked to tobacco use include cardiovascular disease, cancer, chronic lung disease, low birth weight, and other maternal problems. Even passive smoking or environmental tobacco smoke (ETS) is linked to increased heart disease, blood pressure, and respiratory problems (Werner & Pearson, 1998). Cigarettes are most common; however, chewing tobacco, snuff, cigars, and bidis may also be used, and also pose significant health hazards.

Many nurses view tobacco use as an adult issue. While sale of tobacco products to children and advertisements aimed at this age group are forbidden by federal law, many youths obtain and use tobacco. In fact, the statistics are alarming. At a time when tobacco use by adults has dropped, adolescents are at very high risk of adopting this behavior, so their smoking patterns are tracked by the Centers for Disease Control and Prevention. About 35% of twelfth graders, 26% of tenth graders, and 18% of eighth graders in the United States have smoked within the last 30 days. When including children who have ever smoked, the numbers are even larger. About 70% have tried smoking by high school years (MMWR, 2000a). Significant numbers of youth also report using chewing tobacco and cigars in the month prior to being surveyed. (Healthy People 2010, 2000). It is striking to realize that 3,000 youths per day try their first cigarette, and that the major ages for trying tobacco are 9 to 14 years (between sixth and ninth grade). Early initiation of smoking becomes an extremely risky behavior when it is recognized that 82% of current adult smokers began smoking before 18 years of age (MMWR, 2000b). Nicotine is highly addictive, and most people become addicted to the substance in adolescent years.

Certain characteristics contribute to the likelihood of tobacco use. They include increasing age, male gender, ethnic group, ease of obtaining tobacco products, and smoking among family members. Low socioeconomic group membership, access to tobacco products, low price of products, advertising, and lack of parental involvement in the youths' lives are also associated with tobacco use (Healthy People 2010, 2000). Girls commonly cite reasons for smoking as a desire to be slim and to appear mature, while boys more often view smoking as a method to be tough and rebellious. Both genders admit that smoking helps them to feel part of a group (Hanson, 1999) (Figure 7-2 ◆).

Several programs have been developed to encourage youth to avoid tobacco use. In addition, smoking cessation programs are available to assist youth who are already regular smokers, and are successful in achieving the goals of cessation or decrease in tobacco use

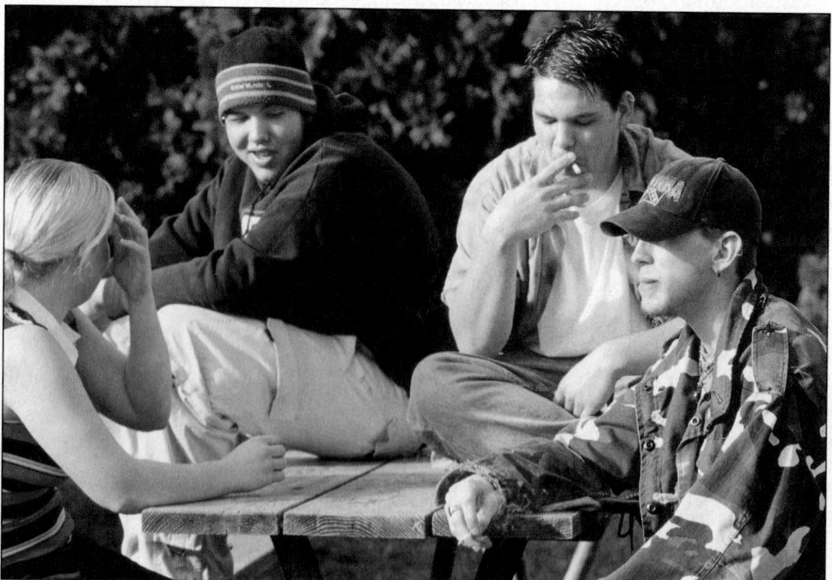

FIGURE 7-2 ◆
About 70% of children have tried smoking by their high school years. Early intervention can begin with discussions about smoking starting at 9–10 years of age.

(Coleman-Wallace, Lee, & Montgomery, et al., 1999). Once a teen is identified as a smoker, using a biological marker such as urine cotinine (a by-product of tobacco) levels can help to identify the frequency of smoking. This information can be used to make suggestions to the teen about the potential outcomes of the behavior and the cessation program which is most likely to be helpful.

CULTURE

Among youth in the United States, white youth are significantly more likely to smoke than either Hispanic or black peers. About 38.6% of white students reported smoking in the previous month, while 32.7% of Hispanic and 19.7% of black students report this behavior (MMWR, 2000). American Indian and Alaska Natives also have high smoking rates, while Asian Americans have low rates (Healthy People 2010, 2000b).

NURSING MANAGEMENT

Nursing Assessment and Diagnosis

Nurses are in a unique position to inquire about the incidence of smoking and other tobacco use among youth. Questions should be inserted into all well-child visits, beginning at about 9 to 10 years of age. Inquire about whether family members (especially parents and siblings) smoke or chew, and ask if some of the child's friends have tried smoking. Determine the child's knowledge and beliefs about the benefits and risks of tobacco use. As the child gets older, more direct and detailed questions are necessary. A nonjudgmental approach will be best to obtain a truthful response. School nurses can make observations about numbers of teens smoking and general attitudes about tobacco use. When children come to hospitals and other health facilities for care, use of tobacco should be part of general admission questions.

The following nursing diagnoses may apply to youth who smoke or show potential for this behavior:

- *Activity intolerance,* related to lowered oxygen supply
- *Impaired gas exchange,* related to ventilation-perfusion imbalance
- *Low self-esteem,* related to negative self-appraisal
- *Knowledge deficit of dangers of tobacco use,* related to developmental focus on present
- *Altered nutrition, less than body requirements,* related to effects of chemical dependence

Planning and Implementation

The roles of nurses in preventing and intervening in youth smoking are to inform youth, identify smokers, and implement programs (Table 7-6). Nurses should provide developmentally appropriate information about the hazards of tobacco use in all settings where youth are present. Posters, flyers, and speakers are particularly useful. Addicted teens who share their stories of difficult withdrawal from tobacco, and adults who have had cancer of the lungs or larynx, may be effective speakers. Find out where teens obtain tobacco products in the community and where they engage in use of the products to target these places.

TABLE 7-6 Nursing Role in Youth Smoking Prevention

INFORM
■ Hang posters, provide brochures, and facilitate presentations about smoking risks in all settings where youth are present. ■ Target smokers with special information about the effects of nicotine on their bodies.
IDENTIFY
■ Ask questions about smoking and other tobacco use at every health encounter beginning at about 9–10 years of age. ■ For users, ask amount and type of tobacco. ■ Learn where youth obtain tobacco and be proactive in stopping sales.
IMPLEMENT
■ Encourage youth tobacco users to quit. ■ Facilitate referral to cessation programs. ■ Arrange positive rewards for youth who are successful in cessation.

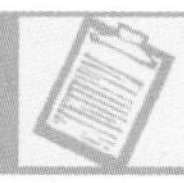

RESEARCH

It is not clear whether smoking cessation efforts for youth should be the same as those aimed at adults. In an attempt to examine the factors associated with adolescent smoking cessation, researchers surveyed 276 youth smokers over a 3-year period, and found that nearly one-third quit smoking. Smoking cessation rate was greatest in those who smoked occasionally versus daily smoking, so researchers suggest that keeping occasional smokers from becoming regular smokers is essential (Sargent, Mott, & Stevens, 1998). Smoking cessation programs may involve use of peer leadership and support, counseling, and computer instruction. When teens have become regular smokers, nicotine replacement therapy may be needed as they are likely addicted to nicotine (Donovan, 2000).

Offer information on available prevention and cessation programs to youth and families in clinics, outpatient surgery centers, community activities, and in hospitals. Use opportunities such as adolescent pregnancy and presence of illness to reinforce the hazardous effects of tobacco on the individual and on those nearby. Speak to young athletes about the effects of tobacco on athletic performance. Show youth the ways in which this product can interfere with their meeting of life goals. Role-play how to tell other youth no when tobacco is offered. Establish programs that increase the sense of self-esteem without tobacco use. Be sure to include parents in the programs so that they see and acknowledge their role in setting an example about tobacco use, and in providing guidelines for the child. Influence of environmental tobacco (secondhand smoke) should be provided.

Adopt a nonjudgmental attitude when asking questions about smoking so that youth who are using tobacco can be identified. Ask questions without parents present and assure youth that the information will not be shared. Encourage youth to cut back and to quit use of tobacco products. Offer assistance to them in these efforts.

Work with the schools and school districts to help establish preventive and cessation programs. There should be clear guidelines about school policies regarding smoking on school grounds. Keeping occasional youth smokers from becoming regular users should be a goal in order to avoid nicotine addiction. Find out what positive incentives can be offered to youth who are successful in quitting smoking. Contract with them to achieve their goals.

Evaluation

Expected outcomes of nursing interventions regarding tobacco use are lowered rates of regular use, delayed initiation of use, and success of cessation programs. Use the following Healthy People 2010 (2000) objectives as guidelines:

- Reduce the proportion of children who are regularly exposed to tobacco smoke at home to 10%.
- Increase smoke-free and tobacco-free environments in schools, including all school facilities, property, vehicles, and school events, to 100%.
- Eliminate tobacco advertising and promotions that influence adolescents and young adults.
- Increase adolescents' disapproval of smoking to 95%.
- Reduce tobacco use by adolescents to 21%.
- Increase the average age of first use of tobacco products from 12 years to 14 years.

SUBSTANCE USE

Substance Abuse Prevention

Substance abuse occurs in children and adolescents of all socioeconomic levels and is a growing health problem. It is important to keep in mind that the use of any drug can pose a serious psychologic and physical risk to children and adolescents.

Although a decline in the daily use of marijuana by adolescents has been reported, abuse of other substances—particularly alcohol, cocaine, crack, and heroin—remains high. The Youth Risk Behavior Surveillance of high school seniors reported the following alarming statistics: 81% have had alcohol to drink, 50% had an alcoholic drink in the month prior to being surveyed, 32% engaged in binge drinking of alcohol, and the average age for beginning alcohol and cigarette use was 12 years (MMWR, 2000a). Prevalence increases with advancing age and grade in school, while 47% of children have had their first drink by 9 years of age (Fetro, Coyle, & Pham, 2001). About 47% of students have used marijuana; 10% have used cocaine; 15% reported inhalant use of glue, paints, or other substances; 9% report methamphetamine use; and 2% used heroin (MMWR, 2000a). Synthetic drugs such as phencyclidine (PCP) (commonly referred to as "designer" drugs) mimic other narcotics, stimulants, and hallucinogens and are also dangerous.

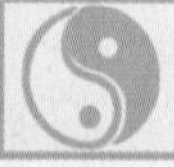

CULTURE

In a study of middle school students, Asian students were least likely to drink alcohol (9%), with African Americans next (23%), followed by Hispanics (26%) and whites (29%) (Fetro, et al., 2001). Nurses can use this information to target groups most at risk of alcohol ingestion, even at these young ages.

Over-the-counter medications are legal substances that are frequently abused. Easily obtainable at grocery stores and drugstores, these drugs include antihistamines, atropine, bro-

TABLE 7-7 Common Contemporary Drugs and Street Names

DRUG	ACTION	STREET NAMES
Methylenediosymethamphetamine (MDMA)	Stimulant; appetite suppressant	Ecstasy, XTC, X, Adam, Clarity, Lover's speed
Gamma-hydroxybutyrate (GHB)	CNS depressant	Grievous Bodily Harm, G., Liquid Ecstasy, Georgia Home Boy
Ketamine	Anesthetic	Special K, K, Vitamin K, Cat Valiums
Rohypnol	Amnesia, sedative	Roffies, Rophies, Roche, Forget-me Pill
Methamphetamine	Stimulant	Speed, Ice, Chalk, Meth, Crystal, Crank, Fire, Glass
Lysergic Acid Diethylamide (LSD)	Hallucinogen	Acid, Boomers, Yellow Sunshines

Note: From National Institute on Drug Abuse. (1999). *Some facts about club drugs.* Bethesda, MD: U.S. Department of Health and Human Services. Adapted.

mides, caffeine, ephedrine, pseudoephedrine, phenylpropanolamine, and amphetamine-like substitutes. Volatile inhalants such as glues are dangerous substances of abuse, and their use appears to be rising among school-age children and adolescents. Anabolic steroids are the drugs of abuse most commonly used by athletes. Some common contemporary drugs and street names are listed in Table 7-7.

COMMON INHALANT AGENTS

Aerosols
Cooking spray
Whipped cream
Spray paint
Cosmetic sprays

Adhesives
Model glues
Rubber cements

Solvents
Nail polish remover
Paint thinner or cleaner
Lighter fluid
Degreaser

Other
Gasoline
Helium

Note: Adapted from Cook, 1999.

Etiology and Pathophysiology

In most cases, substance abuse represents a maladaptive coping response to the stressors of childhood and adolescence. A child may begin using drugs or alcohol to deal with stress because family members or peers do so. Children in families with a history of substance abuse are at higher risk of abusing drugs and alcohol. Other risk factors include rebelliousness, aggressiveness, low self-esteem, dysfunctional parental relationships, lack of adequate support systems, academic underachievement, poor judgment, and poor impulse control.

Initial experimentation with alcohol or drugs may be unpleasant. With continued use, however, the adolescent learns to "achieve the high," an illusion of power and well-being. The adolescent wants the high more frequently and actively seeks alcohol or drugs. Tolerance to the substance occurs with continued use, and ever-increasing amounts are required to achieve a pleasurable high. Physical and psychologic dependence ensues as the body's tissues require the substance to function properly. Withdrawal symptoms occur when the child or adolescent is deprived of the substance.

Clinical Manifestations

Substance abuse in children and adolescents is commonly overlooked and underdiagnosed by health care providers (Pagliaro & Pagliaro, 1996), due in part to the wide range of clinical presentations. These vary according to type of drug abused, amount, frequency, time of last use, and severity of drug dependence.

Common physical manifestations include alterations in vital signs, weight loss, chronic fatigue, chronic cough, respiratory congestion, red eyes, and general apathy and malaise. The mental status examination (refer to Chapter 4) may reveal alterations in level of consciousness, impaired attention and concentration, impaired thought processes, delusions, and hallucinations. Low self-esteem, feelings of guilt or worthlessness, and suicidal or homicidal thoughts are also common.

CLINICAL MANIFESTATIONS OF COMMONLY ABUSED DRUGS

DRUG	POTENTIAL FOR DEPENDENCE	CLINICAL MANIFESTATIONS
Depressants Alcohol, barbiturates (amobarbital, pentobarbital, secobarbital)	*Physical and psychologic:* High; varies somewhat among drugs	*Physical:* Decreased muscle tone and coordination, tremors *Psychologic:* Imparied speech, memory, and judgment; confusion; decreased attention span; emotional lability
Stimulants Amphetamines (e.g., Benzedrine), caffeine, cocaine	*Physical:* Low to moderate *Psychologic:* High; withdrawal from amphetamines and cocaine can lead to severe depression	*Physical:* Dilated pupils, increased pulse and blood pressure, flushing, nausea, loss of appetite, tremors *Psychologic:* Euphoria; increased alertness, agitation, or irritability; hallucinations; insomnia
Opiates Codeine, heroin, meperidine (Demerol), methadone, morphine, opium, oxycodone (Percodan, Oxycontin)	*Physical and psychologic:* High; varies somewhat among drugs; withdrawal effects are uncomfortable but rarely life threatening	*Physical:* Analgesia, depressed respirations and muscle tone (may lead to coma or death), nausea, constricted pupils *Psychologic:* Changes in mood (usually euphoria), drowsiness, impaired attention or memory, sense of tranquility
Hallucinogens Lysergic acid diethylamide (LSD), mescaline, phencyclidine (PCP)	*Physical:* None *Psychologic:* Unknown	*Physical:* Lack of coordination, dilated pupils, hypertension, elevated temperature; severe PCP intoxication can result in seizures, respiratory depression, coma, and death *Psychologic:* Visual illusions and hallucinations, altered perceptions of time and space, emotional lability, psychosis
Volatile Inhalants Glues, typing correction fluid, acrylic paints, spot removers, lighter fluid, gasoline, butane	*Physical and psychologic:* Varies with drug used	*Physical:* Impaired coordination, liver damage (in some cases) *Psychologic:* Impaired judgment, delirium
Marijuana	*Physical:* Low *Psychologic:* Usually low; occasionally moderate to high	*Physical:* Tachycardia, reddened conjunctiva, dry mouth, increased appetite *Psychologic:* Initial anxiety followed by euphoria; giddiness; impaired attention, judgment, and memory

Poor school performance and changes in mood, sleep habits, appetite, dress, and social relationships are nonspecific characteristics of the substance-abusing child.

Clinical Therapy

Multiple psychiatric diagnostic criteria exist for each drug class. Children and adolescents who have other psychosocial disorders commonly use or abuse drugs or alcohol. Treatment should therefore focus not only on the substance use or abuse, but also on the issues underlying the problem. Intervention includes both the family and the substance-abusing child or adolescent.

The primary goal of treatment is to teach the child and other family members to develop and sustain positive coping patterns, and to support them during this process. Most treatment programs offer inpatient and outpatient services, as well as after-care programs. These programs usually consist of peer support focusing on the development of a lifestyle free of drugs or alcohol, healthy family relationships, and positive coping skills. Family involvement is strongly encouraged. Hospitalization is required if the physical dependence is significant and withdrawal places the child at risk for complications such as seizures, depression, or suicidal behavior.

NURSING MANAGEMENT

Nursing Assessment and Diagnosis

Nurses may encounter the substance-abusing child or adolescent in the emergency department or outpatient clinic, in the school and other community settings, or during hospitalization for an injury or other acute problem. Nursing assessment includes taking a thorough history from the parents and child, observing the child's behavior, and performing a physical examination. The history should include the age at which drug use began, pattern of use, length of time the drug has been used, amount of drug used, and psychologic state while on drugs. A history of parental drug use and noninvolvement in parenting the child puts the child at higher risk for substance abuse, reflecting the combined effects of genetic and environmental influences. Two assessment tools provide useful information for the health care provider.

Physiologic Assessment

Look for physical signs and symptoms of substance abuse, including bloodshot eyes, dilated pupils, slurred speech, and weight loss. The adolescent may appear sleepy or restless, or may show signs of clumsiness or inconsistent behavior. Consider all types of substance abuse, including model glue, gasoline, and other sources. Assess for signs of withdrawal and current intoxication effects.

Psychologic Assessment

Changes in social habits may indicate substance abuse. Parents may report a drop in the school-age child's or adolescent's grades or decreased interest in school activities. New friends are not introduced to parents, and the adolescent has less contact with parents, teachers, and other adults who were previously important. The child's current drug use, potential for violence, and motivation to make changes are noted. Assess the degree of family support available.

CLINICAL TIP

PACES provides an easily remembered list of items that is helpful information in identifying risk and protective factors influencing adolescent substance use. How would you phrase questions in each area? (Another tool, known as HEADS, is described in Chapter 6.)

P = Parents, peers
A = Accidents, alcohol/drug use
C = Cigarettes
E = Emotional problems
S = School, sexuality

(Knight, 1997)

CLINICAL TIP

Adolescents who have some or all of the following symptoms may be experiencing alcohol withdrawal: anxiety, headache, tremors, nausea and vomiting, malaise or weakness, insomnia, depressed mood or irritability, and hallucinations.

FAMILIES WANT TO KNOW

Identifying the Youth Who is Abusing Substances

Families are often confused about the behavior of adolescents and unsure whether it represents normal development or abuse of substances. Some characteristics of normal development that help to differentiate these occurrences are listed below. When concerned about possible substance use, the parent can confront the child or talk with school nurses or counselors.

- Many youth are periodically distant with parents at times, but remain involved with peers in school sports and other activities. Withdrawal from all activities and friends may indicate substance abuse.
- Adolescents often complain about school, but when teachers report the student meets expectations and is consistently performing in the classroom this is normal behavior.
- Teens may be weepy on occasion when having a difficult time with friends or not performing as desired. Continued, consistent weepiness is more likely to indicate depression or substance abuse.
- Teens like to stay up late and are frequently tired in the morning, while abusing teens may "nod off" frequently during the day.
- Many adolescents like to achieve a disheveled look in clothing, but the teen who frequently neglects basic hygiene or does not seem to have the energy to wash and dress may be depressed or abusing substances.
- All teens get some infections, but abusing teens may have reddened eyes, oral sores, and constant respiratory discomfort from "snorting" substances.

Following are possible nursing diagnoses for children and adolescents who abuse drugs or alcohol:

- *Impaired social interaction,* related to altered thought processes
- *Self-esteem disturbance,* related to dysfunctional family and social relationships
- *Risk for injury,* related to altered perceptions and sensorium
- *Risk for violence: Self-directed or directed at others,* related to physiologic dependence on drugs, alcohol, and other substances

Planning and Implementation

Care of children and adolescents who abuse drugs, alcohol, and other substances is challenging and often frustrating. Long-term mental health counseling may be necessary to resolve underlying issues and foster lifestyle and behavioral changes.

Prevention is the most desirable intervention. The nurse can play a major role in teaching children and their families about substance abuse. Education should begin in primary school and continue with intensification during middle and high school years. Nurses also can play a major role in community education. Various prevention programs have been developed by federal and private organizations. Referral to support organizations may be beneficial for the child, parents, and other family members. Self-help groups, which are available in most communities, include Alcoholics Anonymous, Narcotics Anonymous, Al-Anon, Nar-Anon, and Ala-Teen. Parents may receive support from a group such as Parents Anonymous.

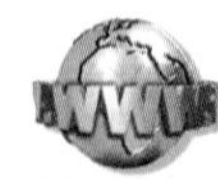

Substance Abuse Support Resources

The youth's protective factors can be identified and used in planning appropriate interventions. For example, a child with goals related to a future career can be helped to see the way in which substance use will interfere with goal attainment. Identifying a strong role model through a program like Big Brothers or Big Sisters can assist children who lack that strength in their families.

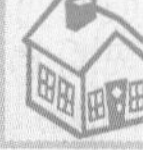

HOME CARE

Children and adolescents spend an average of almost 3 hours/day watching television. This is 20–30 hours weekly, and may extend to 50 hours weekly for some children. When video game and computer time is added to this, the media total average is 6.5 hours daily (Committee on Public Education, American Academy of Pediatrics, 2001).

Children who watch 4 or more hours of television daily get significantly less physical activity and have poorer sports performance than those who watch 1 hour or less (Anderson, Crespo, & Bartlett, et al., 1998). There is often a high intake of fatty snacks during television viewing. Nurses should address this in all health visits with children by asking parents and children what a typical day is like and asking specific questions about television, computers, and video games. Suggest strategies to lessen the hours spent with media such as increased physical activity and family meals.

Evaluation

Expected outcomes of nursing intervention regarding substance abuse include the following:

- abstention from alcohol and street drugs
- successful participation in substance abuse programs
- developmentally normal social interactions
- school performance at level of potential
- absence of injury

PHYSICAL INACTIVITY

In the past few decades, children have become increasingly physically inactive. This decrease is a reflection of lifestyles in which car travel is valued, computers and televisions are part of daily life, neighborhoods are sometimes unsafe places for play activities, and schools do not routinely require daily physical education classes (Figure 7-3 ◆). Physical inactivity leads to many health concerns. A primary outcome is overweight or obesity (see Chapter 3). Other outcomes can be an increased rate of type II diabetes (see Chapter 22), increased exposure to television/computer game violence and sexual activity at early ages, and early progression of cardiovascular disease (see Chapter 14).

On the other hand, patterns of physical activity established in childhood can increase exercise behaviors in adulthood and contribute to lower rates of low back pain, overweight, osteoporosis, heart disease, diabetes, colon cancer, high blood pressure, and a more positive self-image.

Although many children demonstrate low levels of physical activity, a profound decrease in vigorous activity is common in grades 9 through 12. Boys who do remain active generally engage in team sports and weight training, while girls more commonly enjoy aerobics and dance classes (Healthy People 2010, 2000).

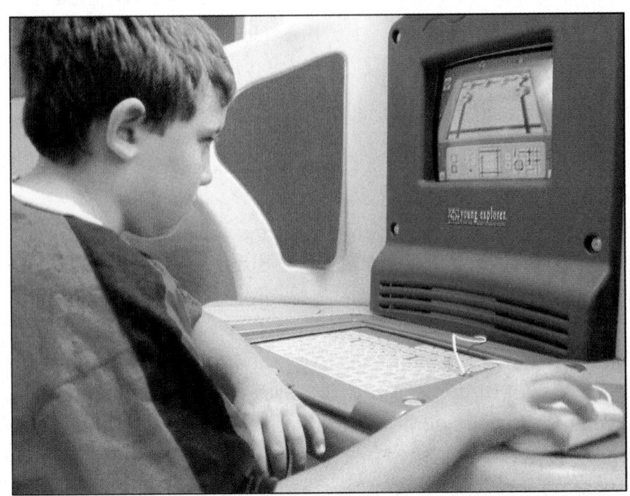

A

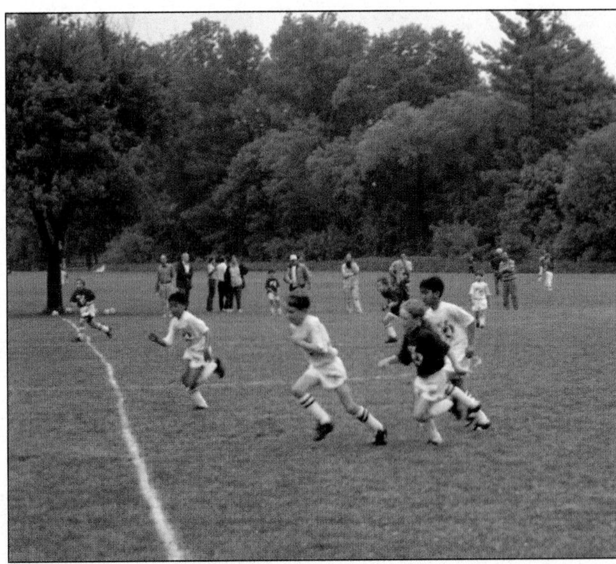

B

FIGURE 7-3 ◆
Physical inactivity is a growing problem among children, and can contribute to poor health. It is important to balance sedentary activities, such as playing computer games, with physical and social activities. Sports are an excellent way for children to develop their psychosocial, cognitive, and motor skills.
Soccer photo courtesy of Rebecca Scheirer, Kensington, Maryland.

Health professionals can integrate assessment of physical activity into all health care, and make recommendations to children and families that will help to increase opportunities for physical activity. Nurses can assess height, weight, and body mass index to look for signs of overweight (see Chapter 3). Children should be asked about how they like to spend free time. Community and school activities should be encouraged and rewarded. Examples include fun runs, walks of benefit causes, aerobics classes, team sports, roadside cleanups, and fairs and carnivals. Help parents and children learn what they can do for physical fitness. Work with school physical education personnel to plan activities both in and out of physical education class that promote lifelong exercise routines.

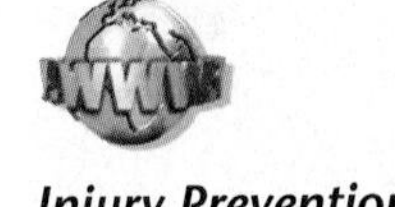

Injury Prevention

INJURY AND PROTECTIVE EQUIPMENT

In the discussion of causes of childhood and adolescent morbidities and mortalities in Chapter 1, unintentional injuries are listed as a common problem. In fact, 72% of all deaths

FAMILIES WANT TO KNOW

Physical Activity Guidelines for Youth

- Engage in moderate physical activity (bike riding, walking, baseball, roller blading) at least 30 minutes 5 times weekly.
- Engage in vigorous physical activity that causes sweating and hard breathing (soccer, running, ice hockey) at least 20 minutes 3 times weekly.
- Encourage schools to offer physical education to all students, and have students sign up when this is an elective.
- Encourage walking and bike riding to friends' homes and stores when safe.
- Plan physical activities together as a family.
- Get a pet and plan to walk the pet daily.
- Limit television and other similar sedentary activities to no more than 2 hours daily.
- On days home, allow the child to watch television for up to 1 hour, and then insist that 1 hour of reading, 1 hour of physical activity, and 1 hour of socializing with others take place before returning to more television.

SAFETY PRECAUTIONS

A recent increase in scooter use led to over 28,000 emergency room visits in 2000 for scooter-related injury. Many injuries could be avoided with use of helmet, knee and elbow pads, riding only on smooth surfaces in areas without cars, and avoiding riding after dark (MMWR, 2000c).

TABLE 7-8 Sports and Activities Requiring Safety Gear

■ Roller blading	■ Soccer
■ Skate boarding	■ Baseball
■ Roller hockey	■ Scooters
■ Ice hockey	■ Skiing or snow boarding fast or using jumps
■ Football	

from age 10 years onward result from four causes—motor vehicle crashes, other unintentional injury, homicide, and suicide (MMWR, 2000a). Chapter 2 discusses the frequent injuries seen in children at different developmental ages, and safety precautions to avoid injuries from car crashes, falls, poisonings, and other developmentally related injuries. Many common injuries are preventable with simple use of protective gear and following of safety guidelines (Figure 7-4 ◆). Sixteen percent of youth rarely or never wear seat belts in automobiles and 38% of those who ride motorcycles do not wear helmets (MMWR, 2000a). The use of safe automobile and motorcycle behaviors must be emphasized again in adolescence, with the recognition that risks increase if driving is combined with use of alcohol and controlled substances. Adolescents sometimes engage in practices that put them at particular risk and nurses should be alert for activities in their communities. Examples include car surfing (standing on the trunk, hood, or roof of a moving vehicle) (Geiger, Drongowski, & Lenni, 2001) or street racing (racing cars down a street at extremely high speed).

Many children ride bicycles, but only about 15% are protected by helmet use, contributing to 23,000 bicycle-related head injuries annually. Bike helmets could prevent up to 88% of serious brain injuries from bicycle crashes (Committee on Injury and Poison Prevention, American Academy of Pediatrics, 2001). Strategies to make helmet use more attractive to children and adolescents are needed. Nurses can play a major role in programs to educate and reward children for helmet use, and can assist families to find helmets at a price they can afford (Behrman, 2000). Other risky behaviors that require protective gear are listed in Table 7-8.

Nurses can be active in identifying behaviors in youths in specific communities and working with schools and other community groups to establish educational programs. Efforts should also include adequate conditioning for sports, proper treatment of injuries, and prevention of overuse injuries (Committee on Sports Medicine and Fitness, American Academy of Pediatrics, 2001).

BODY ART

Body art in the form of painting, tattooing, and piercing has been donned by humans throughout history. There is a resurgence of interest in this decorative art by teens in recent years. Many adolescents have multiple body piercings and tattoos and may even resort to performing these decorations on themselves or friends.

From 10% to 25% of adolescents have tattoos, and even more have at least one body piercing (Armstrong & Kelly, 2001). In some states, teens must be 18 years of age or have parental permission to obtain body art, but students often report that it is easy to have an adult present who signs and claims to be a parent. Only in some states are tattoo and body piercing businesses required to be licensed and comply with certain regulations. Remember that Amy, who is described in the opening scenario, had her piercing done by a friend. Amy demonstrates some common characteristics of teens who choose to use body art. It may be seen as a way to establish individualism and independence, and helps some teens to feel part of a peer group. Multiple tattoos and piercings are common, as is the case with Amy (Figure 7-5 ◆).

Body art is a common source of infections with skin pathogens, as well as hepatitis B and C. Body piercing is a major method of transmission of hepatitis C, a disease that may not even become manifested until years later. It can be a source of HIV if proper techniques are not followed. Piercings in parts of the body such as the mouth or navel are most prone to bacterial infection and continued redness and irritation.

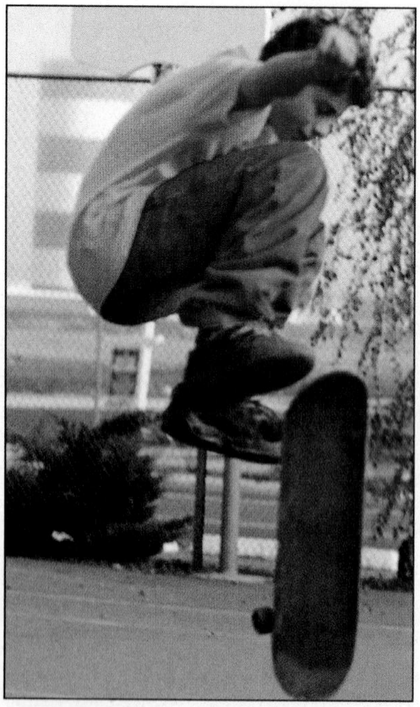

FIGURE 7-4 ◆
What protective gear should children use for skate boarding? How would you convince them to use the protection?

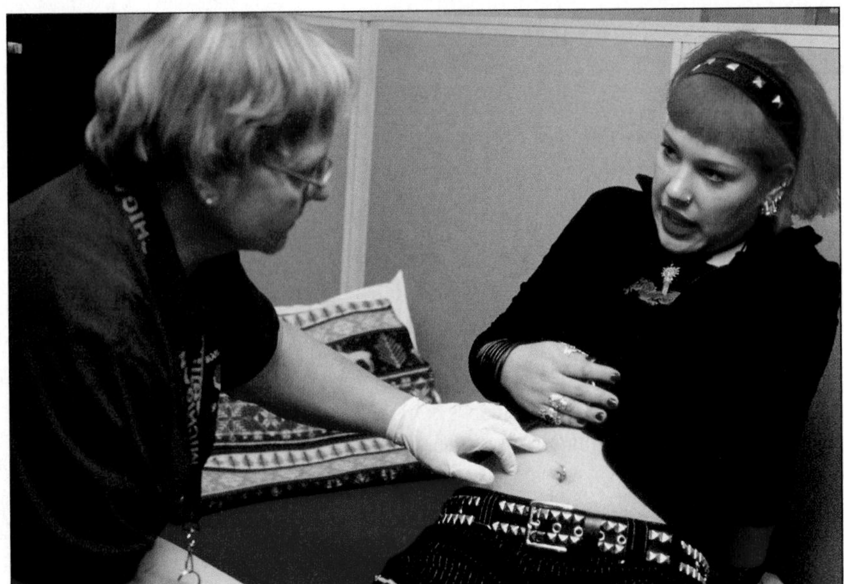

FIGURE 7-5 ◆
Talk openly with adolescents about their health and teach them to avoid health risks connected with tattoos and piercing.

Since teens may choose to obtain body art even if parents object and if there are state laws to prohibit or make it difficult, nursing care must focus on providing information to the teen, assessing sites, identifying infections, and referring if needed (see page 240). Care is almost always provided in community settings such as clinics or schools. Ask teens if they are considering body art, because they often do not seek advice before obtaining the art, and may therefore not get adequate teaching (Montgomery & Parks, 2001).

MINORITY SEXUAL PRACTICES

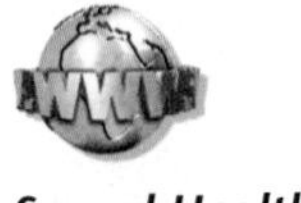

Sexual Health

Adolescence is a time of identifying emerging sexuality. Most teens establish relationships with members of the opposite sex and learn how to interact in ways that are guided by their peer group, family, and culture. For some youth, the transition into adult sexuality is more challenging, as they feel emotional and sexual attraction to people of the same sex (**homosexuality**). The term **gay** is often used for homosexual males and **lesbian** for homosexual females. Other youth are **bisexual,** or attracted to both men and women, and some are **transgendered,** an imprecise term for individuals who cross gender lines. The initials LGBT are sometimes used to refer to these minority sexuality choices. From 1% to 10% of youth self-identify as homosexual (Kreiss & Patterson, 1997).

Alternate sexual attractions and practices are not deviant, but may be viewed as part of a continuum of sexual expression. No gene, early life experience, or other event causes homosexuality.

LGBT youth are at risk for a variety of problems related to emotional and physical health. These include rejection by family members and peers, verbal harassment, sexual abuse and physical assault, a high rate of suicide, substance abuse, high rate of homelessness, and sexual risks of HIV and other sexually transmitted diseases (Stevens & Morgan, 2001). Their health risks need to be identified and appropriate care provided.

Nurses can provide health care for LGBT youth in a variety of settings. School nurses and clinics can display a sign to demonstrate that they are accepting of persons with minority sexual preferences. Terminology in assessment should be gender free. Ask the youth, "Do you have one or more sexual partners?" rather than "Do you have a boyfriend?" When youth identify as LGBT, usual care of all kinds should be provided, including preventive care such as immunizations, sports assessments, and injury prevention teaching. Be alert that the youth may have additional health challenges. Ask about peer and parental support; refer to support groups if needed. Provide resources when the teen is homeless, depressed, or suicidal (see Chapter 24). Perform testing for sexually transmitted diseases if sexual contact is occurring and teach preventive measures. Foster a positive sense of self-esteem through encouraging positive activities such as sports, music, and friendships with peers.

FAMILIES WANT TO KNOW

Care for Tattoos and Body Piercings

BEFORE THE PROCEDURE

- Visit several studios to make comparisons of technique, quality, and cleanliness.
- Ask to watch a tattoo or piercing done on someone else.
- What are the sterilization and hygiene practices of the artist?
- Is the artist licensed? Trained?
- Look at pictures of completed art and talk with former clients.
- Insist that new, sterile equipment be opened in front of the person to be decorated.
- Consider if this permanent body decoration is desired for a lifetime.
- Consider what the tattoo or piercing will look like in several years.
- Consider the possible side effects of infection, dislike for the art, allergy to dyes or metals.
- Be sure that hepatitis B vaccination is completed before the procedure.
- Be aware that no immunization is available to protect against the health risks of hepatitis C and HIV.

CARE AFTER THE PROCEDURE

- Touch the area only after carefully handwashing.
- Keep the area elevated and use ice for the first 2 days to minimize swelling.
- Avoid contact with other person's bodily fluids until well healed.
- Turn the piercing jewelry gently several times daily using washed hands.
- Use antibacterial mouthwash, cleaner, or ointment as recommended.
- Avoid pressure and rubbing on the site (such as belts on navel piercings).
- Watch carefully for signs of infection and report them to a health care provider:
  - Increased redness
  - Swelling
  - Pain
  - Hot feeling
  - Discharge
- Ask the artist how long healing will take. It varies from 2 months in the mouth to 6–8 months in the navel.
- Metal is dangerous during some medical procedures such as magnetic resonance imaging (MRI) or during surgery. Be sure to tell doctors and nurses about the piercings when hospitalized or receiving medical care, especially if they are not readily visible.

If you decide to remove a piece of jewelry soon after placement, then the skin may heal with only a slight scar.

EFFECTS OF VIOLENCE

Violence is a threatened or actual use of physical force that leads to potential or actual physical or emotional trauma (Hennes, 1998). In the past several years, adults and children alike have been shocked by the violent episodes in schools. Although these incidents had much media coverage, they are just one type of violence to which children may be exposed on a regular basis. Children can be the recipients of violence during child abuse and homicides, and they themselves can perform acts of violence on others. They may be touched by violence when parents are killed in gang conflicts, in terrorist attacks, or in wars. The effects of violence are far-reaching and ongoing; they permeate the victim's entire lifetime. This section explores certain types of violence affecting children.

SCHOOLS AND COMMUNITIES

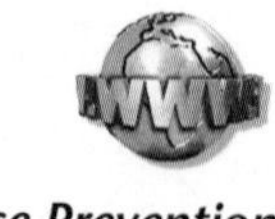

Violence Prevention

At a time when firearm deaths are decreasing overall, unintentional deaths and suicides have increased among children. About 75% of these deaths are committed with firearms found in the home. Forty percent of households with children have guns and in 25% of those homes the firearms are stored loaded or are not secured under lock (Society for Pediatric Nurses, SPN Public Policy Committee, 2000).

Homicide among children has gained attention in past years due to several shootings at schools. Although homicide is an extreme example, other types of violence exist. Children report being threatened verbally and with guns or knives at home, in schools, and neighborhoods. They may be beaten up, bullied, or harassed. They may view domestic violence in their own homes. They may be subjected to dangerous situations in their neighborhoods or during times of homelessness. About half of youths report experiencing serious threats to their well-being (Pratt & Greydanus, 2000). Date rape or other sexual violence is reported by up to 15% of teens (Spencer & Bryant, 2000).

Risk factors have been identified as more commonly seen in situations when violence has been committed against children (see Table 7-9). In addition, children who commit violence more commonly have ready access to firearms, are exposed to violence in the home or community, engage in violent media viewing, and have poor self-esteem or depression.

Realizing the impact of violence on and by children, several federal health care initiatives have begun to assist in lowering violence. Some programs have been helpful and incidents of homicides and most other violence has begun to decrease. Programs that are most successful include individual children, parents, schools, and communities. Health school professionals are instructed to identify signs of violence (Table 7-10). Provide resources for families and children to decrease violence.

NURSING ALERT

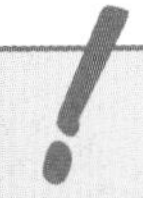

When a group of children is attacked or killed in a school shooting, this tragic occurrence gains media attention. Little do many realize that this tragedy is really part of daily life. Nearly 12 children are killed by a firearm every day in the United States, or a classroom full every other day (Children's Defense Fund, 2000). Every 2 hours a child is killed. Nurses must intervene in this national tragedy.

NURSING ALERT

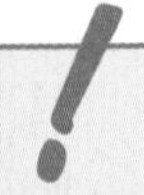

Nurses in school settings can be aware of the practice of bullying. These behaviors seek to harm or disturb the victim, and include such activities as hitting, verbal abuse, name calling, threats, or spreading rumors. About 16% of children in a large national survey had suffered bullying, most commonly in grades 6 through 8, and more frequently among males. Children who are socially isolated are more commonly bullied (Nansel, Overpeek, & Pilla, et al., 2001). Nurses can be active in setting up school policies about bullying. Programs should inform students that the behavior is not tolerated, teach what to do when bullying is experienced or witnessed, and set up peer support for those who are victims.

TABLE 7-9 Risk Factors Common in Families with Child Victims of Violence

- History of mental illness, domestic violence, incarceration, or substance abuse in the home
- Family stresses
- Inadequate child care or supervision
- Inadequate family social support
- Use of corporal punishment for the child
- Child abuse
- Access to firearms
- Gang membership in family or neighborhood
- High exposure to media violence
- Child hyperactivity and other developmental behavioral disorders

Note: From Task Force on Violence, American Academy of Pediatrics. (1999). The role of the pediatrician in youth violence prevention in clinical practice and at the community level. *Pediatrics, 103,* 173–181. Adapted.

TABLE 7-10 Assessment Questions to Identify Violence Risk and Protective Factors

MICROSYSTEM

- Have you been hurt by your parents or anyone else at home?
- When was the last time you were teased or bullied at school? What did you do?
- Have you ever brought a gun, knife, or other weapon to school?
- Do you have access to guns and knives at home? At friends' houses?
- What stresses are there in your family now?
- Tell me about school—what do you like and dislike?

MESOSYSTEM

- Do your parents attend school meetings? Talk with your teachers?
- Do you participate in any church, synagogue, or mosque services?
- Do you participate in any community activities?

EXOSYSTEM

- What stresses do your parents have at work, in their families, with their health or finances?
- Do you feel like your school helps to keep you safe?
- Are there plans for handling violent episodes at your school if they were to occur?
- Do you feel safe in your neighborhood?
- Where would you go or who would you call if you felt unsafe or were hurt and no one was at home?

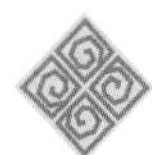

NURSING MANAGEMENT

Nursing Assessment and Diagnosis

Nurses are in key positions to identify children who are at risk of being recipients and victims of violence. The ecological framework can be used to assess children. Some questions that can be asked are listed in Table 7-10. It is important to detect both the risks that lead to vulnerability and the protective factors that can promote resilience and safety. Questions should be adapted to each age group and inserted in every health care encounter.

Nursing care for violence is discussed in the nursing care plan on the following pages. These additional nursing diagnoses may be appropriate:

- *Risk for violence: Self-directed,* related to history of violence
- *Chronic low self-esteem,* related to history of abuse
- *Altered family processes,* related to situational crises
- *Altered growth and development,* related to environmental deficiencies

Planning and Intervention

Nurses intervene with individual children, with families, and in schools and communities to increase safety and decrease violence. Children and families are assisted in meeting basic needs and accessing resources to assist with finances, respite care, domestic violence, and other issues. Education is a key element of intervention.

PROVIDING INFORMATION

The nurse can teach family members about the dangers of firearms and the necessity for use of gun locks, locked cabinets, storing guns unloaded, and storing guns and ammunition in separate places. Suggest alternative activities to minimize child exposure to violence in the media. Inform parents about rating systems for television and other media, and about lockout mechanisms for televisions and computers. Harmful effects of verbal and physical abuse to the child or other family members are discussed and alternatives explored.

FAMILIES WANT TO KNOW

Rating Systems for Media

Television Rating	Television MA Categories	Video & Computer	Movies
TV-Y: for all	FV: fantasy violence	E: for everyone	G: general audience
TV-Y7: for older children	L: language	T: for teen	PG: parental guidance suggested
G: general audience	V: violence	M: mature user	PG13: parents strongly cautioned
TV-PG: parental guidance suggested	S: sexual situation	AO: adults only	R: restricted to above 18 years without adult
TV-14: parents strongly cautioned	D: sexual dialogue		NC17: no one under 18 years admitted
TV-MA: mature audience			

NURSING CARE PLAN The Child and Violent Behavior

GOAL	INTERVENTION	RATIONALE	EXPECTED OUTCOME
1. Risk for violence: Directed at others related to history of family violence			
	NIC Priority Intervention: **Environmental Management: Violence Prevention:** Monitoring and manipulation of the environment to decrease the potential for violent behavior directed toward self, others, or the environment		NOC Suggested Outcome: **Impulse Control:** Ability to restrain compulsive or impulsive behavior in child and others
The child demonstrates impulse control	■ Identify violent behaviors in the child ■ Provide a safe place for exploration of feelings by referral to school or other counseling, support groups and other resources ■ Provide strategies for managing anger, alternative ways for coping with problems	■ Violence in the child usually develops over time ■ The child needs an opportunity to explore feelings and vulnerability ■ Coping strategies can be learned from others and can help in dealing with a stressful home or community situation	The child expresses ability to manage problems in acceptable ways
The child is secure in a safe environment	■ Perform thorough assessment of hazards to physical and emotional state in the child's home, neighborhood, and school ■ Institute actions that will result in removal of child from unsafe situations ■ Use community resources to provide respite care, teaching for families, and safety instruction for the child	■ Hazards to physical and emotional health promote violence to and from the child ■ Removal from family, community or school may be needed to ensure child safety ■ Stress reduction measures may help to decrease violent behaviors	The child expresses a sense of physical and emotional safety in daily life
2. Impaired Home Maintenance Management related to insufficient family organization			
	NIC Priority Intervention: **Home Maintenance Assistance:** Helping the family to maintain the home as a safe place to live		NOC Suggested Outcome: **Role Performance:** Congruence of an individual's role behavior with role expectations
Family members are able to meet role expectations	■ Provide information on child's developmental needs ■ Provide on-going assessment in the home via home health care visits ■ Assist the family in identifying hazards in the environment that can impair the child's growth and development ■ Evaluate ability of adults to provide a safe, secure, nurturing environment	■ Parents need to understand the developmental progression of their children ■ Early identification of hazards can lead to proper interventions to protect against harm to the child ■ Families may need respite care, information about child needs, financial assistance, or other resources in order to meet the needs of the child	Family members meet role expectations, contributing to making the home a safe and secure place for the child
3. Hopelessness related to long-term family stress			
	NIC Priority Intervention: **Hope Instillation:** Facilitation of the development of a positive outlook in the given situation		NOC Suggested Outcome: **Hope:** Presence of internal state of optimism that is personally satisfying and life supporting

(continued)

NURSING CARE PLAN The Child and Violent Behavior (continued)

GOAL	INTERVENTION	RATIONALE	EXPECTED OUTCOME
3. Hopelessness related to long-term family stress (continued)			
The child will have adequate food, sleep, and express satisfaction with life	■ Monitor child's nutritional state and growth and daily patterns ■ Monitor child's developmental status ■ Determine adequacy of relationships and support systems	■ The child's nutrition, sleep, and other patterns provide clues to the family's ability to perceive hope and provide care for the child ■ The child needs close personal relationships in order to grow and learn	The child demonstrates normal growth patterns and meets expected developmental outcomes
The family will identify resources to achieve life goals	■ Monitor the family's decision making ability ■ Provide information on community resources ■ Refer for psychiatric and other services if needed ■ Assist in goal setting	■ Feeling overwhelmed by daily life events leads to an inability to set goals and make decisions to meet the goals ■ Resources can assist the family members in setting and achieving realistic goals	The family establishes realistic goals for growth and development of its members, and takes steps to meet the goals
4. Risk for Injury related to physical or psychological conditions in the environment			
	NIC Priority Intervention: **Safety Behavior:** Family actions to minimize risk of physical or emotional trauma		NOC Suggested Outcome: **Parenting: Social Safety:** Parental actions to avoid social relationships that might cause harm or injury; **Risk Control:** Actions to eliminate or reduce actual, personal, and modifiable health risks
Risk for physical and emotional injury to the child is decreased	■ Identify physical and psychological factors that affect child's safety ■ Assist family to deal with issues such as mental status challenges, fatigue, financial concern, substance abuse, lack of adequate child care resources, and other factors ■ Instruct family on methods of keeping the child safe	■ Multiple factors in the family can contribute to risk of violence and lack of safety for the child ■ Families need information about the impact of unsafe settings on the child and methods that can decrease risk of injury	The child is not injured in physical or emotional ways in the home or other immediate settings
5. Post-Trauma Syndrome related to physical or psychosocial abuse			
	NIC Priority Intervention: **Counseling:** Use of an interactive helping process focusing on the needs, problems and feelings of the child who is a victim of abuse or other violence.		NOC Suggested Outcome: **Abuse/Violence Recovery:** Healing of psychologic and physical wounds of abuse or violence
The child demonstrates abuse or violence recovery	■ Assess the child's affect and behaviors ■ Evaluate social interactions and sense of trust in others ■ Assist the child in identifying feelings and coping strategies by providing counseling, art therapy, and other strategies	■ Disturbed child behaviors can demonstrate a sense of mistrust and insecurity ■ Establishment of close interactions with others demonstrates reestablishment of a sense of trust ■ A child who has experienced abuse or other violence needs a therapeutic relationship with a counselor to deal with the trauma and begin to rebuild trust, respect, and to learn coping mechanisms	The child identifies feelings related to violent episode(s) and expresses healing of the self

The school-age child and adolescent are presented with information about bullying and strategies for dealing with the problem. School and community resources are provided concerning where the child can go if there are threats of any kind. Date rape and violence are topics for discussion for all teens, as is the importance of reporting the situations when they occur.

Care in the Community

Both in schools and community settings, nurses can plan peer mentoring to provide assistance to children at high risk of experiencing violence. School and community programs for children can be linked and coordinated by nurses to provide for parent involvement and child support. Discuss safety issues, both risks and protective actions, in schools and community groups. Report children who are at risk. Work to establish extended programs for children so that they are safe after school. Help children learn behaviors that will help them to be safe in their communities and at home. Teach positive problem solving and conflict management techniques to children and parents.

Evaluation

The expected outcomes of nursing care for violence prevention include a decrease in incidents of homicides, firearm injuries, abuse, date rape, and other violence among children. Additional outcomes are establishment of programs to decrease violence and verbalization by all children of what to do if violence occurs, and how to solve problems without becoming violent.

CHILD ABUSE

One of the most common types of violence against children is child abuse. This type of violence can have implications for both the physical and mental health of children, and can influence their health status long after the abuse has occurred. Awareness of the problem of child abuse is increasing. More cases are being reported; however, these are probably only a small percentage of the total. Approximately 10% to 20% of children between the ages of 3 and 17 years—about 2.8 million children—are physically abused each year (Murry, Baker, & Lewin, 2000).

Physical abuse is only one part of a larger problem. The definition of child abuse has expanded over the past 10 years to include physical neglect, emotional abuse and neglect, verbal abuse, and sexual abuse, as well as physical abuse. Many children who are sexually abused are under the age of 5 years, some as young as 3 months. The average age for sexual molestation is 4 years. The perpetrator is the parent or another person legally responsible who:

- Inflicts or allows another to inflict physical or emotional pain or injury, or
- Creates or allows another to create a significant risk of serious physical or emotional pain or injury, or
- Commits or allows another to commit an act of sexual abuse, as defined by law, against the child.

Abuse generally involves an act of commission, that is, actively doing something to a child physically, emotionally, or sexually, such as hitting, belittling, or molesting. Neglect more often involves an act of omission, such as not providing adequate nutrition, emotional contact, or necessary physical care. Because the evidence is often not visible, emotional abuse and neglect are more difficult to identify and prove than physical abuse or neglect. Risk factors for abuse and neglect are listed in Table 7-11.

PHYSICAL ABUSE

Physical abuse is the deliberate maltreatment of another individual that inflicts pain or injury and may result in permanent or temporary disfigurement or even death. Common methods of physical abuse in children are listed in Table 7-12.

TABLE 7-11 Risk Factors for Child Abuse and Neglect

FACTORS INCREASING RISK FOR PHYSICAL ABUSE	FACTORS INCREASING RISK FOR SEXUAL ABUSE
Poverty Violence in the family Prematurity Unrelated male primary caretaker Parents who were abused as children Age less than 3 years Handicap or condition that requires a great deal of care (e.g., mental retardation, attention deficit hyperactivity disorder) Parental substance abuse or social isolation	Absence of natural father or having a stepfather Being female Mother's employment outside the home Poor relationship with parent Parental relationship characterized by conflict Parental substance abuse or social isolation

TABLE 7-12 Methods of Physical Abuse in Children

Hitting, slapping, kicking, or punching
Whipping with belts, shoes, or electrical cords **(1)**
Inflicting burns with a lit cigarette or lighter **(2)**
Immersing child or body part in scalding water (commonly legs, perineal area, hands, or feet; see Figure 23–12)
Shaking the child violently ("shaken child" syndrome)
Tying the child to a fence, bed, tree, or other object
Throwing the child against a wall, down stairs, or against a window
Choking or gagging the child
Fracturing the legs, arms, ribs, or skull
Deliberately administering excessive doses of prescribed or nonprescribed drugs
Deliberately withholding prescribed medication

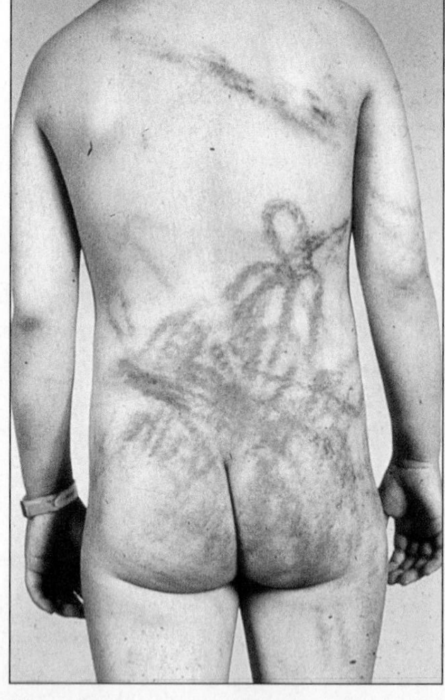

(1)

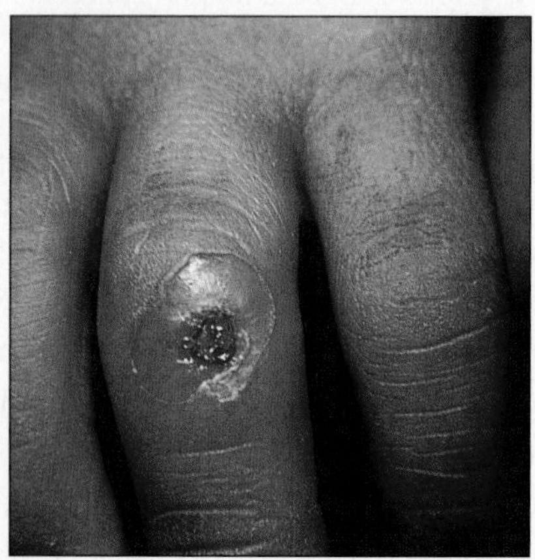

(2)

Used with permission of the American Academy of Pediatrics, Visual Diagnosis of Child Abuse Slide Kit. Photographs Copyright © AAP/Kempe.

PHYSICAL NEGLECT

Physical neglect is the deliberate withholding of or failure to provide the necessary and available resources to the child. Behaviors constituting physical neglect include failure to provide for the following basic needs: adequate nutrition and hydration, hygiene (e.g., clean diapers and clothes, bathing and toileting facilities), shelter (e.g., warmth in winter), and appropriate health care (e.g., immunizations, dental care, medications, eyeglasses).

EMOTIONAL ABUSE

Emotional abuse usually involves shaming, ridiculing, embarrassing, or insulting the child. It can also include the destruction of a child's personal property, such as tearing up the child's favorite family photographs or letters or harming, killing, or giving away the child's pet. These actions are frequently used as a means of frightening or controlling the child.

Verbal abuse is a common method of emotional abuse. Words can be a violent and volatile weapon against a child, eroding the child's fragile sense of self and destroying self-esteem. Common examples of verbal abuse include yelling obscenities at the child, calling the child names, threatening to "put the child away" or to give away or kill the child's pet, telling the child "I wish you were never born" or "You're worthless," and using words to humiliate, shame, or degrade the child.

EMOTIONAL NEGLECT

Emotional neglect is characterized by the caretaker's emotional unavailability to the child. The usual style of interaction is cold and lacking in sensitive personal attention. The child suffers from a lack of nurturance and failure of the parent or caretaker to meet basic dependency needs.

SEXUAL ABUSE

Child sexual abuse is the exploitation of a child for the sexual gratification of an adult. Between 100,000 and 500,000 children in the United States are sexually abused each year. Of child sexual abusers, 75% to 80% are immediate family members, other relatives, friends, or neighbors. Male perpetrators are 92% to 98% of all abusers (Murray, Baker, & Lewin, 2001; Frederickson, 1999). Abusers often threaten to harm or kill the child or another family member if the child discloses the abuse.

COMMON FORMS OF SEXUAL ABUSE

- Oral–genital contact
- Fondling and caressing the genitals
- Anal intercourse
- Sexual intercourse
- Rape
- Sodomy
- Prostitution

Etiology and Pathophysiology

Regardless of the type of abuse, the most common abuser is the child's parent or guardian or the male friend of the child's mother. Risk factors associated with abusive behavior in adults include the following:

- Psychopathology, such as drug addiction or alcoholism, low self-esteem, poor impulse control, and other personality disorders
- Poor parenting experiences, such as abuse in the abuser's own childhood, rejection by the abuser's own parent(s), lack of knowledge of alternative methods of discipline, strong belief in or family tradition of harsh discipline, and lack of parental affection
- Marital stressors and problems with partners, such as hostile-dependent, abusive, or nonsupportive relationships, and one-sided decision making
- Environmental stressors, such as legal, financial, medical, or housing problems
- Social isolation, such as few friends and limited use of sitters, family, or other resources
- Inappropriate expectations for the developmental level of the child

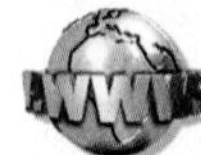

Child Abuse Prevention and Resources

Clinical Manifestations

Clinical manifestations of physical abuse are listed on page 248. Behaviors inconsistent with developmental stage may be apparent. For example, the toddler or preschooler may be indiscriminately friendly with unfamiliar adults, including health care providers, rather than demonstrating shyness or anxiety. For the infant or young child with "shaken baby syndrome" or "shaken child syndrome," the symptoms are those of central nervous system injury from repeated coup and contrecoup injury (see Chapter 20) and include vomiting, irritability, fatigue, poor feeding, bradycardia, apnea, enlarged fontanel, and seizures. Bruises are usually not present (Castiglia, 2001).

Manifestations of physical neglect include undernourishment (evidenced by constantly feeling hungry, hoarding or stealing food, and being underweight), unclean clothes and body, poor dental health (extensive cavities or generally poor condition of teeth), and inappropriate clothing for the season.

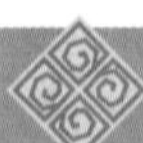

CLINICAL MANIFESTATIONS OF CHILD ABUSE

- Multiple bruises in various stages of healing
- Scald burns with clear lines of demarcation and in a glove or stocking distribution (see Figure 23–19A)
- Rope, belt, or cord marks, usually seen on the mouth, buttocks, back, legs, and arms (see Figure 1 in Table 7-12)
- Burn scars in various stages of healing
- Multiple fractures in various stages of healing
- Shortness of breath and distress upon being moved, indicating chest contusions and possible rib fractures
- Sedation from overmedication
- Exacerbation of chronic illness (such as diabetes or asthma) because of withholding of medication

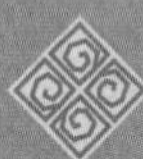

CLINICAL MANIFESTATIONS OF SEXUAL ABUSE IN CHILDREN AND ADOLESCENTS

- Vaginal discharge
- Blood-stained underpants or diaper
- Genital redness, pain, itching, or bruising
- Difficulty walking or sitting
- Urinary tract infection
- Sexually transmitted disease
- Somatic complaints, such as headaches or stomachaches
- Excessively seductive behavior
- Sleeping problems, such as nightmares or night terrors
- Bedwetting
- Unwillingness to go to babysitter, family member, neighbor, or other person
- Fear of strangers
- New or excessive sexual curiosity or play
- Constant masturbation
- Curling into fetal position
- Phobias about particular places, people, or things
- Abrupt changes in school performance and attendance
- Changes in eating habits
- Abrupt changes in behavior (especially withdrawal)
- Child or adolescent female acts like a wife or mother

RESEARCH

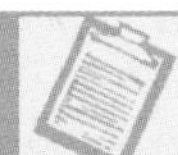

The impact of childhood sexual abuse is long lasting. Persons experiencing such abuse may present with posttraumatic stress syndrome (PTSD). There is also a high rate of substance abuse among those with a history of childhood sexual abuse (Walker, Scott, & Koppersmith, 1998).

Manifestations of emotional abuse, verbal abuse, and emotional neglect include fear, poor physical growth, and failure to meet appropriate developmental milestones. The child may have difficulty relating to adults, impaired communication skills, and developmental delays. Behavioral manifestations include anxiety, fear, shame, aggression, delinquency, and depression (Frederickson, 1999).

Children who have been sexually abused may exhibit a variety of physical and behavioral signs and symptoms. However, sexual abuse does not always result in apparent injury. Among the many long-term consequences of child sexual abuse are ongoing feelings of shame, guilt, anger, and hostility; decreased self-esteem, which leads to increased self-destructive behavior and risk of suicide; recurrence of victimization experiences; substance abuse; and eating disorders. Factors associated with greater psychologic harm to the child include (1) a long period of abuse, (2) use of violent force or threat of violence, (3) abuse involving penetration (intercourse or oral–genital sex), and (4) abuse involving family members, especially the father or stepfather.

Clinical Therapy

Diagnosis of abuse is made on the basis of a careful history and thorough physical examination. X-ray studies may be ordered to identify signs of recurrent abuse such as healed fractures. Some children are admitted directly to the hospital with the diagnosis of suspected abuse or neglect. Less obvious as a victim of abuse is the child admitted with a skull fracture who parents say fell off a chair.

Neglect, which is more difficult to define and identify, frequently requires hospitalization with a comprehensive medical, social, and psychiatric evaluation. Five basic categories must be considered when attempting to diagnose neglect: (1) medical care neglect (lack of necessary medical care), (2) gross safety neglect (lack of appropriate supervision), (3) physical neglect (lack of food and shelter), (4) emotional neglect, and (5) educational neglect.

All 50 states have extensive and complex statutes regarding reporting of child abuse and neglect. A specialist must be consulted, especially if the child's testimony will be used in court.

Children do not routinely make false allegations of abuse. If indeed there is reason to believe the allegations are false, a child and adolescent therapist (psychiatrist, psychologist,

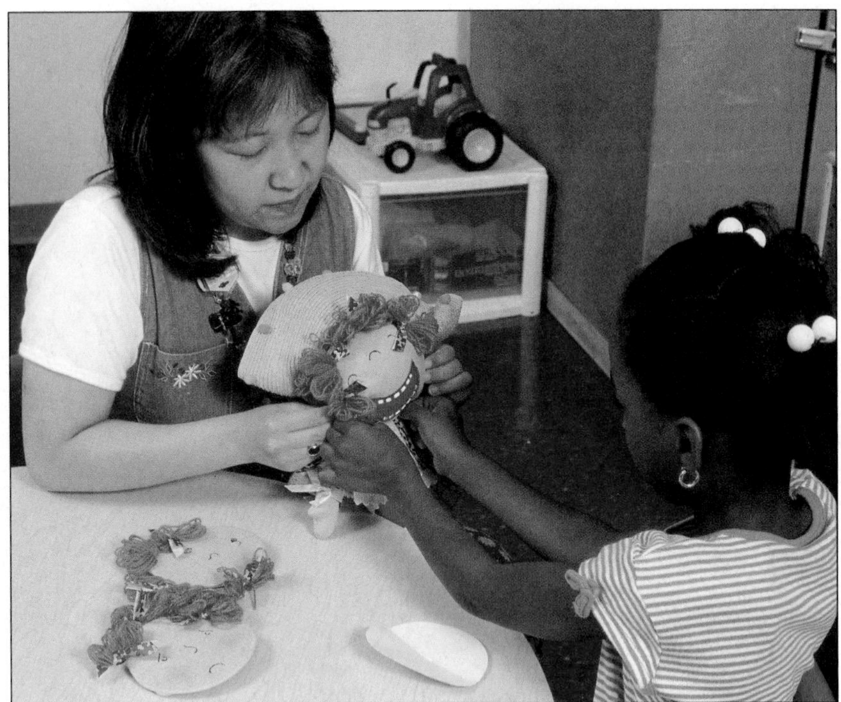

FIGURE 7-6 ◆
Therapeutic strategies with young children involve various methods of communication, such as dramatic play and art.

psychiatric clinical nurse specialist, or social worker) with special expertise should be consulted to determine the truth. Keep in mind that children who withdraw their accusations have often been threatened or coerced into doing so. Because children who have been physically, emotionally, or sexually abused are at risk for major depression, they require skilled care by mental health professionals who are specially trained in this area. Initially the treatment goals include prevention of self-destructive or other dangerous acts. Children must be encouraged to express their fears and feelings in a safe and supportive environment. Equally important is the child's need to build coping skills and self-esteem. The child must be reassured and convinced that he or she is in no way responsible or to blame for what happened.

Individual treatment with art therapy is often used initially because it is the least threatening method in the early stages of treatment, it can easily be tailored to meet the child's individual needs, and it prepares the child for other forms of treatment such as family and group therapy (Figure 7-6 ◆). Family or group therapy may be of benefit in exploring the child's concerns and feelings. Anger is common, especially in children who were abused by a trusted adult such as the father or stepfather.

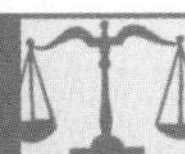

LAW & ETHICS

Every state has a child abuse law specifying the particular behaviors that define every type of abuse. Any professional who works with children and reasonably suspects that a child has been abused is required to report this suspicion to the local agency for child protective services. Reports made in good faith are not liable to countersuits; however, professionals who suspect abuse and do not report it may be held responsible by the courts.

NURSING MANAGEMENT

Nursing Assessment and Diagnosis

Nursing assessment in instances of suspected child abuse or neglect requires a comprehensive history and physical examination, with documentation of findings. Consultation with social service agencies in the community is important if the family is receiving services.

Obtaining the history can be stressful for both the nurse and the parent. Use of therapeutic communication techniques and a quiet, unhurried environment are helpful. Maintaining a nonjudgmental attitude at all times is essential. It is important to differentiate true child abuse from cultural variations that might inaccurately be assumed to indicate abuse (Figures 7–7A and B ◆). Obtaining information about abusive and neglectful behaviors requires the nurse to establish a trusting relationship with parents, who are often afraid to trust any professional.

The health history sequence should include (1) parental concerns, (2) general family history, and (3) specific child history. This sequence begins with nonthreatening topics and allows the nurse to demonstrate concern before asking abuse-related questions. Obtain details about how injuries occurred. The parents' and child's own words should be

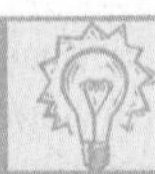

CLINICAL TIP

The nurse should communicate in an open manner. A clear statement of purpose is needed, for example, "Hello, Mr. S. My name is Joan T. I'm Jonathan's nurse. I will be talking with you and asking you some questions about his overall health."

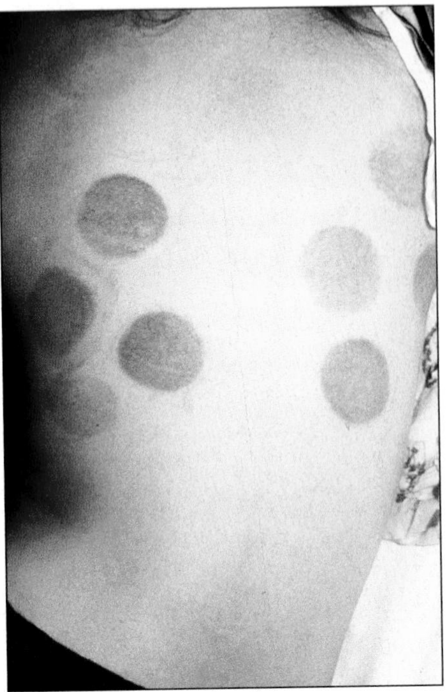
A

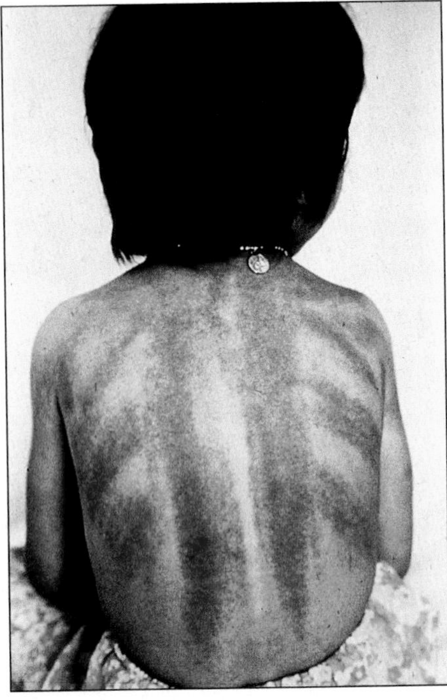
B

FIGURE 7-7 A & B ◆
It is important to differentiate cultural practices such as cupping A, and coining B, from signs of child abuse. Used with permission of the American Academy of Pediatrics, Visual Diagnosis of Child Physical Abuse Slide Kit. Photographs copyright © AAP/Kempe.

documented verbatim using quotation marks. Compare reports obtained from each family member for lack of consistency and details that change over time.

It is desirable to interview the parent and child both separately and together. Parent–child interaction during an intensive history-taking session provides an opportunity to observe the child's behavior and the parent's method of handling and responding to the child.

Data gathered during history-taking are particularly important in light of physical findings. Are there discrepancies between the history and physical assessment data? Do the parents give a history of an uncontrollable, inattentive toddler when the nurse observes a child who is attentive throughout a 15-minute examination? Assess the child's general appearance, including dress and behavior during the assessment. How do the child's affect, behavior, and development compare with those of other children the same age? Be alert for the signs of shaken child syndrome; this most often appears as a subtle neurological condition. Measure head circumference and perform a neurological examination (see Chapter 4).

Documentation of findings is important in all situations, but is essential in cases of suspected child abuse and neglect. Record physical findings as observed. Draw diagrams to document skin injuries. Document the location, nature, and extent of injuries with photographs.

Following are nursing diagnoses that may be appropriate for the physically abused or neglected child:

- *Defensive coping* related to psychological impairment
- *Pain,* related to inflicted injuries
- *Impaired skin integrity,* related to inflicted injuries
- *Altered growth and development,* related to lack of supportive parenting and environment
- *Altered nutrition: Less than body requirements,* related to inadequate caloric intake
- *Altered health maintenance,* related to lack of parental provision of child's essential needs
- *Fear,* related to actual physical harm or repeated risk of injury
- *Risk for injury,* related to physical abuse
- *Risk for violence (parent),* related to inability to manage anger

CULTURE

Traditional treatment practices are sometimes mistaken for signs of physical abuse. The Chinese practice of cupping, which involves heating a bamboo cup and placing it on the skin, is a traditional treatment for headaches or abdominal pain. The Vietnamese practice of caogio (rubbing out the wind), in which a coin or the fingers are forcefully rubbed on the chest, back, or neck, is used to treat minor ailments.

LAW & ETHICS

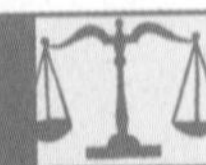

Each person who handles a laboratory specimen or other item (e.g., clothing soiled with semen) in cases of suspected child abuse must be identified in the patient's record, and the specimen must never be left unattended. This documented chain of possession is necessary to ensure the admissibility of the evidence in court.

Additional diagnoses that may apply to the emotionally abused or neglected child include the following:

- *Defensive coping,* related to psychological impairment
- *Chronic low self-esteem,* related to lack of appropriate emotional support from parents
- *Ineffective family coping: Disabling,* related to dysfunctional family dynamics and pattern of physical abuse

Diagnoses that may apply to the sexually abused child include the following:

- *Anxiety,* related to potential separation from parent
- *Rape-trauma syndrome,* related to sexual exploitation
- *Altered role performance,* related to domestic violence
- *Personal identity disturbance,* related to disturbance of usual activities of childhood

Planning and Implementation

Nursing care focuses on helping to remove the child from an abusive environment, preventing further injury, providing supportive care, and reinforcing the importance of follow-up care and counseling.

Prevent Further Injury

Work with social services and community agencies to assess the child's home environment, individuals living in the home, and the actions surrounding the abuse. Assist in removing the child from the home to temporary custody of the court or foster care of another relative, if indicated. Counsel family members about abuse and refer for appropriate therapy.

Provide Supportive Care

Protect and treat the child's injuries (e.g., fractures, burns). Include parents in the child's treatment plan and keep them informed about the child's progress. Even if suspected of inflicting injuries to the child, the parent is still the child's primary caretaker. Talk with the parent as you would with any parent. Be supportive of any guilt expressed. Encourage the parent to assist with the child's care. Observe parent–child interactions and document supportive behaviors and the child's response to the parent versus other care providers.

Interacting nonjudgmentally with a parent suspected of abusing his or her child can be difficult. Talk with a colleague about anger you feel toward the parents or about the child's injuries or specific actions surrounding the abuse. Use team meetings to develop strategies that enable you to work with the parents and child.

Home Care Teaching

If there is any question about the child returning to a potentially dangerous situation, support the child's removal from the situation. The child may receive supervised care in the home by court order. Child care, home nursing, and social worker visits may need to be arranged. Parents should be referred to parent effectiveness classes, family therapy, and support groups as necessary. If a neighbor or friend is the abuser, then the family may need support and legal advice when a term of incarceration is finished and the perpetrator returns to the community. Some states and communities have sexual offender laws which require that the presence of an offender on parole within neighborhoods be publicized.

Encourage the family to inform other care providers when the child's abuse history may affect a response to care. They should be alert to signs of PTSD in order to seek assistance if the child has continuing problems (see Chapter 24).

CLINICAL TIP

When children have been abused, they are often frightened in new situations. Sexually abused children may resist removing clothes for a physical examination or medical test. They may want to wear undergarments to the surgical suite. Members of the gender that abused them may be distrusted. When aware of a history of abuse, ask the parents or guardians how to best facilitate the child's health care. Be sensitive to fears and allow the child to wear clothing, have a support person present, or whatever may provide a sense of security.

Evaluation

Expected outcomes of nursing care for the child who has been abused or neglected include maintenance of normal growth and development, establishment of a positive sense of self-esteem, provision of parenting information and stress relief for parents, provision of a nurturing environment for the child, and absence of episodes of abuse.

MUNCHAUSEN SYNDROME BY PROXY

Munchausen syndrome by proxy is a potentially deadly form of child abuse that involves the fabrication of signs and symptoms of a health condition in a child. Usually it is the mother who creates these fictitious signs in her child (the proxy). The victim is usually under 6 years, and commonly under 1 year of age (Paulk, 2001). Frequently the child's symptoms of illness are used to gain entry into the medical system to meet the abuser's own needs.

The issues of abuse are multidimensional. The child is a victim of the feigned illness, repeated hospitalizations, and invasive procedures. Equally disruptive is the deprivation of the child's daily routine caused by the periodic medical crises.

Munchausen syndrome by proxy should be suspected when unexplained, recurrent, or extremely rare conditions occur; illness is unresponsive to treatment; and the history and clinical findings are inconsistent. The most commonly reported signs and symptoms are central nervous system dysfunction, apnea, diarrhea, vomiting, fever, seizures, signs of bleeding (in urine or stool), and rashes. The parent may overdose the child on medications, such as nonprescription drugs and even syrup of ipecac, causing a variety of side effects. The symptoms occur in the presence of the same caretaker and disappear when the child is separated from that caretaker.

The child often appears uncooperative, extremely anxious, fearful, and negative. The caretaker, who in contrast appears very cooperative, competent, and loving, often expresses a desire for the child to recover. The caretaker may even suggest diagnostic procedures to try to determine "what's wrong." Characteristically the caretaker thrives in the health care environment.

The cause of Munchausen syndrome by proxy is often complex and rooted in the caretaker's own abusive or neglectful childhood. The disorder occurs in all socioeconomic classes. Often the perpetrator has some type of health care background, such as nursing or another allied health profession. The abuser is often young, married, and of the middle socioeconomic class (Paulk, 2001)

A suspicion of Munchausen syndrome by proxy requires a coordinated evaluation by an interdisciplinary team. Members of the team must organize and communicate a strategic plan regarding collection of evidence, confrontation of the abuser, and management of the hospitalized child. The child's safety is the ultimate concern. The case must also be reported to the appropriate child protective services.

Nursing Management

Special care should be taken to maintain a trusting relationship with the caretaker so that he or she does not become suspicious and leave the hospital. Often the best person on the team to function in the role of "trusted other" is a member of the psychiatric consultation team.

Careful documentation of parent–child interactions, presence or absence of symptoms, and other pertinent observations is essential. The child must be closely monitored. If blood is present in the child's urine, stool, or vomitus, careful documentation is needed about whether the nurse was present or whether the sample was provided by the parent. Covert video surveillance may be ordered by the hospital when the syndrome is highly suspected in a particular situation. Expert consultants may be needed to ensure legal requirements for investigation are met. When enough evidence is collected to prove Munchausen syndrome by proxy, the caretaker is confronted by the physician or another member of the psychiatric team.

EATING AND ELIMINATION DISORDERS

A number of eating and elimination disorders affect children and adolescents. The conditions described in this section are clearly linked to lifestyles common in the United States, contributing to an incidence greater than that seen in developing countries or in past decades. The conditions should be examined in light of current stresses, media images, and other environmental forces in order to implement strategies for clinical therapy.

Because food is intricately connected with emotional health, these disorders are often associated with both physiologic and psychologic causes and outcomes. They can impair nutritional status and cause increasing difficulty in family and social relationships for the child or adolescent. The results may be poor nutritional status, depression, isolation and withdrawal, and other self-destructive behaviors.

Eating symbolizes many things. On a basic level, eating represents parental nurturing. The act of being fed or cared for by a parent is the model for all future intimate relationships. For some individuals, however, eating creates anxiety related to a negative association with unpleasant or unsatisfactory parent–child interactions. Elimination, as the outcome of eating, can reflect the same anxieties connected with food intake.

A multidisciplinary team, including a pediatrician, pediatric mental health specialist (psychiatrist, child psychologist, clinical nurse specialist, or social worker), family therapist, and nutritionist, assesses the child's physical, developmental, mental health, familial, and nutritional status. Because nutritional deficiencies often accompany eating and elimination disorders, physical assessment focuses on identifying possible associated problems (e.g., anemia). The overall strengths and weaknesses of the child and family must be evaluated to identify the various factors contributing to the child's inadequate or excessive caloric intake and expenditure. Treatment is then designed to address these factors. Anorexia nervosa and bulimia nervosa, recurrent abdominal pain, irritable bowel syndrome, and encopresis are discussed in the following section. See Chapter 3 for a discussion of eating disorder of infancy and childhood (failure to thrive) and for a discussion of overweight. Other bowel syndromes are discussed in Chapter 17.

ANOREXIA NERVOSA

Anorexia nervosa is a potentially life-threatening eating disorder that occurs primarily in teenage girls and young women, affecting an estimated 5% of young women and 1% of young men in the United States (American Dietetic Association, 2001). The typical patient is white and from a middle- to upper middle-class family. Age at onset varies, and incidence peaks at 12 to 13 years and again at 17 to 18 years.

Etiology and Pathophysiology

Many causes are now thought to contribute to the onset of anorexia. Cultural overemphasis on thinness may contribute to the overconcern with dieting, body image, and fear of becoming fat that is experienced by many adolescents. Chemical changes have been found in the brain and blood of anorectic patients, leading to theories about a biologic cause. Often a significant life stress, loss, or change precedes the onset of anorexia. Stress hormones are commonly elevated in anorectics and immune system function may be disturbed (Brambilla, 2001).

Many authorities view family issues as contributory to anorexia. Intrafamilial conflicts and dysfunctional family patterns may occur when parents are overcontrolling and perfectionistic. The adolescent's eating behaviors may be an attempt to exercise independence and resolve internal psychologic conflicts.

The adolescent may engage in lengthy and vigorous exercise (up to 4 hours daily) to prevent weight gain. Laxatives or diuretics may be used to induce weight loss. As the disorder progresses, the adolescent perceives the ever-thinner body as becoming more beautiful. Youth may share weight loss techniques with anorectic friends and search out Internet sites positive about anorexia. The body responds to the abnormal eating behaviors as if starvation were occurring. Leukopenia, electrolyte imbalance, and hypoglycemia develop as a result of protein–calorie malnutrition. Once the body mass decreases below a critical level, menstruation ceases.

Clinical Manifestations

Anorectic adolescents are characterized by extreme weight loss accompanied by a preoccupation with weight and food, excessive compulsive exercising, peculiar patterns of eating and handling food, and distorted body image. They may prepare elaborate meals for others but eat only low-calorie foods. Characteristically, the fear of becoming fat does not decrease with continued weight loss. Accompanying signs and symptoms of depression, crying spells, feelings of isolation and loneliness, and suicidal thoughts and feelings are common. The disorder is often associated with mental illness such as obsessive-compulsive disorder, anxiety disorders (see Chapter 24), and history of abuse (Herpertz-Dahlmann, Muller, & Herpertz, et al., 2001).

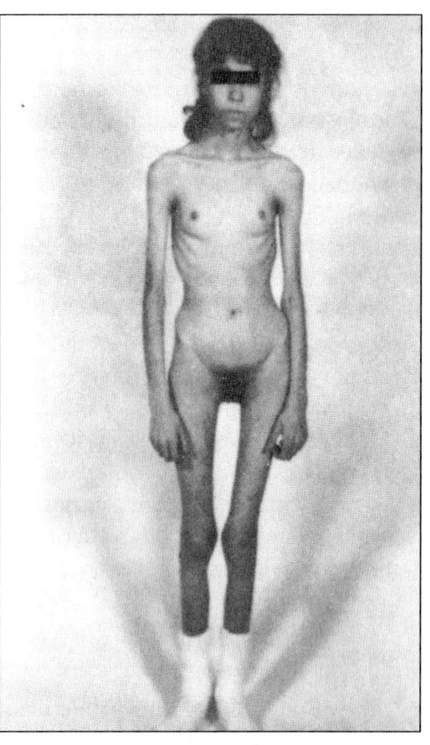
A

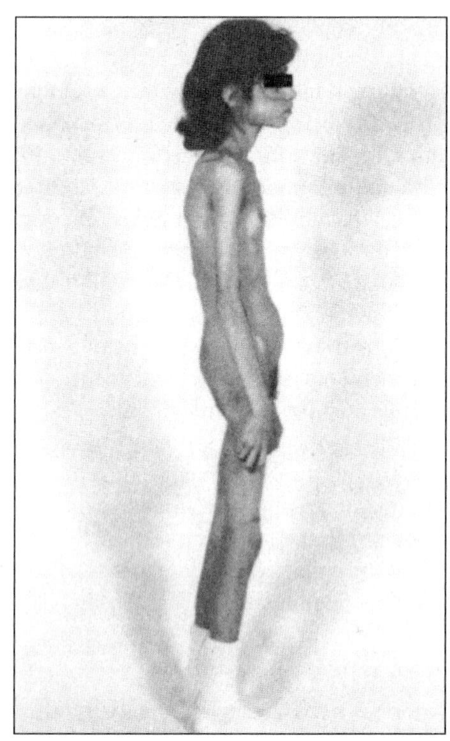
B

FIGURE 7-8 A & B ◆
Characteristic physical appearance of an adolescent girl with anorexia nervosa.
From Rawlings, R. P., Williams, S. R., & Beck, C. K. (1992). *Mental-health psychiatric nursing* (3rd ed.). St. Louis: Mosby-Year Book.

TABLE 7-13 DSM-IV Criteria for Anorexia Nervosa

A. Refusal to maintain body weight at or above a minimally normal weight for age and height (e.g., weight loss leading to maintenance of body weight less than 85% of that expected; or failure to make expected weight gain during period of growth, leading to body weight less than 85% of that expected).
B. Intense fear of gaining weight or becoming fat, even though underweight.
C. Disturbance in the way in which one's weight or shape is experienced, undue influence of body weight or shape on self-evaluation, or denial of the seriousness of the current body weight.
D. In postmenarcheal females, amenorrhea, i.e., the absence of at least three consecutive menstrual cycles. (A woman is considered to have amenorrhea if her periods occur only following hormone, e.g., estrogen administration.)

Note: Reprinted with permission from the *Diagnostic and Statistical Manual of Mental Disorders,* Fourth Edition, Text Revision. Copyright 2000. American Psychiatric Association.

Physical findings include cold intolerance, dizziness, constipation, abdominal discomfort, bloating, irregular menses, and malnutrition (Figure 7-8A and B ◆). Hypothalamic suppression can lead to disturbances of gynecologic function, osteoporosis, decreased bone density, and fractures (Seidenfeld & Rickert, 2001). Lanugo (fine, downy body hair) may be present. Fluid and electrolyte imbalances, especially potassium imbalances, are common. The child or adolescent is usually energetic despite significant weight loss. Extreme weight loss often leads to cardiac arrhythmias (bradycardia).

Clinical Therapy

Diagnosis is based on a comprehensive history, physical examination revealing characteristic clinical manifestations, and the DSM-IV criteria included in Table 7-13.

The goal of treatment is to address the physiologic problems associated with malnutrition, as well as the behavioral and cognitive components of the disorder. A firm focus is placed on reaching a targeted weight with a gradual weight gain of 0.1 to 0.2 kg/day (0.25 to 0.5 lb/day). Enteral feedings or total parenteral nutrition (TPN) may be necessary to replace lost fluid, protein, and nutrients, although the adolescent often perceives these feedings as a punitive measure.

Individual treatment and family therapy are used to address dysfunctional family patterns and assist the family to accept and deal with the adolescent as an independent and less than perfect individual. Family involvement is crucial to effect a lasting change in the adolescent.

Long-term outpatient treatment, in either an individual or a group setting, is frequently necessary. Counseling may be continued for 2 to 3 years to ensure that weight gain and self-image are maintained. Antidepressant drugs such as imipramine (Tofranil) or desipramine (Norpramin) may be prescribed for coexisting conditions such as depression, anxiety, or obsessive-compulsive disorders.

Indications for hospitalization include loss of 25% to 30% of body weight, fluid and electrolyte imbalances or arrhythmias, or the need to provide a more intense period of therapy if outpatient treatment fails to produce improvement. Behavior modification techniques are used extensively in combination with counseling and other methods in care of the hospitalized anorectic adolescent.

NURSING MANAGEMENT

Nursing Assessment and Diagnosis

Obtain a thorough individual and family history. Ask about usual eating patterns, daily caloric intake, exercise patterns, and menstrual history. Ask about medication use; include prescription, nonprescription, and herbal products. Is there a family history of eating disorders? Assess for signs of malnutrition. Obtain height and weight measurements and compare with norms for the general population. Because the anorectic patient often wears layers of clothes when being weighed, strive to obtain an accurate measurement.

Nursing diagnoses for the adolescent with anorexia nervosa may include the following:

- *Altered nutrition: Less than body requirements,* related to inadequate intake
- *Risk for fluid volume deficit,* related to inadequate fluid intake or fluid volume loss from overuse of laxatives and diuretics
- *Risk for altered body temperature,* related to excessive weight loss and absence of subcutaneous fat
- *Constipation,* related to inadequate food intake and overuse of laxatives
- *Body image disturbance,* related to distorted perception of body size and shape
- *Self-esteem disturbance,* related to dysfunctional family dynamics
- *Ineffective family coping: Compromised or disabling,* related to parental tendency to be overcontrolling and perfectionistic

NURSING ALERT

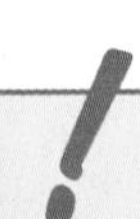

In an attempt to lose weight, anorectics and bulimics use products to bring about anorexia, vomiting, and diarrhea. Many herbal products are used for these purposes. One example is ephedra or ma huang. This Chinese herb is used for asthma, coughs, and flu and it is present in some weight-loss remedies in the United States. It is a chemical source of ephedrine and pseudoephedrine, and in large enough doses can cause increased blood pressure and heart rate, and stimulate the central nervous system (Swerdlow, 2000). Consider that some symptoms seen in those with eating disorders may be related to drugs and herbal products.

Planning and Implementation

Nursing care centers on meeting nutritional and fluid needs, preventing complications, administering medications, and providing referral to appropriate resources. Specific treatment measures vary depending on physical complications, length and degree of illness, emotional symptoms accompanying the disorder, and family dynamics. Resistance to treatment is common, and nurses who care for anorectic adolescents must deal with their own feelings of frustration and anger.

Meet Nutritional and Fluid Needs

Monitor nutritional and fluid intake, encourage consumption of food, and observe eating behaviors at mealtime. Elimination patterns may be altered as a result of increased intake during hospitalization. Monitor for possible problems, including abdominal distention, constipation, or diarrhea. Daily monitoring of serum electrolytes is necessary.

If TPN is administered, watch for complications such as circulatory overload, hyperglycemia, or hypoglycemia. Use strict aseptic technique when changing tubing or dressings.

Administer Medications

Monitor vital signs if the adolescent is receiving antidepressants. Watch for signs of hypertension and tachycardia. Administering medications after meals helps to prevent gastric irritation.

PROVIDE REFERRAL TO APPROPRIATE RESOURCES

Eating Disorder Resources

Refer parents and other family members to the American Anorexia and Bulimia Association, National Anorectic Aid Society, and National Association of Anorexia Nervosa & Associated Disorders for further information about the disorder and a list of support groups in their area.

Evaluation

Expected outcomes for nursing care include weight gain, maintenance of adequate fluid volume, beginning of positive sense of self-esteem, intake of nutritionally balanced diet, and use of psychologic counseling to understand the disorder.

BULIMIA NERVOSA

Bulimia nervosa is an eating disorder characterized by binge eating (a compulsion to consume large quantities of food in a short period of time). Usually the episodes of bingeing are followed by various methods of weight control (purging), such as self-induced vomiting, large doses of laxatives or diuretics, or a combination of methods. Like anorexia, bulimia affects mainly adolescent girls and young women who are white and in the higher socioeconomic classes. It affects 5% or more of young women. The disorder usually begins in middle to late adolescence, frequently emerging during college.

Etiology and Pathophysiology

Causes of bulimia nervosa are similar to those of anorexia nervosa: sensitivity to social pressure for thinness, body image difficulties, and long-standing dysfunctional family patterns. Families may be chaotic and distant from the girl, rather than overinvolved as with the anorectic. Many bulimic individuals experience depression. It is not clear whether the depression is a cause or a result of the bulimic individual's inability to control the bingeing and purging cycles. A bulimic adolescent often binges after any stressful event.

Bingeing usually occurs in secret for several hours until the individual is stopped by abdominal discomfort, by another person, or by vomiting. At first the episodes of binge eating are pleasurable. Immediately following the binge episode, however, feelings of guilt, shame, anger, depression, and fear of loss of control and weight gain arise. As these feelings intensify, the bulimic adolescent becomes increasingly anxious. This usually initiates the purge behaviors.

Purging eliminates the discomfort from bloating and also prevents weight gain. This relieves the feelings of depression and guilt, but only temporarily. Adolescents with bulimia commonly practice the binge–purge cycle many times a day, losing their ability to respond to normal cues of hunger and satiety.

Clinical Manifestations

Bulimic adolescents, like anorectics, are preoccupied with body shape, size, and weight. They may appear overweight or thin and usually report a wide range of average body weight over the years. Physical findings depend on the degree of purging, starvation, dehydration, and electrolyte disturbance. Erosion of tooth enamel, increased dental caries, and gum recession, which result from vomiting of gastric acids, are common findings. The back of a hand can have callouses from inducing vomiting. Abdominal distention is often seen. Esophageal tears and esophagitis may also occur.

Clinical Therapy

A comprehensive history is necessary because most bulimic adolescents appear normal in weight or only slightly underweight. Laboratory evaluation may identify signs of altered electrolyte and hematologic status. The diagnosis is confirmed by the presence of specific DSM-IV criteria (Table 7-14).

Treatment includes management of physiologic problems, behavior modification, and psychotherapy. Behavior modification focuses on modifying the dysfunctional eating patterns and restoring a normal pattern. Until the episodes of bingeing and purging are under control, feelings of discouragement and hopelessness prevail. Thus, the focus early in treatment is on initiating an immediate behavioral change. Once initial interventions have been

TABLE 7-14 DSM-IV for Bulimia Nervosa

A. Recurrent episodes of binge eating. An episode of binge eating is characterized by both of the following:
  1. Eating, in a discrete period of time (e.g., within any 2-hour period), an amount of food that is definitely larger than most people would eat during a similar period of time and under similar circumstances
  2. A sense of lack of control over eating during the episode (e.g., a feeling that one cannot stop eating or control what or how much one is eating)

B. Recurrent inappropriate compensatory behavior in order to prevent weight gain, such as self-induced vomiting; misuse of laxatives, diuretics, enemas, or other medications; fasting; or excessive exercise.

C. The binge eating and inappropriate compensatory behaviors both occur, on average, at least twice a week for 3 months.

D. Self-evaluation is unduly influenced by body weight and shape.

E. The disturbance does not occur exclusively during episodes of anorexia nervosa.

Note: Reprinted with permission from the *Diagnostic and Statistical Manual of Mental Disorders,* Fourth Edition, Text Revision.

successful, group therapy sessions work well for persons with anorexia or bulimia. Specific treatment measures may include the following:

- Educating the adolescent about good nutrition (including food choice and caloric content)
- Encouraging the adolescent to keep a log or food journal and assisting the adolescent to make connections between emotional states and stress and the impulse to binge or purge
- Setting up a daily dietary routine of three meals and three snacks a day (using the same foods for each meal and snack every day to change misconceptions about the weight-gaining potential of certain foods and to decrease anxiety about what food must be eaten at the next meal)

Once these initial measures have been taken, the underlying psychosocial issues are explored. The goals of therapy are to provide the bulimic adolescent with adaptive coping skills and to improve self-esteem.

Most bulimic adolescents do not require hospitalization. Serious abnormalities in fluid and electrolyte levels caused by uncontrollable cycles of bingeing and vomiting, accompanied by depression or suicidal activity, are indications of the need for hospitalization. The prognosis is good with long-term therapy.

NURSING MANAGEMENT

Nursing Assessment and Diagnosis

Obtain a thorough individual and family history, including daily dietary intake and weight fluctuations. Inquire about problems such as abdominal pain or distention, which may indicate an abnormal eating or elimination pattern. Assess the oral mucosa for signs of damage to tooth enamel caused by purging; examine hands for evidence of vomiting-induced callouses.

Following are nursing diagnoses that may be appropriate for the adolescent with bulimia nervosa:

- *Altered nutrition: Less than or more than body requirements,* related to inadequate intake
- *Risk for fluid volume deficit,* related to fluid volume loss
- *Altered oral mucous membrane,* related to chemical effects of vomited gastric acids
- *Knowledge deficit (child),* related to health risks of excessive use of laxatives and diuretics
- *Anxiety,* related to discomfort with weight and eating patterns
- *Self-esteem disturbance,* related to dysfunctional family dynamics
- *Ineffective individual coping,* related to life stressors

CLINICAL TIP 

Monitor bulimic adolescents for at least 30 minutes after each meal to ensure that they do not attempt purging behaviors. If hospitalized, they should not be allowed to go to their rooms alone; have them sit at the nursing desk. When at home or school, they need to remain with other family members or peers and teachers during the allotted time.

Planning and Implementation

Nursing care includes monitoring nutritional intake and elimination patterns, preventing complications, and providing appropriate referrals.

During hospitalization, the patient should keep a food diary. Be alert to the adolescent who hides, gives away, or discards food from the tray or who exits to use the bathroom after meals. Withdrawal from laxatives and diuretics is managed with careful observation for alterations in fluid and electrolyte status. Cardiac monitoring may be necessary if potassium levels are seriously altered. Esophageal tearing or esophagitis is treated to promote mucosal healing. Medications such as antidepressants may be administered. Encourage continuation of group and other therapy sessions.

Bulimic adolescents and their families can be referred to various organizations for assistance and information about the disorder.

Evaluation

Expected outcomes for nursing care for the adolescent with bulimia include healthy mucous membranes and skin, adequate intake of fluids and food, balanced food intake, maintenance of normal weight, and absence of bingeing and purging.

RECURRENT ABDOMINAL PAIN

Recurrent abdominal pain is a frequent problem among young children and adolescents, particularly girls of school age. Although there may be organic causes such as motility problems, constipation, or inflammatory bowel disease, in most cases an organic cause cannot be found. This disorder is associated with the high-stress lifestyles common in contemporary society and has a strong environmental component. However, parents and health care professionals should not dismiss the child's pain just because the cause is unknown or unidentified (Kaufman, Cromer, & Deleiden, et al., 1997).

The pain is generally located in the periumbilical area and occurs on a regular basis. A thorough history and physical examination are necessary to rule out organic causes. Children with recurrent abdominal pain often have little independence and feel controlled by their parents. The history should explore the pressures and stresses in the child's life, the child's temperament or methods of coping, bowel elimination patterns, and history of sexual abuse.

Laboratory studies such as a complete blood count may be ordered to rule out other illness. Gastrointestinal studies may be performed in an outpatient setting. Children are occasionally hospitalized when their condition is severe and not treatable at home.

When no organic cause can be identified, treatment of recurrent abdominal pain focuses on providing outlets for the release of stress within the family and in other settings in the child's life, enhancing the child's coping methods, and promoting dietary changes that encourage regular bowel movements.

Nursing Management

Nursing care includes supporting the child during assessment and diagnostic testing. The child can be taught relaxation techniques and methods for coping with stress. Identify what life events are stressors for the child and ask about specific worries of the child. Methods for giving more independence to the child in the family are explored. The importance of eating a high-fiber diet and maintaining a regular elimination pattern is taught. The child and family may need explanations to understand the pain, which can be compared with neck pain or a headache as an outcome of stress. Children with continuing or recurrent abdominal pain should be referred to a mental health professional.

IRRITABLE BOWEL SYNDROME

Irritable bowel syndrome occurs in 6% of middle school and 14% of high school students. It is characterized by abdominal pain, with episodes of both diarrhea and constipation. The pain is reduced by defecation. The disorder is believed to be related to recurrent abdominal pain (as described above), because symptoms and causes are similar, and children with recurrent abdominal pain frequently suffer from irritable bowel syndrome as they get older. Studies have shown sections of disorganized motility in the bowel (Youssef & DiLorenzo, 2001). In contrast with Crohn's disease and inflammatory bowel disease (see Chapter 17), irritable bowel syndrome shows no structural or metabolic abnormalities. It is believed that the syndrome is closely related to stress, and that individuals with the abnormality have a heightened autonomic nervous system response to stressful events, leading to hypermotility of sections of the gastrointestinal tract.

Most children with irritable bowel syndrome receive only symptomatic treatment (Fass, Longstreth, & Pimentel, et al., 2001). Antispasmodic medicines are sometimes prescribed but may have limited usefulness. Management of stress may be the best solution. Children can be encouraged to exercise, use relaxation techniques, and find other methods of decreasing stress. Ensuring regular bowel movements by use of fresh fruits, vegetables, grains, and fluids can help to reduce the pressure in the gastrointestinal tract.

ENCOPRESIS

Encopresis is an abnormal elimination pattern characterized by the recurrent soiling or passage of stool at inappropriate times by a child who should have achieved bowel continence. It occurs in approximately 1% of school-age children. Children with primary encopresis have never achieved bowel control. Children with secondary encopresis have been continent of stool for several months.

Encopresis is usually associated with voluntary or involuntary retention of stool in the lower bowel and rectum, leading to constipation, dilation of the lower bowel, and incompetence of the inner sphincter. The retention of stool is usually a result of being "too busy"; the child puts off going to the bathroom because there are activities occurring and it would be an inconvenience to leave. The retention of stool leads to constipation that is untreated and chronic (Nowicki & Bishop, 1999). Loose stool leaks around the hard feces, and the child becomes unaware of a need to eliminate. Soiling may occur during the day or night. Bowel movements are irregular, painful, small, and hard. The child may be ridiculed by peers because of his or her offensive body odor. This rejection leads to withdrawal and behavioral problems, often resulting in altered school performance and attendance. The child continues to hold stool because the passage has become painful. Parents commonly seek health care, believing that the child has diarrhea or constipation.

The underlying constipation that leads to encopresis may be caused by the stress of environmental changes (birth of a sibling, moving to a new house, attending a new school), issues of anger and control related to bowel training, diet, a full schedule of activities, or a genetic predisposition.

A thorough history, physical examination, and diagnostic studies (possibly including barium enema) are necessary to rule out organic causes and anatomic abnormalities. Examination of mental health and cognitive functioning may be indicated. Information about the child's toilet-training habits and parents' attitudes concerning those habits is obtained. A dietary history, including eating habits and types of foods eaten, is often helpful. Physical examination sometimes reveals a nontender mass in the lower abdomen.

Treatment may include behavior modification techniques, dietary changes, use of lubricants to clear the bowel of impacted stool and encourage normal defecation, and psychotherapy. Behavior modification programs that reward and reinforce appropriate toileting habits can be successful. Dietary changes include incorporating high-fiber foods such as fruits, vegetables, and whole grain cereals into the diet. Limiting intake of refined and highly processed foods and dairy products also may be helpful. Drugs such as mineral oil, bulk-forming laxatives, and stool softeners are used temporarily to empty the bowel. The child should sit on the toilet for several minutes after morning and evening meals. It takes several months for the bowel to be retrained to respond to sphincter stimulation. Psychotherapy involving the child and family may be indicated in instances of dysfunctional parent–child relationships.

Nursing Management

Prevention of encopresis is a nursing goal. Teach toilet-training techniques to parents, emphasizing the child's developmental readiness (see Chapter 2). Parents should praise the child for successes and avoid punishment and power struggles. Encourage high-fiber diets and regular times for elimination. Nursing care when a child has encopresis centers on educating the child and parents about the disorder and its treatment and providing emotional

CLINICAL TIP

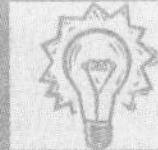

Children with encopresis and constipation need to increase fiber in the diet. A good goal is the child's age + 5 to 6 grams = daily fiber recommendation. Thus, a 5-year-old should have about 10–11 grams of fiber daily. Use dietary lists to learn the fiber content in common foods; make lists of those with high fiber. Have parents include at least one or two of these foods in each meal. Some common high-fiber foods are pears, apples, berries, beans, corn, tomatoes, potatoes, and whole grains. Dry oatmeal and other grains can be sprinkled on cereals and puddings and added to shakes.

support. Explain the treatment plan, including dietary changes and use of laxatives or stool softeners. Reassure the child that he or she has a healthy body and, with treatment, will achieve normal functioning. The child should be followed by the nurse for at least 6 months to be certain new patterns have been established.

Chapter Highlights

- Many of the major morbidities and mortalities of childhood and adolescence are related to social and environmental factors.
- The theory of ecological development provides a framework to use in assessing the interactions of children with factors in their environments.
- The theory of resilience examines risk and protective factors of children in order to formulate interventions to assist the child dealing with health problems related to social conditions.
- Poverty is a pervasive and important risk factor that influences many health outcomes.
- Tobacco use is high among youths, and the most common time for initiation of tobacco use is middle school years.
- Tobacco prevention and cessation programs are needed throughout the school years.
- Substance abuse of many types occurs in childhood and adolescence and compounds many health risks.
- A major contributor to overweight and other health problems is the lack of physical activity among children.
- Protective equipment can reduce the number and severity of injuries during risky physical activities.
- Teens need information about body art safety procedures if they choose this method of self-expression.
- Violence can be directed at children, and children can be the perpetrators of violence.
- All families should be regularly assessed for violence and prevention strategies applied when needed.
- The most common eating disorders of adolescents are anorexia and bulimia.
- A combination of behavioral management, counseling, and medication is often used in treatment programs for eating disorders.

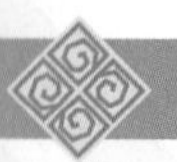

EXPLORE MediaLink

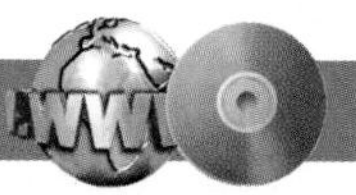

- NCLEX review, case studies, and other interactive resources for this chapter can be found on the Companion Website at **http://www.prenhall.com/ball.** Click on Chapter 7 to select the activities for this chapter.
- For animations, more NCLEX review questions, and an audio glossary, access the accompanying CD-ROM in this textbook.

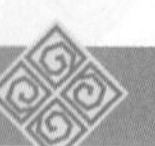

References

1. American Dietetic Association. (2001). Position of the American Dietetic Association. Nutrition intervention in the treatment of anorexia nervosa, bulimia nervosa, and eating disorders not otherwise specified (EDNOS). *Journal of the American Dietetic Association, 101,* 810–819.
2. Anderson, R. E., Crespo, C. J., Bartlett, S. J., Cheskin, L. J., & Pratt, M. (1998). Relationship of physical activity and television watching with body weight and level of fatness among children: Results from the third National Health and Nutrition Examination Survey. *Journal of the American Medical Association, 279,* 938–942.
3. Armstrong, M. L. & Kelly, L. (2001). Tattooing, body piercing, and branding are on the rise: Perspectives for school nurses. *Journal of School Nursing 17,* 12–23.
4. Behrman, R. E. (ed.). (2000). *The future of children: Unintentional injuries in childhood.* Los Altos, CA: The David and Lucille Packard Foundation.
5. Board on Children, Youth and Families, National Research Council and Institute of Medicine. (2001). *From neurons to neighborhoods.* Washington, DC: National Academy Press.
6. Brambilla, F. (2001). Social stress in anorexia nervosa: A review of immuno-endocrine relationships. *Physiology and Behavior, 73,* 365–369.
7. Castiglia, P. T. (2001). Shaken baby syndrome. *Journal of Pediatric Health Care, 15,* 78–80.
8. Children's Defense Fund. (2000). *The state of America's children.* Washington, DC: Author.
9. Coleman-Wallace, D., Lee, J. W., Montgomery, S., Blix, G., & Wang, D. T. (1999). Evaluation of developmentally appropriate programs for adolescent tobacco cessation. *Journal of School Health, 69,* 314–319.
10. Committee on Injury and Poison Prevention, American Academy of Pediatrics. (2001). Bicycle helmets. *Pediatrics, 108,* 1030–1032.
11. Committee on Public Education, American Academy of Pediatrics. (2001). Children, adolescents and television. *Pediatrics, 107,* 423–426.
12. Committee on Sports Medicine and Fitness, American Academy of Pediatrics. (2001). Risk of injury from baseball and softball in children. *Pediatrics, 107,* 782–784.
13. Cook, K. R. (1999). Assessment of potential inhalant use by students. *Journal of School Nursing, 15* (20), 20–23.
14. Crook, W. P. (1998). The new sisters of the road: Homeless women and their children. *Journal of Family Social Work, 3*(4), 49–64.

15. Donovan, K. A. (2000). Smoking cessation programs for adolescents. *Journal of School Nursing, 16* (4), 36–43.
16. Elkind, D. (1998). *The hurried child: Growing up too fast too soon.* Reading, MA: Perseus Books.
17. Ensign, J., & Santelli, J. (1998). Health status and service use. *Archives of Pediatric and Adolescent Medicine, 152,* 20–24.
18. Fass, R., Longstreth, G. F., Pimentel, M., Fullerton, S., Russak, S. M., Chiou, C. F., Reyes, E., Crane, P., Eisen, G., McCarberg, B., & Ofman, J. (2001). Evidence- and consensus-based practice guidelines for the diagnosis of irritable bowel syndrome. *Archives of Internal Medicine, 161,* 2081–2088.
19. Federal Interagency Forum on Child and Family Statistics. (2000). *America's children: Key national indicators of well-being 2000.* Washington, DC: U.S. Government Printing Office.
20. Fetro, J. V., Coyle, K. K., & Pham, P. (2001). Health-risk behaviors among middle school students in a large majority-minority school district. *Journal of School Health, 71,* 30–37.
21. Fields, J., Smith, K., Bass, L. E., & Lugaila, T. (2001). *A child's day: Home, school, and play (selected indicators of child well-being).* Washington DC: U.S. Department of Commerce.
22. Frederickson, D. (1999). Maltreatment of children. *Journal of Child and Family Nursing, 2,* 393–401.
23. Friedman, M. M. (1998). *Family nursing*(4th ed.). Stamford, CT: Appleton & Lange.
24. Geiger, J. D., Drongowski, R. A., & Lenni, J. L. (2001). Car surfing: An underreported mechanism of serious injury in children and adolescents. *Journal of Pediatric Surgery, 36,* 232–234.
25. Hanson, M. (1999). Which straw will break the camel's back? *American Journal of Nursing, 99,* 63–69.
26. (2000). Healthy People 2010. Washington DC: U.S. Department of Health and Human Services. Retrieved April 13, 2001 from the world wide web: http://www.health.gov/healthypeople/document/html.
27. Hennes, H. (1998). A review of violence statistics among children and adolescents in the United States. *Pediatric Clinics of North America, 45,* 269–280.
28. Herpertz-Dahlmann, B., Muller, B., Herpertz, S., Heussen, N., Hedebrand, J., & Remschmidt, H. (2001). Prospective 10-year follow-up in adolescent anorexia nervosa—course, outcome, psychiatric comorbidity, and psychosocial adaptation. *Journal of Child Psychology and Psychiatry, 42,* 603–612.
29. Kaufman, K. L., Cromer, B., Deleiden, E. L., Zaron-Aqua, A., Aqua, K., Greeley, T., & Li, B. U. (1997). Recurrent abdominal pain in adolescents: Psychosocial correlates of organic and nonorganic pain. *Children's Health Care, 26,* 15–30.
30. Knight, J. R. (1997). Adolescent substance use: Screening, assessment, and intervention. *Contemporary Pediatrics, 14,* 45, 51–56, 61–72.
31. Kreiss, J. L., & Patterson, D. L. (1997). Psychosocial issues in primary care of lesbian, gay, bisexual, and transgender youth. *Journal of Pediatric Health Care, 11,* 266–274.
32. Lackey, N., & Walker, B. L. (1998). An ecological framework for family nursing practice and research. In B. Vaughan-Cole, M. A. Johnson, J. A. Malone, & B. L. Walker, *Family nursing practice.* (pp. 38–48). Philadelphia: WB Saunders.
33. Malone, J. A. (1998). The resiliency model of family stress, adjustment, and adaptation. In B. Vaughan-Cole, M. A. Johnson, J. A. Malone, & B. L. Walker, *Family nursing practice.* (pp. 49–60). Philadelphia: WB Saunders.
34. Melnyk, B. M., & Alpert-Gillis, L. J. (1997). Coping with marital separation: Smoothing the transition for parents and children. *Journal of Pediatric Health Care, 11,* 165–174.
35. Menke, E. M. (1998). The mental health of homeless school-age children. *JCAPN, 11,* 87–98.
36. MMWR. (2000a). Youth Risk Behavior Surveillance—United States, 1999. *Morbidity and Mortality Weekly Report, 49* (SS5), 1–94.
37. MMWR. (2000b). Youth Tobacco Surveillance—United States, 1998–1999. *Morbidity and Mortality Weekly Report, 49* (SS10), 1–94.
38. MMWR. (2000c). Unpowered scooter-related injuries—United States, 1998–2000. *Morbidity and Mortality Weekly Report, 49,* 1108–1110.
39. Montgomery, D. F., & Parks, D. (2001). Tattoos: Counseling the adolescent. *Journal of Pediatric Health Care, 15,* 14–19.
40. Murray, S. K., Baker, A. W., & Lewin, L. (2000). Screening families with young children for child maltreatment potential. *Pediatric Nursing, 26,* 47–54.
41. Nansel, T. R., Overpeck, M., Pilla, R. S., Ruan, W. J., Simons-Morton, B., & Scheidt, P. (2001). Bullying behaviors among US youth: Prevalence and association with psychosocial adjustment. *JAMA, 285,* 2094–2100, 2131–2132.
42. National Institute of Child Health and Human Development. (1997). The effects of infant child care on infant-mother attachment security. *Child Development, 68,* 860–879.
43. National Institute on Drug Abuse. (1999). *Some facts about club drugs.* Bethesda, MD: U.S. Department of Health and Human Services.
44. Nowicki, M. J., & Bishop, P. R. (1999). Organic causes of constipation in infants and children. *Pediatric Annals, 28,* 293–300.
45. Pagliaro, A. M., & Pagliaro, L. A. (1996). *Substance abuse among children and adolescents.* New York: John Wiley & Sons.
46. Paulk, D. (2001). Munchausen syndrome by proxy. *Clinician Reviews, 11* (8), 51–56.
47. Pratt, H. D., & Greydanus, D. E. (2000). Adolescent violence: Concepts for a new millennium. *Adolescent Medicine, 11,* 103–125.
48. Santrock, J. (1999). *Life-span development.* Boston: McGraw-Hill.
49. Seidenfeld, M. E., & Rickert, V. I. (2001). Impact of anorexia, bulimia and obesity on the gynecologic health of adolescents. *American Family Physician, 64,* 445–450.
50. Sargent, J. D., Mott, L. A., & Stevens, M. (1998). Predictors of smoking cessation in adolescents. *Archives of Pediatric and Adolescent Medicine, 152,* 388–393.
51. Society for Pediatric Nurses, SPN Public Policy Committee. (2000). Gun accidents, suicides increase among children. *SPN News, 9,* 6.
52. Spencer, G. A., & Bryant, S. A. (2000). Dating violence: A comparison of rural, suburban, and urban teens. *Journal of Adolescent Health, 27,* 302–305.
53. Stein, R. E. K. (1997). Health Care for Children. NY: United Hospital Fund of New York.
54. Stevens, P. E., & Morgan, S. (2001). Health of lesbian, gay, bisexual, and transgender youth. *Journal of Pediatric Health Care, 15,* 24–34.
55. Stewart, M., Reid, G., & Mangham, C. (1997). Fostering children's resilience. *Journal of Pediatric Nursing, 12,* 21–31.
56. Swerdlow, J. L. (2000). Nature's medicine: Plants that heal. Washington, DC: National Geographic Society.
57. Task Force on Violence, American Academy of Pediatrics. (1999). The role of the pediatrician in youth violence prevention in clinical practice and at the community level. *Pediatrics, 103,* 173–181.
58. Thompson, P. (1998). Adolescents from families of divorce: Vulnerability to physiological and psychological disturbances. *Journal of Psychosocial Nursing, 36,* 34–39.
59. Vostanis, P., Grattan, E., & Cumella, S. (1998). Mental health problems of homeless children and families: A longitudinal study. *British Medical Journal, 346,* 899–902.
60. Walker, G. C., Scott, P. S., & Koppersmith, G. (1998). The impact of child sexual abuse on addiction severity and analysis of trauma processing. *Journal of Psychosocial Nursing, 36* (3), 10–18.
61. Wallerstein, J., & Kelly, J. (1996). *Surviving the breakup.* New York: Harper Collins.
62. Wallerstein, J., Lewis, J., & Blakeslee, S. (2000). *The unexpected legacy of divorce: A 25-year landmark study.* New York: Hyperion.
63. Wallerstein, J. S., Corbin, S. B., & Lewis, J. M. (1988). Children of divorce: A ten-year study. In E. M. Hetherington & J. B. Arasteh (eds.), *Impact of divorce, single parenting, and stepparenting on children.* Hillsdale, NJ: Erlbaum Publishers.
64. Werner, R. M., & Pearson, T. A. (1998). What's so passive about passive smoking? *Journal of the American Medical Association, 279,* 157–158.
65. Youssef, N. N., & DiLorenzo, C. (2001). The role of motility in functional abdominal disorders in children. *Pediatric Annals, 30,* 24–30.

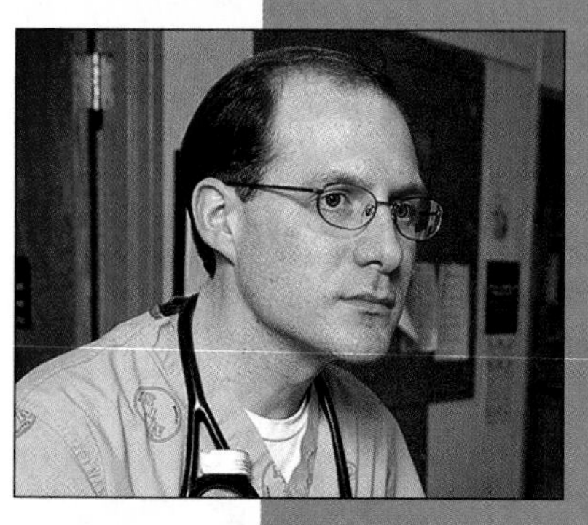

"CONTINUOUS, CAREFUL ASSESSMENT IS NEEDED TO MAKE SURE THE CHILD ADMITTED INTO THE INTENSIVE CARE UNIT HAS A PLAN FOR COMPREHENSIVE NURSING CARE. IN JEREMIAH'S CASE, IT IS SO IMPORTANT TO MAINTAIN THE AIRWAY AND OXYGENATION TO PREVENT HIM FROM DEVELOPING MAJOR COMPLICATIONS."

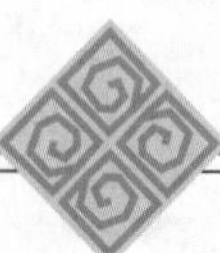

The telephone in the pediatric intensive care unit (PICU) rings at 8:30 a.m. A referring hospital is calling to request the transport of an unstable 12-year-old boy, Jeremiah, who is in status epilepticus. Jeremiah has a seizure disorder that is usually controlled with medications, but several days ago he decided to stop taking them. So many seizure medications have been given in the emergency department at the referring hospital to try to stop the seizures that Jeremiah is now unconscious and must be intubated until he can maintain his airway.

The transport team is in the air within minutes and arrives at the rural community hospital 25 minutes later. After stabilizing Jeremiah and receiving reports from the medical and nursing teams, the transport team meets briefly with his parents, answers a few questions, and is back in the air.

Jeremiah is admitted directly to the PICU, where the unit team has been preparing for his arrival. He is connected to cardiorespiratory and noninvasive blood pressure monitors, while his existing intravenous lines and endotracheal tube are evaluated for patency. Team members quickly complete a head-to-toe assessment. The unit clerk enters Jeremiah's room to say that his parents have arrived in the emergency department and are being escorted to the PICU.

CHAPTER

8

THE CHILD WITH A LIFE-THREATENING ILLNESS OR INJURY

KEY TERMS

coping The cognitive and behavioral responses that manage specific internal and external demands exceeding a person's resources, enabling the person to solve problems and to respond emotionally.

death anxiety A feeling of apprehension or fear of death.

death imagery Any reference to death or death-related topics, such as going away, separation, funerals, and dying, given in response to a picture or story that would not usually stimulate other children to discuss death-related topics.

family crisis An event occurring when a family encounters problems that for a time seem insurmountable and with which the family is unable to cope in its usual ways.

hospice care A philosophy of care that focuses on helping persons with short life expectancies to live their remaining lives to the fullest—without pain and with choices and dignity.

palliative care Active and compassionate therapies intended to comfort and support those with short life expectancies.

stranger anxiety Wariness of strange people and places, often shown by infants between 6 and 18 months of age.

support systems The extended network of family, friends, and religious and community contacts that provide nurturance, emotional support, and direct assistance to parents.

MediaLink 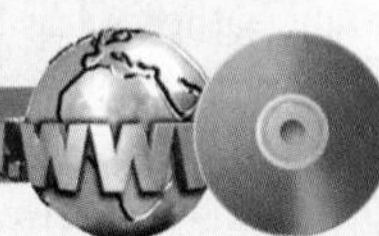

http://www.prenhall.com/ball

Resources for this chapter can be found on the CD-ROM accompanying this textbook, and on the Companion Website at http://www.prenhall.com/ball. Click on Chapter 8 to select the activities for this chapter.

CD-ROM

Audio Glossary

NCLEX Review

COMPANION WEBSITE

Web Links

NCLEX Review

MediaLink Applications

Helping Families Grieve

What stressors do children like Jeremiah face after admission to the PICU? What strategies can you use to help such critically ill or injured children cope with the experience? What stressors will parents face during the initial period when you work with them? How can you intervene to help them in this crisis? What strategies should be used to help siblings understand what has happened to their brother or sister? This chapter will enable you to answer these questions and will assist you in providing supportive care to critically ill and injured children like Jeremiah and to their families.

The intense emotional and physical demands placed on the critically ill or injured child present a challenge to nurses' attempts to provide developmentally appropriate care. The child's parents and siblings are confronted with a stressful situation. A family-centered model of nursing practice offers a framework for performing interventions that help to minimize stress and enhance coping by parents, siblings, and the ill or injured child.

LIFE-THREATENING ILLNESS OR INJURY

A threat to a child's life may be expected, as in a chronic illness or progressive disabling disease, or unexpected, as in an unintentional injury. How children, parents, and siblings cope with the threat will depend on the anticipated or unanticipated nature of the event and the conditions surrounding the child's admission to the hospital.

When death results from a chronic disease or terminal illness, the child and family have time to adjust to the impending death. Parents can become involved in the child's therapy as integral members of the treatment team. Emergency admission for an acute illness or unintentional injury, on the other hand, brings with it sudden stressors as the child and family are thrust into an unfamiliar environment, confronted with frightening or invasive procedures, and faced with an uncertain outcome.

Nursing care of children and families coping with specific chronic diseases or terminal illnesses such as cancer, cystic fibrosis, or muscular dystrophy is discussed elsewhere in this book. The following discussion focuses on care of children with life-threatening illnesses or injuries and care of the dying child.

CHILD'S EXPERIENCE

Admission to the hospital, emergency department, or PICU is one of the most frightening experiences a child can have. The critically ill child may appear extremely anxious and fearful, or withdrawn, solemn, and preoccupied with his or her physical condition. The illness or injury often brings pain, decreases energy, and changes the child's level of consciousness. Younger children may be unable to understand what is happening to them. The environment appears overwhelming, fast paced, and frightening. The child's normal sleep patterns can be disrupted because of the lack of day–night patterns in many intensive care units. Being cared for by strangers produces anxiety in the child. The child's limited ability to move intensifies feelings of powerlessness and vulnerability. An increased incidence of posttraumatic stress disorder (PTSD) has been noted in children with life-threatening illnesses and injuries (see Chapter 24).

Children's responses to stress are influenced by their developmental levels, past experiences, types of illness, coping mechanisms, and available emotional support. Nurses must consider how the child's developmental level and coping skills will influence his or her ability to deal with the PICU experience. Successful coping can provide the child with the skills to handle difficult situations in the future.

> **RESEARCH**
>
> Injured children requiring hospitalization for injury are at risk for posttraumatic stress disorder (PTSD). Variables predictive of PTSD include child acute stress, parental stress, and the degree of the psychological trauma exposure. One study reported 12.5% of injured children met diagnostic criteria for PTSD at 1 month after the injury (Daviss et al., 2000).

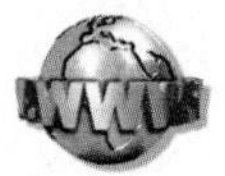

Resources for Critically Ill Children

STRESSORS TO THE CHILD

The four most significant stressors for hospitalized children of all ages are (1) separation from parents or the primary caretaker, (2) loss of self-control, autonomy, and privacy, (3) being subjected to multiple painful and invasive procedures, and (4) fear of bodily injury and disfigurement. Table 8-1 highlights key stressors of hospitalization for children at each developmental stage.

In addition to dealing with these stressors, the critically ill child experiences an intense emotional and physical threat to his or her well-being.

TABLE 8-1 Stressors of Hospitalization for Children in Various Developmental Stages

STAGES	RESPONSES
Infant	
Separation anxiety	Has disrupted sleep–awake cycle
Stranger anxiety	Has disrupted feeding routines
Painful, invasive procedures	Shows excessive irritability
Immobilization	
Sleep deprivation, sensory overload	
Toddler	
Separation anxiety	Is frightened if forced to lie supine
Loss of self-control	Associates pain with punishment
Immobilization	Wonders why parents don't come to the rescue
Painful, invasive procedures	
Bodily injury or mutilation	
Fear of the dark	
Preschooler	
Separation anxiety and fear of abandonment	Has difficulty separating reality from fantasy
Loss of self-control	Fears ghosts and monsters
Bodily injury or mutilation	Fears body parts will leak out
Painful, invasive procedures	Fears that tubes are permanent
Fear of the dark, ghosts, and monsters	Shows withdrawal, projection, aggression, regression
School-Age Child	
Loss of control	Shows increased sensitivity to the environment
Loss of privacy and control over bodily functions	Has detailed recall of events to self and other patients
Bodily injury	
Painful, invasive procedures	
Fear of death	
Adolescent	
Loss of control	Shows denial, regression, withdrawal
Fear of altered body image, disfigurement, disability, and death	Shows intellectualization, projection, displacement
Separation from peer group	
Loss of privacy and identity	

An unanticipated admission places the child at emotional risk for several reasons, including the lack of preparation for the experience, the uncertainty and unpredictability of events that follow, the unfamiliarity of the environment, and the heightened anxiety of parents. An admission for exacerbation of a disease such as cystic fibrosis or leukemia can provoke feelings of depression or hopelessness.

Infant

After 3 months of age, most infants have started to develop a sense of object permanence (the knowledge that an object or person continues to exist when not seen, felt, or heard) and corresponding trust in parents and familiar caretakers. This makes separation from parents an anxiety-producing experience (see Chapter 5). In addition to separation anxiety, infants between 6 and 18 months of age may display **stranger anxiety** (wariness of strangers) when confronted with health care professionals. Other stressors to the infant include painful procedures, immobilization of extremities, and sleep deprivation caused by disruption of normal rhythms and patterns (Figure 8-1 ◆).

Toddler

Toddlers are the group most at risk for a stressful experience as a result of illness. They lack cognitive ability to understand the reason for hospitalization. Separation from parents is extremely distressing to toddlers, and they protest vigorously when their parents depart. The

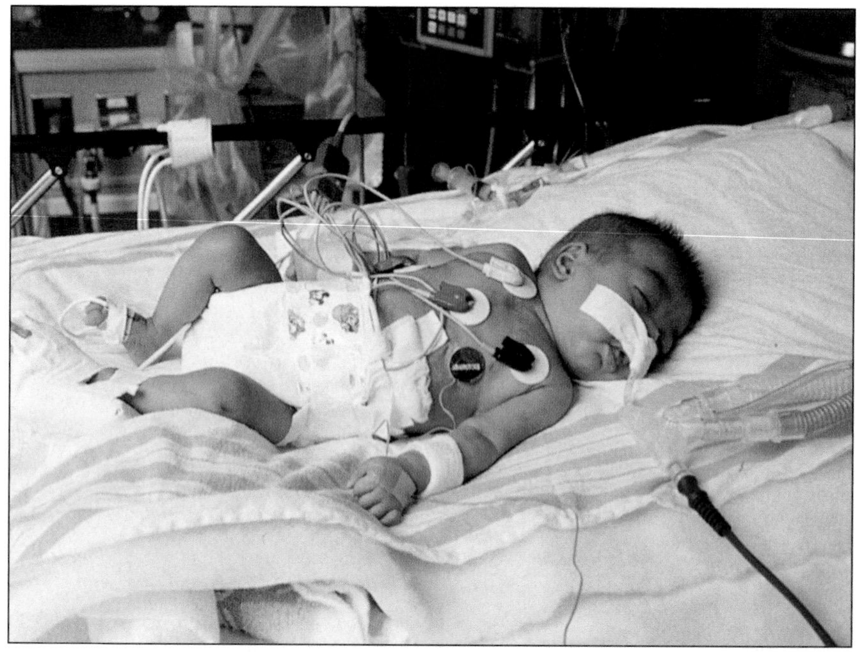

FIGURE 8-1 ◆
Jooti feels pain, hears noises, has her sleep disrupted, and has limited mobility because of all the equipment attached to her. What care and comfort can you offer parents who see their child like this?

toddler often becomes upset when known routines are altered. Having activities limited and being confined especially threaten children in this age group. Fear of pain, fear of the dark, and fear of invasive procedures and mutilation are common.

Preschooler

The greatest stressors to preschoolers are fear of being alone, fear of the dark, fear of abandonment, fear of loss of self-control related to the body and emotions, and fear of bodily injury or mutilation. They may feel guilty about getting sick. Waking up in the PICU and feeling the presence of an endotracheal, nasogastric, or chest tube, along with intravenous, arterial, and urinary catheters, is terrifying to the preschooler.

School-Age Child

Major sources of stress for school-age children are loss of control related to bodily functions, privacy issues, fear of bodily injury, and concerns related to death. School-age children attempt to maintain their composure during painful or invasive procedures but generally still require a great deal of support.

Adolescent

Major stressors to adolescents are separation from the peer group, issues of control and related dependency, privacy, changes in body image, disability, and death. Adolescents often try to maintain rigid self-control when undergoing painful and invasive procedures.

GROWTH & DEVELOPMENT 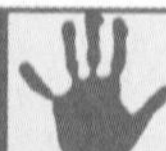

Coping behavior is influenced by maturation, cognitive development (increased attention span, problem-solving ability, and understanding of cause and effect), and increased impulse control. Young children use more behavioral strategies and ventilate feelings (Ryan-Wenger, 1996).

COPING MECHANISMS

Coping refers to the cognitive and behavioral responses that manage specific internal and external demands exceeding a person's resources, thus enabling the person to solve problems and to respond emotionally. The child may mirror the parents' behaviors and responses, which may help or hinder the child's response to stress. The child's temperament, previous coping experiences, and availability of support systems all combine to influence his or her ability to cope with the current experience.

The nature and severity of the illness and an emergency admission to the hospital stress a child's coping capabilities. Defense mechanisms displayed by children in these situations include regression, or return to an earlier behavior (a common reaction to stress), denial, repression (involuntary forgetting), postponement, and bargaining.

NURSING MANAGEMENT

Nursing Assessment and Diagnosis

Nursing assessment involves, in addition to physiologic parameters, skilled observation of the child's psychosocial and emotional needs. It is important for the nurse to understand normal psychosocial and cognitive development in order to plan developmentally appropriate interventions. Assessment should include the child's response to illness, the environment, coping strategies, and the need for information and support.

The accompanying nursing care plan includes common nursing diagnoses for the child who is coping with a critical illness or injury. The following nursing diagnoses may also be appropriate:

- *Impaired verbal communication* related to the effects of endotracheal intubation and mechanical ventilation
- *Impaired social interaction* related to separation from family and friends
- *Spiritual distress* related to the crisis of illness or suffering
- *Ineffective family coping: compromised,* related to the critical illness of the child
- *Impaired physical mobility: level 2,* related to trauma, musculoskeletal impairment, and pain
- *Sleep pattern disturbance* related to circadian asynchrony, excessive stimulation, pain, and anxiety caused by the critical care unit environment
- *Diversional activity deficit* related to forced inactivity
- *Altered growth and development* related to critical illness or injury, and multiple caretakers
- *Body image disturbance* related to loss of body function, severe trauma, or invasive procedures
- *Self-esteem: situational low,* related to hospitalization, or loss of independence and autonomy
- *Hopelessness* related to critical illness, deteriorating physical condition, or prolonged activity restrictions creating isolation
- *Anticipatory grieving* related to potential loss of body function or impending death of self

Planning and Implementation

Nursing care focuses on promoting a sense of trust, providing education about the illness or injury, preparing the child for procedures, facilitating the use of play, and promoting a sense of control. Children admitted to a PICU are presented with a traumatic experience for which they need support. Nurses play a key role in providing developmentally appropriate support to the child. Nursing interventions are directed at building a trusting relationship, minimizing the stressors experienced by the child, and promoting coping. Ongoing reassessment of progress in meeting the child's needs is critical. Honesty in all discussions is key to building trust with the child. The accompanying nursing care plan also summarizes nursing care for the child who is coping with a life-threatening illness or injury.

Promote a Sense of Security

For children of all ages, feeling secure depends on a sense of physical and psychologic safety. A sense of physical security is difficult to attain within the PICU because of the constant barrage of procedures that are part of the child's treatment plan. A sense of psychologic safety is best achieved by the presence of parents. An open visitation policy that enables parents to be at the bedside is optimal. Including parents as partners in the child's care provides comfort and reassurance to the child. Children whose parents have high anxiety levels pick up their parents' emotional cues and become more anxious. Interventions to lower the parents' anxiety may benefit the child (Melnyk & Alpert-Gillis, 1998). Consistency of staff is invaluable in developing familiarity and a trusting relationship with the child.

NURSING CARE PLAN The Child Coping with a Life-Threatening Illness or Injury

GOAL	INTERVENTION	RATIONALE	EXPECTED OUTCOME
1. Anxiety (child) related to separation from parents, foreign environment, strangers as caretakers, invasive procedures			
	NIC Priority Intervention: **Anxiety Reduction:** Minimizing apprehension, dread, foreboding, or uneasiness related to an unidentified source of anticipated danger.		NOC Suggested Outcome: **Anxiety Control:** Ability to eliminate or reduce feelings of apprehension and tension from unidentified source.
The child will exhibit or express an increased sense of security.	■ Encourage parents to remain at bedside (open visitation) and to participate in the child's care by touching, talking to, reading to, and singing to the child. ■ Talk with the child. Avoid discussions at bedside that the child should not overhear. ■ Offer to arrange a visit from the chaplain or other spiritual support. ■ Provide the child with developmentally appropriate explanations when possible, encourage the child to ask questions, and express concerns. ■ Prepare child in advance for procedures using developmentally appropriate techniques. ■ Make the child's bedside more personal and familiar by encouraging parents to bring in security objects, family photos, and favorite toys from home. ■ Involve the child in play appropriate to developmental age (see Chapter 5). ■ Provide care using a primary nursing care model.	■ Presence of parents is comforting to the child. ■ The child may overhear and remember, even if unconscious. ■ Spiritual support often provides comfort and sustenance in a time of crisis. ■ Information reduces anxiety and builds trust. ■ Preparation decreases anxiety related to the unknown. ■ Security objects decrease foreignness of hospital environment. The child derives comfort from presence of personal items. ■ Play provides familiarity, decreases fantasy, and provides motor activity. ■ Consistency in caregivers helps to build the child's trust.	■ The child appears more relaxed, acknowledges parents' presence, and behavioral manifestations of anxiety are absent.
2. Powerlessness (moderate) related to inability to communicate, and control relinquished to the health care team			
	NIC Priority Intervention: **Self-esteem Facilitation:** Encouraging a patient to assume more responsibility for own behavior.		NOC Suggested Outcome: **Health Beliefs: Perceived Control:** Personal conviction that one can influence an outcome.
The child or adolescent will have an increased sense of control over the situation.	■ Provide opportunities for choices when possible. ■ Encourage participation in self-care. ■ Prepare the child or adolescent in advance (timing dependent on developmental level) for procedures. Describe the sensations that will be experienced. Allow some choice in timing or method of pain relief.	■ Such opportunities provide sense of control and autonomy through decision making. ■ Information provides anticipatory guidance and a sense of involvement and value to the child.	The child or adolescent expresses satisfaction over ability to control some elements of situation.

(continued)

NURSING CARE PLAN The Child Coping with a Life-Threatening Illness or Injury (continued)

GOAL	INTERVENTION	RATIONALE	EXPECTED OUTCOME
2. Powerlessness (moderate) related to inability to communicate, and control relinquished to the health care team (continued)			
	■ Provide routines for the child both within a 24-hour period and for scheduled care. Tell the child before the procedure (timing is dependent upon developmental level), repeat explanation of why procedure is necessary, complete procedure in a consistent manner, and offer praise or a special story when completed. When possible, incorporate rituals from home. ■ Encourage play as a means of expressing feelings. ■ Provide other means of communication to the intubated child (e.g., a word board or finger board). ■ For the child requiring restraints, use as seldom as possible, provide appropriate explanations, and release at regular intervals. Wrapping IV lines well and using armboards can help maintain lines and avoid restraints.	■ Self-control is maintained through rituals. ■ Play is a normal activity for children and provides freedom of expression. ■ Maintaining communication provides autonomy and independence for the child. ■ Release from restraints helps diminish the sense of powerlessness that accompanies their use.	
3. Pain related to injuries, invasive procedures, surgery			
	NIC Priority Intervention: **Pain Management:** Alleviation of pain or a reduction in pain to a level of comfort that is acceptable to the patient.		NOC Suggested Outcome: **Comfort Level:** Feelings of physical and psychologic ease.
The child will experience reduced pain and improved comfort.	■ Assess the child's pain: location, intensity, what makes it better or worse. ■ If appropriate, use pain assessment scale (see **Chapter 9**). ■ Prepare the child for procedures. Be honest in explanations and use developmentally appropriate language and format. Describe the sensations that the child will feel, smell, taste, or see. Comfort the child after the procedures. Provide rest periods between procedures. ■ Provide optimal pain relief with prescribed analgesics. Provide comfort measures—position changes, backrubs, etc. Provide diversional activities as appropriate or possible. Incorporate the family in pain relief modality.	■ Assessment provides baseline information from which a plan of care can be developed. ■ Use of scale provides continuity and consistency in monitoring of the child's pain. ■ Information reduces anxiety and fear associated with the unknown and helps the child maintain self-control. ■ Physiologic and psychologic methods of pain control can be used in combination to maximally improve outcomes.	The child experiences a perceived or actual improvement in comfort level.

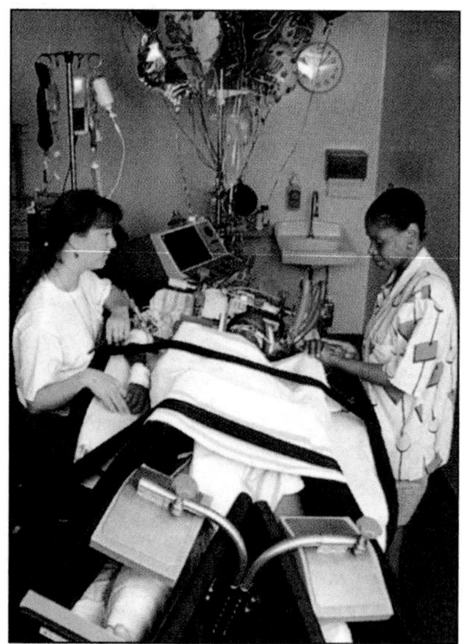

FIGURE 8-2 ◆
By their very nature, PICUs are ominous and sterile. To lessen this effect, it can help to personalize the child's space. Being there with the child and parent, answering questions, or just talking can be a comfort to both.

Personalizing the child's bedside can promote comfort and a sense of security for the child. Pictures from home, a favorite blanket or toy, music tapes, or posters can make the environment friendlier and more familiar to the child (Figure 8-2 ◆). Religious or spiritual icons may also provide psychological support.

Provide Education About the Illness or Injury and Prepare the Child for Procedures

Children's understanding of the cause of the illness and its therapy depends on their cognitive abilities. Explain to younger children that illness and hospitalization are not punishments.

Preparation for procedures is important at all ages, even for the unconscious or sedated child. The timing of this preparation depends on the child's cognitive level. Generally, the younger the child, the shorter the interval should be between the time of the teaching and the actual procedure (see Chapter 5).

Children often are able to feel and hear even when unconscious, so touch and verbal interchanges are important. Toddlers will benefit from being talked to, soothed, and touched during and after the procedure. Provide preschoolers, school-age children, and adolescents with an explanation of the sensations they can expect to experience (temperature, vibrations, sounds, smells, tastes, sight). This information may reduce their stress more than complete details about the procedures (LaMontagne, 1993). In any explanations to the child, avoid medical jargon; use simple language appropriate to the child's developmental level.

Facilitate the Use of Play

The use of play is important in alleviating stress and helping children to prepare for procedures. It is also another way for the nurse to assess the child's developmental level. Therapeutic play adds familiarity, diminishes fantasies, provides motor activity, and helps the child develop a sense of mastery (see Chapter 5). Children who are immobilized by tubes and restraints can still feel a sense of accomplishment, for example, by completing a puzzle, even if the nurse points to each piece and, through nods and gestures, indicates where it should be placed. Play can help children work through a painful situation, making it more tolerable.

Promote a Sense of Control

Children between toddlerhood and adolescence experience a loss of control during a life-threatening illness. This loss of control may be related to the body, emotions, normal routines, or privacy. Nursing interventions should promote a sense of control over these areas.

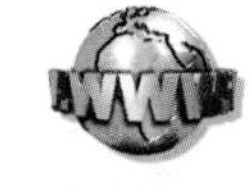

Restraint Use

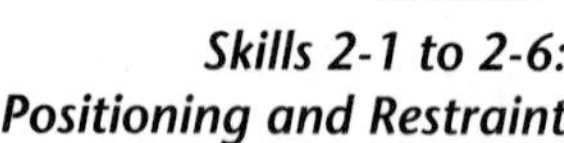

Skills 2-1 to 2-6: Positioning and Restraint

Allow the child choices when possible. Even the simple choice of which arm will receive a new intravenous line can help the child feel in control. Scheduling routine activities and treatments at the same time each day adds predictability and lessens anxiety. Limited mobility and the use of restraints, although sometimes necessary, contribute to the child's sense of powerlessness. The Joint Commission on Accreditation of Health Care Organizations requires that hospitals have policies and procedures in place for the use of restraints. If restraints must be used, plan to release them regularly for short periods. Restrain all children as little as possible, and explain the rationale for restraints, emphasizing that they are not a punishment. Provide diversional activities for the child, for example, by reading stories, playing music, or watching videotapes (see Chapter 5).

Enhance the child's coping skills by teaching the child and family a combination of relaxation, visual imagery, or distraction techniques, and comforting self-talk phrases such as, "This will be over soon. If I stay calm, it will be all right. It will be over faster and then I can do something fun." Help the parents become the child's coping coaches.

Evaluation

Expected outcomes of nursing care include the following:

- A trusting relationship is developed with the child and family.
- The child's social interactions, coping, and growth and development are promoted through diversional activites.
- The child's and family's coping is promoted through education and preparation for procedures.

PARENTS' EXPERIENCE

Families have different reactions and coping mechanisms when challenged. Children who are hospitalized for a critical illness cannot be adequately cared for if their families' needs are not met. Not only will parents find it difficult to support the child if their own needs are not met, but they also can transmit their anxiety to the child, who then becomes even more anxious.

WHAT MAKES A PROBLEM A CRISIS?

A **family crisis** occurs when a family encounters a problem that seems insurmountable and with which the family cannot cope in its usual ways. The critical care environment and the implications of a life-threatening illness or injury are far removed from the everyday experiences of most families. The unfamiliarity of the environment and the uncertainty and seriousness of the illness or injury create a crisis for the family.

Unexpected illness or injury adds another dimension of stress, as families have little time to prepare for the experience. A sudden admission threatens family integrity, causing enormous stress and separation from loved ones. The interruption of the unique parent–child relationship can be more stressful to parents than the physical PICU environment. Stresses are intensified when divorce, separation, and stepparenting are involved. Other current family stresses such as financial problems, long distance from home to hospital, or another family member with an illness can add to the state of crisis.

REACTIONS TO LIFE-THREATENING ILLNESS OR INJURY

How do parents react to a threat to their child's life? What parental behaviors might nurses see when a child is critically ill or injured? Parents typically progress through stages that might include shock and disbelief; anger and guilt; deprivation and loss; anticipatory waiting; and readjustment or mourning.

Shock and Disbelief

The universal reaction of parents is shock and disbelief. As the familiar is disrupted, parents experience a loss of control, an inability to regain their bearings, and feelings of immobility. The hospital environment, emergency department, or PICU may seem unreal. The emotions parents experience initially are intensified by the physical appearance of their child (particularly after traumatic injury); the presence of monitors, tubing, and equipment; and the actual injury or illness (Figure 8-3 ◆). As the mother of a 5-year-old trauma patient said, "I felt distanced, in a daze, in and out of it that first day after the accident."

The stage of shock and disbelief begins in the first few moments after hearing the "news" and can last for days. The shock helps postpone the full impact of the crisis. For most parents,

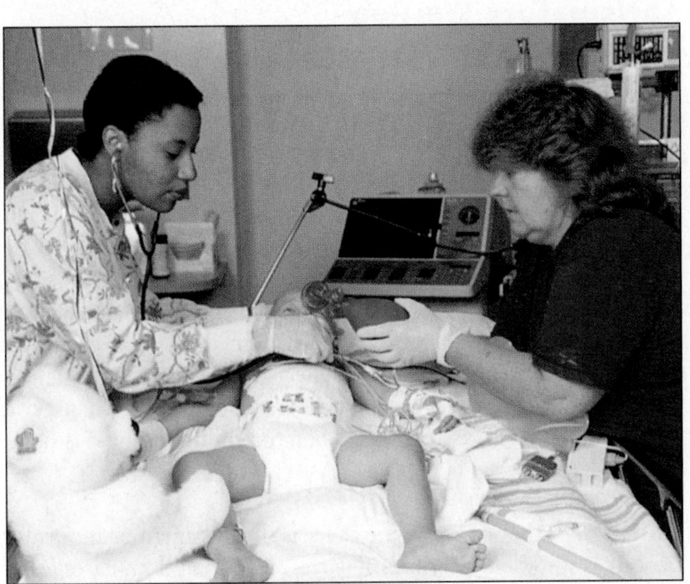

FIGURE 8-3 ◆ Procedures done in the PICU, such as mechanical ventilation, are frightening for parents. Treat the child first, but also remember the needs, fears, and anxieties of the parents and other family members. Anticipating the family's needs and keeping them informed will help them adjust.

however, the overwhelming sense of shock passes during the first 24 hours. During this period, parents grope for answers and explanations about the illness or injury. Information must be repeated many times to parents, since in this stage they are often unable to assimilate information easily.

Anger and Guilt

Anger and guilt surface as parents become more aware of their child's illness or injury. Their anger may be directed toward themselves, each other, health care providers, or other children or parents, as in the case of a motor vehicle crash involving a group of teenagers. Parents may also be angry with their child. This anger may be a result of injuries the child sustained when breaking known rules such as drinking and driving, playing with matches, or riding a bike without a helmet. Lastly, the anger may not be directed at anyone specifically. Injuries caused by natural disasters such as an earthquake, flood, or hurricane provoke just as much anger as those that result from the actions of people. This may create a challenge to the parents' spiritual beliefs.

Parents typically react to their child's illness or injury with some degree of guilt. This reaction may be magnified in the intensive care environment. The fact that the guilt usually has no basis in real events does not lessen the feeling. A question parents frequently ask at this stage is, "Why not me instead of my child?" Parents' feelings of guilt may have one of two causes:

1. *They may feel responsible for causing the illness or injury.* Statements such as, "If only I hadn't sent him to the store on his bike, this wouldn't have happened," or, from the father of a 2-year-old who nearly drowned, "Maybe if I hadn't been working, he would have been in my care and this wouldn't have happened," reflect feelings of guilt for causing or failing to prevent the injury.
2. *They may feel guilty about not noticing the onset of an illness or disregarding earlier symptoms of an illness.* The mother of a 1-year-old with *Haemophilus influenzae* meningitis repeatedly said, "I shouldn't have waited so long to take her to the doctor!"

Deprivation and Loss

As the shock slowly recedes, parents enter a stage of deprivation and loss related to their parental role. Within minutes or hours, parents have gone from the familiar role of being a parent of a healthy child to the unexpected and unfamiliar role of being a parent of a critically ill child. Parents have compared this deprivation and loss to that experienced when a family member dies.

Parents' difficulties and ambivalence in releasing to strangers a part of their responsibility as the child's primary caretakers can threaten their self-esteem and self-control. Moreover, if parents cannot participate in the child's care, they may feel helpless or worthless.

Anticipatory Waiting

Once the child's condition is stabilized and survival seems likely, parents often move into a period of anticipatory waiting. This stage is characterized as "life suspended in time." Parents spend a great deal of time waiting: for test results, for explanations, for their child to become conscious, or for surgery to be over. Parents may fear leaving the area because they may miss an important procedure, physician visit, or decisions or changes in treatment. Lack of mobility decreases the parents' use of typical coping mechanisms, so anxiety and the sense of powerlessness may increase. A pager system has been adopted in some facilities to give parents freedom to take breaks away from the child's bedside, knowing they will be alerted to important events (Ashenberg, Lambert, & Maier, et al., 1996).

Parents may have a preoccupation with medical details. During this period, parents may ask questions about the long-term effects of the illness or injury on the child, about the potential for brain damage, or about the need for additional surgeries. Parents may place demands on staff and be frustrated when the child's progress is slow.

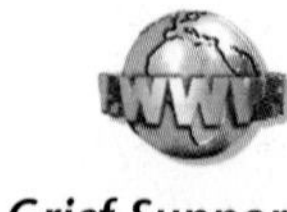

Grief Support

Readjustment or Mourning

The last stage that parents experience is readjustment or mourning. Readjustment is experienced as the child recovers, improves steadily, and prepares for transfer and discharge. In

TABLE 8-2 Parental Needs During Hospitalization of a Critically Ill or Injured Child

INFORMATION (THE MOST IMPORTANT IDENTIFIED NEED)
■ Information and frequent updates about the child's condition. Repeat the information and provide other materials frequently as parents forget or cannot concentrate on details with all their stress ■ Explanations they can understand about the child's condition, equipment being used, and procedures of care ■ Discussion with a physician or care manager daily ■ General information about unit policies, team members, phone numbers, etc.
PROXIMITY
■ Permission to remain at the bedside ■ Permission to touch and speak with the child ■ Open, flexible visiting hours
REESTABLISHMENT OF THE PARENTAL CONTROL
■ Recognition as important to the child's recovery ■ Recognition as the decision maker of the child's treatment options
PARTICIPATION IN THE CHILD'S CARE
■ Performance of care (bathing, diaper changes, feeding, range of motion exercises, massages, hair care) ■ Provision of comfort measures (reading, singing, telling stories, touching, talking) ■ Explanation of equipment and procedures to the child to decrease the child's fears
CONFIDENCE IN THE TREATMENT PLAN AND CAREGIVERS
■ Continuity in staffing and health care contacts ■ Evidence that staff care about the child ■ Assurance that the child is receiving appropriate treatment and pain management
PSYCHOLOGIC SUPPORT
■ Acknowledgment that the situation is difficult ■ Help to focus on the positive or unchanged aspects of the child's appearance ■ Rest and nutrition to maintain physical resources necessary for coping ■ Space and privacy as needed ■ Hope—an essential component of coping ■ Choice of other family members to be present ■ Preparation for responses of siblings and the long-term emotional responses of the child patient

contrast, parents of the child who dies reenter the cycle of emotions characteristic of grief. Mourning also occurs when the child remains seriously ill or unresponsive, when the outcome remains uncertain for an extended period, or when long-term care is required. Table 8-2 lists the most important needs of parents during a child's critical illness or injury.

NURSING MANAGEMENT

Nursing Assessment and Diagnosis

Nurses who work with families of critically ill children have a unique opportunity to help them adapt and to promote family functioning. They begin by assessing the family's reaction to the illness, coping skills, stressors, and needs. This initial assessment provides a baseline of information for developing a care plan and strategies to meet the psychosocial and physiologic needs of families.

Several nursing diagnoses may apply to parents who are dealing with their child's critical illness or injury. They include the following:

- *Ineffective denial* related to knowledge deficit of the child's critical condition and uncertain prognosis
- *Altered family processes* related to the impact of a critically ill child on the family system

- *Parental role conflict* related to the child's critical illness or injury and PICU policies
- *Spiritual distress* related to the child's critical illness, suffering, or death
- *Disabling ineffective family coping* related to the child's severe or fatal illness
- *Family coping: potential for growth,* related to constructive crisis management
- *Fatigue* related to extreme stress, sleep deprivation, and crisis
- *Hopelessness* related to the child's deteriorating physiologic condition
- *Caregiver role strain* related to illness severity of the child
- *Anticipatory grieving* related to potential death of the child or loss of body functions

CLINICAL TIP 

Explain to the child and parents, in easy-to-understand terms, the purpose of equipment that is being used. Answer alarms quickly. Follow with an explanation of why alarms sound.

RESEARCH 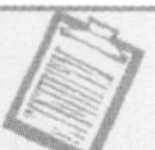

Several studies have revealed that many parents have strong preferences to be present during invasive procedures. One study found that parent preference to be present for specific procedures was as follows: 97.5% for venipuncture, 94.0% for laceration repair, 86.5% for lumbar puncture, and 80.9% for endotracheal intubation. Parents also expressed significant preference to be present during major resuscitation: 80.7% if the child is conscious, 71.4% if the child is unconscious, and 83.4% if the child is likely to die. Strategies to support family presence for these procedures must be developed (Boie, Moore, Bruimmett, & Nelson, 1999).

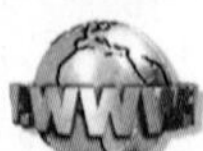

Coping and Respite

CLINICAL TIP 

Encourage parents to take time for themselves to be alone, alternating times to be away for a short time. Suggest places they can go such as a lounge, chapel, or courtyard. Provide parents with a beeper, if possible, to reduce anxiety when they are away from the unit.

Planning and Implementation

Nursing care focuses on providing information and building trust, promoting parental involvement, providing for physical and emotional needs, facilitating positive staff–parent relationships and communication, and maintaining or strengthening family support systems. Ongoing reassessment provides a measure with which to evaluate the family's ability to manage the crisis. The best way to meet the needs of families, minimize stress, and enhance family coping is to provide care using a family-centered approach (Hazinski, 1999; also see Table 1–1). The challenge to nurses is to blend and balance technology with caring.

Provide Information and Build Trust

The information given to parents must be provided frequently and accurately. Information on the child's illness, condition, and plan of care should be delivered in a manner and language readily understandable to parents. Upon admission, parents need to be given an idea of what to expect in the days ahead and be prepared for special procedures or major changes in therapy that may become necessary.

Honesty in discussions with parents is extremely important. If parents feel misled or that information is being withheld, a trusting relationship will be impossible. Informed parents, on the other hand, will feel that they are active participants in decision making and care planning for their child. Trust is facilitated when parents believe that the staff truly cares about the child and sees him or her as an individual, special child.

Parents also need a sense of hope regarding their child's illness to help them cope. Focus on the positives as the child progresses through the different phases of the critical illness.

Promote Parental Involvement

An important role of nurses is to encourage and strengthen parents in their parenting role. The parents' place when possible is at the bedside—their very presence can comfort the child, minimize fears, and reduce the child's experiences with pain during invasive procedures. They provide continuity and may notice subtle changes that a newly assigned nurse may miss (Giganti, 1998). Parents' needs are best met when they are encouraged to participate in their child's care (Scott, 1998).

If the child is in the PICU, parents need to be prepared before they see their child for the first time. Tell them what tubes and monitors are present and how their child will look and react. Throughout the child's hospitalization, parents will continue to need reassurance and encouragement. Open visitation by parents is important to maintain their parenting role.

Provide for Physical and Emotional Needs

The experience of having a child with a critical illness drains parents' physical and emotional reserves. Parents often need encouragement to take care of themselves. A statement such as, "It is important for you to eat and rest because Jeremiah is really going to need you when he wakes up," helps parents to realize that becoming exhausted benefits neither them nor the child.

Orienting parents to the hospital, as well as to the unit routines, helps them to adapt to their surroundings. Many communities now have Ronald McDonald houses—an inexpensive but warm and supportive environment for parents of ill children (Figure 8-4 ◆). When financial burdens are a consideration, family and social service referrals may be needed.

Parents are often at different levels of coping during a crisis. The child's critical illness may foster cohesion between the couple and build a stronger relationship. Unfortunately, the reverse may also be true—differences in styles or levels of coping may foster a sense of isolation, placing a strain on the couple's relationship. Nurses should be alert to family dynamics and refer the family for counseling or therapy, if indicated.

Facilitate Positive Staff–Parent Relationships and Communication

Given the intensity of the parents' experience when their child is critically ill, it is easy to see how problems can arise between staff and parents. Each health care team member must be aware of the child's current status so that parents receive the same information from all staff. Consistency in the message can instill confidence. Provide explanations geared to the parents' level of understanding, using language the parents can understand.

Parents need to know who has the overall responsibility for the care of their child. They should be introduced to the nurse and physician who are responsible for the child's care. This is especially important in teaching hospitals that have rotating staff. The staff physician with the overall responsibility should meet with parents as often as necessary to talk about changes in the child's condition or treatment plan and to allow time for parents to ask questions (Figure 8-5 ◆). Encourage parents to keep a daily log or notebook to record information on the child's care, progress, and needs. Family care conferences can be helpful when a large number of team members provide care.

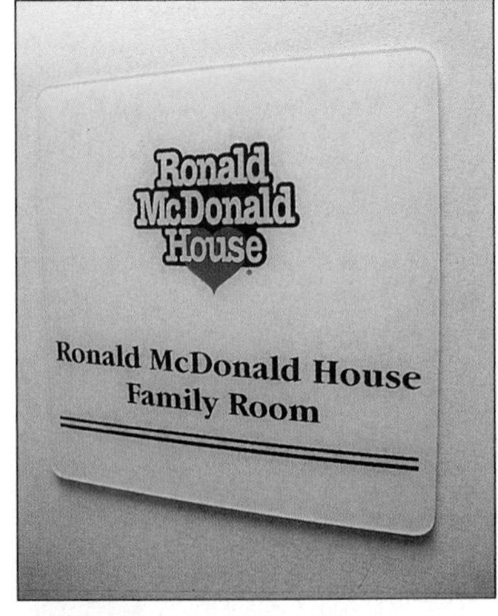

FIGURE 8-4 ◆
A Ronald McDonald family room in a large metropolitan hospital provides a comfortable setting where families of seriously ill children can go to get away from the high-tech hospital atmosphere while remaining near the ill child.

Maintain or Strengthen Family Support Systems

Support systems are the extended network of family, friends, and religious and community contacts that provide nurturance, emotional support, and direct assistance to parents, thus enabling them to cope with overwhelming problems and crises. Most parents indicate that having family or friends nearby is crucial as a support system.

Parents may need to be reassured that it is all right to ask for help from family, friends, or community services. They may be uncomfortable asking for help, instead attempting to handle multiple responsibilities themselves, often to the point of exhaustion. Some parents are unable to respond to offers of help because it requires too great a mental effort on their part.

Nurses may need to intervene on parents' behalf when they have inappropriate support (Tomlinson & Mitchell, 1992). Parents may be frustrated by people who come to visit unannounced, stay too long, or visit too often, and may find it difficult to tell well-meaning but

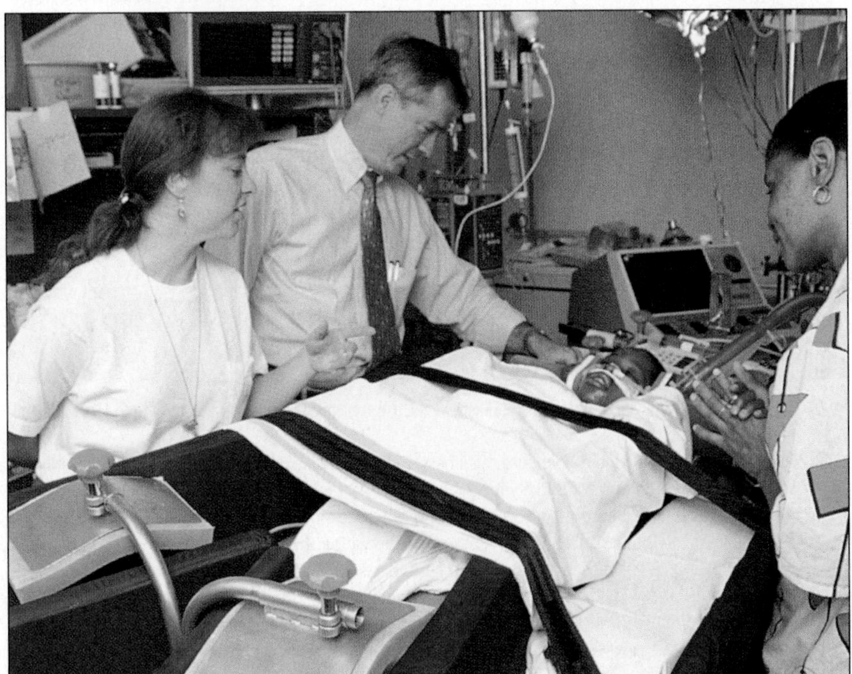

FIGURE 8-5 ◆
In times of crisis, everyone likes to know that someone is in charge and who that person is. The parents should meet and talk with the staff physician in charge and the nurses as often as possible. Parents need to know that someone is responsible, even if different people are providing care.

insensitive friends that they cannot deal with visitors right now. In these situations, offering to serve as a gatekeeper may be helpful.

Families of critically ill or dying children often have emotional needs beyond the support capabilities of the nurse caring for the child. Referrals to family and support services or pastoral care may be beneficial in these instances.

Evaulation

Expected outcomes of nursing care include the following:

- The nurse establishes a trusting relationship and effective communication with the family.
- Parents participate in their child's care as much as desired.
- Family members receive emotional support and nurturance needed to sustain them through their child's illness.

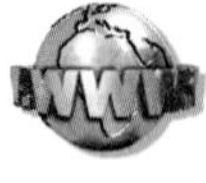

Support for Siblings

SIBLINGS' EXPERIENCE

As the parents' focus shifts to the critically ill child, they may need support in dealing with the healthy siblings. Siblings also need care and may feel left out when everyone's attention is focused on the ill child. Siblings of critically ill children may demonstrate behaviors ranging from jealousy or envy to resentment, guilt and hostility, anger, insecurity, regression, and fear. Recognize that siblings may fear becoming ill themselves or believe that they played a role in the child's illness. Siblings often have nightmares about the illness or injury their brother or sister has sustained and about the ill child dying.

Tell siblings about their brother or sister using language and concepts appropriate to their ages and developmental levels. As appropriate, siblings should be allowed to visit. Such a visit should be encouraged if the child could potentially die, to allow the sibling to say good-bye. These visits often help to lift the spirits of the ill child. Because children's fantasies are often worse than reality, unfounded fears may be relieved by a visit.

Preparation for the visit is important. Before the visit, talk with the siblings about what to expect and describe how their brother or sister will look. If the ill child acts, moves, talks, or looks different than usual, provide an explanation beforehand. Describe the hospital environment, including equipment, sounds, and smells. Using a doll, drawing pictures, or showing an actual picture of the child can help prepare the siblings. Table 8-3 summarizes strategies for working with siblings of an ill or injured child.

During the visit, demonstrate how to talk to and touch the ill child and encourage the siblings to do the same (Figure 8-6 ◆). After the visit, discuss with siblings what they saw and felt, and answer any questions they may have. When a sibling cannot visit, contact with the ill child can be maintained by sending pictures, drawings, cards, and messages recorded on audiotapes or videotapes (Figure 8-7 ◆).

If parents are staying at the hospital with the ill child, encourage them to call the siblings at home at a regular time each night. Allowing the siblings at home the opportunity to share their day, and to receive an update on the ill child, provides a feeling of connectedness. The

TABLE 8-3 Strategies for Working with Siblings of an Ill or Injured Child

- Be truthful. Tell why the child is hospitalized, what the treatment involves, and how long the hospitalization is expected to last.
- Assure siblings that they did not cause the illness and that the ill child did nothing wrong. If a sibling had some involvement in or responsibility for the health crisis, referral for psychological counseling is needed.
- Allow siblings to ask questions and state fears and other feelings.
- Allow siblings to visit if possible. Cover tubes and wires with a sheet. Wash off blood or cover bloody bandages if possible. Prepare them for any equipment, dressing, and procedures they might see.
- Warn siblings if the ill child is not speaking. Say something like, "John can't talk now. He seems to be sleeping deeply. He may be able to hear, though, so you can touch him and talk to him."
- Encourage siblings to express their feelings related to the disruptive effect of the child's hospitalization on family life.

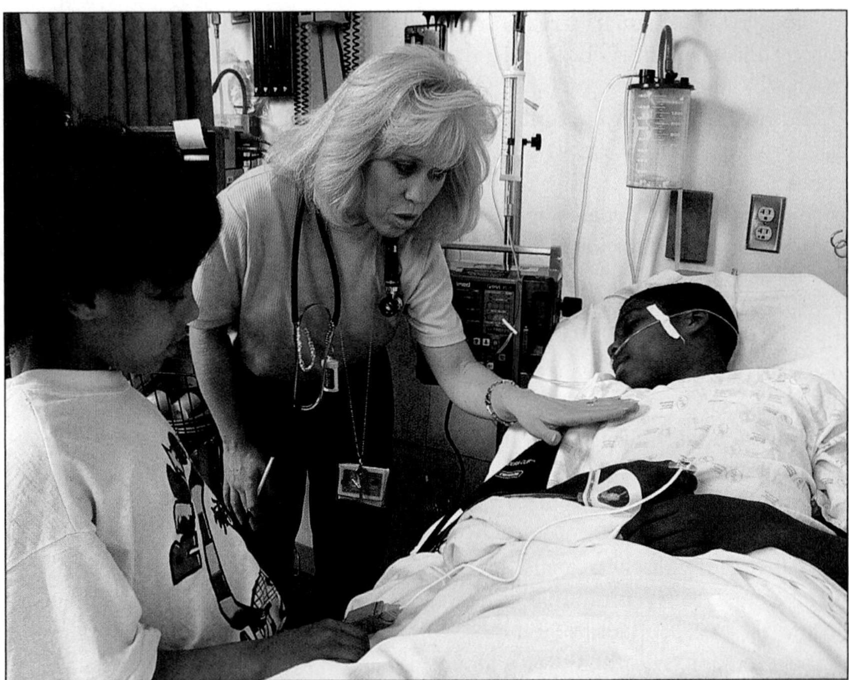

FIGURE 8-6 ◆
During the sibling's visit to the ill child, it is important to talk with the sibling and answer any questions asked in an honest manner at a level the child can understand.

phone call offers siblings a consistent link to the parent as well as the reassurance that they are important and loved.

BEREAVEMENT

PARENTS' REACTIONS

The death of one's child is probably the most painful experience for a parent. When the loss is sudden and unexpected, the abruptness adds a dimension of shock that may last for 4 to 5 weeks. The goal of the nurse in these situations is to provide comfort and support for the dying child and the family (Table 8-4). Staff education must be built on the premise that grief and mourning are normal, necessary processes.

Grief is painful, individualized, and exhausting. Many factors influence the parents' grief responses, including their perception of the preventability of the illness or injury, the suddenness and other circumstances of the death, the nature of their attachment to the child,

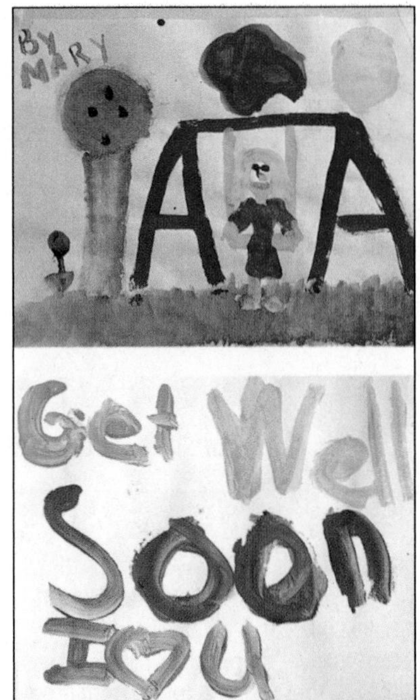

FIGURE 8-7 ◆
It is important that parents and siblings feel comfortable communicating with the seriously ill child. If siblings cannot visit, they should be encouraged to paint or record messages. They need to be able to express themselves and to feel that they are helping.

TABLE 8-4 Strategies for Working with Parents Whose Child Dies Suddenly

- Identify a spokesperson for the medical team to keep the family informed during resuscitation efforts. Have both parents present if possible.
- Provide private space with telephone access.
- Create time for families to assimilate the child's worsening status by providing several updates during the resuscitation. Prepare them for what is to come.
- Offer to telephone clergy, family, and friends.
- After the death, prepare the body for viewing.
- Provide time and a place for the family to say good-bye.
- Sit close, make eye contact. Share your emotions with the family. Accept whatever emotions family members express.
- Convey information to the family about the cause of death, autopsy, funeral preparations, and the normal grief process.
- Arrange for family follow-up to see how they are responding to the child's loss and to review autopsy findings.

Note: From "Helping parents cope with sudden death," by J.E. Anderson, 1996, *Contemporary Pediatrics, 13* (12), 42–57. Adapted.

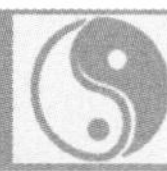

CULTURE

Many culturally influenced rules and customs surround dying. For instance, the Hmong belief system holds that children will live in eternity in the same state in which they existed at the time of death. Therefore it is important that the child's body be intact at death.

CLINICAL TIP

Questions to use with families whose child has died (Shaefer, 1999):

- I am sorry for your loss. How can I help?
- What are your traditions when an infant or child dies?
- Is there someone I can call for you?
- Has your family ever had this experience before?
- How did they handle it?
- Do you have a funeral service? Is it helpful?

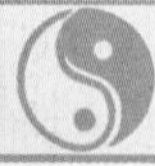

CULTURE

Always ask the parent before cutting a lock of the child's hair. Some cultures and religions, including Native American groups, forbid it (Nelson, 1995).

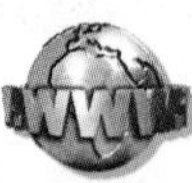

National Support Groups

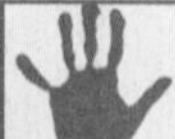

GROWTH & DEVELOPMENT

Children need to understand the finality of death—that all body functions have stopped. Simple statements that can be told to children include, "Adam's heart will never beat again," "He will never get cold or hungry," and "He will never come home again." These simple statements may need to be repeated several times, as young children will test to see if the same answers are given each time (Mahan, 1994).

previous losses, spiritual or religious orientation, and culture. Suicide produces agonizing anger, guilt, and confusion. The fact that the child ended his or her own life compounds the feelings of guilt.

Although parents progress through distinct stages of grief, the time line and nature of the grief process differ for each individual. The intense pain and shock initially felt by parents gradually give way to feelings of anger, guilt, depression, and loneliness. Very slowly, and with much support, energy returns and parents again begin to enjoy life experiences. Spouses may need additional support when they are at different levels of grieving to prevent a sense of loneliness and isolation.

Work closely with the family when the child's death is imminent, since they will remember the experience for the rest of their lives. Prepare the family for changes in the child's appearance and the events to follow. Providing parents with a room in which to be alone with the child ensures privacy at this extremely personal time. Ask the family in a nonjudgmental, supportive manner what is important to them in the last moments or hours of their child's life and what will be important to them in the grief process. Certain religious or cultural practices may need to be planned. Holding the child is a universal request and should be permitted. Many families find that saying good-bye as a group is helpful. Allowing the family to hold, kiss, and talk to the dying child can help grieving (Nelson, 1995). Encourage parents to continue in their parental role by continuing with caregiving activities such as bathing or dressing the child for the last time. See Table 8-5 for more common mourning and after-death rituals.

After the child's death, allow the family to spend as much time as they need with the child's body. Never rush family members who are saying good-bye to the child. Save all of the child's personal items—especially in the case of an infant, whose parents may have few mementos. A lock of hair, hand or foot prints, the infant's identification band, the child's weight and height, the last clothes or patient gown worn by the child sealed in a plastic bag to retain the child's scent, or a picture of the infant can be sources of comfort and remembrance for families. It may be traumatic to receive the child's possessions, and placing them in a plastic garbage bag is insensitive. When possible, a special container should be used for this purpose.

Parents may need direction about resources available to help with a memorial service or funeral. Information about organ and tissue donation, as well as the need for an autopsy, if required, needs to be discussed. Acknowledge with parents that certain dates—such as the day of the week the child died, the child's birthday, or family holidays—will be difficult and may trigger intense sadness again. Parents may benefit from keeping a journal of their thoughts and memories, or writing letters or poems to or about their child.

Emphasize to parents that although the period surrounding their child's death is difficult, caring for themselves physically and mentally is important. Parents may experience friction due to differing rates and intensity of grief. A list of appropriate support groups, books, and articles can be given to parents for later use. Parents can be referred to national organizations, such as the Candlelighters Foundation or Compassionate Friends, and to local support groups for bereaved parents or siblings. Some institutions have formal follow-up programs for bereaved parents to encourage a healthy progression through the grieving process.

SIBLINGS' REACTIONS

Siblings who experience the death of a brother or sister require supportive and compassionate care. In the course of the child's illness the siblings probably will have received less attention from parents. They may fear that they caused their brother or sister to be injured or become ill, or worry that bad thoughts on their part brought on the illness. They need help in adapting to their parents' distraction, grief, and increased protectiveness of them (McIntier, 1995; Schonfeld, 1993). Siblings need to hear that their parents' grief in no way diminishes the love they have for them. Table 8-6 highlights children's understanding of death at different developmental stages and some of the possible behavioral responses.

When talking with the siblings of a dying child, honesty is most important. Provide explanations in language that is developmentally appropriate. Reassure siblings that they did not cause their brother or sister to die and that death was not a punishment for wrongdoing. Allow the siblings to ask questions. Acknowledge the emotions they are feeling and emphasize that it is all right for them to be sad, angry, frightened, or tearful. Ask how they feel about

TABLE 8-5 Cultural Traditions in Mourning and After-Death Rites

RELIGIOUS GROUP	RITUALS YOU MIGHT OBSERVE	ORGAN DONATION OR AUTOPSY BELIEFS
American Indians	■ Beliefs and practices vary widely ■ Navajo do not touch the deceased or their belongings	Varies among tribes
Buddhism	■ Last-rite chanting at bedside ■ Cremation common	Organ donation considered act of mercy, autopsy individual choice
Catholicism	■ Sacrament of the sick ■ Obligated to take ordinary but not extraordinary means to prolong life ■ Burial usual	Autopsy, organ donation acceptable
Christian Science	■ Unlikely to seek medical help to prolong life ■ Disposal of body and parts decided by family	Individual decides about organ donation
Hinduism	■ No restrictions to right-to-die issue ■ Religious prayers chanted before and after death ■ Cremation common ■ Men and women display outward grief ■ Thread tied around wrist signifies a blessing, do not remove	Autopsy, organ donation acceptable
Islam	■ Attempts to shorten life prohibited ■ Body is washed only by Muslim of same gender	Organ donation acceptable Autopsy only for medical or legal reasons
Jehovah's Witness	■ Use of extraordinary means to prolong life is individual choice ■ Burial determined by family preference	Autopsy if required by law Organ donation forbidden
Judaism	■ If death is inevitable, no new procedures needed, but must continue those ongoing ■ Body ritually washed ■ Burial as soon as possible, all body parts must be buried together ■ Seven-day mourning period	Autopsy permitted in certain circumstances, organ donation is a complex issue
Mennonite	■ Do not believe life must be continued at all cost	Autopsy and organ donation acceptable
Mormonism	■ If death inevitable, promote a peaceful and dignified death ■ Burial in "temple clothes"	Autopsy permitted with permission of next of kin, organ donation is permitted
Protestantism	■ Burial or cremation is individual decision	Organ donation and autopsy are individual decisions
Seventh Day Adventist	■ Follow ethic of prolonging life ■ Disposal of body and burial are individual decisions	Autopsy, organ donation acceptable

Note: From *Cultural diversity in health and illness* (5th ed.), by R.E. Spector, 2000, Upper Saddle River, NJ: Prentice Hall Health, pp. 137–138, 144–149. Adapted.

saying good-bye to the dying child, and provide physical and emotional support. Prepare the siblings before they see the dying child by briefly explaining what they may see, feel, hear, and smell. Answer questions truthfully. You may have to repeat information several times.

As appropriate and comfortable, siblings should be permitted to participate in planning the child's memorial or funeral service. Use the same amount of energy and concern in acknowledging their grief as provided to adults. Being able to grieve as a family provides siblings with a sense of connectedness to parents and provides security at a vulnerable time. If siblings attend the funeral, prepare them for what to expect and provide a support person. Keep the family together as much as possible.

As with their parents, sibling bereavement is a lifelong process. Make sure other caregivers and teachers know about the sibling's loss. Let the child express feelings other than sadness (e.g., guilt and anger). Encourage them to express grief through art, stories, and writing. They may conceal their feelings and suppress their questions to protect their parents (Davies, 1997).

GROWTH & DEVELOPMENT

Children must also complete a grieving process. This is usually accomplished in three stages (Baker, Sedney, & Gross, 1992).

- Early stage: They understand the death occurred, while using self-protective mechanisms to block the full emotional impact of the loss.
- Middle stage: They accept and rework the loss while experiencing the intense psychologic pain.
- Late stage: They integrate the loss experience into their identity and resume age-appropriate developmental progress.

CULTURE

Depending on the family's cultural and religious beliefs, a chaplain or other health care professional who specializes in working with terminally ill children and families may help reduce a child's spiritual fears and promote peace and comfort among family members.

DYING CHILD

Care of the dying child presents one of the greatest challenges to the nurse, requiring the utmost sensitivity and compassion. A child's understanding of death varies according to developmental stages, as described in Table 8-6.

Children as young as 5 years of age can sense when they are seriously ill. A child's awareness of death develops more rapidly when he or she is experiencing the progression of a disease and related medical treatment. Children with life-threatening illnesses often learn about death and their own illness from exposure to other seriously ill and dying children when they are receiving treatment during hospitalization or clinic visits.

Preschool children can see their body deteriorate and feel the toxic effects of chemicals during disease progression and treatment. Changes in self-concept occur as they perceive

TABLE 8-6 Children's Understanding of Death and Possible Behavioral Responses

UNDERSTANDING OF DEATH	POSSIBLE BEHAVIORS
Infant	
■ Lacks understanding of concept of death ■ May sense caregivers are tense, routines are altered	■ May show sadness by turning away from your gaze ■ Resists cuddling and eats less, crying, clinging ■ Sleeps more
Toddler	
■ Unable to distinguish fact from fantasy ■ No understanding of true concept of death ■ Aware someone is missing—separation anxiety ■ Unable to distinguish death from temporary separation or abandonment	■ Clingy, refuses to let parent out of sight ■ Stops walking and talking ■ Shows distress by biting, hitting, tears ■ Fearfulness ■ Problems eating and sleeping
Preschooler	
■ Believes death is reversible, temporary ■ Believes bad thoughts cause death ■ Believes magical thinking can bring dead person back or can cause death to occur with thoughts ■ Has beginning experience with death of animals and plants	■ May fear going to sleep, has nightmares, afraid of dark ■ Out-of-control behavior, hyperactivity, tantrums, regression ■ Problems with bowel and bladder control ■ Crying spells ■ Seems morbidly fascinated with death ■ Asks lots of questions ■ Displays anger at failure to keep person "alive," breaks toys, is aggressive to friends
School-Age Child	
■ Acquires more realistic understanding of death ■ By 8–10 years, understands that death is permanent and irreversible, and that people die from internal and external causes ■ Believes that death is universal and will happen to him or her ■ May have exaggerated concerns about death	■ May deny sadness by hiding tears and acting more like adults ■ Difficulty concentrating on schoolwork ■ Psychosomatic complaints—tummy ache or headache ■ Acting-out behavior, anger at being abandoned ■ May try to comfort parents by taking over tasks
Adolescent	
■ Intellectually capable of understanding death ■ Has a better grasp of association between illness and death ■ Sense of invincibility conflicts with fear of death ■ Able to recognize effect of death on others	■ Same as school-age child ■ May have severe depression ■ Acting-out behavior—risk-taking behavior, delinquency, suicide attempts, promiscuity, pseudo-indifference

these body changes. They often describe their illness in terms of mutilation to their body. They may realize that they are dying because of these physical changes.

School-age children also have subtle fears about body integrity and anxieties about the seriousness of their illness. This greater preoccupation with illness is considered by many professionals as the child's version of **death anxiety,** a feeling of apprehension or fear of death. Death anxiety occurs in children even though they are unable to conceptualize or describe death at an adult's level of understanding. It can develop from the perception of loneliness associated with a separation from the known world. Children may express death anxiety as a concern with treatments that invade the body or interfere with normal body functions.

Even if children have not been told they are dying, they know their condition is worsening. They are undergoing treatments, not feeling well, and picking up cues from their parents. They usually do not have the same fears about dying that adults do. Some children keep most of their thoughts about death to themselves. If they have not been told that they are dying, they may feel isolated and get the message not to discuss their condition. They may fear that the family members will abandon them emotionally. Displays of anger often are avoided, since children fear desertion more than death. They may also believe that expressing their awareness of death and their fears will place added emotional burdens on family members that could be unbearable to the family. Parents may not recognize the child's death anxiety because of their own fears, concerns, and feelings of helplessness.

Waechter's (1987) classic study of hospitalized and fatally ill children revealed that children who were given an opportunity to discuss issues related to death openly did not have greater anxiety about death. The permission to discuss any aspect of the illness made the child feel less isolated and alienated from the parents. The child felt that the illness was not too terrible to discuss.

Adolescents have a mature understanding of death, but the normal developmental milestones of adolescence add to their problems in facing a terminal illness. They are struggling to establish their own identity and plans for the future. At a time when body image is extremely important, they may be faced with the possibility of mutilation and disfigurement. Dying teens are often isolated from their peers during a period when peers are the most essential social group. Adolescents with terminal illnesses may be angry because they recognize their loss when the whole world is opening up to them.

Do not expect adolescents to handle feelings in the same way as adults. Adolescents often avoid expressing anger against the family, seeking to control and direct these feelings elsewhere. They often become angry at changes in treatment procedures, lack of explanations, and threats to their independence. As death nears, the adolescent may permit comforting and support and may accept care from warm and loving family members, as long as he or she is not treated condescendingly.

LAW & ETHICS

Some parents ask that their child not be told he or she is dying. Do you abide by the parents' wishes when the child asks you about death? Tell the parents that the child asked the question. Offer to set up a meeting with the care team to discuss their fears and concerns about telling their child the truth. Offer words and phrases they can use to talk with their child about his or her death.

NURSING MANAGEMENT

Make a commitment to children while they are living—to promote growth and development and to foster relationships with family and peers. Help children maintain contact with peers on the hospital unit as long as the child has energy to benefit from the companionship. The comfort of peers reduces the child's feelings of isolation.

Provide opportunities for fantasy play, drawings, and storytelling, without emphasizing or reinforcing death themes. Listen to what children tell you about themselves and their lives. **Death imagery,** references to death or death-related topics (going away, separation, and funerals), or anticipated experiences with treatment, may be themes of their stories. These themes are expected and do not reflect repression or other pathology. Table 8-7 presents strategies for talking with a dying child.

Parents may feel incapable of dealing directly with the child's questions about dying. They may fear that they will be unable to cope with their own feelings during a frank discussion of the possibility of the child's imminent death. The types of questions that children most frequently ask include the following:

- What will death be like?
- What will happen to me when I die?
- Will I be punished for the bad things I have done?

LAW & ETHICS

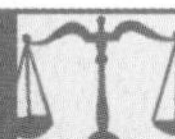

The Patient Self-Determination Act of 1990 (PSDA) supports the rights of persons 18 years of age or older in decisions about their medical care and when they should be admitted to a medical facility. Although many adolescents younger than age 18 have the cognitive skills necessary for decision making and are involved in decisions concerning their care, the PSDA limits their legal rights. Creative strategies are needed to develop a model of decision-making rights and responsibilities for adolescents that is built on the PSDA.

LAW & ETHICS

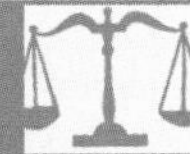

The American Disabilities Act of 1990 and the Education for All Handicapped Children Act mandate that all disabled children—including those with terminal illnesses—are entitled to the same education as other students. This has led to policy challenges in the school setting related to hospice care and Do Not Resuscitate orders (Ramer-Chrastek, 2000).

TABLE 8-7 Strategies for Talking with a Dying Child

- Be flexible.
- Recognize that some children communicate best through nonverbal means (e.g., art or music). The child may be willing to talk through a puppet or a stuffed animal.
- Respect the child's need to be alone and his or her desire to share. Allow communication, but do not force it.
- Be receptive when children initiate a conversation.
- Be specific and literal in explanation of death.
- Acknowledge that a child's life can be complete, even if it is brief. Let dying children know they will always be loved and remembered. Help them find a sense of accomplishment and purpose in the lives they have led.
- Empower children as much as possible in circumstances concerning their deaths. Reassure them of continued love and physical closeness.

Note: From "Talking about death with a dying child," by K.W. Faulkner, 1997, *American Journal of Nursing, 97* (6):64–69.

- When will I be with [person(s) closest to child] again?
- Will my parents be all right?
- Will I experience much pain?

Some parents need help in understanding and answering the child's questions at a developmentally appropriate level for the child. Provide guidance about appropriate methods and words to use that will support the child. Some parents may prefer that the child's questions be answered honestly by another professional. A professional who has special training in bereavement counseling can assist children and families with discussions.

When caring for adolescents, remember that outbursts of anger are common but not personally directed at you. Provide activities to help teens channel their feelings. Continue providing support in spite of their behavior. This approach may encourage teens to accept comforting without losing face. Be available to listen when the teen wants to talk and express feelings and frustrations. Promote friendships with other teens having similar interests or problems.

CLINICAL TIP

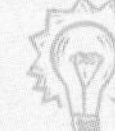

Pediatric palliative care is receiving more attention. The American Academy of Pediatrics recently issued care guidelines for children with life-threatening and terminal illnesses. At this time, only 1% of children with life-threatening illnesses are receiving hospice care. New federal demonstration programs may help improve end-of-life care for children (Stephenson, 2000).

Hospice & Palliative Care

Provide teens with as much independence and control over their situation as possible. Give them a voice in decisions. Answer questions honestly without using a condescending tone.

Palliative care combines active and compassionate therapies intended to comfort and support persons with a short life expectancy. It may be combined with therapies aimed at reducing or curing the illness and treating symptoms more aggressively than hospice care. **Hospice care** helps persons with short life expectancies to live their remaining lives to the fullest—alert, without pain, and with choices and dignity. It does not seek to prolong life. Families often delay contact with hospice care, as it is an admission of death; they may need help to see it as a focus on the time left with the child. In pediatric hospice, the family learns to focus on the quality of life by keeping communication open between the child and family members. Encourage the family to participate in the child's physical and emotional care. Families need to cry together and to tell each other how much they will miss each other. They need to be assured that the vigil with the child is important, so the child does not feel isolated or abandoned as death approaches.

STAFF REACTIONS TO THE DEATH OF A CHILD

Children are highly valued by society because of their potential future contributions. Children are expected to have a normal life span, and the death of a child is often viewed as a tragedy. Caring for dying children is especially stressful and demanding for health care professionals. Nurses involved in long-term relationships with children experience severe grief when these children die (Davies, Cook, & O'Loane, et al., 1996). Nurses often cope by distancing themselves socially from the dying child and family to maintain composure and a professional demeanor. Waechter reported that the total time nurses spent with children decreased as death became more imminent (Davies & Eng, 1993).

Caring for the dying child may be especially difficult for nurses with young children of their own. They tend to identify with the child, making it more likely that they will have dif-

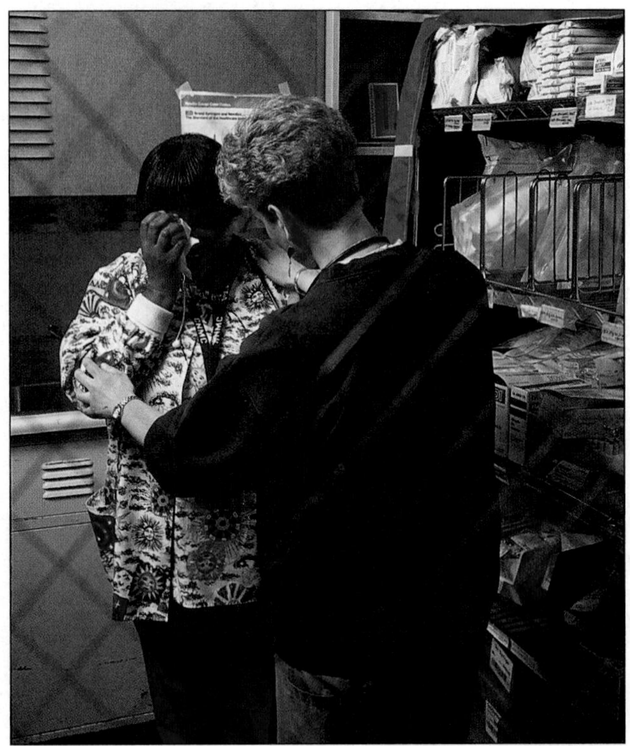

FIGURE 8-8 ◆
Nurses need to express grief in a supportive environment after a child's death. Sharing the sadness and grief or futility of resuscitation efforts with colleagues can often help nurses continue to provide supportive care to the next families who need compassionate care.

ficulty dealing with the death in a professional manner. Nurses may not be able to recognize the dying child's anxiety and fears because of their own personal defenses against their sense of helplessness to alter the course of the child's disease.

Nurses who work with terminally ill children and their families need special preparation to meet the needs of these individuals and to manage personal stress simultaneously. Mentorship with experienced hospice nurses, as well as additional educational experiences, may help promote professional nursing care. Nurses who work with dying children and families must learn to cope effectively with grief and develop empathy, competence, and confidence in their ability to provide more humane and effective nursing care.

Nurses who work in emergency departments caring for children who die suddenly, or in hospice settings and hospital units caring for terminally ill children, need support systems to help balance the stresses of working with dying children. The workplace should acknowledge the stress nurses experience when working with terminally ill children. Support systems may include discussions with peers or debriefing group sessions with mental health professionals that provide an opportunity to discuss their feelings and concerns (Figure 8-8 ◆). Participating in team decisions regarding the dying child's plan of care (palliative rather than curative) helps many nurses manage their distress.

LAW & ETHICS

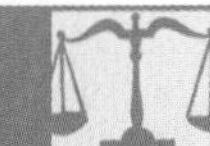

Nurses who have recognized the inevitability of a child's death experience moral distress with feelings of anger, frustration, sadness, and powerlessness when asked to carry out treatments that cause pain and suffering to the child. Discuss these feelings with members of the care team to determine when curative efforts will stop and the focus of attention will shift to palliative care (Davies, 1996).

Chapter Highlights

- A life-threatening illness or injury places intense emotional and physical demands on the child and family due to the unfamiliar environment of the PICU, frightening or invasive procedures, and an uncertain outcome.
- The four most significant stressors for hospitalized children are separation from parents or the primary caretaker; loss of self-control, autonomy, and privacy; being subjected to multiple painful and invasive procedures; and fear of bodily injury and disfigurement.
- The child's developmental stage, temperament, previous coping experiences, and support system influence how he or she will cope with the current experience.
- When the child is hospitalized, work to meet the family members' needs so they can manage their anxiety and support the child.
- Parents typically progress through the stages of shock and disbelief; anger and guilt; deprivation and loss; anticipatory waiting; and readjustment or mourning when their child has a life-threatening illness or injury.

- Make sure siblings get information about their critically ill or injured brother or sister and regular messages from the parents to help them control feelings of jealousy, guilt, fear, and insecurity.
- Work closely with the family when a child's death is imminent, helping to provide the support and services most important to them in the last moments or hours of their child's life.
- Children with life-threatening illnesses often learn about death and their own illness through exposure to other ill and dying children. Even if they have not been told they are dying, they will know their condition is worsening with extra treatments, feeling ill, and cues from their parents.
- Palliative care combines therapies to comfort and support persons with a short life expectancy, by providing therapies to improve the quality of remaining life.
- Caring for a dying child is difficult, and nurses need special preparation to meet the needs of the child and family while managing their own personal stress.

EXPLORE MediaLink

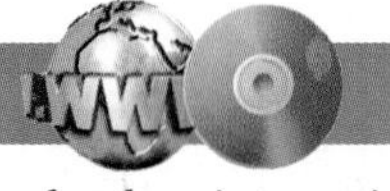

- NCLEX review, case studies, and other interactive resources for this chapter can be found on the Companion Website at **http://www.prenhall.com/ball.** Click on Chapter 8 to select the activities for this chapter
- For animations, more NCLEX review questions, and an audio glossary, access the accompanying CD-ROM in this textbook.

References

1. Ashenberg, M. D., Lambert, S. A., Maier, N. P., & McAliley, L. G. (1996). Easing the wait: Development of a pager program for families. *Pediatric Nursing, 22*(2), 103–107.
2. Baker, J. E., Sedney, M. A., & Gross, E. (1992). Psychological tasks for bereaved children. *American Journal of Orthopsychiatry, 62*(1), 105–116.
3. Boie, E. T., Moore, G. P., Briummett, C., Nelson, D. R. (1999). Do parents want to be present during invasive procedures performed on their children in the emergency department? A survey of 400 parents. *Annals of Emergency Medicine, 34*(1), 70–74.
4. Davies, B. (1997). Commentary on Van Riper's article on sibling bereavement. *Pediatric Nursing, 23*(6), 594–595.
5. Davies, B., & Eng, B. (1993). Factors influencing nursing care of children who are terminally ill: A selective review. *Pediatric Nursing, 19*, 9–14.
6. Davies, B., Cook, K., O'Loane, M., Clarke, D., MacKenzie, B., Stutzer, C., Connaughty, S., & McCormick, J. (1996). Caring for dying children: Nurses' experiences. *Pediatric Nursing, 22*(6), 500–507.
7. Daviss, W. B., Mooney, D., Racusin, R., Ford, J. D., Fleischer, A., & McHugo, G. J. (2000). Predicting posttraumatic stress after hospitalization for pediatric injury. *Journal of American Academy of Child and Adolescent Psychiatry, 39*(5), 576–583.
8. Giganti, A. W. (1998). Families in pediatric critical care: The best option. *Pediatric Nursing, 24*(3), 261–265.
9. Hazinski, M. F. (1999). Psychosocial aspects of pediatric critical care. *Manual of Pediatric Critical Care* (pp. 14–43). St. Louis: Mosby.
10. LaMontagne, L. L. (1993). Bolstering personal control in child patients through coping mechanisms. *Pediatric Nursing, 19*(3), 235–237.
11. Mahan, M. M. (1994). Death of a sibling: Primary care interventions. *Pediatric Nursing, 20*(3), 293–295, 328.
12. Melnyk, B. M., & Alpert-Gillis, L. J. (1998). The COPE program: A strategy to improve outcomes of critically ill young children and their parents. *Pediatric Nursing, 24*(6), 521–527.
13. Nelson, L. (1995). When a child dies: Practical, sensitive advice for helping parents through their worst nightmare. *American Journal of Nursing, 95*(3), 61–64.
14. Ramer-Chrastek, J. (2000). Hospice care for a terminally ill child in the school setting. *Journal of School Nursing, 16*(2), 52–56.
15. Ryan-Wenger, N. A. (1996). Children, coping, and the stress of illness: A synthesis of research. *Journal of the Society of Pediatric Nurses, 1*(3), 126–138.
16. Schonfeld, D. J. (1993). Talking with children about death. *Journal of Pediatric Health Care, 7*(6), 269–274.
17. Scott, L. D. (1998). Perceived needs of parents of critically ill children. *Journal of the Society of Pediatric Nursing, 3*(1), 4–11.
18. Shaefer, J. (1999, July). When an infant dies: Cross-cultural expressions of grief and loss. *NFIMR Bulletin* (pp. 1–19). Washington, DC: National Fetal and Infant Mortality Review Program.
19. Stephenson, J. (2000). Palliative and hospice care needed for children with life-threatening conditions. *Journal of the American Medical Association, 284*(19), 2437–2438.
20. Tomlinson, P. S., & Mitchell, K. E. (1992). On the nature of social support for families of critically ill children. *Journal of Pediatric Nursing, 7*(6), 386–394.
21. Waechter, E. H. (1987). Children's reactions to fatal illness. In T. Krulik, B. Holaday, & I. M. Martinson (Eds.), *The child and family facing life-threatening illness.* Philadelphia: Lippincott.

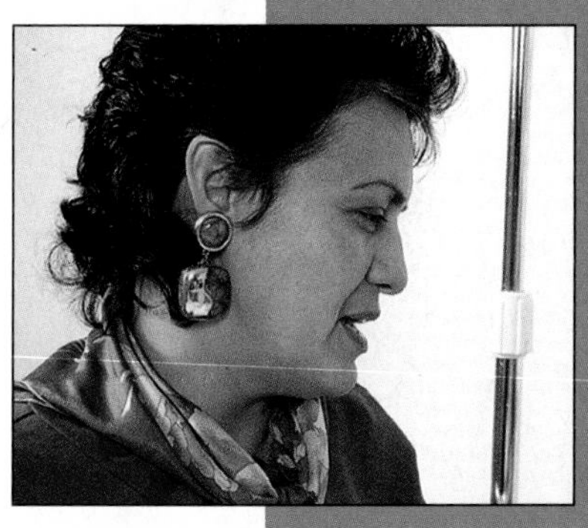

"FELICIA MUST BE IN PAIN SO SOON AFTER HER SURGERY. I KNOW I WOULD HAVE PAIN IF IT WERE ME. CAN SHE GET PAIN MEDICINE WITHOUT GETTING ANOTHER NEEDLE?"

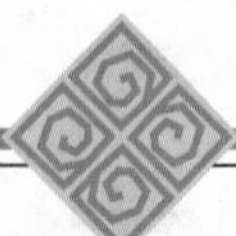

Felicia, who is 5 years old, was struck by a car. Six hours ago she had surgery to repair a liver laceration. After spending 3 hours in the postanesthesia unit, she was moved to the pediatric inpatient unit. She has an intravenous line in place, as well as a nasogastric tube for suction. Her abdominal dressing is clean and dry.

Felicia's mother is rooming in with her during her hospital stay. Because Felicia is thrashing around, her mother thinks she is in pain. She asks the nurse to give her some pain medication. When the nurse enters Felicia's room, she is napping and her facial expression indicates that she is not in pain. When the nurse attempts to straighten her position in bed, she moans. The nurse asks Felicia if she hurts, and Felicia shakes her head no. According to her chart, Felicia received pain medication just before her transfer from the postanesthesia unit 3 hours ago. Her physician has ordered pain medication every 3 to 4 hours as needed.

How do you know whether Felicia is in pain? Can you expect her to tell you if she feels pain? Is any additional assessment needed to justify giving Felicia more pain medication? What other pain relief measures could reduce or help to control her pain?

CHAPTER

9

PAIN ASSESSMENT AND MANAGEMENT

KEY TERMS

acute pain Sudden pain of short duration, associated with a tissue-damaging stimulus.

anxiolysis Sedation by medication.

chronic pain Persistent pain lasting longer than 6 months, generally associated with a prolonged disease process.

conscious sedation Light sedation during which the child maintains airway reflexes and responds to verbal stimuli.

deep sedation A controlled state of depressed consciousness or unconsciousness in which the child may experience partial or complete loss of protective reflexes.

distraction The ability to focus attention on something other than pain, such as an activity, music, or a story.

electroanalgesia A method of delivering electrical stimulation to the skin, to compete with pain stimuli for transmission to the spinal cord; also known as transcutaneous electrical nerve stimulation (TENS).

equianalgesic dose The amount of a drug, whether administered orally or parenterally, needed to produce the same analgesic effect.

NSAIDs Nonsteroidal anti-inflammatory drugs, used for the treatment of pain.

opioids Synthetic narcotic drugs used for the treatment of pain.

pain An unpleasant sensory and emotional experience associated with actual or potential tissue damage. Pain exists when the patient says it does.

patient-controlled analgesia (PCA) A method for administering an intravenous analgesic, such as morphine, using a computerized pump that the patient controls.

tolerance An altered state of response to an opioid or other pain agent in which increasing amounts of the drug are needed to produce or maintain the same level of pain relief or sedation effect.

withdrawal The physical signs and symptoms that occur when a sedative or pain drug is stopped suddenly in a patient who is physically tolerant.

MediaLink

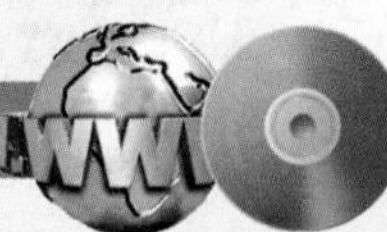

http://www.prenhall.com/ball

Resources for this chapter can be found on the CD-ROM accompanying this textbook, and on the Companion Website at http://www.prenhall.com/ball. Click on Chapter 9 to select the activities for this chapter.

CD-ROM

Audio Glossary

NCLEX Review

COMPANION WEBSITE

Web Links

NCLEX Review

MediaLink Applications

- Implementing Pain Management for Bone Marrow Aspiration
- Managing Conscious Sedation
- Calculating Opioid Dosage

PATHOPHYSIOLOGY ILLUSTRATED

Pain Perception

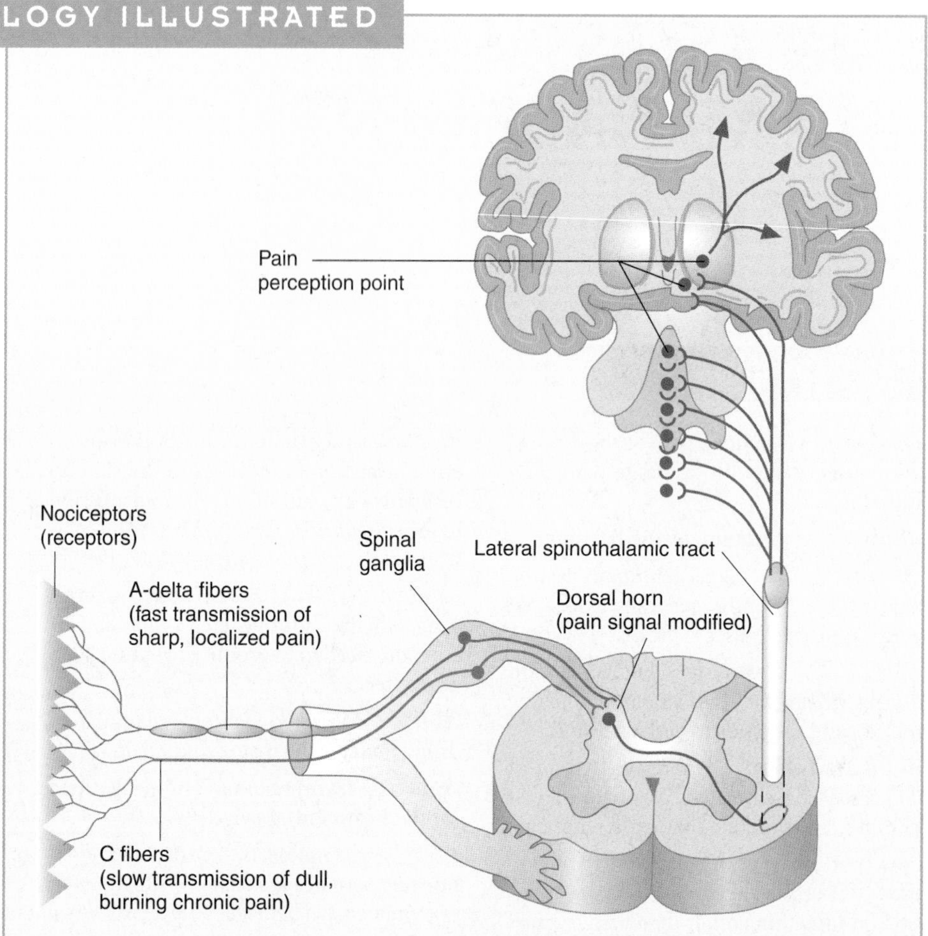

FIGURE 9-1 ◆
Nociceptors (free nerve endings at the site of tissue damage) transmit information by specialized nerve fibers to the spinal cord. Nociceptors are stimulated by mechanical, thermal, and chemical injury. Biochemical mediators (bradykinin, prostaglandin, leukotrienes, and substance P) are produced in response to tissue damage. These substances either activate the pain response or sensitize nerve endings. C fibers slowly transmit dull, burning, diffuse pain as well as chronic pain. A-delta fibers quickly transmit sharp, well-localized pain. After the sensory information reaches the dorsal horn of the spinal cord, the pain signal may be modified depending on the presence of other stimuli, from either the brain or the periphery. The pain signal is then transmitted to the brain through the spinothalamic and reticulospinal nerve pathways, where perception occurs. Once the sensation reaches the brain, emotional responses may increase or decrease the intensity of the pain perceived.

Everyone has his or her own perception of pain. A neurologic response to tissue injury, **pain** is an unpleasant sensory and emotional experience associated with actual or potential tissue damage (Figure 9-1 ◆). Effective pain management is every child's right.

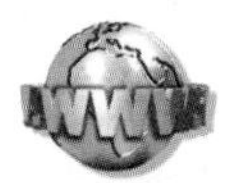

Understanding Pain

Pain exists when the patient says it does (McCaffery & Pasero, 1999). Pain may be either acute or chronic. **Acute pain** is sudden pain of short duration that may be associated with a single event, such as surgery, or an acute exacerbation of a condition such as a sickle-cell crisis. **Chronic pain** is persistent pain lasting longer than 6 months that is generally associated with a prolonged disease process such as juvenile rheumatoid arthritis.

LAW & ETHICS

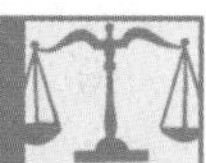

In 2001, the Joint Commission on Accreditation of Health Care Organizations introduced standards for the assessment and management of pain in patients in accredited hospitals and other health care organizations.

- Standard RI.1.2.8: Patients have the right to appropriate assessment and management of pain.
- Standard PF.3.4: Patients are educated about pain and managing pain as part of treatment, as appropriate.

OUTDATED BELIEFS ABOUT PAIN IN CHILDREN

In the past, children did not receive adequate treatment for pain. Undertreatment still occurs (Kachoyeanos & Zollok, 1995). Health care professionals once believed that children feel less pain than adults (Table 9-1). In fact, most physicians did not prescribe pain medication for children or ordered it only as needed. This undertreatment was based on the attitudes of health care professionals about pain, the difficulty and complexity of pain assessment in children, and inadequate research.

Research has shown that past beliefs about children's perception of pain were incorrect. Neonates and infants do feel and remember pain. By 6 months of age, children demonstrate anticipatory fear of pain when taken to a location where they once experienced pain (Lutz, 1986). Health care professionals now recognize that children do not complain of pain because they are afraid that the injection to relieve pain will hurt more than the pain already does.

TABLE 9-1 Outdated Beliefs about Pain and Pain Medication in Children

- Children without obvious physical reasons for pain are not likely to have pain.
- Neonates do not feel pain.
- Children do not feel pain with the same intensity as adults because a child's nervous system is immature.
- Children tolerate discomfort well. They become accustomed to pain after having it for a while.
- Children tell you if they are in pain. They do not need medication unless they appear to be in pain.
- Children are not in pain if they can be distracted or they are sleeping.
- Children recover more quickly than adults from painful experiences such as surgery.
- Parents exaggerate or aggravate their child's pain.
- Children have no memory of pain.
- Narcotics are dangerous for children because they can cause respiratory depression and addiction.
- The best route for giving analgesics is intramuscular.
- After surgery, children should not receive the next analgesic dose until they show obvious signs of pain.
- As-needed medication orders mean that medication should be given as infrequently as possible.

CULTURE

The cultural experiences of health care professionals often contribute to their outdated attitudes about pain experienced by children. For example, health care workers may believe that being in pain for a little while is not so bad, that pain helps build character, or that using pain medication is a sign of a weak character.

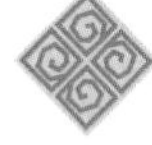

CLINICAL MANIFESTATIONS OF PAIN

PHYSIOLOGIC INDICATORS

Acute pain stimulates the adrenergic nervous system and results in physiologic changes, including tachycardia, tachypnea, hypertension, pupil dilation, pallor, and increased perspiration. Changes in these signs demonstrate a complex stress response. As the body adapts physiologically, vital signs return to near normal and perspiration decreases after several minutes. Thus changes in vital signs are not a reliable indicator of pain in children because they last such a short time.

Chronic pain of long duration permits physiologic adaptation so normal heart rate, respiratory rate, and blood pressure levels are often seen (Leo & Huether, 1998).

BEHAVIORAL INDICATORS

Children in acute pain behave in many of the same ways as children who show signs of fear and anxiety (Hazinski, 1999; Tesler, Holzemer, & Spreker, 1999). These behaviors include the following:

- Restless and agitated or hyperalert and vigilant
- Short attention span (child is difficult to distract)
- Irritability (child is difficult to comfort)
- Facial grimacing, biting or pursing lips (Figure 9-2 ◆)
- Posturing (guarding a painful joint by avoiding movement), remaining immobile, or protecting the painful area
- Drawing up knees, flexing limbs, massaging affected area
- Anorexia
- Lethargy, remaining quiet, or withdrawal
- Sleep disturbances

The nurse evaluating Felicia, the 5-year-old girl described in the opening vignette, would observe for such behavioral indicators of pain.

Preverbal children may show conflicting signs of pain (increased or decreased vital signs, agitation or withdrawal, grimacing, crying, or anger), thus making assessment and monitoring of pain management more challenging.

Children often suffer additional emotional distress and fear that the discomfort will worsen. Depression and/or aggressive behavior are frequently overlooked as indicators of pain.

Behavioral indicators of chronic pain and pain of long duration include posturing and inactivity to avoid pain, depression, difficulty sleeping, and an inability to concentrate (Shapiro, 1995).

GROWTH & DEVELOPMENT

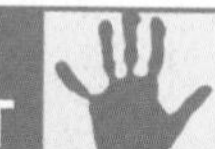

Even neonates feel pain. Cutaneous sensation is actually present by 20 weeks' gestation. Brain centers necessary for pain perception develop toward the end of gestation. Nerve and biochemical pathways associated with pain transmission are functional at birth, but myelination (further development of the myelin sheath) continues during infancy. Although pain conduction may be slower in neonates, the distance that pain stimuli must travel is much shorter than in adults. Because of their immature nervous systems, young children may actually have a lower pain threshold and pain tolerance. Premature infants may be even more sensitive to pain than full-term infants (Anand & Carr, 1989).

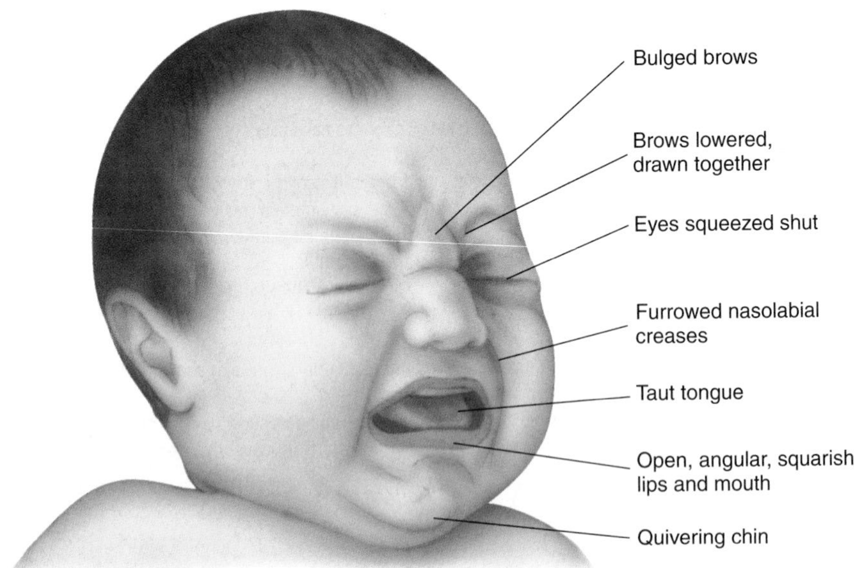

FIGURE 9-2 ◆
Neonatal characteristic facial responses to pain include: bulged brow, eyes squeezed shut, furrowed nasolabial creases, open lips, pursed lips, stretched mouth, taut tongue, and a quivering chin.
Redrawn from Carlson, K. L., Clement, B. A., & Nash, P. (1996). Neonatal pain: From concept to research questions and the role of the advanced practice nurse. *Journal of Perinatal Neonatal Nursing, 10(1),* 64–71.

TABLE 9-2 Physiologic Consequences of Unrelieved Pain in Children

RESPONSES TO PAIN	POTENTIAL PHYSIOLOGIC CONSEQUENCES
Respiratory Changes	
Rapid shallow breathing	Alkalosis
Inadequate lung expansion	Decreased oxygen saturation
Inadequate cough	Retention of secretions
Neurologic Changes	
Increased sympathetic nervous system activity	Tachycardia, change in sleep patterns, increased blood glucose and cortisol levels
Metabolic Changes	
Increased metabolic rate with increased perspiration	Increased fluid and electrolyte losses

Note: Adapted from Eland, J. M. (1990). Pain in children. *Nursing Clinics of North America, 25,* 871–884; and "Postoperative pain management in preverbal children: The prescription and administration of analgesia with and without caudal analgesia," by L. Altimier, S. Norwood, M. J. Dick, et al. (1994). *Journal of Pediatric Nursing, 9*(4), 226–232.

CONSEQUENCES OF PAIN

Unrelieved pain is stressful and has many undesirable physiologic consequences (Table 9-2). For example, the child with acute postoperative pain takes shallow breaths and suppresses coughing to avoid more pain. These self-protective actions increase the potential for respiratory complications. Unrelieved pain may also delay the return of normal gastric and bowel functions and cause a stress ulcer. Anorexia associated with pain may delay the healing process. The long-term effects of pain on the child's physical or psychologic condition are unknown.

PAIN ASSESSMENT

No laboratory tests are routinely used to assess pain. Prolonged, severe pain produces a physiologic stress response that includes the chemical release of catecholamines, cortisol, aldosterone, and other corticosteroids. Insulin secretion also decreases, leading to increased amounts of glucose and severe hyperglycemia (Hazinski, 1999). Existing conditions such as infection, trauma, and anemia can cause the vital sign changes seen with sudden pain.

The goal of pain assessment is to provide accurate information about the location and intensity of pain and its effects on the child's functioning. When assessing pain in children, keep the following questions in mind:

- What is happening in tissues that might cause pain? Assume that children who have had surgery, injury, a vaso-occlusive episode, or illness are experiencing pain, since these events also cause pain in adults.
- What external factors could be causing pain? For example, is the cast too tight or is the child poorly positioned in bed?
- Are there any indicators of pain, either physiologic or behavioral?
- How is the child responding emotionally?
- How does the child or parent rate the pain?

CLINICAL TIP

The presence of physiologic symptoms such as nausea, fatigue, dyspnea, bladder and bowel distention, and fever may influence the intensity of pain felt by a child. The child's behavior or responses to pain stimuli may also be affected by fear, anxiety, separation from parents, anger, culture, age, or a previous pain experience.

PAIN HISTORY

Parents can provide a great deal of information about the child's response to pain, such as the following:

- How the child typically expresses pain, both verbally and behaviorally. Children and parents use similar terms to describe pain. Some examples of words used are a *hurt, owie, boo-boo, stinging, sore, cutting, burning, itching, hot,* and *tight.* Knowing the appropriate word to use makes communicating with the child easier.
- The child's previous experiences with painful situations.
- How the child copes with pain. The child with several past pain experiences may not exhibit the same types of stressful behaviors as the child with few pain experiences.
- The parent's and child's preferences for analgesic use.

Older children may be able to give a history of painful procedures. When attempting to obtain information about the child's pain experiences and present level of pain, ask the child and parent similar open-ended questions. Sample questions are given in Table 9-3. Many children modify their pain descriptions depending on the type of questions asked and what they expect will happen as a result of their response.

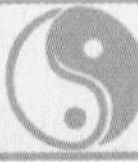

CULTURE

The terms *pain, hurt,* and *ache* have been found to describe pain intensity across cultures. Pain is most intense, hurt is less severe, and ache is least severe (Gaston-/Johansson, Albert, & Fagan, et al., 1990).

The term *tender* or *tenderness* may be confusing for some families in which English is a second language. Tender or tenderness is more commonly associated with caring or romance or with meat rather than soreness or pain.

TABLE 9-3 Pediatric Pain History for Children and Parents

QUESTIONS FOR CHILDREN	QUESTIONS FOR PARENTS
Past Pain Experiences	
Tell me what pain is.	What word(s) does your child use to describe pain?
Tell me about the hurt you have had before.	How would you describe pain experiences your child has previously had?
Do you tell others when you hurt? Who?	Does your child tell you or others when he or she is in pain?
What do you do for yourself when you are hurting?	How do you know when your child is in pain?
What helps the most to take your hurt away?	How does your child usually react to pain?
What do you want others to do for you when you hurt?	What do you do for your child when he or she is in pain?
What don't you want others to do for you when you hurt?	What does your child do to manage pain?
Is there anything special you want me to know about when you hurt? What?	What works best to reduce or take away your child's pain?
	Is there anything special you would like me to know about your child and pain?
Present Pain Experiences	
Where is the pain?	Tell me about the pain your child is having now. Where is it and what does it feel like?
What does it feel like?	
What do you think is causing the pain?	
What would you like me to do for you?	What would you like me to do for your child?

Note: Adapted from "Assessment and management of pain in children" by N. O. Hester & C. S. Barcus, 1986, *Pediatrics: Nursing Update,* 1, 2–8.

CLINICAL TIP

When help in describing pain is needed, give the child over 6 years of age some words to select from, such as *sharp, dull, aching, pounding, cold, hot, burning, throbbing, stinging, tingling,* or *cutting.*

CULTURE

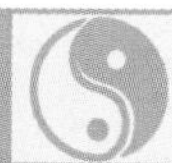

Some ethnic groups, such as Asian, Anglo-Saxon–Germanic, and Irish, do not openly express pain. People of Italian and Jewish descent are more likely to use both verbal and nonverbal methods to express pain freely. However, children have individualized responses, and younger children have had less time to acquire culturally learned behaviors.

RESEARCH

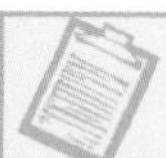

Children do not exhibit distress in direct proportion to their pain intensity. Thus, behavioral measures may not match the child's self-report of pain intensity. Older children often appear calm, expressionless, and limit movement following surgery, but report pain of moderate to severe levels (Tesler, 1999).

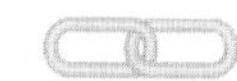

Skill 9-1: Selected Pediatric Pain Scales

Children with recurrent episodes of pain can be asked to keep a diary or log to describe the characteristics, timing, activities, and potential triggers of their pain, as well as their response to pain treatment measures. This record can help improve pain management.

CULTURAL INFLUENCES ON PAIN

Children's culture and social learning have a tremendous influence on their expression of pain. Cultural traditions often guide children about self-control, coping, and enlisting the assistance of others (Leo & Huether, 1998). Children learn directly and indirectly from their parents about how to respond to pain. By showing approval and disapproval, parents teach their children how to behave when in pain. This instruction includes the following:

- How much discomfort justifies a complaint
- How to express the complaint
- How and when to stop complaining
- Whom to approach for pain relief

For example, boys in the United States are usually encouraged to hide their pain by acting brave and not crying. Girls are often encouraged to express their pain openly. Children also observe other family members in pain and imitate their responses (Abu-Saad, 1984).

PAIN ASSESSMENT SCALES

A child's responses to and understanding of pain depend on the child's age, stage of development, and other situational factors (McGrath, 1995) (Tables 9-4, 9-5, and 9-6). For example, neonates cannot anticipate pain and may not demonstrate typical behavior associated with a painful response. Young children are unable to give a detailed description of their pain because of their limited vocabulary and pain experiences. Depending on their developmental stage, children use different coping strategies, such as escape, postponement or avoidance, diversion, and imagery, to deal with pain.

Various pain scales have been developed to assess pain in children (see Table 9-7). Physical and behavioral indicators are used to quantify pain in children. Some pain assessment

TABLE 9-4 Behavioral Responses and Verbal Descriptions of Pain by Children of Different Developmental Stages

AGE GROUP	BEHAVIORAL RESPONSE	VERBAL DESCRIPTION
Infants		
< 6 months	Generalized body movements, chin quivering, facial grimacing, poor feeding	Cries
6–12 months	Reflex withdrawal to stimulus, facial grimacing, disturbed sleep, irritability, restlessness	Cries
Toddlers		
1–3 years	Localized withdrawal, resistance of entire body, aggressive behavior, disturbed sleep	Cries and screams, cannot describe intensity or type of pain
Preschoolers		
3–6 years (preoperational)	Active physical resistance, directed aggressive behavior, strikes out physically and verbally when hurt, low frustration level	Can identify location and intensity of pain, denies pain, may believe his or her pain is obvious to others
School-Age Children		
7–9 years (concrete operations)	Passive resistance, clenches fists, holds body rigidly still, suffers emotional withdrawal, engages in plea bargaining	Can specify location and intensity of pain and describe its physical characteristics
10–12 years (transitional)	May pretend comfort to project bravery, may regress with stress and anxiety	Able to describe intensity and location with more characteristics, able to describe psychologic pain
Adolescents		
13–18 years (formal operations)	Want to behave in a socially acceptable manner (like adults), show a controlled behavioral response	More sophisticated descriptions as experience is gained

TABLE 9-5 Children's Understanding of Pain by Developmental Stage

DEVELOPMENTAL STAGE	UNDERSTANDING OF PAIN
Infants	
< 6 months	No apparent understanding of pain; infants do have memory of pain; neonates exposed to repeated painful experiences in intensive care unit demonstrate memory of pain by breathholding when approached by care providers
6–12 months	Anticipate a painful event such as an immunization with fear
Toddlers	
1–3 years	Demonstrate a fear of painful situations; use common words for pain such as "owie" and "boo-boo"
Preschoolers	
3–6 years (preoperational)	Pain is a hurt; do not relate pain to illness but may relate pain to an injury; often believe pain is punishment; do not believe an injection takes pain away
School-Age Children	
7–9 years (concrete operations)	Can understand simple relationships between pain and disease but have no clear understanding of the cause of pain; can understand the need for painful procedures to monitor or treat disease; may recognize psychologic pain related to grief and hurt feelings
10–12 years (transitional)	Have a more complex awareness of physical and psychologic pain, such as moral dilemmas and mental pain
Adolescents	
13–18 years (formal operations)	Have a capacity for sophisticated and complex understanding of the causes of physical and mental pain; can relate to the pain experienced by others; pain has both qualitative and quantitative characteristics

TABLE 9-6 Situational Factors Influencing Pain in Children

COGNITIVE FACTORS

- Understanding of pain source
- Ability to control what will happen
- Expectations about the quality and strength of pain
- Whether attention is focused on painful event or distractor

BEHAVIORAL FACTORS

- Use of a pain-control strategy
- Response of parents and health care personnel
- Whether or not restrained
- Ability to continue usual activities

EMOTIONAL FACTORS

- Fear
- Anxiety
- Frustration
- Anger
- Depression

Note: From "Pain in the pediatric patient: Practical aspects of assessment," by P. A. McGrath, P. A., 1995, *Pediatric Annals, 24*(3), 126–138. Adapted.

TABLE 9-7 Pain Assessment Scales*

SCALE AND AGE GROUP	ADMINISTRATION	USE
NIPS Preterm and full-term infant to 6 weeks after birth (see Table 9-9)	Observe the neonate's facial expression, cry quality, breathing patterns, arm and leg position, and state of arousal	Useful in measuring pain or pain-elicited distress in infants; overall status of infant and the infant's environment must be factored into the assessment
CHEOPS 1–7 years	Observe the child's cry, facial expression, torso position, leg position, touch-painful area, and verbal complaints; select the numerical score for each category after 5 seconds	Primarily behavioral assessment for postoperative pain or following painful procedures; researchers have no specific score indicating pain in need of medication; in preverbal children scale may measure nonspecific stress rather than only pain
Eland Color Tool 4–9 years	Child picks a crayon color to represent the most severe pain, then a color for the next most severe pain, until four crayons have been selected; child then colors in an outline of the body to indicate the location of the areas that hurt by level of pain	You need six crayons: black, purple, blue, red, green, and orange; no one color is most often selected by children as representing the most pain; limited reliability and validity of data[a]
Oucher Scale 3–7 years	Child selects a face that best fits his or her level of pain; older child can select a number between 0 and 10	Useful in hospital settings; child must understand concepts of higher/lower and more/less; cultural versions available; tool has been successfully tested for reliability and validity in some age groups[a,b]

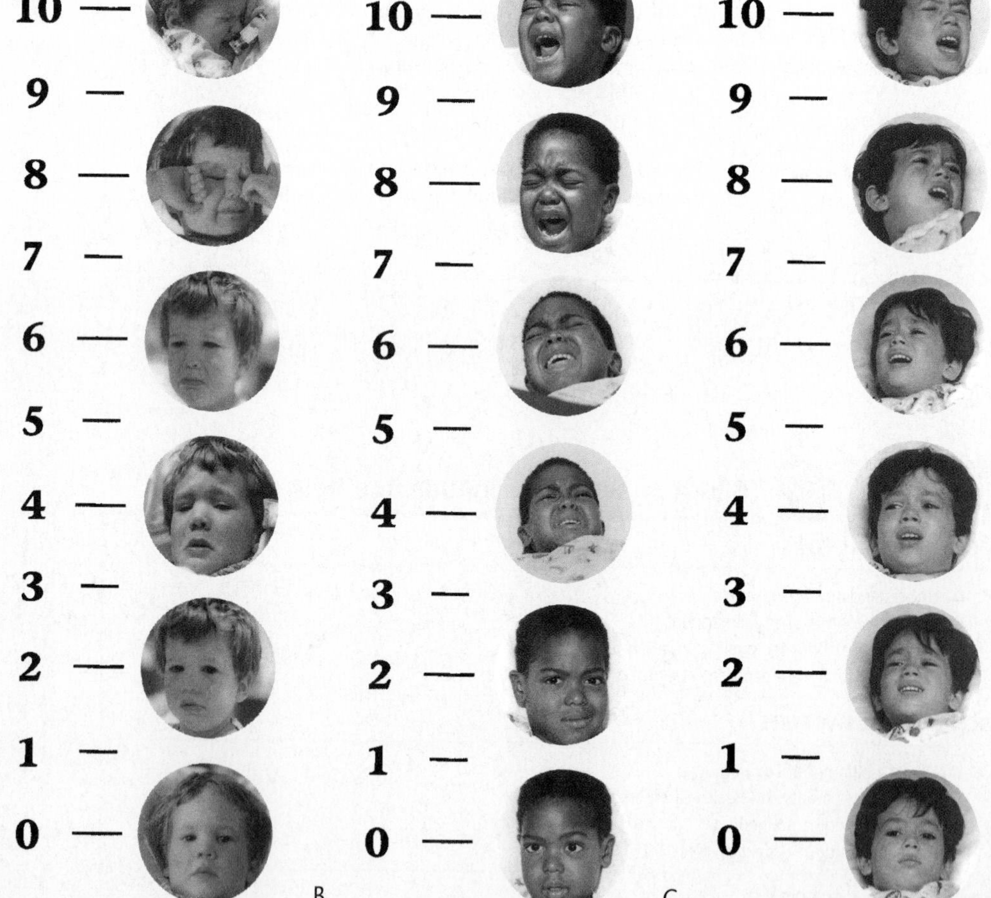

*In the form presented in this book, the Oucher is for educational purposes only and cannot be used for patient care.
[a]Reliability is the extent to which the same score is obtained when an instrument or scale is used either by different persons or by the same person at different times. Validity is the extent to which an instrument or scale measures what it is supposed to measure.
[b]A, The Caucasian version of the Oucher, developed and copyrighted by Judith E. Beyer, RN, Ph.D., 1983. B, The African-American version of the Oucher, developed and copyrighted by Mary J. Denyes, RN, Ph.D., and Antonia M. Villarruel, RN, Ph.D., 1990. Cornelia P. Porter, RN, Ph.D. and Charlotta Marshall, RN, MSN, contributed to the development of the scale. C, The Hispanic version of the Oucher, developed and copyrighted by Antonio M. Villarruel, RN, Ph.D., and Mary J. Denyes, RN, Ph.D., 1990. www.oucher.org

(continued)

TABLE 9-7 Pain Assessment Scales (continued)

SCALE AND AGE GROUP	ADMINISTRATION	USE
Poker Chip Scale 3–7 years	Child selects the number of chips or checkers that matches level of hurt (1 = a little hurt, 5 = the most hurt)	Useful in hospital settings; child must have number concepts from 1 to 5; you can then obtain a measure of child's perception of pain

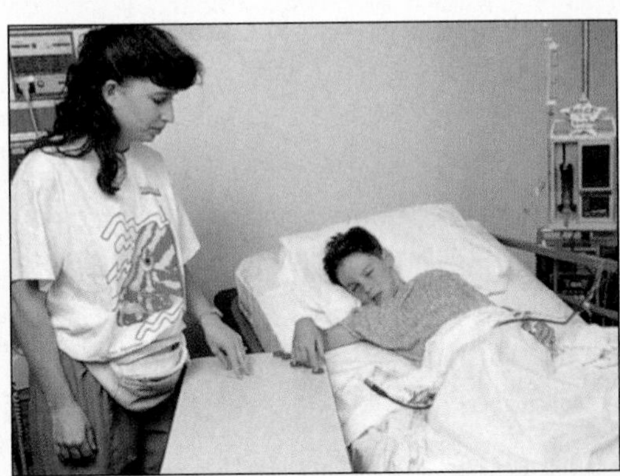

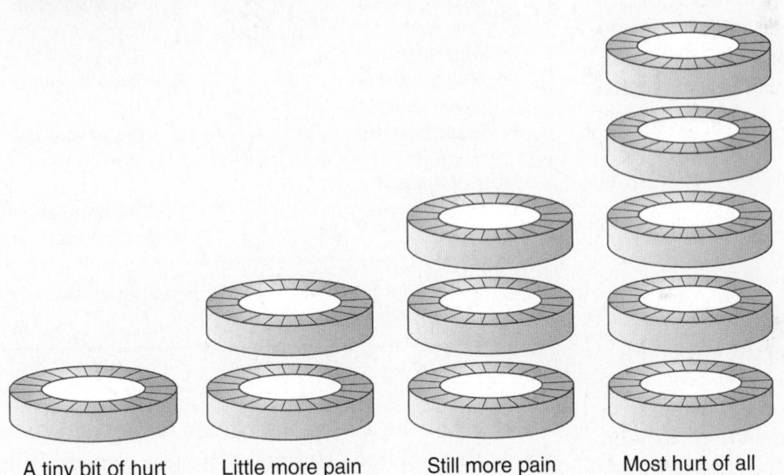

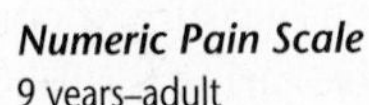

SCALE AND AGE GROUP	ADMINISTRATION	USE
Numeric Pain Scale 9 years–adult	Ask child to rate pain felt on a line with 10 marks (1 = a little pain, 10 = the most pain)	Child must be verbal; easy to carry tool to patient

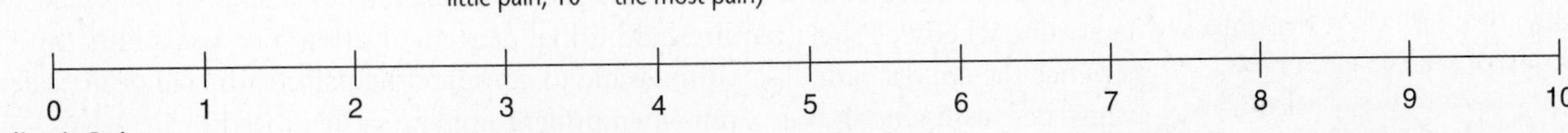

SCALE AND AGE GROUP	ADMINISTRATION	USE
Pediatric Pain Questionnaire[c]	Child selects pain descriptors from checklist, rates current and average pain intensity with visual analog scale and uses own color choices to identify different pain intensities on pain map of body	Parent, child and adolescent forms exist; parent form provides information about history of pain problem and its management; useful for chronic pain

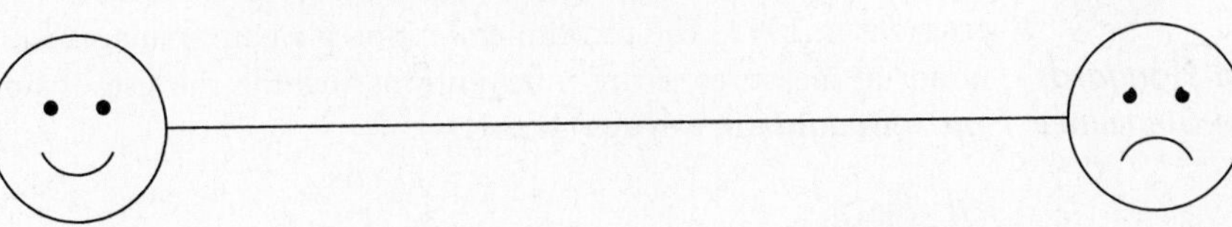

[c]From Varni, J. W., Thompson, K. L., & Hanson V. (1987). The Varni/Thompson pediatric pain questionnaire: Chronic musculoskeletal pain in juvenile rheumatoid arthritis, *Pain, 28,* 27–38.

GROWTH & DEVELOPMENT

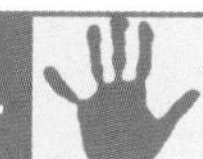

Identify the child's stage of development for readiness to use pain scales.

- Assess the child's language skills (ability to use words in sequence, follow simple directions, and answer simple questions).
- Ask the child to count his or her fingers or up to 10.
- Determine whether the child can understand concepts such as more or less and higher or lower.

RESEARCH

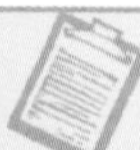

Comparison of faces pain scales has revealed that those scales with a smiling face as the indicator of no pain resulted in significantly higher pain ratings by children and parents than scales using a neutral expression face as an indicator of no pain (Chambers, Gresbrecht, Craig, et al., 1999).

CLINICAL TIP

Surgery and trauma can result in multiple sites of pain (e.g., incision or laceration, cut or bruised muscles, interrupted blood supply, nasogastric tube placement, insertion sites of intravenous lines). When using pain scales in the assessment of a verbal child, attempt to identify all sites of pain. Then evaluate the intensity of pain at each site.

TABLE 9-8 Neonatal Infant Pain Scale (NIPS)

CHARACTERISTIC	SCORING CRITERIA
Facial Expression	
0 = Relaxed muscles	■ Restful face with neutral expression
1 = Grimace	■ Tight facial muscles; furrowed brow, chin, and jaw (Note: At low gestational ages, infants may have no facial expression.)
Cry	
0 = No cry	■ Quiet, not crying
1 = Whimper	■ Mild moaning, intermittent cry
2 = Vigorous cry	■ Loud screaming, rising, shrill, and continuous (Note: Silent cry may be scored if infant is intubated, as indicated by obvious facial movements.)
Breathing Patterns	
0 = Relaxed	■ Relaxed, usual breathing pattern maintained
1 = Change in breathing	■ Change in drawing breath; irregular, faster than usual, gagging, or holding breath
Arm Movements	
0 = Relaxed/restrained (with soft restraints)	■ Relaxed, no muscle rigidity, occasional random movements of arms
1 = Flexed/extended	■ Tense, straight arms; rigid; or rapid extension and flexion
Leg Movements	
0 = Relaxed/restrained (with soft restraints)	■ Relaxed, no muscle rigidity, occasional random movements of legs
1 = Flexed/extended	■ Tense, straight legs; rigid; or rapid extension and flexion
State of Arousal	
0 = Sleeping/awake	■ Quiet, peaceful, sleeping; or alert and settled
1 = Fussy	■ Alert and restless or thrashing; fussy

Note: From "The development of a tool to assess neonatal pain," by J. Lawrence, D. Alcock, D., P. McGrath, et al., 1993, *Neonatal Network, 12*(6), 61.

scales rely on the nurse's observation of the child's behavior if the child is nonverbal, for example, the Children's Hospital of Eastern Ontario Pain Scale (CHEOPS) (see Table 9-7) and the Neonatal Infant Pain Scale (NIPS) (Table 9-8). These scales can provide only an indirect estimate of pain intensity from the child's behaviors or physical states. Most scales depend on the child's report of pain intensity (Table 9-7). Facial scales may be a measure of emotional distress because they reflect the unpleasantness of pain. The nurse caring for Felicia might use a pain scale such as the CHEOPS, Eland, Oucher, poker chip, or faces scale to help determine whether Felicia requires additional pain medication. Because adults cannot experience the child's pain, it is not possible to compare the pain felt by children and adults using these assessment tools, even when undergoing the same procedures.

CLINICAL THERAPY FOR PAIN

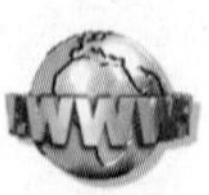

Pain Control Standards and Guidelines

Current guidelines for pain management build upon those published by the U.S. government in 1992. The recommendations for pain management include both drug and nondrug measures. Drug interventions include the use of **opioids** and **nonsteroidal anti-inflammatory drugs** (**NSAIDs**).

OPIOIDS

Opioids such as morphine and codeine may be administered by oral, subcutaneous, intramuscular, and intravenous routes. Administration of opioids by an oral route is as effective as by intramuscular and intravenous routes when the drug is given in an **equianalgesic dose** (the amount of drug, whether given by oral or parenteral routes, needed to produce the

TABLE 9-9 Opioid Analgesics and Recommended Doses for Children and Adolescents*

DRUG	APPROXIMATE EQUIANALGESIC ORAL DOSE	APPROXIMATE EQUIANALGESIC PARENTERAL DOSE	RECOMMENDED STARTING DOSE (ADULTS > 50 KG) ORAL	RECOMMENDED STARTING DOSE (ADULTS > 50 KG) PARENTERAL	RECOMMENDED STARTING DOSE (CHILDREN & ADULTS < 50 KG) ORAL	RECOMMENDED STARTING DOSE (CHILDREN & ADULTS < 50 KG) PARENTERAL
Morphine	30 mg	10 mg	15–30 mg q 3–4 hr	10 mg q 3–4 hr	0.3 mg/kg q 3–4 hr	0.1 mg/kg q 3–4 hr
Codeine	130 mg	75 mg IM or subcutaneous	30–60 mg q 3–4 hr	60 mg q 2 hr	0.5–1 mg q 3–4 hr[a]	NR
Hydromorphone (Dilaudid)	7.5 mg	1.5 mg	4–8 mg q 3–4 hr	1.5 mg q 3–4 hr	0.06 mg/kg q 3–4 hr	0.015 mg/kg q 3–4 hr
Levorphanol (Levo-Dromoman)	4 mg (acute) 1 mg (chronic)	2 mg (acute) 1 mg (chronic)	2–4 mg q 6–8 hr	2 mg q 6–8 hr	0.04 mg/kg q 6–8 hr	0.02 mg/kg q 6–8 hr
Meperidine (Demerol)	300 mg	100 mg	NR	100 mg q 3 hr	NR	0.05–1.5 mg q 2–4 hr
Methadone (Dolophine, others)	20 mg (acute) 2–4 mg (chronic)	10 mg (acute) 2–4 mg (chronic)	5–10 mg q 6–8 hr	10 mg q 6–8 hr	0.2 mg/kg q 6–8 hr	0.1 mg/kg q 6–8 hr
Oxycodone	30 mg	NA	5–10 mg q 3–4 hr	NA	0.1–0.2 mg/kg q 3–4 hr[a]	NA
Fentanyl	NA	0.01 mg	5 mcg/kg Lozenge	1 mcg/kg	5–15 mcg/kg Oralet[b]	1 mcg/kg

NR = Not recommended NA = Not available
*For all parenteral opioids, start with the low dose and titrate to effective pain control.
[a]Caution: Doses of aspirin and acetaminophen in combination with opioid/NSAID preparation must also be adjusted to the patient's body weight.
[b]Oralet is not widely used because of nausea and vomiting side effects.
Resources: American Pain Society (1999). *Principles of analgesic use in the treatment of acute pain and cancer pain,* 4th ed., Glenview, IL: Author: pp. 6–8, 14–15, 20; Hazinski M.F., (1999). Analgesia, sedation, and neuromuscular blockage in pediatric critical care. In Hazinski, M. F. *Manual of Pediatric Critical Care,* St. Louis: Mosby, pp. 44–72.; and Acute Pain Management Guideline Panel (1992). *Acute pain management in infants, children, and adolescents: Operative and medical procedures. Quick reference guide for clinicians.* (AHCPR Pub. No. 92-0020). Rockville, MD: Agency for Healthcare Policy and Research, U.S. Public Health Service, Department of Health and Human Services.

same analgesic effect) (Table 9-9). Rectal preparations of some opioids are also available. The optimal analgesic dose varies widely among patients in all age groups (American Pain Society, 1999).

Common side effects include sedation, nausea, vomiting, constipation, and itching. Potential complications of opioids include respiratory depression, cardiovascular collapse, and addiction. When the child's condition is unstable, as in trauma or critical illness, the dosage of opioids must be carefully calculated to match the child's cardiorespiratory status, although infants and children are no more likely than adults to develop respiratory depression following administration of a weight-specific dose of narcotics (Holder & Patt, 1995). Addiction is a rare complication in adults treated for painful conditions, and the same holds true for children.

Avoid use of opioid agonists such as nalbuphine (Nubain), pentazocine (Talwin), and butorphanol (Stadol) as first-line drugs for pain. These drugs were developed to exert effects on one opioid receptor and antagonize a second receptor. Although this mixed agonist/antagonist action may limit potential side effects such as respiratory depression, the drugs have a ceiling to analgesia. They are inappropriate for escalating pain (Hazinski, 1999).

NURSING ALERT

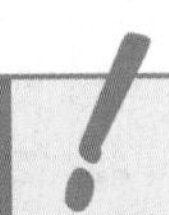

Respiratory depression (unresponsiveness and a respiratory rate less than 12 breaths/min in children less than 2 years of age) may progress to respiratory arrest and is the major life-threatening complication of opioid administration. Respiratory depression is most likely to occur when the child is sleeping. This augments the depressant effect on the respiratory center and potential airway obstruction by the tongue (American Pain Society, 1999). Identify the time interval before drug-specific peak respiratory depression occurs, and then carefully monitor the child's vital signs during that period to detect respiratory depression.

NONSTEROIDAL ANTI-INFLAMMATORY DRUGS

NSAIDs such as aspirin and acetaminophen, which are primarily given orally, are effective for the relief of mild to moderate pain and chronic pain. Table 9-10 presents recommended dosages of these drugs. They are most commonly used for bone, inflammatory, and connective tissue conditions. An NSAID may be prescribed in combination with an opioid to

TABLE 9-10 Recommended Doses of NSAIDs for Children and Adolescents

ORAL NSAID PEAK ACTION TIME	USUAL ADULT DOSE	USUAL PEDIATRIC DOSE	COMMENTS
Acetaminophen 0.5–2 hr	500–1000 mg q 4–6 hr	10–15 mg/kg q 4–6 hr	Lacks the peripheral anti-inflammatory activity of other NSAIDs; rectal suppository available
Aspirin 1–2 hr	650–975 mg q 4–6 hr	10–15 mg/kg q 4 hr	Do not use in children under 12 years with possible viral illness; may cause gastric upset and bleeding; rectal suppository available
Choline magnesium trisalicylate (Trilisate) 2 hr	1000–1500 mg q 12 hr	25 mg/kg q 12 hr	Does not increase bleeding time like other NSAIDs; also available as oral liquid
Ibuprofen (Motrin, others) 0.5 hr	200–400 mg q 4–6 hr	10 mg/kg q 6–8 hr	Available as oral suspension
Naproxen (Naprosyn) 2–4 hr	500 mg initial dose followed by 250 mg q 6–8 hr	5 mg/kg q 12 hr	Available as oral liquid

Resources: American Pain Society (1999). *Principles of analgesic use in the treatment of acute pain and cancer pain,* 4th ed., Glenview, IL: Author; pp. 6–8, 14–15, 20; Hazinski, M.F., (1999). Analgesia, sedation, and neuromuscular blockage in pediatric critical care. In Hazinski, M.F. *Manual of Pediatric Critical Care,* St. Louis: Mosby, pp. 44–72.; and Acute Pain Management Guideline Panel (1992). *Acute pain management in infants, children, and adolescents: Operative and medical procedures. Quick reference guide for clinicians* (AHCPR Pub. No. 92-0020). Rockville, MD: Agency for Healthcare Policy and Research, U.S. Public Health Service, Department of Health and Human Services.

Skill 9-2: Administering Patient-Controlled Analgesia (PCA) Pumps

increase the effectiveness of the narcotic drug. This combination may ultimately reduce the amount of opioids needed for pain relief.

DRUG ADMINISTRATION

Pain from surgery, major trauma, or cancer will be present for predictable periods because of the effects of tissue damage. Pain relief should be provided *around the clock.* Every effort should be made to give the child analgesics without causing more pain. The preferred routes of administration are intravenous, local nerve block, and oral.

Continuous-infusion analgesia, which eliminates the peaks and valleys in pain control, is recommended to keep drug levels constant in children with continuous or persistent severe pain. Analgesics may also be given intravenously on a scheduled basis (e.g., every 3–4 hours). Delays in giving analgesics on a scheduled basis increase the chances of breakthrough pain and the subsequent anticipation of pain. Giving analgesics on an as-needed basis for acute pain also results in the *loss of pain control.* More medications are often needed to restore pain control than would have been required for continuous infusion analgesia.

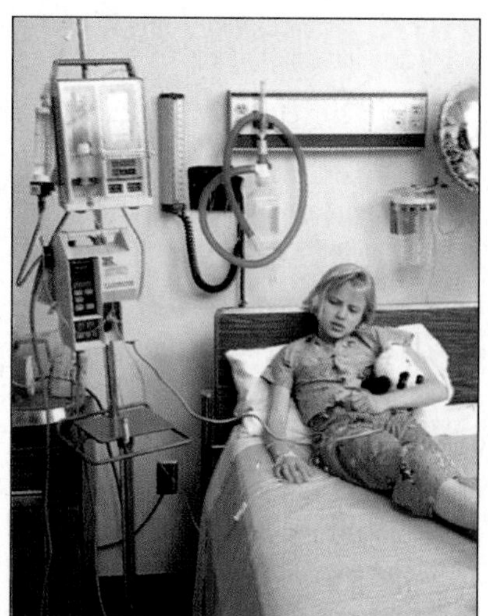

FIGURE 9-3 ◆
By using patient-controlled analgesia, the older child is able to regulate the intake of an intravenous analgesic such as morphine.

Patient-controlled analgesia (PCA) is a method of administering an intravenous or epidural analgesic, such as morphine, using a computerized pump that is programmed by the health care professional and controlled by the child (Figure 9-3 ◆). This technique is especially useful for pain control in the first 48 hours after surgery when oral pain management is not possible. PCA is prescribed mostly for children 5 years and older (Holder & Patt, 1995). Children selected for PCA should be able to push the injection button and should understand that pushing the button will give them medication to relieve pain. Parents are sometimes given responsibility for pushing the injection button for younger children or those with disabilities.

After initial pain control has been achieved with an IV infusion by the nurse, the child presses a button to receive a smaller analgesic dose for episodic pain relief. The PCA moni-

FAMILIES WANT TO KNOW

Patient-Controlled Analgesia (PCA)

- What is PCA? Analgesia means pain relief: You get to control the amount of medicine you receive by using the machine.
- The machine gives the medicine by passing it through the tube that is connected to your intravenous line. When you push the button, the machine pumps pain medicine into the intravenous line to make you feel better.
- The machine limits the amount of medicine you can get to what the doctor orders. You can get any amount up to the maximum by pushing the button repeatedly. The push button will not let you make a mistake if you drop it or roll on it.
- Whenever you feel pain, hurt, or discomfort, push the button to get more medicine. You should be the only one to push the button.
- No needles for pain shots are needed as long as the intravenous line is in place.
- The PCA may not relieve all of your pain, but it should make you feel comfortable. Let the nurse know if you think your PCA is not working.
- The PCA will be used until you can take pills or drink liquid pain medicine.

tor can be set up with or without a continuous infusion of opioid drug in addition to the dose administered when the child pushes the button. A continuous infusion prevents a recurrence of pain during long sleeping periods. Additional pain medication is often ordered as needed to supplement the continuous and patient-administered infusion when pain control is not maintained.

Children and adolescents benefit from PCA by receiving continuous pain control and having the ability to control their comfort level with no trauma from injections. Several studies have documented the maintenance of pain relief without an increase in narcotic side effects (Holder & Patt, 1995). Once children can take oral analgesics, PCA is discontinued.

Epidural pain control provides selective analgesia and has become more common for postoperative pain management. A catheter is inserted into either the lumbar or the caudal space. Only minute doses of drugs are needed because of the high concentration achieved at the opioid receptors in the spinal cord's dorsal horn (Holder, 1995).

Local nerve blocks, such as a popliteal block for anesthesia and analgesia of a lower extremity are used more frequently for pain control after surgery. A subcutaneous catheter is inserted into the local area for infusion of the analgesia. Pain control is achieved without systemic side effects from the medication.

SAFETY PRECAUTIONS

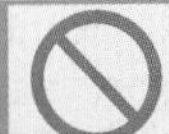

To prevent overdoses, the PCA computerized pump has safety features that include the ability to set the maximum number of infusions per hour and the maximum amount of drug received in a given time period.

NURSING MANAGEMENT OF PAIN

Nursing Assessment and Diagnosis

Nurses have an ethical obligation to relieve a child's suffering not only because of the consequences of unrelieved pain but also because appropriate pain management may have benefits such as earlier mobilization, shortened hospital stays, and reduced costs. To provide effective nursing management of children in pain, anticipate the presence of pain and recognize the child's right to pain control. Assess the child using an appropriate assessment tool (see Tables 9-3 to 9-7).

Examples of nursing diagnoses for children in pain include the following:

- *Moderate sharp knee pain* related to injury and orthopedic surgery
- *Moderate dull chronic hand pain* related to arthritic joint degeneration
- *Anxiety* related to anticipation of pain from an invasive procedure
- *Sleep pattern disturbance* related to inadequate pain control
- *Ineffective individual management of therapeutic regimen* related to self-management of pain control, and use of nonpharmacologic pain control measures
- *Ineffective breathing pattern: potential for,* related to opioid overdose
- *Risk for constipation* related to opioid pain medication and limited activity

LAW & ETHICS

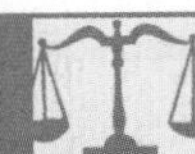

Most children are unaware of their right to pain relief. Nurses and health care institutions have a duty to prevent and alleviate suffering. Pain management should be an institutional priority with a standard of care. Nurses have an ethical responsibility to monitor implementation of that standard (Kachoyeanos & Zollok, 1995).

NURSING CARE PLAN — THE CHILD WITH POSTOPERATIVE PAIN

GOAL	INTERVENTION	RATIONALE	EXPECTED OUTCOME
1. Severe abdominal pain related to surgery and injury			
	NIC Priority Intervention: **Pain Management:** Alleviation of pain or a reduction in pain to a level of comfort that is acceptable to the patient.		NOC Suggested Outcome: **Comfort Level**: Feelings of physical and psychologic ease.
The child will report reduced pain.	■ Give analgesic by a pain-free method. ■ Have the child select a pain scale and rate the amount of pain perceived before and 30–60 minutes after analgesia is given to ensure pain relief. ■ Reposition the child every 2 hr to maintain good body alignment. Provide therapeutic touch or massage.	■ The child may deny pain to avoid analgesia by painful route. ■ The child's pain rating is the best indicator of pain. Maintenance of pain control requires less analgesia than treating each acute pain episode. ■ Anxiety increases perception of pain. New positions decrease muscle cramping and skin pressure.	The child reports reduced pain after administration of analgesia.
2. Sleep pattern disturbance related to inadequate pain control			
	NIC Priority Intervention: **Sleep Enhancement**: Facilitation of regular sleep/wake cycles.		NOC Suggested Outcome: **Sleep**: Extent and pattern of sleep for mental and physical rejuvenation.
The child will experience fewer disruptions of sleep by pain.	■ Give analgesia by continuous infusion or every 3–4 hr around the clock.	■ Pain breakthrough occurs even during sleep.	The child's sleep is undisturbed by pain. Child sleeps for age-appropriate number of hours per day.
3. Ineffective individual management of therapeutic regimen related to self-management of pain control and use of nondrug pain control measures			
	NIC Priority Intervention: **Self-Modification Assistance:** Reinforcement of self-directed change initiated by the patient to achieve personally important goals.		NOC Suggested Outcome: **Treatment Behavior Pain Control**: Personal actions to palliate or eliminate pain.
The child and family will effectively use patient-controlled analgesia (PCA) and nondrug pain control measures.	■ Teach the child how the PCA works and when to push the button. ■ Teach the family and the child how to use age-appropriate imagery, distraction, relaxation techniques, and other nondrug pain relief measures.	■ The child must know that pushing the PCA button will keep pain under control. ■ Nondrug pain control measures reduce amount of analgesia needed.	The child's pain rating stays low. The child and family independently use nondrug pain control measures.

(continued)

Planning and Implementation

Nursing management involves the following actions to increase and maintain patient comfort:

- Recognition of pain and formulation of a nursing diagnosis
- Pharmacologic intervention
- Nonpharmacologic intervention
- Monitoring and documenting the effectiveness of pain control measures to provide optimal comfort
- Patient education

NURSING CARE PLAN — THE CHILD WITH POSTOPERATIVE PAIN (continued)

GOAL	INTERVENTION	RATIONALE	EXPECTED OUTCOME
3. ***Ineffective individual management of therapeutic regimen*** **related to self-management of pain control and use of nondrug pain control measures** (continued)			
The child and family will use appropriate analgesia after discharge.	■ Discuss appropriate pain control to use at home after discharge.	■ The family and child may be anxious about pain management at home.	The family understands pain relief measures for use at home and knows where to call if help is needed.
4. ***Risk for ineffective breathing pattern*** **related to opioid overdose**			
	NIC Priority Intervention: **Respiratory Monitoring**: Collection and analysis of patient data to ensure airway patency and adequate gas exchange.		NOC Suggested Outcome: **Vital Signs Status:** Temperature, pulse, respirations, and blood pressure within expected range for the individual.
The child will maintain adequate ventilations.	■ Verify that correct dose of opioid analgesia is given. ■ Monitor vital signs and depth of inspirations before analgesic is administered and at time of peak drug action. ■ Calculate agonist dose ordered by physician to be sure it will reverse respiratory depression, not counteract effect of analgesia.	■ Respiratory depression is a significant complication of opioid analgesia. ■ Respiratory depression episode must not progress to respiratory arrest. All opioids act on brainstem center which decreases responsiveness to CO_2 tension. ■ Valuable time will be saved if agonist is needed for episode of respiratory depression.	There is no episode of respiratory depression associated with analgesia.
5. ***Constipation*** **related to opioid administration and decreased motility of gastrointestinal tract**			
	NIC Priority Intervention: **Constipation Management**: Prevention and alleviation of constipation.		NOC Suggested Outcome: **Bowel Elimination**: Ability of gastrointestinal tract to form and evacuate stool effectively.
The child will have minimal constipation.	■ Palpate the abdomen, and assess bowel sounds and abdominal distention. ■ Request physician order for stimulating laxative and stool softener. ■ Provide fluids of choice to increase fluid intake when IV fluids are decreased. ■ Inform family and child of possible medication induced constipation.	■ Signs of constipation must be anticipated and identified. ■ Opioids increase the transit time of feces and interfere with bile enzymes needed for evacuation. ■ Extra fluids will counteract opioid action of increasing the absorption of water from the large intestine. ■ Parents can become partners in managing fluid intake and monitoring bowel movements.	The child has bowel movements at least every 2 days while on opioid pain control.

The accompanying nursing care plan summarizes nursing care for the child with postoperative pain.

Pharmacologic Intervention

Give analgesics as ordered by the physician, ensuring that the dose is appropriate for the child's weight. When administering an opioid by intravenous infusion or PCA, monitor the flow rate and the site for infiltration. Make sure analgesic antagonists such as naloxone are available should complications develop. Naloxone may be used to treat respiratory depression caused by an opioid drug at a dose and slow infusion rate that does not reverse the pain control effects of the narcotic. A continuous infusion or repeated doses may be needed for severe overdoses.

CLINICAL TIP

Clinical signs that predict the development of respiratory depression include sleepiness, small pupils, and shallow breathing. Children at particular risk for respiratory depression induced by an opioid are those with an altered level of consciousness, an unstable circulatory status, a history of apnea, or a known airway problem.

SAFETY PRECAUTIONS

Use caution when ambulating a child with a regional nerve block in an extremity. Protect the extremity from injury because the child has reduced feeling in the limb.

LAW & ETHICS

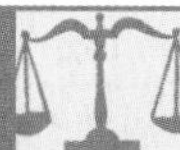

There is growing consensus that placebo use to assess and manage pain should be avoided, especially without consent. Studies suggest that placebos tend to be used for patients who are disliked, with whom staff have conflicts, or who have failed to respond to standard treatment. Placebo use involves deception. Respect the patient's right to be informed of treatment (Rushton, 1995).

Monitor the child's vital signs for complications related to opioids, such as respiratory depression. Other vital signs (heart rate and blood pressure) may not change in response to effective analgesia when infection, trauma, or other stressors keep them elevated. Check for the presence of other side effects of analgesics, such as sedation, nausea, vomiting, itching, urinary retention, and constipation.

When a regional nerve block is used, the analgesic effect does not recede for several hours after the catheter is removed. Monitor the child for tingling of fingers or toes, an indication that the analgesic effect is receding. Effective oral analgesia should be initiated to maintain pain control.

Evaluate the child's level of pain at frequent intervals to determine whether the analgesic eliminated the pain and to identify any increase in pain intensity. Use information collected from the child and parent, as well as from an appropriate pain scale. Dramatic reductions in pain should occur, although not all pain may disappear. Many children sleep after receiving an analgesic. This sleep is not a side effect of the drug or a sign of an overdose, but the result of pain relief. Pain interrupts sleep, and once pain is relieved, the child can sleep comfortably. On the other hand, sleep does not always indicate pain control. A child in pain may fall asleep in exhaustion. Look for other symptoms of pain, such as excess movement or moaning. Be certain to record results of pain control measures to guide future nursing actions. A flowsheet should be used to document assessments and medication administration during the postoperative period.

Become an advocate for children when the dose or type of analgesic ordered is inadequate. **Tolerance** is a decrease in a drug's effect over time or the need for increasing amounts of the drug to produce or maintain the same level of pain relief or sedation effect. This may occur when children with severe pain have been taking opioids or sedatives for several days. Breakthrough pain occurs, and an increase in dosage is needed to achieve the previous level of pain relief. Tolerance can be delayed with effective use of pain scales to allow appropriate drug dosing, and often less analgesia is needed. Magnesium may also slow the development of tolerance (Tobias, 2000). Before asking the physician to change the analgesia, review the child's record for documentation that the prescribed drug has been given at the appropriate dose and frequency and that the child's pain relief is ineffective despite the drug administration. After verifying the record, provide the physician with information about the characteristics of the child's pain and ask that the medication be changed. **Withdrawal** is the physical signs and symptoms that occur when a sedative or pain drug is stopped suddenly in a patient who is physically tolerant. Weaning may take 2 to 4 weeks to prevent withdrawal symptoms. See Table 9-11 for signs and symptoms of withdrawal.

Oral NSAIDs are generally ordered for less severe pain or chronic pain. These drugs may mask fever. Be alert to the potential complication of gastrointestinal hemorrhage in critically ill children who have increased gastric acids as physiologic stress response to pain.

TABLE 9-11 Signs and Symptoms of Opioid or Sedative Withdrawal

SYSTEM	SIGNS AND SYMPTOMS
Central nervous system	Irritability, increased wakefulness, tremulousness, hyperactive deep tendon reflexes, clonus, inability to concentrate, frequent yawning, sneezing, delirium, hypertonicity, visual or auditory hallucinations
Gastrointestinal system	Feeding intolerance with vomiting, diarrhea, uncoordinated suck and swallow
Sympathetic nervous system	Tachycardia, tachypnea, increased blood pressure, nasal stuffiness, sweating, fever

Note: From "Tolerance, withdrawal, and physical dependency after long term sedation and analgesia of children in the pediatric intensive care unit," by J. D. Tobias, 2000, *Critical Care Medicine, 28*(6), 2122–2132. Adapted.

Nonpharmacologic Intervention

Use nonpharmacologic methods of pain control with or without analgesics. One or more of these methods may provide adequate pain relief when the child has low levels of pain. When used with analgesics, nonpharmacologic techniques often increase the effectiveness of the analgesic or reduce the dosage required. When used in association with a medical procedure, remember to use an intervention before, during, and after the procedure. This gives the child a chance to recover, feel mastery, and remember coping (Fanurik, Koh, Schitz, et al., 1997).

Distraction **Distraction** involves engaging a child in a wide variety of activities to help him or her focus attention on something other than pain and the anxiety associated with the procedure. Examples of distracting activities are listening to music, singing a song, playing a game, watching television or a video, and focusing on a picture while counting. Select activities that are developmentally appropriate for the child. Children in severe pain cannot be distracted; but do not assume the pain is gone if a child can be distracted.

Cutaneous Stimulation Cutaneous stimulation involves gently rubbing the painful area, massaging the skin gently, and holding or rocking the child. Touching provides a stimulus to compete with the pain stimuli that are transmitted from the peripheral nerves to the spinal cord. These actions may reduce the pain felt by the child.

Swaddling and blanket rolls may calm a distressed neonate by decreasing tactile stimulation and containing gross motor behaviors (Lynn, Ulma, & Spreker, 1999).

Electroanalgesia Also known as transcutaneous electrical nerve stimulation (TENS), **electroanalgesia** delivers small amounts of electrical stimulation to the skin by electrodes. This stimulation may interfere with the transmission of pain from the peripheral nerves to the spinal cord. TENS may be used for both acute and chronic pain management.

Imagery Imagery is a cognitive process that encourages the child to focus on and explore a favorite place, event, or funny story unrelated to the pain process. This method is most effective in children over 6 years of age. Ask the child to think about all the sights, sounds, smells, tastes, and feelings that will help him or her to experience the favorite place. Imagery is a form of self-hypnosis, and it is most effective when preceded by a relaxation exercise.

Relaxation Techniques Relaxation techniques are used to reduce muscle tension. Pain is often aggravated when muscles are tensed. Relaxation methods include rhythmic breathing (repeatedly taking a deep breath and slowly releasing it), alternately tensing and relaxing selected muscle groups for 10 seconds each. Progressively move from specific muscle groups to more central muscles. Relaxation is enhanced if the child is encouraged to focus attention on something pleasant.

Hypnosis An altered state of consciousness occurs when appropriate suggestions distort perception, memory, and mood in the child. Children who respond to hypnotic suggestions are often more relaxed and experience less pain.

Clinical Tip

Assemble a pain management kit to promote distraction, imagery, and relaxation in children. Items that might be included are magic wands, pinwheels, bubble liquid, a slinky spring toy, a foam ball, party noisemakers, and pop-up books. It may also be helpful to include items for therapeutic play such as syringes, adhesive bandages, alcohol swabs, and other supplies from a medical kit. The pain management kit may be especially helpful for children who are being prepared for surgery or for painful procedures and need to be distracted.

Families Want to Know

Helping a Child Cope with Pain

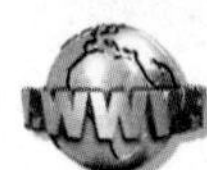

Parents are the single most powerful nonpharmacologic method of pain relief available to children. A parent's presence greatly reduces the anxiety associated with pain and hospitalization (Broome, 2000). Children often feel more secure telling their parents about their pain and anxiety. Parents can help the child to cope with mild or moderate pain using a variety of distraction methods that match the child's developmental stage and individual interests:

- Infants: holding, cuddling, sucking a pacifier
- Preschoolers: engaging in play, watching television or a video
- School-age children: talking about pleasant experiences, playing games, listening to radio, watching television or a video
- Adolescents: having visitors, playing games, watching television, listening to radio or tape player

Application of Heat and Cold Heat application promotes dilation of blood vessels. The increased blood circulation permits the removal of cell breakdown debris from the site. Heat also promotes muscle relaxation, breaking the pain–spasm–pain cycle. To reduce edema, do not apply heat in the first 24 hours after an injury.

The application of cold is believed to slow the ability of pain fibers to transmit pain impulses. Cold also controls pain by decreasing edema and inflammation, and by causing partial or complete anesthesia or numbness of the skin. When cold is applied, assess the skin for redness or signs of irritation. Care should be taken to avoid causing thermal injury. Discontinue cold applications immediately if the skin alternately blanches and reddens afterwards or if blisters or redness do not subside between applications.

Discharge Planning and Home Care Teaching

Children are frequently discharged from the hospital with oral analgesics following surgery, injury, or treatment of acute medical conditions. Teach parents and children about the dosage and frequency of administration and the side effects of the analgesic ordered. Make sure parents know that a sudden increase in pain intensity indicates the development of a complication requiring medical attention.

Educate school-age children and adolescents about pain that may occur with elective procedures, the use of pain scales, and the methods available for pain relief, both pharmacologic and nonpharmacologic. Encourage children and parents to use the techniques that work best for them.

Children with chronic conditions (arthritis, sickle-cell disease) or recurrent painful episodes (headaches, recurrent abdominal pain) often need long-term pain management (Table 9-12). For example, children with severe, long-term pain that is associated with cancer may be cared for at home with intravenous analgesics. These children are often managed by a home health care team. Educate parents thoroughly regarding intravenous care and analgesic administration.

Remember that many common health problems (otitis media, pharyngitis, and urinary tract infection) have pain as one of their presenting symptoms. Often the only medication prescribed is an antibiotic to clear the infection. This may leave the child in pain for 48 to 72 hours until the antibiotic brings the infection under control. Give parents recommendations for pain control and comfort measures during this period.

HOME CARE 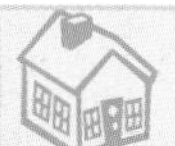

Parents have the responsibility to provide adequate pain control for their child after day surgery. Because of cultural values, some parents may feel the child should learn to tolerate some amount of pain. Provide guidance to help parents assess their child's pain and directions for giving pain medications. Take the time to discuss the importance of pain management and its benefits in promoting the child's healing.

Evaluation

Expected outcomes of nursing care include the following:

- The child's pain level is assessed frequently and pain management is effective in improving the child's comfort.
- The child successfully uses a PCA pump to control acute pain.
- Age-appropriate nonpharmacologic methods of pain management enhance the comfort provided by medications.

TABLE 9-12 Strategies for Chronic Pain Management

- Explain and validate the pain and its causes.
- Define treatment goals, including medications.
- Use distraction, relaxation, self-hypnosis, TENS, and exercise.
- Develop strategies for functional restoration.
- Give guidelines for a gradual increase in activity.
- Have a plan for sudden painful episodes.
- Explore stressors and potential pain triggers.
- Consider whether the child uses manipulatory behaviors for attention or secondary gain.
- Refer to a mental health professional or pain management team as needed.

Note: From "Treatment of chronic pain in children and adolescents," by B. S. Shapiro, 1995, *Pediatric Annals, 24*(3), 148–156. Adapted.

PAIN ASSOCIATED WITH MEDICAL PROCEDURES

Children undergo a wide variety of painful diagnostic and treatment procedures in the hospital and in outpatient settings. Procedures rated the most painful by children in one study included chest tube insertion, arterial puncture, lumbar puncture, bone marrow aspiration, insertion of a central or peripheral intravenous line, and venipuncture for drawing blood (Wong & Baker, 1988). The anticipation of these procedures causes anxiety and emotional distress that can lead to greater intensity of pain. Children who have experienced severe pain in the past may be unwilling to cooperate with health care personnel.

CLINICAL THERAPY

Procedures such as burn debridement, laceration repair, bone marrow aspiration, and fracture reduction are associated with so much pain and anxiety that children need premedication with analgesia and **anxiolysis,** or administration of sedatives.

A local anesthetic such as lidocaine buffered by sodium bicarbonate is often injected to provide analgesia for emergent invasive procedures. Lidocaine can also be injected subcutaneously in a small area to reduce the pain of deeper needle insertion.

Topical anesthetics can be used to reduce the pain associated with the first needle stick. Eutetic mixture of local anesthetics (EMLA) cream, a mixture of 2.5% lidocaine and 2.5% prilocaine in an emulsion is effective if applied 1 to 2 hours before a needle stick procedure on intact skin (Figure 9-4 ◆). Alternatively, Numby Stuff (2% lidocaine with 1:100,000 epinephrine) can be applied by iontophoresis, electric DC type current, to transport the ionizable drugs across intact skin in about 13 minutes (Squire, Kirchoff, & Hissong, 2000).

Conscious sedation is a light sedation during which the child maintains airway reflexes and responds to verbal stimuli (Table 9-13). It can be used on a cooperative child. With conscious sedation, children have minimal anxiety, less pain, and often no memory of the

DRUGS FOR SEDATION
Diazepam (Valium)
Midazolam (Versed)
Lorazepam (Ativan)
Ketamine
Popofol (Diprivan)

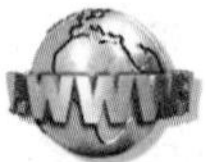

Pain Management for Procedures

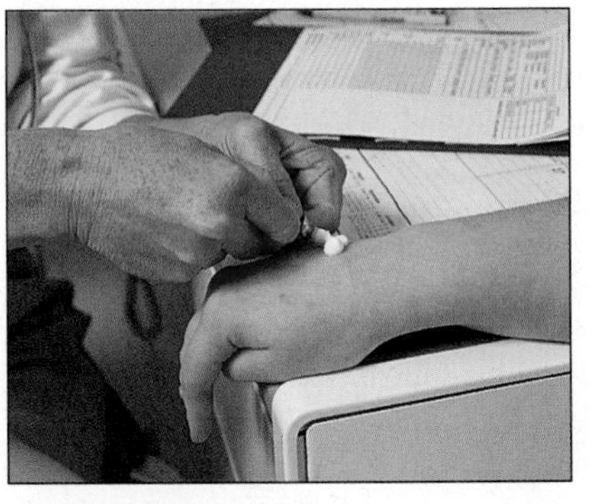

A

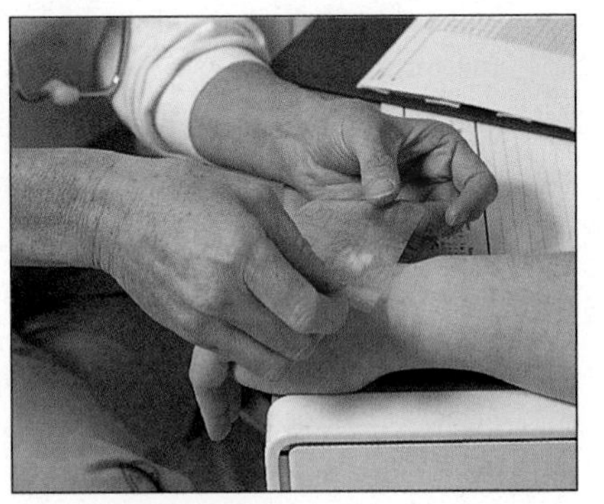

B

FIGURE 9-4 ◆

When painful procedures are planned, use EMLA cream to anesthetize the skin where the painful stick will be made. A, Apply a thick layer of cream over intact skin (1/2 of a 5-g tube). B, Cover the cream with a transparent adhesive dressing, sealing all the sides. The cream anesthetizes the dermal surface in 45–60 minutes.

TABLE 9-13 Characteristics of Conscious Sedation and Deep Sedation

ASSESSMENT FACTORS	CONSCIOUS SEDATION	DEEP SEDATION
Airway	Able to maintain airway independently and continuously	Unable to maintain airway independently or continuously
Cough and gag reflexes	Reflexes intact	Partial or complete loss of reflexes
Level of consciousness	Easily aroused with verbal or gentle physical stimulation	Not easily aroused, may not respond purposefully to verbal or gentle physical stimulation

Note: From Zimmerman, S. (1993). *Conscious sedation in the Emergency Medical Trauma Center.* Washington, DC: Children's National Medical Center.

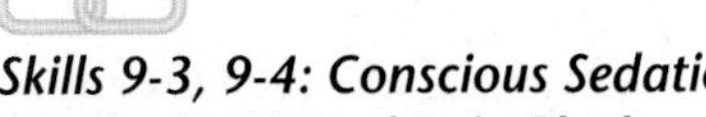

Skills 9-3, 9-4: Conscious Sedation Monitoring; Local Pain Blocks

procedure (Litman, 1995). Analgesia must be given in association with sedation as the sedated child can still feel pain but not communicate its presence. With the combined effects of analgesia and sedatives, the child must be carefully monitored for respiratory depression and **deep sedation,** a controlled state of depressed consciousness or unconsciousness.

NURSING MANAGEMENT

Make every effort to increase the child's comfort during painful procedures. Help the child cope with a painful procedure by telling the child what sensations to expect and what will happen during the procedure. This reduces stress more effectively than just providing information about the procedure (Broome, 1990). Chapter 5 gives methods for preparing children of different developmental ages for procedures.

Drugs may not be used for quick procedures, such as a dressing change, or an unexpected intravenous insertion, injection, or venipuncture. For a planned injection, intravenous insertion, or venipuncture, EMLA or other local anesthetic medication can be placed on the skin. Nonpharmacologic measures, especially imagery, relaxation techniques, and distraction, may reduce the anxiety associated with the anticipation of the procedure. Teach parents and children to use these interventions before procedures. Help children to control their anxiety through therapeutic play.

When pharmacologic pain management is used for a procedure, the nurse's responsibilities include the following:

- Treat anticipated procedure-related pain prophylactically. For example, give an analgesic before a bone marrow aspiration or fracture reduction. Permit time for the drug to become effective.
- Manage preexisting pain before beginning a procedure such as scrubbing a burn.
- When possible, administer drugs by a nonpainful route (oral, transmucosal, intravenous). Avoid intramuscular injections.
- When procedures must be repeated (e.g., bone marrow aspirations for children with leukemia), give optimal analgesia for the first procedure to reduce anxiety about future procedures.
- To prevent increased anxiety, avoid delays in performing procedures.
- Document the results of pain management.

When the child receives conscious sedation, monitoring the child's status is important. Nursing assessments include heart and respiratory rates, blood pressure, pulse oximetry, level of consciousness (response to verbal and physical stimulation), and color. Vital signs must be checked every 15 minutes until the child regains full consciousness and level of functioning. If conscious sedation progresses to deep sedation, airway management is essential, and vital signs should be checked every 5 minutes.

SAFETY PRECAUTIONS

When conscious sedation is given, be sure to have the resources available to monitor the child's vital signs and to provide advanced life support if the child should progress to deep sedation. All health care facilities have special protocols for management of children receiving conscious sedation.

If complications occur, the following equipment should be immediately available: suction apparatus, a bag-valve mask for assisted ventilation with capability of 90% to 100% oxygen delivery, an oxygen supply (5 l/min for more than 60 minutes), and antagonists to sedative medication.

CLINICAL TIP

Help children manage the pain from immunizations by "blowing away the shot pain." As a form of distraction and imagery, have the child repeatedly blow out air during the injection as if blowing bubbles.

Chapter Highlights

- Pain is an unpleasant sensation that is either acute or chronic, perceived in response to tissue damage.
- Research has revealed that infants and children feel pain, like adults, despite past beliefs to the contrary.
- Pain behaviors in children are similar to the behaviors of fearful and anxious children.
- Every infant, child, and adolescent has the right to adequate pain control.
- The goal of pain assessment is to provide accurate information about the location and intensity of the child's pain and how the child responds to it.
- Learning how the child expresses pain, both verbally and behaviorally, will help the nurse make a better assessment.
- Children learn how and when to seek help for pain and how to cope with pain by observing other family members.
- Numerous tools have been developed and validated to assess pain in infants and children.
- Pharmacologic interventions for pain control include opioids and nonsteroidal anti-inflammatory drugs (NSAIDs).
- Opioids are equally as effective when given orally, intramuscularly, and intravenously when an equianalgesic dose is used.

- Analgesia for continuous or severe pain should be given around the clock to maintain pain control. Patient-controlled analgesia is one method of administering a continuous infusion of an opioid medication and allowing the child to infuse additional small doses for episodic pain.
- Epidural and regional nerve blocks are pain control methods gaining acceptance because they do not have the side effects associated with systemic medications.
- Nonpharmacologic methods of pain management include the following: parental presence, distraction, cutaneous stimulation, electroanalgesia, imagery, relaxation techniques, hypnosis, and application of heat and cold.
- Parents need education and preparation to provide pain control for children who are discharged home following surgery and injuries. Children with chronic conditions often need long-term pain management.
- Many diagnostic and therapeutic procedures cause pain and anxiety in children. Provide optimal prophylactic pain management to reduce the anxiety associated with future procedures.
- Conscious sedation is used to reduce the child's anxiety associated with painful procedures. Analgesia is usually given in association with sedation when the procedure would cause pain or discomfort in an alert child.

EXPLORE MediaLink

- NCLEX review, case studies, and other interactive resources for this chapter can be found on the Companion Website at **http://www.prenhall.com/ball.** Click on Chapter 9 to select the activities for this chapter.
- For animations, more NCLEX review questions, and an audio glossary, access the accompanying CD-ROM in this textbook.

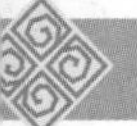

References

1. Abu-Saad, H. (1984). Cultural components of pain: The Asian-American child. *Children's Health Care, 13,* 11–14.
2. American Pain Society. (1999). *Principles of analgesic use in the treatment of acute pain and cancer pain* (4th ed). Glenview, IL: Author.
3. Anand, K. J. S., & Carr, D. B. (1989). The neuroanatomy, neurophysiology, and neurochemistry of pain, stress, and analgesia in newborns and children. *Pediatric Clinics of North America, 36*(4), 795–822.
4. Broome, M. E. (1990). Preparation of children for painful procedures. *Pediatric Nursing, 16,* 537–541.
5. Broome, M. E. (2000). Helping parents support their child in pain. *Pediatric Nursing, 26*(3), 315–317.
6. Chambers, C. T., Gresbrecht, K., Craig, K. D., Bennett, S. M., & Huntsman, E. (1999). A comparison of faces scales for the measurement of pediatric pain: Chidren's and parent's ratings. *Pain, 83,* 25–35.
7. Fanurik, D., Koh, J., Schitz, M., & Brown, R. (1997). Pharmacobehavioral intervention: Integrating pharmacologic and behavioral techniques for pediatric procedures. *Children's Health Care, 26*(1), 1–13.
8. Gaston-Johansson, F., Albert, M., Fagan, E., & Zimmerman, L. (1990). Similarities in pain descriptions of four different ethnic-culture groups. *Journal of Pain and Symptom Management, 5*(2), 94–100.
9. Hazinski, M. F. (1999). Analgesia, sedation, and neuromuscular blockage in pediatric critical care. In M. F. Hazinski, *Manual of pediatric critical care,* (pp. 44–72) St. Louis: Mosby.
10. Holder, K. A., & Patt, R. B. (1995). Taming the pain monster: Pediatric postoperative pain management. *Pediatric Annals, 24*(3), 164–168.
11. Joint Commission on the Accreditation of Health Care Organizations. (2001). *Pain standards for 2001.* Oakbrook Terrace, IL: Author, *www.jcaho.org.*
12. Kachoyeanos, M. K., & Zollok, M. B. (1995). Ethics in pain management of infants and children. *American Journal of Maternal Child Nursing, 20,* 142–147.
13. Leo, J., & Huether, S. E. (1998). Pain, temperature regulation, sleep, and sensory function. In K. L. McCance & S. E. Huether (Eds.), *Pathophysiology: The biologic basis for disease in adults and children* (3rd ed., pp. 422–432). St. Louis: Mosby.
14. Litman, R. S. (1995). Recent trends in management of pain during medical procedures in children. *Pediatric Annals, 24*(3), 158–163.
15. Lutz, W. J. (1986). Helping hospitalized children and their parents cope with painful procedures. *Journal of Pediatric Nursing, 1,* 24–32.
16. Lynn, A. M., Ulma, G. A., & Spreker, M. (1999). Pain control in very young infants: An update. *Contemporary Pediatrics, 16*(11), 39–66.
17. McCaffrey, M., & Pasero, C. (1999). *Pain: Clinical manual* (2nd ed.). St. Louis: Mosby.
18. McGrath, P. A. (1995). Pain in the pediatric patient: Practical aspects of assessment. *Pediatric Annals, 24*(3), 126–138.
19. Rushton, C. H. (1995). Placebo pain medication: Ethical and legal issues. *Pediatric Nursing, 21*(2), 166–168.
20. Shapiro, B. S. (1995). Treatment of chronic pain in children and adolescents. *Pediatric Annals, 24*(3), 148–156.
21. Squire, S. J., Kirchoff, K. T., & Hissong, K. (2000). Comparing two methods of topical anesthesia used before intravenous cannulation in pediatric patients. *Journal of Pediatric Health Care, 14*(2), 68–72.
22. Tesler, M. D., Holzemer, W. L., & Spreker, M. (1999). Pain behaviors: Postsurgical responses of children and adolescents. *Journal of Pediatric Nursing, 13*(1), 41–47.
23. Tobias, J. D. (2000). Tolerance, withdrawal, and physical dependency after long-term sedation and analgesia of children in the pediatric intensive care unit. *Critical Care Medicine, 28*(6), 2122–2132.
24. Wong, D. L., & Baker, C. M. (1988). Pain in children: Comparison of assessment scales. *Pediatric Nursing, 14,* 9–16.

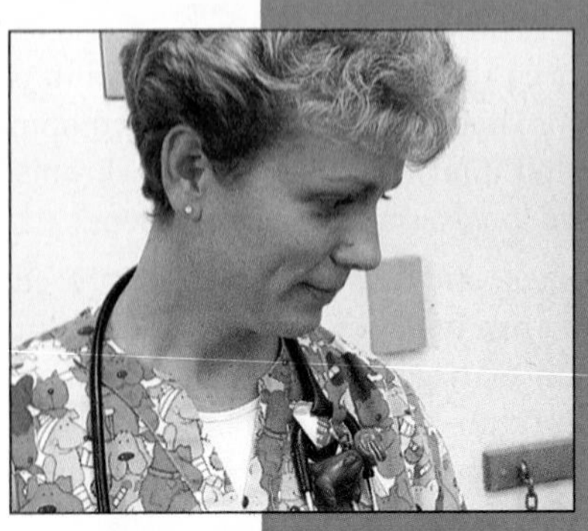

"So few parents realize how important proper hydration is in children. Such a large percentage of children's body weight is water that when they become dehydrated it can cause serious problems."

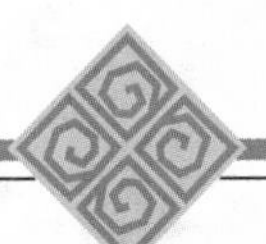

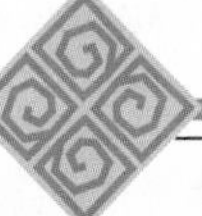

Vernon is 18 months old. Several days ago he developed vomiting and diarrhea. His parents tried to get him to eat, but he had little appetite. He drank a little water and a few sips of juice, but the next morning he was listless and would not drink anything. The diarrhea continued.

His mother has brought him to the urgent care center. Vernon is irritable on arrival, and his mother reports that he has been alternately irritable and lethargic. His mucous membranes and tongue appear dry, and skin turgor over the abdomen is slightly decreased. His mother notes that Vernon has had only two wet diapers today and says the urine in his diapers was dark in color. She also reports that he weighed 12 kg (26 lb) at the clinic last week. However, when the nurse weighs him, the scale reads only 11 kg (24 1/2 lb). Vernon is moderately dehydrated. He needs rapid replacement of the proper type of fluids.

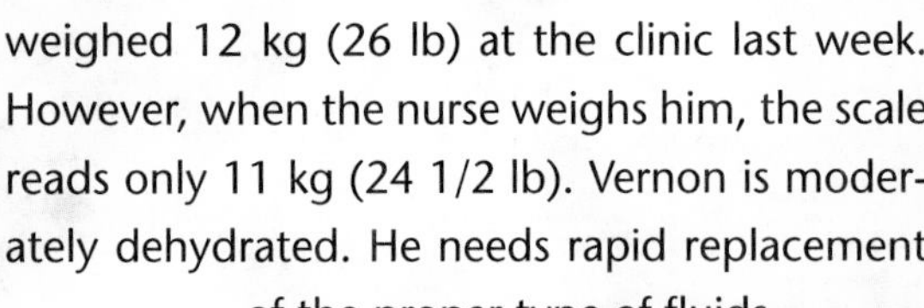

What happens inside the body when dehydration occurs? How can a nurse recognize dehydration? What types of fluid does Vernon need? What nursing management is important for his recovery? Why are young children at greater risk for dehydration than adults? What do parents need to be taught to prevent and manage dehydration? This chapter presents information that will enable you to answer these questions.

CHAPTER

10

ALTERATIONS IN FLUID, ELECTROLYTE, AND ACID–BASE BALANCE

KEY TERMS

acidemia Decreased blood pH.

acidosis Condition caused by excess acid in the blood.

alkalemia Increased blood pH.

alkalosis Condition caused by too little acid in the blood.

body fluid Body water that has substances (solutes) dissolved in it.

buffer Related acid-base pair that gives up or takes up hydrogen ions as needed to prevent large changes in the pH of a solution.

dehydration The state of body water deficit.

electrolytes Charged particles (ions) dissolved in body fluid.

extracellular fluid The fluid in the body that is outside the cells.

filtration Movement into or out of capillaries as the net result of several opposing forces.

hypertonic fluid Fluid that is more concentrated than normal body fluid.

hypotonic fluid Fluid that is more dilute than normal body fluid.

interstitial fluid That portion of the extracellular fluid that is between the cells and outside the blood and lymphatic vessels.

intracellular fluid The fluid in the body that is inside the cells.

intravascular fluid That portion of the extracellular fluid that is in the blood vessels.

isotonic fluid Fluid that has the same osmolality as normal body fluid.

Kussmaul respirations Increased rate and depth of respirations (hyperventilation).

oncotic pressure The part of the blood osmotic pressure that is due to plasma proteins; also called blood colloid osmotic pressure.

osmolality The amount of concentration of a fluid, technically, the number of moles of particles per kilogram of water in the solution.

osmosis Movement of water across a semipermeable membrane into an area of higher particle concentration.

pH Negative logarithm of the hydrogen ion concentration; used to monitor the acidity of body fluid.

saline A mixture of salt and water; normal saline refers to the mixture of salt and water in equal concentration in body fluids.

MediaLink 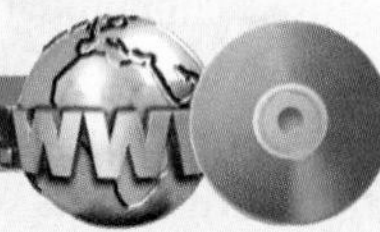

http://www.prenhall.com/ball

Resources for this chapter can be found on the CD-ROM accompanying this textbook, and on the Companion Website at http://www.prenhall.com/ball. Click on Chapter 10 to select the activities for this chapter.

CD-ROM

Animations
- Dehydration
- Edema
- Acid-Base Balance

Audio Glossary

NCLEX Review

COMPANION WEBSITE

Web Links

NCLEX Review

MediaLink Applications
- Calculating Degree of Dehydration and Fluid Excess
- Identifying Intravenous Fluids
- Understanding School-Age Athletes and Fluid Needs
- Care Planning for Hyponatremic Dehydration in Breastfeeding
- Interpreting Blood Gases

A thorough understanding of fluid, electrolyte, and acid–base homeostasis and imbalances is essential when providing nursing care to pediatric patients like Vernon, in the preceding scenario. This chapter presents information about the processes that maintain fluid and electrolyte balance, and describes the common imbalances that may occur in children. It also describes how the body regulates acid–base status and explains the management of acid–base imbalances.

Many health conditions cause changes in body fluids that must be regulated and managed. Sometimes management of fluid status in the home or in a short-term ambulatory facility can prevent more serious illness or hospitalization.

ANATOMY AND PHYSIOLOGY OF PEDIATRIC DIFFERENCES

Infants and young children differ physiologically from adults in ways that make them vulnerable to fluid, electrolyte, and acid–base imbalances.

Fluid in the body is in a dynamic state. In persons of all ages, fluid continuously leaves the body through the skin, in feces and urine, and during respiration. Much of the human body is composed of water. **Body fluid** is body water that has solutes dissolved in it. Some of the solutes are **electrolytes**, or charged particles (ions). Electrolytes such as sodium (Na^+), potassium (K^+), calcium (Ca^{++}), magnesium (Mg^{++}), chloride (Cl^-), and inorganic phosphorus (Pi) ions must be present in the proper concentrations for cells to function effectively.

In persons of all ages, body fluid is located in several compartments. The two major fluid compartments contain the **intracellular fluid** (fluid inside the cells) and the **extracellular fluid** (fluid outside the cells). The extracellular fluid is made up of **intravascular fluid** (the fluid within the blood vessels) and **interstitial fluid** (the fluid between the cells and outside the blood and lymphatic vessels) (Figure 10-1 ◆). Extracellular fluid accounts for about one third of total body water and intracellular fluid for about two thirds (Jospe & Forbes, 1996). The concentrations of electrolytes in the fluid differ depending on the fluid compartment. For example, extracellular fluid is rich in sodium ions; intracellular fluid, by contrast, is low in sodium ions but rich in potassium ions (Table 10-1).

Fluid moves between the intravascular and interstitial compartments by a process called filtration. Water moves into and out of the cells by the process of osmosis. These processes are discussed later in the chapter.

The percentage of body weight that is composed of water varies with age. The percentage is highest at birth (and higher in premature than in full-term infants) and decreases with age (Figure 10-2 ◆). Neonates and young infants have a proportionately larger extracellular fluid volume than older children and adults because their brain and skin (both rich in interstitial fluid) occupy a greater proportion of their body weight. Much of our extracellular fluid is exchanged each day (Davenport, 1996). During infancy, there is a high daily fluid requirement with little fluid volume reserve; this makes the infant vulnerable to dehydration. As an infant grows, the proportion of water inside the cells increases (Figure 10-3 ◆).

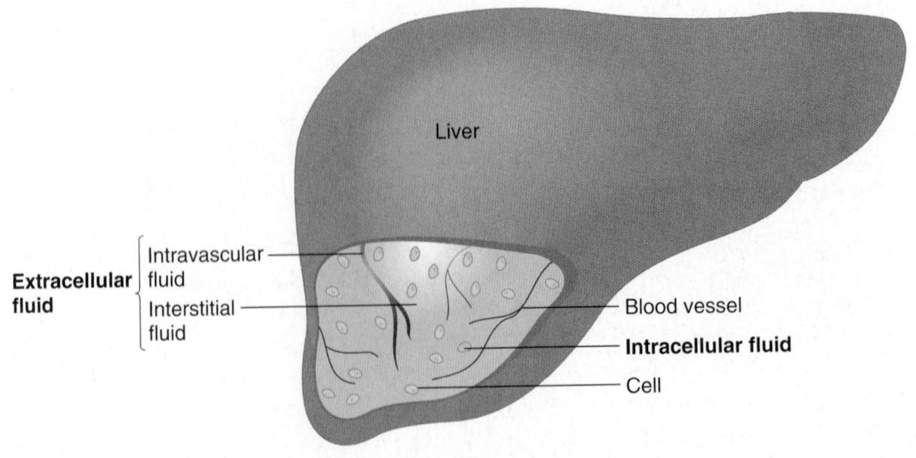

FIGURE 10-1 ◆
The major body fluid compartments. Extracellular fluid is composed mainly of *vascular fluid* (fluid in blood vessels) and *interstitial fluid* (fluid between the cells and outside the blood and lymphatic vessels). Intracellular fluid is that within cells.

TABLE 10-1 Electrolyte Concentrations in Body Fluid Compartments

	EXTRACELLULAR FLUID (ECF)		INTRACELLULAR FLUID (ICF)
Components	*Vascular*	*Interstitial*	
Na^+	High	High	Low
K^+	Low	Low	High
Ca^{++}	Low	Low	Low (higher than ECF)
Mg^{++}	Low	Low	High
Pi	Low	Low	High
Cl^-	High	High	Low
Proteins	High	Low	High

FIGURE 10-2 ◆ The percentage of water in the body varies with age. (ECF = extracellular water; ICF = intracellular fluid)

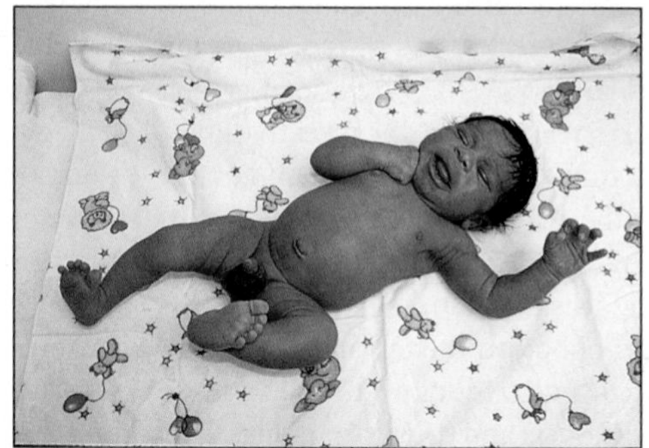

Full-term neonate, 75% water by weight: ECF = 45%, ICF = 30%

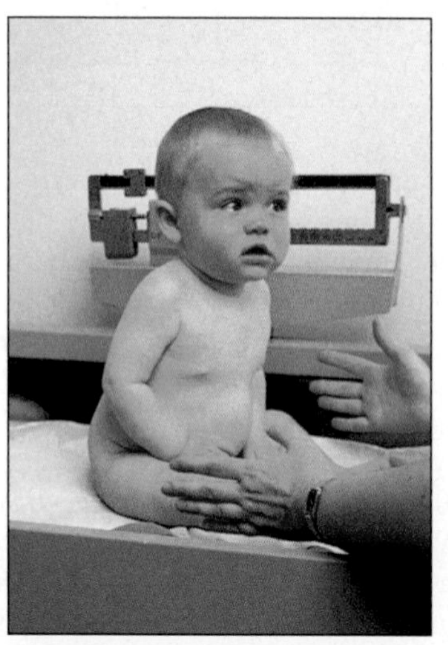

6-month infant, 65% water by weight: ECF = 25%, ICF = 40%

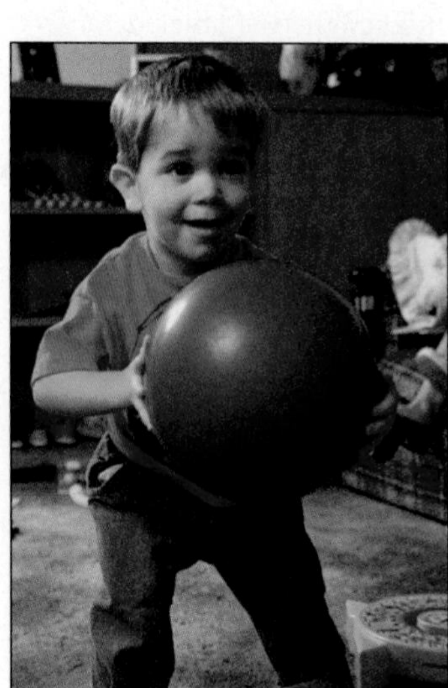

2-year old child, 60% water by weight: ECF = 20%, ICF = 40%

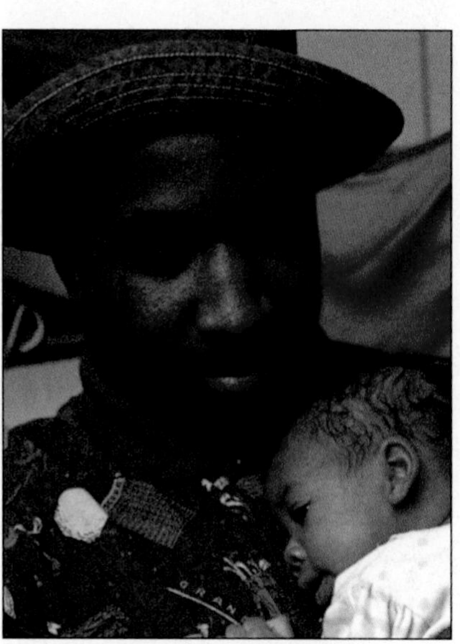

Adult male, 55% water by weight: ECF = 10–15%, ICF = 40%

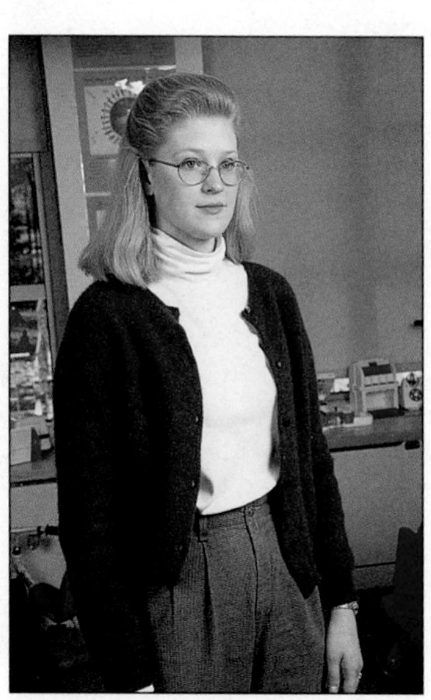

Adult female, 50% water by weight: ECF = 10–15%, ICF = 40%

AS THEY GROW Fluid Proportions

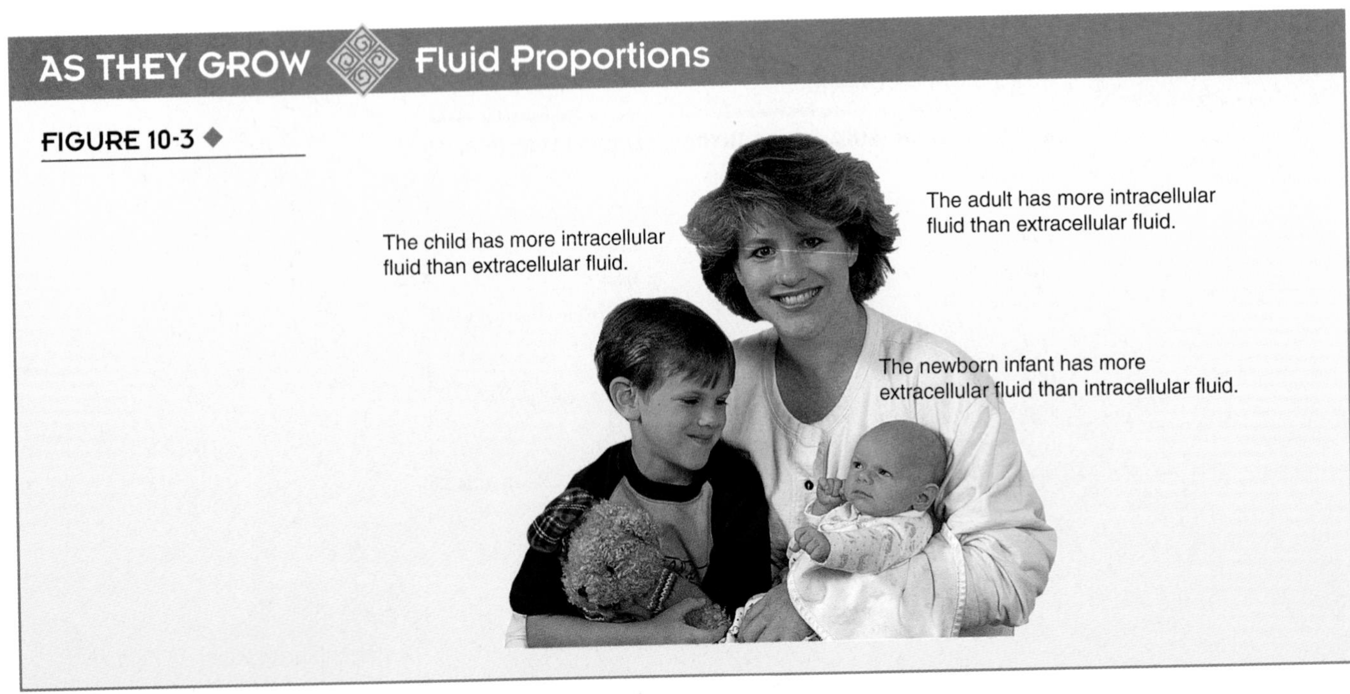

FIGURE 10-3 ◆

Infants and children under 2 years of age lose a greater proportion of fluid each day than older children and adults and are thus more dependent on adequate intake. They have a greater amount of skin surface or body surface area (BSA) and thus have greater insensible water losses through the skin. Because of this large BSA, they are also at greater risk when burned. In addition, respiratory and metabolic rates are high during early childhood. These factors lead to greater water loss from the lungs and greater water demand to fuel the body's metabolic processes (Figure 10-4 ◆). Due to these factors, the exercising child dehydrates easily and must consume more fluid during physical activity, particularly during hot weather (Committee on Sports Medicine and Fitness, 2000).

When fluid status is compromised, a number of body mechanisms are activated to help restore balance. Several of these mechanisms occur in the kidney. The kidneys conserve water and needed electrolytes while excreting waste products and drug metabolites. In children un-

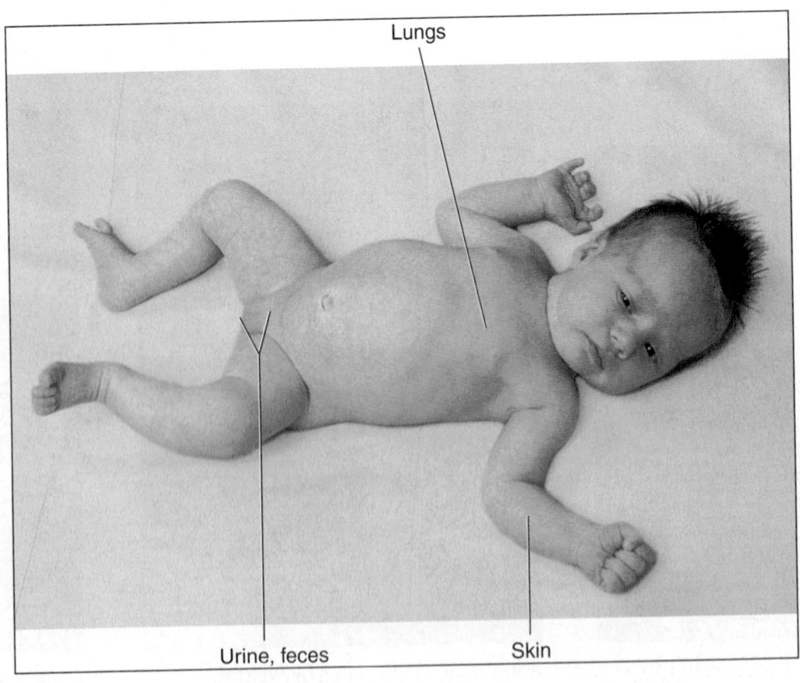

FIGURE 10-4 ◆ Normal routes of fluid excretion from infants and children.

TABLE 10-2 Health Conditions Contributing to Fluid Imbalance

- Radiant heat (phototherapy) used to treat hyperbilirubinemia increases insensible water loss through the skin.
- The increased respiratory rate in some illnesses leads to excessive water loss from lungs.
- Fever increases the metabolic rate and, therefore, water demands of metabolism (for each degree of Celsius increase above 37 degrees, 0.42 mL/kg/hr of additional fluid is needed).
- Vomiting and diarrhea increase fluid and electrolyte losses from the gastrointestinal system.
- Fistulas, blood loss, and drainage tubes contribute to fluid deficits.

der 2 years of age, however, the glomeruli, tubules, and nephrons of the kidneys are immature. They are thus unable to conserve or excrete water and solutes effectively (see Chapter 18). Because more water is generally excreted, the infant and young child can become dehydrated quickly or develop electrolyte imbalances. In addition, infants have a weaker transport system for ions and bicarbonate, placing them at greater risk for acidosis and acid–base imbalances. Children under 2 years of age also have difficulty regulating electrolytes such as sodium and calcium. Renal response to high solute loads is slower and less developed, with function improving gradually during the first year of life (Hewitt-Taylor, 1999).

Finally, in addition to the immaturity of physiologic processes, many health conditions make young children more vulnerable to fluid deficit (Table 10-2).

FLUID VOLUME IMBALANCES

When fluid excretion and losses are balanced by the proper volume and type of fluid intake, fluid balance will be maintained. If, however, fluid output and intake are not matched, fluid imbalance may occur rapidly. The major types of fluid imbalances are extracellular fluid volume deficit (dehydration), extracellular fluid volume excess, and interstitial fluid volume excess (edema).

EXTRACELLULAR FLUID VOLUME IMBALANCES

Extracellular Fluid Volume Deficit (Dehydration)

Extracellular fluid volume deficit occurs when there is not enough fluid in the extracellular compartment (vascular and interstitial). Because sodium is generally lost along with water, hyponatremia can also be present. (Hyponatremia is described later in the chapter, on page 327.) The state of body water deficit is called **dehydration**.

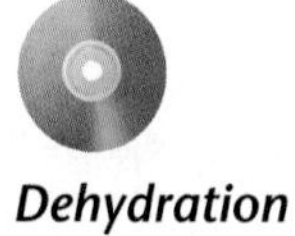

Dehydration

ETIOLOGY AND PATHOPHYSIOLOGY Extracellular fluid volume deficit is usually caused by the loss of sodium-containing fluid from the body. The situations that most often cause loss of fluid containing sodium are vomiting, diarrhea, nasogastric suction, hemorrhage, and burns. Vomiting and diarrhea are common manifestations of disease in children throughout the world, and each year up to 5 million children die from dehydration related to diarrhea. About 300 to 500 die annually in the United States from this problem; about 220,000 are hospitalized; and many more receive care on an outpatient basis (Shamir, Zahavi, Abramowich, et al., 1998).

Another cause of extracellular fluid volume deficit in infants is increased water loss in low-birth-weight infants who are kept under radiant warmers to maintain heat (Figure 10-5 ◆). Less frequently, adrenal insufficiency, accumulation of extracellular fluid in a "third space" such as the peritoneal cavity, and overuse of diuretics may be the cause. The latter etiology is most often seen in bulimic adolescents for weight control (see Chapter 7).

CLINICAL MANIFESTATIONS The signs of dehydration relate to the severity or degree of the body water deficit (Table 10-3). They are a result of both the decreased fluid (e.g., diminished turgor and mucous membrane moisture) and the body's response to the fluid deficit (e.g., pulse and blood pressure changes) (Table 10-4).

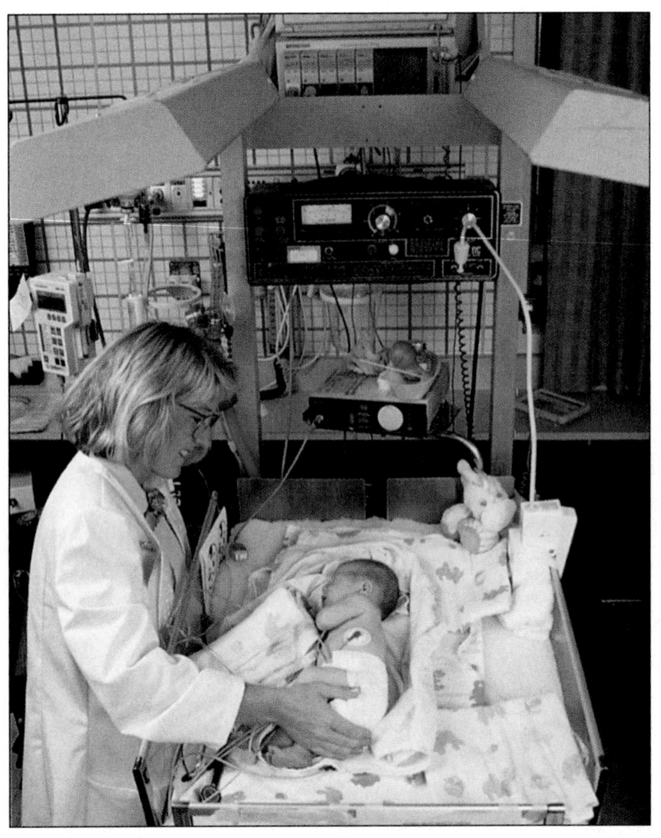

FIGURE 10-5 ◆
Use of an overhead warmer or phototherapy increases insensible fluid excretion through the skin, thus increasing the fluid intake needed.

TABLE 10-3 Severity of Clinical Dehydration

CLINICAL ASSESSMENT	MILD	MODERATE	SEVERE
Percent of body weight lost	Up to 5% (40–50 mL/kg)	6%–9% (60–90 mL/kg)	10% or more (100 + mL/kg)
Level of consciousness	Alert, restless, thirsty	Irritable or lethargic (infants and very young children); alert, thirsty, restless (older children and adolescents)	Lethargic to comatose (infants and young children); often conscious, apprehensive (older children and adolescents)
Blood pressure	Normal	Normal or low; postural hypotension (older children and adolescents)	Low to undetectable
Pulse	Normal	Rapid	Rapid, weak to nonpalpable
Skin turgor	Normal	Poor	Very poor
Mucous membranes	Moist	Dry	Parched
Urine	May appear normal	Decreased output (< 1 mL/kg/hr) dark color; increased specific gravity	Very decreased or absent output
Thirst	Slightly increased	Moderately increased	Greatly increased unless lethargic
Fontanel	Normal	Sunken	Sunken
Extremities	Warm; normal capillary refill	Delayed capillary refill (>2 sec)	Cool, discolored; delayed capillary refill (> 3–4 sec)
Respirations	Normal	Normal or rapid	Changing rate and pattern

TABLE 10-4 Clinical Manifestations of Extracellular Fluid Volume Deficit

SIGNS AND SYMPTOMS	PHYSIOLOGIC BASIS
Weight loss	Decreased fluid volume; 1 L of fluid weighs 1 kg
Postural blood pressure drop (older children)	Inadequate circulating blood volume to offset the force of gravity when in upright position
Increased small-vein filling time	Decreased vascular volume
Delayed capillary refill time	Decreased vascular volume
Flat neck veins when supine (older children)	Decreased vascular volume
Dizziness, syncope	Inadequate circulation to brain
Oliguria	Inadequate circulation to kidneys
Thready, rapid pulse	Cardiac reflex response to decreased vascular volume
Sunken fontanel (infants)	Decreased fluid volume
Decreased skin turgor	Decreased interstitial fluid volume

Mild dehydration is hard to detect, because children appear alert and have moist mucous membranes. Infants may be irritable and older children are thirsty. In moderate dehydration, the child is often lethargic and sleepy, but there may be periods of restlessness and irritability, especially in infants. Skin turgor is diminished, mucous membranes appear dry, and urine is dark in color and diminished in amount. Pulse rate is usually increased and blood pressure can be normal or low. Vernon, described at the beginning of this chapter, was displaying symptoms of moderate dehydration. His urine output was decreased, and he had lost about 8% of his body weight. What other signs and symptoms of moderate dehydration can you identify in the opening scenario? What additional assessments would you want to perform on Vernon?

Severe dehydration is manifested by increasing lethargy or nonresponsiveness, markedly decreased blood pressure, rapid pulse, poor skin turgor, dry mucous membranes, and markedly decreased or absent urinary output.

GROWTH & DEVELOPMENT

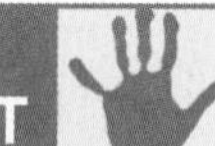

Urine specific gravity may increase in older children who are dehydrated; but due to the inability of the child under 2 years of age to concentrate urine effectively, a rising specific gravity may not be seen in the younger dehydrated child.

CLINICAL THERAPY Medical management depends on accurate identification of the degree of dehydration. In addition to physical signs and symptoms (Table 10-3), elevated blood urea nitrogen (>25 mg/dL) and serum bicarbonate (>17 mEq/L) are useful to identify moderate and severe diarrhea (Eliason & Lewan, 1998; Vega & Avner, 1997). The treatment of extracellular fluid volume deficit is administration of fluid containing sodium. This may be accomplished by oral rehydration therapy or by intravenous fluids.

Oral rehydration therapy has been used for a number of years in developing countries without an accessible supply of intravenous fluids. More recently, the benefits of using this therapy early to prevent severe dehydration and to treat mild and moderate dehydration in children in developed countries has been recognized. The therapy is successful in treating the dehydration caused by many gastrointestinal illnesses and prevents hospitalization for many infants and young children (Armon, Stephenson, MacFaul et al., 2001). It is the treatment of choice for children with diarrhea who have mild to moderate dehydration (Provisional Committee on Quality Improvement, 1996). Solutions are available commercially that contain water, carbohydrate (sugar), sodium, potassium, chloride, and lactate (Table 10-5). Some clinicians allow lactose-free milk, breast milk, or half-strength milk to be given in addition to oral rehydration therapy solution. The WHO/UNICEF solution was developed for use with cholera and is not generally used for diarrhea treatment in the United States, as its sodium and chloride loads are higher than that of other commercial solutions.

CLINICAL TIP

Assessing skin turgor takes skill and practice. In moderate dehydration, the skin may have a doughy texture and appearance. Later, in severe dehydration, the more typical "tenting" of skin is observed. Diminished turgor is most easily assessed in infants or children with little subcutaneous fat; it is more difficult to assess in those with larger amounts of fat.

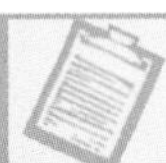

RESEARCH

How accurate are clinical observations of children by health professionals in assessing the degree of dehydration? In an attempt to make more accurate decisions, some clinicians have tried to combine laboratory studies with clinical observations. A rising blood urea nitrogen has been used by some, but other studies have found that increased serum bicarbonate is a better laboratory study to predict degree of dehydration (Vega & Avner, 1997; Liebelt, 1998).

Skill 5-3: Weight Measurement
Skill 5-10: Blood Pressure Measurement
Skill 5-22: Intake and Output Measurement

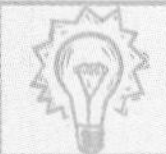

CLINICAL TIP

To calculate the percentage of weight loss:

- Subtract the child's present weight from the original weight to find the loss.
- Divide the loss by the child's original weight.

EXAMPLE: In the opening scenario, Vernon weighed 12 kg (26 lb) at the clinic last week. However, when he is weighed today, the scale reads only 11 kg (24 1/2 lb). In this case, subtracting 11 kg from 12 kg yields 1 kg of weight loss. Dividing 1 kg by his original weight of 12 kg reveals that he has lost approximately 8% of his body weight, which indicates moderate dehydration.

CLINICAL TIP

To obtain urine from an infant for testing specific gravity, place two cotton balls in the diaper. When they are wet, push them into a 10-mL syringe and squeeze out the urine with the plunger.

TABLE 10-5 Oral Rehydration and Maintenance Fluids for Mild and Moderate Dehydration

Pedialyte	Nutralyte	Ricelyte
Infalyte	Hydralyte	Rehydralyte
Resol	Lytren	WHO/UNICEF oral rehydration solution

When the child is severely dehydrated, intravenous fluid will be given, often accompanied with oral rehydration. The intravenous fluid is often Ringer's lactate followed by or accompanied with dilute saline, such as one half or one quarter normal saline (Aker & O'Sullivan, 1998). The fluid combination replenishes the extracellular fluid volume and adds solutes to return the body fluid to normal. The child may be hospitalized or treated with intravenous fluids in a short-stay unit until the dehydration is controlled. Once hydration is completed, the child may resume an age-appropriate diet (Burkhart, 1999).

NURSING MANAGEMENT

Nursing Assessment and Diagnosis

Weigh the child daily with the same scale and without clothing. Compare to past weights and calculate weight loss. Carefully measure intake and output, urine specific gravity, level of consciousness, pulse rate and quality, skin turgor, mucous membrane moisture, quality and rate of respirations, and blood pressure. Compare the blood pressure when the child is supine with the pressure when the child is sitting with legs hanging down or standing. If the child is dehydrated, the sitting or standing blood pressure will be lower than the supine blood pressure, because blood accumulates in the dependent legs. The nurse will obtain samples of urine and blood as needed for dehydration evaluation.

The nursing diagnosis *fluid volume deficit* applies to all children who have an extracellular fluid volume deficit. Other diagnoses depend on the severity of the condition and the age of the child. Several nursing diagnoses that might be appropriate for the mildly to severely dehydrated child are included in the accompanying nursing care plan. Additional care of the child with dehydration from gastroenteritis can be found in Chapter 17. Specific examples of nursing diagnoses include the following:

- *Fluid volume deficit* related to active fluid volume loss or failure of regulatory mechanisms
- *Risk for altered peripheral tissue perfusion* related to hypovolemia
- *Risk for injury* related to postural hypotension

Planning and Implementation

Nursing care of the dehydrated child focuses on providing oral rehydration fluids, teaching parents oral rehydration methods, and, if necessary, administering intravenous fluids to restore fluid balance. The accompanying nursing care plan summarizes care of the child with mild to severe dehydration.

PROVIDE ORAL REHYDRATION FLUIDS

In mild or moderate dehydration, oral rehydration fluid is the first intervention (see Table 10-5). It is given in frequent small amounts; for example, 1 to 3 teaspoons of fluid every 10 to 15 minutes is a useful guideline for starting oral rehydration. For the first 2 to 4 hours of treatment, 50 mL of fluid for each kg of the child's weight should be the target intake (Endsley & Galbraith, 1998; Larson, 2000). Instruct parents to continue to administer the 1 teaspoon every 2 to 3 minutes even if the child vomits, as small amounts of the fluid may still be absorbed. Table 10-6 provides guidelines for oral rehydration therapy.

TEACH PARENTS ORAL REHYDRATION METHODS

Instruct parents about the types of fluids and amounts to be given. Begin teaching with parents of all newborns and reinforce teaching at each well-child visit. Advise parents to continue

NURSING CARE PLAN The Child with Mild or Moderate Dehydration

GOAL	INTERVENTION	RATIONALE	EXPECTED OUTCOME
1. Ineffective management of theapeutic regimen related to knowledge deficit about diarrhea and vomiting			
	NIC Priority Intervention: **Family Involvement:** Facilitate family participation in care of the child.		NOC Suggested Outcome: **Participation: Health Care Decisions:** Personal involvement in selecting health care options.
Parents will describe appropriate home management of fluid replacement for diarrhea and vomiting.	■ Explain how to replace body fluid with an oral rehydration solution. Encourage parents to keep the solution at home and begin use with the first sign of diarrhea. ■ Teach parents to continue the child's normal diet in addition to providing replacement fluids for diarrhea. ■ Provide verbal and written instructions to parents at each well-child visit.	■ Use of an oral rehydration solution can enable successful treatment of vomiting and diarrhea at home. ■ Diet plus fluid supplementation leads to faster recovery. ■ Parents are provided with a reference for later use.	Parents are successfully able to treat the child's diarrhea and vomiting at home.
2. Knowledge deficit (parent) related to causes of dehydration			
	NIC Priority Intervention: **Teaching:** Teach causes of dehydration.		NOC Suggested Outcome: **Knowledge:** Extent of understanding conveyed about treatment regimen
Parents will state common causes of childhood dehydration.	■ Teach parents childhood conditions that commonly lead to dehydration.	■ If parents recognize situations that can lead to dehydration, they will be more alert to its appearance.	Parents recognize conditions of risk for dehydration in children.
3. Risk for fluid volume deficit related to worsening of child's condition			
	NIC Priority Intervention: **Fluid Management:** Promote fluid balance.		NOC Suggested Outcome: **Fluid Balance:** Balance of water in extra- and intracellular compartments of body.
Parents will seek health care for the child's worsening condition.	■ Teach parents to seek care when the child's vomiting or diarrhea worsens, or the child's mental alertness changes.	■ Severe dehydration may occur if milder forms are not successfully treated.	Parents seek prompt attention for the child's worsening condition, preventing the development of severe dehydration.

the child's normal diet in addition to providing the rehydration solution. Cereals, starches, soups, fruits, and vegetables are allowed. Tell parents to avoid simple sugars, which can worsen diarrhea because of osmotic effects, including soft drinks (if used, they should be diluted with equal parts of water), undiluted juice, Jell-O, and sweetened cereal.

Repeated vomiting of large volumes of fluid or a worsening of the child's condition can indicate the need for intravenous therapy. Teach parents when to seek further medical care. If the child's condition worsens or does not improve after 4 hours of oral rehydration therapy, parents should contact a health care professional.

SAFETY PRECAUTIONS

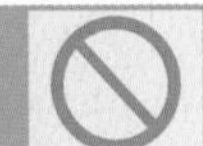

Sugar facilitates the absorption of sodium in oral rehydration fluids. Tell parents not to give diet beverages for oral rehydration, because they contain no sugar and will not be effectively absorbed.

Monitor Intravenous Fluid Administration

The hospitalized child usually requires administration of intravenous fluids. Be sure that the amount of fluid administered corresponds with the diagnosed dehydration state of the child (Table 10-7). Usually, about half of the 24-hour total maintenance and replacement needs will be given in the first 6 to 8 hours, with a slower rate infused for the remainder of the 24 hours. During the first 1 to 3 hours, the infusion rate may be highest to rapidly expand the

NURSING CARE PLAN The Child with Severe Dehydration

GOAL	INTERVENTION	RATIONALE	EXPECTED OUTCOME
1. Fluid volume deficit related to excess losses and inadequate intake			
	NIC Priority Intervention: **Fluid Management:** Promote fluid balance.		NOC Suggested Outcome: **Fluid Balance**: Balance of water in extra- and intracellular components of the body.
The child will return to normal hydration status and will not develop hypovolemic shock.	■ Monitor weight daily. Assess intake and output every shift. Assess heart rate, postural blood pressure, skin turgor, small-vein filling time, capillary refill time, fontanel (infant), and urine specific gravity every 4 hours or more frequently as indicated. ■ Administer intravenous fluids as ordered. Monitor for crackles in dependent portions of the lungs.	■ Frequent assessment of hydration status facilitates rapid intervention and evaluation of the effectiveness of fluid replacement. ■ Replace fluid lost from the body. Excessive replacement of sodium-containing fluids could cause extracellular fluid volume excess.	The child has signs of normal hydration.
2. Risk for injury related to decreased level of consciousness			
	NIC Priority Intervention: **Fall Prevention**: Institute special precautions.		NOC Suggested Outcome: **Fall Prevention**: Minimize risk factors that precipitate falls.
The child will not experience injury.	■ Raise the side rails of the bed. Ensure that a small child does not become tangled in bed covers. ■ Monitor level of consciousness every 2–4 hours or more often as indicated. ■ Monitor serum sodium concentration daily or more often. ■ Have the child sit before rising from bed and assist to stand slowly.	■ Safety measures protect the child. ■ Frequent assessment provides evidence of the need for safety interventions and of the effectiveness of therapy. ■ Elevated serum sodium concentration causes brain cell shrinkage and decreased level of consciousness. ■ Slow adjustment to upright posture reduces light-headedness from decreased blood volume.	The child does not fall or suffer other injury.
3. Activity intolerance related to bedrest/immobility			
	NIC Priority Intervention: **Activity Therapy**: Plan activities to meet child's developmental needs.		NOC Suggested Outcome: **Energy Conservation**: Manage energy to sustain activity.
The child will engage in normal activity for age.	■ Plan activities appropriate for the age of the child that can be done in bed. ■ Group nursing interventions to provide time for the child to rest. ■ Provide assistance during meals and other activities as needed.	■ Activities will provide distraction and promote recovery. ■ The child will require more rest than usual. ■ Prevention of overexertion will conserve body fluid and promote healing.	The child engages in normal developmental activities and receives adequate rest.

TABLE 10-6 Oral Rehydration Therapy Guidelines

- Children with diarrhea and no dehydration should be continued on age-appropriate diets.
- For mild dehydration, give 50 mL/kg oral rehydration therapy in 4 hours in addition to replacing fluids lost in stool and emesis. (Measure emesis and give 10 mL/kg of fluid for each diarrheal stool.)
- For moderate dehydration, give 100 mL/kg oral rehydration therapy in 4 hours in addition to replacing fluids lost as described above.
- For severe dehydration, the child is hospitalized and treated with intravenous fluids. When hydrated adequately or concurrently with intravenous rehydration, begin oral rehydration therapy with 50–100 mL/kg of fluid in 4 hours and stool replacement as described above.
- When rehydration is complete, resume normal diet.

Note: From Provisional Committee on Quality Improvement, Subcommittee on Acute Gastroenteritis (1996). Practice parameter: the management of acute gastroenteritis in young children. *Pediatrics, 97*, 424–436. Adapted.

TABLE 10-7 Calculation of Intravenous Fluid Needs

1. First, calculate the *maintenance* fluid needs of the child, according to the following guideline:

USUAL WEIGHT	MAINTENANCE AMOUNT
Up to 10 kg	100 mL/kg/24 hr
11–20 kg	1000 mL + (50 mL/kg for weight above 10 kg)/ 24 hr
> 20 kg	1500 mL + (20 mL/kg for weight above 20 kg)/ 24 hr

Example: Vernon's weight is 12 kg. He needs 1000 mL + (50 × 2), or 1100 mL/24 hr for maintenance fluid.

2. Next, calculate *replacement* fluid for that lost:

Example: Vernon has lost 1 kg (8%) of his body weight. Multiplying the percentage of body weight × 10 yields the mL/kg/24 hr required:

$$8 \times 10 = 80 \text{ mL/kg/24 hr}$$
$$80 \text{ mL/kg} \times 12 \text{ kg} = 960 \text{ mL}$$

Thus, Vernon's replacement fluid needs are 960 mL/24 hr.

3. Finally, calculate continued *losses* and add to the total maintenance and replacement needs.

vascular space. Rapid infusion of 20 to 30 mL/kg over 1 to 2 hours is sometimes used in outpatient settings, followed by oral fluids. When oral fluids are maintained, the decision for discharge can be made and hospitalization avoided (Reid & Bonadio, 1996).

Maintain the intravenous line carefully so fluid infusion can be kept on schedule (refer to the Skills Manual). Use a pump to prevent inadvertent, rapid infusion, which can lead to fluid overload and electrolyte imbalance. Play with the toddler and preschool child frequently and use diversionary methods, as necessary, to distract the child from the intravenous line. Monitor the child carefully and implement safety precautions as necessary. Once the child begins to tolerate some oral fluids, oral rehydration therapy is substituted for intravenous fluid administration and frequent administration of appropriate fluids is needed.

DISCHARGE PLANNING AND HOME CARE TEACHING

Prior to discharge, parents need instructions about types of fluids and amounts to encourage. Teach the signs of dehydration (see Table 10-3) so that if the child does not take in adequate fluids, parents can seek help immediately. Instruct them to begin the child's normal diet once hydration is complete, determined by adequate urinary output and normal behaviors. Review methods of minimizing the child's chance of acquiring gastrointestinal infections (e.g., avoiding contact with other children who are infected; using careful handwashing and dishwashing procedures when a child in the home is affected). During well-child visits, encourage all parents to keep oral rehydration fluids at home in case they are needed at some time; they are available in most grocery stores and pharmacies. Address the need for increasing fluids in hot weather and when the child is exercising.

NURSING ALERT

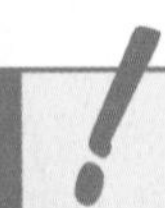

If an oral rehydration solution is too concentrated, it can worsen the diarrhea. Juice and cola are highly concentrated and should be diluted to half strength when given to a child who has diarrhea. Encourage parents to keep an oral rehydration solution (see Table 10-5 for examples) in liquid or powder form on hand at all times and to use these solutions rather than juice or soda when the child first develops diarrhea (Straughan & English, 1996).

Skill 8-5: Administering IV Fluids

SAFETY PRECAUTIONS

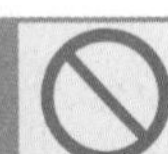

Dizziness and lethargy can be manifestations of dehydration, so interventions to promote safety are important. Keep up the side rails and supervise the child when he or she is getting out of bed.

Evaluation

Expected outcomes of nursing care for the child with dehydration include the following:

- Balance of water and electrolytes in intracellular and extracellular compartments
- Normal urinary output
- Adequate fluid intake for maintenance needs
- Vital signs within normal limits

Extracellular Fluid Volume Excess

Extracellular fluid volume excess occurs when there is too much fluid in the extracellular compartment (vascular and interstitial). This imbalance may also be called saline excess or extracellular volume overload. If this disorder occurs by itself (without saline disturbance), the serum sodium concentration is normal. There is simply too much extracellular fluid, even though it has a normal concentration.

Infants and children who develop an extracellular fluid volume excess have a condition that causes them to retain **saline** (sodium and water) or they have been given an overload of sodium-containing isotonic intravenous fluid (Figure 10-6 ◆). What conditions cause retention of saline? The hormone aldosterone is secreted by the adrenal cortex. One of its normal functions is to cause the kidneys to retain saline in the body (Figure 10-7 ◆). Saline excess can be caused by any condition that results in excessive aldosterone secretion, such as adrenal tumors that secrete aldosterone, congestive heart failure, liver cirrhosis, and chronic renal failure (Figure 10-8 ◆). Most glucocorticoid medications (such as prednisone) have a mild saline-retaining effect when taken long term.

CLINICAL TIP

A normal saline solution is a salt solution that has the same percentage of salt as the human body. This is a 0.9% solution of sodium chloride. The term *normal* indicates that there is the same weight, in grams, of sodium and chloride in the solution. There are 154 mEq/L of sodium and 154 mEq/L of chloride in normal saline.

Because fluid has weight, extracellular fluid volume excess is characterized by weight gain. An overload of fluid in the blood vessels and interstitial spaces can cause clinical manifestations such as bounding pulse, distended neck veins in children (not usually evident in infants), hepatomegaly, dyspnea, orthopnea, and lung crackles. Edema is the sign of overload of the interstitial fluid compartment. In an infant, edema is often generalized. Edema in children with extracellular fluid volume excess occurs in the dependent parts of the body, that is, in the parts closest to the ground. Thus, edema is evident in sacral areas in a child supine in bed. Edema that develops from other causes is described in the next section of this chapter.

CLINICAL TIP

You can tell if a child's weight gain is due to normal growth or to the development of extracellular fluid volume excess by looking at the speed with which the increase develops. Sudden weight gain (e.g., 0.5 kg [1 lb] in 1 day) is due to the accumulation of fluid. Gain of 0.5 kg overnight is due to retention of about 500 mL of saline.

Intravenous fluid volume regulation is important, especially in young children. Either inaccurate calculation of needed fluid or inadvertent infusion of excess fluids can cause overload.

The clinical therapy for extracellular fluid volume excess focuses on treating the underlying cause of the disorder. For example, a child who has congestive heart failure is given medications to strengthen the heart's ability to contract. Managing the cause also helps to

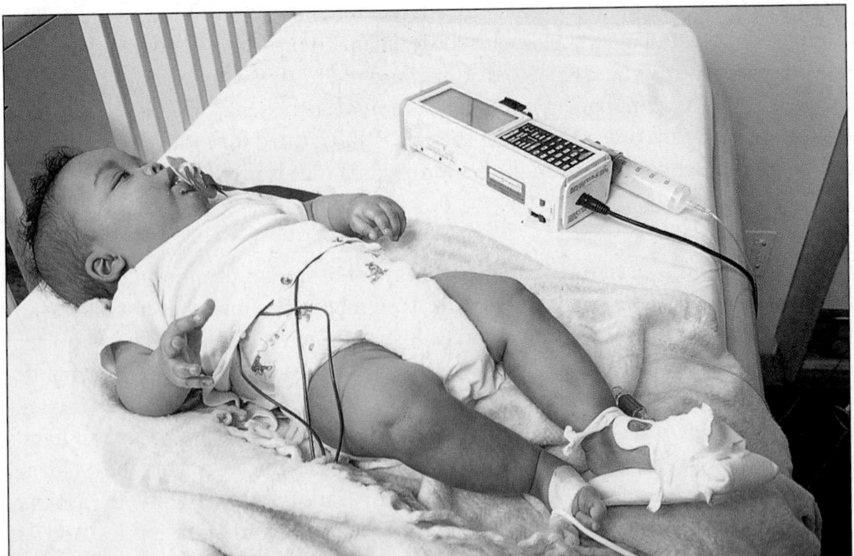

FIGURE 10-6 ◆
If isotonic fluid containing sodium is given too rapidly or in too great an amount, an extracellular fluid volume excess will develop. It is important to monitor fluid intake, excretion, and retention in children.

PATHOPHYSIOLOGY ILLUSTRATED

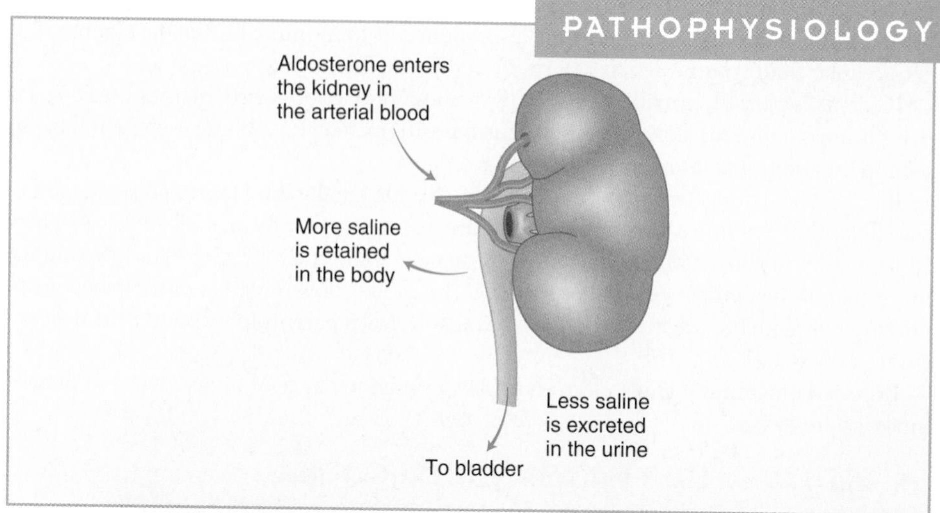

Aldosterone Effects

FIGURE 10-7 ◆
Aldosterone has a saline-retaining effect. Increased aldosterone secretion can be caused by adrenal tumors or congestive heart failure.

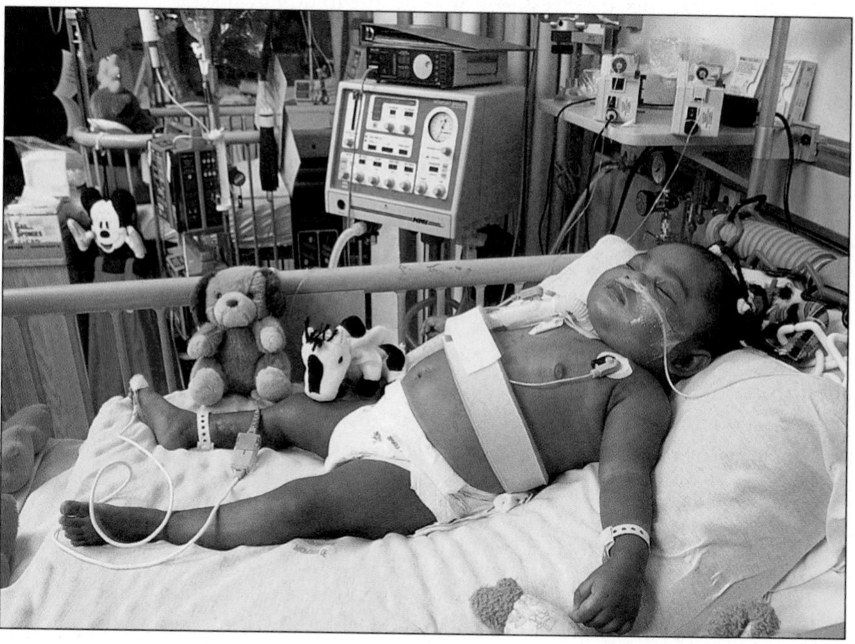

FIGURE 10-8 ◆
This infant with congenital heart disease has signs of generalized edema. Note the fluid retention in the face and abdomen.

CLINICAL TIP

An infant's urine output can be approximated by weighing diapers before and after use. The difference in grams is the urine volume in milliliters. Change the diaper frequently to minimize loss from evaporation.

reduce the extracellular fluid volume excess. Diuretics may be given to remove fluid from the body, thus reducing the extracellular fluid volume directly.

NURSING MANAGEMENT Rapid weight gain is the most sensitive index of extracellular fluid volume excess. Therefore, daily weighing is an important nursing assessment. Measure the child's intake and output. When treatment is successful, output is greater than intake. Assess the character of the pulse and observe for neck vein distention when the child is sitting (usually visible only in older children). Monitor for signs of pulmonary edema (an indication of severe imbalance) by listening to lung sounds in the dependent lung fields (crackles) and assessing for respiratory distress (rapid respiratory rate, use of accessory muscles of respiration). Observe for edema.

The potential for a child to develop a fluid overload is present whenever an isotonic intravenous solution containing sodium is being administered. Therefore, monitor the infusion rate frequently and carefully and use a pump when possible to aid in accurate administration (Figure 10-9 ◆).

If an excess of fluid has already developed, administer the medical therapy as prescribed and monitor for any complications of the therapy. For example, many diuretics increase potassium excretion in the urine, an increase that may lead to an abnormally low plasma

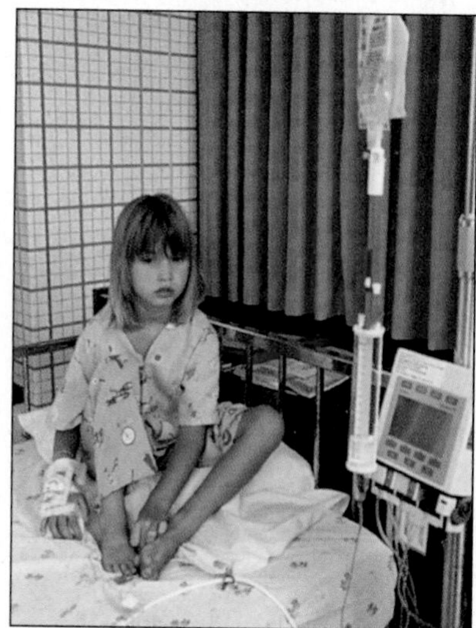

FIGURE 10-9 ◆
The use of a volume control device with an intravenous saline infusion is important to prevent a sudden extracellular fluid volume overload.

CULTURE

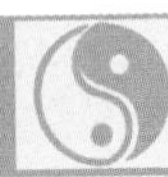

To adapt teaching about low-sodium diets to the cultural practices of a family, ask them what types of food they usually eat. Help them to choose low-sodium foods from their diets and to avoid high-sodium foods. This approach is more effective than giving the same list of restricted foods to each family.

SAFETY PRECAUTIONS

Occasionally intravenous fluid is infused too rapidly, endangering the fluid and electrolyte status of a young child. The nurse can take the following measures to minimize this risk:

- Use small bags of fluid, so if the fluid were to infuse quickly, the amount infused would be limited.
- Always use infusion pumps when available so that the rate is programmed and monitored.
- Check and double-check the machine after setting to be sure it was properly programmed.
- Have another nurse check your calculation of rates and total fluid to be infused until you are certain of your skill in this area.
- Finally, remember that even mechanical pumps can have faulty performance so check the intravenous line, bag, and rate frequently.

ISOTONIC INTRAVENOUS FLUIDS CONTAINING SODIUM

Normal saline (0.9% NaCl)
Ringer's solution
Lactated Ringer's solution

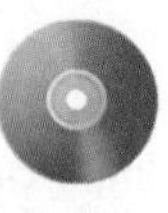

Edema

potassium concentration unless potassium intake is increased. (Refer to the discussion of hypokalemia later in this chapter.) It is also important to monitor for the development of extracellular fluid volume deficit as a result of diuretic therapy.

If edema is present, provide careful skin care and protection for edematous areas. Teach parents how to provide skin care and perform position changes at home. See the following section for additional interventions related to edema.

If a child has a long-term condition such as chronic renal failure that predisposes to extracellular fluid volume excess, a dietary sodium restriction may be prescribed (see Chapter 18 for further detail). Teach parents how to manage sodium restriction. Plan low-sodium meals that fit the family's cultural practices. If the child is old enough to participate, incorporate games into the teaching. If a scale is available, teach parents to take and record an accurate daily weight.

Expected outcomes include electrolyte balance, maintenance of intact skin, and dietary intake as prescribed.

INTERSTITIAL FLUID VOLUME EXCESS (EDEMA)

Edema is an abnormal increase in the volume of the interstitial fluid. It may be caused by an extracellular fluid volume excess or it may be due to other causes.

The causes of edema are best understood in the context of normal capillary dynamics. Fluid moves between the vascular and interstitial compartment by the process of **filtration.** Filtration is the net result of forces that tend to move fluid in opposing directions. The strongest forces will determine the direction of fluid movement.

At the capillary level, two forces (blood hydrostatic pressure and interstitial osmotic pressure) tend to move fluid from the capillaries into the interstitial fluid, while two other forces (blood colloid osmotic pressure and interstitial fluid hydrostatic pressure) tend to move fluid in the opposite direction (from the interstitial fluid into the capillaries). The net result of these forces usually moves fluid from the capillaries into the interstitial compartment at the arterial end of the capillaries and fluid from the interstitial compartment back into the capillaries at the venous end of the capillaries. This process brings oxygen and nutrients to the cells and removes carbon dioxide and other waste products.

Edema occurs if the balance of these four forces is altered so that excess fluid either enters or leaves the interstitial compartment (Figure 10-10 ◆). This may occur through (1) increased blood hydrostatic pressure, (2) decreased blood colloid osmotic pressure, (3) increased interstitial fluid osmotic pressure, or (4) blocked lymphatic drainage. Various clinical conditions are associated with these altered forces (Table 10-8), as described here.

1. *Increased blood hydrostatic pressure.* When extracellular fluid volume excess occurs, the increased fluid volume in the vascular compartment congests the veins. The pressure against the sides of the capillary is increased and more fluid then enters the interstitial compartment.
2. *Decreased blood colloid osmotic pressure.* Much of the osmotic pressure that pulls fluid into the capillaries is due to the presence of albumin and other plasma proteins made by the liver. The part of the blood osmotic pressure that is due to plasma proteins is often called **oncotic pressure** or blood colloid osmotic pressure. Any condition that decreases plasma proteins will decrease blood colloid osmotic pressure and cause edema. For example, if a clinical condition causes large amounts of albumin to leak into the urine, the liver will not be able to make albumin fast enough to replace it. As a result, the plasma protein level will fall, decreasing the blood osmotic pressure. Without this pulling force to return fluid to the capillaries, edema will occur. This is the cause of the edema that occurs in children who have nephrotic syndrome (see Chapter 18).
3. *Increased interstitial fluid osmotic pressure.* Ordinarily, only a few small proteins enter the interstitial fluid, and the interstitial fluid osmotic pressure is small. If the capillary becomes abnormally permeable to proteins, however, the influx of large amounts of proteins into the interstitial fluid causes a dramatic increase in interstitial fluid osmotic pressure. This increased pulling force keeps an abnormal amount of fluid in the interstitial compartment. This mechanism plays an important part in the edema caused by a bee sting or a sprained ankle. It occurs to a greater extent in

PATHOPHYSIOLOGY ILLUSTRATED

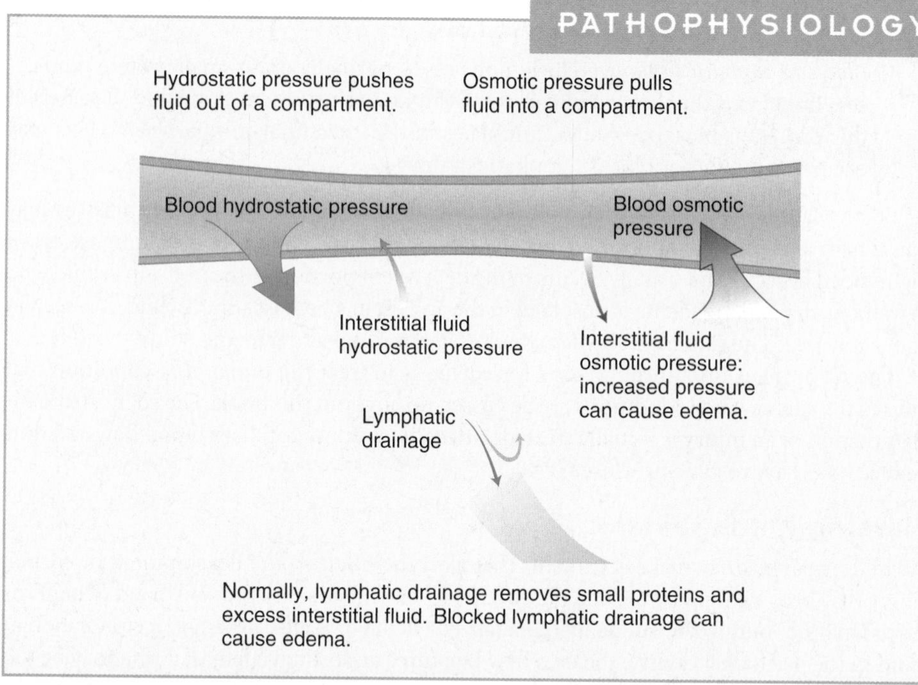

Capillary Dynamics and Edema

FIGURE 10-10 ◆
With normal capillary dynamics, fluid moves out of the compartment by the force of hydrostatic pressure in the blood vessel and is pulled out by interstitial osmotic pressure. Fluid is forced into the compartment by interstitial hydrostatic pressure and pulled in by compartment osmotic pressure. Abnormal capillary dynamics cause edema.

TABLE 10-8 Clinical Conditions That Cause Edema

EDEMA DUE TO INCREASED BLOOD HYDROSTATIC PRESSURE
Increased Capillary Blood Flow Inflammation Local infection ***Venous Congestion*** Extracellular fluid volume excess Right heart failure Venous thrombosis External pressure on vein Muscle paralysis
EDEMA DUE TO DECREASED BLOOD OSMOTIC PRESSURE
Increased Albumin Excretion Nephrotic syndrome (albumin leaks into urine) Protein-losing enteropathies (excess albumin in feces) ***Decreased Albumin Synthesis*** Kwashiorkor (low-protein, high-carbohydrate starvation diet provides too few amino acids for liver to make albumin) Liver cirrhosis (diseased liver unable to make enough albumin)
EDEMA DUE TO INCREASED INTERSTITIAL FLUID OSMOTIC PRESSURE
Increased Capillary Permeability Inflammation Toxins Hypersensitivity reactions Burns
EDEMA DUE TO BLOCKED LYMPHATIC DRAINAGE
Tumors Goiter Parasites that obstruct lymph nodes Surgery that removes lymph nodes

burns, leading to swelling at the same time that there is a great loss of fluid volume through the burned skin (see Chapter 23).

4. *Blocked lymphatic drainage.* The lymph vessels normally drain small proteins and excess fluid from the interstitial compartment and return them to the blood vessels. If this process is blocked, fluid accumulates in the interstitial compartment. This may occur when a tumor blocks lymphatic drainage.

Edema causes swelling, which may be localized or generalized. The swelling of tissue may cause pain and restrict motion. Edema that is due to extracellular fluid volume excess or right-sided heart failure usually occurs in the dependent portion of the body. In a child who is walking, dependent edema is observed in the ankles; in a bedfast supine child, it is seen in the sacral area. The skin over an edematous area often appears thin and shiny.

The main focus of clinical therapy for edema is to treat the underlying condition that caused the edema. Such conditions are discussed throughout this book. The edema from inflammation of an injury is initially treated with cold to reduce capillary blood flow and thus reduce blood hydrostatic pressure.

Nursing Management

A child or parent may make comments that alert the nurse to the development of edema. Shoes may become tight by the end of the day (dependent edema); the waistband of pants or a skirt may be "outgrown" suddenly (generalized edema or ascites, which is accumulation of fluid in the peritoneal cavity); the eyes may be puffy (periorbital edema); a ring may be too tight; fingers may "feel like sausages." In many cases visual inspection is sufficient to recognize edema. Observe for the presence of pitting edema. To detect changes in the amount of swelling, measure around the edematous part (Figure 10-11 ◆). If the edema is caused by extracellular fluid volume excess, daily measurements of weight and intake and output are a necessary part of the daily assessment. Nursing assessment should also focus on the integrity of the skin, presence of pain, restricted motion, and alterations in the child's body image.

Elevation of an area of localized edema helps to reduce the swelling. The skin over an edematous area needs extra care because it is fragile (Figure 10-12 ◆). Carefully position an infant or child who is on bedrest and turn frequently to prevent pressure sores. Turning must be performed carefully to avoid skin abrasion by rubbing against the sheets. Pat the skin dry after cleansing rather than rubbing it. Trim the child's fingernails smooth to prevent scratching. Teach parents skin care for the child at home. Teach older children to inspect their skin carefully to identify areas needing special care.

If restricted mobility is a problem, specific plans to help the child manage activities are needed. For example, if an edematous finger restricts the motion of a hand, food can be cut into bite-size portions before the meal is served, so that the child can still eat independently.

Discomfort from edema may require creative interventions by the nurse. Distraction with toys or activities appropriate to the child's developmental level can be useful. Interventions to treat the underlying problem can also reduce the edema and its accompanying

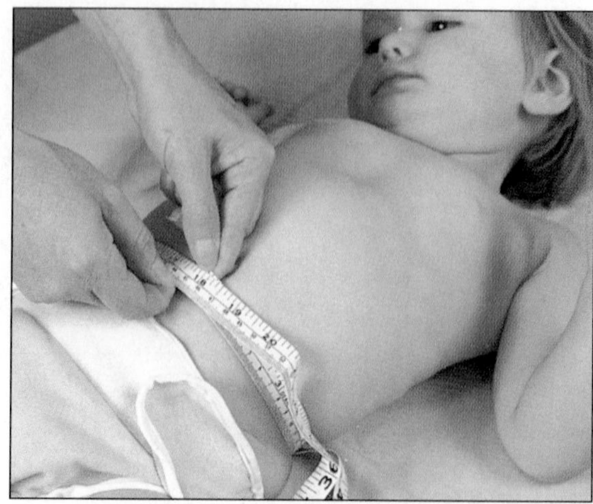

FIGURE 10-11 ◆
Finding the same location each day for measuring circumference to assess edema can be accomplished by use of a reference point. An indelible marker may be used to mark the measurement location on the skin, if this is acceptable to the child and parents.

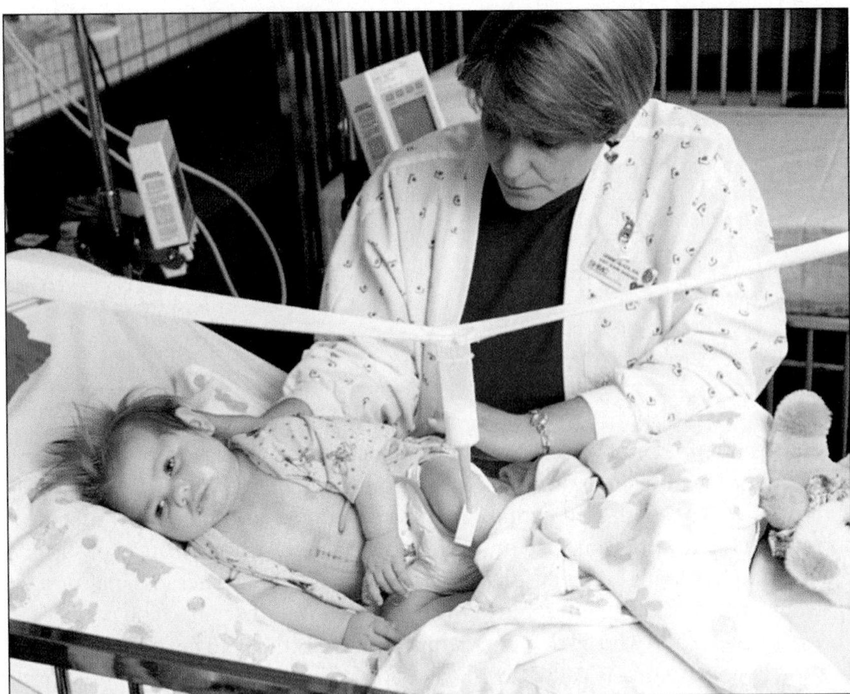

FIGURE 10-12 ◆ Edematous tissue is easily damaged. It must be kept clean and dry and free of pressure.

discomfort. Interventions for edema should be added to the nursing management of the underlying condition that causes the edema. Administration of the prescribed medical therapy and observation for the complications of therapy are nursing responsibilities.

Discuss with school-age children and adolescents feelings of embarrassment about the edematous appearance. They need to understand the reason for edema and be able to explain it to peers. Arrange for the child to meet other children with similar concerns.

Desired outcomes of care include maintenance of intact skin, normal respiratory sounds and effort, and normal weight patterns.

ELECTROLYTE IMBALANCES

All body fluids contain electrolytes, although the concentration of those electrolytes varies, depending on the type and location of the fluid. When a serum electrolyte value is reported from the laboratory, it provides information about the concentration of that electrolyte in the blood. It may not necessarily reflect the concentration of the electrolyte in other body compartments. Refer to Table 10-1 to see which electrolytes are highest and lowest concentration in the blood and other fluid compartments.

Electrolytes are normally gained and lost in relatively equal amounts so the body remains in balance. However, when a child has an abnormal route of loss, such as vomiting, wound drainage, or nasogastric suction, electrolyte balance can be disturbed. Monitoring for signs of imbalance becomes important.

SODIUM IMBALANCES

The serum sodium concentration reflects the **osmolality** of body fluids, that is, their degree of concentration or dilution. It refers to the number of moles of the substance per kilogram of water in the solution. Serum sodium concentration reflects the proportion of water and sodium in the extracellular compartment. When the osmolality of body fluids becomes abnormal, the cells swell or shrink. These cell size changes are due to **osmosis**, the movement of water across a semipermeable membrane into an area of higher particle concentration.

Hypernatremia

Hypernatremia is a condition of increased osmolality of the blood. The body fluids are too concentrated, containing excess sodium relative to water. A serum sodium level above 148 mmol/L in children (146 mmol/L in newborns) is diagnostic of hypernatremia.

NORMAL SERUM SODIUM CONCENTRATION

Newborns: 133–146 mmol/L
Children: 135–148 mmol/L

TABLE 10-9 Causes of Hypernatremia

LOSS OF RELATIVELY MORE WATER THAN SODIUM	GAIN OF RELATIVELY MORE SODIUM THAN WATER
Diabetes insipidus (not enough antidiuretic hormone)	Inability to communicate thirst
Diarrhea or vomiting without fluid replacement	Limited or no access to water
Excessive sweating without fluid replacement	High solute intake without adequate water (e.g., tube feedings)
High solute intake without adequate water (causes kidneys to excrete water)	Intravenous hypertonic saline

Hypernatremia results from conditions that cause the body to lose relatively more water than sodium or to gain relatively more sodium than water (Table 10-9). Special circumstances in which a high solute intake may occur without adequate water include an infant formula that is too concentrated or one that is prepared with salt instead of sugar. A breast-fed baby not receiving adequate breast milk who has normal water loss may develop hypernatremic dehydration (Livingstone, Willis, & Abdel-Wareth, et al., 2000).

An infant or child who has hypernatremia is generally thirsty. The urine output is small unless the hypernatremia is caused by diabetes insipidus. A decreased level of consciousness manifested by confusion, lethargy, or coma results from shrinking of the brain cells. Seizures can occur when hypernatremia occurs rapidly or is severe. Severe hypernatremia can be fatal.

Hypernatremia is treated by intravenous administration of **hypotonic fluid**, or fluid that is more dilute than normal body fluid. This therapy dilutes the body fluids back to normal concentration. If a child is dehydrated, **isotonic fluids** (those with the osmolality of body fluids) may be ordered first to replenish the volume, followed by hypotonic fluid to correct the osmolality. The underlying cause of the disorder is also treated.

NORMAL SPECIFIC GRAVITY OF URINE

Infants to 2 years: 1.001–1.018
Children > 2 years: 1.010–1.030
Note: Specific gravity compares the density of urine with the density of water (density of water is 1.000). The infant's kidney is less able to concentrate urine.

NURSING MANAGEMENT Monitor serum sodium level and measure intake and output and urine specific gravity. Specific gravity changes toward normal levels as therapy progresses. Frequently assess responsiveness to monitor the effect of hypernatremia on brain cells. As the concentration of body fluids returns to normal, the child will become more alert and responsive. Watch for rebound hyponatremia while monitoring the fluid replacement. Implement safety interventions such as raised bed rails for protection. Ensure adequate rest and introduce developmentally appropriate activities when the child is alert.

Water deprivation is a form of child neglect or abuse. In neglect, the parents simply do not provide adequate water for the child. A form of child abuse that sometimes includes water deprivation is Munchausen syndrome by proxy (see Chapter 7). A small child who is hospitalized with hypernatremia that does not have a detectable cause may be subject to water deprivation. Assess the child's general condition, developmental tasks, the family dynamics, and parent's understanding of formula preparation and the child's fluid intake needs.

Teaching can prevent many cases of hypernatremia. Be sure the breast-feeding mother has instruction and resources about lactation before discharge after delivery. If discharged soon after birth, be sure the infant has an appointment to have weight checked within the first few days, and alert the parents to expected output of at least six wet diapers daily. By about 10 days, infants should have regained the birth weight.

CLINICAL TIP

Careful teaching about how to mix powdered formula so that it is not too concentrated can help prevent hypernatremia. Pictures are an important teaching tool if the parents are not able to read labels or instructions.

When an infant is sick or developing slowly, parents sometimes want to feed the infant more concentrated formula to build the child's strength. Parents and caregivers of bottle-fed babies should be taught never to give undiluted formula concentrate or evaporated milk. Parents should be cautioned to keep salt out of reach, because eating handfuls of salt has caused hypernatremia. Teach parents to offer extra fluids during hot weather. Teach oral rehydration therapy for use at home during mild vomiting and diarrhea (see p. 319).

Nurses can prevent hypernatremia in hospitalized infants and children by administering water between tube feedings, keeping water available, and offering it frequently. Offering frequent small amounts and using popsicles and other creative interventions can increase children's intake.

Desired outcomes of treatment for hypernatremia include balance of electrolytes and fluid in the intracellular and extracellular compartments, and alert level of consciousness.

Hyponatremia

In hyponatremia, the osmolality of the blood is decreased. The body fluids are too dilute, containing excess water relative to sodium. Hyponatremia is the most common sodium imbalance in children (Dabbagh, Ellis, & Gruskin, 1996). A serum sodium level below 135 mmol/L in children (133 mmol/L in newborns) is diagnostic of hyponatremia.

ETIOLOGY AND PATHOPHYSIOLOGY Hyponatremia results from conditions that cause gain of relatively more water than sodium or loss of relatively more sodium than water (Table 10-10). Oral intake of water causes hyponatremia in unusual conditions such as forced fluid intake. More commonly, parents feed an infant only water or dilute formula to save money instead of regular-strength formula or breast milk. Excessive swallowing of swimming pool water by an infant can have the same effect. Infants are vulnerable to the type of hyponatremia caused by water intoxication, because they have a poorly developed thirst mechanism and may continue to drink, and then are unable to excrete excess water quickly due to immature kidney function (Fann, 1998).

CLINICAL MANIFESTATIONS The child who has hyponatremia has a decreased level of consciousness, which results from swelling of brain cells. This can be manifested as anorexia, headache, muscle weakness, decreased deep tendon reflexes, lethargy, confusion, or coma. If hyponatremia arises rapidly or is extreme, seizures may occur. Hyponatremia is a frequent cause of seizures in infants under 6 months of age who have a low body temperature (Farrar, Chande, & Fitzpatrick, 1995). Nausea and vomiting also occur in some children. Severe hyponatremia can be fatal.

CLINICAL THERAPY In most cases, hyponatremia is treated by restricting the intake of water. This therapy allows the kidneys to correct the imbalance by excreting excess water from the body. If a child is having seizures from hyponatremia, intravenous **hypertonic fluid** (more concentrated than body fluid) may be administered. Use of this concentrated saline is a way to rapidly increase body fluid concentration, but it must be monitored carefully because it can easily cause rebound hypernatremia.

NURSING MANAGEMENT

Nursing Assessment and Diagnosis

Monitor serum sodium level and measure intake and output. If an infant with hyponatremia has normal antidiuretic hormone (ADH) levels, and other causes have been ruled out, careful questioning about proper preparation of formula and feeding practices is needed. A toddler or school-age child may be subjected to forced fluid intake as a form of child abuse. Sensitive interviewing and a caring manner on the part of the nurse can help identify such problems in a family.

Because hyponatremia is characterized by decreased level of consciousness, frequent assessment of responsiveness will be necessary to monitor the response to therapy. The child will become more alert and responsive as the concentration of body fluids returns to normal.

TABLE 10-10 Causes of Hyponatremia

GAIN OF RELATIVELY MORE WATER THAN SODIUM	LOSS OF RELATIVELY MORE SODIUM THAN WATER
Excessive intravenous D5W (5% dextrose in water) Excessive tap water enemas Irrigation of body cavities with distilled water Excessive antidiuretic hormone Forced excessive oral intake of tap water	Diarrhea or vomiting with replacement by tap water only instead of fluid containing sodium

The highest priority nursing diagnosis for hyponatremia addresses the *risk for injury* related to the child's decreased level of consciousness. The following diagnoses might also apply:

- *Self-care deficit* related to weakness and tiredness
- *Altered health maintenance* related to parental information misinterpretation about infant formula
- *Ineffective breastfeeding* related to inadequate sucking by infant or inadequate milk production

Planning and Implementation

Nurses can prevent hyponatremia in hospitalized children by using normal saline instead of distilled water for irrigations and by avoiding tap water enemas. It is important to help the child comply with prescribed fluid restrictions (Table 10-11). Allow the child to choose favorite fluids to drink. Teach parents to replace body fluids lost through diarrhea or vomiting with oral electrolyte solutions (see p. 319).

Evaluation

Expected outcomes of nursing care for hyponatremia include the following:

- Avoidance of injury
- Balance of fluid and electrolytes
- Establishment of adequate intake of formula and/or breast milk

POTASSIUM IMBALANCES

Potassium is an essential electrolyte that performs many necessary functions in the body. Potassium intake in healthy children comes from potassium-rich foods such as fruits and vegetables. Potassium is absorbed easily from the intestine. A normal potassium distribution is important for proper function.

A potassium imbalance arises when the serum potassium concentration rises or falls outside the normal range. Potassium imbalances are caused by alterations in potassium intake, distribution, or excretion; or by loss of potassium through an abnormal route such as burns, emesis, or renal failure.

Most of the potassium ions in the body are found inside the cells. The sodium-potassium pump in cell membranes moves potassium ions into cells to maintain the high intracellular potassium concentration. Potassium ions can be shifted into or out of cells by various physiologic factors (Figure 10-13 ◆). Potassium is excreted from the body through urine, feces, and sweat. The hormone aldosterone increases potassium excretion in the urine.

NORMAL SERUM POTASSIUM CONCENTRATION

Premature infants: 4.5–7.2 mmol/L
Full-term newborns: 3.7–5.2 mmol/L
Children: 3.5–5.8 mmol/L

Hyperkalemia

Hyperkalemia is an excess of potassium in the blood. It is reflected by a level above 5.8 mmol/L in children or above 5.2 mmol/L in newborns.

TABLE 10-11 Nursing Interventions for a Child Who Has a Fluid Restriction

(Modify according to child's developmental level)

- Give cold rather than lukewarm fluids.
- Use an insulated glass that looks bigger than it is.
- Be sure that extra fluids are removed from meal trays before the child sees them.
- Have the child swish fluids around in the mouth before swallowing to relieve thirst.
- Provide frequent oral care.
- Suggest eating meals dry and drinking between meals.
- Provide a chart so an older child can keep intake records.

PATHOPHYSIOLOGY ILLUSTRATED

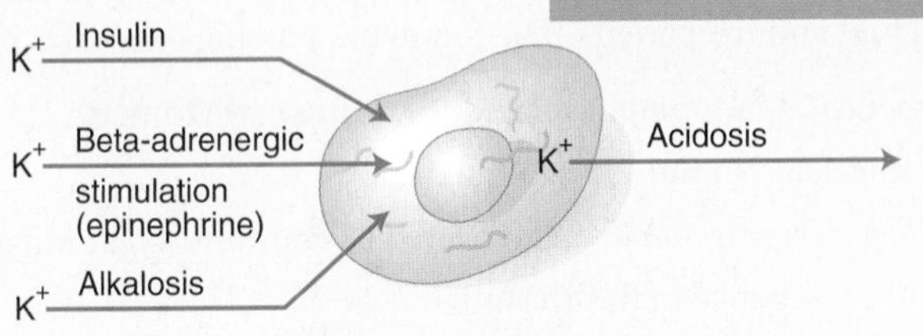

Potassium Ions

FIGURE 10-13 ◆
Factors that shift potassium ions into or out of cells.

ETIOLOGY AND PATHOPHYSIOLOGY Hyperkalemia is caused by conditions that involve increased potassium intake, shift of potassium from cells into the extracellular fluid, and decreased potassium excretion. Increased potassium intake is usually due to intravenous potassium overload. Excessive or too rapid intravenous administration of potassium-containing solutions can occur if potassium requirement is overestimated or if the intravenous infusion runs in too fast.

Blood transfusion is another source of potassium intake that may cause hyperkalemia. Potassium ions leak out of red blood cells that are stored in a blood bank. The longer the blood is stored, the more potassium leaks out of cells and accumulates in the fluid portion of the transfusion. Hyperkalemia from administration of stored blood arises when multiple units are transfused, as when infants receive exchange transfusions or children receive multiple blood transfusions after a serious injury or in surgery.

Shift of potassium from cells into the extracellular fluid occurs when there is massive cell death, as with a crush injury, in sickle-cell anemia (hemolytic crisis), or when chemotherapy for a malignancy is rapidly effective. In these situations, the dead cells release their high-potassium contents into the extracellular fluid. Potassium ions also shift out of cells in metabolic acidosis caused by diarrhea and in diabetes mellitus when insulin levels are low.

Decreased potassium excretion occurs with acute or chronic oliguria during renal failure, severe hypovolemia, and conditions that decrease the secretion of aldosterone by the adrenal cortex (lead poisoning, Addison's disease, hypoaldosteronism). Several medications can cause hyperkalemia.

DRUGS THAT MAY CAUSE HYPERKALEMIA

- Potassium-containing preparations
- Cytotoxic agents
- Potassium-sparing diuretics
- Angiotensin-converting enzyme inhibitors
- Nonsteroidal anti-inflammatory analgesics

CLINICAL TIP 

If an infant's hyperkalemia was diagnosed using blood obtained from a heel stick, intracellular fluid may have contaminated the sample. A venous sample should be obtained.

CLINICAL MANIFESTATIONS All clinical manifestations of hyperkalemia are related to muscle dysfunction because potassium plays a vital role in muscle activity. Hyperactivity of gastrointestinal smooth muscle causes intestinal cramping and diarrhea in some children. The skeletal muscles become weak, beginning typically with leg weakness and ascending. Weakness can progress to flaccid paralysis. The child is often lethargic. Dysfunction of cardiac muscle causes cardiac arrhythmias such as tachycardia and may result in heart failure and cardiac arrest. Abnormalities in the electrocardiogram include a prolonged QRS complex, a peak in T waves, and prolonged PR intervals (White, 1997).

CLINICAL THERAPY Hyperkalemia is treated by management of the underlying condition that caused the imbalance. If the serum potassium concentration is very high or is causing dangerous cardiac arrhythmias, treatment to decrease the serum potassium level may be ordered. These treatments may remove potassium from the body or drive it from the extracellular fluid into the cells. Potassium is removed from the body by peritoneal dialysis or hemodialysis, by potassium-wasting diuretics, or with a cation exchange resin (Kayexalate) that is administered orally or rectally. Medical treatments that drive potassium ions into cells are intravenous bicarbonate, intravenous insulin, and glucose.

GROWTH & DEVELOPMENT 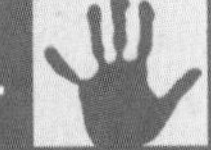

The nursing diagnoses for hyperkalemic children will prompt a nurse to provide safety measures appropriate to the child's developmental level and to assist the child with activities that muscle weakness makes difficult. It is important to provide play and diversional activities that take into account both the child's degree of muscle strength and the appropriate developmental level.

NURSING MANAGEMENT

Nursing Assessment and Diagnosis

Monitor serum potassium levels. Ongoing assessment of muscle strength is important, because the muscle weakness may progress to flaccid paralysis. (This paralysis is reversible on correction of the potassium imbalance.) Diarrhea can occur in infants and children. An older child may complain of intestinal cramping. Monitor the pulse rate carefully.

Nursing diagnoses for a child who has hyperkalemia depend on the severity of the clinical manifestations. The cause of the imbalance may also lead to useful diagnoses that guide teaching for the child and the parents. The following nursing diagnoses may apply:

- *Risk for decreased cardiac output* related to cardiac arrhythmias
- *Risk for injury* related to muscle weakness
- *Self-care deficit: Hygiene and dressing* related to neuromuscular impairment
- *Anxiety* related to change in health status
- *Altered health maintenance* related to parental lack of exposure to potassium intake in chronic renal failure
- *Ineffective management of therapeutic regimen* related to complexity of therapy

Planning and Implementation

Nursing care includes measures to prevent hyperkalemia from developing in hospitalized children. If hyperkalemia does develop, care shifts to administering intravenous solutions, monitoring cardiopulmonary status, ensuring safety, promoting adequate nutrition, and preparing the child and family for discharge.

Prevent Hyperkalemia

Any child who is receiving an intravenous infusion that contains potassium is at risk for hyperkalemia. Check that urine output is normal before administering intravenous potassium solutions. Intravenous solutions to which potassium has been added should be turned over several times to mix the contents thoroughly before they are connected to the infusion tubing.

Be sure blood or packed red blood cells are fresh, especially for the child receiving multiple transfusions, and for all neonates. Use a cardiac monitor during infusion of these products to watch for arrhythmias.

Administer Intravenous Solutions

Once a child is diagnosed as hyperkalemic, ensure that any infusions with added potassium are stopped. Several infusions may need to be managed, including glucose, bicarbonate, and calcium gluconate. Maintain the infusion at the ordered rate and monitor the child's condition frequently.

Skill 10-4: Placement of ECG Electrodes

Monitor Cardiopulmonary Status

Upon diagnosis of hyperkalemia, an electrocardiogram is performed and a cardiac monitor applied. Monitor for any changes in cardiac status and for cardiac arrhythmias. Report abnormal rate and character of pulse as well as shortness of breath.

Ensure Safety

Since the child is weak, side rails should be raised. Position the child carefully. Assist the child with activities requiring leg muscle strength, such as climbing into bed or pushing up in bed. Encourage quiet activities with frequent rest periods. Document and report any change in muscle weakness.

Promote Adequate Nutritional Intake

Adequate caloric intake is necessary to prevent tissue breakdown and the resultant potassium release from cells. Offer the child nourishing snacks if his or her appetite is decreased. Restrict potassium-rich foods.

Discharge Planning and Home Care Teaching

If the child has chronic renal failure or another condition that decreases aldosterone secretion, parents and the child need to be taught to restrict foods that are high in potassium. Most oral rehydration solutions, including Pedialyte, contain potassium and should not be used to provide fluid for the child. Instruct the family not to use salt substitutes, which commonly contain potassium. Parents should check with the care provider and pharmacist before giving even over-the-counter products to the child, as some of these medications contain potassium. Management of renal failure at home with frequent visits for dialysis and other treatments can be challenging. Refer to Chapter 18 for further suggestions to help parents handle this condition.

Evaluation

Expected outcomes of nursing care for hyperkalemia include the following:

- Return to a state of fluid and electrolyte balance
- Maintenance of safety
- Adequate nutritional intake to provide essential potassium
- Normal cardiac rate and rhythm

Hypokalemia

Hypokalemia occurs when the serum potassium concentration is too low. Total body potassium may be decreased, normal, or even increased when the serum level is low, depending on the cause of the imbalance. Serum potassium levels below 3.5 mmol/L in children (3.7 mmol/L for newborns) are diagnostic of hypokalemia.

ETIOLOGY AND PATHOPHYSIOLOGY Hypokalemia is caused by conditions that involve increased potassium excretion, decreased potassium intake, shift of potassium from the extracellular fluid into cells, and loss of potassium by an abnormal route.

Increased potassium excretion is a major cause of hypokalemia in children. In addition to diuretics and other medications, causes of increased urinary potassium excretion are osmotic diuresis (glucose present in urine), hypomagnesemia, increased aldosterone (hyperaldosteronism, congestive heart failure, nephrotic syndrome, cirrhosis), and increased cortisol (Cushing's disease and syndrome). Eating large amounts of black licorice increases renal excretion of potassium. Diarrhea causes potassium to be excreted in the feces. In the chapter opening vignette, Vernon had increased potassium excretion through diarrhea.

Decreased potassium intake will lead to hypokalemia slowly, or more rapidly if combined with increased excretion or loss of potassium. Hospitalized children may be placed on NPO status and receive prolonged intravenous therapy without potassium. Adolescents concerned about weight loss or those with anorexia nervosa may embark on diets low in potassium and may take medications that induce diuresis or diarrhea.

Shift of potassium from the extracellular fluid into cells occurs in alkalosis and hypothermia (unintentional or induced for surgery). Hyperalimentation often causes hypersecretion of insulin, which also shifts potassium into cells.

DRUGS THAT MAY CAUSE HYPOKALEMIA

- Beta-adrenergic agonists
- Insulin
- Potassium-wasting diuretics
- Parenteral penicillins
- Glucocorticoids
- Aminoglycoside antimicrobials
- Systemic antifungals
- Antineoplastics
- Laxatives

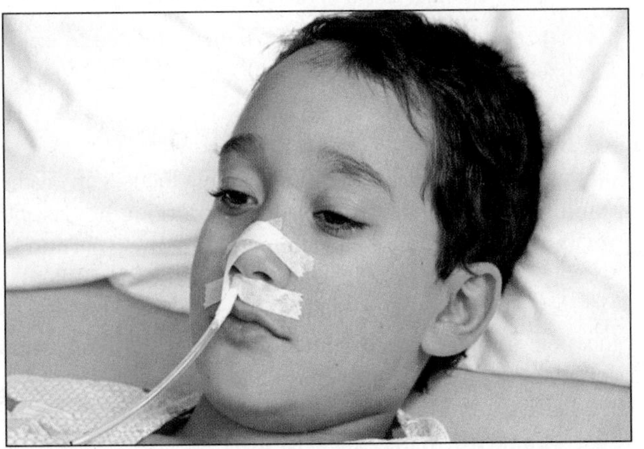

FIGURE 10-14 ◆ Because this child has a nasogastric tube in place that requires suctioning, it is important to monitor his potassium levels.

Loss of potassium by an abnormal route occurs through vomiting. Self-induced vomiting in bulimia is an example of this cause. Nasogastric suctioning (Figure 10-14 ◆) and intestinal decompression can cause potassium loss. Hypokalemia can also be caused by several medications.

CLINICAL MANIFESTATIONS Since the ratio of intracellular to extracellular potassium determines the responsiveness of muscle cells to neural stimuli, it is not surprising that the clinical manifestations of hypokalemia involve muscle dysfunction. Gastrointestinal smooth muscle activity is slowed, leading to abdominal distention, constipation, or paralytic ileus. Skeletal muscles are weak and unresponsive to stimuli, and weakness may progress to flaccid paralysis. The respiratory muscles may be impaired. Cardiac arrhythmias can occur. Polyuria results from changes in the kidney caused by hypokalemia.

CLINICAL THERAPY Medical management of hypokalemia focuses on replacement of potassium while treating the cause of the imbalance. Potassium replacement may be given intravenously or orally.

NURSING MANAGEMENT

Nursing Assessment and Diagnosis

Monitor serum potassium levels. Observe for muscle weakness, which is frequently detected first in the legs. Parents may report that muscle weakness restricts the child's activities and impairs interactions with peers. Skeletal muscle strength can be difficult to assess if the child is lethargic, as shown with Vernon at the beginning of the chapter.

Muscle weakness may affect the respiratory muscles. Assess the child frequently to determine the need for assisted ventilation. Cardiac monitoring is important for continued assessment of hypokalemia-associated arrhythmias.

Assess for diminished bowel sounds. Ask the parents if the child has recently been awakening to use the toilet at night or has begun bedwetting after previously being dry at night. These may be symptoms of polyuria associated with chronic hypokalemia.

The most important nursing diagnoses in the child with severe hypokalemia relate to cardiac arrhythmias and respiratory muscle weakness. The following nursing diagnoses may apply:

- *Risk for decreased cardiac output* related to cardiac dysrhythmias
- *Ineffective breathing pattern* related to respiratory musculoskeletal impairment
- *Risk for injury* related to muscle weakness
- *Self-care deficit: Hygiene and dressing* related to neuromuscular impairment
- *Constipation* related to decreased motility
- *Anxiety* related to change in health status
- *Altered health maintenance* related to management of potassium supplements or high-potassium diet
- *Ineffective management of therapeutic regimen* related to complexity of potassium therapy
- *Nutrition: Less than body requirements* related to lack of basic nutritional knowledge regarding safe weight-loss diet

Planning and Implementation

Nursing care of the child with hypokalemia focuses on ensuring adequate potassium intake, monitoring cardiopulmonary status, promoting normal bowel function, ensuring safety, providing dietary counseling, and preparing the child and family for discharge.

ENSURE ADEQUATE POTASSIUM INTAKE

Since potassium is excreted from the body every day, daily potassium intake is necessary to prevent hypokalemia. A hypokalemic child who is able to eat should be given a high-potassium diet. Teach parents (and the child if old enough) which foods are high in potassium and how to incorporate them into the daily diet.

POTASSIUM-RICH FOODS	
Apricots	Orange juice
Bananas	Peaches
Cantaloupe	Potatoes
Cherries	Prunes
Dates	Raisins
Figs	Strawberries
Molasses	Tomato juice

Children who have no oral intake for a period of time should receive intravenous fluids that contain potassium. Calculate the dosage to ensure accuracy, and be sure that the infusion runs on schedule. Sometimes the child will complain of burning along the vein when potassium is infused. The infusion may need to be slowed temporarily to allow it to continue. Check serum potassium for high or low potassium levels. Monitor urine output. An oliguric child can develop hyperkalemia when receiving supplements.

GROWTH & DEVELOPMENT

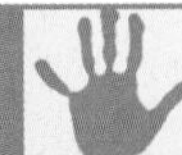

Bradycardia occurs at a different level for children of various ages. For infants, a pulse rate below 100 is considered bradycardia. For young children, 80 may be the identified number, whereas for adolescents, a pulse below 60 is bradycardia. Look at the child's age and normal pulse range to find changes that indicate bradycardia.

Monitor Cardiopulmonary Status

Hypokalemia potentiates digitalis toxicity. A hypokalemic child who is receiving digitalis needs careful surveillance for digitalis toxicity, which is manifested as anorexia, nausea, vomiting, and bradycardia. Observe for these effects. Take the pulse rate and rhythm regularly. Monitor respirations and ease of breathing to watch for decreased respiratory muscle activity.

Promote Normal Bowel Function

Ensure adequate fluids and fiber in the diet. Monitor and record the number of stools and report inadequate stools.

Ensure Safety

Keep side rails up. Assist the child as needed to move into and out of bed. Reposition the child frequently to preserve skin integrity of limbs that are not moved regularly. Perform passive range of motion if the child is not moving. Use supportive pillows to position the child properly.

Provide Dietary Counseling

The adolescent who is trying to lose weight and not consuming a nutritious diet needs dietary teaching. More intensive treatment will be needed for teens who are anorexic or bulimic (see Chapter 7 for interventions in these cases).

Discharge Planning and Home Care Teaching

Teach parents how to give potassium supplements, if prescribed. Liquid or powdered potassium supplements can be mixed with juice or sherbet to improve the bitter taste. The parent should call the mixture "medicine" so that the child does not learn to dislike all juices. Teach the parents signs of both hypokalemia and hyperkalemia and whom to call to report these symptoms. The signs must be reported promptly so medications can be adjusted.

Evaluation

Expected outcomes of nursing care during hypokalemia include the following:

- Normal rate and rhythm of heart and respiratory system
- Regular bowel movements
- Maintenance of safety
- Knowledge of child and family regarding food sources of potassium

THE THREE FORMS OF CALCIUM IN PLASMA

Calcium bound to protein
Calcium bound to small organic ions (e.g., citrate)
Free ionized calcium (Ca^{++}), the only physiologically active form

CALCIUM IMBALANCES

A normal serum calcium concentration is important for many physiologic functions, including muscle and nerve function, secretion of hormones, bone formation and strength, and clotting of the blood.

Calcium imbalances are caused by alterations in calcium intake, absorption, distribution, or excretion. Calcium absorption requires vitamin D for maximum efficiency and is greatest in the duodenum. Calcium distribution involves calcium entry into and exit from bones and the distribution of different forms of calcium in the plasma. Excretion of calcium occurs in urine, feces, and sweat (Figure 10-15 ◆).

Parathyroid hormone is the major regulator of the plasma calcium concentration. It increases this concentration by increasing calcium absorption, increasing calcium withdrawal

NORMAL SERUM CALCIUM CONCENTRATION

Premature infants: 3.5–4.5 mEq/L (1.7–2.3 mmol/L)
Full-term newborns: 4–5 mEq/L (2–2.5 mmol/L)
Children: 4.4–5.3 mEq/L (2.2–2.7 mmol/L)

PATHOPHYSIOLOGY ILLUSTRATED

Calcium Imbalance

FIGURE 10-15 ◆

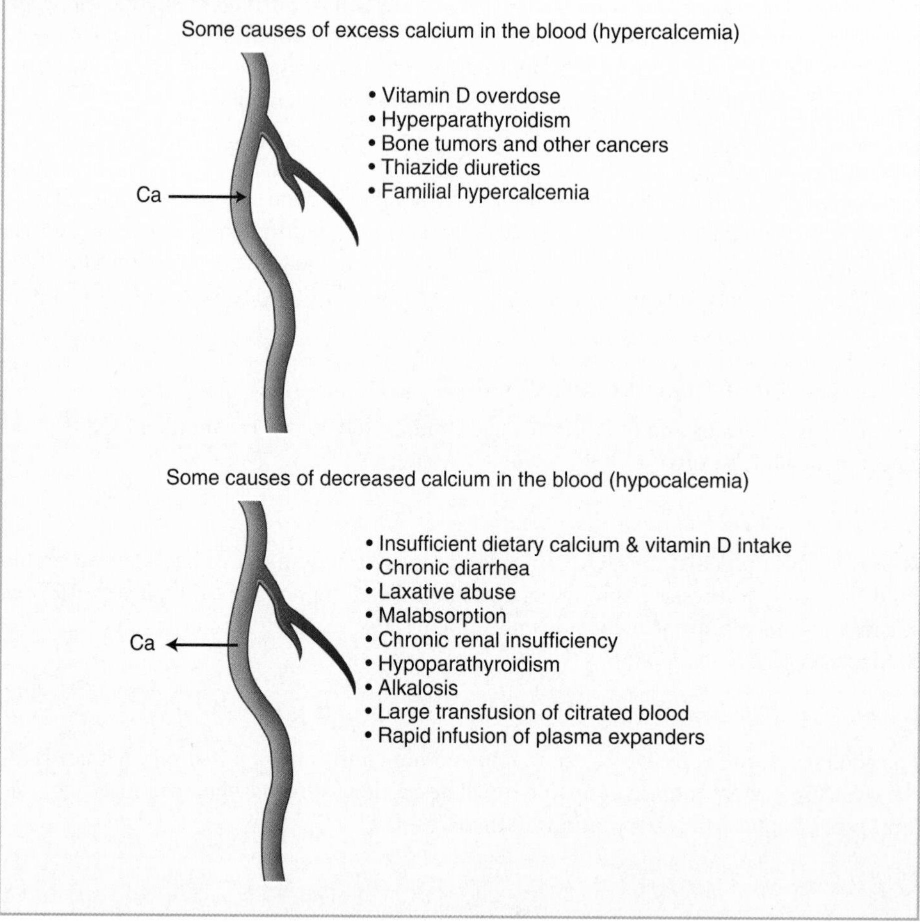

from bones, and decreasing calcium excretion in the urine. The plasma calcium concentration has an important influence on cell membrane permeability and influences the threshold potential of excitable cells. For this reason, calcium imbalances alter neuromuscular irritability.

Hypercalcemia

Hypercalcemia refers to a plasma excess of calcium (above 5.3 mEq/L [2.7 mmol/L] in children or 5 mEq/L [2.5 mmol/L] in newborns). Because so much calcium is stored in the bones, however, the serum levels of calcium may not reflect body stores.

ETIOLOGY AND PATHOPHYSIOLOGY Hypercalcemia is caused by conditions that involve increased calcium intake or absorption, shift of calcium from bones into the extracellular fluid, and decreased calcium excretion. Hypercalcemia due to increased calcium intake or absorption may occur if an infant is fed large amounts of chicken liver (source of vitamin A) or is given megadoses of vitamin D or vitamin A, or if a child or adolescent consumes large amounts of calcium-rich foods concurrently with antacids (milk-alkali syndrome). Infants with very low birth weight can develop hypercalcemia if they have inadequate phosphorus intake, as bone phosphorus and calcium will be resorbed. Hypercalcemia may also occur when children receiving total parenteral nutrition are given doses of calcium that are too high.

Most cases of hypercalcemia in children are due to a shift of calcium from bones into the extracellular fluid. The excessive amounts of parathyroid hormone produced in hyperparathyroidism cause calcium withdrawal from bones. Prolonged immobilization also causes withdrawal of calcium from bones. Often, the excess calcium ions are excreted in the urine. However, if calcium is withdrawn from bones faster than the kidneys can excrete it, hypercalcemia results. Hypercalcemia also occurs with many types of malignancies such as leukemias. The malignant cells produce substances that circulate in the blood to the bones and cause bone resorption. The calcium from the bones then enters the extracellular fluid, causing hypercalcemia. Bone tumors and chemotherapy destroy bone directly, leading to the release of calcium. Familial hypercalcemia and infantile hypercalcemia are rare congenital disorders.

Thiazide diuretics (e.g., thiazide and hydrochlorthiazide) decrease calcium excretion in the urine and may contribute to development of hypercalcemia.

CLINICAL MANIFESTATIONS Hypercalcemia may have nonspecific symptoms, making diagnosis difficult. Many of the signs and symptoms of hypercalcemia are manifestations of decreased neuromuscular excitability. Constipation, anorexia, nausea, and vomiting can occur. Fatigue and skeletal muscle weakness predominate. Confusion, lethargy, and decreased attention span are common, and polyuria develops. Severe hypercalcemia may cause cardiac arrhythmias and arrest. Neonates with hypercalcemia have flaccid muscles and exhibit failure to thrive. Hypercalcemia increases sodium and potassium excretion by the kidneys and can lead to polyuria and polydipsia.

CLINICAL THERAPY Hypercalcemia is treated by increasing fluids and administering the diuretic furosemide (Lasix) to increase excretion of calcium in the urine. Treatment to decrease intestinal absorption of calcium involves effective use of glucocorticoids. Bone resorption can be decreased by administration of glucocorticoids and calcitonin. Phosphate is sometimes given to treat hypercalcemia, but it may cause dangerous precipitation of calcium phosphate salts in body tissues. Dialysis may be used, if necessary.

NURSING MANAGEMENT

Nursing Assessment and Diagnosis

Nursing assessment of a child with hypercalcemia includes monitoring serum calcium levels, level of consciousness, gastrointestinal function, urine volume, specific gravity, cardiac rhythm, and pH. With chronic hypercalcemia, assessment of activity tolerance and developmental level becomes important.

Many nursing diagnoses are appropriate for children who have hypercalcemia. Diagnoses that address cardiac and neuromuscular manifestation are especially important. The following nursing diagnoses may apply:

- *Risk for decreased cardiac output* related to dysrhythmia
- *Risk for injury* related to decreased level of response
- *Risk for injury* related to neuromuscular impairment
- *Risk for injury* related to possibility of spontaneous fractures
- *Self-care deficit: Hygiene and dressing* related to neuromuscular impairment
- *Anxiety* related to change in health status
- *Constipation* related to decreased motility
- *Risk for altered nutrition: Less than body requirements* related to anorexia and nausea
- *Risk for altered urinary elimination* related to renal calculi

Planning and Intervention

Carefully calculate calcium in total parenteral nutrition and other solutions, administer these solutions with caution, and use cardiac monitoring to prevent hypercalcemia in hospitalized children.

Interventions to increase fluid intake are important for children with hypercalcemia or those who are immobilized. A large fluid intake, appropriate to the child's age, is necessary to keep the urine dilute and to help reduce constipation (a common symptom of hypercalcemia). An acidic urine helps to keep calcium from forming stones. Because urinary tract infections may cause the urine to be alkaline, nursing interventions to prevent urinary tract infection are necessary. Thiazide diuretics, which decrease calcium excretion, should not be given to the hypercalcemic child. Provide a high-fiber diet to help reduce constipation.

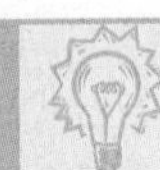

CLINICAL TIP

To decrease calcium intake in hypercalcemia, restrict intake of milk, ice cream, and other dairy products. Nondairy fruit-based desserts are acceptable alternatives.

Increasing mobility through assisted weight bearing helps to decrease the withdrawal of calcium from bones that is caused by immobility. If the hypercalcemia is caused by withdrawal of calcium from bones, the child is at risk for fractures with minor trauma and must be handled with special care. See Chapter 21 for further discussion of care following fractures and prolonged casting.

Teach parents to avoid giving calcium-rich foods and calcium antacids (e.g., Tums) to children with hypercalcemia. Vitamin D supplements should be avoided as they increase calcium absorption from the gastrointestinal tract.

Evaluation

Expected outcomes of nursing care include the following:

- Cardiac pump effectiveness
- Safety
- Normal bowel excretion
- Adequate nutritional status.

Hypocalcemia

Hypocalcemia is a serum deficit of calcium (below 4.4 mEq/L [2.2 mmol/L] in children or 4 mEq/L [2 mmol/L] in newborns). Remember that serum calcium levels may not reflect body stores of this mineral, as most of the body's calcium is stored in bone.

ETIOLOGY AND PATHOPHYSIOLOGY Hypocalcemia is caused by conditions that involve decreased calcium intake or absorption, shift of calcium to a physiologically unavailable form, increased calcium excretion, and loss of calcium by an abnormal route.

Decreased calcium intake or absorption causes hypocalcemia in children with chronic generalized malnutrition, or with a diet that is low in vitamin D and calcium. Female adolescents trying to lose or maintain a low weight often decrease foods that contain calcium and may develop chronic hypocalcemia. In these cases, premature bone loss and inadequate bone formation occur. (See Chapter 3 for further discussion of calcium intake during adolescence.) This deficit cannot be made up later in life, thus increasing the risk of osteoporosis.

Even with a normal calcium intake, hypocalcemia occurs if the mineral is not absorbed. If a child does not have enough vitamin D, calcium is not absorbed efficiently from the duodenum. Sunlight speeds formation of vitamin D in the skin. Children who are institutionalized without access to sunlight (e.g., severely developmentally delayed children), those with very dark skin, or children kept well covered when outside may become hypocalcemic because of the lack of vitamin D (see Chapter 3). Uremic syndrome is another cause of vitamin D deficiency. It interferes with the kidney's ability to activate vitamin D. High phosphate intake can cause hypocalcemia. Chronic diarrhea and steatorrhea (fatty stools) also reduce calcium absorption from the gastrointestinal tract.

The shift of calcium into a physiologically unavailable form occurs when calcium shifts into bone or free ionized calcium in plasma binds to proteins or small organic ions in the plasma. Too much calcium shifts into bones in various types of hypoparathyroidism, including DiGeorge syndrome (congenital absence of the parathyroid glands). Hypomagnesemia impairs parathyroid hormone function and may cause hypocalcemia. Some types of neonatal hypocalcemia are associated with delayed parathyroid hormone function or hypomagnesemia. Calcium shifts rapidly into bone when rickets is treated. A high plasma phosphate concentration causes plasma calcium to decrease. Ionized hypocalcemia, which is due to an increased binding of plasma ionized calcium, occurs very rapidly. The ionized hypocalcemia persists until the alkalosis resolves or the citrate is metabolized by the liver. Children who receive liver transplants are hypocalcemic for several days because of impaired citrate metabolism.

Increased calcium excretion occurs in steatorrhea, when calcium secreted into the gastrointestinal fluid binds to the fecal fat in addition to the dietary calcium that is bound in the feces. A similar situation occurs in acute pancreatitis.

Loss of calcium by an abnormal route may contribute to hypocalcemia as calcium is lost from the body through burn or wound drainage or sequestered in acute pancreatitis. Many different medications can cause hypocalcemia.

CAUSES OF IONIZED HYPOCALCEMIA

Alkalosis, which causes more calcium to bind to plasma proteins
Citrate in transfused blood products, which binds calcium

DRUGS THAT MAY CAUSE HYPOCALCEMIA

Antacids (if overused)
Laxatives (if overused)
Oil-based bowel lubricants
Anticonvulsants
Phosphate-containing preparations
Protein-type plasma expanders during rapid infusion
Antineoplastics

CLINICAL MANIFESTATIONS The signs and symptoms of hypocalcemia are manifestations of increased muscular excitability (tetany). In children they include twitching and cramping, tingling around the mouth or in the fingers, carpal spasm, and pedal spasm. Laryngospasm, seizures, and cardiac arrhythmias are more severe manifestations of hypocalcemia and may be fatal. Hypocalcemia may cause congestive heart failure, especially in neonates.

Although these symptoms are diagnostic of acute calcium deficiency, a more common state in children and adolescents is chronic low intake of calcium. This may be manifested by spontaneous fractures in infants and in adolescents who exercise excessively.

CLINICAL THERAPY Hypocalcemia is treated by oral or intravenous administration of calcium. The original cause of the imbalance is also treated. If the hypocalcemia is due to hypomagnesemia, the magnesium must be replenished before the calcium replacement can be successful. When the cause is chronic low dietary intake, counseling is needed about high-calcium foods, and perhaps the necessity for vitamin D intake or supplements.

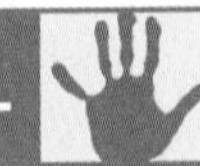

GROWTH & DEVELOPMENT

Hypocalcemia in infants is more frequently manifested as tremors, muscle twitches, and brief tonic–clonic seizures.

CLINICAL TIP

To test for Trousseau's sign, apply a blood pressure cuff to the arm and leave inflated for 3 min. If a carpal spasm occurs, the Trousseau's sign is positive. To test for Chvostek's sign, tap the skin lightly just in front of the ear (over the facial nerve). If the corner of the mouth draws up because of muscle contraction, the Chvostek's sign is positive.

NURSING MANAGEMENT

Nursing Assessment and Diagnosis

Carefully assess growth in the young female who is trying to diet. When an adolescent female is very thin, be sure to ask about excessive sports and other activities, and about regularity of menstrual periods. If periods are irregular or not occurring, collect additional dietary information to help determine whether the girl is lacking in intake of calcium, calories, and other nutrients. These assessments are needed even if serum calcium values are normal. Look for signs of inadequate nutrition such as fat and muscle wasting, dry hair, and cold hands and feet (Johnson, 1994). Assess for muscle cramps, stiffness, and clumsiness; grimacing caused by spasms of facial muscles and twitching of arm muscles; and laryngospasm. Increased neuromuscular excitability may be detected by testing for Trousseau's sign or Chvostek's sign. Many healthy newborns have a positive Chvostek's sign; however, this assessment should be reserved for children over several months of age. Monitor serum calcium levels and perform cardiac monitoring to observe for cardiac arrhythmias.

The effects of increased neuromuscular excitability in the child with hypocalcemia are the basis for the following nursing diagnoses:

- *Risk for injury* related to potential for fractures
- *Risk for ineffective breathing pattern* related to laryngospasm
- *Risk for decreased cardiac output* related to cardiac arrhythmias
- *Sensory/perceptual alteration* related to electrolyte imbalance
- *Altered nutrition: Less than body requirement* related to lack of basic nutritional knowledge of sources and recommended amounts of calcium intake

HIGH-CALCIUM FOODS

Milk
Cheese
Yogurt
Pudding
Egg yolks
Legumes
Nuts
Figs
Chicken
Salmon (canned with bones)
Grains (Cream of Wheat, farina, bran muffins)
Sardines (canned)
Tofu
Fruit drinks with added calcium

Planning and Implementation

To correct calcium deficiency in the hospitalized child, give oral or intravenous calcium as ordered. Monitor for complications of calcium supplementation. A 10% calcium gluconate solution should be readily available for emergency use in severe hypocalcemia. Calcium is never given intramuscularly because it causes tissue necrosis.

Take measures to ensure safety for the child who is hospitalized with hypocalcemia. Seizure precautions may be necessary. Explain the cause of muscle cramps to parents and older children.

Counsel the family about dairy products and nondairy foods rich in calcium. For the adolescent female whose weight and menstrual patterns show irregularities, total calories and calcium intake should be increased. Teaching may also be needed about proper calcium intake and its importance both to athletic performance and to prevention of osteoporosis. Encourage three glasses of nonfat milk per day (Snow-Harter, 1994). Teach ways to use milk in the diet. For example, sprinkle nonfat dry milk on cereal and other foods. If the child is lactose intolerant, emphasize nondairy sources of calcium and advise parents to purchase

COMPLICATIONS OF CALCIUM SUPPLEMENTS

Oral calcium
Constipation
Intravenous calcium
Tissue sloughing with infiltration
Elevated serum calcium
Decreased serum phosphate

special milk treated with lactase. This milk is more costly, and inadequate family finances may be an impediment to its use. If a child has a health condition leading to chronic diarrhea, encourage increased intake of calcium-rich foods. Calcium supplements in the form of calcium carbonate tablets may be used.

Evaluation

Expected outcomes of nursing care for hypocalcemia include the following:

- Ingestion of recommended dietary allowances for calcium
- Absence of discomfort related to calcium imbalance
- Freedom from injury

MAGNESIUM IMBALANCES

Magnesium is necessary for enzyme function in cells, acetylcholine release, glycolysis, stimulation of ATPases, and bone formation. Magnesium is a component of chlorophyll; thus, magnesium intake is aided by eating dark green leafy vegetables. Nuts and grains are also good sources of this mineral. Magnesium is absorbed primarily from the terminal ileum. It is distributed among the extracellular fluid (small amounts), the cells (larger amounts), and the bones (largest amounts). Magnesium excretion occurs in urine, feces, and sweat.

Magnesium imbalances are caused by alterations in magnesium intake, distribution, or excretion; by loss through an abnormal route; or by a combination of these factors. The plasma magnesium concentration influences the release of acetylcholine at neuromuscular junctions. Thus, magnesium imbalances are characterized by alterations in neuromuscular irritability.

Hypermagnesemia

NORMAL SERUM MAGNESIUM CONCENTRATION

1.5–2.4 mg/dL (0.62–0.99 mmol/L)

Hypermagnesemia occurs when the plasma magnesium concentration is too high (above 2.4 mg/dL [0.99 mmol/L]). Keep in mind that the serum levels measured in the laboratory may not reflect body magnesium stores, because most of the magnesium in the body is located in the bones and inside the cells.

Hypermagnesemia is caused by conditions that involve increased magnesium intake and decreased magnesium excretion. Impaired renal function leading to decreased magnesium excretion is the most common cause of hypermagnesemia in children. In both oliguric renal failure and adrenal insufficiency, magnesium ions that cannot be excreted in the urine accumulate in the extracellular fluid.

DRUGS THAT MAY CAUSE HYPERMAGNESEMIA

Magnesium-containing cathartics
Magnesium antacids

Less frequently, increased magnesium intake may cause hypermagnesemia. Magnesium sulfate (MgSO4) given to treat eclampsia in the mother before delivery causes hypermagnesemia in the newborn. Abnormally high amounts may also be taken in magnesium-containing enemas, laxatives, antacids, and intravenous fluids. Aspiration of seawater, as in near-drowning, is an uncommon but potentially serious source of excessive magnesium intake. Children with Addison's disease can have abnormally high magnesium levels.

Clinical manifestations of hypermagnesemia include decreased muscle irritability, hypotension, bradycardia, drowsiness, lethargy, and weak or absent deep tendon reflexes. In severe hypermagnesemia, flaccid muscle paralysis, fatal respiratory depression, cardiac arrhythmias, and cardiac arrest occur.

Hypermagnesemia is managed primarily by increasing the urinary excretion of magnesium. This is usually accomplished by increasing fluid intake (except in oliguric renal failure) and by the administration of diuretics. Dialysis may sometimes be necessary.

HOME CARE 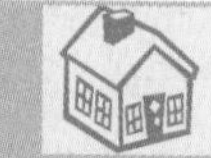

Instruct parents of a child with chronic renal failure to read labels to detect magnesium in antacids and cathartics.

NURSING MANAGEMENT Monitor serum magnesium levels. Take the child's blood pressure (to watch for hypotension), heart rate and rhythm (to monitor for bradycardia and cardiac arrhythmias), respiratory rate and depth (to watch for respiratory depression), and deep tendon reflexes (to check muscle tone and paralysis or movement). Keep the side rails of the bed raised. Children with hypermagnesemia or oliguria should not be given magnesium-containing medications or sea salt.

Teach parents of children with chronic renal failure that these children should never be given milk of magnesia, antacids that contain magnesium, or other sources of magnesium.

When hypermagnesemia is treated with diuretics, monitor potassium levels to watch for hypokalemia.

Expected outcomes of nursing care include maintenance of electrolyte balance, normal neuromuscular tone, safety, and regular heart rate and rhythm.

Hypomagnesemia

Hypomagnesemia refers to a plasma magnesium concentration that is too low (below 1.5–1.7 mg/dL [0.62–0.70 mmol/L]). Remember that the serum levels of magnesium may not reflect body stores, as most of the magnesium in the body is found in cells and bones.

Hypomagnesemia is caused by conditions that involve decreased magnesium intake or absorption, shift of magnesium to a physiologically unavailable form, increased magnesium excretion, and loss of magnesium by an abnormal route.

Decreased magnesium intake or absorption can occur if a child who is not eating has prolonged intravenous therapy without magnesium. Chronic malnutrition is another cause of decreased magnesium intake. Magnesium absorption is decreased in chronic diarrhea, short bowel syndrome, malabsorption syndromes, and steatorrhea.

A shift of magnesium to a physiologically unavailable form may occur after transfusion of many units of citrated blood products, because magnesium bound to the citrate is not physiologically active. Such transfusions cause prolonged hypomagnesemia in liver transplant patients who have impaired citrate metabolism. Magnesium shifts rapidly into bones that have been deprived of adequate stores.

Increased magnesium excretion in the urine occurs with diuretic therapy, the diuretic phase of acute renal failure, diabetic ketoacidosis, and hyperaldosteronism. Chronic alcoholism, occasionally seen in adolescents, increases urinary magnesium excretion. Magnesium contained in gastrointestinal secretions is bound to fat and excreted in the stool.

Loss of magnesium by an abnormal route occurs with prolonged nasogastric suction and through sequestration of magnesium in acute pancreatitis. Several medications may cause hypomagnesemia.

Hypomagnesemia is characterized by increased neuromuscular excitability (tetany). The clinical manifestations are hyperactive reflexes, skeletal muscle cramps, twitching, tremors, and cardiac arrhythmias. Seizures can occur with severe hypomagnesemia.

Hypomagnesemia is managed by administering magnesium and treating the underlying cause of the imbalance.

NURSING MANAGEMENT In addition to monitoring serum magnesium levels, nursing assessment of hypomagnesemia includes monitoring deep tendon reflexes, testing for Trousseau's and Chvostek's signs (see p. 000), monitoring cardiac function, and observing for muscle twitching. Children who are able to talk will report muscle cramping. Because magnesium levels are not routinely measured in many settings, request the test for any child who has risk factors and early manifestations of hypomagnesemia. When intramuscular or intravenous magnesium is ordered, administer carefully as directed and monitor vital signs. Electrocardiogram and renal studies may precede drug administration. Have resuscitative drugs and equipment readily available during drug administration.

Teach parents of a child with hypomagnesemia or continuing risk factors such as chronic diarrhea to include magnesium-rich foods in the diet. Before administering magnesium supplements, verify that the child's urine output is adequate. Monitor deep tendon reflexes if intravenous magnesium is given, and observe for complications of magnesium supplementation.

Expected outcomes for nursing care include restoration and maintenance of electrolyte balance.

DRUGS THAT MAY CAUSE HYPOMAGNESEMIA

Magnesium-wasting diuretics
Antineoplastics
Systemic antifungals
Aminoglycoside antimicrobials
Laxatives

MAGNESIUM-RICH FOODS

Whole-grain cereal
Dark green vegetables
Soy
Almonds
Peanut butter
Bananas
Egg yolk

COMPLICATIONS OF MAGNESIUM SUPPLEMENTS

Oral magnesium
Diarrhea
Intravenous magnesium
Flushing, warmth
Elevated serum magnesium
Cardiac arrhythmias
Decreased deep tendon reflexes

CLINICAL ASSESSMENT OF FLUID AND ELECTROLYTE IMBALANCE

How can you assess children appropriately for fluid and electrolyte imbalance without thinking through the clinical manifestations of every possible disorder one after the other? First, perform a rapid risk factor assessment on each child to see which factors are present (Tables 10–12 and 10–13).

TABLE 10-12	Risk Factor Assessment for Fluid Imbalances
ISOTONIC FLUID (EXTRACELLULAR FLUID VOLUME IMBALANCES) ■ Source of increased intake? ■ Aldosterone secretion increased or decreased? ■ Source of loss from the body?	
WATER ■ Source of increased intake? ■ Antidiuretic hormone secretion increased or decreased? ■ Source of unusual loss from the body?	

TABLE 10-13	Risk Factor Assessment for Electrolyte Imbalances
ELECTROLYTE INTAKE AND ABSORPTION ■ Increased? ■ Decreased?	
ELECTROLYTE SHIFTS ■ From electrolyte pool to plasma? ■ From plasma to electrolyte pool?	
ELECTROLYTE EXCRETION ■ Increased? ■ Decreased?	
ELECTROLYTE LOSS BY ABNORMAL ROUTE ■ Vomiting? ■ Diarrhea? ■ Nasogastric suction? ■ Wound? ■ Burn? ■ Excessive sweating?	

A risk factor assessment may be performed mentally during routine tasks. Look for factors that alter the intake, retention, and loss of isotonic fluid and water. This information is used to evaluate which fluid imbalance is most likely to occur in a particular child. Next, look for factors that alter electrolyte intake and absorption, distribution between plasma and other electrolyte pools, excretion, and abnormal routes of electrolyte loss. This information is used to evaluate which electrolyte imbalances are most likely to occur in the child. A review of pathophysiology is important to understand the role of the other electrolytes and substances, such as phosphorus, in the body.

After evaluating possible imbalances for the child, perform a clinical assessment. Assessment of fluid imbalances is performed by assessing weight changes, vascular volume, interstitial volume, and cerebral function (Table 10-14). Assessment of electrolyte imbalances is performed by assessing serum electrolyte levels, skeletal muscle strength, neuromuscular excitability, gastrointestinal tract function, and cardiac rhythm (Table 10-15). Next, check for other manifestations that are specific to a particular high-risk imbalance (e.g., polyuria in hypokalemia). Evaluate any serum laboratory values available. This method of risk factor assessment followed by clinical assessment provides a rapid yet thorough approach to assessment for fluid and electrolyte imbalances.

NORMAL VALUES OF ARTERIAL BLOOD PH

Infants: 7.36–7.42
Children: 7.37–7.43
Adolescents: 7.35–7.41

PHYSIOLOGY OF ACID–BASE BALANCE

Normal acid–base balance is necessary for proper function of the cells and the body. The number of hydrogen ions (H^+) present in a fluid determines its acidity. Increasing the hydrogen ion concentration makes a solution more acidic. Because the hydrogen ion concen-

TABLE 10-14 Summary of Clinical Assessment of Fluid Imbalances

ASSESSMENT CATEGORY	SPECIFIC ASSESSMENTS	CHANGES WITH FLUID IMBALANCES
Rapid changes in weight	Daily weights	Weight gain—extracellular volume excess Weight loss—extracellular volume deficit; clinical dehydration
Vascular volume	Small-vein filling time	Increased—extracellular volume deficit; clinical dehydration
	Capillary refill time	Increased—extracellular volume deficit; clinical dehydration
	Character of pulse	Bounding—extracellular volume excess Thready—extracellular volume deficit; clinical dehydration
	Postural blood pressure measurements	Postural drop—extracellular volume deficit; clinical dehydration
	Lung sounds in dependent portions	Crackles—extracellular volume excess
	Central venous pressure	Increased—extracellular volume excess Decreased—extracellular volume deficit; clinical dehydration
	Tenseness of fontanel (infants)	Bulging—extracellular volume excess Sunken—extracellular volume deficit; clinical dehydration
	Neck vein filling (older children)	Full with upright—extracellular volume excess Flat when supine—extracellular volume deficit; clinical dehydration
Interstitial volume	Skin turgor	Skin tents—extracellular volume deficit; clinical dehydration
	Presence or absence of edema	Edema—extracellular volume excess
Cerebral function	Level of consciousness	Decreased—clinical dehydration

TABLE 10-15 Summary of Clinical Assessment of Electrolyte Imbalances

ASSESSMENT CATEGORY	SPECIFIC ASSESSMENTS	CHANGES WITH ELECTROLYTE IMBALANCES
Skeletal muscle function	Muscle strength	Weakness, flaccid paralysis—hyperkalemia; hypokalemia
Neuromuscular excitability	Deep tendon reflexes	Depressed—hypercalcemia; hypermagnesemia Hyperactive—hypocalcemia; hypomagnesemia
	Chvostek's sign (not infants)	Positive—hypocalcemia; hypomagnesemia
	Trousseau's sign	Positive—hypocalcemia; hypomagnesemia
	Paresthesias	Digital or perioral—hypocalcemia
	Muscle cramping or twitching	Present—hypocalcemia; hypomagnesemia
Gastrointestinal tract function	Bowel sounds	Decreased or absent—hypokalemia
	Elimination pattern	Constipation—hypokalemia; hypercalcemia Diarrhea—hyperkalemia
Cardiac rhythm	Arrhythmia	Irregular—hyperkalemia; hypokalemia; hypercalcemia; hypocalcemia; hypermagnesemia; hypomagnesemia
	Electrocardiogram	Abnormal—hyperkalemia; hypokalemia; hypercalcemia; hypocalcemia; hypermagnesemia; hypomagnesemia
Cerebral function	Level of consciousness	Decreased—hyponatremia; hypernatremia

tration in body fluids is very low, acidity is expressed as **pH** (the negative logarithm of the hydrogen ion concentration) rather than as the hydrogen ion concentration itself. The range of possible pH values is 1 to 14. A pH of 7 is neutral. The lower the pH, the more acidic the solution. A pH above 7 is basic. The higher the pH, the more basic the solution. Body fluids are normally slightly basic.

The pH of body fluids is regulated carefully to provide a suitable environment for cell function. The pH of the blood influences the pH inside the cells. **Acidemia** is a term that refers to a decreased blood pH below normal levels, whereas **alkalemia** is an increased blood pH. For the enzymes outside the cells to function optimally, the pH must be in the normal range. If the pH inside the cells becomes too high or too low, then the speed of chemical reactions becomes inappropriate for proper cell function. Cell protein function relies on the correct level of hydrogen ions. Thus acid–base imbalances result in clinical signs and symptoms, and, in severe cases, they may cause death.

EXAMPLES OF METABOLIC ACIDS

- Pyruvic acid
- Sulfuric acid
- Acetoacetic acid
- Lactic acid
- Hydrochloric acid
- Beta-hydroxybutyric acid

In the course of their normal function, all cells in the body produce acids. Cells produce two kinds of acids: carbonic acid (H_2CO_3) and metabolic (noncarbonic) acids. These acids are released into the extracellular fluid and must be neutralized or excreted from the body to prevent dangerous accumulation. They can be neutralized to some degree by the buffers in body fluids. Carbonic acid is excreted by the lungs in the form of carbon dioxide and water. Metabolic acids are excreted by the kidneys.

BUFFERS

The maintenance of hydrogen ions within normal range relies heavily on buffers. A **buffer** is a compound that binds hydrogen ions when their concentration rises and releases them when the concentration falls (Figures 10–16A and B ◆). Several kinds of buffers are present in the body (Table 10-16). Various body fluids have buffers to meet their special needs (Halperin & Goldstein, 1994). The bicarbonate buffer system neutralizes metabolic acids (Figure 10-17 ◆); however, it cannot neutralize carbonic acid.

All buffer systems have limits. For example, if there are too many metabolic acids, the bicarbonate buffers become depleted. The acids then accumulate in the body until they are

PATHOPHYSIOLOGY ILLUSTRATED

Buffer Responses to Acid Base

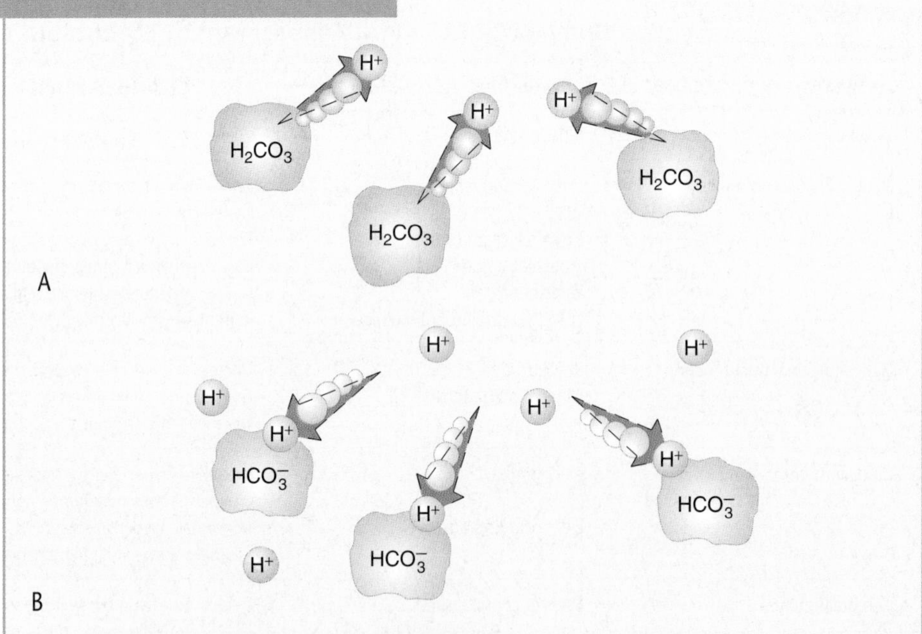

FIGURE 10-16 ◆
A, How buffers respond to an excess of base. If the blood has too much base, the acid portion of a buffer pair (e.g., H_2CO_3 of the bicarbonate buffer system) releases hydrogen ions (H^+) to help return the pH to normal. B, How buffers respond to an excess of acid. If the blood has too much acid, the base portion of a buffer pair (e.g., HCO_3^-) of the bicarbonate buffer system) takes up hydrogen ions (H^+) to help return the pH to normal.

TABLE 10-16 Important Buffers

BUFFER	MAJOR LOCATIONS IN THE BODY
Bicarbonate	Plasma; interstitial fluid
Protein	Plasma; inside cells
Hemoglobin	Inside red blood cells
Phosphate	Inside cells; urine

PATHOPHYSIOLOGY ILLUSTRATED

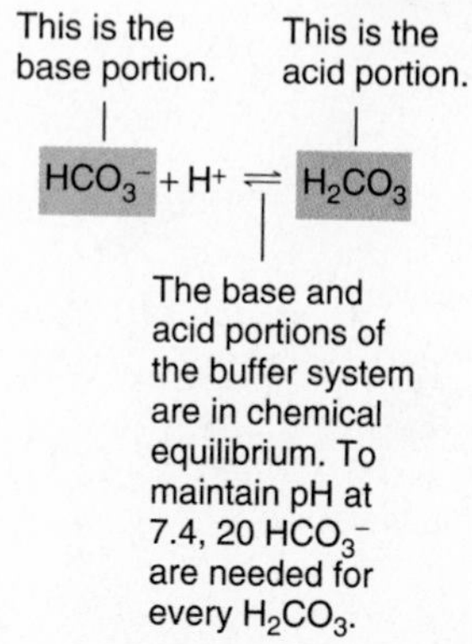

This is the base portion.

This is the acid portion.

$HCO_3^- + H^+ \rightleftharpoons H_2CO_3$

The base and acid portions of the buffer system are in chemical equilibrium. To maintain pH at 7.4, 20 HCO_3^- are needed for every H_2CO_3.

The Bicarbonate Buffer System

FIGURE 10-17 ◆

excreted by the kidneys. Clinically, this is seen as a decreased serum bicarbonate concentration and decreased blood pH.

ROLE OF THE LUNGS

The lungs are responsible for excreting excess carbonic acid from the body. A child breathes out carbon dioxide and water, the components of carbonic acid, with each breath. With faster and deeper breaths, more carbonic acid is excreted. Since carbonic acid is converted in the body to carbon dioxide and water by the enzyme carbonic anhydrase, an indirect laboratory measurement of carbonic acid is P_{CO_2}.

Although a child can voluntarily increase or decrease the rate and depth of respirations, they are usually involuntarily controlled. The P_{CO_2} and pH of the blood are monitored by chemoreceptors in the hypothalamus of the brain and in the aorta and carotid arteries. These arteries also monitor the P_{O_2} of the blood. The input from the chemoreceptors is combined with other neural input to change breathing according to needs. Rate and depth increase or decrease according to the amount of carbonic acid that needs to be excreted.

If a child has a condition that decreases the excretion of carbonic acid or causes breathing to be too slow or shallow (such as overmedication following surgery), carbonic acid accumulates in the blood. Clinically, this is seen as an increased blood P_{CO_2}. The reverse will also be true.

CARBONIC ACID

Carbonic acid = carbon dioxide + water
$H_2CO_3 = CO_2 + H_2O$

P_{CO_2} NORMAL ARTERIAL

Blood Values
Infants: 27–41 mm Hg (3.6–5.5 pKa)
Children: 32–48 mm Hg (4.3–6.4 pKa)

ROLE OF THE KIDNEYS

The kidneys excrete metabolic acids from the body in two ways. They reabsorb filtered bicarbonate and form bicarbonate when needed to restore balance. Bicarbonate is formed when acids and ammonium combine with extra ions (Hanna, Scheinman, & Chan, 1995). The blood bicarbonate concentration is an indicator of the amount of metabolic acids present, because bicarbonate is used in buffering the acids. When the concentration is normal, metabolic acids are present in usual amounts (Figures 10–18A and B ◆).

In a healthy child, the result of these renal processes is excretion of metabolic acids and maintenance of blood bicarbonate concentration within normal limits. However, a child whose kidneys are not producing enough urine may be unable to excrete metabolic acids effectively. Accumulation of these acids uses up many of the available bicarbonate buffers, resulting in a decreased serum bicarbonate concentration.

NORMAL CONCENTRATIONS OF ARTERIAL BLOOD BICARBONATE

Infants: 19–24 mmol/L
Children: 18–25 mmol/L
Adolescents: 23–25 mmol/L

ROLE OF THE LIVER

The liver also plays a role in maintaining acid–base balance by metabolizing protein, which produces hydrogen ions. It also synthesizes proteins needed to maintain osmotic pressures in the fluid compartments.

PATHOPHYSIOLOGY ILLUSTRATED

The Kidneys and Metabolic Acids

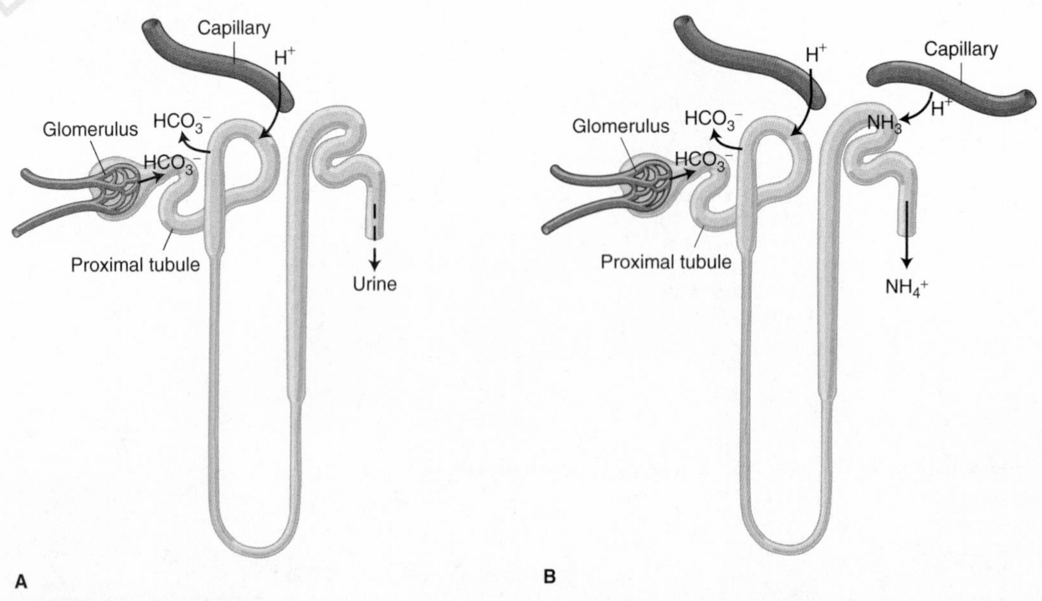

FIGURE 10-18 ◆
A, Recycling of bicarbonate by the kidneys. Bicarbonate ions that are in the blood are filtered into the renal tubules at the glomerulus. In the proximal tubules, bicarbonate ions are reabsorbed into the blood at the same time that hydrogen ions are transported from the blood into the renal tubular fluid. B, Secretion and buffering of hydrogen ions in the kidneys. If the urine is too acidic, the cells that line the urinary tract could be damaged. To prevent this problem, hydrogen ions secreted into the distal tubules are neutralized by phosphate buffers or bound to ammonia and excreted in the form of ammonium ions.

ACID–BASE IMBALANCES

Acid-Base Balance

There are four acid–base imbalances. Two are the result of processes that cause too much acid in the body and are referred to as **acidosis**. The other two imbalances are the result of processes that cause too little acid in the body and are called **alkalosis** (Noble, 1999). An acid–base disorder caused by too much or too little carbonic acid is called a respiratory acid–base imbalance. A disorder caused by too much or too little metabolic acid is called a metabolic acid–base imbalance.

Arterial blood gas measurements (ABGs) provide a laboratory evaluation of a child's current acid–base status. Table 10-17 provides a method that can help to interpret the pH, P_{CO_2}, and bicarbonate concentrations, which are the most important acid–base measures. End-tidal CO_2 can provide a continuous noninvasive measurement. (Remember that P_{CO_2} reflects carbonic acid status and bicarbonate concentration reflects the metabolic acid status.)

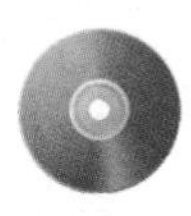

ACID–BASE IMBALANCES

Acidosis: Relatively too much acid in the body
- Respiratory acidosis: Relatively too much carbonic acid
- Metabolic acidosis: Relatively too much metabolic acid

Alkalosis: Relatively too little acid in the body
- Respiratory alkalosis: Relatively too little carbonic acid
- Metabolic alkalosis: Relatively too little metabolic acid

RESPIRATORY ACIDOSIS

Respiratory acidosis is caused by the accumulation of carbon dioxide in the blood. Since carbon dioxide and water can be combined into carbonic acid, respiratory acidosis is sometimes called carbonic acid excess. The condition can be acute or chronic. It is controlled by the lungs.

Etiology and Pathophysiology

Any factor that interferes with the ability of the lungs to excrete carbon dioxide can cause respiratory acidosis. These factors may interfere with the gaseous exchange within the lungs,

TABLE 10-17 How to Interpret Arterial Blood Gas Measurements

Ask the following questions to analyze blood gas results.

1. **What is the pH?** If the pH is normal, the child has no imbalance or has compensated for an imbalance. If the pH is below normal, the child has acidosis. If the pH is above normal, the child has alkalosis.
2. **What is the Pco_2?** If the Pco_2 is normal, the child does not have an acid–base imbalance. If the Pco_2 is above normal, the child has respiratory acidosis. This may be the primary disorder or may be a compensatory response to metabolic alkalosis. Looking at the bicarbonate concentration helps you decide. If the Pco_2 is below normal, the child has respiratory alkalosis. Again, this can be the primary disorder or may be a compensatory response to metabolic acidosis.
3. **What is the bicarbonate concentration?** If the bicarbonate concentration is within normal range, the child does not have a metabolic acid–base imbalance. If the bicarbonate is above normal, the child has metabolic alkalosis. This can be a primary disorder or can be compensatory in respiratory acidosis. When bicarbonate is below normal, the child has metabolic acidosis, either as a direct disorder or as a compensatory response to respiratory alkalosis.
4. **What do the results together tell you?** If the pH is abnormal and either the Pco_2 or bicarbonate concentration is normal, there is an uncompensated acid–base disorder. If all three values are abnormal, the child has a partially compensated disorder and the pH will provide the definitive answer. If Pco_2, pH, and bicarbonate are all decreased, then partially compensated metabolic acidosis is most likely. If pH is normal and Pco_2 and bicarbonate are abnormal, there is a fully compensated acid–base disorder.
5. **What are the child's history and clinical signs?** Does your interpretation fit with what you know about the child's medical condition and with assessments you are making? This last step helps you to integrate laboratory data with the clinical picture to strengthen your nursing care of the child with an acid–base imbalance.

may impair the neuromuscular pump that moves air in and out of the lungs, or may depress the respiratory rate (Table 10-18; Figure 10-19 ◆).

As the Pco_2 begins to increase, the pH of the blood begins to decrease. Compensatory mechanisms begin to act in the form of nonbicarbonate buffers, additional hydrogen ion excretion by the kidneys, and formation and decreased bicarbonate excretion by the kidneys. These compensatory mechanisms take several days to become active so the child manifests a changing clinical situation, depending on the underlying cause and the amount of compensation occurring (Table 10-19).

Clinical Manifestations

Acidosis in the brain cells causes central nervous system depression, manifested by confusion, lethargy, headache, increased intracranial pressure, and even coma. Acute respiratory acidosis can lead to tachycardia and cardiac arrhythmias. The child's arterial blood gases always show an increased Pco_2, the laboratory sign of increased carbonic acid. Serum pH can be decreased or normal.

TABLE 10-18 Causes of Respiratory Acidosis

FACTORS AFFECTING THE LUNGS	FACTORS AFFECTING THE NEUROMUSCULAR PUMP	FACTORS AFFECTING CENTRAL CONTROL OF RESPIRATION
Aspiration	Flail chest	Sedative overdose
Spasm of the airways	Pneumothorax or hemothorax	General anesthesia
Laryngeal edema	Mechanical underventilation	Head injury
Epiglottitis	Hypokalemic muscle weakness	Brain tumor
Croup	High cervical spinal cord injury	Central sleep apnea
Pulmonary edema	Botulism	
Atelectasis	Tetanus	
Severe pneumonia	Kyphoscoliosis	
Cystic fibrosis	Poliomyelitis	
Bronchopulmonary dysplasia	Muscular dystrophy	
Pulmonary embolism	Congenital diaphragmatic hernia	
	Guillain-Barré syndrome	

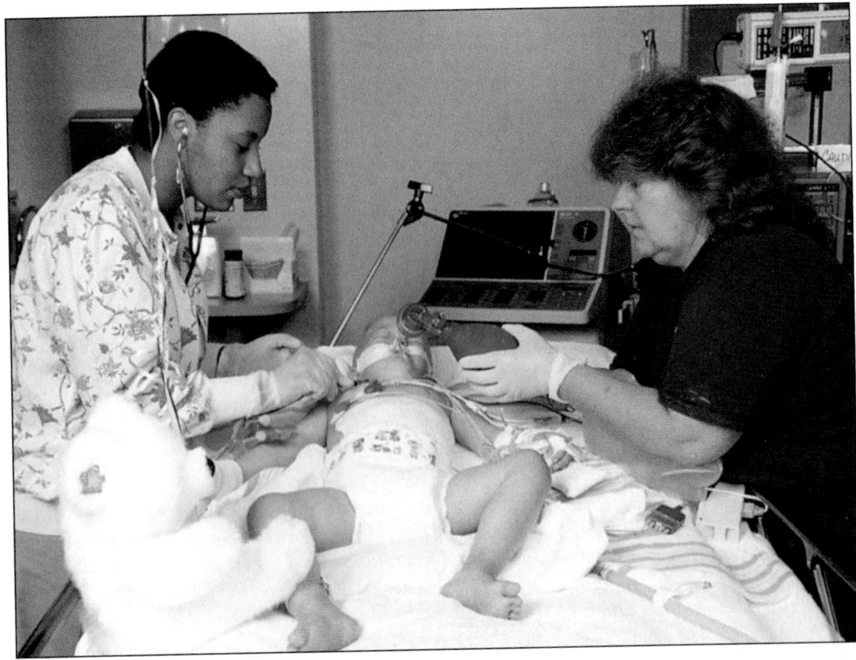

FIGURE 10-19 ◆
This child may develop respiratory acidosis or respiratory alkalosis. If the tidal volume is set too low during mechanical ventilation, carbon dioxide (carbonic acid) will accumulate in the body (respiratory acidosis) because it is not being excreted by the lungs. If the tidal volume is set too high, carbon dioxide will be depleted in the body (respiratory alkalosis) because it is being excreted in great quantities.

TABLE 10-19 Laboratory Values in Uncompensated and Compensated Respiratory Acidosis

	Pco_2	pH	HCO_3^-
Uncompensated	Increased	Decreased	Normal
Partially compensated	Increased	Decreasing but moving toward normal	Increasing
Fully compensated	Increased	Normal	Increased

Clinical Therapy

Treatment of respiratory acidosis requires correction of the underlying cause. For example, treatment may include bronchodilators for bronchospasm, mechanical ventilation for neuromuscular defects, decreasing sedative use, or surgery for kyphoscoliosis.

NURSING MANAGEMENT

Nursing Assessment and Diagnosis

Nursing assessment plays a pivotal role in decisions about interventions for respiratory acidosis, especially in chronic conditions such as cystic fibrosis and kyphoscoliosis. Assess respiratory rate, rhythm, and depth carefully. Take the apical pulse and be alert for tachycardia or arrhythmia. A cardiac monitor may be used. Obtain serial arterial blood gas measurements in acute conditions to evaluate changing status. Assess the level of consciousness and energy. Observe for chronic fatigue, headache, or decreased level of consciousness.

Several nursing diagnoses may apply to the child with respiratory acidosis. The most important of these addresses the child's risk for injury. Other nursing diagnoses depend on the specific clinical manifestation and the particular cause of the acidosis. Examples include:

- *Risk for injury* related to decreased level of consciousness
- *Risk for decreased cardiac output* related to cardiac dysrhythmias
- *Ineffective breathing pattern (hypoventilation)* related to neuromuscular impairment
- *Pain (headache)* related to cerebral vasodilation
- *Ineffective management of therapeutic regimen* related to complexity of bronchodilator therapy

GROWTH & DEVELOPMENT

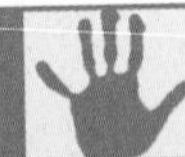

It is usually difficult to get a young child to do deep breathing or to use the "blow bottle" that is often given to older children and adults. To make deep breathing fun, use a pinwheel and have the child turn it during play. Alternatively, give a child a straw and have him or her blow bubbles in a glass of water, or have the child use the straw to blow scraps of paper across the bedside table.

Planning and Intervention

Care in the Community

Teach children at risk for respiratory acidosis and their parents preventive measures to use at home. For the child with a chronic condition such as cystic fibrosis, muscular dystrophy, or kyphoscoliosis, demonstrate deep breathing and encourage its use several times each day. Teach the family signs of infection—including fever, increased respiratory secretions, and discomfort with breathing—so the problems can be treated promptly to prevent further respiratory involvement. Position the child to facilitate chest expansion (Figure 10-20 ◆). Teach parents about proper administration of any necessary medications. For example, the child with cystic fibrosis may receive antibiotics to prevent respiratory infections. Teach parents and older children about home respirator use (Figure 10-21 ◆).

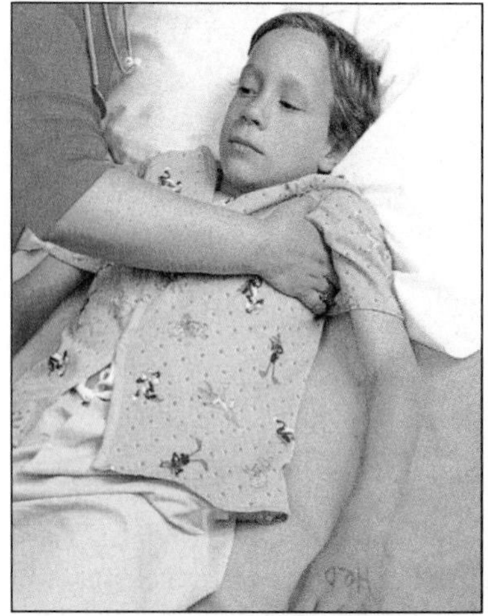

FIGURE 10-20 ◆
Positioning to facilitate chest expansion. If the child is positioned to avoid chest compression or slumping to the side, this will help correct respiratory acidosis.

Hospital-Based Care

For the hospitalized child, the focus is on ensuring safety. Keep side rails raised, and turn and position the child frequently. Evaluate mental status and document and report any changes in alertness. When laboratory values of blood pH and P_{CO_2} are available, evaluate them promptly and report any changes or abnormalities. Administer medications as ordered. Carefully watch the doses of sedatives to avoid further respiratory depression. Provide suctioning and encourage deep breathing.

Evaluation

Expected outcomes of nursing care for the child with respiratory acidosis include the following:

- Maintenance of safety
- Adequate rate and rhythm of respirations
- Management of causative disorders

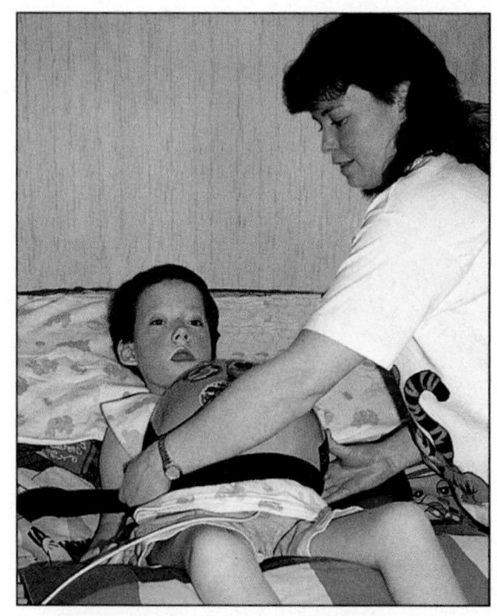

FIGURE 10-21 ◆
This child, who has muscular dystrophy, uses a "turtle" respirator at home to assist with breathing. His parents required instructions from the nurse on use of the respirator. The family has a generator to provide electricity for the respirator during power outages.

RESPIRATORY ALKALOSIS

Respiratory alkalosis occurs when the blood contains too little carbon dioxide. It is sometimes called carbonic acid deficit.

Excess carbon dioxide loss is caused by hyperventilation, in which more air than normal is moved into and out of the lungs. Common causes of hyperventilation are listed in Table 10-20.

In many cases, respiratory alkalosis lasts for several hours only. Renal compensation does not occur, as these compensatory mechanisms take several days to begin action. An example is the hyperventilation that occurs with acute anxiety. If the condition persists, however, the kidneys will begin to retain more acid and excrete more bicarbonate. Hydrogen ions will be released from body buffers to decrease plasma bicarbonate. While the imbalance continues, cellular function is thus protected by returning pH to normal levels (Table 10-21).

Arterial blood gas measurements show a decreased P_{CO_2} in respiratory alkalosis. Blood pH is generally elevated. The lack of carbon dioxide causes neuromuscular irritability and paresthesias in the extremities and around the mouth. Muscle cramping and carpal or pedal spasms can occur. The child may be dizzy or confused.

Medical management focuses on correcting the condition that caused the hyperventilation so that the body's compensatory mechanisms can return carbon dioxide levels to normal.

TABLE 10-20 Causes of Hyperventilation

Hypoxemia	Fever	Encephalitis
Anxiety	Salicylate poisoning	Septicemia caused by gram-negative bacteria
Pain	Meningitis	Mechanical overventilation

TABLE 10-21 Laboratory Values in Uncompensated and Compensated Respiratory Alkalosis

	Pco_2	pH	HCO_3^-
Uncompensated	Decreased	Increased	Normal
Partially compensated	Decreased	Increased but moving toward normal	Decreasing
Fully compensated	Decreased	Normal	Decreased

NURSING ALERT

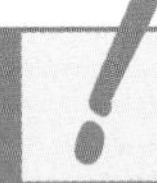

The Po_2 must be checked before any therapy for respiratory alkalosis is started, because it is dangerous to stop hyperventilation if oxygenation is poor.

Nursing Management

Assess the child's level of consciousness and ask if the child feels light-headed or has tingling sensations or numbness in the fingers, toes, or around the mouth. Assess the rate and depth of respirations. Monitor the hospitalized child's Po_2 with serial arterial blood gas measurements to evaluate changes in status. A careful assessment is needed regarding the cause of hyperventilation. Did an occurrence cause anxiety for the child? Is pain present (see Chapter 9)? Has the child received salicylates in any form? Is the child mechanically ventilated? Is there a central nervous system infection such as meningitis?

Nursing care for the child with respiratory alkalosis centers on teaching stress management techniques, maintaining pain control, promoting respiratory function, ensuring safety, maintaining fluid status, and providing health supervision and home care.

TEACH STRESS MANAGEMENT TECHNIQUES When anxiety is the cause of respiratory alkalosis, instruct the child to breathe slowly, in rhythm with your own breathing. Teach stress control techniques such as relaxation and imagery for situations that cause anxiety (Table 10-22).

MAINTAIN PAIN CONTROL Use medications, imagery, distraction, positioning, massage, and other techniques to decrease pain and maintain pain management. Chapter 9 describes these and other measures to assist with pain control.

Skills 10-15 to 10-19: Suctioning

PROMOTE RESPIRATORY FUNCTION Have the child cough, or suction as needed. Be certain that mechanical ventilation systems are working properly.

ENSURE SAFETY Provide a safe environment for the child who has a decreased level of consciousness. Be sure the child is supervised when sitting or standing up. Keep bed rails raised.

REGULATE FLUID STATUS Renal compensation to manage ongoing respiratory alkalosis requires adequate urinary output. Regulate fluid intake to ensure urine output unless fluids are restricted due to medical condition.

CARE IN THE COMMUNITY Teach parents to keep aspirin and other salicylate products out of reach of children, preferably in a locked medicine box. Instruct parents to keep syrup of ipecac in their homes and how to use it. Provide stickers with the number for the Poison Control Center.

TABLE 10-22 Techniques for Reducing Anxiety in Children With Parethesias

INFANT Calming touch, quiet voice, swaddling, holding quietly
TODDLER OR PRESCHOOLER Stuffed toy to hug, singing familiar quiet nursery songs, acknowledging the child's feelings, holding calmly
YOUNG SCHOOL-AGE CHILD Talking quietly about a happy event, telling a familiar story, reading a familiar book together, explaining that the tingling will go away, use of simple guided imagery, supportive listening
OLDER SCHOOL-AGE CHILD OR ADOLESCENT Explaining the reason for the tingling and that it will go away, use of guided imagery, familiar music on tape or radio, asking what the child does when anxious or "scared," and talking about coping strategies

Evaluation

Expected outcomes of nursing care for the child with respiratory alkalosis include the following:

- Normal respiratory rate and rhythm
- Maintenance of safety
- Regulation of fluid status

METABOLIC ACIDOSIS

Metabolic acidosis is a condition in which there is an excess of any acid other than carbonic acid. For this reason, it is sometimes called noncarbonic acid excess.

Etiology and Pathophysiology

Metabolic acidosis is caused by an imbalance in production and excretion of acid or by excess loss of bicarbonate (Table 10-23). Excess accumulation occurs by one of two mechanisms. First, a child can eat or drink acids or substances that are converted to acid in the body. Examples include aspirin, boric acid, and antifreeze. Second, cells can make abnormally high amounts of acid that cannot be excreted. This is the case in ketoacidosis of untreated diabetes mellitus, untreated growth hormone deficiency (Glaser, Shirali, & Styne, 1998), in children with bladder construction that uses part of the bowel (Mundy, 1999), or the starvation that can occur in anorexia or bulimia. A disorder of excretion occurs in conditions such as oliguric renal failure (Figure 10-22 ◆).

Bicarbonate can be lost from the body through the urine or through excessive loss of intestinal fluid. Diarrhea, fistulas, and ileal drainage are all possible sources. Carbonic anhydrase inhibitors can cause loss of excess bicarbonate in the urine.

When the pH of the blood decreases below normal, the chemoreceptors in the brain and arteries are stimulated and respiratory compensation begins. The child's rate and depth of breathing increase and carbonic acid is removed from the body. The blood pH shifts to a more normal range even though the cause is not corrected. The underlying condition and the degree of compensation will alter the clinical laboratory values observed (Table 10-24).

Clinical Manifestations

Laboratory values show decreased blood pH and decreased HCO_3 and Pco_2. An attempt at respiratory compensation causes one of the most important signs of metabolic acidosis, increased rate and depth of respirations (hyperventilation) or **Kussmaul respirations**. Severe acidosis can cause decreased peripheral vascular resistance and resultant cardiac arrhythmias, hypotension, pulmonary edema, and tissue hypoxia. Confusion or drowsiness may result, as well as headache or abdominal pain.

TABLE 10-23 Causes of Metabolic Acidosis

GAIN OF METABOLIC ACID
Ingestion of acids (e.g., aspirin) Ingestion of acid precursors (e.g., antifreeze) Oliguria (e.g., renal failure) Distal renal tubular acidosis Hyperalimentation Diabetic ketoacidosis Starvation ketoacidosis Some inborn errors of metabolism (e.g., maple syrup urine disease) Tissue hypoxia (lactic acidosis)
LOSS OF BICARBONATE
Diarrhea Intestinal or pancreatic fistula Proximal renal tubular acidosis

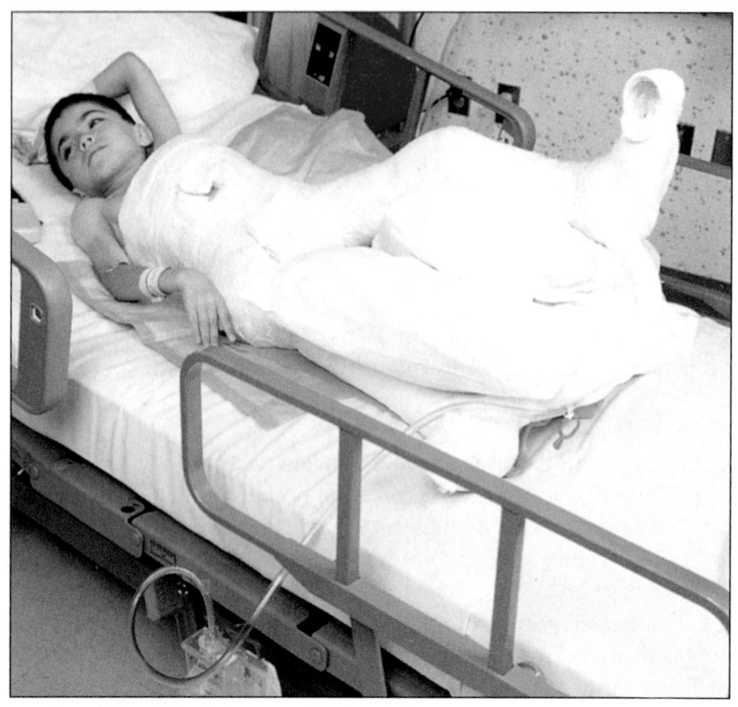

FIGURE 10-22 ◆ With any postoperative or immobilized child, it is important to monitor urine output to detect oliguria. If the kidneys do not produce very much urine, the metabolic acids accumulate in the body and cause metabolic acidosis. Inadequate fluid intake in the postoperative or immobilized child can lead to oliguria and, potentially, metabolic acidosis. Note this child's urine collection device.

TABLE 10-24 Laboratory Values in Uncompensated and Compensated Metabolic Acidosis

	HCO_3^-	pH	Pco_2
Uncompensated	Decreased	Decreased	Normal
Partially compensated	Decreased	Decreased but moving toward normal	Decreasing
Fully compensated	Decreased	Normal	Decreased

Clinical Therapy

Treatment of metabolic acidosis depends on identification and treatment of the underlying cause. In severe metabolic acidosis, intravenous sodium bicarbonate may be used to increase the pH and to prevent cardiac arrhythmias. This treatment is difficult to manage, because renal excretion can cause excess retention of bicarbonate; therefore, intravenous sodium bicarbonate is used only in severe situations, such as prolonged cardiac arrest.

Nursing Management

NURSING ASSESSMENT AND DIAGNOSIS Assess the rate and depth of respirations. Evaluate the child's level of consciousness frequently. Be alert for signs or complaints of headache and abdominal pain. Serial arterial blood gas measurements will usually be obtained to evaluate changes in status.

The following nursing diagnoses can apply to the child with metabolic acidosis:

- *Risk for injury* related to confusion/drowsiness or decreased responsiveness
- *Risk for decreased cardiac output* related to cardiac dysrhythmias
- *Altered tissue perfusion: Cerebral* related to tissue hypoxia
- *Ineffective management of therapeutic regimen* related to complexity of management of diabetes mellitus

PLANNING AND IMPLEMENTATION Ensure safety, taking into account the child's level of consciousness and alertness. Turn the child and change his or her position to prevent pressure on the skin. Limit the child's activities to decrease cardiac workload.

Position the child to facilitate chest expansion. Provide oral care during rapid respirations because the mouth may become dry.

Monitor intravenous solutions and laboratory values indicating acid–base balance. Report changes promptly.

Once the child is stabilized, provide teaching to compensate for knowledge deficits. Teach parents of young children to keep medications and acids locked in a secure place and out of reach to prevent poisoning (Figure 10-23 ◆). This includes medicines with aspirin as well as substances commonly kept in the garage for car maintenance. Teach about home management of diabetes and about early identification and treatment to avoid diabetic ketoacidosis. Expected outcomes of nursing care relate to prevention of acidosis and restoration of normal body balance during disease processes.

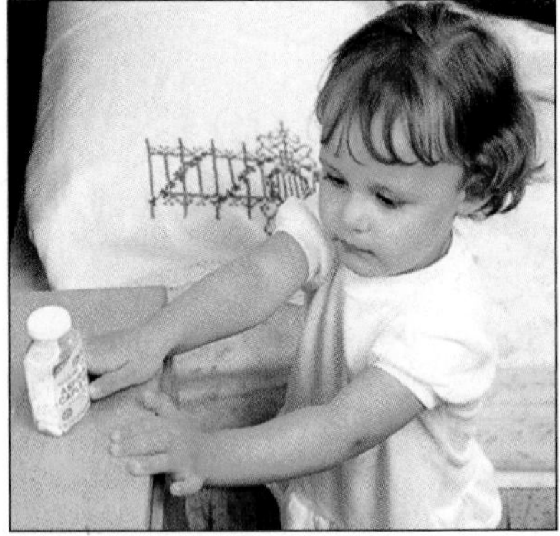

FIGURE 10-23 ◆
Teaching parents to use safety latches on cabinets to keep aspirin away from small children can prevent one cause of metabolic acidosis.

METABOLIC ALKALOSIS

Metabolic alkalosis occurs when there are too few metabolic acids. It is sometimes called noncarbonic acid deficit.

A gain in bicarbonate or a loss of metabolic acid can cause metabolic alkalosis (see Table 10-25). Bicarbonate is gained through excessive intake of bicarbonate antacids or baking soda or through metabolism of bicarbonate precursors such as the citrate contained in blood transfusions. Increased renal absorption of bicarbonate can occur in profound hypokalemia, primary hyperaldosteronism, or extreme deficit in extracellular fluid volume. Acid can be lost through severe vomiting, such as that seen in infants with pyloric stenosis and in continued removal of gastric contents through suction.

When the chemoreceptors in the brain and arteries detect the rising pH of metabolic alkalosis and respirations decrease, carbonic acid is retained in the body. This carbonic acid can neutralize the bicarbonate and return pH toward normal.

Blood pH, bicarbonate, and P_{CO_2} are usually elevated in metabolic alkalosis (Table 10-26). Hypokalemia often occurs simultaneously (refer to p. 331 to review signs of hypokalemia).

TABLE 10-25 Laboratory Values in Uncompensated and Compensated Metabolic Alkalosis

	HCO_3^-	pH	P_{CO_2}
Acute condition; uncompensated	Increased	Increased	Normal
Partially compensated	Increased	Increased but moving toward normal	Increasing
Fully compensated	The need for oxygen drives respirations and limits full compensation for metabolic alkalosis.		

TABLE 10-26 Causes of Metabolic Alkalosis

GAIN OF BICARBONATE
Ingestion of baking soda Ingestion of large quantities of bicarbonate antacids Exchange transfusion or massive transfusion (citrate is metabolized to bicarbonate) Increased renal absorption of bicarbonate
LOSS OF METABOLIC ACID
Prolonged vomiting (e.g., pyloric stenosis) Nasogastric suction Cystic fibrosis Hypokalemia Diuretic therapy Hyperaldosteronism Adrenogenital syndrome Cushing's syndrome

Respiratory rate and depth usually decrease. Increased neuromuscular irritability, cramping, paresthesia, tetany, seizures, and excitation can occur. Finally, this state can progress to weakness, confusion, lethargy, and coma.

Clinical therapy is directed at treating the underlying cause of the condition. Increasing the extracellular fluid volume with intravenous normal saline is used to facilitate renal excretion of bicarbonate.

Nursing Management

Assess the child's level of consciousness frequently. Alertness may decrease after an initial period of excitement, so regular assessments are needed. Monitor neuromuscular irritability. Observe for nausea and vomiting. Assess the rate and depth of respirations carefully. Obtain serial arterial blood gas measurements as ordered.

Facilitate ease of respirations. Ensure safety by keeping bed rails elevated and by turning the child frequently. Position the child on the side to avoid aspiration of vomitus.

If antacids were the cause of the alkalosis, teach the child and parents about correct use of these medications.

MIXED ACID–BASE IMBALANCES

It is possible for two acid–base imbalances to occur simultaneously. For example, a child with cystic fibrosis can develop respiratory acidosis from lung problems and concurrent metabolic alkalosis from vomiting during an illness. Treatment with diuretics may cause concurrent metabolic alkalosis resulting from extracellular volume depletion and hypokalemia in a child with congestive heart failure and chronic respiratory acidosis. In these cases, all underlying causes must be identified and treated. Care of children with mixed acid–base imbalances is often complicated, requiring hospitalization and careful management. Upon discharge, the nurse can teach parents about signs of imbalance that need to be reported and treated to prevent further complications. Evaluation of care is based on outcomes of adequate respiratory ventilation and metabolic balance.

Chapter Highlights

- Young children are at risk for fluid and electrolyte imbalance due to differences in body fluid compartments and regulation systems.
- Extracellular fluid volume deficit manifests as dehydration.
- Extracellular fluid volume excess is due to an excess of saline in the body.
- Interstitial fluid volume excess manifests as edema and weight gain.
- Nurses carefully manage fluid status of young children and teach parents prevention and treatment of fluid imbalances caused by gastroenteritis.
- The most common electrolyte imbalances are hypernatremia and hypokalemia, and thus involve sodium and potassium.
- Normal acid–base balance is necessary for proper function of cells in the body.
- The lungs, kidneys, and liver play a role in maintaining acid–base balance.
- Acid–base imbalance can involve alkalosis or acidosis; either can have a respiratory or metabolic origin.

EXPLORE MediaLink

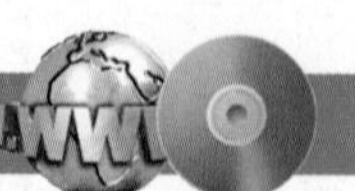

- NCLEX review, case studies, and other interactive resources for this chapter can be found on the Companion Website at **http://www.prenhall.com/ball.** Click on Chapter 10 to select the activities for this chapter.
- For animations, more NCLEX review questions, and an audio glossary, access the accompanying CD-ROM in this textbook.

References

1. Aker, J., & O'Sullivan, C. (1998). The selection and administration of perioperative intravenous fluids for the pediatric patient. *Journal of PeriAnesthesia Nursing, 13,* 172–181.
2. Armon, K., Stephenson., T., MacFaul, R., Eccleston, P. & Werneke, U. (2001). An evidence and consensus based guideline for acute diarrhoea management. *Archives of Diseases in Children* 85, 132–142.
3. Askin, D. F. (1997). Interpretation of neonatal blood gases, Part I: Physiology and acid–base homeostasis. *Neonatal Network, 16,* 17–21.
4. Askin, D. F. (1997). Interpretation of neonatal blood gases, Part II: Disorders of acid–base balance. *Neonatal Network, 16,* 23–29.
5. Bar-Or, O. (1996). Water and electrolyte replenishment in the exercising child. *International Journal of Sport Nutrition, 6,* 93–99.
6. Burkhart, D. M. (1999). Management of acute gastroenteritis in children. *American Family Physician, 60,* 2555–2563.
7. Committee on Sports Medicine and Fitness. (2000). Climatic heat stress and the exercising child and adolescent. *Pediatrics, 106,* 158–159.
8. Davenport, M. (1996). Pediatric fluid balance. *Care of the Chronically Ill Child, 12*(1), 26–28, 30–31.
9. Dabbagh, S., Ellis, D., & Grus Kin, A. B. (1996). In E. K. Motoyama & P. J. Davis (Eds.). Smith's anesthesia for infants and children. (6th ed.) pp. 105–137. St. Louis: Mosby-Year Book.
10. Eliason, B. C., & Lewan, R. B. (1998). Gastroenteritis in children: Principles of diagnosis and treatment. *American Family Physician, 58,* 1769–1776.
11. Endsley, S., & Galbraith, A. (1998). Are you overlooking oral rehydration therapy in childhood diarrhea? *Postgraduate Medicine, 104,* 159–166, 171.
12. Fann, B. D. (1998). Fluid and electrolyte balance in the pediatric patient. *Journal of Intravenous Nursing, 21,* 153–159.
13. Farrar, H. C., Chande, V. T., Fitzpatrick, D. F., & Shema, S. J. (1995). Hyponatremia as the cause of seizures in infants: A retrospective analysis of incidence, severity, and clinical predictors. *Annals of Emergency Medicine, 26,* 42–48.
14. Glaser, N. S., Shirali, A. C., Styne, D. M., & Jones, K. L. (1998). Acid–base homeostasis in children with growth hormone deficiency. *Pediatrics, 102,* 1407–1414.
15. Halperin, M. L., & Goldstein, M. B. (1994). *Fluid, electrolyte, and acid-base physiology* (2nd ed., pp. 69–144). Philadelphia: Saunders.
16. Hanna, J. D., Scheinman, J. I., & Chan, J. C. M. (1995). The kidney in acid–base balance. *Pediatric Clinics of North America, 42,* 1365–1396.
17. Hewitt-Taylor, J. (1999). Children in intensive care: Physiological considerations. *Nursing in Critical Care, 4,* 40–45.
18. Johnson, M. D. (1994). Disordered eating in active and athletic women. *Clinics in Sports Medicine, 13,* 355–369.
19. Jospe, N., & Forbes, G. (1996). Fluids and electrolytes—clinical aspects. *Pediatrics in Review, 17,* 395–404.
20. Larson, C. E. (2000). Safety and efficacy of oral rehydration therapy for the treatment of diarrhea and gastroenteritis in pediatrics. *Pediatric Nursing, 26,* 177–179.
21. Liebelt, E. L. (1998). Clinical and laboratory evaluation and management of children with vomiting, diarrhea, and dehydration. *Current Opinion in Pediatrics, 10,* 461–469.
22. Livingstone, V. H., Willis, C. E., Abdel-Wareth, L. O., Thiessen, P., & Lockitch, G. (2000). Neonatal hypernatremic dehydration associated with breast-feeding malnutrition: A retrospective survey. *Canadian Medical Association Journal, 162,* 647–652.
23. Mundy, A. R. (1999). Metabolic complications of urinary diversion. *Lancet, 353,* 1813–1814.
24. Noble, K. A. (1999, June 28). Putting the puzzle together: Arterial blood gas interpretation. *Advance for Nurses,* 19–22.
25. Provisional Committee on Quality Improvement, Subcommittee on Acute Gastroenteritis. (1996). Practice parameter: The management of acute gastroenteritis in young children. *Pediatrics, 97,* 424–436.
26. Reid, S. R., & Bonadio, W. A. (1996). Outpatient rapid intravenous rehydration to correct dehydration and resolve vomiting in children with acute gastroenteritis. *Annals of Emergency Medicine, 28,* 318–323.
27. Shamir, R., Zahavi, I., Abramowich, T., Poraz, I., Tal, D., Pollak, S., & Dinari, G. (1998). Management of acute gastroenteritis in children in Israel. *Pediatrics, 101,* 892–894.
28. Snow-Harter, C. M. (1994). Bone health and prevention of osteoporosis in active and athletic women. *Clinics in Sports Medicine, 13,* 389–404.
29. Straughn, A., & English, B. (1996). Oral rehydration therapy. *American Journal of Maternal-Child Nursing (MCN), 21,* 144–147.
30. Vega, R., & Avner, J. R. (1997). A prospective study of the usefulness of clinical and laboratory parameters for predicting percentage of dehydration in children. *Pediatric Emergency Care, 13,* 179–182.
31. White, V. M. (1997). Hyperkalemia. *American Journal of Nursing, 97*(6), 35.

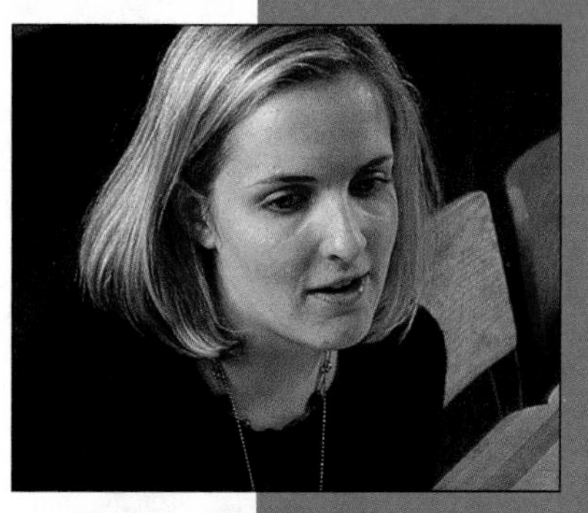

"Raymond's family is learning to deal with the diagnosis of AIDS. They are in a state of shock but want to learn how to best care for him. All of us on the team are trying to give them the support they need now and to prepare them for the future."

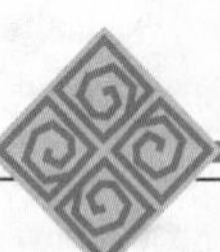
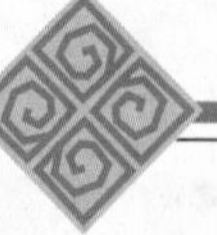

Raymond, a 2-year-old child, has had recurrent infections since he was born. In the last 3 months he has had bronchitis twice, otitis media three times, and several colds. Raymond has had a fever, vomiting, and diarrhea for several days, and does not appear to be improving. His mother brings him to an ambulatory clinic for evaluation.

After a thorough history is taken, blood tests are performed to assess Raymond's immune function. On the basis of an evaluation of Raymond's clinical symptoms and the results of the laboratory tests, he sees a specialist and is diagnosed with acquired immunodeficiency syndrome (AIDS). Raymond is admitted to a special unit of the hospital for children with AIDS so that his treatment can begin. Like many of the other children, Raymond is often irritable and difficult to console. Because he vomits frequently, the nurses pay particular attention to Raymond's nutritional problems, giving him frequent small feedings.

Raymond is diagnosed as having failure to thrive, a common sequela of AIDS. Broad-spectrum antibiotics are given, and he is assessed frequently for the development of new infections. Drugs for treatment of human immunodeficiency virus (HIV) are initiated. A multidisciplinary team, including nurses, physicians, nutritionists, and social services professionals, are involved in planning Raymond's care.

CHAPTER 11

ALTERATIONS IN IMMUNE FUNCTION

KEY TERMS

allergen An antigen capable of inducing hypersensitivity.

antibody A protein capable of reacting to a specific antigen.

antigen A foreign substance that triggers an immune system response.

graft-versus-host disease A series of immunologic responses mounted by the host of a transplanted organ with the purpose of destroying the transplant cells.

hypersensitivity response An overreaction of the immune system, responsible for allergic reactions.

immunodeficiency A state of the immune system in which it cannot cope effectively with foreign antigens.

immunoglobulin A protein that functions as an antibody. Immunoglobulins are responsible for humoral immunity.

opportunistic infection An infection that is often caused by normally nonpathogenic organisms in persons who lack normal immunity.

primary immune deficiency congenital immunodeficiency.

primary immune response The process in which B lymphocytes produce antibodies specific to a particular antigen on first exposure.

secondary immune response The body's response to an antigen at any time other than the initial exposure.

secondary immune deficiency Acquired immunodeficiency.

vertical transmission The passage of disease from the mother to the fetus during the period of pregnancy.

MediaLink

http://www.prenhall.com/ball

Resources for this chapter can be found on the CD-ROM accompanying this textbook, and on the Companion Website at http://www.prenhall.com/ball. Click on Chapter 11 to select the activities for this chapter.

CD-ROM

Audio Glossary

NCLEX Review

COMPANION WEBSITE

Web Links

NCLEX Review

MediaLink Applications

Case Study: Toddler with HIV

What are the signs and symptoms of immunologic disorders in children? Many times they are nonspecific. Raymond's admitting signs and symptoms, described in the opening scenario, are characteristic of several different immunodeficiency disorders. The immune system is one of the few body systems that regulates, either directly or indirectly, all other body functions. Thus, a problem with the immune system can have multisystem consequences and may be life threatening. Allergic reactions to food or frequent episodes of otitis media may indicate a disorder of immune function. Immune conditions can be mild to severe and life threatening. Congenital abnormalities sometimes signal a defect in cellular immunity. In this chapter, we will examine some of the more common disorders of immune function and discuss nursing care of children who have these diseases and their families.

ANATOMY AND PHYSIOLOGY OF PEDIATRIC DIFFERENCES

The function of the immune system is to recognize any foreign substances within the body—in simple terms, to distinguish "nonself" from "self"—and to eliminate foreign substances as efficiently as possible. When the body recognizes the presence of a substance that it cannot identify as part of itself, the body protects itself through the immune response. Normally, the immune system responds to an invasion of foreign substances, or antigens, in numerous ways. It produces **antibodies,** or proteins that work against **antigens,** the foreign substances that trigger the immune response. There are many types of antibodies, which are described later in this section. The immune system also produces other types of cells, such as T lymphocytes and natural killer (NK) cells.

Immunity is either natural or acquired. Natural immune defenses are those an infant has at birth, such as intact skin, body pH, natural antibodies from the mother, and inflammatory and phagocytic properties. Acquired immunity consists of humoral (antibody-mediated) and cell-mediated immunity and is not fully developed until a child is about 6 years of age.

Humoral immunity is responsible for destroying bacterial antigens. B lymphocytes, produced in the bone marrow, develop into plasma cells that produce antibodies. Antibodies are a type of protein called **immunoglobulins,** of which there are five types: IgM, IgG, IgA, IgD, and IgE (Table 11-1). IgM, IgG, and IgA act to control a number of body infections, whereas IgE is useful in combating parasitic infections and is part of the allergic response. The role of IgD is unknown.

Antibodies are found in serum, body fluids, and certain tissues. When a child is first exposed to an antigen, the B lymphocyte system begins to produce antibodies that react specifically to that antigen (Figure 11-1 ◆). It takes approximately 3 days for this process, known as **primary immune response,** to occur. Subsequent encounters with the antigen trigger memory cells, resulting in a **secondary immune response** within 24 hours.

Infants and children have differing amounts of some immunoglobulins. IgG is the only immunoglobulin that crosses the placenta; as a result, a newborn's levels are similar to those of the mother's. This maternal IgG disappears by 6 to 8 months of age. The infant's IgG then increases gradually until mature levels are reached at 7 to 8 years. IgM levels are low at birth, rise markedly at 1 week of age, and continue to increase until adult levels are reached at about 1 year. IgA and IgE are not present at birth. Manufacture of these immunoglobulins begins by 2 weeks of age; however, normal values are not achieved until 6 to 7 years. It is thus

TABLE 11-1 Classes of Immunoglobulins

IgM	Present in intravascular spaces
IgG	Present in all body fluids
IgA	Present in secretions of gastrointestinal, respiratory, and genitourinary tracts
IgD	Presence and function not yet described
IgE	Present in internal and external body fluids

PATHOPHYSIOLOGY ILLUSTRATED

Primary Immune Response

FIGURE 11-1 ◆

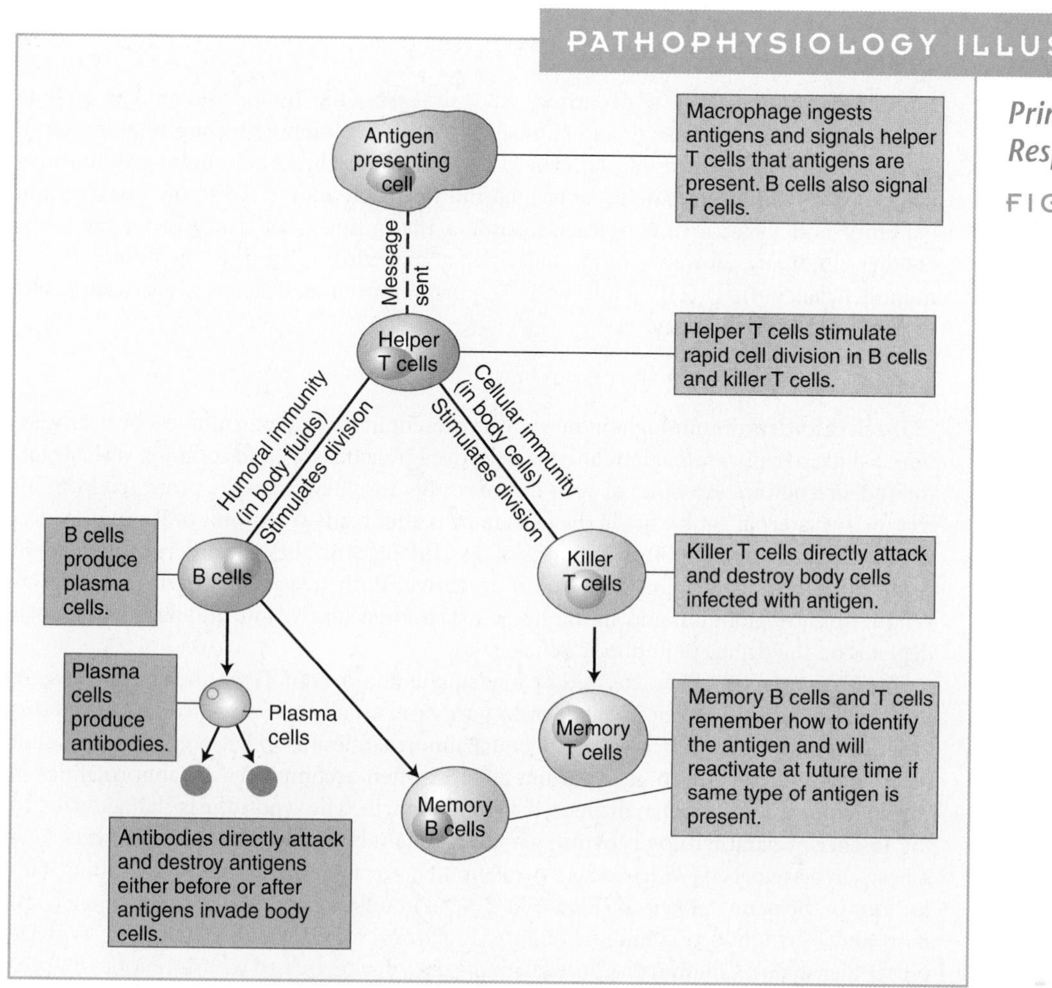

easy to see why children under 6 years of age become ill so often—they do not have a full complement of immunoglobulins.

In contrast, cell-mediated immunity achieves full function early in life. T lymphocytes, produced in the thymus, provide cellular immunity and protect against most viruses, fungi, slowly developing bacterial infections such as tuberculosis, and tumors. In addition, they control the timing of the response in delayed hypersensitivity reactions, such as the purified protein derivative (PPD) test, and they are responsible for the rejection of foreign grafts, such as transplants. For this reason, the blood infused into newborns is generally irradiated to prevent **graft-versus-host disease** (a series of immunologic reactions in response to transplanted cells) from transfused lymphocytes (Stiehm & Ammann, 1997). Specialized types of T lymphocytes include killer T cells, suppressor T cells, and helper T cells. Suppressor T cells inhibit B lymphocytes from differentiating into plasma cells. Helper T cells aid in the proliferation and immunologic function of other cells. T lymphocytes have proteins on their surfaces that can be used to measure the immune activity of these cells. For example, some of the common proteins are CD2, CD3, CD4, CD5, CD7, and CD8. Natural killer (NK) cells (also known as non-B/non-T lymphocytes) originate in the bone marrow and thymus and migrate to the blood and spleen. They play a role in control of viral infection, tumors, and autoimmune disease. Newborns have somewhat lower numbers of NK cells than older children and adults, decreasing their ability to respond to certain antigens.

Complement is a component of blood serum consisting of 11 protein compounds. It is an inactive enzyme that activates in response to antigen–antibody functions, resulting in a generalized inflammatory reaction that kills foreign cells. It also plays a role in causing some autoimmune diseases. The levels of some complement proteins are lower in newborns than in older children and adults, thus delaying and hampering response to certain infections.

IMMUNODEFICIENCY DISORDERS

Immunodeficiency, a state of decreased responsiveness of the immune system, can occur to varying degrees in response to any number of events. Children with congenital immunodeficiency, or **primary immune deficiency,** are born with a failure of humoral antibody formation (B-cell disorder), a deficient cellular immune system (T-cell disorder), or a combination of both defects. In congenital disorders, the immune deficiency is not caused by another condition. However, immunodeficiency may also be acquired, as in human immunodeficiency virus (HIV) infection. Acquired immunodeficiency is also called **secondary immune deficiency.**

B-CELL AND T-CELL DISORDERS

In B-cell disorders, immunoglobulins may be present in inadequate numbers or nearly absent. X-linked hypogammaglobulinemia, selective IgA deficiency, and common variable immunodeficiency are examples of such disorders. Because newborns are protected from infection by maternal antibodies in the first months after birth, symptoms of B-cell disorders usually become apparent after 3 months of age. Infants with these disorders have frequent recurrent bacterial infections and failure to thrive. With treatment, consisting of intravenous immunoglobulins and antibiotics, most children survive into adulthood. Prognosis depends on the degree of antibody deficiency.

T-cell disorders are characterized by inadequate numbers of T lymphocytes or absence of T-cell functions. Isolated T-cell disorders are rare, usually accompanied by a B-cell disorder, and may be associated with congenital abnormalities (as in DiGeorge syndrome) or of unknown cause. DiGeorge syndrome is most often accompanied by abnormalities in chromosome 22, and is often diagnosed soon after birth. The syndrome is characterized by the absence of parathyroid or thymus glands, resultant hypocalcemia, cardiac defects, low-set ears, hypertelorism (widely set eyes), tetany 48 hours after birth, and viral and fungal infections in the neonatal period (Figure 11-2 ◆). Pneumonia and failure to thrive are common, and T-lymphocyte counts are often $< 1500/\text{mm}^3$ for CD3 and $< 1000/\text{mm}^3$ for CD4 cells (Elder, 2000). Children diagnosed with the disorder are treated with antibiotics for prophylaxis against pneumonia from *Pneumocystis carinii,* oral calcium, thymus transplantation, and HLA-identical bone marrow transplantation. Without thymus transplantation, few children survive beyond 5 years.

Immunodeficiency with hyper-IgM is a T-cell disorder that affects mainly males and causes decreased T-cell function, variable abnormal levels of immunoglobulins, and high titers of some antibodies. It is usually X-linked but is autosomal in some cases. Treatment with intravenous immune globulin (IVIG) therapy is helpful although later malignancies and liver disease can occur (Schwartz, 2000).

Table 11-2 compares laboratory values for selected congenital immunodeficiency disorders.

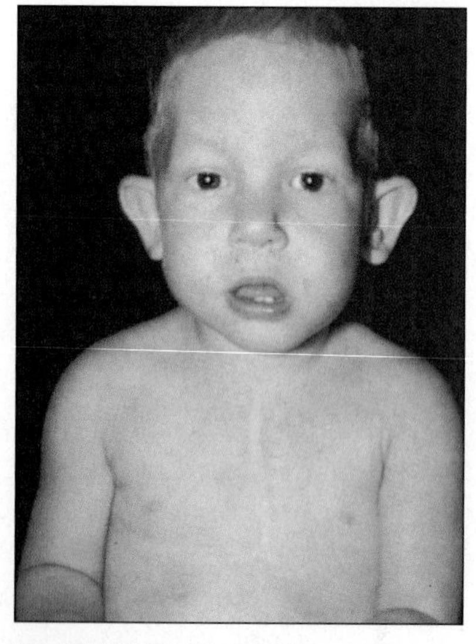

FIGURE 11-2 ◆
This infant has characteristic features of DiGeorge Syndrome. Note the low-set and malformed ears.
From Zitelli, B. J., & Davis, H. W. (Eds.) (1997). *Atlas of Pediatric Physical Diagnosis* (3rd ed., p. 101). St. Louis, MO: Mosby, Inc.

SEVERE COMBINED IMMUNODEFICIENCY DISEASE

Severe combined immunodeficiency disease (SCID) is a congenital condition characterized by absence of both humoral and cellular immunity. SCID occurs in X-linked recessive, autosomal recessive, and sporadic forms. Without appropriate treatment, children born with SCID usually die within the first 2 years of life.

Etiology and Pathophysiology

Severe combined immunodeficiency disease is caused by genetic mutations of cellular receptors to interleukin. The mutations lead to impaired lymphoid development in children with low T and NK cells. The B lymphocytes present may appear normal in number but are defective in performance (Candotti, 2000).

Clinical Manifestations

Symptoms in a child born with SCID develop early in life. The neonate often demonstrates a susceptibility to infection by 3 months of age. The disorder is characterized by chronic infection (such as otitis media or pneumonia), failure to completely recover from infection,

TABLE 11-2 Selected Congenital Immunodeficiency Disorders

DISORDERS	LABORATORY FINDINGS
B cell	
X-linked hypogammaglobulinemia	Reduced IgA, IgM, IgE, IgG (<100 mg/dL), absence of B cells in peripheral blood, normal T cells
Selective IgA deficiency	IgA <10 mg/dL
Common variable immunodeficiency	IgA, IgM reduced; IgG <250 mg/dL
T cell	
DiGeorge syndrome	Lymphopenia; absent T-cell functions, decreased T cells, normal B cells
Immunodeficiency with hyper-IgM	Reduced IgG, IgA; elevated IgM; mutations in T-cell surface proteins
Combined	
Severe combined immunodeficiency syndrome (SCID)	Complete absence of T- and B-cell and NK immunity
Wiskott-Aldrich syndrome	Thrombocytopenia, low platelet volume, nonfunctional B cells, normal IgG, decreased IgM, increased IgA, increased IgE; inability to respond to polysaccharide antigens

frequent reinfection, and infection with viruses such as cytomegalovirus and the bacterium *Pneumocystis carinii.* Often the first infection seen is a resistant oral candidiasis. Children are also highly susceptible to serious infections such as meningitis, skin or organ infection, osteomyelitis, or sepsis. Failure to thrive is a consequence of persistent illness.

Some infants experience graft-versus-host disease as a result of placental transfer of maternal T lymphocytes. If the child receives foreign tissue, for example, in a blood transfusion, signs such as skin rash, fever, hepatosplenomegaly, and diarrhea may occur.

Clinical Therapy

A marked reduction in lymphocyte counts is indicative of SCID. B and T lymphocytes are generally few in number or absent from the peripheral blood and lymphoid tissues. In some cases, the B-lymphocyte count may be elevated, although these cells do not function normally. NK cells are few in number. Immunoglobulin levels are significantly reduced. Refer to Table 11-2 for laboratory findings in SCID. Diagnosis is usually made only after extensive laboratory testing. In addition to a complete blood count, erythrocyte sedimentation rate, and B- and T-cell lymphocyte counts, other studies including IgA, IgG, and IgM antibody titers to immunizations received and neutrophil count may be performed (Table 11-3).

The goal of medical management is to restore immune function. Thymic hormones have been given to some children with limited success. Intravenous immune globulin

TABLE 11-3 Cells Evaluated in Laboratory Studies for Immune Conditions

TEST AND TYPE OF CELL EVALUATED	ACTION	IMPLICATION OF INCREASED OR DECREASED LEVELS
White blood cell (WBC) count		
Neutrophil	Phagocytic cell that defends against bacteria	Increased in bacterial infection, inflammatory processes, and some malignancies
Eosinophil	Associated with antigen–antibody reaction	Increased in allergic reaction; decreased in children receiving corticosteroids
Lymphocytes (T, B, non-B/non-T [NK])	Major components of immune system	Increased in many infections; decreased in children with immune deficiency
Immunoglobulins		
(IgM, IgG, IgA, IgD, IgE)	Many roles in a number of immunologic reactions	Increased in presence of infection or allergic response; decreased in children with immune deficiency

(IVIG) may be administered. Bone marrow transplantation offers hope for children with SCID (see Chapter 16). However, the donor must be a histocompatible donor, such as a sibling. T-cell function is corrected with the marrow transplantation, and new cells appear 3 to 4 months after infusion of the donor marrow. With the identification of the genetic defect for SCID in recent years, gene transfer has been successfully attempted to treat a small number of children. This experimental therapy is expected to be used more often in the future (Candotti, 2000).

Prognosis is poor without aggressive therapy. Some children have survived 10 years after a successful bone marrow transplant.

NURSING MANAGEMENT

Nursing Assessment and Diagnosis

Obtain a thorough history of infections, including age of onset, type of causal organism, frequency, and severity. Take a family history, and find out if the child has had any unusual reactions to vaccines, medications, or foods. Measure the child's height and weight accurately to identify failure to thrive. Look for any evidence of infections involving the skin, subcutaneous tissues, respiratory system, and mucous membranes. Palpate the abdomen for hepatomegaly and the lymph nodes for lymphadenopathy.

Assess family support systems and coping mechanisms when a child is diagnosed with the disorder.

The primary nursing diagnosis for a child with SCID is *risk for infection,* related to immunodeficiency. Other nursing diagnoses may include the following:

- *Risk for altered nutrition: Less than body requirements,* related to chronic illness
- *Risk for impaired skin integrity,* related to immunologic deficit
- *Risk for caregiver role strain,* related to a child with a chronic, life-threatening illness
- *Risk for altered growth and development,* related to physical disability and chronic illness

Planning and Implementation

Nursing care of the immunodeficient child focuses on preventing infection. However, even with the use of environmental controls, such as keeping children inside special units to maintain a sterile environment, these children are prone to **opportunistic infections** (those caused by normally nonpathogenic organisms in persons who lack normal immunity).

Prevent Systemic Infection

Infection Control Methods

Frequent and thorough handwashing is important. Standard precautions are always used, with transmission-based precautions when needed. Use sterile aseptic technique when caring for all sites where needles, catheters, central lines, endotracheal tubes, pressure-monitoring lines, and peripheral intravenous lines enter the child's body. Food and other items entering the hospital room may need special treatment. The child should be placed in a private room, and contact with infectious individuals should be minimized.

Promote Skin Integrity

The skin is the only intact defense that many immunodeficient children have. Provide good skin care, and observe all possible pressure areas closely for signs of breakdown or infection. Turn the child frequently. Encourage range of motion exercises. Avoid any skin trauma.

Manage Medication Therapy

Many of the medications used long term in the treatment of children with SCID have numerous side effects. Monitor closely for side effects of antibiotics, such as overgrowth of resistant organisms (e.g., thrush infections in the mouth, *Clostridium difficile* infections of the gastrointestinal tract) and administer IVIG safely (see Table 11-4).

TABLE 11-4 Nursing Considerations in the Administration of Intravenous Immune Globulin (IVIG)

USED IN TREATMENT OF
■ Immunodeficiency disease, such as severe combined immunodeficiency and acquired immunodeficiency syndrome (AIDS) ■ Antibody deficiency associated with other conditions such as malignancy ■ Kawasaki disease
ADMINISTRATION
■ IVIG must be administered as stated in the package insert. ■ Use separate tubing and do not mix with other medications. ■ Start infusion slowly and increase to recommended rate after 30 minutes if no reaction occurs (see below). ■ Monitor for hypersensitivity reaction (fever, increased pulse or respiration, decreased blood pressure, chest pain, shaking, chills). ■ Schedule immunizations 14 days before or 3 months after IVIG infusion, as immune response will be altered.
POSSIBLE ADVERSE REACTIONS
■ Headache ■ Fever ■ Nausea, vomiting ■ Arthralgia ■ Anaphylaxis
SPECIAL TYPES AVAILABLE
■ RespiGam (helpful in respiratory syncytial virus) ■ CytoGam (enriched with antibodies to cytomegalovirus)
Note: From "IVIG therapy: separating fact from wishful thinking," by H. M. Lederman, 1996, *Contemporary Pediatrics 13*, 75–92. Adapted.

Provide Emotional Support and Referral to Appropriate Support Groups and Services

SCID is a life-threatening and devastating disease. Even with aggressive therapy, the prognosis is poor. Evaluate the family's knowledge about the disease. The parents may be experiencing guilt because of the genetic nature of the disease and the difficulties of treatment. Listen closely to their concerns and encourage them to discuss their fears. Refer them to an appropriate support group or counselor if needed. Genetic counseling should be encouraged if the parents plan to have more children.

The family of a child who undergoes bone marrow transplantation requires additional support and referrals. The transplantation procedure involves surgery for both the ill child and the donor, often another child in the family (refer to the discussion in Chapter 16). After the infusion of the donor marrow, the ill child will be hospitalized for several months until T-lymphocyte levels are sufficient to provide resistance to infection. During this period, parents may need to rely on social services to help manage the family situation, particularly if the child is hospitalized at a medical center far from the family's home. Assess the family's situation and make appropriate referrals to social service and to support groups. Introduce parents to other families undergoing bone marrow transplantation.

Evaluation

Expected outcomes of nursing care include the following:

- Adequate nutritional status as determined by normal growth patterns
- Maintenance of intact skin
- Adaptive coping by family to demands of a chronic illness
- Developmental performance within normal level for age

WISKOTT–ALDRICH SYNDROME

A combined congenital immunodeficiency syndrome, Wiskott–Aldrich syndrome is an X-linked disorder which causes mutation in the WAS gene and changes in the WAS protein (Elder, 2000). It is characterized by thrombocytopenia, eczema, hemorrhagic tendencies, and recurrent infections. Thrombocytopenia with bleeding tendencies appears during the neonatal period. Eczema appears by 1 year of age. Infections involve the middle ear and often lead to chronic otitis media. Children are particularly susceptible to infections from herpes viruses and lymphoreticular malignancies, especially of the lymphatic system.

The diagnosis is made in the early neonatal period on the basis of the thrombocytopenia, which leads to petechiae and bleeding (refer to Table 11-2). How and when Wiskott–Aldrich syndrome manifests itself varies; some children maintain normal lymphocyte levels for years. Treatment is symptomatic and includes antibiotic prophylaxis with platelet infusions and, sometimes, splenectomy. Without bone marrow transplantation, most children die within the first 5 years of life. Survival beyond adolescence is unusual. Infection, bleeding, or malignancy (leukemia or lymphoma) may be the cause of death (Elder, 2000).

Nursing Management

Nursing care is similar to that for the child with SCID. Refer the parents for genetic counseling to help them understand the transmission of the disease and the probability of having another child with the same disorder. Arrange for psychologic support for those parents who may be overwhelmed with guilt from learning that the illness is inherited.

Help the parents and family cope with the knowledge that the child has a chronic and potentially fatal illness. Referral to family counseling may be appropriate. Expected outcomes are a return to normal immunologic function or successful coping with a life-threatening illness.

ACQUIRED IMMUNODEFICIENCY SYNDROME

Soon after acquired immunodeficiency syndrome (AIDS) was recognized in homosexual adults and intravenous drug abusers, cases of AIDS were seen in children. Increasing numbers of children infected with the human immunodeficiency virus (HIV) have been diagnosed, making HIV infection a leading cause of immune disease in infants and children and a major cause of death in children 1 to 4 years of age.

Most cases of HIV in children—and virtually all new cases—are the result of perinatal transmission. Each year in the United States, approximately 6,000 to 7,000 infants are born to HIV-infected mothers (Lindegren, Steinberg, & Byers, 2000). It is expected and hoped that the number will decrease with new therapies for treating infected women during pregnancy and labor/delivery and their infants after birth. Because of the high rate of transfer from mother to infant, HIV counseling and voluntary testing are encouraged for all pregnant women.

The virus affects multiple systems and eventually destroys the child's immune system (Figure 11-3 ◆). An understanding of the natural history of HIV disease is still evolving, as there are several important differences in the disease progression and clinical manifestations of pediatric and adult HIV infection.

PEDIATRIC AIDS STATISTICS

As of June 30, 2001, over 13,200 cases of AIDS had been reported in children and adolescents 19 years of age or younger:

- Under age 5 years: 6,928
- 5–12 years: 2,066
- 13–19 years: 4,219

Over 5,000 deaths had been reported in children under 15 years of age. Sources of exposure in infected children were identified as:

- Hemophilia/coagulation disorder: 2.6%
- Mother with HIV: 91.2%
- Receipt of blood or tissue: 4.2%
- Risk not identified: 1.9%

What age group has the major number of cases? Why?

Data from Centers for Disease Control & Prevention (CDC). Retrieved 3/13/02 from http://www.cdc.gov/hiv/stats.htm cumage

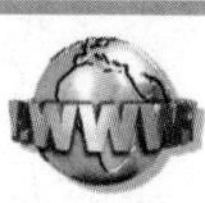

HIV/AIDS Resources

Etiology and Pathophysiology

Acquired immunodeficiency syndrome is caused by the human immunodeficiency virus (HIV-1). Most children acquire HIV in a form of **vertical transmission** from their mothers transplacentally or during delivery. Transmission can occur during birth from blood, amniotic fluid, and exposure to genital tract secretions, and after birth through breast milk from HIV-positive mothers. However, risk for perinatal transmission has been significantly reduced since mothers identified as infected are delivered by C-section, and receive zidovudine (ZDV) during pregnancy (Grosch-Worner, 2000).

HIV has also been transmitted to children through transfusions of infected blood before mandatory screening of blood and blood products was instituted in 1985. Most of these children were infected during treatment of hemophilia. Although 30% of adolescents with AIDS also have hemophilia, with infected blood the expected etiology, adolescents now most commonly acquire the virus through intravenous drug abuse or unprotected sexual activities.

PATHOPHYSIOLOGY ILLUSTRATED

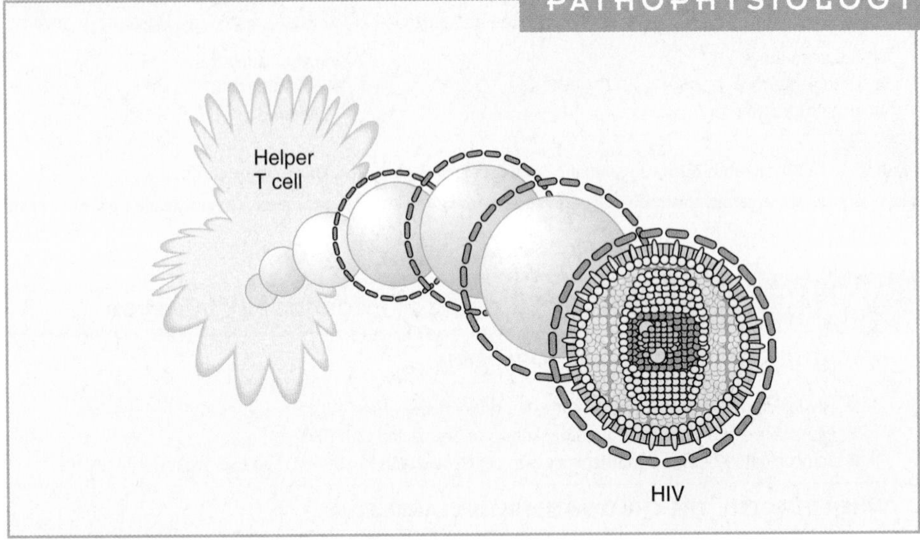

Human Immunodeficiency Virus

FIGURE 11-3 ◆

HIV selectively targets and destroys T cells, thereby decreasing and eventually eliminating cellular immunity. Humoral immunity is also affected. Thus, the child is left unprotected against a myriad of bacterial, viral, fungal, and opportunistic infections, which are ultimately fatal. Every organ system can be affected.

Clinical Manifestations

The interval from HIV infection to the onset of overt AIDS is shorter in children than in adults, and shorter in children infected perinatally than in those infected through transfusion. Most children with AIDS have nonspecific findings, including lymphadenopathy, hepatosplenomegaly, nephropathy, oral candidiasis, failure to thrive and weight loss, diarrhea, chronic eczema and dermatitis, and fever. Raymond, described at the beginning of this chapter, had several of these findings, as well as a history of recurrent, acute infections (bronchitis, otitis media, and colds).

Bacterial and opportunistic infections, such as *Streptococcus, Haemophilus influenzae, Salmonella,* and *Pneumocystis carinii* pneumonia (PCP), as well as malignancies such as lymphomas frequently occur as the disease progresses. Children infected with HIV around the time of birth have a higher cancer risk than other children, with the average age of cancer diagnosis at 5 to 6 years (Caselli, 2000). Lymphocytic interstitial pneumonitis is a common manifestation of pediatric AIDS. Frequently children develop encephalopathy resulting in developmental delay or a deterioration of motor skills and intellectual functioning. Adolescents with HIV infection often are also infected with hepatitis B virus (Rogers, 2000).

Clinical Therapy

Most children with AIDS are diagnosed early in life. Serologic tests for detection of the virus are monitored in infants born to HIV-positive mothers. These tests are performed at birth and repeated at 3 and 6 months. The preferred test is the polymerase chain reaction (PCR); other tests include p24 antigen, or HIV culture (which is not universally available). Any positive result is confirmed by retesting. When the infant has had two negative tests, testing with enzyme-linked immunosorbent assay (ELISA; HIV antibody) should be done at 12, 15, and 18 months. After two consecutive negative results with ELISA, the child is considered free of HIV. In addition, a complete blood count (CBC) and CD4+ T-cell subset is performed at 3 to 6 months. Rapid serologic tests are under study and results are showing promise. Their use in the future may shorten the diagnosis time and promote better follow-up of potential cases (Nielsen & Bryson, 2000).

The Centers for Disease Control and Prevention (CDC) considers children under 13 years of age to be infected if their symptoms meet the CDC criteria for AIDS, if they have HIV in the blood or tissues, or if they have antibodies to HIV. The CDC criteria address two

CLINICAL TIP 

Two types of tests are commonly used to test for HIV infection. One is ELISA, or enzyme-linked immunosorbent assay, and the other is PCR, or polymerase chain reaction. Although the PCR has the greatest sensitivity, it is costly (about $175) and identifies some false positive results. ELISA is less expensive (about $50) but not as sensitive, especially for children under 18 months. For this reason, repeated tests are recommended, especially in the infant who may become HIV positive after birth to an infected mother. In developing countries where expense prohibits repeated tests, the ELISA is often used with astute clinical observations of the child at risk.

CLINICAL MANIFESTATIONS OF HIV

■ Chronic, bilateral otitis media ■ Oral candidiasis (thrush) ■ *Pneumocystis carinii* pneumonia (PCP)	■ Failure to thrive ■ Chronic diarrhea ■ Hepatosplenomegaly	■ Lymphadenopathy ■ Skin disorders ■ Fever

Be alert for the possibility of HIV infection in infants with some combinations of such clinical manifestations, especially in infants known to be at risk.

TABLE 11-5 Clinical Staging of Pediatric HIV Infection

DIAGNOSIS OF HIV INFECTION IN CHILDREN
■ HIV infected (two or more positive tests for HIV or demonstrates AIDS) ■ Perinatally exposed (born to a mother known to be infected with HIV) ■ Seroconverter (born to a mother known to be infected with HIV but has had two negative HIV tests)
WHEN INFECTED, THE CHILD WITH HIV IS CLASSIFIED AS
■ Category N (not symptomatic) ■ Category A (mildly symptomatic) ■ Category B (moderately symptomatic) ■ Category C (severely symptomatic; multiple, recurrent infection)
Note: From "Guidelines for the use of antiretroviral agents in pediatric HIV infection," 1998, *MMWR (RR-4), 1–43.*

issues: the diagnosis of HIV and the clinical classification of children infected with HIV (Table 11-5).

Because of the rapidity of disease progression in perinatally transmitted HIV infection, early identification of infected infants is important to ensure the most effective treatment. HIV-infected mothers should be identified during pregnancy, and their infants should undergo periodic laboratory testing, as described above. Regardless of the results of these tests, all infants of infected mothers should start prophylaxis against PCP (a commonly serious or fatal outcome in infants) by the age of 4 to 6 weeks and continue to 12 months, or until two negative HIV tests have been documented (at 1 and 4 months of age). Drugs used for PCP prophylaxis include trimethoprim-sulfamethoxazpole (Bactrim or Septra), dapsone, or aerosolized pentamidine. In addition, all infected mothers should receive oral zidovudine (ZDV) after the first trimester of pregnancy and intravenous ZDV during labor and delivery; and the newborn should receive 6 weeks of oral ZDV after birth. A CBC with differential is performed at birth, 4 to 6 weeks, and 12 weeks to monitor for drug side effects.

Medical management is supportive, as there is no cure for AIDS. Intravenous immune globulin (IVIG; see Table 11-4) has been used to prevent bacterial infections in children under the age of 2 years. Treatment involves prompt therapy for bacterial and opportunistic infections. Children between 3 months and 12 years of age are given antiretroviral drugs, including nucleoside reverse transcriptase inhibitors such as zidovudine (ZDV), didanosine (DDI), zalcitabine (DDC), lamivudin (3TC), and stavudine (D4T). The protease inhibitors (PIs), ritonavir, and nelfinavir have now been approved for use in children over 2 years, and other PIs are now under investigation (Temple, Koranyi, & Nahata, 2001). The protease inhibitors are most effective when used in combination with nucleoside reverse transcriptase inhibitors, which slow replication of the virus. Recent drug trials have demonstrated reduction of serum HIV load in infants who acquired the infection from their mothers and were treated with a combination of several antiviral drugs (Luzuriaga, Bryson & Krogstad, et al., 1997). The antineoplastic drug hydroxyurea can be used in combination with nucleoside reverse transcriptase inhibitors (Kline, Calles, & Simon, et al., 2000).

The earlier the child develops AIDS, the poorer the prognosis. However, as treatment improves, more children are living longer with the disease. Younger children are more likely to die of pulmonary diseases or infection, while those who survive past 10 years of age are more

MEDICATIONS USED TO TREAT HIV

1. **Nucleoside Analogs** or **Nucleoside Reverse Transcriptase Inhibitors** (inhibit action of viral reverse transcriptase, an enzyme in the conversion of RNA to DNA)
   Examples: zidovudine, didanosine, zalcitabine, stavudine, lamivudine
2. **Protease Inhibitors** (block the function of the enzyme protease needed for viral formation and growth)
   Examples: saquinavir, ritonavir, indinavir, nalfinavir, kaletra (lopinavir/ritonavir combination)
3. **Nonnuceloside Reverse Transcriptase Inhibitors** (bind to viral reverse transcriptase and disrupt the conversion of RNA to DNA)
   Examples: nevirapine, delavirdine

Note: The average cost of annual therapy with a combination of drugs as recommended is about $10,000 (Burpo, 2000). What special financial needs will families have when someone is treated for HIV?

likely to die of cardiac disease, wasting syndrome, encephalopathy, and infection with *Mycobacterium avium* complex. The average age for survival of a child after diagnosis of HIV infection is 8 years (Langston, Cooper, & Goldfarb, et al., 2001).

NURSING MANAGEMENT

Nursing Assessment and Diagnosis

For infants at risk of HIV infection, obtain the HIV test results of the mother if available. When these are positive, the infant will need to be screened numerous times during infancy for HIV infection, as described in the previous section. Facilitate the screening and explain the necessity to the family.

Physiologic Assessment

Assessment centers on observation and evaluation of potential sites of infection. Assess breath sounds, respiratory status, arterial blood gases, level of consciousness, and mental status. Any evidence of lymphocytic interstitial pneumonitis or neurologic abnormalities should be reported. Assess the child's height and weight frequently. Observe for signs of failure to thrive and assess for anemia. Look for *Candida* infections in the mouth and the diaper area. Note any developmental delays in motor skills or intellectual functioning, which could result from encephalopathy and poor nutrition, and can signal the progression from HIV infection into AIDS (Pearson, McGrath, & Nozycs, et al., 2000). These should be reported so that further medical evaluation can be carried out.

Psychosocial Assessment

Assess family support systems and coping mechanisms, as the stressors of caring for a child with AIDS may overwhelm parents. Assess the family's ability to care for the child. If the mother is infected, inquire about the extended family's ability to provide daily care as well as emotional support. Support the family when they decide to inform a school-age child or adolescent of the diagnosis. When assessing an adolescent with AIDS, evaluate the teen's understanding of how AIDS is transmitted and the response to the diagnosis.

The accompanying nursing care plan includes common nursing diagnoses that may apply to a child hospitalized with AIDS. Other nursing diagnoses may include the following:

- *Diarrhea,* related to gastrointestinal infection, malignancy, or drug reactions
- *Impaired gas exchange,* related to pulmonary disease
- *Altered growth and development,* related to chronic infection and poor nutrition
- *Risk for ineffective family coping: Compromised,* related to life-threatening illness

Planning and Implementation

The first step in dealing with HIV infection is prevention. Nurses must be active in evaluating test results and instituting measures to prevent vertical transmission of HIV to the

LAW & ETHICS

The American Academy of Pediatric Committee on Pediatric AIDS recommends that school children and adolescents with HIV be informed of their diagnosis. Telling the child is difficult for parents and they often avoid doing so. Because parents usually want to be the ones to tell the child, they need help to plan how to discuss the issue and ongoing support in the process of communication (Instone, 2000). Nurses can help parents understand the need to discuss the diagnosis with the child, provide information about how to tell the child, and emotionally support them with this difficult task.

NURSING CARE PLAN The Child with Acquired Immunodeficiency Syndrome

GOAL	INTERVENTION	RATIONALE	EXPECTED OUTCOME
1. Risk for Infection related to immunosuppression			
	NIC Priority Intervention: **Infection Control:** Minimizing the acquisition and transmission of infectious agents.		NOC Suggested Outcome: **Risk Control:** Actions to eliminate or reduce actual, personal, and modifiable health threats.
Risk factors for infection will be eliminated as evidenced by infection control.	■ Assess the child every 2–4 hours for fever; lesions in the mouth; redness, inflammation, soreness, and lesions on the skin or around intravenous lines.	■ Fever is one of the few signs of infections in the immunosuppressed child who does not have a sufficient number of white blood cells.	The child has no fever and shows no other signs of infection.
	■ Auscultate for changes in breath sounds every 2 hours. Perform pulmonary toilet (coughing, deep breathing, incentive spirometry) every 2–4 hours.	■ Pneumonia is a likely infection in the child with AIDS.	
	■ Enforce strict handwashing. Allow no fresh flowers, fruits, or vegetables in child's room. Screen visitors for colds or recent exposure to varicella. Use blood and body fluid precautions (refer to the Skills Manual). Practice strict asepsis for dressing changes and suctioning.	■ Control of environmental factors helps prevent infection.	
	■ Coordinate patient care assignments to avoid exposing the child to individuals with recent infections or immunizations.	■ Planning minimizes chances for infection.	
	■ Organize patient care activities to allow for adequate period of rest.	■ Rest periods allow the child to regain energy.	
	■ Follow recommendations of CDC and AAP for immunizing immunosuppressed children. Avoid live oral polio virus vaccine and live varcella vaccine. Perform annual TB testing.	■ Special recommendations consider the child's decreased immune response and the danger of acquiring disease from certain live virus vaccines.	
2. Altered Nutrition: Less Than Body Requirements related to Loss of appetite and decreased absorption of nutrients			
	NIC Priority Intervention: **Nutrition Management:** Assistance with or provision of a balanced dietary intake of food and fluids.		NOC Suggested Outcome: **Nutritional Status:** Nutrient value: adequacy of nutrients taken into the body
The child will demonstrate adequate nutritional status to meet metabolic needs.	■ Encourage frequent small meals to promote nutritional and fluid intake.	■ Additional nutrition is required to rebuild the immune system.	The child eats frequent meals of adequate nutritional content.
	■ Maintain nasogastric tube feeding, if ordered. Hyperalimentation may be necessary to ensure adequate nutrition.		
	■ Eliminate unpleasant stimuli and odors from the environment during meals.	■ Unpleasant stimuli decrease the desire for food.	
	■ Monitor skin turgor every shift.	■ Skin turgor reflects hydration status.	
	■ Involve a nutritionist in planning a diet for the child that includes favorite foods.	■ Including favorite foods encourages intake.	

(continued)

NURSING CARE PLAN The Child with Acquired Immunodeficiency Syndrome (continued)

GOAL	INTERVENTION	RATIONALE	EXPECTED OUTCOME
3. Risk for Impaired Skin Integrity related to skin infection, immobility, or diarrhea			
	NIC Priority Intervention: **Skin Surveillance:** Collection and analysis of patient data to maintain skin integrity.		NOC Suggested Outcome: **Risk Control:** Actions to eliminate or reduce actual, personal, and modifiable health threats.
The child will have structural intactness and normal physiologic function of skin.	■ Observe all pressure areas closely for signs of infection or breakdown. ■ Keep skin clean and dry. Provide perineal care to minimize irritation from diarrhea.	■ Skin care is important in the immunocompromised child. The skin may be the only intact defense the child has. ■ Prevents breaking or cracking of skin.	The child is free of preventable skin breakdown.
4. Risk for Altered Oral Mucous Membrane related to infection			
	NIC priority Intervention: **Oral Health Restoration:** Promotion of healing for a patient who has an oral mucosa lesion.		NOC Suggested Outcome: **Tissue Integrity:** Structural intactness and normal physiologic function of mucous membranes.
The child will have intact oral mucous membranes.	■ Inspect mouth for sign of blistering or lesions. ■ Provide mouth care with normal saline solution or lemon-glycerine swabs every 2–4 hours.	■ Candidal infection is frequently associated with immunodeficiency. ■ Provides comfort and promotes healing.	The child has intact oral mucous membranes.
5. Pain related to infections			
	NIC Priority Intervention: **Pain Management:** Alleviation of pain or a reduction in pain to level of comfort that is acceptable to the patient.		NOC Suggested Outcome: **Comfort Level:** Feelings of physical and psychologic ease.
The child will be free of pain or experience only mild pain/discomfort.	■ Observe for signs of pain and discomfort. ■ Medicate for pain as ordered and document results. ■ Implement general comfort measures (holding, rocking, etc).	■ Pain relief adds to comfort of the child and family.	The child shows evidence of pain relief.
6. Knowledge Deficit (Parent) related to home care of child with AIDS			
	NIC Priority Intervention: **Teaching, Treatment:** Preparing a patient and family to understand and mentally prepare for a treatment.		NOC Suggested Outcome: **Knowledge, Treatment Regimen:** Extent of understanding conveyed about AIDS treatment.
The parent(s) will demonstrate knowledge about home care, measures to prevent infection, and signs and symptoms to report to health care providers.	■ Explain the importance of optimizing the child's health status and reducing risk of complications through diet, rest, and meticulous personal hygiene. Be sure that parents and other family members understand how AIDS is spread and appropriate precautions. ■ Discuss with the parents and the child reasons for protective measures.	■ Knowledge about the disorder and preventive measures is necessary to provide safe and effective home care for the child. ■ Knowledge of rationale increases compliance.	The parent describes appropriate home care and preventive measures for a child with AIDS.

(continued)

NURSING CARE PLAN The Child with Acquired Immunodeficiency Syndrome (continued)

GOAL	INTERVENTION	RATIONALE	EXPECTED OUTCOME
6. Knowledge Deficit (Parent) related to home care of child with AIDS (continued)			
	■ Inform the family about signs and symptoms of infection that should be reported promptly to the physician or nurse (fever, chills, cough, mild erythema).	■ Prompt treatment improves outcome.	
7. Caregiver Role Strain related to anxiety about child's condition and demands of providing care			
	NIC Priority Intervention: **Caregiver Support:** Provision of the necessary information, advocacy, and support to facilitate primary patient care by someone other than a health professional.		NOC Suggested Outcome: **Caregiver Emotional Health:** Feelings, attitudes, and emotions of a family care provider while caring for the child over an extended period of time.
The parent(s) will demonstrate emotional health as evidenced by decreased anxiety related to the child's condition and care.	■ Encourage family members to express fears and concerns regarding the child's prognosis. ■ Advise family about support services or other resources available in the community.	■ Expression of fears helps to decrease anxiety. ■ Provides additional support to help family cope with the child's illness and the dying process, when needed.	The parent states decreased anxiety.

infants of infected mothers. Adequate testing, prophylaxis for HIV and PCP, and follow-up visits for evaluation of general health and development for all infants at risk of the disease is advised. Recent guidelines from the American Academy of Pediatrics recommend that pediatricians offer HIV testing and counseling to adolescents who are sexually active or involved in substance abuse (Committee on Pediatric AIDS, 2001). There are also recommendations for inclusion of HIV and AIDS education into comprehensive health education for students from kindergarten through 12th grade (Committee on Pediatric AIDS, 1998). (See Table 11-6.) Nurses can implement these policies and counsel teens about the dangers and prevention measures for HIV (St. Louis, Levine, & Wasserheit, et al., 1998).

If the child is diagnosed with HIV, close health supervision is needed to ensure medications and examinations are carried out. When HIV progresses to AIDS, nursing care is similar to that of a child with any serious chronic, life-threatening disease. It centers on preventing infection, managing pain, promoting respiratory and other organ function,

TABLE 11-6 Teaching About AIDS

The American Academy of Pediatrics recommends that HIV and AIDS education be part of health education in kindergarten through 12th grade. School nurses should be educated about HIV/AIDS, ethics, testing, and counseling. The particular roles defined for nurses in school settings include:

1. participate in education programs for teachers
2. assist schools and other organizations to develop education programs
3. review, adapt, and develop educational materials
4. participate in public discussions about HIV/AIDS
5. take part in meetings with school administrators, staff, and parents
6. facilitate networking among parents and AIDS community groups

Note: Adapted From Committee on Pediatric AIDS (1998). Human immunodeficiency virus/acquired immunodeficiency syndrome education in schools. *Pediatrics, 101,* 933–935.

promoting adequate nutritional intake, and providing emotional support to the parents and child, while promoting the child's growth and development. The accompanying nursing care plan summarizes nursing care for the child hospitalized with acquired immunodeficiency syndrome.

PREVENT INFECTION

Immunosuppressed children become infected with bacteria as well as other organisms that are common in the environment. Frequent handwashing and limiting exposure of the child to individuals with upper respiratory or other infections are the best interventions to protect the child with HIV from acquiring other infections (Kaplan, Masur, & Holmes, 1997). A modified immunization schedule that avoids exposure to live varicella vaccine should be followed. Live measles-mumps-rubella vaccine is used unless the child is severely affected with AIDS, because the risk of serious outcomes for measles disease is great. Tuberculosis is more common in children with AIDS so annual skin tests that are read by health professionals are recommended (Cohen, Chen, & Sunkle, et al., 2000). Teach sexually active adolescents the importance of practicing safe sex and the ramifications of high-risk sexual behaviors and intravenous drug abuse.

SAFETY PRECAUTIONS 

Health care workers who come in contact with blood or other body fluids of children infected with HIV are at risk for exposure to the virus. Standard precautions should be used in caring for all children, as HIV status and presence of other infections may not be known (refer to the Skills Manual).

PROMOTE RESPIRATORY FUNCTION

Because many children with AIDS develop pneumonia, encourage the child to cough and deep breathe every 2 to 4 hours. Blowing cotton balls with a straw, blowing bubbles, or other games may engage the interest of a younger child. Reposition infants frequently so all areas of the lungs can aerate. Rest periods to conserve energy and lower the body's demand for oxygen are important.

SAFETY PRECAUTIONS 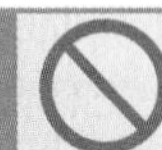

Children with immune disorders, their siblings, or other household contacts should not be immunized with live varicella vaccine because of the risk of transmitting the virus to the immunodeficient child.

PROMOTE ADEQUATE NUTRITIONAL INTAKE

Because many children with AIDS have failure to thrive, nutrition is an important part of their care. (See Chapter 3 for information to include in a detailed nutritional assessment.) A nutritionist should be involved in planning an appropriate diet for the child that provides necessary calories, protein, and other nutrients. Vitamins may be especially lacking in the diets of infected children. Antioxidants (vitamin A, vitamin E, zinc, and selenium) are known to enhance general immune system function and should be consumed at recommended levels. Periodic dietary analysis and teaching are needed. Adequate nutrition is sometimes provided by hyperalimentation.

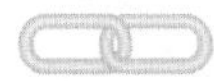

Skill 8-7: Total Parenteral Nutrition

Diarrhea resulting from gastrointestinal infection and lactose intolerance is a common finding in these children and complicates other nutritional disturbances. Antidiarrheal medications may be prescribed, or alternative formulas tried. Keep the child's lips and mouth moist and pay close attention to hydration status. Monitor the skin turgor and urine output, and provide careful perineal skin care to prevent infection.

The frequency of Candida infections leads to blisters, cracking, and discharge involving the oral mucous membranes. Mouth care with a non-alcohol-based solution such as normal saline or lemon–glycerine swabs should be done every 2 to 4 hours.

PROVIDE EMOTIONAL SUPPORT

The family of the child with AIDS is under great strain. The mother and others in the family may also be infected. Integrate social services and support groups into the care of the child as soon as the diagnosis is made. Spend time talking with the family about their fears and feelings. In many parts of the United States, AIDS still carries a tremendous stigma, and the family may not be able to discuss their feelings outside of the health care environment. Safeguard the wishes of the family regarding the privacy of the diagnosis.

Clarify any misconceptions the older child with AIDS may have about the transmission of the disease. Routes of transmission and the need for safe sexual practices must be clearly discussed with adolescents. Providing support for adolescents is particularly important, as the dependence which this chronic and terminal disease brings can make it difficult to meet the developmental task of independence. Adolescents may benefit from contact with other infected peers.

LAW & ETHICS 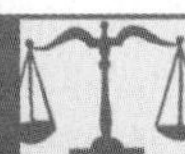

Disclosure of patient information is a breach of confidentiality that may subject a nurse to legal action. Disclosure of confidential information occurs when a patient's condition—for example, a diagnosis of AIDS—is discussed inappropriately with any third party.

SAFETY PRECAUTIONS

Because children with HIV or other bloodborne infections may be enrolled in child care centers, staff in these centers should use standard precautions in handling blood and body fluids. Instruct child care center personnel in use of these precautions. Assist child care centers in establishing procedures to notify all parents when a child with an infectious disease has been at the center. Parents of immunocompromised children can then take any necessary precautions to minimize the chances of their children becoming ill. Parents of HIV-infected children must be very cautious to limit the exposure of their children to infectious diseases.

Discharge Planning

The diagnosis of AIDS is surrounded by strong emotions and fears. Be honest and direct. Education is essential. Explain that there is no evidence that casual contact among family members can spread the infection. For the child who has been hospitalized, home care needs should be identified well in advance of discharge.

Discuss the family's finances as well as health insurance coverage for the child's care. Assess the family's ability to provide nutritious food, required medications, and a supportive environment. Refer to services as needed to ensure provision of quality care for the child after discharge.

Support groups, home health care nursing services, financial assistance, and psychological counseling are usually needed at some point during the child's illness, and the family should be aware of the availability of such services. Help the family deal with guilt feelings about the child's condition.

Care in the Community

Much of the care of the child with HIV infection or AIDS takes place in the community. Evaluate the family and community support systems and provide resources and referrals as needed. Many children with HIV infection are placed in foster homes, and these families need careful instruction to manage this multifaceted illness.

School attendance guidelines for children with AIDS by the American Academy of Pediatrics (AAP) and the CDC recommend unrestricted school attendance for children with AIDS or AIDS-related complex as long as their physician approves. Contraindications to school attendance include lack of control of body secretions, biting, and open wounds that cannot be covered. The nurse often prepares the school personnel with training related to care for children with known and unknown cases of HIV. The nurse also may be responsible for providing medicines or other care for the HIV-infected child at school.

Assist the family to alter the home environment to provide standard precautions during care. Make sure the child and family understand that HIV is transmitted through blood, urine, stool, and other body secretions. Teach family members the importance of careful hygiene. Encourage careful handwashing and tell parents to use precautions when handling body fluids. Explain that they should wear gloves when changing diapers; disposing of urine, stool, and emesis; or treating the child's cuts and scrapes. Instruct parents to use a bleach solution for disinfection of objects when necessary and to avoid contact with persons with infectious illnesses. Precautions to guard against food-borne illness are particularly important for the HIV infected child. Parents will also need instruction on correct administration and side effects of any medications the child is taking. Giving a child a complicated combination of drugs can be challenging for all families, so use teaching that is tailored to the particular family and perform repeated evaluation of the family's success with medication administration.

Emphasize the importance of promoting the child's development. Frequent developmental screening should be performed. Teach the parents how to support the child in achieving developmental milestones. Encourage contact with other children and adults, provide for appropriate toys, teach parents how to encourage the child's communication,

FAMILIES WANT TO KNOW

Food Safety and HIV

The child with HIV infection is more prone to food-borne disease. Instruct parents to practice the following:

1. Use a separate cutting board for meats, and wash it with hot soapy water after use.
2. Wash all utensils with hot soapy water between any uses.
3. Wash and peel fresh fruits and vegetables.
4. Use a disposable cloth or cloth that is washed after each meal to clean dishes. A sponge can harbor organisms and should not be used.
5. Have well water checked for contaminants regularly if that is the source of drinking water.
6. Do not allow the child to eat raw or undercooked meats, fish, eggs, or cookie dough.
7. Bleach solution is the best product for cleaning surfaces in the kitchen.

and praise the family for what the child has already accomplished. Children who manifest decreasing developmental milestones or other neurologic symptoms should be assessed for HIV-induced encephalopathy by the primary care provider. The nurse's record of development will be of great importance in this situation.

The child must receive regular health maintenance care, such as child health supervision visits, immunizations, and care for any other health conditions.

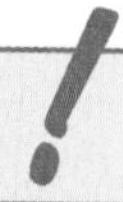

NURSING ALERT

When a child has been diagnosed with HIV, even common childhood infections are a cause for concern. Conditions such as respiratory infection, fever, chickenpox, or gastrointestinal illness can progress rapidly to a life-threatening stage. Teach families to seek prompt treatment at the first sign of illness.

Evaluation

There are many desired outcomes of care for the child with HIV infection or AIDS. Expected outcomes of nursing care include the following:

- Decreased numbers of cases of pediatric HIV due to vertical transmission from known infected mothers
- Prevention of infectious diseases in children with the virus
- Adequate respiratory function and perfusion
- Nutritional intake to support normal growth patterns and prevent malnutrition
- Adequate family coping with the stress of chronic disease
- School attendance and support in the educational process

AUTOIMMUNE DISORDERS

In an immune system damaged by pathologic changes, an immune response may occur to some of the body's own proteins, resulting in the production of autoantibodies. These pathologic conditions in which the body directs the immune response against itself—identifying "self" as "nonself"—are called autoimmune disorders.

The primary feature of autoimmune disorders is tissue injury caused by a probable immunologic reaction of the host with its own tissues. Structural or functional changes occur as immune cells attack other cells in the body.

The autoimmune disorders are grouped into systemic and organ-specific diseases. Systemic diseases, which largely involve more than one organ, include systemic lupus erythematosus and juvenile rheumatoid arthritis. Organ-specific diseases, which primarily affect a single organ, include insulin-dependent diabetes mellitus (IDDM; see Chapter 22) and thyroiditis. Idiopathic (or immune) thrombocytic purpura is an immune disease affecting blood platelets and clotting and is discussed in Chapter 15.

SYSTEMIC LUPUS ERYTHEMATOSUS

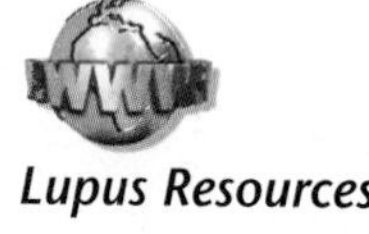

Lupus Resources

Systemic lupus erythematosus (SLE), a generalized disorder seen mainly in females, is a chronic inflammatory disease of unknown origin that involves many organ systems. SLE is more common in African Americans, Hispanics, and Asians than in Caucasians, affecting 4.4 per 100,000 Caucasian females from 10 to 20 years of age, 20 per 100,000 African-American females, 13 per 100,000 Hispanic females, and 31 per 100,000 Asian females (Lehman, 1995). The majority of cases are diagnosed in the teenage and early adult years. A genetic component is suspected as the disease is often more common in certain families.

Etiology and Pathophysiology

The exact etiology of SLE is unknown. It is believed that an outside environmental agent causes the body to initiate an abnormal immune system response to its own tissues. Antigen–antibody complexes are deposited in the vascular system, leading to widespread inflammation and tissue damage. The tissues most likely to be affected are the small blood vessels, glomeruli, joints, spleen, and heart valves. Because many systems can be affected simultaneously, organ damage with subsequent system failure may occur.

Clinical Manifestations

Symptoms depend on the organ involved and the amount of tissue damage that has occurred. Initial symptoms include fever, chills, fatigue, malaise, and weight loss. The most common symptoms are arthritis and skin rash. A butterfly rash on the face, consisting of a

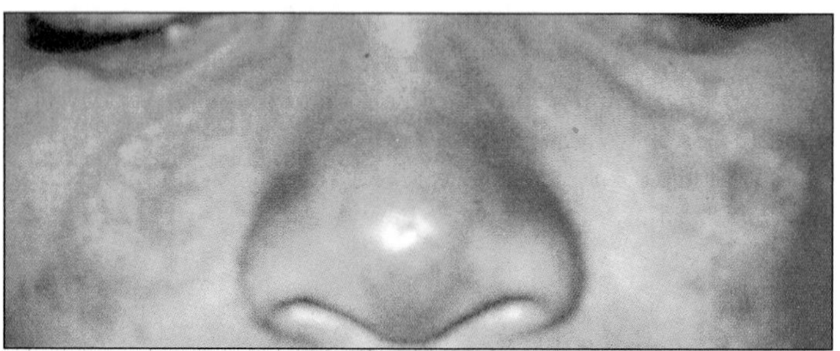

FIGURE 11-4 ◆
This child displays a "butterfly" rash across the cheeks and bridge of the nose. It is often seen in the child with SLE.
From Zitelli, B. J. & Davis H. W. (Eds.) (1997). *Atlas of Pediatric Physical Diagnosis* (3rd ed., p. 192). St. Louis, MO: Mosby, Inc.

pink or red rash over the bridge of the nose extending to the cheeks, is a characteristic finding (Figure 11-4 ◆). Children with SLE may have hemolytic anemia, with a low white blood cell and platelet count; bleeding disorders; hypergammaglobulinemia; and vasculitis.

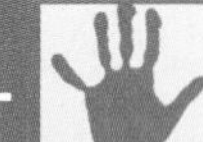

GROWTH & DEVELOPMENT

The side effects of the corticosteroids, immunosuppressants, and antimalarial drugs used in the treatment of children with SLE are significant and include hair loss, susceptibility to infection, "moon face," retinal damage, and bone loss. These are significant side effects for the adolescent who is commonly concerned about appearance. Special teaching, guidance, and support may be needed for teens with SLE.

Clinical Therapy

Blood tests reveal anemia, an elevated blood urea nitrogen (BUN), abnormal plasma proteins, abnormal erythrocyte sedimentation rate (ESR), presence of antinuclear antibodies, and a positive lupus erythematosus (LE) cell reaction, which indicates nonspecific inflammation. The Coombs test is positive. Urinalysis may reveal proteinuria.

The goals of medical management are to create a remission of symptoms and to prevent complications. Corticosteroids, such as prednisone, are prescribed to control inflammation. Antimalarial preparations, such as hydroxychloroquine and chloroquine, are used to treat symptoms associated with skin lesions and renal and arthritic problems. Although the exact action of these drugs on SLE is not known, they often permit continued remission with a lowered dose of steroids. Nonsteroidal antiinflammatory drugs (aspirin, ibuprofen, naproxen) are used to relieve muscle and joint pain. Immunosuppressant drugs, such as cyclosporin and methotrexate, have been used to help control SLE. Diet may be restricted if the child has excessive weight gain or fluid retention from steroids and renal damage.

Prognosis depends on the severity of the disease. The 5-year survival rate now approaches 80% to 90% because of improved treatment measures (Sack & Fye, 1997).

NURSING MANAGEMENT

Nursing Assessment and Diagnosis

Physiologic Assessment

A thorough assessment is needed, as symptoms are widespread. Assess for rash, petechiae, cyanosis, skin ulcers, joint deformity, friction rub, edema, and splenomegaly.

Psychosocial Assessment

Because SLE is a chronic disease that affects primarily adolescents, psychosocial assessment is indicated. Assess family interactions, exploring stressful situations such as divorce or trauma. Treatment-related restrictions and changes in appearance can lead to withdrawal, depression, and suicidal tendencies.

The following nursing diagnoses may apply to the child with SLE:

- *Risk for ineffective management of therapeutic regimen, family,* related to complexity of therapeutic regimen
- *Risk for altered tissue perfusion (renal),* related to interrupted blood flow in kidneys
- *Risk for impaired skin integrity,* related to immunologic deficit
- *Risk for activity intolerance,* related to chronic disease
- *Risk for body image disturbance,* related to side effects of medications and skin alterations
- *Risk of infection,* related to immunosuppressive medications
- *Pain,* related to joint inflammation and injury

Planning and Implementation

The goals of nursing care are to assist the child to manage and cope with a chronic disease, and to facilitate a remission.

Maintain Fluid Balance

Because most children with SLE have renal involvement, it is important to monitor intake and output and frequently evaluate the child's fluid and electrolyte status. Renal dysfunction can manifest itself by edema, muscle cramps, diarrhea, tetany, and convulsions.

Promote Skin Integrity

Presence of the rash on mucous membranes can cause weakening of the tissues, placing the child at increased risk for infection. Encourage the use of good hygienic measures and a mild soap. Recommend that adolescents limit their use of cosmetics. Reinforce the importance of avoiding sunlight as much as possible and the use of sun protection factor (SPF) of 15 or higher at all times when in the sun.

Promote Rest and Comfort

Because of fatigue and joint pain, the child has little energy reserve during acute episodes of the disease. Encourage frequent rest periods and a nutritious diet to maximize energy stores. A physical therapist can plan a program to encourage mobility and increase muscle strength.

Manage Side Effects of Medications

Observe for side effects of medications used for treatment, and teach the child and family about these effects. For example, immunosuppressant drugs can promote infection anywhere in the body; and nonsteroidal antiinflammatory drugs commonly cause gastric distress and bleeding of the gastrointestinal tract. The antimalarial drug hydroxychloroquine can cause serious vision changes; thus, frequent eye examinations are needed.

Provide Emotional Support

Adolescents may have an altered body image as a result of rash, alopecia, arthritic changes in the joints, and chronic disease. Referral to a lupus support group, social services, or counseling may be helpful. The American Lupus Society and the Lupus Foundation of America can provide information to help parents and children adjust to the disease. The Arthritis Foundation also publishes a useful pamphlet, *Meeting the Challenge: A Young Person's Guide to Living with Lupus.*

Evaluation

Successful outcomes of nursing care involve management of this chronic disease. Expected outcomes of nursing care include the following:

- Normal intake and output levels, with demonstrated fluid and electrolyte balance
- Maintenance of intact skin
- A balance of rest and activity to promote development
- Medication management
- Positive body image

JUVENILE RHEUMATOID ARTHRITIS

Juvenile rheumatoid arthritis (JRA) is an autoimmune inflammatory disease that occurs slightly more often in girls than in boys. It usually occurs in children between 2 and 5 or between 9 and 12 years of age, and it may disappear in adolescence or occasionally continue as a chronic disease.

Etiology and Pathophysiology

The cause of JRA is unknown, but it is thought to have an autoimmune basis. Inflammation begins in the joint and leads to pain and swelling. Scar tissue eventually develops, resulting in limited range of motion. There are three types of JRA: pauciarticular, systemic, and polyarticular.

Clinical Manifestations

JRA may be restricted to a few joints or be systemic with involvement of multiple joints. Symptoms can include fever, rash, lymphadenopathy, splenomegaly, and hepatomegaly. The child may develop a limp or obviously favor one extremity over the other. Pain, stiffness, loss of motion, and swelling occur in the large joints such as the knees. Older children may develop symmetric involvement of the small joints of the hand.

Clinical Therapy

Diagnosis is made primarily on the basis of the history and assessment findings, in particular, arthritis having an onset before 16 years of age and persisting for at least 6 weeks, with no other identifiable cause (Gottlieb & Ilowite, 2000). There are no specific laboratory tests for the disease. In some children, rheumatoid factor, human leukocyte antigen (HLA) B27, and antinuclear antibody (ANA) tests are positive.

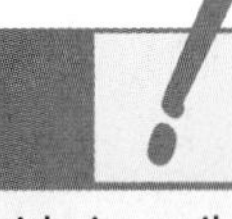

NURSING ALERT

Infants and children with juvenile rheumatoid arthritis who are receiving aspirin therapy are at risk of developing Reye syndrome if they contract influenza. These children should be immunized with influenza vaccine in the fall of each year.

Medical management involves drug therapy, physical therapy, and, when necessary, surgery. The goals of treatment are to relieve pain and prevent contractures. Salicylates (aspirin) or nonsteroidal antiinflammatory drugs (tolmetin sodium, naproxen, diclofenac, ibuprofen) are prescribed to reduce inflammation. Steroids may be used with children who have moderately active disease. Children who do not respond to aspirin or nonsteroidal antiinflammatory drugs may be treated with sulfasalazine and methotrexate. Physical therapy is performed to increase strength and mobility of joints while protecting them from injury. Surgery is occasionally performed to relieve pain and maintain or improve joint function in children with joint contractures.

JRA is a chronic disease that has periods of remission and exacerbation. During its course, the child may experience pain, impaired mobility, and interference with normal growth and development. Seventy percent of children with JRA experience permanent remission of the disease by adulthood. Rarely, the disease is unresponsive to treatment or the child may suffer lasting impairment such as bone and joint changes. Children with early onset have a better prognosis for complete recovery.

NURSING MANAGEMENT

Nursing Assessment and Diagnosis

A careful history is important, as it is sometimes the primary mode of diagnosis. Assess for joint swelling and deformities, fever, nodules under the skin, and enlarged lymph nodes.

The following nursing diagnoses may apply to the child with JRA:

- *Activity intolerance,* related to chronic pain
- *Impaired physical mobility,* related to joint stiffness
- *Anxiety,* related to stress of chronic illness
- *Pain,* related to joint inflammation
- *Body image disturbance,* related to illness

Planning and Implementation

Nursing care focuses on promoting mobility, encouraging adequate nutrition, and teaching the parents and child about the disease and its management. Most care will occur in the community, including physical therapy, with only occasional hospitalizations at the time of an exacerbation of the disease.

PROMOTE IMPROVED MOBILITY

Physical therapists play an essential role in the child's treatment. The goals of physical therapy are to maintain joint function, strengthen muscles, increase tone, maintain body alignment, and prevent permanent deformities such as contractures. Range-of-motion exercises, stretching, hydrotherapy, and swimming help to prevent deformities (Figures 11–5 ◆ and 11–6 ◆). Encourage the child to perform activities of daily living. Medications may be given to reduce joint swelling and inflammation. Warm compresses to the involved joints are soothing.

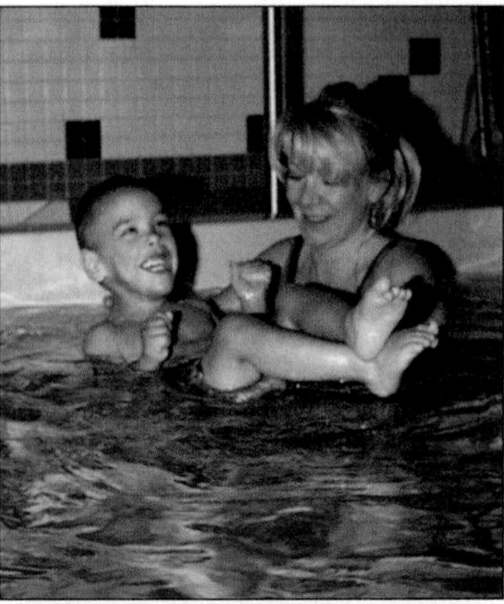

FIGURE 11-5 ◆
The physical therapist uses hydrotherapy to help maintain joint function in a child who has juvenile rheumatoid arthritis.

ENCOURAGE ADEQUATE NUTRITION

Promote general health by encouraging a well-balanced diet. Children with decreased mobility may have reduced metabolic needs, and excess weight causes additional muscle strain.

CARE IN THE COMMUNITY

The child with JRA may never, or rarely, be hospitalized. Most care takes place during visits to health care offices, clinics, and physical therapy. Teach parents about the child's condition and prognosis, and answer their questions about the child's treatment. The child may need support to adjust to the diagnosis of a chronic illness. Encourage the child to maintain contact with peers and to attend school when possible. Explain to the child and parents that overexertion may lead to exacerbation of the disease. Inform parents about possible complications of JRA, such as altered growth related to early closure of epiphyseal plates, small joint contractures, and synovitis. Parents and children can be referred to the Arthritis Foundation and the American Juvenile Arthritis Foundation for further information and support.

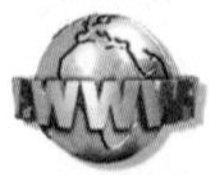

Arthritis Support and Resources

Evaluation

Expected outcomes of nursing care for the child with JRA include the following:

- Maintenance of joint mobility
- Comfort and freedom from pain
- Positive body image
- Aviodance of infection
- Parental understanding and support of the therapeutic process

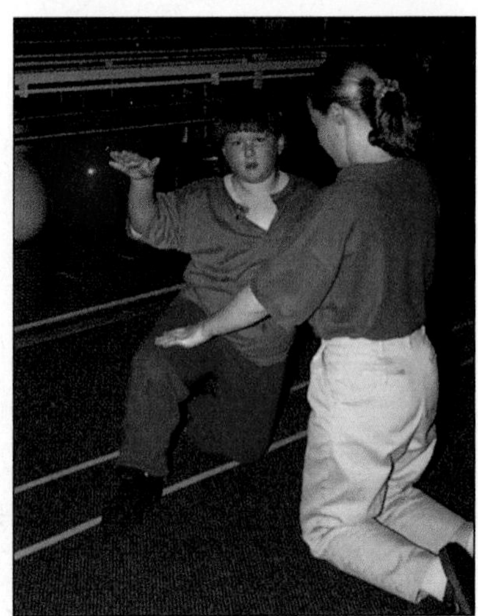

FIGURE 11-6 ◆
Stretching exercises are an important part of physical therapy for a child who has juvenile rheumatoid arthritis.

ALLERGIC REACTIONS

Allergy is one of the major chronic illnesses of children today. Why are some children allergic to cats, for instance, although no one else in the family has allergies? To answer this question, the nurse requires a basic understanding of the mechanisms of allergy.

Allergy is an abnormal or altered reaction to an antigen. Antigens responsible for clinical manifestations of allergy are called **allergens.** Allergens can be ingested in food or drugs or injected or absorbed through contact with unbroken skin. Common allergens in children include medications such as penicillin; animal dander; dust, mites, mold, and plant pollens; and foods such as nuts, seafood, or egg white. An allergic reaction is an antigen–antibody reaction and can manifest itself as anaphylaxis, atopic disease, serum sickness, or contact dermatitis. Therefore, the symptoms can be mild to severe or life threatening, and they can be localized or systemic. Characteristic findings in children with allergies are summarized in Table 11-7.

The **hypersensitivity response,** an overreaction of the immune system, is responsible for allergic reactions. Hypersensitivity reactions have been classified into four types (Table 11-8). Type I hypersensitivity reactions are immediate reactions that occur within seconds or minutes of exposure to the antigen. Symptoms can include a wheal and flare in the skin, edema, spasm of smooth muscle, wheezing, vomiting, diarrhea, or anaphylaxis. The release of chemical substances such as histamine is responsible for the signs and symptoms exhibited. The first time a child is exposed to the allergen, there is no reaction. With every exposure thereafter, however, the allergic child may have a reaction to the allergen.

Type IV reactions are delayed responses that do not appear until several hours after exposure and require 24 to 72 hours to develop fully. A type IV reaction, which is not confined to any specific tissue, is elicited by relatively complex antigens such as those of bacteria and viruses and by simple antigens such as drugs and metals. Symptoms include contact dermatitis, itching, and blistering.

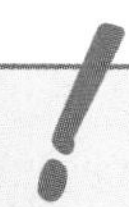

NURSING ALERT

Anaphylaxis is an exaggerated hypersensitivity reaction that may manifest with itching; localized or generalized hives on the hands, feet, or mucosa; soft-tissue swelling; cough; dyspnea; pallor; sweating; and tachycardia. Severe reactions may lead to respiratory distress or death. Nursing roles involve preventing anaphylactic reactions by teaching families how to minimize exposure and by alerting all health care personnel in hospitals and clinics to the child's allergy. In addition, knowledge of emergency procedures is important in all facilities such as schools, homes, and hospitals.

Assessment of the child with allergy includes a complete physical examination; laboratory, x-ray, and pulmonary function studies; tests of nasal function; and skin testing. Treatment generally involves avoidance of the allergen, such as substitution of a different drug when the child has a drug allergy. Desensitization may sometimes be used with increasing doses of the allergen administered intradermally in an office where resuscitation is readily available. This treatment is useful for allergy to bees or some pollens. For skin allergies, the allergen is avoided, skin is kept well lubricated, and topical steroids may be used. Oral antihistamines are sometimes used to treat allergy. When exposure to an allergen occurs, medical care may require treatment of anaphylaxis.

NURSING MANAGEMENT

The child with allergies requires a thorough assessment, including a complete past medical history, family history, personal and social history, and review of symptoms. The history focuses on the following areas:

- What symptoms does the child experience? Encourage the child to describe the difficulty in his or her own words.
- Are the symptoms continuous or intermittent? What are the frequency and duration of episodes?

TABLE 11-7 Characteristic Findings in Children With Allergies

Respiratory system: Asthma, rhinitis (seasonal and perennial), serous otitis media, cough, pneumonia, croup, edema of glottis

Gastrointestinal system: Abdominal pain and colic, stomatitis, constipation, diarrhea, bloody stools, geographic tongue, vomiting

Skin: Angioedema, urticaria, eczema, atopic dermatitis, erythema multiforme, purpura, drug and food rashes, contact dermatitis

Nervous system: Headache, tension, fatigue, convulsions, Ménière syndrome, tremor

Eye: Conjunctivitis, cataract, ciliary spasm, iritis

Blood: Thrombocytopenic purpura, hemolytic anemia, leukopenia, agranulocytosis

Musculoskeletal system: Arthralgia, myalgia, rheumatoid arthritis, torticollis

Genitourinary system: Dysuria, vulvovaginitis, enuresis

Miscellaneous: Anaphylactic shock, serum sickness, autoimmune diseases

TABLE 11-8 Types of Hypersensitivity Reactions

TYPE	MECHANISM OF ACTION	CLINICAL MANIFESTATIONS	EXAMPLES
Type I Localized or systemic reactions (anaphylaxis)	Antibodies bind to certain cells, causing release of chemical substances that produce an inflammatory reaction.	Hypotension, wheezing, gastrointestinal or uterine spasm, stridor, urticaria	Extrinsic asthma, hay fever
Type II Tissue-specific reactions	Antibodies cause activation of complement system, which leads to tissue damage.	Variable; may include dyspnea or fever	Transfusion reaction, ABO incompatibility, hemolytic disease of the newborn
Type III Immune-complex reactions	Immune complexes are deposited in tissues, where they activate complement, which results in a generalized inflammatory reaction.	Urticaria, fever, joint pain	Acute glomerulonephritis, serum sickness
Type IV Delayed reactions	Antigens stimulate T cells that release lymphokines, which cause inflammation and tissue damage.	Variable; may include fever, erythema, itching	Contact dermatitis, tuberculin skin test, graft-versus-host disease, allograft rejection

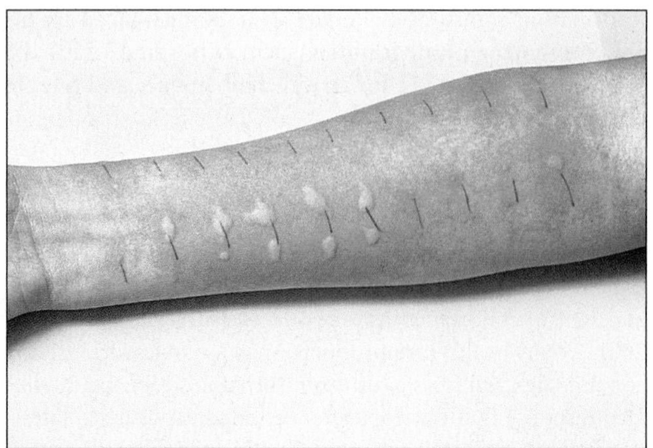

FIGURE 11-7 ◆
Results of intradermal skin testing on the forearm. Injections are given on each side of the markings. Note the positive results marked by induration and erythema in response to certain antigens.
Note: From VU/Southern Illinois University/Visuals Unlimited.

- When did the child first begin to experience symptoms? Did the child have eczema or a feeding problem in infancy or childhood? Did the infant have frequent bouts of colic or skin problems when new foods were introduced? Was there a change in symptoms at puberty? Are the symptoms becoming worse or spontaneously improving?
- What known agents in the environment cause difficulties?
- Are there seasonal variations in symptoms? At what time of the day or night do symptoms usually occur?

The nurse may be responsible for performing intradermal skin tests for allergies (Figure 11-7 ◆). Nursing care focuses on treating the symptoms, alleviating the anxiety of the child and parents, and identifying the allergens. Teaching the child and family how to minimize or avoid exposure to allergens is important. Parents of children who have had severe reactions to bee or wasp stings should be taught how to take precautions and how to provide emergency treatment if the child is stung.

Families may need instructions on allergy-proofing the home. Pets, dust, carpets, fabrics, feather pillows and bedding, and cigarette smoke can all cause allergic reactions. If families are reluctant to give up pets, frequent baths can reduce dander, which is the usual allergen.

When the child has type I reactions to an environmental substance, avoidance of the allergen is most critical. In addition, care providers, families, and school personnel must be able to treat anaphylaxis if exposure to the allergen occurs. Be sure to label the child's chart, bed, and apply a red armband to alert others to allergies when the child is hospitalized. School nurses keep records about children's allergies and inform school personnel about the allergies and cautions that need to be followed. See Chapter 3 for more

SAFETY PRECAUTIONS

If the child has had a severe or systemic reaction in the past to a bee or wasp sting, ensure that the parents know how to handle an anaphylactic reaction if the child is stung again. Kits with syringes of premeasured adrenaline are available on a prescription basis. Instruct family members how to use the kit. Make sure that the kit is properly stored without exposure to sun or high temperature. Have the family check the expiration date of the adrenaline frequently. The child should wear a medical alert bracelet. A kit should be readily available at school, child care or other settings, with someone instructed in its use. An allergy specialist should be consulted to determine whether desensitization injections would be helpful for the child.

FAMILIES WANT TO KNOW

Removing Common Allergens from the Home

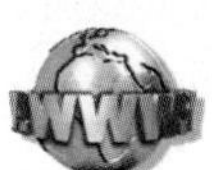

Exposure to the known allergens in the home setting is important. Several measures that families can take to minimize contact with allergens are as follows:

- Remove household pets.
- Control dust by frequent cleaning.
- Clean with moist cloths and mops to remove dust.
- Use plastic covers on mattresses and pillows.
- Avoid carpeting when possible.
- Avoid toys that collect dust (plastic and wood toys are better alternatives than stuffed fabric toys).
- Use high-efficiency air filters.
- Repair homes to prevent entry of water and subsequent molds.
- Consider dehumidification in moist climates.

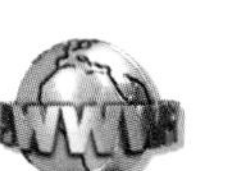

Skills 10-13, 10-14: Cardiopulmonary Resuscitation

information about food allergies. Nurses must be aware of the resuscitation procedures and equipment in all facilities such as hospital units, offices, child care centers, and schools. See Chapter 13 for airway maintenance and refer to the Skills Manual for resuscitation procedures.

LATEX ALLERGY

Latex Allergy Resources

Latex allergy is common among certain occupations, including health care workers, and in patients. For example, about 10% of health care workers, 50% of children with spina bifida, and 34% of children with three or more surgeries are sensitive to latex (Brehler & Kutting, 2001). Many health care products, such as gloves, drains, catheters, and intravenous ports, contain latex, which is a sap from the rubber tree. Latex allergy is caused by an IgE-mediated response that develops after repeated exposure to latex. In some cases, intraoperative deaths have occurred when allergic individuals were exposed to latex products during surgery. A reaction to latex products can be manifested as irritant reaction of the skin, type IV of delayed hypersensitivity, with redness, inflammation, and blisters on the skin, or type I hypersensitivity which is immediate and often has systemic manifestations (itchy eyes, asthma, or anaphylaxis).

Children most at risk for latex allergy include those with myelodysplasia and congenital urinary tract anomalies. Persons who have had repeated surgeries are also at higher risk due to high exposure to latex during surgery. Health care personnel are also at risk for latex allergy because of exposure in the workplace (Table 11-9).

Children and adolescents at high risk should receive allergy testing for latex; the radioallergosorbent test (RAST) is most often used. Health care personnel should use alternative products when caring for those persons at risk.

When a positive skin test has occurred or when the person has had a reaction to latex, all latex products must be removed from the allergic individual's environment. Alternative products, such as nonlatex gloves and catheters, must be used when providing health care. These individuals should also wear a medical identification bracelet at all times, and should have an epinephrine kit readily available at home and school. Be alert for any signs of hypersensitivity when the child is receiving health care, and be prepared with drugs and equipment to treat anaphylaxis. This is especially important in operative settings when acute anaphylaxis is often life threatening (Lee & Kim, 1998). Emphasize to parents and children that many everyday products contain latex, including latex balloons and condoms (Table 11-10).

NURSING ALERT

Starting in September 1998, the Food and Drug Administration ordered that medical products with latex carry a warning label that reads: "Caution: This product contains natural rubber latex, which may cause allergic reactions." Check on the labels of products in your health care facility to find this label. What products do you expect to need the label?

RAST

The RAST is a common laboratory test used to detect IgE antibodies. It measures circulating IgE antibodies to many allergens and generally correlates well with skin test results. It is not as sensitive as skin tests, however, so those tests are generally preferred.

TABLE 11-9 Measures to Protect Against Latex Allergy

Health care personnel are at high risk of developing latex allergy because of intense exposure to products containing latex. An estimated 8% to 12% of health care workers are latex sensitive. You can protect yourself by using the following measures.

- Decrease exposure by using alternative products when available (use synthetic rubbers, polyethylene, nitrile, neoprene, vinyl gloves).
- Use powder-free gloves if using latex gloves (the powder has high amounts of latex, which can be inhaled).
- Avoid use of oil-based hand creams and lotions before putting on latex gloves, as these preparations break down the latex.
- When symptoms of sensitivity to latex occur on exposure (rash, hives, nasal congestion, conjunctivitis, cough, or wheeze), contact the employee health department of your facility.
- If severely allergic, avoid all contact and wear a medical identification bracelet.
- Contact the National Institute for Occupational Safety and Health (NIOSH) at 800-346-4647 or the American Nurses Association at 800-637-0323 for more information.

TABLE 11-10 LATEX in the Hospital Environment

FREQUENTLY CONTAIN LATEX	EXAMPLES OF LATEX-SAFE ALTERNATIVES/BARRIERS
Adhesives, skin (Smith+Nephew) Anesthesia circuits, bags, oxygen masks	Mastisol (Ferndale) Neoprene (Anesthesia Associates, Ohmeda adult), *some* Vital Signs
Bandaids Blood pressure cuff, tubing (J&J) Bulb syringe	Active Strip (3M), CURAD Neon, Readi-Bandages, NHP, *some* Airstrip Cleen Cuff (Vital Signs), nylon (*some* Trimline) *selected* Davol, Medline, Rusch, Premium, Baxter
Casts: Delta-Lite Podiatry, Orthoflex (J&J) Catheters, condom Catheters, indwelling & systems, UDS Catheters, cardiac, vascular, pulmonary Catheters, straight, coude Catheters, feeding CPR manikins & Medical training aids	Scotchcast soft, Delta-Lites, *recent* Conformable (J&J), Caraglas Ultra, liners (Gore) Clear Advantage, ProSys NL, *selected* Coloplast, Rochester, PolyTech (Hollister) *some* Am BioMed, Argyle, Bard, Cook, Dale, Kendall, Lifetech, Mentor, Rochester, Rusch, Vitaid. Adapters & plug (Addto) *some* World Medical, Am BioMed Mentor, RobNel (Sherwood), Coloplast, *selected* Bard, Rusch catheters Accumark feeding catheter (Sims Portex) *most* Laerdal products
Dressings: Dyna-flex, butterfly closures (J&J) BDF Elastoplast, Action Wrap, Coban (3M) Lyofoam (Acme), Spandage (Medi-tech), Telfa	Duoderm, Reston foam (3M), Opsite, Venigard, Comfeel, Sorbaview, Telfa(some) Xeroform, PinCare, Bioclusive, Montg'ry strap (J&J), Webril, Metalline, Selopor, Opraflex, Centurion brief, *some* Airstrips, Rainbow Net (Surgilast), VAC
NOTE: latex in package only: Steri-strip wound closure system, Tegaderm, Tegasorb, Active Strips (3M), Nu-Derm (J&J), CURAD	
Ear Plugs Elastic wrap: ACE, Esmarch, Zimmer Dyna-flex, Elastikon (J&J) Electrode bulbs, pads, grounding Endotracheal tubes, airways Enemas	Grainger (5F767) E-Cotton, CEB elastic(coNco), Champ (Carolon), Adban Adhesive, X-Mark (Avcor) Co-Flex, PowerFlex (Andover), Comprilan (Jobst), Esmark (DeRoyal, NHP) *some* Baxter, Dantec EMG, Conmed, ValleyLab, Vermont Med, Staodyn, Neotrode *selected* Berman, Mallinckrodt, Polamedco, Portex, Rusch, Sheridan, Shiley BabyLax, Theravac, Bowel Man't Tube (MIC), Pharmaseal set, all Fleet Ready-to-use, cone irrigation set (Convatec), silicone retention cuff tip (Lafayette)
G-tubes, buttons Gloves: sterile, clean, surgical, orthodontic	Silicone (Bard, Flexiflo, MIC, Rusch, Stomate) Allergard (J&J), dermaprene (Ansell), N-DEX (Best), Safeskin Nitrile, Neolon, SensiCare, Tru-touch (Maxxim), Nitrex, Tactyl 1,2 (SmartPractice), Duraprene, (Allegiance Healthcare), Elastyren (Hermal, Center Labs), Boston Medical, Masel, Neotech
Incentive deep breathing exerciser **IV access:** injection ports, Y-sites, bags, pumps, buretrol ports, PRN adapters, buretrol ports, PRN adapters, needleless systems	Voldyne 5000 (Sherwood David & Geck), Triflo II **Cover Y-sites and bag ports – do not puncture. Use stopcocks for meds.** Polymer injection caps + burettes + Safsite (Braun), Abbot systems, Walrus, Gemini (IMED), *selected* Baxter (InterLink), Statlock, Ready Med, ConMed, Clave, Alaris, Hudson, *select Sims,* IV boards (Avcor), Terumo Pumps: Mach II, ADS 100; Clic-Open (vial top remover – Sepha Pharm.)
OR/Infection Control masks, hats, shoe covers	*some* by Kimberly Clark, TECNOL; OR & sterile packs (CML, DeRoyal) twill ties
Medication vial stoppers	*some* AmRegent, Astra, Bedford Labs, Fujisawa, Gensia, Glaxo, Lilly, Roche
Miscellaneous items	Soft-Grip fabric clamp covers(Scanlan), Precision Dynamics I.D. bracelets
Penrose drains Pulse oximeters, thermometer probes	Jackson-Pratt, Zimmer Hemovac Nonin oximeters, *selected* Nellcor sensors, Diatec probe covers
Reflex hammers Respirators Resuscitators, manual	Cover with plastic bag Advantage (MSA), HEPA-Tech (Uvex), PFR 95 (Tecnol), 3M 1860 *certain* Ambu, Armstrong, Laerdal, Puriton Bennett, Vital Blue, Respironics, Rusch
Spacer (for metered dose inhalers) Stethescope tubing Suction tubing Syringes, disposable	ACE spacer (Center Labs), OptiHaler (HealthScan) PVC (*some* Littman) cover with ScopeCoat or latex-free stockinette (**Alba**health) PVC (Davol, Laerdal, Mallinckrodt, Superior, Yankauer) Medline, Ballard Terumo Medical, Abbott PCA Abboject, Norm-Ject (Air-Tite), EpiPen, *selected* BD syringes, AdvantaJet (Activa) (continued)

TABLE 11-10 LATEX in the Hospital Environment (continued)

FREQUENTLY CONTAIN LATEX	EXAMPLES OF LATEX-SAFE ALTERNATIVES/BARRIERS
Tapes: pink, Waterproof (3M), Zonas, Moleskin, cloth, Waterproof (J&J), adhesive felt (Acme) Tonopen disposable covers (glaucoma tester) Tourniquets Theraband (also strip, tube), Other OT supplies Tubing, sheeting	Dermicel (J&J), Durapore, Microfoam, Micropore, Transpore (3M) Cath-Strip (Genetic Labs), Ice Tape (P.O.Pak), All-Felt (Universal Foot Care) Children's Medical, Grafco, VelcroPedic, X-Tourn straps(Avcor), Free-Band(Kent) REP Bands & Cords (OPTP), Exercise putty (Rolyan), new Thera-Band Exercisers plastic tubing-Tygon LR-40 (Norton), elastic thread, sheets (JPS Elastomerics)
Vascular stockings (Jobst)	Compriform Custom (Jobst)
Latex in the Home and Community	
Art supplies: paints, glue, erasers, fabric paints	Elmers (School Glue, Glue-All, GluColors, Carpenters Wood Glue, Sno-Drift paste) FaberCastel erasers, Crayola (**except** stamps, erasers), Liquitex paints, DickBlick Tempera & acrylic paints & soap erasers, Play-Doh
Balloons Balls: Koosh balls, tennis balls, bowling balls	Mylar balloons, self-sealing *Myloons* PVC (Headstrom Sports Ball), Nerf Foam Balls
Carpet backing, gym floor, basement sealant Chewing gum Clothes: applique on Tees, elastic on socks, underwear, sneakers, sandals Condoms, contraceptive sponges, diaphragm Crutches: tips, axillary pads, hand grips	Provide barrier – cloth or mat Bubblicious, Trident (Warner-Lambert), Wrigley gums (check new products) Cloth-covered elastic, neoprene (Decent Exposures, NOLATEX Industries) Buster Brown elastic-free socks (Vermont Country Store) Polyurethane (Avanti), female condom (Reality), Wideseal Silicone Diaphragms (Milex), Trojan Supra Condom Cover with cloth, tape
Dental dams, cups, bands, root canal material orthodontic rubber bands Diapers, Incontinence pads, rubber pants	PURO/M27 intraoral elastics (Midwest Orthodontic), wire springs, sealant (Delton) dams (Meer Dental, Hygenic Corp), John O Butler, Earloop masks (Richmond) Huggies, First Quality, Gold Seal, Tranquility, Always, *some* Attends, Drypers Diapers (not training pants), Confidence (Paper-Pak), Pampers, Luvs
Feeding nipples Food handled with latex gloves	Silicone, vinyl (***selected*** Gerber, Evenflo, MAM, Ross, Mead Johnson) Synthetic gloves for food handling
NOTE: Associated allergies are reported to banana, avocado, chestnut, kiwi and other fruits	
Handles on racquets, tools, bicycles	Vinyl, leather handles, or cover with cloth or tape
Infant toothbrush-massager	Soft bristle brush or cloth, Gerber/NUK
Kitchen cleaning gloves	PVC MYPLEX (Magla), cotton liners (Allerderm)
Miscellaneous items	*some* medical stickers by MediBadge, UAL, Cushie Tushie Potty Seat
Newsprint, ads, coupons, lottery scratch tickets	
Pacifiers	Soothies (Children's Med Ventures), ***selected*** Binky, Gerber, Infa, Kip, MAM
Rubber bands, bungee cords	Plasti bands
Toys – Stretch Armstrong, old Barbies	Jurassic Park figures (Kenner), 1993 Barbie, Disney dolls (Mattel), many toys by Fisher Price, Little Tikes, Playschool, Discovery, Trolls (Norfin), Silly-putty
Water toys & equipment: beach thongs, masks, bathing suits, caps, scuba gear, goggles Wheelchair cushions, tires	PVC, plastic, nylon, Suits Me Swimwear Jay, ROHO cushions, Use leather gloves, Sof Care bed/chair cushions (Gaymar)
Zippered plastic storage bags	Waxed paper, plain plastic bags, Ziploc bags

Note: From the Spina Bifida Association of America. www.sbaa.org. 4590 MacArthur Blvd NW, Suite 250, Washington, DC 20001-4226. Used with permission.

Chapter Highlights

- The infant is born with natural immunity from the mother, and develops acquired immunity gradually in the first 6 years of life.
- Acquired immunity is humoral (antibody mediated) and cell mediated.
- B cells, T cells, natural killer (NK) cells, and complement proteins are the major components of a healthy immune system.
- Disorders of the immune system can be due to genetic causes (primary immunodeficiency), or can be acquired (secondary immunodeficiency).
- Severe combined immunodeficiency disease (SCID) is life threatening and requires careful medical and nursing management.
- Human immunodeficiency virus (HIV) can lead to acquired immunodeficiency syndrome (AIDS); care focuses on prevention of this major viral infection.
- When the child is infected with HIV, support for nutrition, infection control, and developmental stimulation is needed.
- Nurses provide support for families of children with severe immune deficiency with a focus on finances, provision of complex medical care, and emotional support.
- Autoimmune disorders such as eczema, juvenile rheumatoid arthritis, and systemic lupus erythematosis occur when the body perceives its own tissue as foreign and mounts a defense against it.
- Although progress is slow, the body may return to normal after manifestation of autoimmune disorder.
- A thorough assessment and careful teaching can help the child with allergies to successfully manage reactions.
- Allergy to latex products is commonly seen in children, health care workers, and the general population.

EXPLORE MediaLink

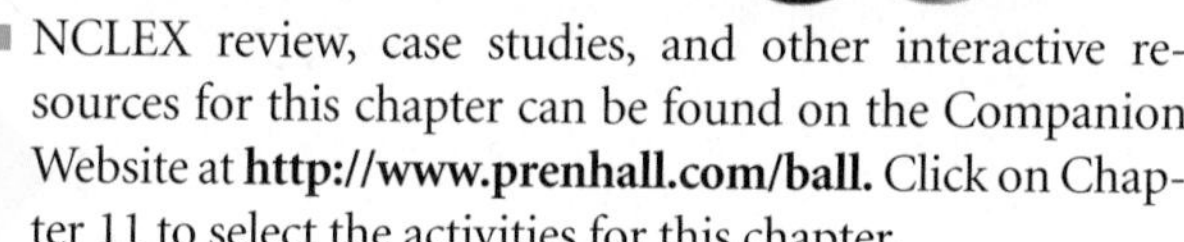

- NCLEX review, case studies, and other interactive resources for this chapter can be found on the Companion Website at **http://www.prenhall.com/ball.** Click on Chapter 11 to select the activities for this chapter.
- For animation, more NCLEX review questions, and an audio glossary, access the accompanying CD-ROM in this textbook.

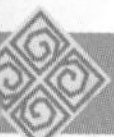

References

1. Brehler, R. & Kutting, B. (2001). Natural rubber latex allergy. Archives of Internal Medicine 161, 1057–1064.
2. Burpo, R. H. (2000). Common antiviral agents used in women's and children's care. Journal of Obstetric, Gynecologic and Neonatal Nursing 29:181–200.
3. Candotti, F. (2000). The potential for therapy of immune disorders with gene therapy. *Pediatric Clinics of North America, 47,* 1389–1408.
4. Caselli, D. (2000). Human immunodeficiency virus–related cancer in children: Incidence and treatment outcome—Report of the Italian Register. *Journal of Clinical Oncology, 18,* 3854–3861.
5. Cohen, H., Chen, X. C., Sunkle, S., Davis, L., Geromanos, K., Xanthos, G., & Shearer, W. (2000). Ability of caregivers to read delayed hypersensitivity skin tests in children exposed to and infected by HIV. *Journal of Pediatric Health Care, 14,* 50–55.
6. Committee on Pediatric AIDS. (1998). Human immunodeficiency virus/acquired immunodeficiency syndrome education in schools. *Pediatrics, 101,* 933–935.
7. Committee on Pediatric AIDS and Committee on Adolescence. (2001). Adolescents and human immunodeficiency virus infections: The role of the pediatrician in prevention and intervention. *Pediatrics, 107,* 188–190.
8. Elder, M. E. (2000). T-cell immunodeficiencies. *Pediatric Clinics of North America, 47,* 1253–1274.
9. Gottlieb, B. S., & Ilowite, N. T. (2000). Meeting the challenge of rheumatologic diseases in teens. *Contemporary Pediatrics, 17,* 61–98.
10. Grosch-Worner, I. (2000). An effective and safe protocol involving zidovudine and caesarean section to reduce vertical transmission on HIV-1 infection. *AIDS, 14,* 2903–2911.
11. Instone, S. L. Perceptions of Children with HIV infection when not told for so long: Implications for diagnosis disclosure. *Journal of Pediatric Health Care 14:*235–243.
12. Kaplan, J. E., Masur, H., & Holmes, K. K. (1997). 1997 USPHS/IDSA guidelines for the prevention of opportunistic infections in persons infected with human immunodeficiency virus. *MMWR, 46* (RR-12), 1–46.
13. Kline, M. W., Calles, N. R., Simon, C., & Schwarzwald, H. (2000). Pilot study of hydroxyurea in human immunodeficiency virus–infected children receiving didanasine and/or stavudine. *Pediatric Infectious Disease Journal, 19,* 1083–1086.
14. Langston, C., Cooper, E. R., Goldfarb, J., Easley, K. A., Husak, S., Sunkle, S., Starc, T. J., & Colin, A. A. (2001). Human immunodeficiency virus–related mortality in infants and children: Data from the pediatric pulmonary and cardiovascular complications of vertically transmitted HIV study. *Pediatrics, 107,* 328–338.
15. Lee, M. H., & Kim, K. T. (1998). Latex allergy: A relevant issue in the general pediatric population. *Journal of Pediatric Health Care, 12,* 242–246.
16. Lehman, T. J. A. (1995). A practical guide to systemic lupus erythematosus. *Pediatric Clinics of North America, 42,* 1223–1238.
17. Lindegren, M. L., Steinberg, S., & Byers, R. H. (2000). Epidemiology of HIV/AIDS in children. *Pediatric Clinics of North America, 47,* 1–20.
18. Luzuriaga, K., Bryson, Y., Krogstad, P., Robinson, J., Stechenberg, B., Lamson, M.,

Cort, S., & Sullivan, J. (1997). Combination treatment with zidovudine, didanosine, and nevirapine in infants with human immunodeficiency virus type infection. *New England Journal of Medicine, 336,* 1343–1344.

19. Nielsen, K., & Bryson, Y. J. (2000). Diagnosis of HIV infection in children. *Pediatric Clinics of North America, 47,* 39–64.

20. Pearson, D. A., McGrath, N. M., Nozyce, M., Nichols, S. L., Raskino, C., Brouwers, P., Lifschitz, M. C., Baker, C. J., & Englund, J. A. (2000). Predicting HIV progression in children using measures of neuropsychological and neurological functioning. *Pediatrics, 106* (6), *http://www.pediatrics.org/cgi/content/full/106/6/e76.* Retrieved 1/15/02.

21. Rogers, A. S. (2000). Serologic examination of hepatitis B infection and immunization in HIV-positive youth and associated risks. *AIDS Patient Care and STDs, 14,* 651–657.

22. Sack, K. E., & Fye, K. H. (1997). Rheumatic diseases. In D. P. Stites, A. T. Terr, & T. G. Parslow (Eds.), *Medical immunology* (pp. 456–479). Stamford, CT: Appleton & Lange.

23. Schwartz, S. A. (2000). Intravenous immunoglobulin treatment of immunodeficiency disorders. *Pediatric Clinics of North America, 47,* 1355–1370.

24. St. Louis, M. E., Levine, W. C., Wasserheit, J. N., DeCock, K. M., West, G. R., Holtgrave, D. R., & Valdiserri, R. O. (1998). HIV prevention through early detection and treatment of other sexually transmitted diseases—United States. *MMWR, 47* (RR-12), 1–24.

25. Stiehm, E. R., & Ammann, A. J. (1997). Combined antibody (B-cell) & cellular (T-cell) immunodeficiency disorders. In D. P. Stites, A. I. Terr, & T. G. Parslow (Eds.), *Medical immunology* (pp. 352–363) Stamford, CT: Appleton & Lange.

26. Temple, M. E., Koranyi, K., & Nahata, M. C. (2001). The safety and antiviral effect of protease inhibitors in children. *Pharmacotherapy, 21,* 287–294.

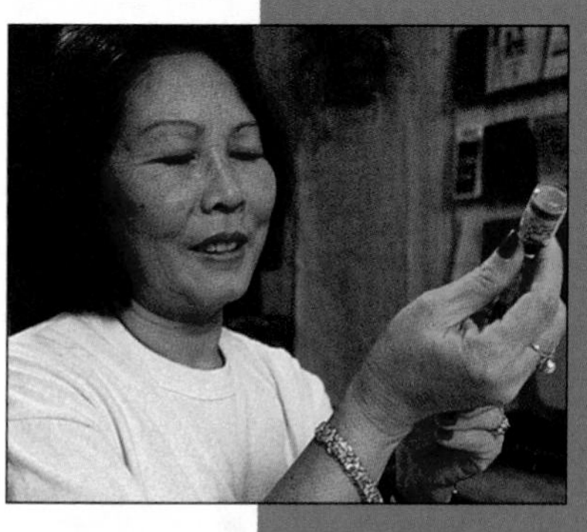

"BOTH LIAN AND CHANG NEED SEVERAL IMMUNIZATIONS, AND WE DON'T WANT TO MISS THIS OPPORTUNITY TO CATCH THEM UP. CHANG WAS FOUND TO HAVE ONLY A MINOR ILLNESS. LIAN WILL BE GOING TO KINDERGARTEN IN THE FALL, SO IT IS VERY IMPORTANT FOR HER TO GET ALL OF THE IMMUNIZATIONS SHE NEEDS NOW."

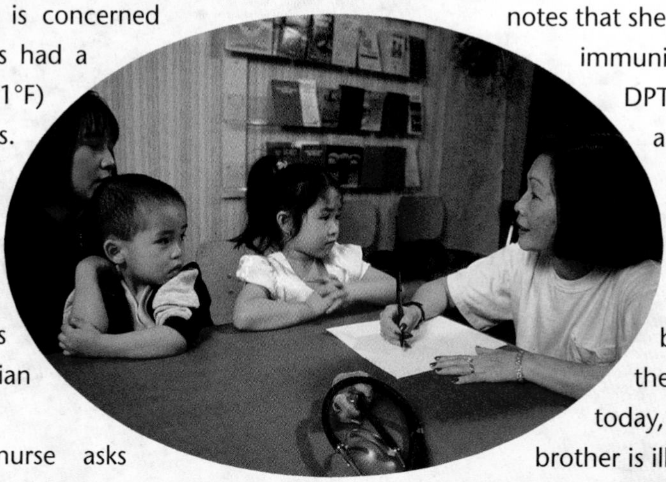

Lian, 5 years old, has accompanied her mother and 2-year-old brother, Chang, to the pediatric clinic. Her mother is concerned because Chang has had a fever of 38.3°C (101°F) for the past 3 days. Chang has been to this office several times in the past few months for health care, but this is the first time Lian has come along.

When the nurse asks about Lian's last visit to the doctor and the status of her immunizations, her mother says Lian has not been seen for about 2 years. She is not sure whether Lian has had all of her shots. In checking Lian's health records, the nurse notes that she is in need of several immunizations, including DPT, polio, varicella, and hepatitis B. Chang needs polio, MMR, and Hib vaccines.

Should Lian be given any of these immunizations today, even though her brother is ill? Which immunizations could be given at the same time? Should Chang also receive any immunizations today?

CHAPTER

12

INFECTIOUS AND COMMUNICABLE DISEASES

KEY TERMS

acellular vaccine A vaccine that uses proteins from the microorganism rather than the whole cell to stimulate the process of active immunity.

active immunity Stimulation of antibody production without causing clinical disease.

communicable disease An illness that is transmitted directly or indirectly from one person to another.

direct transmission The passage of an infectious disease through physical contact between the source of the pathogen and a new host.

endogenous pyrogenes Pyrogens released in response to an invasive organism that travel through the circulatory system to the hypothalamus, where they trigger the production of prostaglandins.

indirect transmission The passage of an infectious disease involving survival of pathogens outside humans before they invade a new host.

infectious disease Illness, caused by a microorganism, that is commonly communicated from one host (human or otherwise) to another.

killed virus vaccine A vaccine that contains a killed microorganism that is still capable of inducing the human body to produce antibodies to the disease.

live virus vaccine A vaccine that contains the microorganism in a live but attenuated, or weakened, form.

nosocomial infection An infection acquired in a health care agency, not present at the time of entrance to the agency.

passive immunity Immunity produced through introduction of specific antibodies to the disease, which are usually obtained from the blood or serum of immune persons and animals. Does not confer lasting immunity.

toxic appearance Lethargy, poor perfusion, hypoventilation or hyperventilation, and cyanosis.

toxoid A toxin that has been treated (by heat or chemical) to weaken its toxic effects but retain its antigenicity.

transplacental immunity Passive immunity that is transferred from mother to infant.

MediaLink 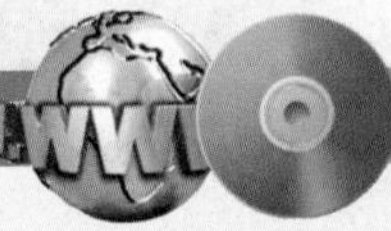 http://www.prenhall.com/ball

Resources for this chapter can be found on the CD-ROM accompanying this textbook, and on the Companion Website at http://www.prenhall.com/ball. Click on Chapter 12 to select the activities for this chapter.

CD-ROM

Audio Glossary

NCLEX Review

COMPANION WEBSITE

Web Links

NCLEX Review

MediaLink Applications

- Immunizations and Older Children
- Vaccine Administration Record
- Families Want to Know: Frequently Asked Questions About Immunizations
- Bioterrorism Preparedness
- Develop an Immunization Schedule: Infant with HIV
- Case Study: Reporting an Adverse Vaccine Event

Young children such as Lian and Chang are particularly susceptible to illnesses that are transmitted among close contacts or through exposure to microorganisms in various settings. Many of these illnesses can be prevented by following the recommended schedule of childhood immunizations. Why are children more vulnerable than adults to infectious and communicable diseases? How do you recognize the common infectious and communicable diseases, and what is the medical and nursing management of these diseases? Using information in this chapter, you will be able to answer these questions.

An **infectious disease** is an illness caused by microorganisms that are commonly communicated from one host (human or otherwise) to another. A **communicable disease** is an illness that is directly or indirectly transmitted from one person to another. Communicable diseases are a major cause of morbidity in infants and children in the United States, and in some cases result in death.

For a communicable disease to occur, the following links need to be present (Figure 12-1 ◆).

- An infectious agent, or pathogen
- An effective means of transmission
- A susceptible host

An effective chain of transmission for infection requires a suitable habitat, or reservoir, for the pathogen. A reservoir may be living or nonliving. Transmission may be direct or indirect. **Direct transmission** involves physical contact between the source of the infection and the new host. **Indirect transmission** occurs when pathogens survive outside humans before causing infection and disease.

A susceptible host is also necessary for the occurrence of an infectious disease. Young children, whose immune systems are not fully developed and who have not yet developed antibodies to many agents, cannot defend themselves against disease as well as older children. Other characteristics, such as immunodeficiency and poor health, may increase a child's risk of contracting an infectious disease.

CULTURE

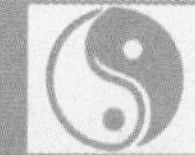

In some cultures infectious diseases are seen as punishment or the result of curses or evil spirits. For example, Native Americans traditionally view illnesses as the result of disharmony or displeasing the spirits. They may not believe in the germ theory of disease causation.

PATHOPHYSIOLOGY ILLUSTRATED

The Chain of Infection

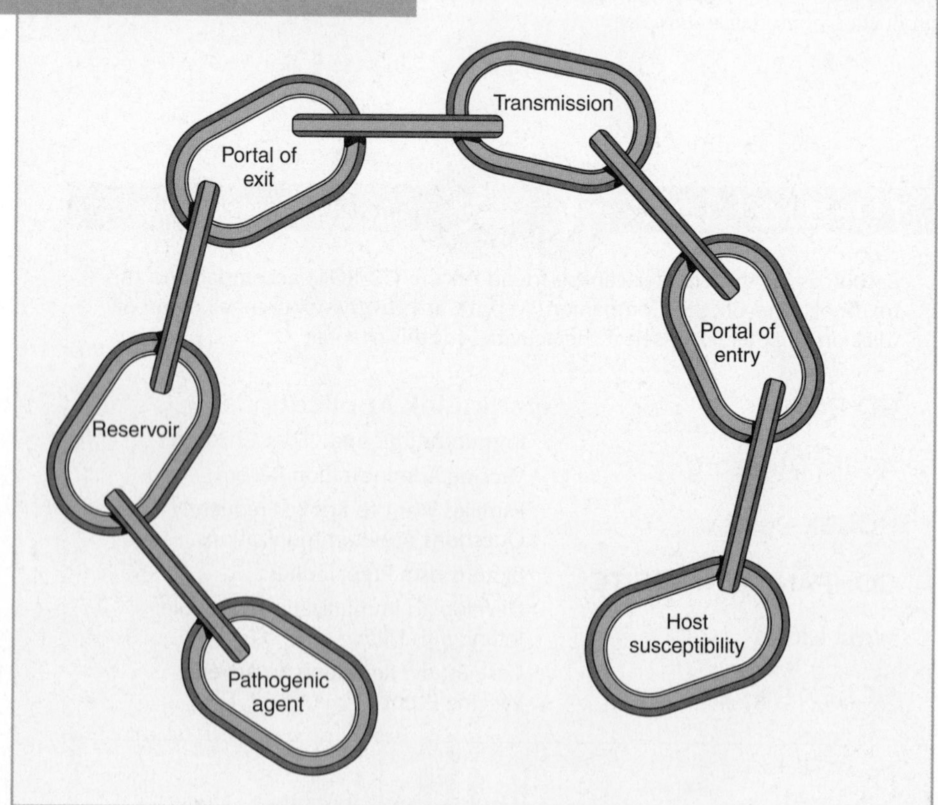

FIGURE 12-1 ◆
To achieve infection control, one of the links in the chain must be broken.

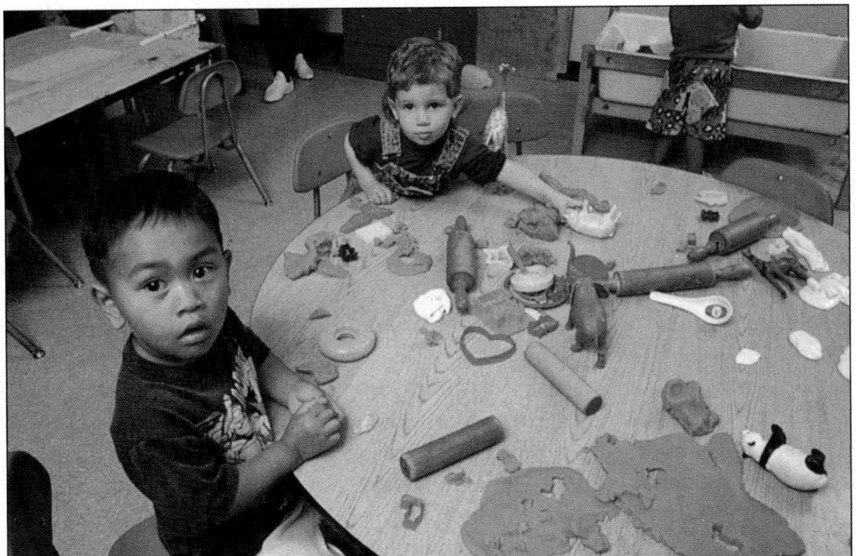

FIGURE 12-2 ◆
Infectious diseases are easily transmitted in setting such as day-care centers where children handle common objects.

Control of infectious diseases is usually directed at interrupting the chain of transmission or eliminating one or more of the habitats or reservoirs (e.g., spraying insecticide to kill mosquitoes that carry malaria). Isolating an infected individual interferes with disease transmission, and killing the pathogen eliminates the causal agent. Public health authorities monitor patterns of disease occurrence, and health care workers are required to report cases of many infectious diseases to state health officials.

As a result of major public health programs and scientific advances such as safer drinking water, better sanitation, improved standards of living, immunizations, and advanced medical treatment, infectious and communicable diseases have decreased in occurrence but remain a significant source of morbidity and mortality in infants and children, especially in developing countries. Special attention is now directed at infectious agents that can become weapons of terrorists and cause disease epidemics.

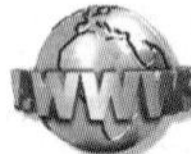

Bioterrorism Preparedness

 SPECIAL VULNERABILITY OF CHILDREN

The capability and function of the immune system, especially of infants, is poorly understood. Infants are particularly vulnerable to infectious diseases for the following reasons:

- Their immune responses are immature.
- Passively acquired maternal antibodies are decreasing.
- Disease protection through immunization is as yet incomplete.

As children grow, they develop immunity through immunization or exposure to the natural disease. As children mature and become more active, they interact more frequently with other children and adults, which increases their exposure to infectious agents (Figure 12-2 ◆). As healthy children are exposed to more infections, they develop antibodies naturally. Thus, subsequent infections with the same type of organism may be less severe or avoided. (Refer to "Anatomy and Physiology of Pediatric Differences" in Chapter 11.)

Transmission of infectious diseases in child care and other close environments is facilitated by the poor hygiene behaviors of young children. The fecal–oral and respiratory routes are the most common sources of transmission in children. Children usually do not wash their hands after toileting unless they are closely supervised. They put toys and their hands in their mouths, and then rub their nose and eyes. They often are unable to care for a runny nose without help. Diapers may leak stool and provide the fecal exposure to organisms. In addition, the staff in child care centers or other persons caring for children may not use proper handwashing techniques (Figure 12-3 ◆). All of these behaviors promote the transmission of infection.

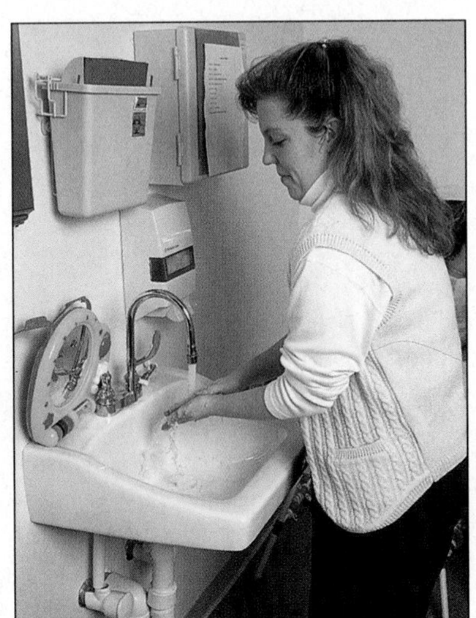

FIGURE 12-3 ◆
Proper handwashing is one of the most effective measures in preventing transmission of microorganisms.

IMMUNIZATION

The development and widespread availability of immunizations has been one of the great breakthroughs of modern medicine. Immunization introduces an antigen (a foreign substance that triggers an immune system response) into the body, allowing immunity against a disease to develop naturally. The person produces antibodies, which are proteins capable of responding to specific antigens.

In **active immunity** (in which antibody production is stimulated without causing clinical disease), an antigen is given in the form of a vaccine. When a child needs antibodies faster than the body can develop them, **passive immunity** may be induced, with antibodies produced in another human or animal host and given to the child. This approach is also used with at-risk children after a single exposure to a disease to prevent the disease from occurring or to reduce its severity. For example, if a child who has never had a tetanus immunization steps on a rusty nail, the child needs immediate protection (passive immunity) from tetanus. Tetanus immune globulin injection is given to combat the tetanus toxin produced by the bacterial spores introduced by the nail. Because passive immunity does not confer lasting immunity, the process of antibody development (active immunity) is then initiated with the administration of a tetanus toxoid vaccine.

TYPES OF VACCINES

- **Killed virus vaccine**—a vaccine that contains a microorganism that has been killed but is still capable of inducing the human body to produce antibodies (e.g., inactivated poliovirus vaccine)
- **Toxoid**—a toxin that has been treated (by heat or chemical) to weaken its toxic effects but retain its antigenicity (e.g., tetanus toxoid)
- **Live virus vaccine**—a vaccine that contains a microorganism in live but attenuated, or weakened, form (e.g., measles vaccine)
- **Recombinant forms**—an organism that has been genetically altered for use in vaccines (e.g., hepatitis B and acellular pertussis vaccine, which is a vaccine that uses proteins from, say, pertussis rather than the whole cell to stimulate the process of active immunity)
- **Conjugated forms**—an altered organism that is joined with another substance to increase the immune response (e.g., the *Haemophilus influenzae* type b (Hib) vaccine is conjugated with a protein carrier such as tetanus toxoid (PRP-T); however, there is no immunity to tetanus conferred by this specific vaccine brand)

Since vaccines were first developed in the late 1800s, many diseases have decreased dramatically in incidence. The introduction of vaccines against childhood diseases such as measles, mumps, rubella, polio, whooping cough, diphtheria, smallpox, *Haemophilus influenzae* type b, hepatitis B, and chickenpox has greatly improved the quality of life for children and adults. Improvements in vaccine technology continue to increase the safety and efficacy of immunization against an increasing number of diseases. Today's vaccines are often produced synthetically by means of recombinant DNA technology or genetic engineering.

Vaccines should be administered at specific ages and intervals. Timing for first immunizations is determined by the age at which **transplacental immunity** (passive immunity transferred from mother to infant) decreases or disappears, and the infant or child develops the ability to make antibodies in response to the vaccine. Scientists continue to study the duration of protection from vaccines. Some vaccines do not confer lifelong immunity.

The recommended schedule for immunization is updated annually to reflect new vaccines and the need for repeat immunization. The Advisory Committee on Immunization Practices (ACIP) of the Centers for Disease Control, the American Academy of Pediatrics (AAP), and the American Academy of Family Practitioners (AAFP) collaborate to recommend a vaccination schedule that is updated annually. The 2002 recommendations are given in Table 12-1. This schedule applies to immunizations all children should receive, and schedules and recommendations vary for children who begin immunizations later in childhood or need catch-up doses. Other immunization recommendations are made for children who recently received blood products or immunosuppressive agents.

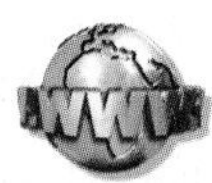

Immunization Schedules

Supplemental immunizations for influenza, meningococcal, and pneumococcal infections are recommended for certain children, as noted in Table 12-2.

The effectiveness of vaccines depends on the proper storage of vaccines and the immunization of all susceptible individuals. An improperly stored or poorly administered vaccine may be rendered ineffective, thus preventing the child from developing immunity. Read the package inserts of vaccines to determine proper storage conditions. Some vaccines are frozen; others are refrigerated. When reconstituting vaccines, it is important to use the solution provided or follow the manufacturer's directions. Write the date and time on the bottle if it is a multidose vial. Many reconstituted vaccines (e.g., varicella vaccine) have a very short shelf life.

CLINICAL TIP

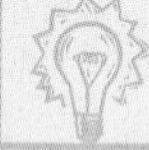

Thimerosol, a preservative that contains ethyl mercury, is contained in trace elements in some vaccines and immune globulins. While there is no evidence that the mercury is harmful to children receiving vaccines, some allergic reactions have been reported. Vaccine manufacturers are working to further reduce or eliminate thimerosol from vaccines. At least one brand of each vaccine does not contain thimerosol (Atkinson, 1999).

Lower immunization rates of children are often associated with economic factors, limited access to health care, the lack of primary care at hours convenient for working parents, inadequate education regarding the importance of immunization, and religious prohibitions. Efforts to administer vaccines and monitor immunization status in children are increasing. For example, managed care organizations require that contracted health care providers comply with the pediatric immunization standards, and patient records are audited to ensure compliance.

TABLE 12-1 Recommended Childhood Immunization Schedule United States, 2002

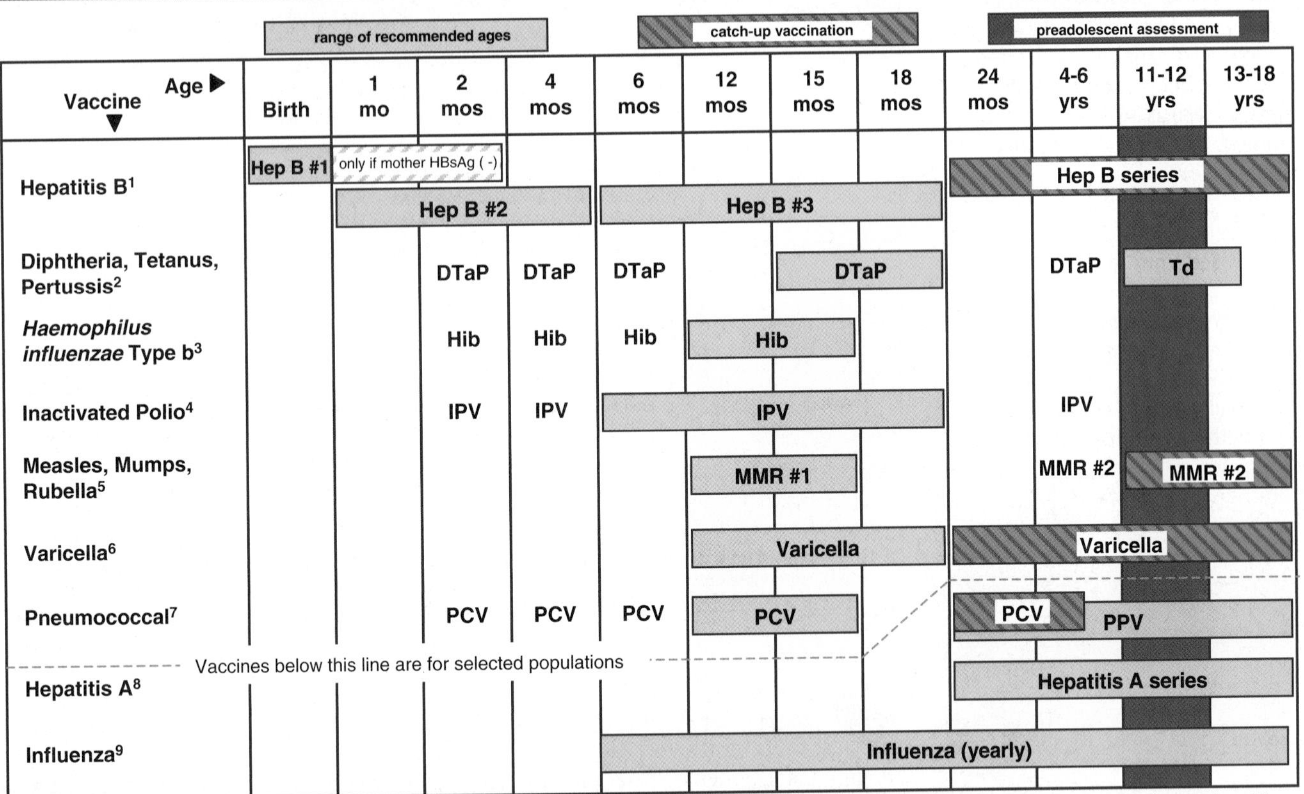

range of recommended ages | catch-up vaccination | preadolescent assessment

Vaccine ▼ / Age ▶	Birth	1 mo	2 mos	4 mos	6 mos	12 mos	15 mos	18 mos	24 mos	4-6 yrs	11-12 yrs	13-18 yrs
Hepatitis B[1]	Hep B #1	only if mother HBsAg (-)							Hep B series			
		Hep B #2			Hep B #3							
Diphtheria, Tetanus, Pertussis[2]			DTaP	DTaP	DTaP		DTaP			DTaP	Td	
Haemophilus influenzae Type b[3]			Hib	Hib	Hib	Hib						
Inactivated Polio[4]			IPV	IPV	IPV					IPV		
Measles, Mumps, Rubella[5]						MMR #1				MMR #2	MMR #2	
Varicella[6]						Varicella			Varicella			
Pneumococcal[7]			PCV	PCV	PCV	PCV			PCV	PPV		
Vaccines below this line are for selected populations												
Hepatitis A[8]									Hepatitis A series			
Influenza[9]					Influenza (yearly)							

This schedule indicates the recommended ages for routine administration of currently licensed childhood vaccines, as of December 1, 2001, for children through age 18 years. Any dose not given at the recommended age should be given at any subsequent visit when indicated and feasible. ▨ Indicates age groups that warrant special effort to administer those vaccines not previously given. Additional vaccines may be licensed and recommended during the year. Licensed combination vaccines may be used whenever any components of the combination are indicated and the vaccine's other components are not contraindicated. Providers should consult the manufacturers' package inserts for detailed recommendations.

Approved by the Advisory Committee on Immunization Practices (www.cdc.gov/nip/acip) the American Academy of Pediatrics (www.aap.org), and the American Academy of Family Physicians (www.aafp.org).

1. **Hepatitis B vaccine (Hep B).** All infants should receive the first dose of hepatitis B vaccine soon after birth and before hospital discharge; the first dose may also be given by age 2 months if the infant's mother is HBsAg-negative. Only monovalent hepatitis B vaccine can be used for the birth dose. Monovalent or combination vaccine containing Hep B may be used to complete the series; four doses of vaccine may be administered if combination vaccine is used. The second dose should be given at least 4 weeks after the first dose, except for Hib-containing vaccine which cannot be administered before age 6 weeks. The third dose should be given at least 16 weeks after the first dose and at least 8 weeks after the second dose. The last dose in the vaccination series (third or fourth dose) should not be administered before age 6 months.

   Infants born to HBsAg-positive mothers should receive hepatitis B vaccine and 0.5 mL hepatitis B immune globulin (HBIG) within 12 hours of birth at separate sites. The second dose is recommended at age 1-2 months and the vaccination series should be completed (third or fourth dose) at age 6 months.

   Infants born to mothers whose HBsAg status is unknown should receive the first dose of the hepatitis B vaccine series within 12 hours of birth. Maternal blood should be drawn at the time of delivery to determine the mother's HBsAg status; if the HBsAg test is positive, the infant should receive HBIG as soon as possible (no later than age 1 week).

2. **Diphtheria and tetanus toxoids and acellular pertussis vaccine (DTaP).** The fourth dose of DTaP may be administered as early as age 12 months, provided 6 months have elapsed since the third dose and the child is unlikely to return at age 15-18 months. **Tetanus and diphtheria toxoids (Td)** is recommended at age 11-12 years if at least 5 years have elapsed since the last dose of tetanus and diphtheria toxoid-containing vaccine. Subsequent routine Td boosters are recommended every 10 years.

3. ***Haemophilus influenzae* type b (Hib) conjugate vaccine.** Three Hib conjugate vaccines are licensed for infant use. If PRP-OMP (PedvaxHIB® or ComVax®[Merck]) is administered at ages 2 and 4 months, a dose at age 6 months is not required. DTaP/Hib combination products should not be used for primary immunization in infants at age 2, 4 or 6 months, but can be used as boosters following any Hib vaccine.

4. **Inactivated poliovirus vaccine (IPV).** An all-IPV schedule is recommended for routine childhood poliovirus vaccination in the United States. All children should receive four doses of IPV at age 2 months, 4 months, 6-18 months, and 4-6 years.

5. **Measles, mumps, and rubella vaccine (MMR).** The second dose of MMR is recommended routinely at age 4-6 years but may be administered during any visit, provided at least 4 weeks have elapsed since the first dose and that both doses are administered beginning at or after age 12 months. Those who have not previously received the second dose should complete the schedule by the visit at age 11-12 years.

6. **Varicella vaccine.** Varicella vaccine is recommended at any visit at or after age 12 months for susceptible children (i.e. those who lack a reliable history of chickenpox). Susceptible persons aged ≥13 years should receive two doses, given at least 4 weeks apart.

7. **Pneumococcal vaccine.** The heptavalent **pneumococcal conjugate vaccine (PCV)** is recommended for all children aged 2-23 months and for certain children aged 24-59 months. **Pneumococcal polysaccharide vaccine (PPV)** is recommended in addition to PCV for certain high-risk groups. See *MMWR* 2000;49(RR-9);1-37.

8. **Hepatitis A vaccine.** Hepatitis A vaccine is recommended for use in selected states and regions, and for certain high-risk groups; consult your local public health authority. See *MMWR* 1999;48(RR-12);1-37.

9. **Influenza vaccine.** Influenza vaccine is recommended annually for children age ≥ 6 months with certain risk factors (including but not limited to asthma, cardiac disease, sickle cell disease, HIV and diabetes; see *MMWR* 2001;50(RR-4);1-44), and can be administered to all others wishing to obtain immunity. Children aged ≤12 years should receive vaccine in a dosage appropriate for their age (0.25 mL if age 6-35 months or 0.5 mL if aged ≥ 3 years). Children aged ≤ 8 years who are receiving influenza vaccine for the first time should receive two doses separated by at least 4 weeks.

Additional information about vaccines, vaccine supply, and contraindications for immunization, is available at www.cdc.gov/nip or at the National Immunization Hotline, 800-232-2522 (English) or 800-232-0233 (Spanish).

CLINICAL TIP

Two major resources provide more extensive information about immunization schedules and specific vaccines, as well as infectious and communicable diseases. The American Academy of Pediatrics *Red Book: Report of the Committee of Infectious Diseases* is updated every few years. The revised immunization schedule is published each January in the American Academy of Pediatrics newsletter and in its journal, *Pediatrics.* The Centers for Disease Control maintains a current website with detailed information about immunizations and infectious and communicable diseases.

TABLE 12-2 Supplemental Immunizations

VACCINE	RECOMMENDATION
Influenza	For children with chronic pulmonary disease, cardiac disease, sickle-cell disease or other hemoglobinopathies, diabetes, metabolic disease, human immunodeficiency virus (HIV) infection, or those undergoing immunosuppressive therapy or chronic aspirin therapy (e.g., for rheumatoid arthritis or Kawasaki disease). Administered annually in autumn. Children with no history of influenza illness or vaccine need two doses 1 mo apart
Meningococcal	For children older than 2 years of age with asplenia. Vaccine duration is 5 years or longer in children older than 4 years at the time of immunization. The vaccine is also suggested for college students. The vaccine should be repeated after 1 year if the child is younger than 4 years at the time of initial immunization.
23-valent Pneumococcal	For children older than 2 years of age with sickle-cell disease, asplenia, chronic cardiovascular and pulmonary disorders, nephrotic syndrome, renal failure, HIV infection, cerebrospinal fluid leaks, or those undergoing immunosuppressive therapy. Repeat the immunization after 3–5 years if the child is younger than 10 years and at severe risk for pneumococcal infection.

Note: Adapted from the American Academy of Pediatrics Committee on Infectious Disease. (2000). *Red Book: Report of the Committee on Infectious Disease* (25th ed.). Elk Grove Village, IL: author.

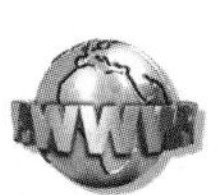
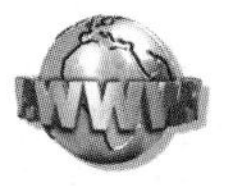

Immunization Information

NURSING MANAGEMENT

Nursing management focuses on informing parents about immunizations and possible side effects, addressing their fears about possible reactions, obtaining consent, and reporting adverse reactions.

Nursing Assessment and Diagnosis

Nurses are responsible for reviewing a child's immunization record and determining whether the child needs immunization. Inquire about the child's preventive care as well as health problems. Make sure you use the most current guidelines for comparison with the child's record. If the child is behind in appropriate immunizations for age, determine the best combination of vaccines to give at this visit to better protect the child. Also take advantage of opportunities to give needed immunizations to siblings accompanying the family on the visit, such as Lian in the opening scenario. A minor illness should not deter the nurse from giving an immunization to a child, such as Lian's brother Chang.

Many missed opportunities to immunize children have been identified. Children (and siblings present) should have their immunization status assessed during all health care visits, hospitalizations, and in schools. To reduce the number of missed opportunities for full immunization of children, use the following guidelines (American Academy of Pediatrics, 2000):

- Several vaccines—diphtheria, tetanus, and acellular pertussis (DTaP); measles, mumps, and rubella (MMR); hepatitis B (HBV); *Haemophilus influenzae* type b (Hib); inactivated polio (IPV); varicella; and heptavalent pneumococcal vaccines—can be given at the same visit.
- Two injections can be given in different sites on the same extremity.
- Immunizations can be given when the child has a minor illness with or without a low-grade fever, and with antibiotic treatment. Recent exposure to an infectious disease is not a reason to defer a vaccine.
- Premature infants have the same requirements for immunizations as full-term infants.
- Immunizations can be given when there was a local reaction to a prior vaccine or a family member had an adverse response.

CULTURE

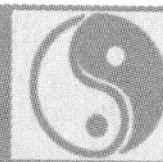

Vietnamese-American children 3 to 18 years have lower rates of hepatitis B vaccination than other ethnic groups. This fact is particularly concerning, as hepatitis B is endemic in those born in Southeast Asia and has a prevalence of 7% to 14% among Vietnamese adults living in the United States. As people with hepatitis B disease can transmit the virus to others and are at increased risk for chronic hepatitis, cirrhosis, and liver cancer, these children should be targeted for special immunization efforts (Jenkins, McPhee, & Wong, et al., 2000).

True contraindications for a vaccine are an anaphylactic reaction to the vaccine or one of its components and a moderate to severe acute illness. Some additional contraindications for specific vaccines may also exist, such as pregnancy and allergy to some components of the vaccine (e.g., neomycin, gelatin, eggs) (see Table 12-3).

Assess the child for potential contraindications to vaccines. Inquire about past reactions to vaccines as well as allergy to key vaccine components such as eggs, gelatin, or neomycin. Determine whether female teens could be pregnant.

Inquire about recent administration of immune globulin or blood products. Antibody response to vaccines may be decreased. Follow guidelines for administration of specific live virus vaccines (e.g., measles, varicella).

The accompanying nursing care plan explores three potential nursing diagnoses that may apply to the child needing immunizations. Additional nursing diagnoses may include the following:

- *Ineffective airway clearance,* related to an obstructed airway
- *Risk for impaired skin integrity,* related to vaccine response
- *Altered health maintenance,* related to cultural beliefs regarding routine immunization

NURSING ALERT

Be prepared for potential vaccine anaphylaxis. Keep epinephrine 1:1000 and resuscitation equipment immediately available. The dose for epinephrine is 0.01 mL/kg per dose and can be repeated every 10–20 minutes until symptoms subside or other emergency care interventions are initiated (American Academy of Pediatrics, 2000).

Planning and Implementation

Nurses should be strong advocates for immunization. Being well informed about immunizations, their potential side effects, and recommended schedules assists immunization efforts (see Table 12-3).

Provide written materials about immunizations to the parents or guardian. When teaching about immunizations, explain the risks and benefits of immunization, risks of disease, and common side effects and treatments. Record the child's history carefully, specifying any previous reactions to immunizations, allergies, and immune diseases.

Some parents have fears about immunization reactions based on stories they have heard. Talk with parents to understand their concerns. Be able to explain the risks and benefits of each immunization. Parents have the right to refuse immunizations for their child on the basis of religious beliefs, but they must sign a waiver noting their decision. If there is a disease outbreak, the nonimmunized child must be kept out of school. Local, city, or state courts decide how to settle any conflicts.

Federal legislation requires consent to be obtained before administering a vaccine. In most institutions, the nurse has the responsibility to inform the parents or the child's legal guardian, supply literature, and obtain written consent before the vaccine is administered. The nurse is required to record the (1) month, day, and year of administration, (2) vaccine given, (3) manufacturer, (4) lot number and expiration date of the immunization given, (5) site and route of administration, and (6) name, title, and address of the person who administers the vaccine. In addition, the nurse must ensure that any severe immunization reaction is reported to the National Vaccine Injury Compensation Program.

Obtain written consent to give the needed vaccines from the parent or guardian. Give the appropriate immunizations to the child as efficiently as possible, while providing support to the child (Figure 12-4 ◆). Anticipate ways to reduce pain and anxiety associated with immunizations. Do not prolong the process of giving immunizations, and give the child honest answers that the needles will cause some pain. Let the child select the arm or leg for the injection and forms of distraction to promote coping. After the injections are completed, let the parent comfort the child. Provide guidelines for managing expected mild reactions at home. Schedule the child's next appointment for a health supervision visit to complete needed immunizations for age.

Certain reactions following immunization are reportable by law to the U.S. Department of Health and Human Services (Table 12-4). The National Childhood Vaccine Injury Act of 1986 provides compensation if a link between immunization and a serious adverse effect is found. This act resulted after serious neurologic adverse reactions from pertussis immunizations were reported, creating significant liability concerns for health care professionals. More recently, reported adverse events to the rotavirus vaccine (intussusception), led to the withdrawal of the

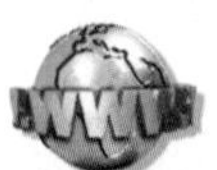

Vaccine Safety

RESEARCH

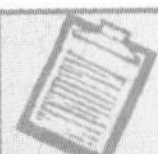

Use of longer needles (25 mm rather than 16 mm) reduces the rates of local reactions and tenderness in infant immunizations. This may ensure that the vaccine is given intramuscularly rather than subcutaneously (Diggle & Deek, 2000).

CLINICAL TIP

Reduce pain and anxiety associated with injections with the following techniques.

- Apply pressure at the site for 10 seconds before the injection.
- Instruct parent how to apply EMLA cream to the site for an hour before the injection.
- Use vapocoolant spray immediately before the injection.
- Give two injections simultaneously in different extremities using two different providers.
- Use age-appropriate distraction techniques (see Chapter 9).

Skill 2-1: Positioning a Child for Intravenous Access/Injection

TABLE 12-3	Common Pediatric Immunizations		
IMMUNIZATION TYPE	**SIDE EFFECTS**	**CONTRAINDICATIONS**	**NURSING CONSIDERATIONS**
Diphtheria and Pertussis Vaccines and Tetanus Toxoid (DTaP) *Route:* Intramuscular *Dosage:* 0.5 mL *Age(s) Given:* 2, 4, 6, 15–18 months; 4–6 years (5 doses) *Storage:* Store in body of refrigerator at 2°–8°C (35°–46°F). Do not freeze. *ACEL*-IMUNE and Tripedia are licensed for all 5 doses. Infanrix and Certiva are licensed for the first 4 doses (Centers for Disease Control, 2000)	*Common:* Redness, pain, swelling, nodule at injection site; temperature up to 38.3°C (101°F); drowsiness, fussiness; anorexia within 2 days of injection. Increase in frequency and magnitude of local reactions with doses 4 and 5 (e.g., entire limb swelling). *Serious:* Anaphylaxis; shock or collapse; fever above 38.8°C (102°F); persistent inconsolable crying.	Occurrence of a serious side effect after previous administration of DTaP, such as anaphylaxis. Administration to be delayed for 1 month after immunosuppressive therapy and until moderate to severe febrile illnesses have resolved. Administration of immune serum globulin within last 90 days.	Use same brand for all doses where feasible. Prior to immunization, ask about previous reactions to immunization. DTaP may coincide with or hasten the recognition of a seizure disorder. In children with a history of seizures with or without fever, give acetaminophen at the time of vaccine and then every 4 hours for 24 hours. Shake vaccine before withdrawing. Solution will be cloudy. If it contains clumps that cannot be resuspended, do not use. When required, simultaneous administration of tetanus immune globulin or diphtheria antitoxin should be given in separate sites with a new needle and syringe. Inform parents of the chance of increased reaction to doses 4 and 5.
Poliovirus Vaccine Inactivated (IPV) *Route:* Subcutaneous *Dosage:* 0.5 mL *Age(s) given:* 2, 4, 12–18 months; 4–6 years (4 doses) *Storage:* Store in body of refrigerator at 2°–8°C (35°–46°F). Do not freeze	*Common:* Swelling and tenderness, irritability, tiredness *Serious:* Anaphylaxis	Hypersensitivity to vaccine components: neomycin, streptomycin, and polymyxin B. Anaphylactic response.	Prior to immunization, ask if the child has an allergy to neomycin, streptomycin, or polymyxin B. Clear, colorless suspension. Do not use if it contains particulate matter, becomes cloudy, or changes color. Recommended for use in all vaccine doses.
Measles, Mumps, Rubella Vaccines (MMR) *Route:* Subcutaneous *Dosage:* 0.5 mL *Age(s) given:* 12–15 months; 4–6 years (2 doses) *Storage:* Store in body of refrigerator at 2°–8°C (35°–46°F). When reconstituted, keep refrigerated and away from light; discard if unused within 8 hours. Diluent is stored at room temperature or in refrigerator. Do not freeze.	*Common:* Elevated temperature 1–2 weeks after immunization; redness or pain at injection site; noncontagious rash; joint pain. *Serious:* Anaphylaxis; encephalopathy; thrombocytopenia purpura, chronic arthritis.	Allergy to neomycin or gelatin. Severely impaired immune system due to malignancy, immune deficiency disease, immunosuppressive therapy. MMR vaccine is recommended for those infected with HIV. Wait at least 3 to 11 months after administration of immune serum globulin or blood products (time determined by the type) before giving vaccine. Pregnancy.	Prior to immunization, ask if child has allergy to neomycin or gelatin. Inquire about immunosuppression. Instruct adolescent girls of childbearing age to avoid pregnancy for 3 months after immunization. Give tuberculosis (TB) skin test at same time as MMR or 4–6 weeks later. Reconstituted vaccine is a clear, yellow solution. Give entire contents of vial even if more than 0.5 mL. As college students are at greater risk due to decreasing immunity, make sure they have received a second MMR dose.
Hepatitis B Vaccine (HB) *Route:* Intramuscular *Dosage:* Engerix-B: 0.5 mL or Recombivax HB: 0.5 mL *Age(s) given:* Birth–2 months, 1 month after first dose; 6 months after first dose *or* Birth–2 months, 1–4 months, 6–18 months (3 doses) *Storage:* Store in body of refrigerator at 2°–8°C (35°–46°F). Do not freeze. Storage out of recommended temperature range decreases potency.	*Common:* Pain or redness at injection site; headache; photophobia; altered liver enzymes. *Serious:* Anaphylaxis	Prior anaphylaxis, liver abnormalities. Serious allergic reaction to past dose.	Prior to immunization, check status of mother's hepatitis B test and presence of other liver disease. Note: If mother has HbsAg+, vaccine must be given to infant within 12 hours of birth along with hepatitis B immune globulin at the same time in another site with new needle and syringe. Shake vaccine before withdrawing. Solution will appear cloudy. Various formulations (pediatric, adult, dialysis) are available in different strengths. Read package insert carefully to determine proper dosage for age for the particular formulation used.

Note: Adapted from the American Academy of Pediatrics. (2000). *Red Book: Report of the Committee on Infectious Disease* (25th ed.). Elk Grove Village, IL: Author; and Bindler, R. M., & Howry, L. B. (1997). *Pediatric drugs and nursing implications* (2nd ed.). Stamford, CT: Appleton & Lange.

(continued)

TABLE 12-3 Common Pediatric Immunizations (continued)

IMMUNIZATION TYPE	SIDE EFFECTS	CONTRAINDICATIONS	NURSING CONSIDERATIONS
Haemophilus influenza Type B (Hib) *Route:* Intramuscular *Dosage:* 0.5 mL *Age(s) given:* 2, 4, 6, 12–15 months (4 doses for HbOC[a] [HibTITER] and PRP-T[a] [ActHIB or OmniHIB]) *or* 2, 4, 12–15 months (3 doses for PRP-OMP[a] [PedvaxHIB]) *Storage:* Store in body of refrigerator at 2°–8°C (35°–46°F). Do not freeze. Use or discard reconstituted ActHIB and OmniHIB within 30 minutes. Refrigerate reconstituted PedvaxHIB and discard within 24 hours.	*Common:* Pain, redness, or swelling at site *Serious:* Anaphylaxis (extremely rare)	Prior anaphylactic reaction to this vaccine.	Prior to immunizations, ask if child is immunosuppressed. Solution is clear and colorless. Since schedules for product preparations of different companies vary, it is important to read package inserts carefully. Use the same vaccine preparation for all doses of the primary series if possible. Some preparations combine Hib with DTaP (TriHIBit), DT (VaxemHIB), and Hep B (Comvax).
Heptavalent Pneumococcal Conjugate Vaccine (PCV) *Route:* Intramuscular *Dosage:* 0.5 mL *Age(s) given:* 2, 4, 6, 12–15 months *Storage:* Store in body of refrigerator at 2°–8°C (35°–46°F). Do not freeze.	*Common:* Soreness, swelling, redness at injection site; mild to moderate fever; irritability, drowsiness, restless sleep, decreased appetite, vomiting and diarrhea, rash or hives. *Severe:* Anaphylaxis	Hypersensitivity to diphtheria toxoid.	Clear, colorless, or slightly opalescent liquid. In addition to infants this vaccine is a priority for children 2–5 years with sickle-cell disease, asplenia, HIV infection, or immunocompromised. The vaccine is also a priority for American Indian and Native Alaskan children 2–5 years because of their increased risk for pneumococcal disease.
Varicella Virus Vaccine (Varivax) *Route:* Subcutaneous *Dosage:* 0.5 mL *Age(s) given:* 12–18 months; or any time up to 12 years of age (1 dose); 13 years or older (2 doses 4–8 weeks apart) *Storage:* Frozen at 5°F or colder. May be stored in refrigerator at 2°–8°C (35°–46°F) up to 72 hours before reconstitution. Once reconstituted, vaccine must be used within 30 minutes or discarded. Do not refreeze. Diluent kept at room temperature.	*Common:* Pain or redness at injection site; fever up to 38.8°C (102°F) in children or up to 37.7°C (100°F) in adults; rash at injection site or generalized. *Severe:* Anaphylaxis	Allergy to neomycin or gelatin. Immunodeficiency or receiving immunosuppression therapy. Administration of immune serum globulin or blood products in last 3–11 months. Active untreated TB. Pregnancy. Moderate or severe febrile illness.	Prior to immunization, ask if child is immunodeficient, is on immunosuppression treatment, or has had an allergy to neomycin or gelatin. Clear, colorless to pale yellow liquid when reconstituted. Give the entire contents of the vial even if more than 0.5 mL. Instruct adolescent girls of childbearing age to avoid pregnancy for 3 months after immunization.
Hepatitis A, inactivated (Hep A) *Route:* intramuscular *Dosage:* 0.5 mL, 1.0 mL over 17 years for Vaqta,[a] 1.0 mL over 18 years for Havrix[a] *Age(s) given:* 2–18 years, 6–12 months after first dose (2 doses) in areas with increased incidence. *Storage:* Store in body of refrigerator at 2°–8°C (35°–46°F). Do not freeze; do not use if frozen.			Shake well, slightly opaque white suspension. Can be given for postexposure prophylaxis against Hepatitis A. Immune globulin and vaccine can be given at the same time in different sites. High incidence areas include the states of Alaska, Arkansas, Arizona, California, Colorado, Idaho, Missouri, Montana, New Mexico, Nevada, Oklahoma, Oregon, South Dakota, Texas, Utah, Washington, and Wyoming. Other high-risk populations to receive vaccine include Native Alaskans and American Indians (Centers for Disease Control, 2001).

[a]Trade names

NURSING CARE PLAN The Child Needing Immunizations

GOAL	INTERVENTION	RATIONALE	EXPECTED OUTCOME
1. Risk for infection related to incomplete immunization series			
	NIC Priority Intervention: **Immunization Administration:** Provision of immunizations for prevention of communicable disease.		NOC Suggested Outcome: **Risk Control:** Actions to eliminate or reduce actual, personal, and modifiable health threats.
The child will become adequately protected from disease-preventable illnesses.	■ Review the child's immunization record for needed vaccines at each health care visit. ■ Identify all due vaccines that can be provided simultaneously. ■ Identify potential contraindications to needed vaccines. Review past reactions to vaccines.	■ Assessment identifies the children who have missed needed immunizations. ■ Many vaccines can be given at the same visit to more adequately protect the child. This also saves health care trips for families. ■ Reduces the risk for the child and other caretakers to have adverse reactions to vaccines.	The child is adequately protected from vaccine-preventable illnesses.
2. Knowledge deficit (parent) related to potential side effects of vaccines			
	NIC Priority Intervention: **Teaching, Prescribed Vaccines:** Preparing a patient to safely take prescribed vaccines and monitor their effects.		NOC Suggested Outcome: **Knowledge:** Vaccine reactions and comfort measures: Extent of understanding conveyed about treatment regimen.
Parents will sign consent for vaccines to be given.	■ Educate the parents about the need for specific vaccines and the risk if not given. Obtain signed consent before giving vaccines.	■ Informed consent is required for all treatments.	The parent(s) complete(s) consent form, which is placed in the child's file.
Parents will state the side effects of vaccines given.	■ Review past reactions to vaccines and describe common potential reactions and why they occur.	■ Parents should expect common reactions and know they indicate the child's body is building protection to the illness.	Parents report all serious side effects to the health care provider.
Parents will manage common side effects of vaccines.	■ Describe serious side effects that should be reported to health care provider.	■ Parents need to be prepared for potential serious side effects so they can obtain care.	The child is given comfort measures after vaccine administration.

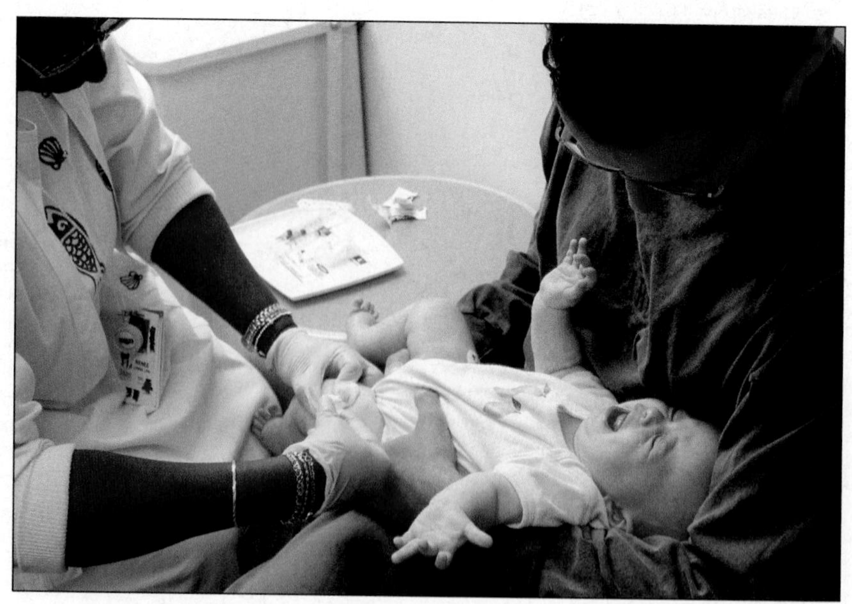

FIGURE 12-4 ◆ Give immunizations quickly and efficiently. Do not prolong the wait and let fear grow. The child will be anxious, especially if more than one injection must be given.

NURSING CARE PLAN The Child Needing Immunizations (continued)

GOAL	INTERVENTION	RATIONALE	EXPECTED OUTCOME
2. Knowledge deficit (parent) related to potential side effects of vaccines (continued)			
	■ Teach parents general comfort measures for children's common side effects, for example: ■ Cool pack to tender leg ■ Acetaminophen for fever and discomfort ■ Rocking and holding the infant ■ Gentle movement of affected extremity	■ Parents will know how to make the child more comfortable during the 24–48 hours after the vaccine is given.	
3. Risk for injury related to vaccine reaction			
	NIC Priority Intervention: **Vaccine Precautions:** Reducing the risk of a systemic reaction to vaccine.		NOC Suggested Outcome: **Risk Control:** Actions to eliminate or reduce actual, personal, and modifiable health threats.
The child's potential vaccine reactions will be safely managed.	■ Prepare for life-threatening reactions by having resuscitation drugs and equipment immediately available. ■ Monitor the child for 15 minutes after the vaccine is given before letting the child go home. ■ Assess the child for extreme anxiety and injection fearfulness. ■ Have the fearful child sit or lie down until symptoms of vasovagal response have disappeared. ■ Report all vaccine-related reactions to the appropriate agency using the standard form.	■ Anaphylactic reactions must be managed quickly and effectively. ■ A life-threatening response will usually become apparent within this time frame. ■ These are potential signs the child may have a vasovagal response to the injection. ■ The child who faints may sustain a head injury. ■ Legal requirements for all health care providers.	The child has no reaction or has a severe reaction to a vaccine that is managed effectively.

vaccine. The Vaccine Adverse Event Reporting System was established in 1988 to track serious vaccine reactions (see Table 12-4). Follow-up of the patient's condition occurs at 60 days and 1 year after the adverse event. Follow guidelines for reporting according to the Vaccine Adverse Event Reporting System. Provide parents with a record of the child's immunizations, and record the vaccines given in the health care agency's official records.

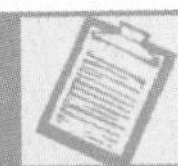

RESEARCH

The Vaccine Safety Datalink project continually evaluates vaccine safety on more than 6 million people. Studies in process are examining the association of immunizations with diabetes mellitus, and of MMR vaccine with inflammatory bowel disease (American Academy of Pediatrics, 2000).

Evaluation

Expected nursing outcomes include the following:

- Parents are fully informed and give consent for immunizations.
- All age-appropriate immunizations are provided for the child at each health visit or catch up immunizations are provided as needed.
- The parents are prepared to manage mild reactions to immunizations at home.

INFECTIOUS AND COMMUNICABLE DISEASES IN CHILDREN

Infectious and communicable diseases cause acute illnesses. These diseases are caused by bacterial, viral, protozoan, or fungal organisms. As noted earlier, infants and children develop infectious and communicable diseases more frequently than adults do. They develop antibodies

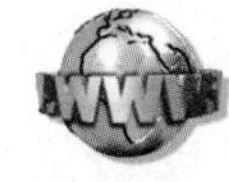

Reporting Infectious Diseases

TABLE 12-4 National Vaccine Injury Compensation Program—Vaccine Injury Table

VACCINE	ILLNESS, DISABILITY, INJURY, OR CONDITION COVERED	TIME PERIOD FOR FIRST SYMPTOM OR MANIFESTATION OF ONSET OR OF SIGNIFICANT AGGRAVATION AFTER VACCINE ADMINISTRATION—FOR COMPENSATION
DTaP, P, DT, Td, DTP-Hib, or Tetanus Toxoid; or any other vaccine containing whole cell pertussis bacteria, extracted or partial cell pertussis bacteria, or specific pertussis antigen(s)	Anaphylaxis or anaphylactic shock Encephalopathy (or encephalitis) Bacterial neuritis Any acute complication or sequela (including death) of above events. Events described in manufacturer's package insert as contraindications of additional doses of vaccine.	0–4 hours 72 hours 2–28 days No limit Not applicable
Measles, mumps, rubella, or any vaccine containing any of the foregoing as a component	Anaphylaxis or anaphylactic shock Encephalopathy (or encephalitis) Events described in manufacturer's package insert as contraindications of additional doses of vaccine.	0–4 hours 5–15 days for measles, mumps, rubella, or any vaccine containing any of the foregoing as a component. Not applicable
Rubella-containing vaccines	Chronic arthritis	7–42 days
Measles-containing vaccines	Thrombocytopenia purpura Vaccine strain measles viral infection in an immunodeficient recipient.	7–30 days 0–6 months
Inactivated polio vaccine	Anaphylaxis or anaphylactic shock Any acute complication or sequela (including death) of above events. Events described in manufacturer's package insert as contraindications of additional doses of vaccine.	0–4 hours No limit Not applicable
Hepatitis B antigen–containing vaccines	Anaphylaxis or anaphylactic shock Any acute complication or sequela (including death) of above events. Events described in manufacturer's package insert as contraindications of additional doses of vaccine.	0–4 hours No limit Not applicable
Haemophilus influenzae type B polysaccharide vaccines (unconjugated, PRP vaccines)	Any early-onset Hib disease Any acute complication or sequela (including death) of above events. Events described in manufacturer's package insert as contraindications of additional doses of vaccine.	0–7 days No limit Not applicable
Haemophilus influenzae type B polysaccharide conjugate vaccine	No condition specified for compensation Events described in manufacturer's package insert as contraindications of additional doses of vaccine.	Not applicable Not applicable
Varicella virus–containing vaccine	No condition specified for compensation Events described in manufacturer's package insert as contraindications of additional doses of vaccine.	Not applicable Not applicable

Note: Used with the permission of the American Academy of Pediatrics. (2000). *Red Book: Report of the Committee on Infectious Disease* (25th ed.). Elk Grove Village, IL: Author.

as they are exposed to infectious organisms, so they frequently become symptomatic after exposure. The epidemiology, clinical manifestations, treatment, prevention, and nursing care of selected infectious and communicable diseases of childhood are detailed in Table 12-5.

CLINICAL MANIFESTATIONS

The child with an infectious or communicable diseases will have several symptoms. Each disease has its own specific cluster of symptoms. Skin rash, poor appetite, malaise, vomiting

PATHOPHYSIOLOGY ILLUSTRATED

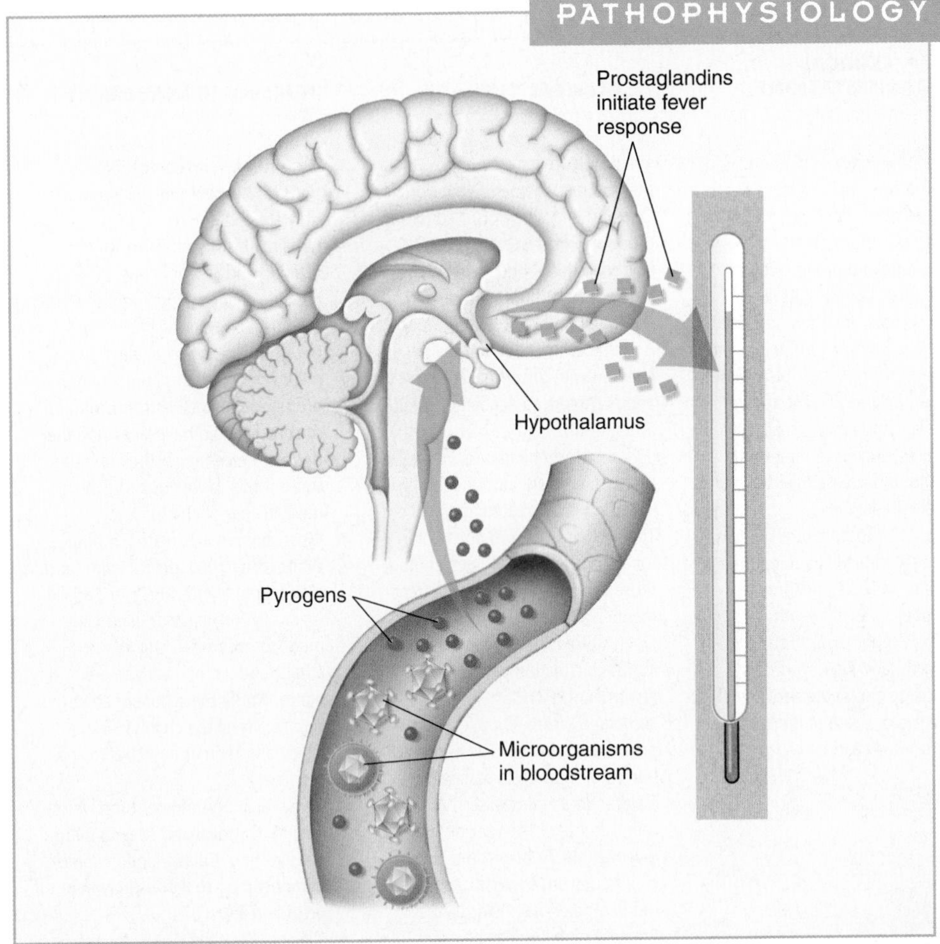

Fever

FIGURE 12-5 ◆

The hypothalamus functions as the body's thermostat, directing the body to conserve or dissipate heat. When microorganisms invade the body, endogenous pyrogens are released into the bloodstream. These substances travel to the hypothalamus, where they trigger the production and release of prostaglandins, which initiate the fever response. Blood is diverted from the extremities to more central vessels. This helps increase the core body temperature by decreasing heat loss. Shivering increases both metabolic action and heat production. The hypothalamus then maintains the temperature at the new set point.

and/or diarrhea, and body aches are some common signs and symptoms. Fever in a child is often a sign of infectious disease. Why does fever develop in response to certain illnesses and infections? What methods can be used to manage fever in children?

CLINICAL TIP

One degree of temperature elevation causes an increase in respiratory rate by four breaths per minute and increases oxygen need by 7%.

Physiology of Fever

The hypothalamus is the control center for the regulation of body temperature and is frequently compared to a thermostat because of its regulatory function (Figure 12-5 ◆). As blood circulates through the hypothalamus, this brain structure regulates body temperature by directing body systems to conserve or dissipate heat, depending on the temperature of the blood.

- If body temperature is lower than normal, vasoconstriction is initiated to conserve heat. The adrenal glands produce epinephrine and norepinephrine, which cause an increase in metabolism, more vasoconstriction, and more heat production.
- Shivering or chills may occur, which in turn may increase heat production.
- When excess heat is produced, the body responds with an increase in temperature. The heart rate and respiratory rate increase.
- Vasodilation occurs and the skin flushes, becoming warm to the touch. As the temperature decreases, the child may start to perspire, and the heart and respiratory rates return to normal.

Endogenous pyrogens (interleukins, interferons, and tumor necrosis factor) are released by macrophages in response to an invasive organism. These pyrogens travel through the circulatory system to the hypothalamus, where they trigger the production of prostaglandins. Prostaglandins are believed to raise the body's thermoregulatory set point, thus causing the fever to occur (Cimpella, Goldman, & Khine, 2000).

TABLE 12-5 Selected Infectious and Communicable Diseases in Children

DISEASE	CLINICAL MANIFESTATIONS	CLINICAL THERAPY	NURSING MANAGEMENT
Chickenpox (Varicella)*† *Causal agent:* Varicella-zoster, human herpesvirus 3. *Epidemiology:* Peak occurrence is in the late fall, winter, and spring. Maternal antibodies disappear 2–3 months after birth. *Transmission:* Direct contact with lesions or airborne spread of secretions. *Incubation period:* 14–21 days *Period of communicability:* As long as 5 days before the onset of the rash to a maximum of 6 days after the appearance of the first group of vesicles, when all lesions have crusted over. This period may be prolonged after passive immunization or in immunodeficient children.	The onset of symptoms is acute. Mild fever, malaise, and irritability occur before and with eruption. The rash begins as a macule on an erythematous base and progresses to a papule, then a clear, fluid-filled vesicle. Lesions are often described as a "teardrop on a rose petal" and may erupt for 1–5 days. Lesions of all stages may be present at any one time. Crusts may remain for 1–3 weeks. Lesions in the mouth may lead to decreased fluid intake and dehydration. *Complications:* Most are rare but can include secondary infection, encephalitis, varicella pneumonia, thrombocytopenia, hepatitis, glomerulonephritis, arthritis, meningitis, and Reye syndrome. This disease may cause very significant illness or death to immunocompromised children.	There is no cure for chickenpox. Medical management is supportive. Oral and IV Acyclovir is used for immunocompromised patients. If started within 24 hours will decrease new lesion formation and the total number of lesions, but this is not recommended for healthy children with uncomplicated chickenpox (American Academy of Pediatrics, 2000). *Prognosis:* Most children recover fully. Children who are immunocompromised must be treated aggressively. This includes children on steroids for asthma and other illnesses, and those on long-term salicylate treatment. The disease is more severe when steroids have been given during the incubation period (Twomey, 1998). *Prevention:* Chickenpox is a vaccine-preventable disease. The immunization may be given to susceptible children at any time after 12 months of age. The vaccine may be given within 72 hours after exposure to prevent or significantly modify the disease. Varicella-zoster immune globulin may be given to exposed immunocompromised children with no history of chickenpox or immunization up to 4 days after exposure.	■ Use airborne and contact precautions for hospitalized children while they are contagious. ■ Obtain a history of varicella immunization and recent exposure in susceptible children upon admission to the hospital. Place all children exposed to varicella in isolation as a means of protecting immunocompromised patients. Nurses caring for the child should have a varicella titer done to be certain of their immune status if they have not had a documented case of chickenpox. ■ Most children are treated at home. While contagious, isolate them from all susceptible individuals, especially medically fragile children and immunocompromised children or adults, and women early in pregnancy. Notify the school or child care facility of the child's illness. ■ Give nonaspirin antipyretics to control fever. ■ Give oral antihistamines for relief of itching. Oatmeal and Aveeno baths are soothing. Caladryl lotion applied in moderation to lesions may also provide relief. ■ Observe the child closely for drowsiness, meningeal signs, respiratory distress, and dehydration. ■ Keep the child's fingernails short and clean. Young children may need to wear soft cotton mittens to prevent infections when itching cannot be controlled. ■ Change bed linens frequently. Linen should be washed in mild soap and rinsed well. ■ Watch for symptoms of complications. ■ Disorientation and restlessness may indicate viral encephalitis. ■ Reassure the child that the lesions are temporary and will go away.

A

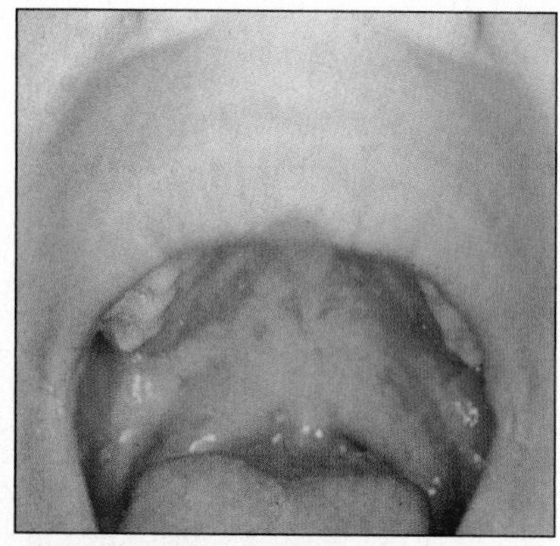

Mouth lesions of chickenpox.
Courtesy of Centers for Disease Control and Prevention, Atlanta, GA.

B

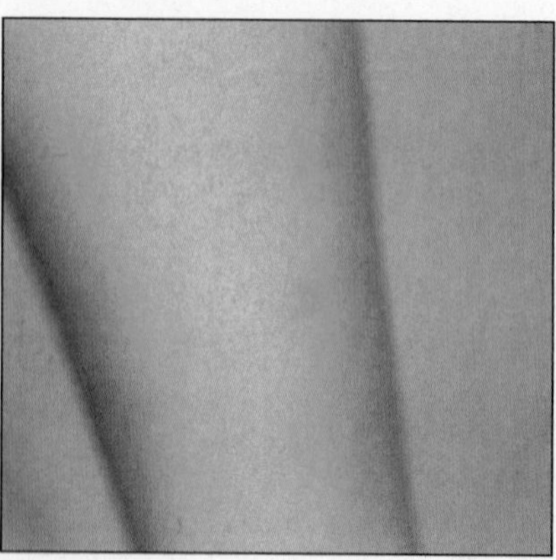

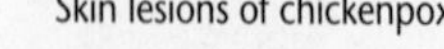

Skin lesions of chickenpox.

NURSING ALERT

Chickenpox can be fatal in immunocompromised children. When undergoing chemotherapy, steroid treatment, or transplant therapy, children should be carefully monitored after exposure to the disease. Varicella-zoster immune globulin is usually administered as soon as possible after exposure. A chickenpox vaccine is available and recommended for use in all children who have not had the disease.

*Indicates that a vaccine or antitoxin is available for use in high-risk or as-needed situations.
†Indicates that the disease has a safe and effective vaccine.

TABLE 12-5 Selected Infectious and Communicable Diseases in Children (continued)

DISEASE	CLINICAL MANIFESTATIONS	CLINICAL THERAPY	NURSING MANAGEMENT
Coxsackievirus *Causal agent:* Coxsackievirus A16 and Enterovirus 71 cause a wide group of acute diseases that range from minor and self-limiting to potentially fatal. *Epidemiology:* Occurs worldwide, most commonly in summer and early fall. Sporadic outbreaks are seen, especially among children in out-of-home settings. Illnesses include the common cold; pharyngitis; pneumonia; hand, foot, and mouth disease; and herpangina. Immunity probably occurs after clinical or subclinical infection, but duration of the immunity is unknown. *Transmission:* Fecal–oral route; probably respiratory route. *Incubation period:* 3–6 days. *Period of communicability:* 2 days before rash to 2 days after it disappears.	Each of the coxsackieviruses is responsible for a different set of manifestations. Herpangina is an acute, self-limiting viral disease characterized by the sudden onset of fever, sore throat, and small, discrete greyish papulovesicular ulcerative pharyngeal lesions that gradually increase in size. In hand, foot, and mouth disease the lesions are more diffuse and may occur on the buccal surfaces of the cheeks, gums, and sides of the tongue. Papulovesicular lesions occur on the hands and feet and last for 7–10 days. Children may be irritable and have a fever, anorexia, dysphagia, malaise, and a sore throat. *Complications:* Enterovirus 71 caused a fatal epidemic in Taiwan in 1998. Of the 90,000 cases of hand, foot, and mouth disease, 78 deaths resulted (Chang, Lin, & Hsu, et al., 1999).	There is no specific treatment. An antiviral medication, pleconaril, is being evaluated for use in immunodeficient children (American Academy of Pediatrics, 2000). *Prognosis:* Recovery is generally good with supportive care. *Prevention:* Avoid contact with infected persons early in the disease.	■ Isolate the child while contagious. Use contact precautions if the child is hospitalized. ■ Apply topical lotions and give systemic medications as ordered to lessen the pain and relieve the irritation. ■ Offer cool drinks and soft, bland foods (no citrus, salty, or spicy foods). Swallowing may be painful. ■ Offer warm saline mouth rinses. ■ Observe for dehydration. ■ Provide reassurance and support to parents. ■ Give nonaspirin antipyretics for fever. Keep the child out of school or child care while the child is febrile.
Diphtheria*† *Causal agent:* Corynebacterium diphtheriae, a bacterium *Epidemiology:* Occurs mostly during colder months in temperate zones in unimmunized, partially immunized, and immunized children with waning immunity. In tropical areas, cases of cutaneous and wound diphtheria occur sporadically. Maternal immunity lasts as long as 6 months after birth. While there are less than 5 cases annually in the United States, the disease is endemic in areas where immunization is no longer routine, such as Russia. *Transmission:* By contact with an infectious patient or carrier's nasal or eye discharge, or skin lesion; or less commonly, indirectly by contact with contaminated articles. Unpasteurized milk has also served as a vehicle. *Incubation period:* 2–7 days, sometimes longer *Period of communicability:* Varies but is usually 2–4 weeks or until 4 days after antibiotics are initiated.	Symptoms can be mild or severe with a gradual onset over 1–2 days. Low-grade fever, anorexia, malaise, rhinorrhea with a foul odor, cough, hoarseness, stridor or noisy breathing, cervical lymphadenitis, and pharyngitis may be present. In more severe cases the membranes of the tonsils, pharynx, and larynx are affected. The characteristic membranous lesion is a thick, bluish white to grayish black patch that covers the tonsils. It can spread to cover the soft and hard palates and the posterior portion of the pharynx. Attempts to remove the membrane result in bleeding. *Complications:* Produces an endotoxin that causes myocarditis and peripheral neuropathy (diplopia, slurred speech, difficulty swallowing, or paralysis of the palate) or ascending paralysis similar to Guillain-Barre syndrome.	Administration of IV antitioxin and antibiotics within 3 days of onset of symptoms. The child must be tested for sensitivity to horse serum before giving the antitoxin. When diphtheria is suspected, antibiotic therapy (penicillin G or erythema) should be initiated without waiting for laboratory results. Removal of membrane may be needed to treat airway obstruction. *Prognosis:* With treatment, prognosis is good. If untreated, diphtheria can cause death from airway obstruction. *Prevention:* Diphtheria is a vaccine-preventable disease. The immunization series is initiated at 2 months of age and is usually given in combination with tetanus and pertussis. Diphtheria-tetanus (Td) is administered to children over 7 years. This is a reportable disease.	■ Use droplet precautions for pharyngeal disease and contact precautions for cutaneous disease. ■ Monitor closely for signs of increasing respiratory distress, as well as cardiac and neurologic complications. Provide humidified oxygen as necessary. ■ Have emergency airway equipment available. ■ Administer antibiotics. Give no medications containing caffeine or other stimulants. ■ Use oral suction gently as necessary. ■ Allow children to use mouthwash if desired. Gargling is not permitted because it can irritate the back of the throat. ■ Encourage liquids as tolerated. Intravenous fluids may be necessary. ■ Provide emotional support to the family. ■ Initiate the trace for contacts with the patient to give antibiotics and immunization boosters.

(continued)

TABLE 12-5 Selected Infectious and Communicable Diseases in Children (continued)

DISEASE	CLINICAL MANIFESTATIONS	CLINICAL THERAPY	NURSING MANAGEMENT
Erythema Infectiosum (Fifth Disease) *Causal agent:* Human parvovirus B19 *Epidemiology:* Occurs worldwide, most often in winter and spring. The disease also occurs in epidemics, with peak activity every 6 years. The incidence is highest in children between the ages of 5 and 14 years. *Transmission:* Respiratory secretions and blood. *Incubation period:* 6–14 days *Period of communicability:* Believed to be the highest before the onset of the disease. Not contagious after rash appears unless in aplastic crisis (Adams & Ware, 1996).	The child first manifests a flulike illness (headache, chills, malaise, nausea, body ache) that lasts 2–3 days; 1 week later, a fiery red rash appears on the cheeks giving a "slapped face" appearance. The rash is accompanied by circumoral pallor. In 1–4 days a lacelike symmetric, erythematous, maculopapular rash appears on the truck and limbs, spreading proximal to distal. During the third stage, which lasts 1–3 weeks, the rash fades but can reappear if the skin is irritated or exposed to sunlight. The rash may be mildly pruritic. *Complications:* Children with hemolytic conditions may have transient aplastic crisis. The child has flulike symptoms but no rash. Arthritis occurs in 10% of children, lasting 1–6 days after the rash (Cherry, 1999).	There is no specific treatment, and recovery is spontaneous. Children with hemolytic conditions may need blood transfusion if aplastic crisis occurs. *Prognosis:* Fetal infection may occur resulting in spontaneous abortion. *Prevention:* Avoid contact with infected persons early in the disease.	■ Children with aplastic crisis are often hospitalized. ■ Isolation is needed only for children with aplastic crisis or when immunosuppressed. Use contact precautions. ■ Nonaspirin antipyretics may be given to control fever. ■ Use soothing oatmeal or Aveeno baths if the rash is pruritic. Antipruritics may also help to relieve itching. ■ Encourage rest and offer frequent fluids. ■ Keep children out of direct sunlight if possible. ■ Provide protective, light, loose clothing if exposure to sunlight cannot be avoided. ■ Provide quiet diversionary activity. There is no reason to keep the child out of school or daycare. ■ Explain the three stages of rash development to parents.

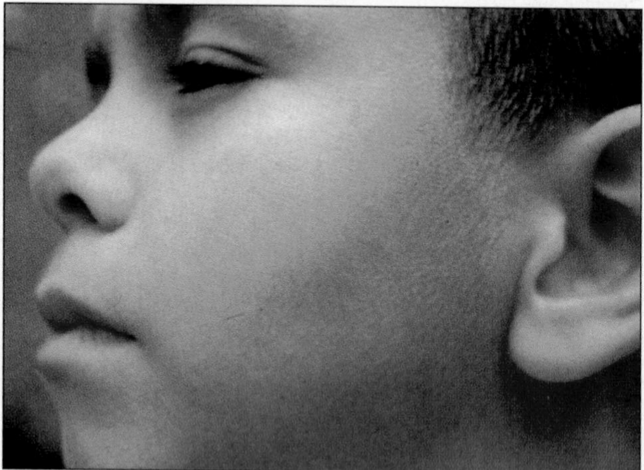

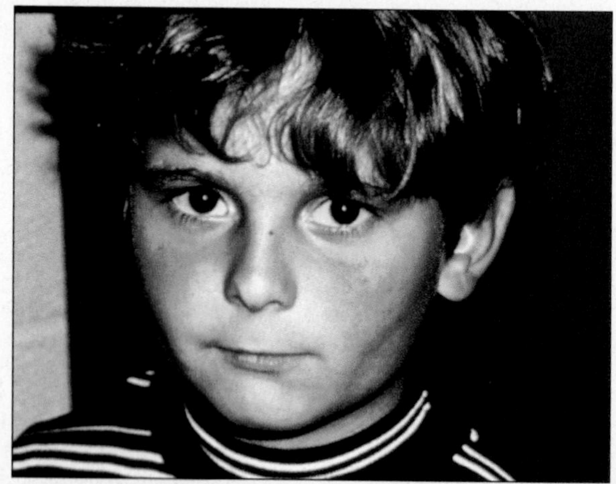

Characteristic facial rash of erythema infectiosum (Fifth disease).
Courtesy of Centers for Disease Control and Prevention, Atlanta, GA.

*Indicates that a vaccine or antitoxin is available for use in high-risk or as-needed situations.
†Indicates that the disease has a safe and effective vaccine.

TABLE 12-5 Selected Infectious and Communicable Diseases in Children (continued)

DISEASE	CLINICAL MANIFESTATIONS	CLINICAL THERAPY	NURSING MANAGEMENT
Haemophilus Influenzae Type B+ (H-Influenzae Type B)			
Causal agent: Coccobacilli *H. influenzae* bacteria, which has several serotypes and can be encapsulated or nonencapsulated. *Epidemiology:* Occurs most often in the spring and summer. Most commonly affected are infants and young children in childcare centers. Low-birth-weight children and children with chronic illnesses also have an increased susceptibility. Invasive disease has decreased 96% in the United States from 1987–1995 due to the vaccine (Kaplan, 1999) *Transmission:* Direct person-to-person contact or droplet inhalation. The organism is frequently asymptomatically colonized in the respiratory tract. *Incubation period:* Unknown. *Period of communicability:* 3 days from onset of symptoms.	*H. influenzae* type B starts with a viral upper respiratory infection. The organism passes through the mucosal barrier to directly invade the bloodstream. It can cause several severe invasive illnesses, including meningitis, epiglottitis, pneumonia, septic arthritis, and cellulitis. It is also a cause of sepsis in infants. Other illnesses include sinusitis, otitis media, bronchitis, and pericarditis. Each disease has very specific clinical manifestations. *Complications:* Illness caused by *H. influenzae* type B responds to antibiotic therapy. Left untreated, severe sequelae and death, especially in young infants, can occur from conditions such as meningitis, epiglottitis, sinusitis, pneumonitis, and cellulitis.	Treatment consists of antibiotic therapy; however, one-third of strains are resistant to ampicillin. Rifampin may be given to unprotected household contacts (not pregnant women), if another child has not completed immunizations, within 1 week after diagnosis. In this case, the infected child also gets rifampin to eliminate nasopharyngeal colonization. *Prognosis:* With rapid diagnosis and treatment, the outlook for recovery is good but highly dependent on the disease the organism has caused. When treatment has been delayed, the prognosis for full recovery becomes much more guarded. *Prevention:* Immunization is now available for *H. influenzae* type B as part of the recommended childhood immunization series beginning at 2 months of age. Other types of *H. influenzae* are not vaccine preventable.	■ Use droplet precautions until 24 hours after the initiation of antibiotics. ■ Antibiotic therapy is administered intravenously for severe infections. Infections such as otitis media can be managed at home with oral antibiotics. ■ Children under the age of 4 years who have not been immunized are at increased risk for developing disease from *H. influenzae.* Specific prophylactic measures for susceptible children may be ordered by the physician. ■ Administer antipyretics to help the child feel more comfortable. ■ Closely monitor IV sites for patency and infiltration. ■ Perform nursing care measures specific to the illness. ■ Inform family members that rifampin turns urine and other body fluids orange.
Hepatitis A, Hepatitis B, and Hepatitis C **See Chapter 17.**			
Lyme Disease*			
Causal agent: Borrelia burgdorferi, a spirochete, which is transmitted by ixodid ticks. *Epidemiology:* Distribution in the United States correlates highly with the distribution of various tick carriers (vectors). It occurs in 49 states and the District of Columbia. Exposure occurs in any outdoor setting where ticks are endemic. Animals such as dogs and cats can also have the disease. Lyme disease occurs yearround, with the highest risk of infection in the summer. Children between 5 and 14 years are at highest risk. Infection does not induce immunity. *Transmission:* Tick bite. The tick transmits the infected spirochete when it draws blood. The tick must feed for 36 hours to transmit the disease. *Incubation period:* 3–32 days after an infected tick bit. A rash in 48 hours is an allergic reaction or infection, not Lyme disease.	The most typical early symptom is a slowly expanding red rash, called erythema migrans, at the site of the bite, often found on the groin, axilla, or thigh. The rash starts as a flat or raised red area and may progress to partial clearing, develop blisters or scabs in the center. The rash may look like a bruise in dark-skinned patients. The rash has a "bull's-eye" appearance and is at least 5 cm in diameter. It resolves spontaneously within 4 weeks. Only 50%–75% of patients have the rash (Wade, 2000). Stage 1 symptoms, lasting 5–21 days, include malaise, fatigue, headache, stiff neck, mild fever, and muscle and joint aches. Stage 2 (early disseminated) occurs 1–4 months after the bite. The most common symptoms of untreated disease are pain and swelling of the joints, most commonly the knee (Lyme arthritis), facial palsy, meningitis, AV block.	Antibiotics are the treatment of choice. Amoxicillin, cefuroxime axetil, or erythromycin are most often used in children 8 years of age or younger. Doxycycline or tetracycline is given to children over the age of 8 years. A 4-week course of oral medication is given. If no response in 2–4 weeks, IV ceftriaxone, cefotaxime, or penicillin G is needed to prevent progression to later phases. (See drug guide for ceftriaxone.) Intravenous antibiotics are often required in the later stages of the disease. Relapse can occur. *Prognosis:* Lyme disease does not cause acute life-threatening illness, but it may result in significant morbidity, especially when chronic.	■ Children with early disease are usually treated at home. Children with progressive symptoms may be hospitalized. Use standard precautions. ■ Educate parents about the need for the long course of medications, informing them that the spirochete can go dormant. ■ Tell parents to have the child avoid sun exposure when taking doxycycline. Nonaspirin analgesics and antipyretics may provide relief of mild fevers, headaches, and muscle and joint aches. ■ Children with Lyme disease may tire easily. Promote rest and avoid vigorous activities that may be difficult. ■ Educate parents and children about the disease and early recognition of the symptoms. Teach them to safely remove ticks.

(continued)

TABLE 12-5 Selected Infectious and Communicable Diseases in Children (continued)

DISEASE	CLINICAL MANIFESTATIONS	CLINICAL THERAPY	NURSING MANAGEMENT
Lyme Disease (continued)	Stage 3 (late disseminated) occurs months later and includes problems such as Lyme arthritis and central nervous system changes. These may become chronic problems. *Complications:* Left untreated, Lyme disease can cause significant neurologic deficits, including arm and leg weakness, Bell's palsy, encephalopathy, meningitis, severe headaches, and cognitive and behavioral changes as well as chronic arthritis, and disorders of the peripheral nerves. The spriochete can cross the placental barrier and infect the fetus (Wade, 2000).	*Prevention:* A vaccine, LYMErix, is approved for high-risk patients 15–70 years. Some clinical trials in younger children appear promising. Avoid areas that are heavily tick infested, and wear protective clothing. Check for ticks (especially hidden in hair) after every outing. Check pets because they can carry home ticks that are then transferred to the child. Remove ticks as soon as possible. There is no acquired immunity.	■ To remove a tick, grasp it gently but firmly with fine-point tweezers where the mouthparts are attached. Pull gently—avoid squeezing of the tick's body—until it releases. Clean the area with soap and water. If any tick parts are left under the skin, take the child to a health care provider for removal. Tell them to mark the date of the tick bite on the calendar and monitor the child's health for flulike symptoms over the next 2 weeks. Encourage them to seek medical attention promptly if symptoms develop. ■ Provide emotional support.

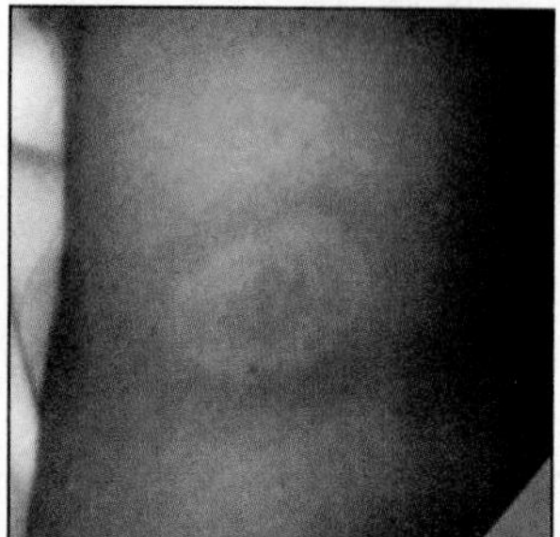

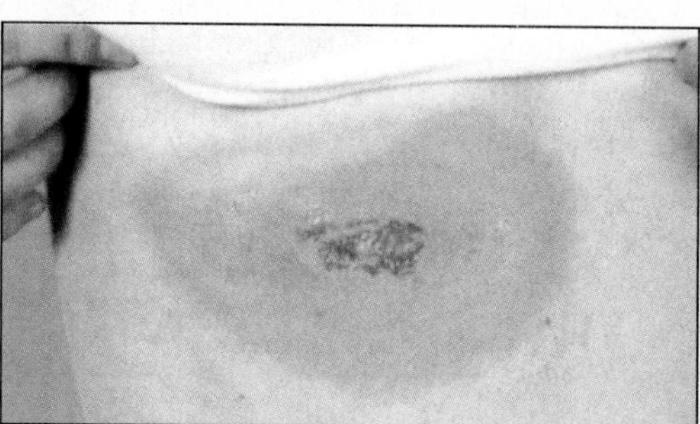

The appearance of erythema migrans rash may vary in early Lyme disease.
From Pfizer Central Research. (1989). Lyme Disease. *Groton: CT: Author.*

LAW & ETHICS

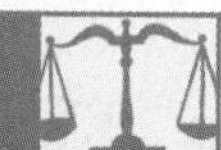

Patients are sometimes denied health insurance coverage for oral and IV medications for long courses of treatment for Lyme disease. Connecticut passed legislation in 1999 requiring insurers to cover treatment. Other states are considering such legislation (Healy, 2000).

DISEASE	CLINICAL MANIFESTATIONS	CLINICAL THERAPY	NURSING MANAGEMENT
Malaria *Causal agent:* Plasmodium, four species (P. falciparum, P. vivax, P. ovale, P. malariae) *Epidemiology:* Occurs in tropical and subtropical regions on four continents (Africa, Americas, Asia, and Oceana). The disease is acquired during travel to an endemic area. *Transmission and incubation:* The bite of an infected female Anopheles mosquito during a nocturnal blood meal permits the parasite to enter the human blood stream. The parasite passes to the liver and infects hepatic cells. During an asymptomatic 5–16-day cycle, the parasite transforms to become a merozoite. The merozoites are released and infect the red blood cells.	Nonspecific signs such as myalgia, malaise, headache, abdominal pain, back pain, diarrhea, nausea, and vomiting are common. Spiking fever occurs at the time red blood cells rupture, becoming a classical cyclic pattern every 48–72 hours. Periods of symptomatic improvement are sometimes seen between spells.	The patient is hospitalized to receive fluid replacement, antipyretics, and anemia management. In severe disease with greater than 5% parasitemia, intensive care and IV treatment is needed. The blood is regularly monitored for parasite density. Quinine sulfate and tetracycline are used for chloroquine-resistant P. falciparum. Hypoglycemia may result from quinine treatment. Sulfadoxine-pyremethamine rather than tetracycline is used for children under 8 years of age. Mefloquine is used for chloroquine-sensitive organisms. Primaquine will cause severe anemia if given to individuals with G6PD disorder (Barat & Zucker, 1999).	■ Use standard precautions for the hospitalized patient. ■ Maintain fluid intake. Monitor intake and output. ■ Monitor blood glucose level and be prepared to respond to sudden hypoglycemia. ■ Observe for signs of increasing illness severity such as confusion, seizures, and shock. Be prepared to protect the patient from injury and provide emergency support with airways and oxygen supplementation until the child can be transferred to intensive care. ■ Monitor the hematocrit and hemoglobin levels. ■ Administer antipyretics to control the fever and promote comfort.

*Indicates that a vaccine or antitoxin is available for use in high-risk or as-needed situations.
†Indicates that the disease has a safe and effective vaccine.

TABLE 12-5 Selected Infectious and Communicable Diseases in Children (continued)

DISEASE	CLINICAL MANIFESTATIONS	CLINICAL THERAPY	NURSING MANAGEMENT
Malaria (continued) *Period of communicability:* Not communicable except by blood or blood product transfusion, or the transplantation of organs from an infected person.	*Complications:* When more than 5% of red blood cells are infected, severe anemia is seen; seizures and cerebral malaria (increased intracranial pressure, confusion, stupor, coma, and sometimes death) are most common in children. Pulmonary edema, respiratory failure, renal failure, spontaneous bleeding, and shock are seen in older children and adolescents. Children with asplenia are at high risk for death. Causes 1–2 million deaths worldwide annually.	*Prevention:* Minimize contact with mosquitoes; use DEET insect repellent, screened rooms, and DEET-treated mosquito netting; and cover the body with clothing when traveling in endemic regions. Antimalarial chemoprophylaxis (mefloquine) should be used 1 week before arrival, weekly during travel, and 4 weeks after leaving the risk area. Doxycycline is sometimes used as an alternate chemoprophylaxis, but must be taken daily.	■ Educate families traveling to endemic areas about the importance of antimalarial chemoprophylaxis. Explain the need to take the medication correctly despite the common side effects of nausea and vomiting. Discuss the need to protect children during nocturnal feeding times of mosquitoes with protective clothing, mosquito repellent, and mosquito netting around the bed.
Measles (Rubeola)*† *Causal agent:* Mobillivirus, a member of the paramyxovirus group. *Epidemiology:* Occurrence peaks in the late winter and early spring. In developed countries, measles occurs mostly in outbreaks among children, which are largely the result of lack of immunization or possibly declining immunity. Many cases are imported from countries without routine immunization. Maternal immunity is active in the infant until the age of approximately 12–15 months. Vaccination induces lifelong immunity. In developing countries, measles remains largely an endemic problem and is a significant cause of infant and child morbidity and mortality. *Transmission:* Airborne, respiratory droplets and contact with infected persons. *Incubation period:* about 8–12 days. *Period of communicability:* Begins during the prodromal phase and ends about 2–4 days after the rash appears.	Children are quite ill in the 3–5-day prodromal phase, with symptoms including high fever, conjunctivitis, coryza, cough, anorexia, and malaise. Small, irregular, bluish white spots on a red background, called Koplik spots, appear on the buccal mucosa about 2 days before and after the onset of the rash. The characteristic red, blotchy, maculopapular rash that becomes confluent usually appears 2–4 days after onset of prodromal phase. The rash begins on the face and spreads to the trunk and extremities. Symptoms gradually subside in 4–7 days. Other symptoms include anorexia, malaise, fatigue, and generalized lymphadenopathy. *Complications:* Diarrhea, otitis media, bronchopneumonia, bronchitis, laryngotracheobronchitis, and encephalitis. Complications and sequelae occur most often in children who are malnourished, medically fragile, and immunosuppressed. The younger the child, the greater the risk for complications.	There is no cure for measles. Treatment is supportive. Antibiotics are used for bacterial secondary infections. *Prognosis:* Recovery is generally good with supportive care. *Prevention:* Measles is a vaccine-preventable disease. The measles vaccine is available alone (M), in combination with the rubella vaccine (MR), or in combination with the rubella and mumps vaccines (MMR). Immune globulin, administered up to 6 days after exposure, may be helpful in preventing the disease in susceptible persons (immunocompromised children, infants less than 1 year of age, pregnant women). All health care workers should have documented immunity. This is a reportable disease.	■ If the child is hospitalized, maintain airborne precautions during the contagious period (5 days after the rash appears). ■ Use a cool-mist vaporizer to help clear respiratory passages. ■ Suction nose and oral cavity very gently as necessary. ■ Give nonaspirin antipyretics for fever and antipruritics for itching. ■ Assess lungs carefully, especially in young children, in whom pneumonias are a common complication. ■ Antitussives may be ordered to control coughing. ■ Keep lights dim, and cover windows if the child has photophobia. ■ Elevate the head of the bed. Keep the room cool with good air circulation. Provide light, nonirritating blankets. ■ Keep skin clean and dry. No soaps should be used. ■ Maintain fluid intake. Offer cool liquids frequently in small amounts. Blended, pureed, and mashed foods are most easily tolerated. ■ Maintain bed rest. ■ Ensure visitors are immune to measles. ■ Provide diversions such as music, stories, and favorite toys.

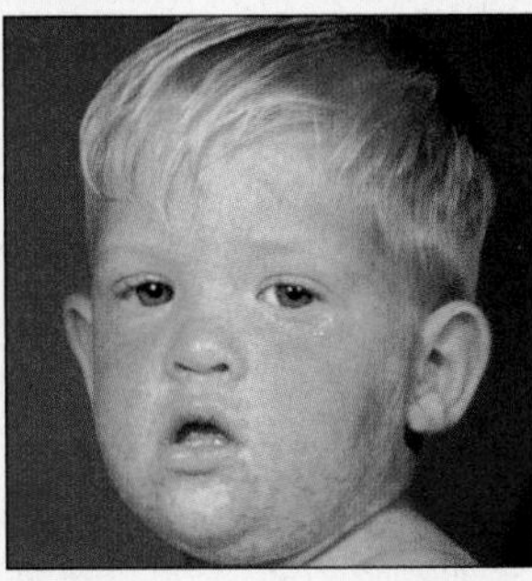
A

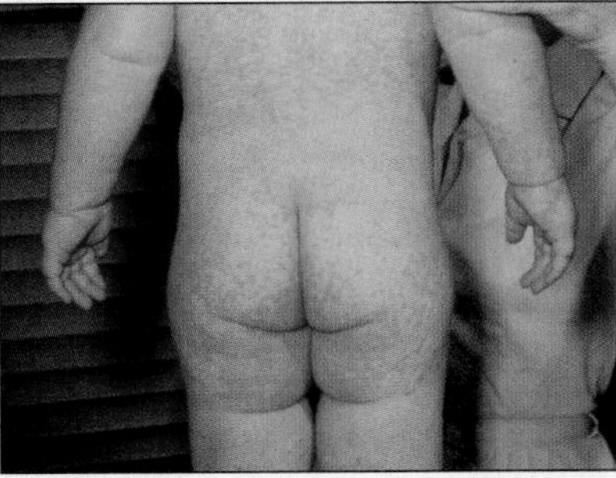
B

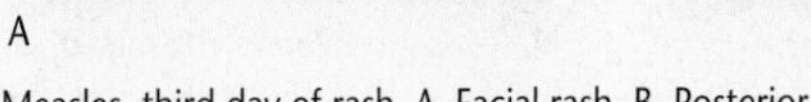
Measles, third day of rash. A, Facial rash. B. Posterior view.

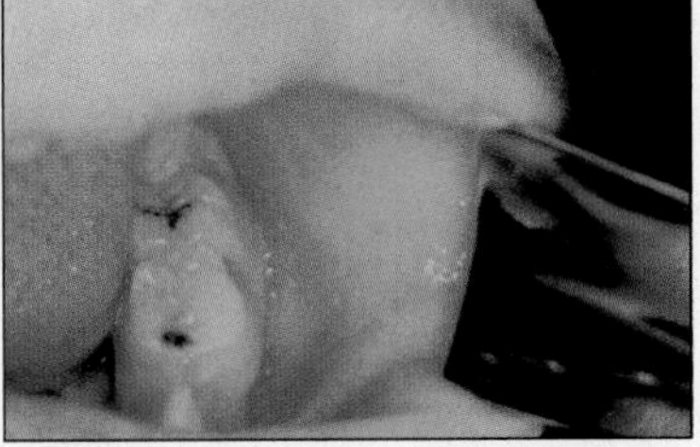
Koplik spots on oral mucosa, fifth day of rash. *Courtesy of Centers for Disease Control and Prevention, Atlanta, GA.*

(continued)

TABLE 12-5 Selected Infectious and Communicable Diseases in Children (continued)

DISEASE	CLINICAL MANIFESTATIONS	CLINICAL THERAPY	NURSING MANAGEMENT
Mononucleosis *Causal agent:* Epstein-Barr virus (EBV), a member of the herpesvirus group. *Epidemiology:* Occurs worldwide. In developing countries, the disease occurs in young children and may be asymptomatic or mild. In developed countries, the disease is more common in older children and adolescents. *Transmission:* Direct contact with infected oropharyngeal and genital tract secretions. EBV can also be transmitted by blood transfusion. *Incubation period:* 30–50 days. *Period of communicability:* Virus is shed for up to 18 months after the clinical course of the disease.	In very young children mononucleosis may cause irritability, but be otherwise asymptomatic. A maculopapular rash may be seen in a few cases. In other children, the disease is characterized by malaise, headache, anorexia, abdominal pain, fatigue, and fever for 2–3 days, followed by lymphadenopathy and a sore throat. Hepatosplenomegaly may occur. Pain from swelling of the tonsils and lymph nodes may be significant. The syndrome typically lasts 2–3 weeks and is self-limited. *Complications:* Rare side effects include central nervous system symptoms such as encephalitis, aseptic meningitis, and Guillain-Barre syndrome. Splenic rupture, respiratory failure, and hematologic complications such as thrombocytopenia can also occur. In immunodeficient children, fatal infections or lymphomas can develop.	There is no specific treatment. Corticosteroids may be used to control tonsillar swelling and pain when there is impending airway obstruction. Antibiotics (penicillin or erythromycin) are used for secondary infections. A rash may develop with antibiotic treatment (Sullivan, 1999). *Prognosis:* After recovery, the virus remains latent in the lymphoid system. It can be reactivated during periods of immunosuppression. The child will be a virus carrier for life. *Prevention:* No known prevention.	■ Children are usually treated at home. Standard precautions should be used. ■ Give antipyretics and analgesics for fever and sore throat. Offer warm saltwater for gargling. Offer soft foods and encourage fluids. ■ Maintain bedrest. ■ Give adolescents a sense of responsibility by involving them in decisions about care whenever possible. Be sure to include parents and adolescents in discussions. ■ Reassure adolescents who may be worried about keeping up with schoolwork that they can return to school when the fever is gone and swallowing is normal. ■ Teens should avoid kissing until the fever has been gone several days. ■ Contact sports should be avoided until the liver and spleen are normal, usually in about 4 weeks.
Mumps (Parotitis)† *Causal agent:* A paramyxovirus. *Epidemiology:* Occurs worldwide in unvaccinated children, most often in winter and spring. Infection and vaccination induce lifelong immunity. Maternal antibodies begin to disappear in infants at the age of 12–15 months. *Transmission:* Saliva droplets and direct contact. *Incubation period:* 12–25 days. *Period of communicability:* 7 days before parotid swelling until 9 days after swelling subsides.	Malaise; low-grade fever; and earache, headache, malaise, pain with chewing, decreased appetite and activity; followed by bilateral or unilateral parotid gland swelling. Swelling peaks around the third day. Meningeal signs (stiff neck, headache, photophobia) occur in about 15% of patients. *Complications:* Orchitis (inflammation of the epidydimis, pain on testicular palpation, and scrotal swelling—most often unilateral) may occur in postpubertal males; sterility is relatively rare (Taber & Demmler, 1999). Oophoritis, pancreatitis, aseptic meningoencephalitis, and unilateral permanent deafness are sometimes seen.	There is no specific treatment. Therapy is supportive, focused on symptom relief. *Prognosis:* Mumps is usually self-limiting. *Prevention:* Mumps is a vaccine-preventable disease. The vaccine is usually administered in combination with measles and rubella vaccines (MMR) at 12–15 months of age and again at either 4–6 years or 11–12 years. This is a reportable disease.	■ Children are generally uncomfortable but are rarely very ill. They are usually cared for at home. ■ Use droplet precautions for hospitalized children while contagious. Avoid exposure to immunocompromised individuals or susceptible persons. ■ Keep children out of school or child care until all symptoms subside. Encourage diversional activities. ■ Give nonaspirin analgesics and antipyretics to control fever and pain. Give steroids if ordered. Encourage fluid intake. Swallowing and chewing may be painful. Offer soft and blended foods. Avoid foods and beverages that increase salivary flow (citrus, spices, and candies) because they cause pain. ■ Talking may be painful. Provide a bell or other attention-getting device. ■ Apply warm or cool compresses, whichever is preferred, to the parotid area. ■ Be alert for signs of complications. Headache, stiff neck, vomiting, and photophobia may indicate meningeal irritation. ■ Provide scrotal supports if testicular swelling occurs. ■ Reassure children who may be upset about the facial swelling that it will go away.

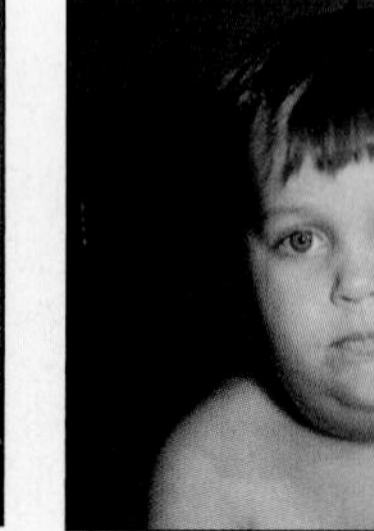

A B

This child has mumps with diffuse lymphedema of the neck. A, Side view. B, Front view.
Courtesy of Centers for Disease Control and Prevention, Atlanta, GA.

TABLE 12-5 Selected Infectious and Communicable Diseases in Children (continued)

DISEASE	CLINICAL MANIFESTATIONS	CLINICAL THERAPY	NURSING MANAGEMENT
Pertussis (Whooping Cough)† *Causal agent:* Bordetella pertussis. *Epidemiology:* Occurs worldwide. Predominantly a childhood disease that is most common in children under 6 months of age. Epidemic cycles occur every 2–5 years. Pertussis also occurs in health care workers or adults who may have weakened or incomplete immunity. Adults may become only mildly ill but can spread the disease to unimmunized children. *Transmission:* Respiratory droplets and direct contact with discharge from the respiratory membranes. *Incubation period:* 7–21 days (commonly 7–10 days). *Period of communicability:* Begins approximately 1 week after exposure. Pertussis is communicable for 5–7 days after the initiation of antibiotic therapy. The disease is most contagious before the paroxysmal cough stage.	The onset is insidious. The disease begins with a runny nose, followed by an irregular, nonproductive cough. The cough becomes more severe at night and changes into spasms of paroxysmal coughing followed by inspiration, stridor, or "whooping." (Young infants do not manifest the "whooping.") The whoop sound results from forceful inhalation and a narrowed glottis. Sucking on a bottle may trigger the coughing spell. May be accompanied by flushing, cyanosis, vomiting, profuse drainage from the nose, eyes, and mouth. Dehydration may result from decreased oral intake. Paroxysmal coughing may last 1–4 weeks or more. *Complications:* Pneumonia, atelectasis, otitis media, and seizures.	Treatment consists of antibiotics (erythromycin and other macrolides), corticosteroids, if ordered, and supportive care. *Prognosis:* The disease is most severe in infants under 1 year of age, and most deaths occur in this age group. *Prevention:* Pertussis is a vaccine-preventable disease. Active immunization should be given in early infancy. Health care professionals who are in close contact with infected children before diagnosis may need antibiotics to prevent transmission. This is a reportable disease.	■ Use droplet precautions until 5–7 days after the initiation of antibiotics. Most hospitalized cases occur in children under the age of 5 years. ■ Closely monitor respirations and oxygen saturation. The smaller the child, the greater the risk for respiratory distress and apnea. ■ Remain with the child during coughing spells, when hypoxic and apneic episodes are most likely. Give oxygen if ordered. Have emergency equipment available. ■ Provide humidification. Gentle suctioning may be necessary. ■ Give nonaspirin antipyretics as needed for fever. ■ Encourage frequent rest periods. ■ Allow the child to eat desired foods. ■ Encourage the child to take fluids. The child may need IV hydration if oral intake is not tolerated. ■ Provide emotional support to parents. ■ Teach parents to watch for signs of respiratory failure and dehydration if the child is managed at home.
Pneumococcal infection† *Causative agent:* Streptococcus pneumoniae, a gram-positive diplococcus. *Epidemiology:* The organism is found in the pharynx of healthy people. Outbreaks occur in the winter and spring when people are more crowded in physical settings. In temperate climates, six serotypes account for most of the infections found in children. The disease is more common in African Americans, American Indians, and Native Alaskans. It occurs most commonly in the 6-month to 2-year age group. Of particular concern is the development of penicillin and multiantibiotic-resistant strains. *Transmission:* Respiratory secretions, and droplets. Upper respiratory infections help the spread. *Incubation period:* 1–3 days. *Period of communicability:* Unknown. Probably less than 24 hours after initiation of effective antibiotic therapy.	The signs and symptoms are related to the focal area of infection. The organism causes otitis media, sinusitis, pharyngitis, laryngotracheobronchitis, pneumonia, meningitis, and bacteremia. In otitis media, upper respiratory infection, fever, ear pain, and decreased appetite are seen. In bacteremia, there is unexplained fever and no localized infection site. In pneumonia, fever, chills, chest pain, dyspnea, malaise, and a productive cough are seen. In meningitis, inconsolable crying, increased irritability, lethargy, refusal to eat, nausea, vomiting, diarrhea, myalgia, photophobia, and seizures are seen. *Complications:* This organism is one of the leading causes of morbidity and mortality. It causes 85% of bacteremia, is the leading cause of meningitis, and is responsible for 40% of acute otitis media (Rennels, 1999). Other complications include septic arthritis, osteomyelitis, endocarditis, and brain abscess.	Penicillin is given for penicillin-sensitive strains, but up to 48% of infections are penicillin resistant. Macrolide antibiotics are used for mild disease if the child is allergic to penicillin. Penicillin-resistant strains are treated with third-generation cephalosporins (cefotaxime or ceftriaxone). Vancomycin and rifampen are used in combination when strains are resistant to antibiotics listed above (American Academy of Pediatrics, 2000). Symptomatic care is also provided. *Prognosis:* With rapid diagnosis and treatment recovery is generally good, but highly dependent on disease the organism caused and resistance of organism to antibiotics. *Prevention:* Many serotypes are preventable with immunization. Active immunization should begin in infancy with the 7-valent vaccine (Prevnar). In studies testing the efficacy of the vaccine, the new pneumococcal conjugate vaccine resulted in significant reduction in pneumonia, meningitis, bacteremia, and otitis media (Rennels, Edwards, & Keyserling, 1998). A 23-valent vaccine is available for older children at high risk of pneumococcal disease.	■ If the child is hospitalized, maintain standard precautions. ■ Provide nonaspirin antipyretics for control of fever and comfort. ■ Encourage fluids, and monitor intake and output. ■ Monitor vital signs and consciousness level to identify signs of worsening condition. ■ Educate parents about the need for the vaccine, as the unimmunized child could become infected with another serotype. ■ Many children with mild disease will be treated at home. Educate parents about signs indicating a need to seek additional medical care, the need for proper medication administration, and comfort measures for the child.

(continued)

TABLE 12-5 Selected Infectious and Communicable Diseases in Children (continued)

DISEASE	CLINICAL MANIFESTATIONS	CLINICAL THERAPY	NURSING MANAGEMENT
Poliomyelitis† *Causal agent:* There are three serotypes of poliovirus. *Epidemiology:* Occurs worldwide. Polio primarily affects children, although some cases involve transmission to immunocompromised or non-polio-protected adults caring for infants who had received live polio virus vaccine. The disease can be mild or severe. The vaccine induces lifelong immunity. The live poliovirus vaccine was associated with paralytic disease and is no longer recommended for routine immunization in the United States. *Transmission:* Primarily by the fecal-oral route, possibly respiratory. *Incubation period:* Usually 7–10 days (range 3–36 days). *Period of communicability:* Unknown. Infectious for up to several weeks before symptoms develop. The virus is shed in pharyngeal secretions for a few days and in the stool for several weeks.	Affects the central nervous system. Less severe infections may be limited to fever and stiffness in the neck and back, headache, vomiting, and sore throat. In other cases, fever, headache, stiff neck, Kernig or Brudzinski sign, decreased deep tendon reflexes, and progressive weakness occur. There may be respiratory difficulties, and an increased respiratory rate that may interfere with the ability to talk because frequent pauses are needed. Onset of paralysis may be sudden, in hours, or gradual over 3–5 days. Paralysis results from damage to neurons. *Complications:* Permanent motor paralysis, respiratory arrest, myocardial failure, aseptic meningitis, and post-polio syndrome.	Treatment is supportive. No chemotherapeutic agents that directly kill the polio virus are available. *Prognosis:* Respiratory complication is life threatening and involves 5%–10% of all cases. Respiratory paralysis may lead to death. *Prevention:* Poliomyelitis is a vaccine-preventable disease. Children should be immunized with the inactivated poliovirus vaccine (IPV) according to the recommended schedule. This is a reportable disease.	■ Use standard and droplet precautions in the hospital and keep the child on strict bedrest. ■ Observe closely for respiratory paralysis (ineffective cough, talking with frequent pauses, shallow and rapid respiratory rate). Have emergency equipment at bedside. Assist ventilations as needed until mechanical ventilation is set up. ■ Administer sedatives and nonaspirin analgesics as ordered to allow for rest and comfort. Most hot packs may relieve discomfort. ■ Encourage fluids. ■ Position the child to promote body alignment. ■ Perform range-of-motion exercises to prevent contractures after the acute phase. ■ Provide emotional support. ■ Patients are alert and aware. Tell them what is happening to them. ■ Long-term orthopedic (physical therapy) support may be needed by some children.
Rabies (Hydrophobia)* *Causal agent:* Rhabdoviridae, two types (urban, in dogs; wild, in wildlife). *Epidemiology:* Occurs worldwide. Urban rabies is generally controlled by vaccination of domestic animals susceptible to the infection, especially dogs and cats. Rabies can occur in many wild animals, particularly bats, foxes, skunks, and raccoons. *Transmission:* Infected saliva from bite of rabid animal. Virus enters the wound and travels along the nerves from point of entry to the brain where it multiplies and migrates along the efferent nerves to the salivary glands.	Children may be free of symptoms during the long incubation period. Initial acute symptoms include pain or paresthesia at the site of exposure along with headache, fever, loss of appetite, and malaise. Painful contractures in the muscles used for swallowing lead to hydrophobia (50% of patients), a reflex contraction at the sight of liquid. Neurologic symptoms such as hallucinations, disorientation, periods of excitability (mania) and quiet, and seizures later occur. Some patients may have confusion with or without agitation with progression to stupor and coma. Symptoms last about 2 weeks.	Immediately wash animal bites thoroughly with soap and water and irrigate well. Suturing should be avoided if possible. Human rabies immune globulin (HRIG) and human diploid cell rabies vaccine (HDCV) should be given to all persons bitten by animals that may be rabid. Half of the HRIG is infiltrated around the wound and the remainder is given IM. HRIG and HDCV can be delayed 48 hours if testing of the animal's brain is done (Phelps, 1997). The vaccine is of no value once rabies symptoms are present. *Prognosis:* If symptoms develop, no drug improves the prognosis.	■ Administer HRIG and HDCV as ordered. Assist family with obtaining help to find and quarantine the animal for observation. ■ Provide emotional support to the family while reinforcing the urgency for the vaccine and the need for a series of injections. ■ Inform parents and the child about the side effects of the vaccine—irritation at the injection site, itching, headache, muscle aches, nausea, and dizziness. ■ If the child acquires rabies, he or she will be hospitalized.

*Indicates that a vaccine or antitoxin is available for use in high-risk or as-needed situations.
†Indicates that the disease has a safe and effective vaccine.

CLINICAL TIP

Any animal suspected of having rabies should be quarantined, if possible (Phelps, 1997). Rabies is diagnosed on the basis of history and clinical symptoms. The importance of history cannot be underestimated. Diagnosis is usually confirmed by fluorescent antibody staining of the dead animal's brain tissue.

TABLE 12-5 Selected Infectious and Communicable Diseases in Children (continued)

DISEASE	CLINICAL MANIFESTATIONS	CLINICAL THERAPY	NURSING MANAGEMENT
Rabies (Hydrophobia)* (continued) *Incubation period:* Highly variable (3–7 weeks); average 6 weeks. This period depends on the amount of virus in the saliva, how close to the brain or major nerves the bite occurred, and how deeply the saliva penetrated the skin.	*Complications:* Usually results in death.	*Prevention:* Postexposure prophylaxis with HRIG and HDCV should be given as soon as possible after exposure. HDCV is repeated on days 3, 7, 14, and 28 after the bite (5 doses). The HDCV series may be stopped if the animal is found free of rabies. Expert advice on the administration of these vaccines is available from state and local health officials. Prevention also includes immunizing all domestic animals against rabies. Teach children to avoid contact with all unknown animals, dead or alive.	■ Institute standard and contact precautions. The virus is transmitted primarily in the saliva and cerebrospinal fluid. ■ Make the child as comfortable as possible. ■ Keep liquids out of sight of the hydrophobic child. ■ Use caution in the late stages of the disease when children are usually combative. Various medications, paralyzing agents, and sedatives may be used to provide relief. Coma and death occur after an exhaustive period of excitement and agitation that may last for days. ■ Provide emotional support to the family of the dying child.
Rocky Mountain Spotted Fever (Tickborne Typhus Fever, Sao Paulo Typhus) *Causal agent: Rickettsia rickettii,* a bacterium that is transmitted by infected ticks. *Epidemiology:* Rocky Mountain spotted fever (RMSF) occurs in most of the United States, southwestern Canada, and Mexico. In the United States, cases are most prevalent in the southeastern region. Nearly half of all cases occur in Oklahoma, North Carolina, South Carolina, and Tennessee, generally between April and September. Most infections occur in children who are less than 15 years of age. Infection induces immunity. *Transmission:* Transmitted by bites of ticks, principally dog ticks. There is no evidence of person-to-person transmission. *Incubation period:* 2–8 days (most commonly 7 days) after bite of an infected tick.	RMSF is a multisystem disease that can be mild, moderate, or severe. Onset may be gradual or rapid. Children may be very ill. Sudden onset is characterized by a moderate-to-high fever (40°C) that ordinarily lasts for 2–3 weeks, significant malaise, deep muscle pain, persistent headache, chills, and conjunctival injection. The characteristic rash, which usually appears between the third and fifth days, starts on the extremities, including the palms and soles, and moves to the trunk. Initially the rash is maculopapular and blanches with pressure. It later becomes petechial and more defined; it is rarely pruritic. The child may have splenomegaly, hepatomegaly, and jaundice. *Complications:* In severe cases bleeding from disseminated intravascular coagulation (DIC) can be significant. Gastrointestinal symptoms often occur early in the disease. Pulmonary complications, especially pneumonitis, are common and can become life threatening. Central nervous system involvement can cause significant encephalitis and overall severe neurologic dysfunction. Cardiac and renal complications can also occur, leading to shock in severe cases.	Treatment consists of antibiotics, such as chloramphenicol and doxycycline. *Prognosis:* Without early recognition and treatment, morbidity is significant and mortality in children is 4%–7% (Feigin & Bloom, 1999). If the rash occurs late or not at all, the disease is likely to be more severe. *Prevention:* Avoid areas that are heavily tick infested, and wear protective clothing. Check for ticks and if found remove promptly. Infected ticks must be attached and feeding for 4–6 hours to transmit the disease. Seek medical attention promptly for a child who has been bitten and becomes symptomatic.	■ Use standard precautions. ■ Children may require prolonged hospitalization, including monitoring in the intensive care unit. ■ Have hemodynamic monitoring equipment and emergency supplies readily available. ■ Administer antibiotics as ordered. ■ Observe for any abnormal bleeding. ■ Make the child as comfortable as possible. If the child is unconscious, support the extremities and keep the eyes closed and lubricated. ■ Provide quiet diversional activities. ■ Provide emotional support, and keep parents informed about the child's condition. 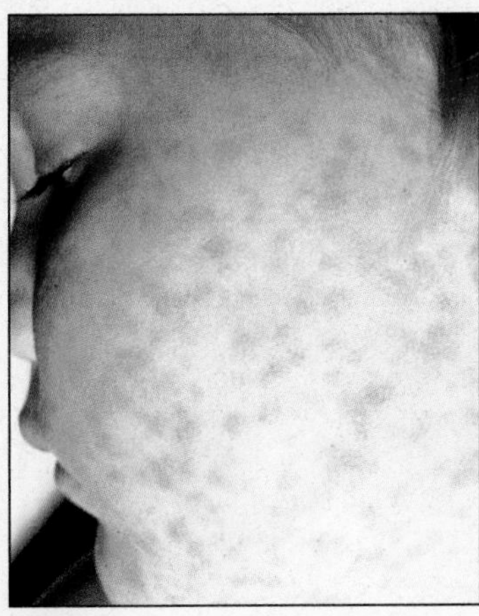 Rash of Rocky Mountain spotted fever.

(continued)

TABLE 12-5 Selected Infectious and Communicable Diseases in Children (continued)

DISEASE	CLINICAL MANIFESTATIONS	CLINICAL THERAPY	NURSING MANAGEMENT
Roseola (Exanthem Subitum) *Causal agent:* Herpesvirus type 6 *Epidemiology:* Occurs worldwide, primarily in children 6–24 months of age during the spring and summer months. Maternal antibodies are present in infants at birth. *Transmission:* Unknown. A latent virus is probably shed by a caregiver in saliva. *Incubation period:* Appears to be 5–15 days. *Period of communicability:* Unknown, probably infectious but person-to-person spread is not reported.	Sudden, high fever up to 40.5°C (105°F) for 3–8 days, during which the child does not appear toxic (normal appetite and behavior). The fever phase is followed by a characteristic pale pink, discrete, maculopapular rash, which starts on the trunk and spreads to the face, neck, and extremities. The rash can last for 1–2 days. The child's appetite is normal. *Complications:* Children may have febrile seizures.	Roseola is self-limiting, and there is no treatment other than supportive care. *Prognosis:* Roseola is benign in most cases. *Prevention:* None	■ Children are rarely hospitalized, but if they are, use standard precautions. ■ Give nonaspirin antipyretics to control fever. ■ Observe closely for any seizure activity, especially during the acute febrile periods. ■ Encourage fluids. ■ Reassure parents that the rash will disappear in a few days.
Rubella (German Measles)† *Causal agent:* An RNA virus, member of the family Togaviridae, genus Rubivirus. *Epidemiology:* Occurs worldwide and is most prevalent in the winter and spring. Children are susceptible after loss of transplacentally acquired maternal antibodies about 6–9 months after birth. Natural infection or vaccination induces lifelong immunity. Most cases occur in the adults older than 20 years. Congenital rubella syndrome is most likely the result of lack of immunization rather than vaccine failure. Rates of congenital rubella syndrome have increased since 1989 because 25% of postpubertal women lack antibody to rubella virus (Taber & Demmler, 1999). *Transmission:* Droplet spread, direct contact with infected persons, or contact with articles soiled by nasal secretions. *Incubation period:* 14–21 days (most commonly 16–18 days). *Period of communicability:* From about 7 days before until about 4 days after the onset of the rash. Infants with congenital rubella may shed the virus for months after birth and should not be exposed or cared for by persons who are not immune to the disease. Discrete maculopapular erythematous rash of rubella.	Rubella is generally a mild disease with a characteristic pink, nonconfluent, maculopapular rash. The rash appears on the face, progresses to the neck, trunk, and legs, and disappears in the same order. Prodromal symptoms occur 1–5 days before the rash and include low-grade fever, headache, malaise, coryza, sore throat, and anorexia. Forschheimer spots (discrete, erythematous pinpoint or larger lesions on the soft palate) are seen during the prodromal phase. Generalized lymphadenopathy involving the postauricular, suboccipital, and posterior cervical areas is common up to 7 days before the rash. *Complications:* Rare, but include arthritis in adolescents, encephalitis, and congenital rubella syndrome. 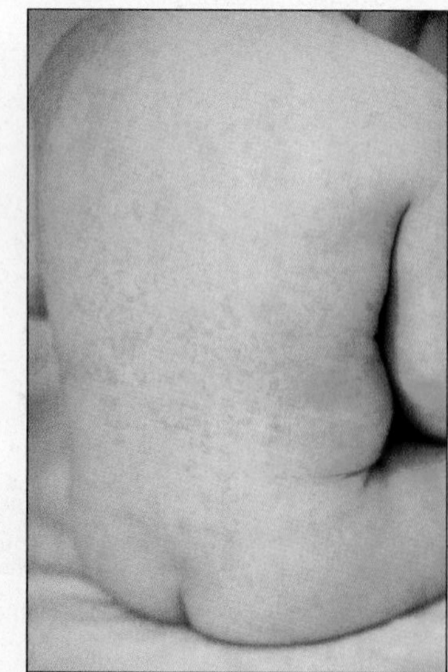	Treatment is supportive. Rubella is generally self-limiting in children. *Prognosis:* Disease is usually mild and benign. Major risk is for fetus if the mother is infected in the first trimester. Spontaneous abortion, stillbirth, or fetal death are common (10% die after birth). Many other anomalies may be present, such as intrauterine growth retardation, cardiac, ear, and eye deficits. *Prevention:* Rubella is a vaccine-preventable disease. It is important that females of childbearing age be immunized because of the severe complications rubella poses to the fetus during the first trimester. All health care workers should have documented immunity.	■ Children are usually treated at home and rarely require hospitalization. They should not attend school or child care while contagious, and they should be isolated from pregnant women. School and child care facilities should be notified of the child's illness. ■ Maintain droplet precautions for contagious children. Maintain contact precautions for infants with congenital rubella syndrome until 1 year of age (American Academy of Pediatrics, 2000). ■ Give nonaspirin analgesics and antipyretics for any pain and fever. ■ Allow children to choose what they would like to eat and drink. Encourage fluids. ■ Provide quiet activities.

TABLE 12-5 Selected Infectious and Communicable Diseases in Children (continued)

DISEASE	CLINICAL MANIFESTATIONS	CLINICAL THERAPY	NURSING MANAGEMENT
Streptococcus *Causal agent:* Group A streptococci (GAS). *Epidemiology:* The illness is caused by various M- protein groups of group A alpha- and beta- hemolytic streptococci. In recent years severe infections have appeared, in some cases threatening life and limb. Different strains are associated with pharyngeal and pyodermal infections. Pharyngeal infections tend to occur more in late fall, winter, and spring. Pyodermal infections tend to occur in warmer seasons because of the association with minor skin trauma and insect bites. *Transmission:* Airborne respiratory droplets, and direct contact. *Incubation period:* Pharyngeal: usually 2–5 days; Pyodermal: usually 7–10 days. *Period of communicability:* For weeks in untreated pharyngeal infections. The child is most contagious during the acute stage of the illness.	*Pharyngeal:* Onset is abrupt, with a sore throat, dysphagia, malaise, high fever, chills, headache, abdominal pain, anorexia, and vomiting. A beefy red pharynx with exudate (strep throat) and tender cervical nodes are present. Palatal petechia may be seen. A characteristic erythematous rash associated with scarlet fever appears in some cases 12–48 hours after onset of symptoms, starting on the neck and spreading to the trunk and extremities. In 3–4 days, the rash begins to fade and the tips of the toes and fingers begin to peel. The classic strawberry tongue is seen on day 4–5. *Pyodermal:* Lesions (impetigo) are honey-colored crusts at the site of open lesions. *Complications:* If untreated, retropharyngeal abscess, cervical lymphadenitis, acute rheumatic fever, acute glomerulonephritis, toxic shock syndrome, bacteremia, and necrotizing fascitis or myositis can occur.	Prompt antibiotic treatment is effective. Penicillin is the drug of choice. Erythromycin is used if the child is allergic to penicillin. The fever decreases after treatment is begun. Uncomplicated impetigo is treated with bacitracin or mupirocin ointment. Invasive strains causing necrotizing fasciitis or myositis need surgical intervention (exploration and debridement of dead tissue). Clindamycin may be needed for toxic shock syndrome and necrotizing fasciitis (McMillan & Feigin, 1999). *Prognosis:* Recovery is usually good with antibiotic therapy. Ten to 20% of school-age children become chronic carriers. *Prevention:* None.	■ Children with uncomplicated streptoccocal infections are usually cared for at home. Promote bedrest during the febrile stage. Give nonaspirin antipyretics to control fever. Teach parents important signs of a worsening condition. ■ For pharyngeal infections, offer warm saltwater for gargling; a soft diet and nonacidic beverages. Encourage fluids. Provide cool, clear liquids. Swallowing may be difficult. ■ Explain to parents the importance of the child's taking antibiotics for the full number of days prescribed. ■ Encourage other family members with sore throats to have throat cultures taken. ■ For impetigo, teach the parents to wash the skin, remove crusts, and apply antibiotic ointment. If the child is hospitalized, maintain droplet precautions for pharyngeal infections and contact precautions for skin lesions for 24 hours after beginning antibiotics. Monitor vital signs, especially temperature. Administer antibiotics as ordered. ■ If the child develops invasive streptococcal infection, use standard precautions. The child with toxic shock syndrome will need intensive care to manage shock and fluid and electrolyte imbalances.

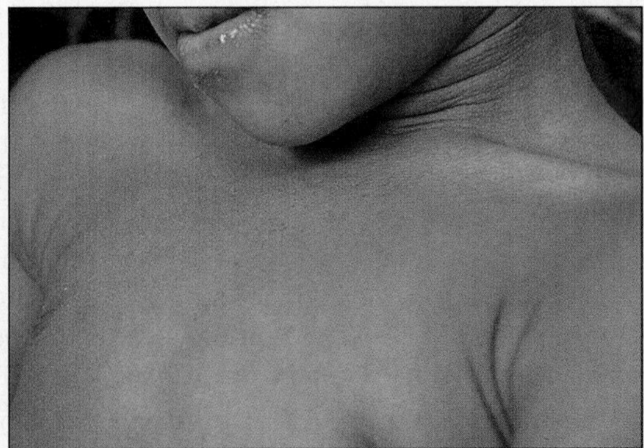

Skin rash of scarlet fever.

*Indicates that a vaccine or antitoxin is available for use in high-risk or as-needed situations.
†Indicates that the disease has a safe and effective vaccine.

(continued)

TABLE 12-5 Selected Infectious and Communicable Diseases in Children (continued)

DISEASE	CLINICAL MANIFESTATIONS	CLINICAL THERAPY	NURSING MANAGEMENT
Tetanus *Causal agent: Clostridium tetani* or tetanus bacillus. *Epidemiology:* The bacillus is common and exists as a spore in soil, dust, and animal excretions. The organism produces an endotoxin that affects the central nervous system. *Transmission:* The organism is transmitted to humans through wounds in the skin from contact with contaminated soil or implements. Newborns can acquire tetanus via the umbilical cord if they are born in an unclean area or if a contaminated implement is used to cut the cord. *Incubation period:* 3 days–3 weeks (average 8 days). *Period of communicability:* Not communicable to other individuals except through skin wounds.	Stiffness of the neck and jaw, with painful facial spasms and difficulty swallowing over a few days. Noise or sudden movement may stimulate spasms. Localized prolonged and painful muscle contraction may occur at the site of the wound, and eventual rigidity of the abdomen and trunk. There is difficulty swallowing the increased oral secretions. Newborns have difficulty with sucking, progressing to an inability to suck, irritability, and nuchal rigidity. *Complications:* Laryngospasm, respiratory distress, death.	Tetanus immune globulin is given to unimmunized persons as soon as possible. Tetanus toxoid is given at the same time in a separate site. Medications are provided to treat muscle spasms. Intensive care is provided with cardiorespiratory monitoring, assisted ventilation, IV metronidazole or penicillin G, nutrition, and supportive care. Survival beyond 4 days indicates an increased chance of recovery. Paroxysms become less frequent and complete recovery may take weeks. *Prognosis:* 30% mortality; much higher in newborns. Intensive care has improved mortality. *Prevention:* Tetanus immunizations are routinely given. They must be updated every 10 years, or, if a potentially contaminated wound occurs, in 5 years. Proper surgical debridement of wounds decreases the chance of infection.	■ Prevent disease by checking immunization records and administering immunizations as necessary. ■ Give immune globulin to unimmunized persons. ■ Assist with wound debridement. ■ The child with tetanus is hospitalized. Use standard precautions. ■ Monitor the child's condition. Handle as little as possible. Reduce stimulation by placing child in a quiet, darkened room. ■ Offer skin and respiratory care. The child may need an endotracheal tube, suctioning, and supplemental oxygen for airway support. ■ Provide feedings via total parenteral nutrition or feeding tube. ■ Maintain hydration with IV fluids and electrolytes. ■ Try to reduce the child's anxiety, as mental status may be unaffected. ■ Prepare the family for a possible poor prognosis.
Tuberculosis **See Chapter 13**			

Skills 5-11 to 5-14: Body Temperature

CLINICAL THERAPY

Diagnostic tests include cultures from sites where the infection may potentially be located (skin, pharynx, blood, urine, feces, cerebrospinal fluid, etc.). In some cases, x-rays or special imaging may be used to identify localized infection in an organ such as the lungs.

For many infectious and communicable diseases, management is supportive. An elevated temperature can be a beneficial physiologic response, helping to eradicate organisms that thrive at lower body temperatures, and mobilizing the immune response. It may also enhance the effect of antibiotics. In addition, fever decreases the plasma iron concentration, which may limit the growth of microorganisms (Cimpella et al., 2000). Fever is not inherently harmful until it reaches 41°C (105.9°F). For this reason, medical management may include postponing treatment of low-grade fevers under 38.9°C (102°F) to promote the body's natural defenses against an infection. If not managed, elevated temperatures can result in febrile seizures, which usually have no long-term sequelae. Thus, fevers greater than 38.9°C (102°F) should be treated, especially if associated with discomfort. Persistent temperatures of 38.3–38.5°C (101–101.5°F) may also benefit from antipyretic treatment. Acetaminophen and ibuprofen are the preferred antipyretics for children. Aspirin is no longer recommended for children because of its association with Reye syndrome.

Administration of antibiotics is often another component of clinical therapy for infectious diseases. Before the introduction of antibiotics, children were often unable to fight infection and died as the result of overwhelming sepsis. Antibiotics have been responsible for decreases in morbidity and mortality from infections among children. However, strains of bacteria have developed resistance to many antibiotics. Children with chronic illnesses such as cystic fibrosis, sickle-cell disease, and acquired immunodeficiency syndrome (AIDS) are particularly susceptible to infection by drug-resistant pathogens.

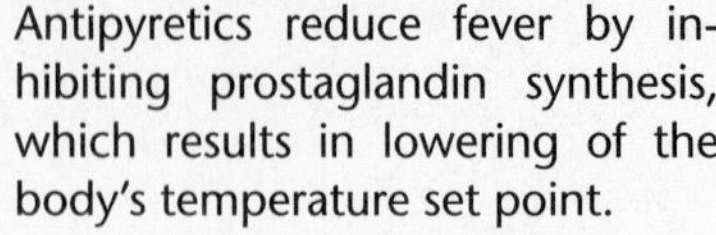

CLINICAL TIP

Antipyretics reduce fever by inhibiting prostaglandin synthesis, which results in lowering of the body's temperature set point.

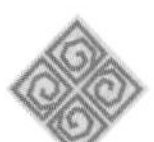

NURSING MANAGEMENT

Nursing Assessment and Diagnosis

Assess the child's hydration status and fluid intake, vital signs, comfort level, and appetite and observe for seizures and for a **toxic appearance** (lethargy, poor perfusion, hypoventilation or hyperventilation, and cyanosis). The child with a fever may be irritable and restless, sleep fitfully, and have nonspecific muscular pain. Identify those children who may be at higher risk for a serious illness in association with a fever, in particular (Thomas, 1995):

- Children having a toxic appearance
- Children less than 28 days of age with a temperature over 38°C (100.4°F)
- Children less than 4 years of age with a temperature over 41°C (105.8°F)
- Children with conditions such as a ventriculoperitoneal shunt, congenital heart disease, asplenia, and sickle-cell anemia

Observe the child for other signs of infection, such as a rash, nausea and vomiting, and/or diarrhea, as well as generalized symptoms of a poor appetite and malaise.

The following nursing diagnoses may be appropriate for children with infectious and communicable diseases:

- *Hyperthermia,* related to infectious disease process
- *Risk for fluid volume deficit,* related to hypermetabolic state
- *Impaired skin integrity,* related to hyperthermia and self-mutilation of skin lesions
- *Altered oral mucous membranes,* related to infectious disease process
- *Fluid volume deficit,* related to repeated episodes of vomiting and diarrhea
- *Ineffective management of therapeutic regimen (family),* related to complexity of therapeutic regimen

Planning and Implementation

Most children with infectious diseases are cared for at home; however, children may be evaluated in various health care settings.

Nursing care of children with infectious diseases in health care settings focuses on preventing the spread of infection. Children with suspicious rashes should be isolated from other children. When possible, hard surfaces in the examining room where the child was seen should be wiped down with antiseptic solution before another child uses the room. Linens are disposed of in appropriately marked linen bags.

Nursing care for treatment of fever includes administering antipyretics, removing unnecessary clothing, and encouraging increased fluid intake. Tepid baths or sponging may be ordered when the child's temperature is greater than 40°C (104°F) while waiting for the antipyretic to work. Use water that is about 26.6°C (80°F).

Children are often admitted to the hospital for treatment of severe infections. In addition, countless numbers of **nosocomial** (hospital-acquired) **infections** occur each year. The fecal–oral and respiratory routes are the most common sources of infections in children. All items with which the infected child comes into contact are considered contaminated (linens, toys, medical equipment, etc.). Transmission-based precautions, including isolation, must be implemented to reduce exposure of other children and staff to the infectious agent. Follow your facility's standard precautions and transmission-based precautions to reduce the spread of infectious diseases to staff and other patients. Bring any questions and concerns to your hospital's infection control nurse. (Refer to the Skills Manual for more detailed information.)

Involve the parents by allowing them to assist with their child's care. Nursing care also includes treating infection, administering antibiotics on schedule, monitoring antibiotic blood levels if indicated to ensure appropriate results, and educating parents.

CLINICAL TIP

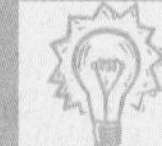

A study comparing methods of fever reduction in febrile children with temperatures of more than 38.9°C (102°F) found no significant differences in temperature reduction over a 2-hour period when the child was given acetaminophen alone or with a 15-minute tepid sponge bath. However, the children who were given sponge baths had significantly higher discomfort scores (Sharber, 1997).

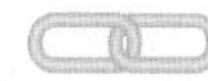

Infection Control Methods

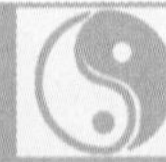

CULTURE

Many Latino and Asian cultures subscribe to the hot and cold theory of disease causation. Fever, a hot condition, is treated by giving the patient cold substances (foods or medicines). "Hot" and "cold" do not refer to temperature but to categories. Cold foods include vegetables, fruits, and fish. Cold medicines include orange flower water, linden, and sage. Ask parents how they think the illness should be treated. Encourage them to use that treatment as long as it is safe. Teach them additional western medicine treatments they can use.

CARE IN THE COMMUNITY

Teach parents to care for their child at home, including how and when to give antipyretics and antibiotics if ordered, what foods and beverages are appropriate, and how to care for rashes and other topical symptoms. Parents often fear fevers and need information and reassurance. Help them to recognize the signs of the child's worsening condition in association with the child's specific disease.

Correct any misconceptions parents and child care workers may have about the occurrence or cause of the infectious disease in their child. The parents and other providers may believe that they have exposed the child to certain germs or bacteria. Teach them that infection control will reduce exposure of other children and family members to the infectious disease. Following are specific infection-control measures that can be taken:

- Good handwashing is one of the best ways to decrease the spread of infection.
- Disinfect hard surfaces such as those touched by the child who has a cold, diaper changing areas, diaper pails, and cribs.
- Tell children not to kiss pets on the mouth.
- Remove toys that the child has mouthed and disinfect them before other children play with them.
- Make sure all children in the house are fully immunized.

Evaluation

Expected outcomes of nursing care include the following:

- Opportunities for spread of infection are minimized between patients and family members.
- The child's fever is effectively managed with antipyretics.

FAMILIES WANT TO KNOW

Guidelines for Evaluating and Treating Fever in Children

CALL YOUR HEALTH CARE PROVIDER IMMEDIATELY IF:

- The child is under 2 months old or has a fever over 40.1°C (104.2°F).
- The child is crying inconsolably or whimpering.
- The child cries when moved or otherwise touched by the parent or other family members.
- The child is difficult to awaken.
- The child's neck is stiff.
- There are any purple spots present on the skin.
- Breathing is difficult and no better after the nose is cleared.
- The child is drooling saliva and is unable to swallow anything.
- The child has a convulsion.
- The child acts or looks very sick.

CALL YOUR HEALTH CARE PROVIDER WITHIN 24 HOURS IF:

- The child is 2 to 4 months old (unless fever occurs within 48 hours of a DTP shot and the infant has no other serious symptoms).
- The fever is higher than 40.1°C (104.2°F) (especially if the child is under 3 years).
- The child complains of burning or pain with urination.
- The fever has been present more than 24 hours without an obvious cause or location of infection.
- The fever went away for more than 24 hours and then returned.
- The fever has been present for more than 72 hours.

TREATING THE FEVER

- Use acetaminophen or ibuprofen to lower a fever.
- Use the correct dose of the medication—drops and syrups do not have the same concentration.
- Ibuprofen lasts 1 to 2 hours longer than acetaminophen, so it may be given less often.
- Remove all but a light layer of the child's clothing to help lower the temperature.

Note: From Hay, W. W., Jr., Groothuis, J. R., Hayward, A. R., & Lewin, M. J. (Eds.). (1997). *Current pediatric diagnosis and treatment* (13th ed.) Stamford, CT: Appleton & Lange. Modified.

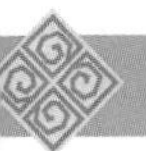

Chapter Highlights

- Infectious and communicable diseases remain a significant source of morbidity and mortality in children, especially in developing countries.
- Infants are especially vulnerable to infectious diseases because their immune system is immature, their passively acquired maternal antibodies are decreasing, and disease protection through immunization is not yet complete.
- For a child to acquire a communicable disease, an infectious agent or pathogen, an effective means of transmission, and a susceptible host need to be present.
- Major public health efforts that have decreased the occurrence of infectious and communicable diseases include safer drinking water, better sanitation, improved standards of living, and increased immunization.
- Vaccines must be given at specific ages and intervals. Immunization timing is related to decreasing maternal antibody protection, to the child's developing ability to make antibodies in response to a vaccine, and whether the vaccine provides lifelong immunity.
- Vaccines must be stored properly and administered appropriately to ensure their effectiveness.
- The National Childhood Vaccine Injury Act of 1986 provides compensation if a link between immunization and a serious adverse effect is found. The Vaccine Adverse Event Reporting System has been established to track serious vaccine reactions.
- Infectious and communicable diseases are caused by bacterial, viral, protozoan, or fungal organisms.
- Fever is often a sign of infectious disease in children. The hypothalamus functions as the body's thermostat, directing the body to conserve or dissipate heat. When microorganisms invade the body, endogenous pyrogens are released into the bloodstream. These substances travel to the hypothalamus, where they trigger the production and release of prostaglandins, which initiate the fever response.
- The child with a toxic or septic appearance has the following signs: lethargy, poor perfusion, tachypnea or bradypnea, and pallor or cyanosis.
- Infection control measures caregivers can take include the following: using good handwashing techniques, disinfecting hard surfaces touched by the child, telling children not to kiss pets, disinfecting toys the child has mouthed before letting other children play with them, and making sure all children are fully immunized.

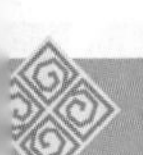

EXPLORE MediaLink

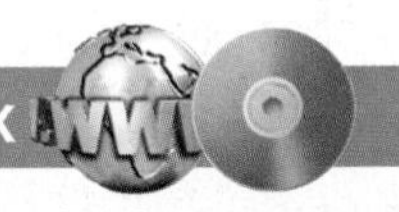

- NCLEX review, case studies, and other interactive resources for this chapter can be found on the Companion Website at **http://www.prenhall.com/ball.** Click on Chapter 12 to select the activities for this chapter.
- For animations, more NCLEX review questions, and an audio glossary, access the accompanying CD-ROM in this textbook.

References

1. Adams, D. M., & Ware, R. E. (1996). Parrovirus B19: How much should you worry? *Contemporary Pediatrics,* 13(4), 85–96.
2. American Academy of Pediatrics Committee on Infectious Disease. (2000). *Red Book: Report of the Committee on Infectious Disease* (25th ed.). Elk Grove Village, IL: Author.
3. Atkinson, W. L. (1999). Thimerosol. *Needle Tips and the Hepatitis B Coalition News,* 9(2), 1, 15.
4. Barat, L. M., & Zucker, J. R. (1999). Malaria. In J. A. McMillan, C. D. DeAngelis, R. D. Feigin, & J. B. Warshaw (Eds.), *Oski's pediatrics: Principles & practice* (3rd ed., pp. 1177–1184). Philadelphia: Lippincott, Williams & Wilkins.
5. Centers for Disease Control Advisory Committee on Immunization Practices. (2000). Use of diphtheria toxoid—tetanus toxoid—acellular pertussis vaccine in a 5-dose series. *Morbidity and Mortality Weekly Reports, 49*(RR-13); 1–7.
6. Centers for Disease Control Advisory Committee on Immunization Practices. (2001). Recommended childhood immunization schedule—United States, 2001, *Morbidity and Mortality Weekly Report, 50*(61), 7–10, 19.
7. Chang, L. Y., Lin, T. Y., Hsu, K. H., Huang, Y. C., Lin, K. L., et al. (1999). Clinical features and risk factors of pulmonary edema after Enterovirus 71–related hand, foot, and mouth disease. *Lancet, 354*(9191), 1682–1686.
8. Cherry, J. D. (1999). Parvoviruses. In J. A. McMillan, C. D. DeAngelis, R. D. Feigin, & J. B. Warshaw (Eds.), *Oski's pediatrics: Principles & practice* (3rd ed., pp. 1098–1100). Philadelphia: Lippincott, Williams & Wilkins.
9. Cimpella, L. B., Goldman, D. L., Khine, H. (2000). Fever pathophysiology. *Clinical Pediatric Emergency Medicine, 1*(2), 84–93.
10. Diggle, L., & Deek, J. (2000). Effect of needle length on incidence of local reactions to routine immunizations in infants aged 4 months: Randomized control trial. *British Medical Journal, 321*(7266), 931–933.
11. Feigin, R. D., & Bloom, M. L. (1999). Rickettsial disease. In J. A. McMillan, C. D. DeAngelis, R. D. Feigin, & J. B. Warshaw (Eds.), *Oski's pediatrics: Principles & practice* (3rd ed., pp. 898–902). Philadelphia: Lippincott, Williams & Wilkins.
12. Healy, T. L. (2000). The impact of Lyme disease on school children. *Journal of School Nursing, 16*(2), 12–18.

13. Jenkins, C. N. H., McPhee, S. J., Wong, C., Nguyen, T., & Euler, G. L. (2000). Hepatitis B immunization coverage among Vietnamese-American children 3 to 18 years old. *Pediatrics, 106*(6), 1–8.

14. Kaplan, S. L. (1999). Haemophilis influenzae. In J. A. McMillan, C. D. DeAngelis, R. D. Feigin, & J. B. Warshaw (Eds.), *Oski's pediatrics: Principles & practice* (3rd ed., pp. 969–973). Philadelphia: Lippincott, Williams & Wilkins.

15. McMillan, J. A., & Feigin, R. D. (1999). Group A streptococcal infections. In J. A. McMillan, C. D. DeAngelis, R. D. Feigin, & J. B. Warshaw (Eds.), *Oski's pediatrics: Principles & practice* (3rd ed., pp. 1012–1017), Philadelphia: Lippincott, Williams & Wilkins.

16. Phelps, R. (1997). Rabies: Confronting the continuing threat. *Contemporary Pediatrics, 14*(7), 137–150.

17. Rennels, M. B. (1999). Resistant pneumococcal disease: Treatment and prevention. *Contemporary Pediatrics.* (Suppl. 3), 4–10.

18. Rennels, M. B., Edwards, K. M., & Keyserling, H. L. (1998). Safety and immunogenicity of heptavalent pneumococcal vaccine conjugated to CRM in United States infants. *Pediatrics, 101*(4), 604–611.

19. Sharber, J. (1997). The efficacy of tepid sponge bathing to reduce fever in young children. *American Journal of Emergency Medicine, 15*(2), 211–213.

20. Sullivan, J. L. (1999). Epstein-Barr virus infection in children. In J. A. McMillan, C. D. DeAngelis, R. D. Feigin, & J. B. Warshaw (Eds.), *Oski's pediatrics: Principles & practice* (3rd ed., pp. 1107–1110). Philadelphia: Lippincott, Williams & Wilkins.

21. Taber, L. H., & Demmler, G. J. (1999). Mumps. In J. A. McMillan, C. D. DeAngelis, R. D. Feigin, & J. B. Warshaw (Eds.), *Oski's pediatrics: Principles & practice* (3rd ed., pp. 1141–1142). Philadelphia: Lippincott, Williams & Wilkins.

22. Taber, L. H., & Demmler, G. J. (1999). Rubella (German Measles). In J. A. McMillan, C. D. DeAngelis, R. D. Feigin, & J. B. Warshaw (Eds.), *Oski's pediatrics: Principles & practice* (3rd ed., pp. 1134–1137). Philadelphia: Lippincott, Williams & Wilkins.

23. Thomas, D. O. (1995). Fever in children: Friend or foe? *RN, 58*(4), 42–47.

24. Twomey, J. (1998). Varicella exposure in a child at risk of being immunosuppressed. *Pediatric Nursing, 23*(5), 459–464.

25. Wade, C. F. (2000). Keeping Lyme disease at bay: An integrated approach to prevention. *American Journal of Nursing, 100*(7), 26–31.

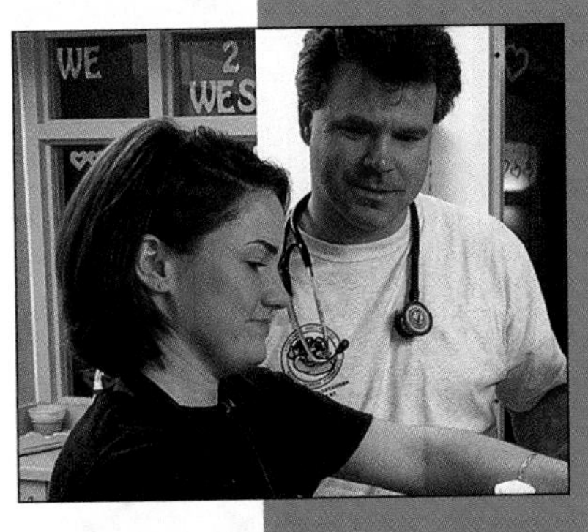

"DURING THE TRANSPORT, WE WILL BE MONITORING EMILY FOR SIGNS OF INCREASED RESPIRATORY DISTRESS THAT COULD BE CAUSED BY EXCESSIVE SECRETIONS OR A WORSENING CONDITION. IT IS SAFER TO TRANSPORT A CHILD WITH THESE PROBLEMS WITH ALL OF THE TREATMENT RESOURCES AT HAND, RATHER THAN LET THE MOTHER TAKE HER TO THE HOSPITAL BY CAR."

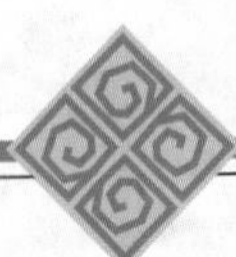

Emily, an 8-month-old infant with bronchopulmonary dysplasia, is cared for at home by her mother. She has a tracheostomy and receives humidification. When Emily develops a fever, more secretions than usual in the tracheostomy, and labored breathing, her mother arranges for an urgent care visit to the pediatrician. Emily's mother knows how important it is to obtain prompt treatment for her daughter's respiratory problems.

When Emily is seen by the pediatrician, her temperature is 38.8°C (102°F), her respiratory rate is 50, and her heart rate is 130. Intercostal and substernal retractions are visible, and crackles can be heard over the lower right lobe. The pediatrician decides that a chest x-ray is needed. Because of the potential for Emily's respiratory difficulty to worsen, he plans to have her observed in the hospital's 23-hour unit. Intravenous antibiotics may be needed if an infection is confirmed by x-ray. The hospital's transport team is called to take Emily from the office to the hospital.

The transport team takes Emily to the hospital in a car safety seat strapped to a stretcher. This promotes safe travel and provides the proper position to assist breathing. Oxygen is administered to prevent hypoxia. Suction is available if needed. The trip by ambulance to the hospital takes only 20 minutes.

Why are infants with bronchopulmonary dysplasia at higher risk for respiratory problems? What are the signs of respiratory distress? What nursing care is required when an infant experiences respiratory distress?

CHAPTER 13

ALTERATIONS IN RESPIRATORY FUNCTION

KEY TERMS

adventitious Breath sounds that are not normally heard, such as crackles and rhonchi.

airway resistance The effort or force needed to move oxygen through the trachea to the lungs.

alveolar hypoventilation The condition in which the volume of air entering the alveoli during gas exchange is inadequate to meet the body's metabolic needs.

apnea Cessation of respiration lasting longer than 20 seconds.

dysphonia Muffled, hoarse, or absent voice sounds.

dyspnea Shortness of breath; difficulty in breathing.

hypercapnia Greater than normal amounts of carbon dioxide in the blood.

hypoxemia Lower than normal amounts of oxygen in the blood.

hypoxia Lower than normal amounts of oxygen in the tissues.

laryngospasm Spasmodic vibrations of the larynx, which create sudden, violent, unpredictable, involuntary contraction of airway muscles.

paradoxical breathing Severe respiratory distress in which the chest falls and the abdomen rises on inspiration.

periodic breathing Pauses in respiration lasting less than 20 seconds; a normal breathing pattern in infancy and childhood.

retractions A visible drawing in of the skin of the neck and chest, which occurs on inhalation in infants and young children in respiratory distress.

stridor An abnormal, high-pitched musical respiratory sound caused when air moves through a narrowed larynx or trachea.

tachypnea An abnormally rapid rate of respiration.

trigger A stimulus that initiates an asthmatic episode; a substance or condition, including exercise, infection, allergy, irritants, weather, or emotions.

MediaLink 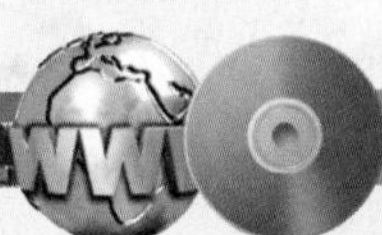 http://www.prenhall.com/ball

Resources for this chapter can be found on the CD-ROM accompanying this textbook, and on the Companion Website at http://www.prenhall.com/ball. Click on Chapter 13 to select the activities for this chapter.

CD-ROM

Audio Glossary

NCLEX Review

COMPANION WEBSITE

Web Links

NCLEX Review

MediaLink Applications

Teaching Plan: Metered Dose Inhaler

This chapter explores several special factors in the child's respiratory system that create ongoing threats to respiratory function and overall health. Most respiratory problems in children produce mild symptoms, last a short time, and can be managed at home. Nevertheless, acute respiratory problems are the most common cause of illness requiring hospitalization in infants and children under 15 years of age (Health Resources and Services Administration, 2000).

Pediatric respiratory conditions may occur as a primary problem or as a complication of nonrespiratory conditions and may be life threatening or have long-term implications. Nurses must learn to assess the child's current respiratory status quickly, monitor progress, and anticipate potential complications (Table 13-1).

Respiratory problems may be a result of structural problems, functional problems, or a combination of both. Structural problems involve alterations in the size and shape of parts of the respiratory tract. Functional problems involve alterations in gas exchange and threats to this normal process from irritants (such as large particles and chemicals) or invaders (such as viruses or bacteria). Alterations in other organ systems, especially the immune and neurologic systems, may also threaten respiratory function. As you read this chapter, keep the distinction between structural and functional problems in mind to help you understand what is normal and what is abnormal about the child's maturing respiratory system. Refer to Chapter 19 for information on upper respiratory tract infections.

TABLE 13-1 Assessment Guidelines for a Child in Respiratory Distress[a]

QUALITY OF RESPIRATIONS

- Inspect the rate, depth, and ease of respirations.
- Identify the signs of respiratory distress: tachypnea (abnormally rapid rate of respirations), retractions, nasal flaring, inspiratory stridor, expiratory grunting.
- Note lack of simultaneous chest and abdominal rise with inspiration (paradoxical breathing).
- Auscultate breath sounds: bilateral, diminished or absent, **adventitious** (sounds that are not normally heard, such as wheezes, crackles, rhonchi).

QUALITY OF PULSE

- Assess the rate and rhythm: tachycardia may indicate hypoxia.
- Compare pulse sites (apical to brachial) for strength and rate.

COLOR

- Observe overall color: with respiratory distress, color progresses from pallor to mottled to cyanosis; central cyanosis is a late sign of respiratory distress.
- Compare peripheral and central color: assess capillary refill and nailbed color and inspect mucous membranes; central cyanosis in mucous membranes is more ominous.
- Note whether crying improves or worsens color.

COUGH

- Quality: note whether dry (nonproductive), wet (productive, mucousy), brassy (noisy, musical), croupy (barking, seal-like).
- Effort: note whether forceful or weak; weak cough may indicate an airway obstruction or fatigue from prolonged respiratory effort (not valid in neonates).

BEHAVIOR CHANGE

- Note level of consciousness: alert or lethargic
- Restlessness and irritability are associated with hypoxia.
- Watch for abrupt behavior changes (restlessness, irritability) and lowered level of consciousness, which indicate increasing hypoxia.

SIGNS OF DEHYDRATION

- Inspect for dry mucous membranes, lack of tears, poor skin turgor, and decreased urine output, which indicate that fluid needs are not being met.

[a]Refer to Chapter 4 for the actual techniques of assessment mentioned in this table.

ANATOMY AND PHYSIOLOGY OF PEDIATRIC DIFFERENCES

The child's respiratory tract constantly grows and changes until about 12 years of age. The young child's neck is shorter than an adult's, resulting in airway structures that are closer together.

UPPER AIRWAY DIFFERENCES

The child's airway is shorter and narrower than an adult's. These differences create a greater potential for obstruction (Figure 13-1 ◆ and Table 13-2). The infant's airway is approximately 4 mm in diameter, about the width of a drinking straw, in contrast to the adult's airway diameter of 20 mm. The upper airway primarily increases in length rather than diameter during the first 5 years of life.

The child's narrower airway causes an increase in **airway resistance,** the effort or force needed to move oxygen through the trachea to the lungs. As air moves from the child's nares down the trachea to the distal airways (alveoli), it must flow through a relatively small area. Friction and increasing resistance are generated as air passes through the airway. When edema and swelling occur in response to a virus, bacterium, or other irritant, the airway is

CLINICAL TIP

The diameter of a child's trachea closely approximates the diameter of the child's little finger. This "rule of finger" can be used for quick assessment of airway size.

AS THEY GROW ◆ Comparison of Airway Structures

FIGURE 13-1 ◆

It is easy to see that a child's airway is smaller and less developed than an adult's airway, but why is this important? An upper respiratory tract infection, allergic reaction, positioning of the head and neck during sleep, and the small objects children play with can have serious consequences in the child.

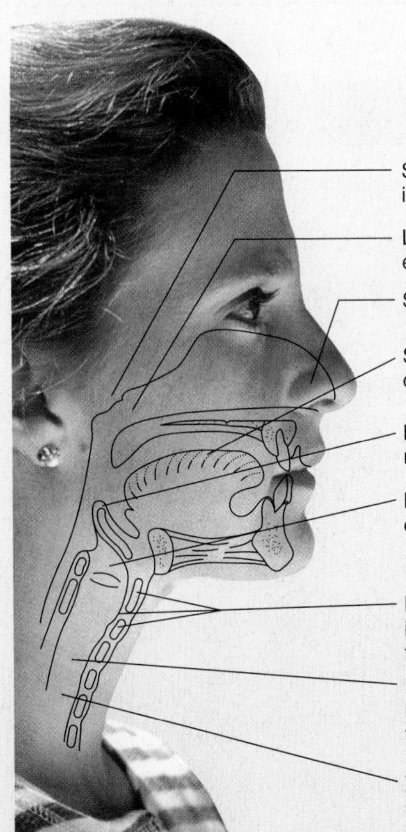

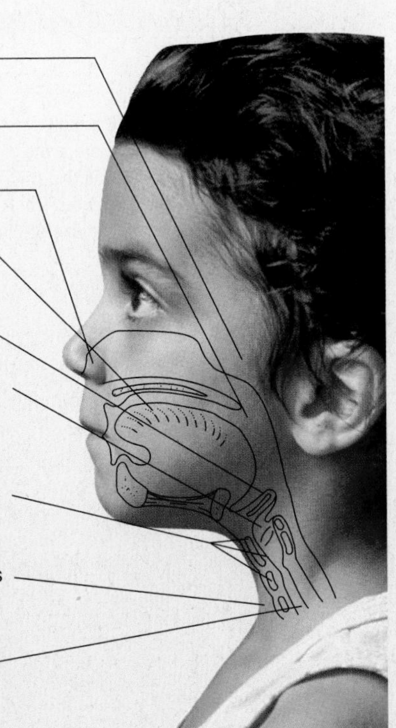

GROWTH & DEVELOPMENT

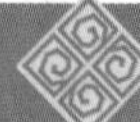

Airway resistance in infancy is 15 times greater than in adults (Webster & Huether, 1998).

further narrowed, increasing airway resistance even more. The trachea in a child is higher and at a different angle than the adult's (Figure 13-2 ◆).

Physiologically the upper airway is the port for inspiration of oxygen and expiration of carbon dioxide. Infants, children, and adults can breathe through either the nose or the mouth. Until 4 weeks of age, newborns are obligatory nose breathers. The coordination of mouth breathing is controlled by maturing neurologic pathways; thus, young infants do not automatically open the mouth to breathe when the nose is obstructed. The only time a newborn breathes through the mouth is when he or she is crying. Nasal patency in newborns is therefore essential for such activities as breathing and eating.

TABLE 13-2 Summary of Upper Airway Differences Between Children and Adults

DIFFERENCE IN CHILDREN	SIGNIFICANCE
Small oral cavity and large tongue	Increases risk of obstruction; nasal patency is critical in infants
Rapid growth of lymph tissue (tonsils and adenoids) during early childhood, atrophy after age 12	Larger tissues in smaller pharyngeal structures; infection can easily cause obstruction of upper airway as lymph tissues swell in response
Larynx and glottis high in neck	Increases chance of aspiration
Thyroid, cricoid, and tracheal cartilages immature and incomplete	Easily collapse when neck is flexed, further narrowing airway; less protective of glottis
Large amount of soft tissue and loosely anchored mucous membranes lining length of airway	Increases likelihood of airway edema and obstruction
Long, floppy epiglottis	Vulnerable to swelling with resultant obstruction
Fewer functional muscles in the airways	Less able to compensate for edema, spasm, and trauma; may swallow more mucus than able to sneeze or cough out

AS THEY GROW 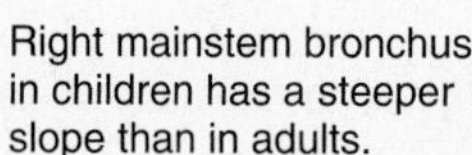 Trachea Position

FIGURE 13-2 ◆

In children, the trachea is shorter and the angle of the right bronchus at bifurcation is more acute than in the adult. When you are resuscitating or suctioning, you must allow for the differences. Do you think that this difference is significant in respiratory infection? Why?

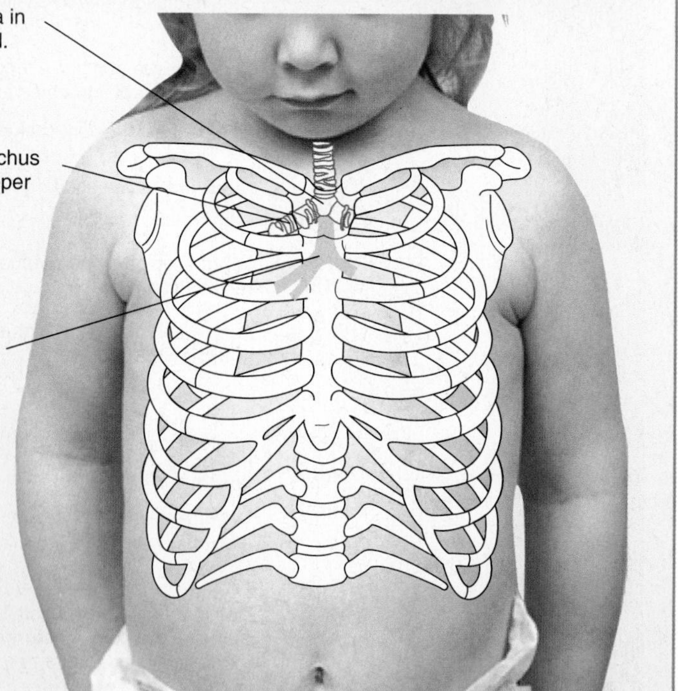

LOWER AIRWAY DIFFERENCES

The child's lower airway is also constantly growing. The developing alveoli change size and shape, and their numbers increase until respiratory maturity is attained at age 12 years. This alveolar growth increases the area available for gas exchange. At birth the distal (peripheral) bronchioles that extend to the alveoli are narrow and fewer in number than in an adult. The child's overall growth can be correlated to the increased branching of the peripheral bronchioles as the alveoli continue to multiply. The taller the child, the greater the lung surface area.

The bronchi and bronchioles are lined with smooth muscle. The newborn does not have enough smooth muscle bundles to help trap airway invaders. By 5 months of age, however, sufficient muscles exist to react to irritants by bronchospasm and muscle contraction. Smooth muscle development is complete and comparable to that of an adult by 1 year of age (Webster & Huether, 1998).

The lungs, which have no muscles of their own, rely on the diaphragm and intercostal muscles to power respiration. Children up to 6 years are primarily diaphragmatic breathers. Because the intercostal muscles are immature and the ribs are primarily cartilage and very flexible, their efficiency in assisting ventilation is reduced. The chest wall is so flexible that the negative pressure created by the downward movement of the diaphragm draws in air, but in cases of respiratory distress causes the chest wall to be drawn inward, causing **retractions.** By 6 years of age, the child begins to use the intercostal muscles more effectively for breathing (Figure 13-3 ◆).

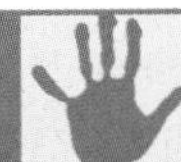

GROWTH & DEVELOPMENT

At birth the lung tissue contains only 25 million alveoli, which are not fully developed. The number of alveoli increases to 300 million by 8 years of age, after which these structures begin increasing in size and complexity until puberty (Webster & Huether, 1998).

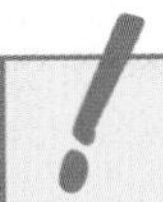

NURSING ALERT

The depth and location of retractions is associated with the severity of respiratory distress. Isolated intercostal retractions indicate mild distress. Subcostal, suprasternal, and supraclavicular retractions indicate moderate distress. These retractions accompanied by use of accessory muscles indicate severe distress.

URGENT RESPIRATORY THREATS

From the moment a child is born, airway integrity is threatened because of the immaturity of the respiratory muscles and neurologic system. Learn to recognize the early signs of respiratory compromise so that you will be able to intervene quickly to assist the infant in distress.

APNEA

Infants normally breathe with an irregular rhythm and may have pauses of up to 20 seconds between breaths. This **periodic breathing** should not be confused with apnea. **Apnea,** by

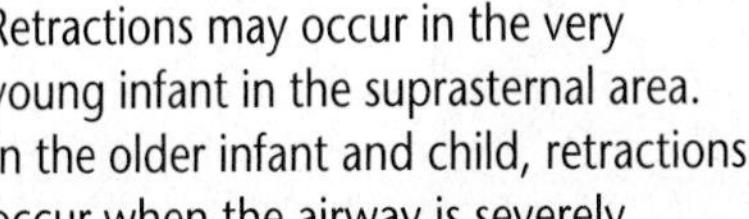

Supraclavicular
Suprasternal
Intercostal
Substernal
Subcostal
Subcostal

Retraction Sites

FIGURE 13-3 ◆

Retractions may occur in the very young infant in the suprasternal area. In the older infant and child, retractions occur when the airway is severely obstructed, as in croup.

NURSING ALERT

These signs and symptoms signal the body's response to increased metabolic demands for oxygenation as a result of stress or impending illness:

- Increasing restlessness, irritability, unexplained sudden confusion
- Rapid heart rate accompanied by rapid respiratory rate

definition, is cessation of respiration lasting longer than 20 seconds, or any pause in respiration associated with cyanosis, marked pallor, hypotonia, or bradycardia. Apnea may be the first major sign of respiratory dysfunction in the neonate.

There are two types of apnea: apnea of prematurity (AOP) and an apparent life-threatening event (ALTE). AOP occurs in preterm infants, usually as a result of immaturity. ALTE (sometimes referred to as apnea of infancy) occurs in near-term or term infants. In the past, both AOP and ALTE were often called "near-miss sudden infant death" or "aborted crib death." These terms erroneously implied a close association between such episodes and sudden infant death syndrome (SIDS). SIDS should not be confused with apnea and is discussed later in this chapter.

Apnea of Prematurity

AOP is a pathologic apnea with no definable cause in infants less than 37 weeks gestational age. It usually presents between 2 and 7 days of life, and its incidence increases with lower gestational age. It often resolves in most infants by 40 weeks postconceptional age (Theobald, Botwinski, & Albanna, et al., 2000). It may be caused by neurologic and immunologic immaturity, or immature muscle development and coordination.

APPARENT LIFE-THREATENING EVENT

ALTE is defined as an episode of apnea accompanied by a color change (cyanosis, pallor, or occasionally ruddiness), limp muscle tone, choking, or gagging occurring in a near-term or term infant who is greater than 37 weeks' gestation. These episodes may occur during sleep, wakefulness, or feeding. A variety of identifiable diseases and conditions can cause ALTE. See the clinical manifestations table on p. 423. In 50% of cases, however, no cause is identified (Loughlin & Carroll, 1999).

ALTE can frighten the parent or observer, who often fears the infant has died. Emergency resuscitation is usually required.

Skills 10-2 to 10-4: Cardiorespiratory Monitoring

Nursing Management

After AOP or ALTE, infants are usually admitted to the hospital for evaluation and cardiorespiratory monitoring. Nursing care includes collecting a detailed history of the event, observing and monitoring cardiorespiratory status, providing supportive care to the infant and family, and anticipating the need for emergency resuscitation and for the diagnostic process.

MONITOR CARDIORESPIRATORY STATUS Cardiorespiratory monitoring records heart rate and respiratory rate while the infant is awake and asleep (Figure 13-4 ◆). Transcutaneous Po_2 (oxygen saturation or oximetry) monitoring provides continuous evaluation of the infant's oxygenation status.

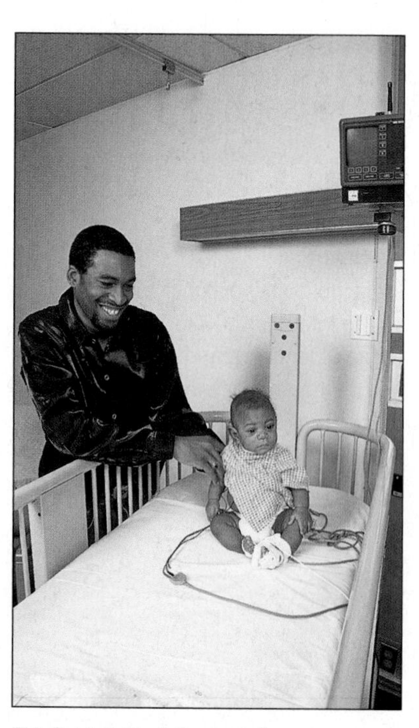

FIGURE 13-4 ◆
Infants who experience an episode of apnea are usually admitted to the hospital for cardiorespiratory monitoring.

PROVIDE EMOTIONAL SUPPORT Establishing rapport and open communication with the parents is essential for creating a sense of trust. To obtain further information about the episode, use open-ended questions and active listening skills. Do not give parents the impression that their parenting skills are being judged or questioned. Parents experience fear and anxiety about the infant's prognosis. Explanations of tests and treatment help to decrease their anxiety and increase their understanding of the situation.

During hospitalization the infant should be held and cuddled to provide a sense of security and well-being. Encouraging parents' participation in the infant's care helps to meet these needs and promotes family bonding. Often parents are afraid to touch the infant because they might disconnect the monitoring cable. Wrapping the cable inside the infant's blanket helps secure the wires, thus increasing parents' feelings of confidence when handling the infant.

PROVIDE TACTILE STIMULATION Tactile stimulation, such as rubbing the infant's back or feet, often is enough to halt an apneic episode. Continuous stimulation from an oscillating waterbed reduces the frequency of apneic episodes in some infants (Theobald et al., 2000). Both methods of stimulation remind the infant to take a breath.

ADMINISTER MEDICATIONS Methylxanthines (aminophylline, caffeine) or doxapram may be administered to stimulate the respiratory center in the brain. Infants have immature

CLINICAL MANIFESTATIONS OF APPARENT LIFE-THREATENING EVENTS

ETIOLOGY	CLINICAL MANIFESTATIONS	CLINICAL THERAPY
Functional or structural airway problem or immaturity	Apnea of 20 sec or longer; accompanied by bradycardia or cyanosis	Cardiorespiratory monitoring, sleep study, pneumogram, sepsis workup
Aspiration as a result of dysfunctional swallowing or gastroesophageal reflux	Choking, coughing, cyanosis, vomiting	Barium swallow, esophageal pH probe
Cardiac problems	Tachycardia, tachypnea, dyspnea	Cardiorespiratory monitoring, electrocardiogram, echocardiogram, arterial blood gases
Drug toxicity or poisoning; maternal history of ingestion	Central nervous system depression, hypotonia	Serum magnesium level, toxicity screen
Environmental, thermoregulation problem	Lethargy, tachypnea, hypothermia or hyperthermia	Cardiorespiratory and temperature monitoring, environmental temperature level (ambient air temperature)
Impaired oxygenation, respiratory disease (pulmonary edema, atelectasis, pneumonia)	Cyanosis, tachypnea, respiratory distress, anemia, choking, coughing	Oximetry, chest radiograph, arterial blood gases, complete blood count, upper airway evaluation, sleep study, serum electrolytes
Acute infection (sepsis, meningitis, necrotising enterocolitis)	Feeding intolerance, lethargy, temperature instability	Complete blood count, cultures when appropriate, C-reactive protein, chest and abdominal radiographs
Intracranial pathology (intraventricular hemorrhage, ventricular dilation, CNS anomalies, meningitis)	Abnormal neurologic examination, seizures	Cranial ultrasound, computed tomography scan, electroencephalogram, magnetic resonance imaging, cerebrospinal fluid evaluation
Metabolic disorders	Jitteriness, poor feeding, lethargy, central nervous system depression or irritability, hypotonia	Serum electrolytes (potassium, sodium, chloride), glucose, calcium, arterial blood gases

Note: Modified from Theobald, K., Botwinski, C., Albanna, S., & McWilliam, P. (2000). Apnea of prematurity: Diagnosis, implications for care, and pharmacologic management, *Neonatal Network, 19*(6), 17–24; and Eichenwald, E., & Stark, A. (1992). Apnea of prematurity: Etiology and management. *Tufts University School of Medicine Reports on Neonatal Respiratory Diseases, 2*(1), 1–11.

hepatic and renal systems, so the rate and efficiency of drug absorption and excretion are affected. Serum drug levels should be monitored frequently because the metabolism and distribution of the drug can be unpredictable.

ANTICIPATE EMERGENCY RESUSCITATION Because the infant who has had AOP or ALTE continues to be at risk for cardiopulmonary arrest, emergency resuscitation equipment and drugs should be readily accessible at all times.

DISCHARGE PLANNING AND HOME CARE TEACHING Home care needs should be identified and addressed well in advance of discharge. Parents need to be taught how to operate an apnea monitor, what to do when the infant has an apneic episode, and how to perform cardiopulmonary resuscitation (CPR) and choking-intervention techniques.

CLINICAL TIP

Caffeine is preferred because it enhances diaphragmatic contraction, has a longer action time, fewer side effects, and more stable plasma concentration.

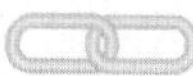

Skill 10-13: Performing Infant Cardiopulmonary Resuscitation

SUDDEN INFANT DEATH SYNDROME

Sudden infant death syndrome (SIDS) has been defined as the sudden death of an infant under 1 year of age that remains unexplained after a complete autopsy, a death scene investigation, and review of the history. It remains a leading cause of death in infants between 1 month and 1 year of age, with 90% of cases occurring before 6 months of age (American

FAMILIES WANT TO KNOW

Home Care Instructions for the Infant Requiring Apnea Monitoring

APNEA EQUIPMENT

- Understand monitor type, lead wires, placement of skin electrodes or chest belt, battery power, manual for troubleshooting.

EMERGENCY PREPARATION

- Notify telephone company, electric company, local rescue squad, local emergency department (establishes priority status).
- Post phone numbers of rescue squad, physician, equipment company, power company, emergency number, cardiopulmonary resuscitation (CPR) guidelines, other important numbers (neighbor, parents' work numbers) in at least two places in the home; have at least one added extension phone.
- Keep the apnea monitor battery fully charged.

SAFETY PRECAUTIONS

- Place monitor on firm surface; keep away from other appliances (television, microwave oven) and water.
- Ensure that alarms are audible from all locations.
- Double-check that monitor is *on* before going to bed.
- Thread cable and wires through lower end of infant's clothes.
- Ensure integrity of leads, monitor cable, power cord (replace if frayed).

ROUTINE CARE

- Understand reasons for apnea monitor and frequency of use.
- Be able to attach and detach infant chest leads and belt.
- Evaluate skin for irritation or breakdown from electrode placement and give skin care (no oils or lotion; move patches correctly).

EMERGENCY CARE

- Develop plan for respiratory failure and power failure.
- Demonstrate CPR and back blows and chest thrusts for airway obstruction.
- Understand how to respond to alarms for apnea, bradycardia, or loose lead.

APNEA ALARM

- Observe infant's respiratory movement.
- If respiration is absent or infant is lethargic, stimulate by calling name and gently touching, proceeding to vigorous touch if needed.
- If no response, proceed with CPR.

BRADYCARDIA ALARM

- Stimulate infant; infant should respond quickly.

LOOSE LEAD

- Check electrode patch. Is it loose? Dirty? Belt loose?
- Check wires from electrode or monitor cable.
- Check power supply. Is battery low? Power failure? Monitor-malfunctioning?

Academy of Pediatrics Committee on Child Abuse and Neglect, 2001). SIDS occurs rarely in infants less than 2 weeks. It is currently unpredictable and unpreventable. The first symptom is cardiopulmonary arrest.

SIDS is referred to as a "syndrome" because of the many and varied autopsy and clinical findings that characterize most infants who die of the disorder. The autopsy typically does not identify a disease process that caused the death. Clinical findings include evidence of a struggle or change in position and the presence of frothy, blood-tinged secretions from the mouth and nares. SIDS occurs more often in the fall and winter and during periods of sleep. Most deaths are unobserved. Typically parents find the infant dead in the crib in the morning and report having heard no cries or disturbances during the night. A mild respiratory illness often precedes the death.

The current thinking about the etiology of SIDS is that an abnormality of the arcuate nucleus of the brainstem causes a delayed development of arousal, cardiorespiratory control, or cardiovascular control (Parnigrahy, Filiano, & Sleeper, et al., 1997). Other proposed

TABLE 13-3 Risk Factors for Sudden Infant Death Syndrome

INFANT

- Prematurity
- Low birth weight
- Twin or triplet birth
- Race (in decreasing order of frequency): most common in Native American infants, followed by African American, Hispanic, white, and Asian infants
- Gender: more common in males than females
- Age: most common in infants between 2 and 4 months of age
- Time of year: more prevalent in winter months
- Exposure to passive smoke
- History of cyanosis, respiratory distress, irritability, and poor feeding in the nursery
- Sleeping prone

MATERNAL AND FAMILIAL

- Maternal age less than 20 years
- History of smoking and illicit drug use (increases incidence 10 times)
- Anemia
- Multiple pregnancies, with short intervals between births
- History of sibling with SIDS (increases incidence 4 to 5 times)
- Low socioeconomic status; crowding
- Poor prenatal care, low weight gain

causes include H. pylori gastrointestinal infection, and a cardiac dysrhythmia called long QT syndrome. Several infant, maternal, and familial factors appear to place infants at risk for SIDS (Table 13-3). SIDS has not been found to be associated with newborn apnea or immunizations for diphtheria, tetanus, and pertussis (DTP). Child abuse or homicide may be associated with 1% to 5% of SIDS cases (American Academy of Pediatrics, 2001).

Nursing Management

The sudden, unexpected nature of the infant's death is confirmed in the emergency department. The nurse's role is to be empathetic and provide support during one of the greatest crises a family must face. The focus is on supporting the family during the acute grieving period (Table 13-4).

Reassure the parents that they are not responsible for the infant's death and assist them in contacting other family members and mobilizing support. Older children may need reassurance that SIDS will not happen to them. They may also believe that bad thoughts or wishes about their baby brother or sister caused the death. Support groups can help parents, siblings, and other family members express these fears and work through their feelings about the infant's death. The SIDS Alliance and SHARE are organizations that can help families locate a support group in their geographic area.

Nurses can play an important role in educating the public about the link between SIDS and infant positioning during sleep. Hospitalized infants should be placed to sleep in supine position rather than side-lying or prone.

RESPIRATORY FAILURE

Respiratory failure occurs when the body can no longer maintain effective gas exchange. An inflammatory response and alveolar capillary damage lead to respiratory failure. Other body systems may also contribute directly or indirectly to an increased workload, causing the respiratory system to fail. The clinical manifestations of respiratory failure are signs of respiratory distress: **hypoxemia** (lower than normal blood oxygen level) and **hypercapnia** (an excess of carbon dioxide in the blood).

The physiologic process that ends in respiratory failure begins with **alveolar hypoventilation.** Alveolar hypoventilation occurs when any of these factors exist: (1) oxygen need exceeds actual oxygen intake; (2) the airway is partially occluded; or (3) the transfer of oxygen

CLINICAL TIP

Guidelines for the support of families experiencing SIDS should include baptism services, religious support, grief counseling, assistance with funeral arrangements, and counseling on cessation of breastfeeding and sibling reactions.

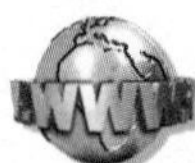

SIDS Resources for Parents and Providers

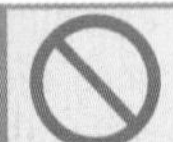

SAFETY PRECAUTIONS

The American Academy of Pediatrics recommends that infants be placed on their back to sleep. The dramatic decrease in SIDS deaths, from 67% of postneonatal deaths in 1993 to 28% in 1998, is believed to be related to the success of educational campaigns about infant sleep position. Recent findings indicate that infants placed to sleep on their stomach who typically sleep on their backs have an increased incidence of SIDS. This is believed to be a factor in the rising incidence of SIDS found in child care settings (Cote, Gerez, & Brouillette, et al., 2000; and Moon, Patel, & Shaefer, 2000).

LABORATORY VALUES: RESPIRATORY FAILURE

Arterial blood gas levels indicative of respiratory failure are a Po_2 level less than 50 mm Hg and a Pco_2 level greater than 50 mm Hg. See Appendix C for expected laboratory values by age.

TABLE 13-4 Supportive Care for the Family of an Infant with Sudden Infant Death Syndrome (SIDS)

NURSING INTERVENTIONS	RATIONALE
1. Provide parents with a private area and a support person who reinforces that the infant's death was not their fault.	1. Parents need to be able to express their grief in their own way and be told that they are not being blamed for the infant's death.
2. Prepare the family for the viewing of the infant. Describe how the infant will look and feel.	2. You can say "Paul's (use the infant's name) skin will feel cool. He will be very still and his eyes will be closed." They probably know this, but a gentle explanation demonstrates empathy. Explain that pooling of blood on the dependent areas will look like bruises.
3. Allow parents to hold, touch, and rock the infant if desired.	3. Viewing the infant allows parents a chance to say good-bye. Before bringing the infant to parents, wrap in a clean blanket, comb the hair, wash the face, swab the mouth clean, and apply Vaseline to lips.
4. Reinforce the physician's explanation about the need for an autopsy.	4. An autopsy is required for all unexplained deaths. You can say to parents, "It is the only way we can be sure of what caused your baby's death."
5. Answer parents' questions and provide them with sources for further information. Provide literature and a name of the local contact for a SIDS support group, as well as for the national foundation.	5. Parents may not be able to take in all of your answers. Many emergency departments and pediatric units have a social worker who provides ongoing contact with the family. Provide names of resource persons and phone numbers for SIDS support groups.
6. Advise parents that surviving siblings may benefit from psychological support.	6. Siblings often require emotional support in the weeks and months after the death. Social workers can help the family obtain counseling and support for all members.
7. Provide parents with a lock of hair, footprints, and handprints, if they desire.	7. Personal items can be placed in a memory book. This reaffirms the child's existence for many parents.

CLINICAL TIP

Grunting slows the expiratory flow and increases the lung volume and alveolar pressures. This sign of severe disease suggests the onset of respiratory failure (Margolis & Gadomski, 1998)

and carbon dioxide in the alveoli is disrupted. This disruption may occur either because of a malfunction of respiratory center stimulation (the alveoli do not receive the message to diffuse) or because the alveolar membrane is defective (a structural problem).

Alveolar hypoventilation results in hypoxemia and hypercapnia. When the blood levels of oxygen and carbon dioxide reach abnormal levels, **hypoxia** (lower than normal oxygen in the tissues) occurs and respiratory failure begins. Signs of impending respiratory failure include irritability, lethargy, cyanosis, and increased respiratory effort such as **dyspnea** (difficulty breathing), **tachypnea** (increased respiratory rate), nasal flaring, and intercostal retractions. Any signs of respiratory failure should be reported immediately.

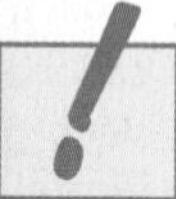

Skills 5-8 to 5-14: Assessing Vital Signs

Nursing Management

Early recognition of impending respiratory failure is the most important aspect of care for a child with any signs of respiratory compromise. The child who has even a slight degree of respiratory distress should immediately be placed in an upright position (by elevating the head of the bed). Assess respiratory quality and rate, followed by apical pulse rate and temperature. Oxygen saturation and end-tidal CO_2 monitoring are also helpful. Oxygen administration equipment and respiratory emergency equipment should be kept at the child's bedside. Ensure that an order for oxygen is obtained or that oxygen is administered. Monitor the child for changes in vital signs, respiratory status, and level of responsiveness. Be prepared to assist ventilations if respiratory status deteriorates.

NURSING ALERT

When the child has a chronic respiratory condition, development of respiratory failure may be gradual. Signs will be subtle. Be particularly alert to behavior changes in addition to respiratory signs. Serial blood gases may be needed to monitor the child.

USING ARTIFICIAL AIRWAYS Respiratory problems that do not respond to oxygen therapy, medications, or position changes require the insertion of an artificial airway. As the child's level of responsiveness deteriorates, the ability to keep the airway open decreases. Endotra-

CLINICAL MANIFESTATIONS OF RESPIRATORY FAILURE AND IMMINENT RESPIRATORY ARREST

PHYSIOLOGIC CAUSE	CLINICAL MANIFESTATIONS
These signs occur because the child is attempting to compensate for oxygen deficit and airway blockage. Oxygen supply is inadequate; behavior and vital signs reflect compensation and beginning hypoxia.	*Respiratory failure -Initial signs* Restlessness Tachypnea Tachycardia Diaphoresis
The child attempts to use accessory muscles to assist oxygen intake; hypoxia persists and efforts now waste more oxygen than is obtained.	*Respiratory failure - Early decompensation* Nasal flaring Retractions Grunting Wheezing Anxiety and irritability Mood changes Headache Hypertension Confusion
These signs occur because oxygen deficit is overwhelming and beyond spontaneous recovery. Cerebral oxygenation is dramatically affected; central nervous system changes are ominous.	*Imminent respiratory arrest-Severe hypoxia* Dyspnea Bradycardia Cyanosis Stupor and coma

cheal intubation is a short-term, emergency measure to stabilize the airway by placing a tube in the trachea. A tracheostomy is the creation of a surgical opening into the trachea through the anterior neck at the cricoid cartilage. Surgeons prefer to perform this procedure in the operating room; however, a tracheostomy may also be performed in an emergency department or other setting when the situation dictates immediate intervention. These children usually require admission to the intensive care unit (ICU) for monitoring and ventilatory support.

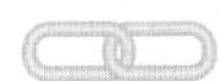

Skill 10-10: Endotracheal Tube Care

Because endotracheal and tracheostomy tubes prevent vocal cord vibration, intubated children cannot cry or talk. Infants and young children often express initial frustration when they realize they cannot communicate verbally. They often develop other noise-making behaviors, such as striking the mattress to gain attention. When time permits, the nurse should teach the parents and child what to expect before insertion of the endotracheal or tracheostomy tube. A communication board can be used with older children.

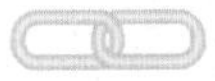

Skills 10-8, 10-9: Tracheostomy General Guidelines and Care

Many children are discharged from the hospital and cared for at home for an extended period with a tracheostomy tube in place. It is essential to teach parents how to maintain the airway, clean the tracheostomy site, and change the tube. A home health care nurse can provide follow-up care and support for the child and family.

REACTIVE AIRWAY DISORDERS

Reactive airway disorders occur when airway tissue reacts to invasion by a virus, bacterium, allergen, or irritant. These invaders cause airway tissue to respond with inflammation, edema, increased mucous production, and bronchospasm. Reactive airway disorders are reversible, usually self-limiting, and generally responsive to supportive therapies. They occur in either upper or lower airways and include croup syndromes, asthma, and bronchiolitis.

CROUP SYNDROMES

Croup is a term applied to a broad classification of upper airway illnesses that result from swelling of the epiglottis and larynx. The swelling usually extends into the trachea and bronchi. Included under the classification of croup syndromes are viral syndromes, such as

PATHOPHYSIOLOGY ILLUSTRATED

Airway Changes with Croup

FIGURE 13-5 ◆
There are two important changes in the upper airway in croup: the epiglottis swells, thereby occluding the airway, and the trachea swells against the cricoid cartilage, causing restriction.

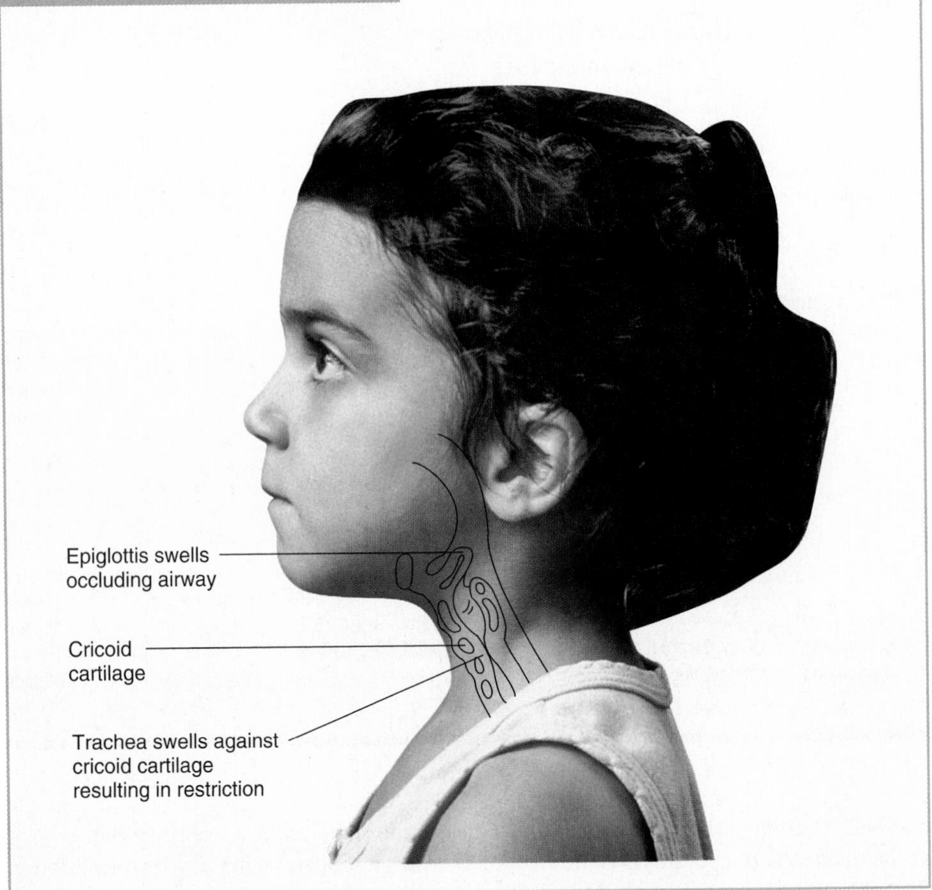

spasmodic laryngitis (spasmodic croup), laryngotracheitis, and laryngotracheobronchitis (LTB), and bacterial syndromes, such as bacterial tracheitis and epiglottitis (Figure 13-5 ◆ and Table 13-5).

LTB, epiglottitis, and bacterial tracheitis are referred to as the "big three" of pediatric respiratory illness because they affect the greatest number of children across all age groups in both sexes. The initial symptoms of all three conditions include inspiratory **stridor** (a high-pitched, musical sound that is created by narrowing of the airway), a seal-like barking cough, and hoarseness. LTB is the most common disorder, but epiglottitis and bacterial tracheitis are more serious.

Laryngitis and laryngotracheitis are mild illnesses that can be managed at home. LTB is the most serious type of viral croup, frequently necessitating an emergency department visit for infants and children under 6 years of age.

Laryngotracheobronchitis

Although the term *croup* is applied to several viral and bacterial syndromes, it is most often used to refer to LTB, a viral invasion of the upper airway that extends throughout the larynx, trachea, and bronchi. Table 13-5 compares LTB and other croup syndromes.

ETIOLOGY AND PATHOPHYSIOLOGY Acute viral LTB is most common in children 3 months to 4 years of age but can occur up to 8 years of age. Boys are affected more often than girls. LTB is of greatest concern in infants and children under the age of 6 years, because of potential airway obstruction. The causative organism is usually parainfluenza virus type I, II, or III, which appears during winter months in clustered outbreaks (Kaditis & Wald, 1998).

TABLE 13-5 Summary of Croup Syndromes

	VIRAL SYNDROMES			BACTERIAL SYNDROMES	
	Acute Spasmodic Laryngitis (Spasmodic Croup)	*Laryngotracheitis*	*Laryngotracheo-bronchitis*	*Bacterial Tracheitis*	*Epiglottitis (Supraglottitis)*
Severity	Least serious	Most common[a]	Most serious; progresses if untreated	Guarded; requires close observation	Most life threatening (medical emergency)[a]
Age affected	3 months to 3 years	3 months to 8 years	3 months to 8 years	1 month to 13 years[a]	2 years to 8 years
Onset	Abrupt onset; peaks at night, resolves by morning (recurs)[a]	Gradual onset; starts as URI, progresses to moderate respiratory difficulty	Gradual onset; starts as URI, progresses to symptoms of respiratory distress	Progressive from URI (1–2 days)	Progresses rapidly (hours)[a]
Clinical manifestations	Afebrile; mild respiratory distress; barking-seal cough	*Early:* mild fever [<39.0°C (102.2°F)]; hoarseness; barking-seal, brassy, croupy cough; rhinorrhea; sore throat; stridor; apprehension (inspiratory) *Progressing to* labored respirations	*Early:* mild fever; [<39.0°C (102.2°F)]; barking-seal, brassy, croupy cough; rhinorrhea; sore throat; stridor (inspiratory); apprehension; restless/irritable *Progressing to* retractions (progressive); increasing stridor; cyanosis	High fever [>39.0°C (102.2°F)]; URI appears as viral croupy cough; croup initially; stridor (tracheal); purulent secretions	High fever [>39.0°C (102.2°F)]; URI; intense sore throat; dysphagia[a], drooling[a]; increased pulse and respiratory rate; prefers upright position (tripod position with chin thrust)[a]
Etiology	Unknown; suspect viral with allergic/emotional influences	Parainfluenza, types I and II, RSV, or influenza	Parainfluenza, types I and II, RSV, or influenza	*Staphylococcus*	*Haemophilus influenzae*

[a]Classic parameter or key point (distinguishes condition).

Airway tissues respond to the invading virus by producing copious, tenacious secretions and swelling, which increase the child's respiratory distress. The laryngeal inflammation causes the airway diameter to narrow in the subglottic area, the narrowest part of the airway. Even small amounts of mucus or edema can quickly obstruct the airway (see Figure 13-5). Both the large and small airways can be affected.

CLINICAL MANIFESTATIONS Most children brought to the emergency department with LTB have been ill for a couple of days with upper respiratory symptoms. These symptoms progress to a cough and hoarseness. Fever may or may not be present. Common presenting signs are tachypnea, inspiratory stridor, and a seal-like barking cough.

CLINICAL THERAPY Diagnosis is often made by clinical signs. Pulse oximetry is used to detect hypoxemia. If the diagnosis of LTB is in question, anteroposterior (AP) and lateral x-rays of the upper airway are taken; these may show symmetric subglottic narrowing called a steeple sign.

Medical management consists of maintaining and improving respiratory effort with humidification, medications, and supplemental oxygen when the saturated oxygen level is less than 92%.

Children with a good response to medications are often sent home from the emergency department after an observation period. Children with moderate to severe symptoms after medications are admitted for further observation and treatment. Airway obstruction is a potential complication of LTB. The child may require intubation and transfer to the ICU to maintain airway patency if obstruction is imminent. Most children, however, respond positively to the medications and oxygen therapy and are discharged within 48 to 72 hours.

NURSING ALERT

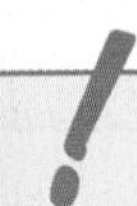

Throat cultures and visual inspection of the inner mouth and throat are contraindicated in children with LTB and epiglottitis. These procedures can cause **laryngospasms** (spasmodic vibrations that close the larynx) to occur as a result of the child's anxiety or of probing this reactive and already compromised area.

Skill 10-2: Pulse Oximetry

MEDICATIONS USED FOR SYMPTOMATIC TREATMENT OF LARYNGOTRACHEOBRONCHITIS

Medication	Action/Indication	Nursing Considerations
Beta-agonists and beta-adrenergics (e.g., albuterol, racemic epinephrine): aerosolized through face mask	Rapid-acting bronchodilator, decreases bronchial and tracheal secretions and mucosal edema, used to decrease symptoms of moderate to severe respiratory distress; and constriction of subglottic mucosa and submucosal capillaries.	Provides only temporary relief; improvement in 30 minutes which lasts about 2 hours, giving time for the steroid to work; the child may experience tachycardia (160–200 beats/min) and hypertension; dizziness, headache, and nausea may necessitate stopping medication; reduces the need for artifical airway.
Corticosteroids (e.g., dexamethasone): IM, PO, Nebulized budesonide	Anti-inflammatory, used to decrease edema; has a long half-life of 36–54 hours	The child may experience cardiovascular symptoms (hypertension): requires close observation for individual response; children less frequently need emergency airways; stridor resolves faster

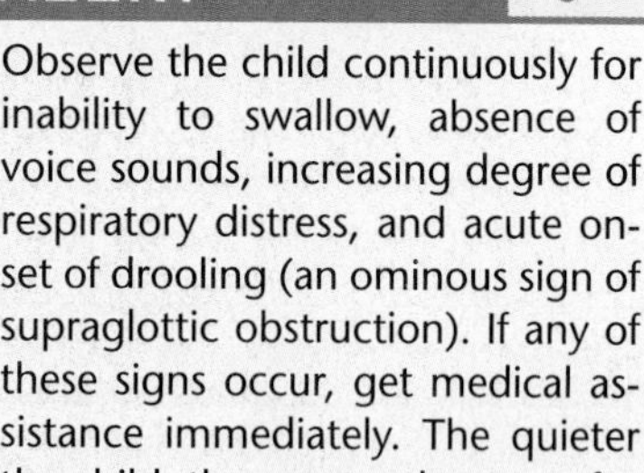

NURSING ALERT

Observe the child continuously for inability to swallow, absence of voice sounds, increasing degree of respiratory distress, and acute onset of drooling (an ominous sign of supraglottic obstruction). If any of these signs occur, get medical assistance immediately. The quieter the child, the greater the cause for concern.

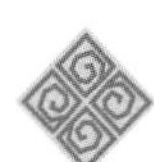

NURSING MANAGEMENT

Nursing Assessment and Diagnosis

The initial and ongoing physical assessment of the child with LTB focuses on adequacy of respiratory functioning. Close monitoring is required to identify changes in airway patency. The child should be continuously monitored in the emergency department observation area or the ICU. When the child's condition stabilizes, monitoring can be less frequent (Tables 13-6 and 13-7).

Particular attention should be paid to the child's respiratory effort, breath sounds, and responsiveness. Physical exhaustion can diminish the intensity of retractions and stridor. As the child uses the remaining energy reserve to maintain ventilation, breath sounds may

TABLE 13-6 Nursing Assessment of Child With a Reactive Airway Disorder

NURSING ACTION	RATIONALE
Assess heart rate and respiratory rate	Tachypnea and tachycardia indicate increasing respiratory effort
Check position of the child (sitting? prone? supine?)	Upright or semi-Fowler's promotes airway patency; the child's change to a more upright position may signal increased distress
Assess overall quality of respiratory effort: Determine inspiratory and expiratory breath sounds, ability to speak, and presence of stridor, cough, refractions, nasal flaring, cyanosis	Reflects overall adequacy of airway and respiratory function
Initiate croup score (Table 13-7) and continue scoring every 2–4 hours or more frequently if distress increases; initiate nursing actions appropriate for croup score	Provides consistent and objective assessment data with quantitative score for future comparison
Attach cardiorespiratory monitor and pulse oximeter	Provides continuous assessment data as part of ongoing physiologic monitoring

TABLE 13-7 Croup Scale to Identify the Severity of Croup

	SEVERITY SCORE			
Signs	*0*	*1*	*2*	*3*
Stridor	None	Mild	Moderate at rest	Severe, on inspiration and expiration
Retractions	None	Mild	Suprasternal, intercostal	Severe, may see sternal retractions
Color	Normal	—	—	Dusky or cyanotic
Breath	Normal sounds	Mildly decreased	Moderately decreased	Markedly decreased
Level of consciousness	Normal	Restless when disturbed	Anxious, agitated	Lethargic

Scoring: To quantify the severity of croup, add the individual scores for each of the sign categories. A score between 0 and 15 is possible. The rating of mild, moderate, and severe is as follows: 4–5 is mild, 6–8 is moderate, >8 or any sign in the severe category is severe.
Note: Modified from Davis, H. W., Gartner, J. C., Galvis, A. G., Michaels, R. H., and Mestad, P. H. (1981). Acute upper airway obstruction: Croup and epiglottitis. *Pediatric Clinics of North America, 28*(4), 859–880.

actually diminish. Noisy breathing (audible airway congestion, coarse breath sounds) in this situation verifies adequate energy stores. Responsiveness will decrease as hypoxemia increases.

The following nursing diagnoses might be appropriate for the child with acute LTB:

- *Ineffective breathing pattern,* related to tracheobronchial obstruction, decreased energy, and fatigue
- *Risk for fluid volume deficit,* related to inadequate fluid intake prior to admission
- *Fear (child),* related to unfamiliar surroundings, procedures, and separation from support system

GROWTH & DEVELOPMENT

Infants and preverbal toddlers with laryngotracheobronchitis require constant supervision to monitor respiratory status. A means of communication (sign language or simple word cues) must be established to enable the older child to alert nursing staff to respiratory difficulty.

Planning and Implementation

Skillful nursing care can greatly assist children with LTB and their families to cope with the symptoms of the illness. Nursing care focuses on maintaining airway patency, promoting fluid balance, reducing stress, and teaching the family how to care for the child at home.

Maintain Airway Patency

Supplemental oxygen with humidity may be needed for hypoxemia. High-humidity mist tents are rarely used as studies have not demonstrated any improvement in symptoms. Allow the child to assume a position of comfort.

An important developmental consideration is the child's ability to communicate reliably. The nurse must be immediately available to attend to the child's respiratory needs. The child should be roomed near the nurses' station and emergency resuscitation equipment kept at the bedside.

Meet Fluid and Nutritional Needs

The illness preceding the emergency department visit may have compromised the child's fluid status. Recognizing fluid deficit and monitoring the child's hydration and nutritional status are essential. Fluids promote liquification of secretions and provide calories for energy and metabolism. Parents can be encouraged to participate in gaining the child's cooperation in taking oral fluids. An intravenous infusion may be necessary to rehydrate the child, maintain

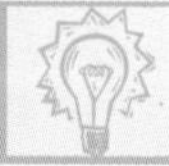

CLINICAL TIP

Children with laryngotracheobronchitis usually prefer cool, noncarbonated, nonacidic drinks such as apple juice or fruit-flavored drinks. Remember that gelatin, ice, and fruit-flavored ice pops are also fluids. Oral rehydration fluids may also be used.

fluid balance, or provide emergency access. The child should be observed closely for difficulty in swallowing, which may be an early sign of epiglottitis or bacterial tracheitis.

Discharge Planning and Home Care Teaching

During the child's observation period, nurses should take every opportunity to assess the parents' knowledge of symptoms of LTB and discuss actions to take if symptoms recur. For example, instruct parents to call the child's physician if the following occurs.

- Mild symptoms do not improve after 1 hour of humidity and cool air treatment.
- The child's breathing is rapid and labored.

Evaluation

Expected outcomes of nursing care include the following:

- The child responds to medications with decreased respiratory distress.
- The child's fear and anxiety are managed with family support and explanations about care.

Epiglottitis (Supraglottitis)

Epiglottitis (also known as supraglottitis) is an inflammation of the epiglottis, the long narrow structure that closes off the glottis during swallowing (see Figure 13-5◆). Because edema in this area can rapidly (within minutes or hours) obstruct the airway by occluding the trachea, epiglottitis is considered a potentially life-threatening condition. (Table 13-5 compares epiglottitis and other croup syndromes.)

Epiglottitis is caused by bacterial invasion of the soft tissue of the larynx by streptococcus and staphylococcus, and by *Haemophilus influenzae* type B (Hib) in unimmunized children. The resulting inflammation and edema in the tissues and surrounding the epiglottis lead to airway obstruction. Fortunately, since use of the Hib vaccine has become widespread, the number of cases of epiglottitis has decreased significantly.

THE FOUR DS OF EPIGLOTTITIS

The four classic signs of epiglottitis, in order of their appearance are:

- Dysphonia
- Dysphagia
- Drooling
- Distressed respiratory effort

Characteristically, a previously healthy child suddenly becomes very ill. The child initially develops a high fever (greater than 39°C [102.2°F]), with a sore throat, **dysphonia** (muffled, hoarse, or absent voice sounds), and **dysphagia** (difficulty in swallowing). As the larynx becomes obstructed, inspiratory stridor develops. The child resists normal swallowing of saliva because of intense throat pain and swelling, resulting in drooling. To fully open the airway and improve air intake, the child sits up and leans forward with the jaw thrust forward in the classic "sniffing" or tripod posture and refuses to lie down.

Diagnosis is often based on a lateral neck x-ray (Figure 13-6 ◆), which reveals a narrowed airway and an enlarged, rounded epiglottis, seen as a mass at the base of the tongue.

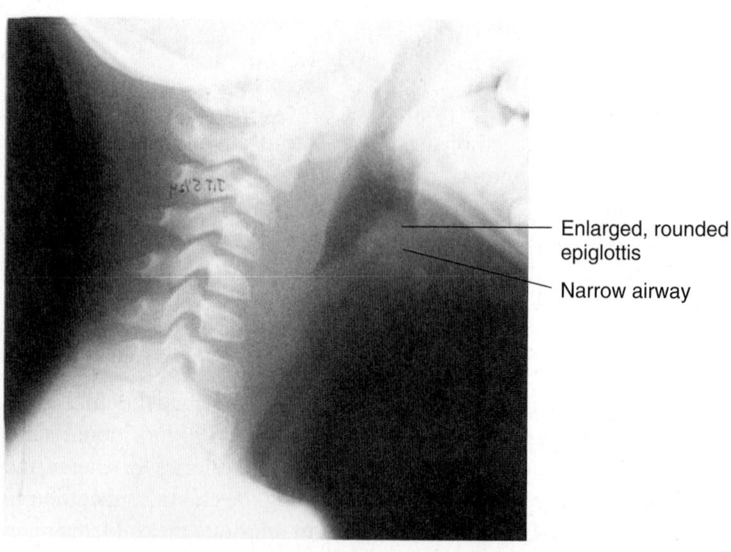

FIGURE 13-6 ◆
The phrase "thumb sign" has been used to describe this enlargement of the epiglottis. Recall the trachea's usual "little finger" size. Do you see the stiff, enlarged "thumb" above it in this lateral neck x-ray?

A blood culture may be taken after the child is stabilized. Laryngospasm and airway obstruction can occur as a result of the severe irritation and hypersensitivity of the airway muscles. For this reason, visual inspection of the mouth and throat is contraindicated in children with suspected epiglottitis until immediate intubation or tracheostomy can be performed (Eichelberger, Ball, & Pratsch, et al., 1998).

Immediate clinical therapy usually involves insertion of an endotracheal tube to maintain the airway. Antibiotics effective for gram-positive organisms and *H. influenzae* are given until blood culture sensitivities are available. Antipyretics (acetaminophen, ibuprofen) may be useful in managing fever and sore throat pain.

NURSING ALERT

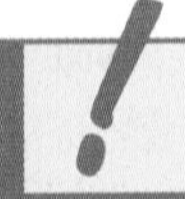

Because infants and preverbal toddlers cannot alert the nurse if they have respiratory distress, they must not be left alone during the acute phase of epiglottitis.

NURSING MANAGEMENT Nursing management consists of airway management, drug therapy, hydration, and emotional and psychosocial support of the child and parents. Until the endotracheal tube is removed, the child is usually managed in the intensive care unit to ensure continual observation.

Until intubated, allow the child to sit upright or assume a position of comfort to maintain the airway and breathe more easily. Supplemental humidified oxygen may be used initially to reverse hypoxemia. The child's respiratory and airway status should be observed closely and often. Provide a quiet environment with as little stress as possible to decrease anxiety and crying. Crying stimulates the airway, increases oxygen consumption, and can precipitate laryngospasm; the calmer the child, the better the respiratory function (Eichelberger et al., 1998).

Skill 10-1: Using Oxygen Delivery Systems

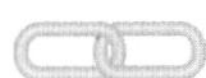

Skill 10-10: Endotracheal Tube Care

Administer antibiotics to treat the infection and provide fluids to provide hydration. Because the child was febrile with a sore throat before admission, fluid intake may have been compromised.

The loss of voice, or even the inability to create sounds, can be frightening to a child. The unfamiliar hospital environment and strange equipment can create stress for child and parent alike. The nurse reassures the parents that the child's voice loss is temporary and explains the need for the various pieces of equipment.

Most children show rapid improvement once cool mist and oxygen, antibiotics, and fluid therapy are started. The endotracheal tube can usually be removed within 24 to 36 hours (Hazinski, 1999). Home care may involve completing the course of antibiotics. Parents need instructions on proper administration and potential problems of drug therapy.

Bacterial Tracheitis

Bacterial tracheitis is a secondary infection of the upper trachea after viral laryngotracheitis that is most often caused by group A streptococcus or *Haemophilus influenzae.* The disorder starts with croupy cough and stridor but progresses to include a high fever greater than 39°C (102.2°F), which persists for several days (Bank & Krug, 1995). Table 13-5 compares bacterial tracheitis and other croup syndromes.

Because of the similarity of symptoms, bacterial tracheitis is often misdiagnosed initially as LTB. Instead of improving with therapy, however, the child's condition becomes worse. Children generally prefer lying flat to sitting up. This seems to be a position of comfort that allows the child to conserve energy. Diagnosis is often made by blood cultures after the child is found unresponsive to usual LTB management. Antibiotics are given for a full 10-day course. Most children need a secured artificial airway and ventilatory support.

NURSING MANAGEMENT Nursing management involves the following:

- Careful airway assessment and support
- Airway maintenance (Artificial airway assistance is often required because of the thick tracheal secretions that pool high in the upper airway.)
- Suctioning as needed (Mechanical suction enables easier removal of secretions and helps maintain a patent airway.)
- Administration of humidified oxygen
- Administration of antibiotics
- Preparation for resuscitation

The earlier section on epiglottitis discusses other nursing care interventions that may also be appropriate for the child with bacterial tracheitis.

ASTHMA

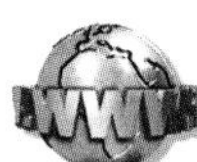

National Asthma Statistics and Prevention Programs

Asthma (also called bronchial asthma) is a chronic inflammatory disorder of the airway with airway obstruction that can be partially or completely reversed, and increased airway responsiveness to stimuli (Kieckhefer & Ratcliffe, 2000). It affects about 5 million children in the United States. Affected children have about 10 days of school absenteeism and 20 days of restricted activity per year (Sydnor-Greenberg & Dokken, 2000). Most children with asthma experience their first symptoms before the age of 5 years. Asthma occurs more frequently in boys than girls until the teen years, when the incidence equalizes (Kieckhefer & Ratcliffe, 2000).

Asthma is a chronic condition with acute exacerbations or persistent symptoms. Children require continuous coordinated care to control sudden symptoms and minimize long-term airway changes. Although unusual in the past, severe persistent asthma is more common now. Mortality from asthma in children rose 31% between 1980 and 1987, and continues to rise (National Education and Prevention Program, 1997). How does this chronic condition pose a threat to children?

PASSIVE SMOKE EXPOSURE

Research has confirmed that passive smoke exposure (secondhand smoke) contributes significantly to the development of respiratory problems in children. Passive smoke exposure has been linked specifically to an increase in asthma symptoms, emergency department visits, and hospital admissions in children of parents who smoke. It is believed to be responsible for thousands of new cases of asthma in children each year. In addition, children exposed to tobacco smoke in utero have a higher rate of asthma. It is thought that the increased number of women smokers may have contributed to the increased rates of asthma (Gilliland, Yu-Fen, & Peters, 2001).

Etiology and Pathophysiology

The respiratory difficulties of an asthma attack result from inflammation that contributes to airway obstruction (Richman, 1997). The inflammation causes the normal protective mechanisms of the lungs (mucous formation, mucosal swelling, and airway muscle contraction) to react excessively in response to a stimulus.

The stimulus, more correctly termed a **trigger,** that initiates an asthmatic episode can be inflammatory or noninflammatory. Triggers increase the frequency and severity of smooth muscle contraction, and airway responsiveness is enhanced through inflammatory mechanisms. During the acute reaction, an antigen binds to the specific immunoglobulin E surface on the mast cell, and histamine is released along with intercellular chemical mediators resulting in bronchospasm. Inflammation peaks in 12 to 24 hours (Kieckhefer & Ratcliffe, 2000). Asthmatic triggers include exercise, viral or bacterial agents, allergens (mold, dust, or pollen), food additives, pollutants, weather changes (humidity and temperature), and emotions. The reactive airway responses to stimuli are present *before* the trigger initiates the physiologic sequence that results in an asthma attack.

Airway narrowing results from airway swelling and production of copious amounts of mucus. Mucus clogs small airways, trapping air below the plugs (Figure 13-7 ◆). The airways swell, creating muscle spasms that often become uncontrolled in the large airways. With time, repeated episodes of bronchospasm, mucosal edema, and mucous plugging can damage the respiratory cells that line the airway. This process leaves the airway chronically irritated and scarred and results in air trapping, called hyperinflation.

The psychologic sequence of events during an asthmatic episode starts with moderate anxiety as the episode begins. The anxiety becomes severe as the episode intensifies. Severe anxiety, in turn, intensifies physical responses and symptoms, and a vicious cycle is established. Recognizing and addressing the child's fear and panic are essential for reestablishing normal respirations.

Clinical Manifestations

Asthma is characterized by airway inflammation, airway obstruction or narrowing, and airway hyperreactivity. The sudden appearance of breathing difficulty is often referred to as an asthma "attack" or "episode."

During an acute attack, respirations are rapid and labored and the child often appears tired because of the ongoing exertion of breathing. Nasal flaring and intercostal retractions may be visible. The child exhibits a productive cough and expiratory wheezing, use of accessory muscles, decreased air movement, and respiratory fatigue. The resulting hypoxia, as well as the cumulative effect of previously administered medications, contributes to behaviors ranging from wide-eyed agitation to lethargic irritability.

In children who have repeated acute exacerbations, a barrel chest and the use of accessory muscles of respiration are common findings (see Figure 13-12, p. 445).

PATHOPHYSIOLOGY ILLUSTRATED

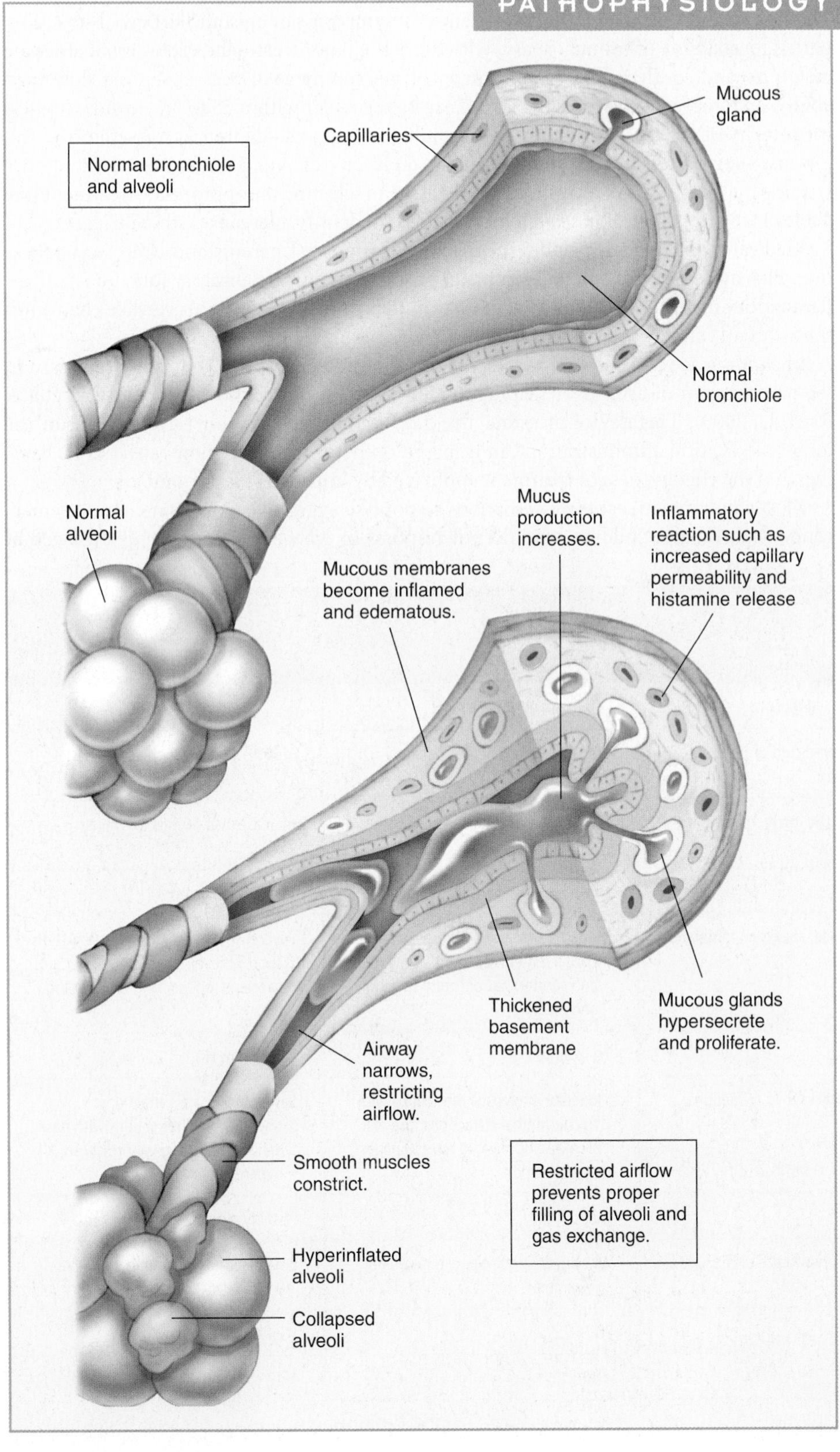

Asthma Attack

FIGURE 13-7 ◆
What can cause an asthma attack? Some asthma triggers are exercise, infection, and allergies. Shown is how asthma obstructs airflow through constriction and narrowing of the airway along with increased production of mucus.

Skill 10-5: Using a Peak Expiratory Flow Meter

Clinical Therapy

The diagnosis of asthma has four key elements: symptoms of episodic airflow obstruction; partial reversibility of bronchospasm with bronchodilator treatment; exclusion of alternate diagnosis; and confirmation by spirometry of measurement of peak expiratory flow variability. A spirometer measures the forced expiration of air within 25 to 75 seconds to assess the severity of airway obstruction. Because the test requires children to cooperate and follow instructions, it is usually administered to children over 4 or 5 years of age. Findings determine the extent of airway restriction and assist in selecting the appropriate treatment (see Tables 13-8 and 13-9). Skin testing may be used to identify allergens (asthma triggers).

Medical management includes medications, support of parents and child, and education. Pharmacologic treatment attempts to promote optimal respiratory function. Anti-inflammatory medications should begin early in the course to prevent irreversible changes in the asthmatic airway (Steinbach, 2000).

In children as young as 4 to 5 years, the use of a peak expiratory flow meter can assist in the management of asthma by helping to identify when obstruction occurs (Kieckhefer & Ratcliffe, 2000). This device measures the child's ability to push air forcefully out of the lungs. Medication administration can be based on peak expiratory flow rate (PEFR) readings and the effectiveness of treatment confirmed by improved PEFR numbers.

Most children with acute exacerbations respond to aggressive management in the emergency department. Children who do not respond or who are already being managed at

CLINICAL TIP

Bechlomethaone is available in a new aerosol metered-dose inhaler that uses hydrofluoroalkane as a propellant, replacing chlorofluorocarbon (CFC) propellant. This permits asthma control at a lower dose than inhalants with CFC.

CLINICAL MANIFESTATIONS OF ASTHMA IN CHILDREN BY SEVERITY OF ACUTE EXACERBATIONS

ASSESSMENT CRITERIA	MILD	MODERATE	SEVERE
PEFR[a]	70%–90% predicted or personal best	50%–70% predicted or personal best	<50% predicted or personal best
Respiratory rate, resting or sleeping	Normal to 30% increase above the mean	30%–50% increase above mean	Increase over 50% above mean
Alertness	Normal	Normal	May be decreased
Dyspnea[b]	Absent or mild; speaks in complete sentences	Moderate; speaks in phrases or partial sentences; infant's cry softer and shorter; has difficulty sucking and feeding	Severe; speaks only in single words or short phrases; infant's cry softer and shorter; stops sucking and feeding
Pulsus paradoxus[c]	<10 mm Hg	10–20 mm Hg	20–40 mm Hg
Accessory muscle use	No intercostal to mild retractions	Moderate intercostal retractions with tracheosternal retractions; use of sternocleidomastoid muscles; chest hyperinflation	Severe intercostal retractions, tracheosternal retractions with nasal flaring during inspiration; chest hyperinflation
Color	Good	Pale	Possibly cyanotic
Auscultation	End-expiratory wheeze only	Wheeze during entire expiration and inspiration	Breath sounds becoming inaudible
Oxygen saturation	>95%	90%–95%	<90%
Pco_2	<35	<40	>40

Note: Within each category, the presence of several parameters, but not necessarily all, indicate the general classification of the exacerbation.
[a]For children 5 years of age or older.
[b]Parents or physicians' impressions of degree of children's breathlessness.
[c]Pulsus paradoxus does not correlate with phase of respiration in small children.
Note: From National Asthma Education and Prevention Program. (1994). *Acute exacerbations of asthma: Care in a hospital-based emergency department* (p. 13). Bethesdo, MD: National Heart, Lung, and Blood Institute, National Institutes of Health.

TABLE 13-8 Assessing Peak Expiratory Flow Rate (PEFR)

ZONE	PEFR (BEST OR PREDICTED FOR AGE)	ACTION
Green	80–100%	Continue regular management plan.
Yellow	50–80%	Implement action plan provided by physician.
Red	<50%	**Medical Alert:** Implement action plan predeter mined by physician. Call provider if PEFR does not return to yellow or green zone.

The child's personal best is determined after reviewing the recorded PEFRs measured two to four times a day for 2–3 weeks. The child should be optimally treated with medications during the day so the best reading is obtained (Richman, E. 1997). Asthma diagnosis and management: New severity classifications and therapy alternatives. *Clinician Review's,* 7(8), 76–112.

TABLE 13-9 Revised Asthma Severity Classification

CLASSIFICATION (STEPS)	DESCRIPTION	CLINICAL THERAPY
Step 1: Mild intermittent	Brief exacerbations with symptoms no more often than twice a week. Nighttime symptoms less than twice a week. PEFR ≥80% of predicted with variability <20%.	Quick relief bronchodilator as needed. If needed more than twice a week, move to next level.
Step 2: Mild persistent	Exacerbations more than twice a week, but less than once a day. May affect activity. PEFR ≥80% of predicted.	Daily anti-inflammatory medication. Quick relief bronchodilator as needed.
Step 3: Moderate persistent	Daily symptoms. Daily use of inhaled short-acting beta-agonist. Exacerbations at least twice a week that may last for days; nighttime symptoms more than once per week. Affects activity. PEFR >60% but <80% of predicted with variability >30%.	Daily anti-inflammatory medication, medium dose. Bronchodilator as needed up to three times a day.
Step 4: Severe persistent	Continuous symptoms, limited physical activity. Frequent exacerbations and frequent nighttime symptoms. PEFR ≤60% of predicted with variability >30%.	Daily anti-inflammatory medication, high dose. Systemic corticosteroid. Bronchodilator as needed for symptoms up to three times a day.

Note: From National Asthma Education and Prevention Program. (1997). *Expert panel report II: Guidelines for the diagnosis and management of asthma* (NIH Publication No. 97-4051, pp. 45–48). Bethesda, MD: National Institutes of Health.

home on corticosteroids have a greater chance of being admitted. Some children will need mechanical ventilation. Support of the parents and child should focus on helping them to cope with and understand the diagnosis and the need for daily management to promote near-normal respiratory function while the child continues to grow and develop normally.

NURSING MANAGEMENT

Nursing Assessment and Diagnosis

The nurse usually encounters the child and family in the emergency department or nursing unit. Acute care has become necessary because the child's level of respiratory compromise

CLINICAL TIP

Spacers with valves are often used with metered-dose inhalers (MDI) for children who cannot coordinate inspiration with medication release. The spacer captures the aerosol released by the MDI in a reservoir for the child to breathe in over a couple of minutes. This provides a benefit similar to nebulizer treatment, but it takes less time and is less expensive (Steinbach, 2000).

MEDICATIONS USED TO TREAT ASTHMA

Medication	Action/Indication	Nursing Considerations
Bronchodilators		
Beta$_2$-agonists (short acting and long acting) Albuterol, metaproterinal, terbutaline, or salmeterol: SQ, PO, aerosol	Relax smooth muscle in airway, resulting in rapid bronchodilation within 5–10 minutes; drugs of choice for acute or daily therapy (inhaled route); used for nocturnal symptoms and exercise-induced bronchospasm.	Have some side effects (tachycardia, nervousness, nausea and vomiting, headaches), but these are usually dose related; repetitive or excessive use can mask increasing airway inflammation and hyperresponsiveness
Methylxanthines Theophylline (related to caffeine): PO	Relax muscle bundles that constrict airways; dilate airway; provide continuous airway relaxation; sustained release for prevention of nocturnal symptoms.	Used later in the treatment course for moderate to severe symptoms. Used for long-term control, so continuous administration is needed; works best when a specific amount is maintained in the bloodstream (therapeutic serum level, 10–20 μ g/L); requires serum level checks and dose adjustment; have many and varied side effects (including tachycardia, dysrhythmias, restlessness, tremors, seizures, insomnia, hypotension, severe headaches, vomiting, and diarrhea)
Anti-inflammatory Agents		
Cromolyn sodium: aerosol only Nedocromil: aerosol only	Preventive medications, best taken daily to stop chemicals associated with producing asthma; controls seasonal, allergic, and exercise-induced asthma; may be used for unavoidable allergen exposure.	Less effective in older children; prophylactic medications, once wheezing starts, these medications are ineffective. Short courses of IV corticosteroids used to gain control and speed resolution of moderate to severe asthma.
Corticosteroids: IV, PO, or aerosol Bechlomethasone, triamcinolone, prednisone	Effectively reduce mucosal edema in airways; usually combined with other asthma medications for prompt control.	Side effects (such as abnormalities in glucose metabolism, increased appetite, fluid retention, weight gain, moon face, mood alteration, and hypertension) may be severe if used long term; if used on daily basis, lowest therapeutic dose should be given; growth suppression possible with long-term use.
Leukotriene Modifiers		
Montelukast: PO	Steroid-sparing adjunct for exercise-induced asthma to prevent bronchospasm. Alternate therapy to low doses of inhaled corticosteroids. Improves pulmonary function, but less effective than corticosteroids; enhances effect of corticosteroids and may permit lowering of dosage.	Increased risk of diarrhea, laryngitis, pharyngitis, nausea, otitis, sinusitis; give at bedtime once a day for easier compliance. Infrequent adverse effects of mild headache and gastrointestinal disturbances.
Other		
Hyposensitization (allergy shots), SQ	Series of injections that can reduce sensitivity to unavoidable allergens (e.g., environmental organisms—mold, pollen); gradual dose increase over time (called a buildup) increases the child's tolerance to allergic substances; has been of help in some children.	Use is controversial; some question about actual effect.

cannot be managed at home. What needs to be done first? What is the nurse's role during an acute asthmatic episode?

PHYSIOLOGIC ASSESSMENT

Skills 5-1 to 5-21: Performing a Physical Assessment

Identify the child's current respiratory status first by assessing the airway, breathing, and circulation (see clinical manifestations table on p. 436). If the child is moving air or talking, assess the quality of breathing. Is the child wheezing? Is stridor present? Are retractions visible (see Figure 13-3, p. 421)? What is the respiratory rate? What is the quality of breath sounds? Observe the child's color and assess the heart rate. Oxygen saturation is obtained via pulse oximeter. Only after no life-threatening respiratory distress is found should the assessment move on to other systems. Assess PEFR, skin turgor, intake and output, and spe-

TABLE 13-10 Psychosocial Assessment of the Child With an Acute Respiratory Illness

CHILD
■ Assess for indications of anxiety or fear that may have an impact on respiratory status. ■ For young children, inquire about security objects (such as a blanket or doll), the child's reaction to strangers, and reaction to absence of parents. ■ For older children, ask whether this is the first hospital stay and what previous illness and hospital experiences have meant to the child.
PARENTS
■ Assess parents' reactions: Are they anxious? Fearful? Verbal or quiet? Asking appropriate questions? ■ Observe for nonverbal cues. Often parents have financial worries (cost of hospital stay, lost work and wages) and personal worries (siblings at home who are ill) that they may not readily share with staff.

cific gravity. Because asthma can be a symptom of another illness, a head-to-toe assessment should be performed to identify other associated problems (see Tables 13-1 and 13-6).

Psychosocial Assessment

Is the child anxious? Crying? (See Table 13-10.) In an older child whose asthma was previously diagnosed, have the asthmatic episode and hospitalization created guilt about doing something the child thinks he or she should have avoided or about forgetting to take medication? The nurse should look for clues to hidden stress and self-blaming.

Common nursing diagnoses for the child experiencing an acute asthmatic episode include the following:

- *Ineffective airway clearance,* related to airway compromise, copious mucous secretions, and coughing
- *Impaired gas exchange,* related to airway obstruction, possible additional respiratory illness, and poor response to medication
- *Anxiety/fear (child or parents),* related to change in health status, difficulty in breathing
- *Ineffective management of therapeutic regimen (family),* related to acute and daily medical management of chronic disease

CLINICAL TIP 

To help toddlers learn how to use a peak flow meter, have them practice by blowing into party favors (i.e., noisemakers). To use a metered-dose inhaler, let the child learn to breathe in slowly with straws.

NURSING ALERT 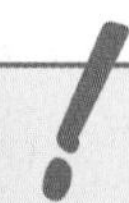

The infant or child who has had episodes of frequent coughing or frequent respiratory infections (especially pneumonia or bronchitis) should also be evaluated for asthma. The cough is the warning signal that the child's airway is very sensitive to stimuli; it may be the only sign in "silent" asthma.

Planning and Implementation

Pharmacologic and supportive therapies are used to reverse the airway obstruction and promote respiratory function. Nursing interventions center on maintaining airway patency, meeting fluid needs, promoting rest and stress reduction for the child and parents, supporting the family's participation in care, and providing the family with information to enable them to manage the child's acute asthmatic episodes and ongoing needs.

Maintain Airway Patency

If the child is exhibiting breathing difficulty, supplemental oxygen is required. Oxygen is best administered by nasal cannula or face mask. Humidified oxygen should be used to prevent drying and thickening of mucous secretions. The child should be placed in a sitting (semi-Fowler's) or upright position to promote and ease respiratory effort. The effectiveness of positioning and oxygen administration is evaluated by transcutaneous oxygen monitoring (pulse oximeter) and by observing for improved respiratory status.

The respiratory distress and need for supplemental oxygen can be stressful for parents and child alike (Figure 13-8 ◆). Encouraging the parents' presence can be reassuring for the child. The parents should be kept informed of procedures and results, and their input should be obtained in developing the treatment plan.

Skill 10-1: Using Oxygen Delivery Systems

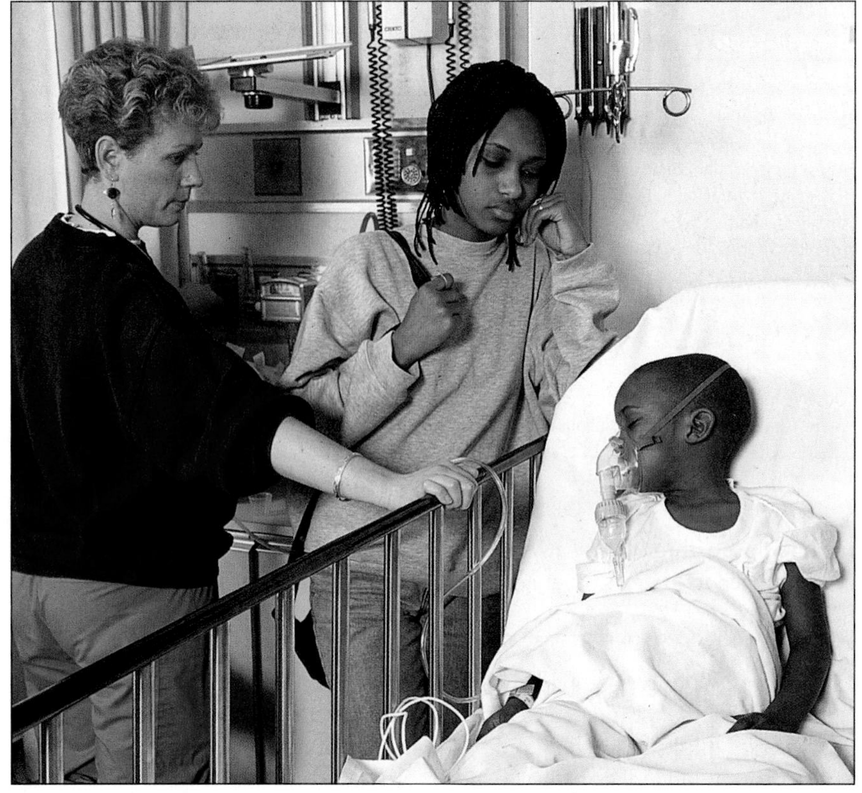

FIGURE 13-8 ◆
Acute exacerbations of asthma may require management in the emergency department. The child is positioned in a semi-sitting position to facilitate respiratory effort. Providing support to both the child and parent is an important part of nursing care during these acute episodes. The mother is exhausted after a sleepless night of caring for her son.

Many medications are given by the aerosol route (Figure 13-9 ◆). The advantages of aerosol are that the medication acts quickly, enabling the pulmonary blood vessels to absorb the inhaled medication; systemic effects are minimized; and the inhaled droplets provide the added benefit of moisture. Because the medication is quickly absorbed, continuous aerosol treatments may be implemented. Monitor the child for side effects. The frequency of vital sign assessment is related to the severity of symptoms.

Skill 7-10: Administering Nebulizer Aerosol Therapy

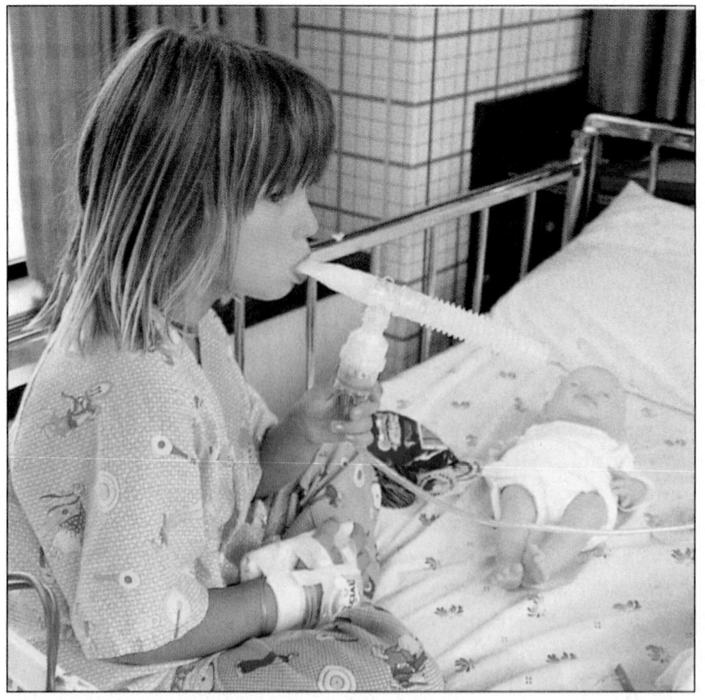

FIGURE 13-9 ◆
Medications given by aerosol therapy allow children the freedom to play and entertain themselves.

Meet Fluid Needs

Fluid therapy is often necessary to restore and maintain adequate fluid balance. Adequate hydration is essential to thin and break up trapped mucous plugs in the narrowed airways. An adequate oral intake may not be possible with the child's compromised respiratory status. An intravenous infusion may be needed, and this route also may be used for administering medications and providing glucose. Overhydration must be avoided to prevent pulmonary edema in severe asthma attacks.

As respiratory difficulty diminishes, oral fluids can be offered slowly. Intake and output are monitored and specific gravity is assessed frequently to evaluate the child's hydration status. Involving parents in feeding can help gain the child's cooperation in taking oral fluids. The child's fluid preferences should be determined and choices provided where possible.

SAFETY PRECAUTIONS

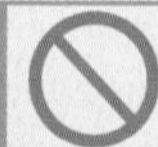

Iced beverages precipitate bronchospasms in some children with asthma. It is safest to offer the asthmatic child room temperature or slightly cooled fluids without ice.

Promote Rest and Stress Reduction

The child who has had an acute asthmatic episode is usually very tired when admitted to the nursing unit. Labored breathing and low oxygen status have left the child exhausted. The child should be placed in a quiet, private room if possible, to promote relaxation and rest. By grouping tasks, nurses can avoid repeatedly disturbing the child.

Support Family Participation

The parents may stay with the child, but may be exhausted after hours of their child's respiratory distress. Give parents the option of assisting with the child's treatments, rather than expecting them to do it in addition to comforting the child. Provide frequent updates about the child's condition and encourage the parents to take breaks as needed.

Length of hospitalization depends on the child's response to therapy. Any underlying or accompanying health problem, such as preexisting lung disease or pneumonia, can complicate and extend the child's hospital stay. Communicate with the family of the hospitalized child at least once a day about the child's condition.

Discharge Planning and Home Care Teaching

Parents need a thorough understanding of asthma—how to prevent attacks and use treatment to maintain the child's health and avoid unnecessary hospitalization. When possible, educate parents when they are rested. Provide a written treatment plan about how to manage asthma on a daily basis and in a crisis. *Pediatric Asthma: Promoting Best Practice* is a good resource for families and is available from the American Academy of Asthma, Allergy, and Immunology. Through printed educational materials and referral to a local support group, parents gain additional knowledge and confidence that enable them to help their child lead a normal life (National Education and Prevention Program, 1997) (Figure 13-10 ◆). Special summer camps for asthmatic children are also available.

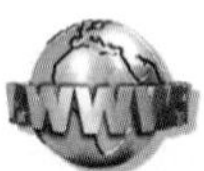

Asthma at Home

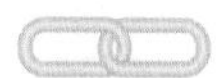

Skill 7-11: Using a Metered Dose Inhaler

Discharge planning for the asthmatic child focuses on increasing the family's knowledge about the disease, medication therapy, and the need for follow-up care according to guidelines of the National Asthma Education and Prevention Program. The required lifestyle changes may be difficult for the child and parents. The need to modify the home by removing a loved pet, for example, may create stress. The nurse can play a role in keeping lines of communication open and can facilitate discussion and clarification of ways to prevent asthmatic episodes. Teach the family how to measure peak expiratory flow and necessary medications to manage asthma attacks early on. The family should be reassured that most children with asthma can lead a normal life with some modifications.

CULTURE

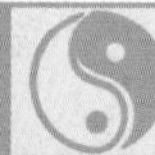

Parents of children from different cultures may have concerns about daily medication regimens. Some prefer to use folk medicines such as rubbing oils or Vicks preparations on the child's chest. Learn about the family's cultural beliefs and practices (Sydnor-Greenberg & Dokken, 2000).

Care in the Community

Nurses provide care to children with asthma in pediatricians' offices, specialty asthma clinics, schools, and summer camps. Once the stress of the acute episode has passed, opportunities exist to provide more extensive education (Figure 13-11 ◆).

If the child has severe asthma and uses high doses of aerosol or oral glucocorticoids to control asthma attacks, monitor the child's growth every 6 months as the disease and medications may affect overall growth. Review the family's daily plan for monitoring the child's

ASTHMA TRIGGERS ABOUND
Everyday life is filled with the allergens and other precipitating factors that can kick off an attack
ALLERGIC REACTIONS
• Pollens • Feathers
• Molds • Animals
• Some Foods
• House Dust
VIGOROUS EXERCISE
SLEEP
(Nocturnal Asthma)
INFECTIONS
• Common Cold
• Influenza
COLD AIR
HOUSEHOLD PRODUCTS
• Paint • Cleaners
• Sprays
STRESS
EMOTIONAL STRESS AND EXCITEMENT
OCCUPATIONAL DUSTS AND VAPORS
• Plastics • Grains
• Metals • Wood
DRUGS
• Aspirin, Ibuprofen
• Some Heart Medications
AIR POLLUTION
• Cigarette Smoke
• Ozone
• Sulfur Dioxide
• Auto Exhaust

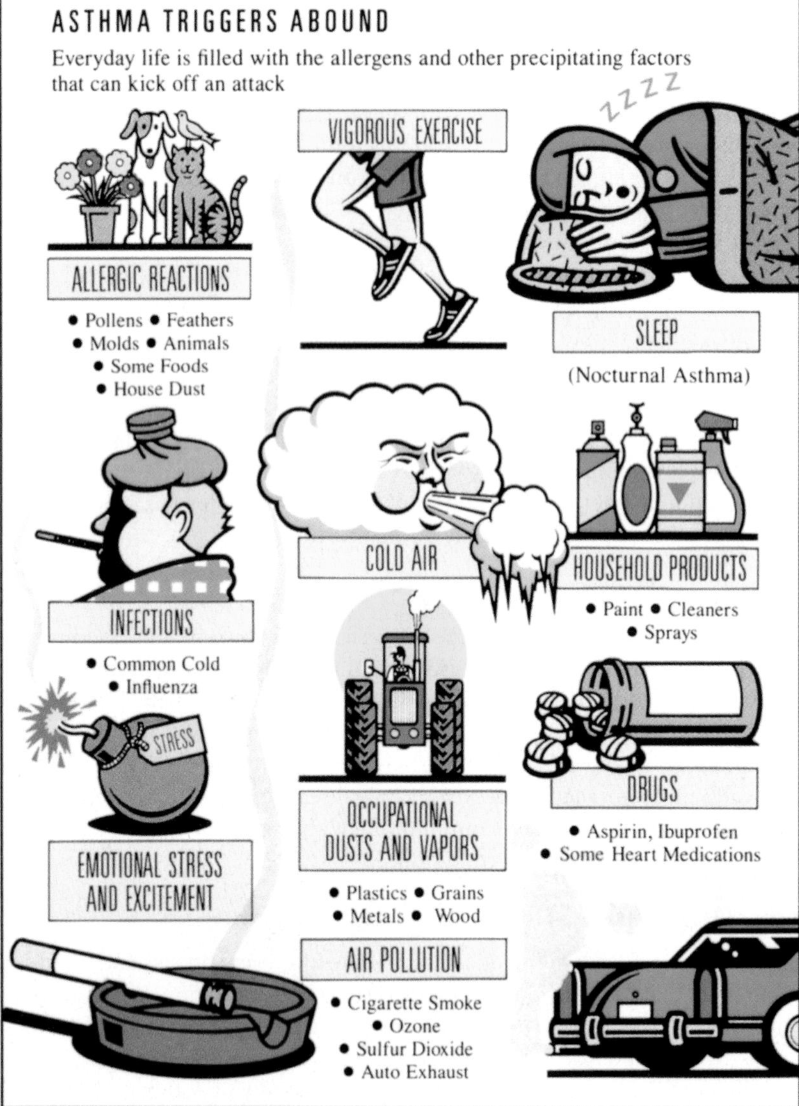

FIGURE 13-10 ◆
This educational piece from the American Lung Association explains what triggers an asthma attack. The required lifestyle changes for the child and family will be significant, so be sensitive to the family's situation and needs. Culture sometimes plays a significant part in exposure to life-style triggers.
Reprinted with permission ©2002 American Lung Association. For more information on how you can support to fight lung disease, the third leading cause of death in the U.S., please contact the American Lung Association at 1-800-LUNG-USA (1-800-586-4872) or log on to the website at www.lungusa.org.

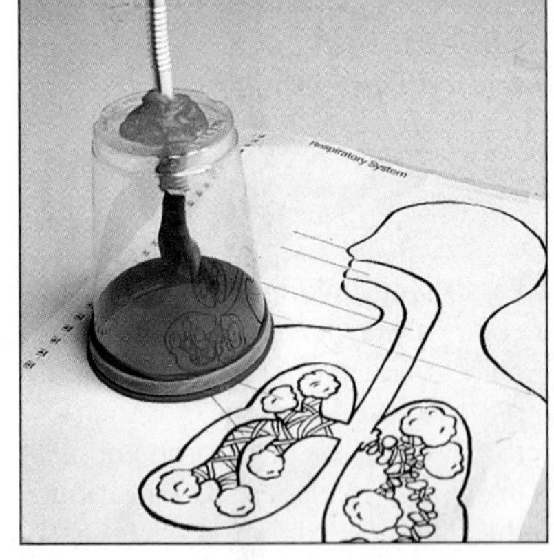

FIGURE 13-11 ◆
School-age children can be taught how the lung functions using simple activities such as this project, in which a "lung" is made using a plastic cup, a straw, and balloons. The school nurse who organized the asthma club described in Chapter 1 uses this activity to illustrate how the lung takes in air, expanding and contracting during breathing.

respiratory status. Evaluate the child's technique for PEFR and the parent's ability to identify the timing and type of stepped-up care needed to manage worsening symptoms. The goal is to bring asthma attacks under control with stepped-up care before a significant episode occurs. This can be achieved only with daily monitoring (Table 13-11).

Environmental control is an important part of asthma management. When possible, pets should not be kept in the home (and never in the child's bedroom). Cockroaches and dust mites should be eliminated or controlled. Smoke from cigarettes, wood stoves, and fireplaces has the potential to trigger an asthma attack.

Help the child learn the signs of early respiratory distress so that treatment can be obtained before signs get more serious. Parents should communicate with school personnel regarding the child's condition, and have an individual school health plan developed to ensure that medications are given as needed, even in preparation for exercise. Make sure the child has a supply of medications at school or child care as well as at home.

Refer to the nursing care plan for the child with asthma in the community setting, in Chapter 6, for additional information.

Evaluation

Expected outcomes of nursing care include the following:

- The child recognizes asthma symptoms and uses rescue medications before severe respiratory distress occurs.

FAMILIES WANT TO KNOW

Home Care Instructions for the Child with Asthma

IDENTIFY PARENTS' KNOWLEDGE ABOUT THE CONDITION:

a. Review why asthma occurs and assess parents' understanding of the physiologic process. Ask:
   - Do you understand what happens in your child's lungs during an asthma attack?
   - Do you know the early warning signs of an asthma episode in your child?
   - What are your child's symptoms and how does he or she respond to them? Does your child use the peak expiratory flow meter to evaluate symptoms?
b. Identify asthma triggers and assess parents' understanding of how to prevent, avoid, or minimize their effect in a timely manner. Ask:
   - Do you know your child's personal asthma triggers? (Suggest that the parents and child keep a notebook to track episodes so they can learn more about these triggers.)
   - What steps can you take to minimize or eliminate your child's exposure (quitting smoking, environmental control, etc.)?

SET UP A SCHEDULE FOR PARENTS TO LEARN ASTHMA MANAGEMENT. ASK:

- Do you know when and where to seek emergency medical help?
- What actions can you take before seeking medical assistance?

REVIEW PARENTS' UNDERSTANDING OF MEDICATION THERAPY:

- Provide information about medications: name, type of drug, dose, method of administration, expected effect, possible side effects.
- Evaluate the child's technique for the use of an inhaler and peak flow meter.

ADDRESS ASSOCIATED ISSUES:

- Do parents know how to store and properly transport medications?
- What are the financial considerations of medication cost and lifestyle changes?
- Has the child's school or teacher been notified? What arrangements have been made for the child's use of medications at school?
- Has a medical identification bracelet or medallion been obtained for the child to facilitate assistance when away from home?

IDENTIFY NEED FOR FOLLOW-UP CARE:

- Do parents know when to see a physician? When drug levels need to be checked?
- Does the child need to see an allergist?
- Do the child and parents have special emotional needs?
- Would a self-help group or camp experience be helpful for the child?

TABLE 13-11 Markers of Good Asthma Control

- Prevents chronic and troublesome symptoms of cough, wheeze, difficulty breathing, and chest tightness
- Maintains normal or near-normal pulmonary function
- Maintains normal activity levels including physical exercise
- Prevents recurrent exacerbations and minimizes the need for urgent care or hospitalization
- Provides optimal pharmacotherapy with minimal or no adverse effects
- Meets patient's and family's expectations of asthma care and maintains their satisfaction with care

Note: From National Asthma Education and Prevention Program. (1997). *Expert panel report II: Guidelines for diagnosis and management of asthma* (NIH Publication No. 97-4051). Bethesda, MD: National Institutes of Health.

- The child and family implement a daily treatment plan for asthma and reduce the number of asthma attacks the child has.
- The child with a serious asthma attack responds to oxygen, fluids, and medication therapy, avoiding hospital admission.

GROWTH & DEVELOPMENT

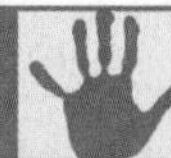

For young school-age children, make sure their teachers can help recognize respiratory distress and can reduce their fear of going to the nurse for rescue medications.

STATUS ASTHMATICUS

Status asthmaticus is unrelenting, severe respiratory distress and bronchospasm in an asthmatic child, which persists despite pharmacologic and supportive interventions. Without immediate intervention the child with status asthmaticus may die. The child is placed in an intensive care unit and may require endotracheal intubation with assisted ventilation. The section on respiratory failure earlier in the chapter gives additional information on the nurse's role in providing emergency respiratory care.

LOWER AIRWAY DISORDERS

The lower airway, or bronchial tree, lies below the trachea and includes the bronchi, bronchioles, and alveoli. Lower airway disorders occur because a structural or functional problem interferes with the lungs' ability to complete the respiratory cycle. Lower airway disorders include neonatal respiratory distress syndrome, bronchopulmonary dysplasia, bronchitis, bronchiolitis, pneumonia, tuberculosis, and cystic fibrosis.

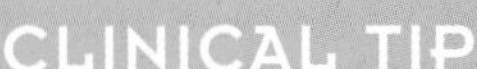

CLINICAL TIP

An alveolus can be thought of as a small balloon filled with water. When the balloon is emptied, the water droplets that remain inside the balloon cause the surface tension to increase. As a result, the sides of the balloon stick together. The increased surface tension makes reinflation almost impossible.

NEONATAL RESPIRATORY DISTRESS SYNDROME

Neonatal respiratory distress syndrome (RDS) manifests during the first hours of life in newborn infants with severely compromised respiratory systems. It may be caused by hyaline membrane disease or meconium aspiration. RDS is the most common cause of respiratory failure during the first days after birth, but due to improved technology, 80% to 90% of affected infants survive (Tooley, 1996).

RDS results from inadequate or inactivated pulmonary surfactant. Surfactant is a substance that lowers the surface tension of the alveoli by keeping the alveoli inflated and preventing the interior walls from adhering. Without sufficient surfactant, the alveoli collapse and cannot reinflate.

In utero, the fetal lungs are filled with fluid. When the infant takes the first breath after birth, this fluid is expelled from the alveoli. If insufficient surfactant is present, the alveolar walls adhere to each other. As a result, oxygen and carbon dioxide cannot be exchanged, which creates a threat to life. The alveoli themselves become damaged and die, creating thick scar tissue (the hyaline membrane tissue) in the alveolar space. The alveoli are replaced with fibrous nonfunctional tissue that stiffens the lung (Tooley, 1996).

Clinical manifestations include tachypnea (70 to 120 breaths/min), retractions, grunting, rales, cyanosis, slow capillary refill, **paradoxical breathing** (in which the chest falls and the abdomen rises on inspiration), decreased breath sounds, and labored breathing.

Diagnosis usually occurs in the newborn nursery. A chest x-ray showing air in the bronchial tree, atelectasis, and decreased lung volume confirms the diagnosis. Medical management focuses on adequate resuscitation at birth, good temperature control, and assisted ventilation to expand the alveoli and preserve respiratory function. Intravenous fluid therapy and medications (primarily theophylline and dexamethasone) are administered to support function of the respiratory and other body systems. Synthetic surfactant given within 24 hours of birth has decreased mortality, but it has not changed the development of chronic inflammation (Gross, 1999). Blood products may be administered to expand blood volume, thus increasing oxygen capacity. Ventilatory support is provided by constant positive airway pressure (CPAP) or intubation with ventilation.

Nursing Management

The respiratory status of the infant with RDS is closely monitored. Nursing assessment focuses on identifying changes in respiratory status, such as quality of respirations and pulse, overall color, signs of dehydration, and changes in the infant's behavior. Pulse oximetry and blood gases are monitored to aid in assessment.

Care of the infant is organized to eliminate any unnecessary physical stimulation, as this additional stress contributes to respiratory compromise. The infant is usually placed in a warmer to reduce metabolic demands. Provide fluids and nutrition to help meet metabolic demands. Position the infant to facilitate breathing. Parents need clear explanations about the infant's health status and planned interventions. By remaining available to parents and answering their questions, the nurse establishes a positive relationship and facilitates essential communication.

Skill 10-13: Performing Infant Cardiopulmonary Respiration

Because of the potential for respiratory distress and chronic lung disease after discharge, parents should be taught CPR. The infant is also monitored at home for apnea, and medical follow-up should be continuous. Parents may benefit from a referral to a support group.

BRONCHOPULMONARY DYSPLASIA

Bronchopulmonary dysplasia (BPD) is an acute lung injury in which an abnormal radiograph is found and oxygen is required at 36 weeks postconceptional age. It is the most prevalent and serious chronic respiratory disorder that begins during infancy. Premature infants are affected more often than full-term infants, and morbidity is greater in males than in females. The incidence is increasing due to advances in medical technology that permit very-low-birth-weight infants to survive (Daigle & Cloutier, 1997).

BPD is a direct result of the treatment provided to premature and term infants with such conditions as RDS, congenital heart disease, meconium aspiration, patent ductus arteriosis, and fluid overload and edema in newborns. The sequence of events is an immature lung leading to respiratory failure requiring mechanical ventilation resulting in barotrauma, oxygen toxicity, inflammation, cellular damage, and death. Fibrosis and edema of the bronchioles along with smooth muscle hypertrophy follow (Harvey, 2000).

The infant with BPD has persistent signs of respiratory distress: tachypnea, wheezing, crackles, irritability, nasal flaring, grunting, retractions, pulmonary edema, and failure to thrive. Cyanosis may be seen in severe cases. Normal activities, such as feeding, can create increased oxygen demands that are difficult for the compromised infant to meet.

The chest x-ray is the best indicator of lung changes and is the key to medical diagnosis. There may be cystic changes or fine lacy densities with or without hyperinflation (Harvey, 2000). The air trapping persists and in time causes the chest to assume a barrel shape (Figure 13-12 ◆). Medical management focuses on symptomatic treatment that supports respiratory function and on good nutrition, which helps to accelerate lung maturity. Supplemental oxygen with humidity is used to keep the SaO_2 more than 90% to 92% even during sleep and feeding. Chest physiotherapy and medications (diuretics, bronchodilators, anti-inflammatories, and inhaled corticosteroids) are also used. With improvement and adequate weight gain, the child is weaned off of oxygen, diuretics, and bronchodilators. Long-term sequelae include asthma and respiratory infections with frequent rehospitalization rates.

Nursing Management

Nursing management focuses on promoting respiratory function and preparing the family for home care needs. Nursing assessment includes close monitoring of respirations, pulse, color, behavior changes, and vital signs. The infant with chronic BPD may become acutely ill at any time.

COMMUNITY CARE

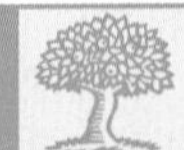

Potential long-term outcomes of BPD include:

- Developmental delays
- Growth retardation
- Continuing airway obstruction
- Persistent airway hyperactivity

PATHOPHYSIOLOGY ILLUSTRATED

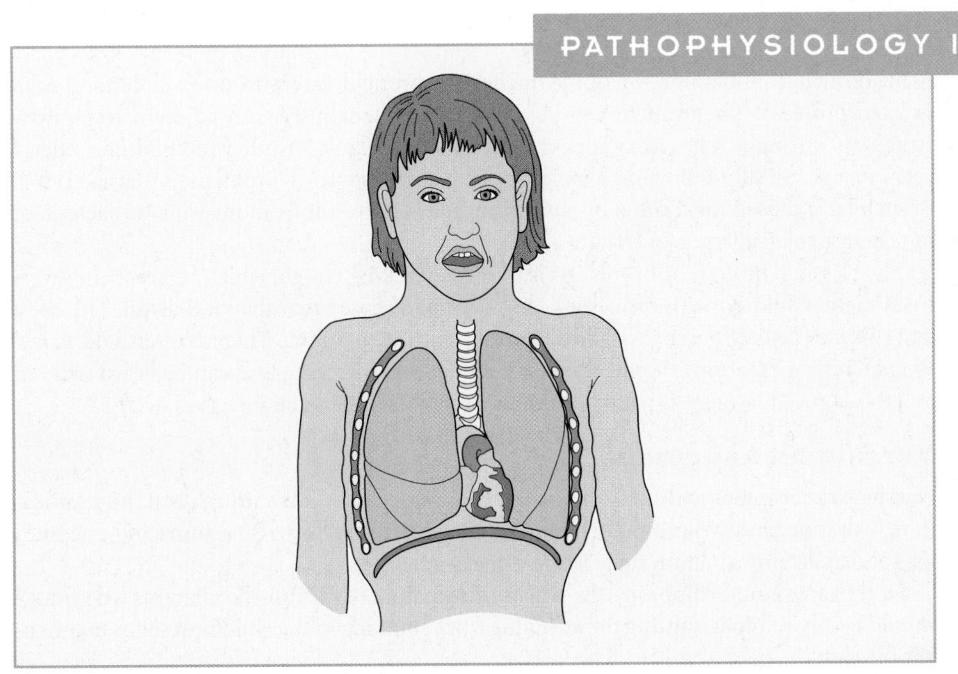

Barrel Chest

FIGURE 13-12 ◆
A barrel chest may result from chronic respiratory conditions such as bronchopulmonary dysplasia or asthma, in which air trapping or hyperinflation of the alveoli occur.

MEDICATIONS USED TO TREAT BRONCHOPULMONARY DYSPLASIA

Medication	Action/Indication
Bronchodilators (beta$_2$-adrenergics, anticholinergics, theophylline, albuterol nebulizer)	Decreases airway resistance, increases expiratory flow in small airways, stimulates mucous clearance; different drugs work together for best response.
Anti-inflammatory agents (corticosteroids, inhaled cromolyn, becholmethasone)	Reduces pulmonary edema and inflammation in small airways, enhances effect of bronchodilators, helps decrease the need for other drugs and oxygen; for moderate disease only
Diuretics (furosemide, chlorothiazide, spironoloactone)	Helps remove excess fluid from lungs, decreases pulmonary resistance and increases pulmonary compliance; may cause electrolyte imbalances
Potassium chloride	Prevents electrolyte imbalances associated with diuretics
Antibiotics	Low-dose prophylactic therapy prevents severe illness; specific treatment for identified organisms
RSV immune globulin	Prevents respiratory syncytial virus

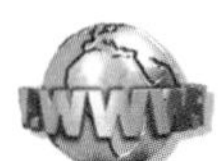

BPD Support Online

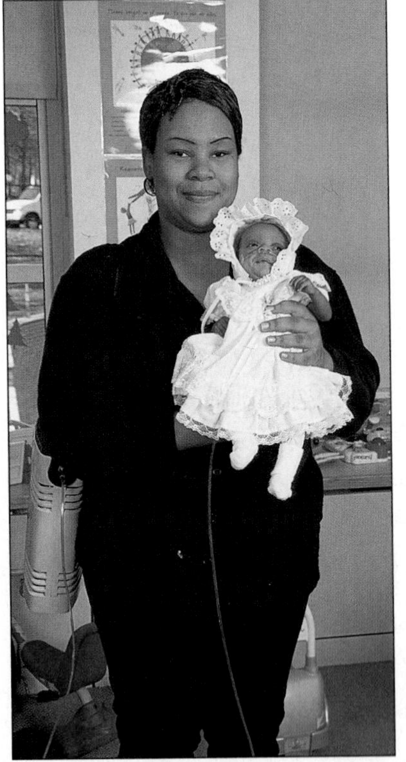

FIGURE 13-13 ◆
Many children with BPD are cared for at home, with the support of a home care program to monitor the family's ability to provide airway management, oxygen, and support. This premature infant girl, who is now 4-months old but weighs only about 5 pounds, requires respiratory support, which is provided by a portable oxygen tank.

Once home, many infants need ventilation therapy, oxygen respiratory support, and drug therapy (Figure 13-13 ◆). Frequent rehospitalization may be necessary because, although the lungs may function adequately, they remain vulnerable throughout childhood to common respiratory illnesses. Infants with BPD do not have the same respiratory reserve as healthy infants, and they can become very ill very quickly. This was illustrated by the case of Emily, described in the vignette at the beginning of this chapter. Nutritional requirements to support growth must be balanced with fluid restrictions. A formula supplemented with carbohydrates and medium chain triglycerides may be given to promote weight gain. Some children need nasogatric or gastrostomy tube feedings to get adequate nutrition when cyanosis is noted with feeding. Electrolytes must be monitored monthly.

It is important to provide for the infant's normal development through rest, nutrition, stimulation, and family support. Including parents in the infant's care early on promotes bonding and prepares them for home care responsibilities. Some families require home nursing assistance. Referrals for needed respiratory supplies, medications, an early intervention program, and follow-up care must be carefully planned and coordinated well in advance of the infant's discharge date.

BRONCHITIS

Acute bronchitis, inflammation of the trachea and bronchi, rarely occurs in childhood as an isolated problem. The bronchi can be affected simultaneously with adjacent respiratory structures during a respiratory illness. Bronchitis occurs most often in children under 4 years of age, usually following a mild upper respiratory tract problem (D'Auria, 1997). Bronchitis is caused most often by a virus but may also result from invasion of bacteria or in response to an allergen or irritant.

The classic symptom of bronchitis is a coarse, hacking cough, which increases in severity at night. Children with bronchitis look tired and report that they feel awful. The chest and ribs may be sore because of the deep and frequent coughing. There is often a deep, rattling quality to breathing. Some children have audible wheezing that can be heard without a stethoscope. Treatment is palliative unless a secondary bacterial infection occurs.

Nursing Management

Nursing management includes supporting respiratory function through rest, humidification, hydration, and symptomatic treatment. Refer to the sections on asthma and pneumonia for detailed information on treatment measures.

Home care should emphasize the self-limiting nature of the disorder. Parents who smoke should be advised that quitting or refraining from smoking in the child's presence may benefit the child.

BRONCHIOLITIS

Bronchiolitis is one of the most frequent causes of hospitalization in infants and poses one of the greatest threats to the respiratory system of infants and small children (Webster & Huether, 1998). Although some infants and children have mild symptoms that are easily managed at home, others become acutely ill with severe respiratory distress that can become a life-threatening emergency. What makes bronchiolitis such a potential threat?

Bronchiolitis is a lower respiratory tract illness that occurs when an infecting agent (virus or bacterium) causes inflammation and obstruction of the small airways, the bronchioles. Infection occurs most frequently in toddlers and preschoolers. Infection is most severe in infants under 6 months of age. Infants under 2 months of age are particularly vulnerable, and they are routinely hospitalized when bronchiolitis is diagnosed.

Etiology and Pathophysiology

Viral, bacterial, and mycoplasmal organisms may cause bronchiolitis; however, infection with respiratory syncytial virus (RSV) is the most common cause. RSV is transmitted through direct or close contact with respiratory secretions of infected individuals. Viruses, acting as parasites, are able to invade the mucosal cells that line the small bronchi and bronchioles. The invaded cells die when the virus bursts from inside the cell to invade adjacent cells. The resulting cell debris clogs and obstructs the bronchioles and irritates the airway. In response, the airway lining swells and produces excessive mucus. Despite this protective effort by the bronchioles, the actual effect is partial airway obstruction and bronchospasms.

The cycle is repeated throughout both lungs as the airway cells are invaded by the virus. The partially obstructed airways allow air in, but the mucus and airway swelling block expulsion of the air. This creates the wheezing and crackles in the airways. Air trapped below the obstruction also interferes with normal gas exchange. The child with RSV is therefore at risk for respiratory failure as the oxygen level decreases and the carbon dioxide level increases. Apnea and pulmonary edema may occur.

As the airflow continues to decrease, breath sounds diminish. Thus the noisier the lungs, the better, as this indicates that the child is still able to move air in and out of the lungs.

RESPIRATORY SYNCYTIAL VIRUS

Respiratory syncytial virus (RSV) occurs in annual epidemics from October to March. Nearly all children have been infected with RSV by 2 years of age, and reinfection (via siblings or close family contacts) throughout life is common (National Respiratory and Enteric Virus Surveillance System, 2000). It is the most common cause of lower respiratory tract infections in infants and children. RSV causes severe or fatal illness in infants with conditions such as congenital heart disease, bronchopulmonary dysplasia (BPD), prematurity, and immunosuppression. Health care workers should follow principles of good handwashing, as the virus is easily transmitted and can survive on the hands for 1 hour.

Clinical Manifestations

The infant or child with bronchiolitis may have been ill with upper respiratory symptoms such as nasal stuffiness, cough (not usually noted in infants), and fever (less than 39°C [102.2°F]) for a few days. As the illness progresses and the lower respiratory tract becomes involved, symptoms increase and include wheezing; a deeper, more frequent cough; and more labored breathing. Respirations are rapid, shallow, and accompanied by nasal flaring and retractions (signs of severe distress). Parents report that the infant or child is acting more ill—appearing sicker, less playful, and less interested in eating. Infants, especially, may refuse to feed or may spit up what they do eat along with thick, clear mucus.

Clinical Therapy

The history and physical examination provide the data needed to diagnose bronchiolitis. Chest x-rays show nonspecific findings of inflammation.

Viral cultures or antigen testing of an immunofluorescence stain of respiratory secretions obtained by either a nasal swab in special culture medium or a nasopharyngeal wash confirm the presence of RSV. Children who test positive for RSV are isolated, roomed together, or placed on the same ward to minimize the spread of the virus to other hospitalized children. Medical management is frequently supportive, especially when the causative agent is unknown and the condition is mild to moderate in severity (Table 13-12). The child may be intubated and ventilated for apnea or respiratory failure. Ribavirin is the only antiviral drug available for treatment, but because studies have not confirmed its effectiveness, it is reserved for life-threatening cases (Margo & Shaughnessy, 1998).

Skills 6-13, 6-14: Collecting Respiratory Secretions

There is evidence that bronchiolitis in infancy may increase the chances of childhood wheezing and asthma. It also may be a major risk factor for chronic obstructive pulmonary disease later in life (Webster & Huether, 1998).

TABLE 13-12 Clinical Therapy for Bronchiolitis

CLINICAL THERAPY	RATIONALE
Cardiorespiratory monitor and pulse oximetry	Enable provider to follow course and assess need for specific therapies
Humidified oxygen therapy via hood or face tent, tent, or nasal cannula	Delivery method determined by desired concentration of oxygen, degree of moisture, and child's response
Intubation and assisted ventilation	Used when the child becomes too fatigued to breathe effectively
Hydration via intravenous or oral fluids	Provider must consider insensible fluid loss, decreased intake, the child's current electrolyte and hydration status, and risk for pulmonary edema
Aerosol medications	Bronchodilators, steroids, and beta-antagonists act directly on inflamed and obstructed airways; bronchodilators help prevent apnea episodes in premature infants; ribavirin (RSV antiviral agent) reduces the severity of the illness, improves oxygenation, and decreases inflammatory injury
Pulmonary hygiene (postural drainage and chest physiotherapy)	Helps to further loosen trapped mucus
Systemic medications	Symptomatic treatment may include antipyretics (acetaminophen or ibuprofen preferred; no antibiotics are given unless evidence of secondary bacterial infection such as otitis media is present)
High-Risk Infant or Child[a] Respigam (RSV immune globulin) IV Palivizumab IM	Give for 5 consecutive months during RSV season to high-risk children. May prevent RSV bronchiolitis. Both are expensive, but less than hospitalization.

[a]Defined as a child with congenital heart disease, bronchopulmonary dysplasia, chronic lung problems, or cystic fibrosis or who is premature or severely ill and less than 6 weeks old.

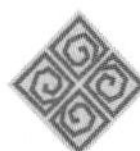

NURSING MANAGEMENT

Nursing Assessment and Diagnosis

Physiologic Assessment

Assess airway and respiratory function carefully. Good observation skills are important to ensure timely interventions for worsening respiratory symptoms and prevention of respiratory distress (see Table 13-1 and the clinical manifestations table on p. 427). A decreased oxygen saturation level is the best indicator of the severity of the disease.

Psychosocial Assessment

Children and their parents should be observed for signs of fear and anxiety (see Table 13-10). The unfamiliar hospital environment and procedures can increase stress. Parents' questions, as well as their nonverbal cues, help direct nursing interventions during admission and throughout hospitalization.

Developmental Assessment

Observe for signs of stranger and separation anxieties, which are common in the age group most often hospitalized for bronchiolitis (infants and small children). Involving parents in procedures and care, when appropriate, can promote emotional security.

The accompanying nursing care plan lists common nursing diagnoses for the child with bronchiolitis. The following diagnoses might also be appropriate:

- *Ineffective airway clearance,* related to increased airway secretions, fatigue from coughing and dyspnea, and air trapping
- *Activity intolerance,* related to imbalance between oxygen supply and demand
- *Risk for fluid volume deficit,* related to inability to meet fluid needs and increased metabolic demands (insensible loss, fever, thickened or increased respiratory secretions)

Planning and Implementation

Nursing management focuses on maintaining respiratory function, supporting overall physiologic function and hydration, reducing the child's and family's anxiety, and preparing the family for home care. Refer to the accompanying nursing care plan, which summarizes nursing care for the child with bronchiolitis.

Maintain Respiratory Function

Close monitoring is essential to evaluate the child's improvement or to spot early signs of deterioration. Oxygen and pulmonary care therapies are administered. High humidity and supplemental oxygen may be provided with a mist tent if the child requires only moisture and minimal oxygen. If more concentrated oxygen is required, it can be given via nasal cannula, hood, or tent. Pulse oximetry is used to evaluate oxygenation.

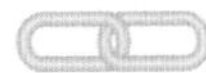

Skill 10-1: Using Oxygen Delivery Systems

Patent nares are important to promote oxygen intake. A bulb syringe is a helpful tool that can quickly and easily clear the nasal passages. The head of the bed should be elevated to ease the work of breathing and drain mucus from the upper airways. Pulmonary hygiene and nebulized medications are usually administered by a respiratory therapist. Maintenance of a nebulizer for medications may be needed.

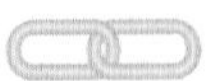

Skill 10-15: Using a Bulb Syringe

Support Physiologic Function

The grouping of nursing tasks promotes the child's physiologic function by decreasing stress and promoting rest. Rest is a key component in improving the child's breathing and overall health. Medications may be administered to control temperature and promote comfort as needed. An intravenous infusion may be ordered to rehydrate and maintain fluid balance until the child is capable of taking sufficient oral fluids.

Reduce Anxiety

The need for hospitalization and assistive therapies creates anxiety and fear in the child and parents. An important part of nursing care is anticipating, recognizing, and acting to decrease the child's and parents' anxiety. Provide parents with thorough explanations and daily updates, and encourage their participation in the child's care.

The presence of parents and their ability to calm the infant or child can be helpful in the child's recovery. The parents may themselves be frightened by the child's continued respiratory difficulty and the presence of assistive equipment at bedside. They should be reassured that holding or touching the child will not dislodge wires or tubing.

If the child has been ill for a few days before admission, the parents are likely to be tired. Acknowledging parents' physical and emotional needs facilitates a spirit of caring and enhances communication between staff and family. The parents should be encouraged to take turns at the child's bedside and to take breaks for meals and rest.

Discharge Planning and Home Care Teaching

Children are discharged once they show sufficient stability in maintaining adequate oxygenation (as evidenced by easing of respiratory effort, decreased mucous production, and absence of coughing). In most children, symptoms abate within 24 to 72 hours; however,

NURSING CARE PLAN The Child with Bronchiolitis

GOAL	INTERVENTION	RATIONALE	EXPECTED OUTCOME
1. Ineffective Breathing Pattern related to increased work of breathing and decreased energy (fatigue)			
	NIC Priority Intervention: **Respiratory monitoring:** Collection and analysis of patient data to ensure airway patency and adequate gas exchange.		NOC Suggested Outcome: **Vital signs status:** Temperature, pulse, respiration, and blood pressure within expected range for the child's age
The child will return to respiratory baseline. The child will not experience respiratory failure.	■ Assess respiratory status (Table 13-1) a minimum of every 2–4 hours or more often as indicated for a decreasing respiratory rate and episodes of apnea. Cardiorespiratory monitor and pulse oximeter attached with alarms set, if ordered. Record and report changes promptly to physician.	■ Changes in breathing pattern may occur quickly as the child's energy reserves are depleted. Assessment and monitoring baseline reveal rate and quality of air exchange. Frequent assessment and monitoring provides objective evidence of changes in the quality of respiratory effort, enabling prompt and effective intervention.	The child returns to respiratory baseline within 48–72 hours.
The child's oxygenation status will return to baseline.	■ Administer humidified oxygen via mask, hood, or tent.	■ Humidified oxygen loosens secretions and helps maintain oxygenation status and ease respiratory distress.	The child's respiratory effort eases. Pulse oximetry reading remains >94% oxygen saturation during treatment.
	■ Note child's response to ordered medications (nebulizer treatments).	■ Medications act systemically and locally (on respiratory tissue) to improve oxygenation and decrease inflammation.	The child tolerates therapeutic measures with no adverse effects.
	■ Position head of bed up or place child in position of comfort on parent's lap, if crying or struggling in crib or bed.	■ Position facilitates improved aeration and promotes decrease in anxiety (especially in toddlers) and energy expenditure.	The child rests quietly in position of comfort.
2. Risk for Fluid Volume Deficit related to inability to meet body requirements and increased metabolic demand			
	NIC Priority Intervention: **Fluid management:** Promotion of fluid balance and prevention of complications resulting from abnormal or undesired fluid levels.		NOC Suggested Outcome: **Hydration:** Amount of water in intracellular and extracellular compartments of body.
Child's immediate fluid deficit is corrected.	■ Evaluate need for intravenous fluids. Maintain IV, if ordered.	■ Previous fluid loss may require immediate replacement.	Child's hydration status is maintained during acute phase of illness.
Child will be adequately hydrated, be able to tolerate oral fluids, and progress to normal diet.	■ Maintain strict intake and output monitoring and evaluate specific gravity at least every 8 hours.	■ Monitoring proves objective evidence of fluid loss and ongoing hydration status.	Child takes adequate oral fluids after 24–48 hours to maintain hydration.

(continued)

resolution of all symptoms may take weeks. The same supportive therapies implemented in the hospital may be needed at home:

- Use of the bulb syringe to suction the nares of an infant under 1 year of age
- Fluid intake to thin respiratory secretions (making them easier to clear) and provide glucose for energy (since the child's appetite may not return to normal for several days)
- Rest

Children are usually capable of recognizing their own activity limits. However, parents should encourage active toddlers to nap and take rest periods. Teach the parents proper administration of medications. Acetaminophen may be prescribed for persistent low-grade

NURSING CARE PLAN — The Child with Bronchiolitis (continued)

GOAL	INTERVENTION	RATIONALE	EXPECTED OUTCOME
2. Risk for Fluid Volume Deficit related to inability to meet body requirements and increased metabolic demand (continued)			
	■ Perform daily weight measurement on the same scale at the same time of day. Evaluate skin turgor.	■ Further evidence of improvement of hydration status.	Child's weight stabilizes after 24–48 hours; skin turgor is supple.
	■ Assess mucous membranes and presence of tears. Report changes promptly to physician.	■ Moist mucous membranes and tears provide observable evidence of hydration.	Child shows evidence of improved hydration.
	■ Offer clear fluids and incorporate parent in care. Offer fluid choice when tolerated.	■ Choice of fluid offered by parent gains the child's cooperation.	The child accepts beverage of choice from parent or nursing staff.
3. Anxiety (Child and Parent) related to acute illness, hospitalization, uncertain course of illness and treatment, and home care needs			
	NIC Priority Intervention: **Anxiety reduction:** Minimizing apprehension, dread, foreboding, or uneasiness related to an unidentified source of anticipated danger.		NOC Suggested Outcome: **Anxiety control:** Ability to eliminate or reduce feelings of apprehension and tension from an unidentifiable source.
Child and parents will demonstrate behaviors that indicate decrease in anxiety.	■ Encourage parents to express fears and ask questions; provide direct answers and discuss care, procedures, and condition changes.	■ Provides opportunity to vent feelings and receive timely, relevant information. Helps reduce parents' anxiety and increase trust in nursing staff.	Parents and child show decreasing anxiety and decreasing fear as symptoms improve and as child and parents feel more secure in hospital environment.
	■ Incorporate parents in the child's care. Encourage parents to bring familiar objects from home. Ask about and incorporate in care plan the home routines for feeding and sleeping.	■ Familiar people, routines, and objects decrease the child's anxiety and increase parents' sense of control over unexpected, uncertain situation.	*Parent* freely asks questions and participates in the child's care. The *child* cries less and allows staff to hold and/or touch him or her.
Parents will verbalize knowledge of symptoms of bronchiolitis and use of home care methods before the child's discharge from the hospital.	■ Explain symptoms, treatment, and home care of bronchiolitis.	■ Anticipate potential for recurrence. Assist family to be prepared should respiratory symptoms recur after discharge.	Parent accurately describes respiratory symptoms and initial home care actions.
	■ Provide written instructions for follow-up care arrangements as needed.	■ Written and oral instructions reinforce knowledge. Parents may not "hear" and remember the particulars of home care if presented only orally.	

fevers and general discomfort. Advise parents that RSV infection can recur; therefore, they need to know how to recognize symptoms and when to call the physician.

Evaluation

Expected outcomes of nursing care are provided on the accompanying nursing care plan.

PNEUMONIA

Pneumonia is an inflammation or infection of the bronchioles and alveolar spaces of the lungs. It occurs most often in infants and young children. Pneumonia in children often

FAMILIES WANT TO KNOW

Discharge Teaching for Bronchiolitis

Advise parents to call the physician if the following occurs:

- Respiratory symptoms interfere with sleep or eating.
- Breathing is rapid or difficult.
- Symptoms persist in a child who is less than 1 year old, has heart or lung disease, or was premature and had lung disease after birth.
- The child acts sicker—appears tired, less playful, less interested in food (parents just "feel" the child is not improving).

resolves much sooner than in adults. The key is early recognition, enabling the child to be managed at home rather than in the hospital.

Pneumonia may be viral, mycoplasmal, or bacterial in origin. Common organisms causing pneumonia include RSV, parainfluenza virus, adenovirus, enterovirus, and pneumococcus. Children who are immunosuppressed are susceptible to many other bacterial, parasitic, or fungal infections. Regardless of the causative agent, symptoms include elevated temperature, rhonchi, crackles, wheezes, cough, dyspnea, tachypnea, restlessness, and decreased breath sounds if consolidation exists.

What physiologic process occurs to precipitate the symptoms? Bacterial and viral invaders act differently within the lungs. Bacterial invaders circulate through the bloodstream to the lungs, where they damage cells. Bacteria tend to be distributed evenly throughout one or more lobes of a single lung, a pattern termed *unilateral lobar pneumonia.* Viral or mycoplasma invaders, on the other hand, are parasites of cells. Viruses frequently enter from the upper respiratory tract, infiltrating the alveoli nearest the bronchi of one or both lungs. There they invade the cells, replicate, and burst out forcefully, killing the cells and sending out cell debris. They rapidly invade adjacent areas, distributing themselves in a scattered, patchy pattern referred to as bronchopneumonia. The end result of bacterial, viral, or mycoplasma invasion is the presence of exudate resulting from cell death, which fills the alveolar spaces, pooling and clumping in dependent areas of the lung to create areas of consolidation.

Diagnosis is made by chest x-ray, which shows an abnormal density of tissue, such as a lobar consolidation. There is no clinical way to differentiate bacterial and viral cause. The child's age, severity of symptoms, and presence of an underlying lung, cardiac, or immunodeficiency disease can create varying responses.

Clinical management for all types of pneumonia includes symptomatic therapy (pain and fever control) and supportive care through airway management, fluids, and rest. Mycoplasma and other bacterial pneumonias are treated with organism-sensitive antibiotics; viral pneumonias usually improve without antibiotics. Some children need oxygen and anti-inflammatory medications.

Nursing Management

Nursing care incorporates supportive measures and medical therapies as appropriate. Nursing measures used to manage the child with bronchiolitis are generally applicable to the child with pneumonia.

CLINICAL TIP

Teach the child and parent how to splint the chest, by hugging a small pillow, teddy bear, or doll, to make coughing less painful.

In addition to ongoing respiratory assessment and supportive therapies (pulmonary care, antibiotics, hydration), the child may need relief from pain when coughing and deep breathing. Pain medication (acetaminophen or ibuprofen) can provide the added benefits of temperature control and may aid in sleep. Hospitalization is reserved for seriously ill children.

The goal of nursing care is to restore optimal respiratory function. Discharge planning should be addressed early in the hospital stay. Medications, especially antibiotics, must be taken at prescribed intervals and for the full course. Parents should be taught the proper administration of drugs and any side effects. Follow-up may include a chest x-ray to see if the lungs are clear. Symptoms of pneumonia usually disappear long before the lungs are completely healed. Some children continue to have worsening reactive airway problems or abnormal results on pulmonary function tests. Most children, however, recover uneventfully.

Preventive measures against pneumonia are limited. An immunization against pneumococcal bacteria is recommended for children over 2 years of age who are immunosuppressed or have chronic diseases (see Chapter 12).

TUBERCULOSIS

Tuberculosis (TB) is caused by the organism *Mycobacterium tuberculosis,* which is transmitted through the air in infectious particles called droplet nuclei. Since 1988, the incidence of TB has been on the rise, particularly among immigrants, minorities, and children younger than 15 years (Brashers & Davey, 1998). An estimated 15 million people are infected in the United States, creating a large reservoir for infection in children. The risk of developing TB is greatest during the first 2 years of life (American Thoracic Society and Centers for Disease Control and Prevention, 2000). Adults with active laryngeal or pulmonary TB may transmit the disease to children.

By coughing, sneezing, speaking, or singing, a person with active TB sends out tiny droplets of moisture that remain in the air. If these droplets are inhaled, the bacillus is small enough to travel directly to the alveoli. Frequently, however, the organism is trapped in the upper airway, preventing infection. Pulmonary infection occurs only when the bacillus reaches the alveoli.

Once the organism reaches the alveoli, an immune response is initiated to combat the invader. The immune system sends macrophages to surround and wall off the bacillus in small hard capsules, called tubercles. There the bacillus can remain dormant (inactive) indefinitely or can progress to active TB. In young children, the disease develops as an immediate complication of the primary infection. Children with HIV infection or immunosuppression may have more rapidly progressive disease. If the tubercle extends into a blood vessel, the bacillus may spread through the bloodstream to affect the liver, spleen, bone marrow, or meninges (tubercular meningitis). This systemic form of TB (meningeal or miliary tuberculosis) may lead to serious illness or death. Miliary tuberculosis is not, however, transmissible; only active pulmonary TB has the potential to infect another individual.

Clinical manifestations of TB in infants include a persistent cough, weight loss or failure to gain weight, and fever. Wheezing and decreased breath sounds may be present. Older children may be asymptomatic.

Several tests may be required to confirm the diagnosis (Table 13-13). Medical management focuses on diagnosis and treatment of active TB with antitubercular drug therapy. Drugs used to treat TB include isoniazid, rifampicin, pyrazinamide, ethambutol, and streptomycin. Challenges to treatment have occurred with the development of multidrug-resistant TB. Up to 90%

CLINICAL TIP

In suspected cases of tuberculosis, the child, immediate family, and supposed carrier should be skin tested for TB. Intradermal testing using purified protein derivative (PPD, the Mantoux test) is considered the most accurate test. A control skin test verifies the response status of the immune system. High-risk children who should receive a TB skin test include those with a TB contact, travel to a TB endemic area, contact with adults at high risk of TB, and positive HIV status (Ozuah, Ozuah, & Stein, et al., 2001).

TABLE 13-13 Diagnostic Tests for Tuberculosis

TEST	INDICATION
Mantoux test (intradermal injection of purified protein derivative [PPD])	Confirms infection with the TB organism (3–12 weeks after exposure)
Chest x-ray examination (anteroposterior and lateral views)	Confirms presence of pulmonary tuberculosis (small, seedlike opacities may be visible)
Blood cultures for *Mycobacterium tuberculosis*	Proves diagnosis; defines specific drug sensitivity
Gastric washings (early morning after overnight fast; 3 consecutive days)	Confirms pulmonary tuberculosis (active form of tuberculosis). Used in children under 12 years as they do not produce sputum.
Sputum cultures (expectorated or from bronchoscopic examination)	Confirms active pulmonary tuberculosis
Pleural biopsy for culture and tissue examination	Taken when pleural effusion is present
Lumbar puncture	Confirms meningeal tuberculosis (inactive form of tuberculosis)

LAW & ETHICS

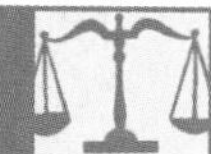

By law, cases of tuberculosis must be reported immediately to the public health department so that disease contacts can be traced. For every child infected with TB, an adult who has active disease and requires treatment is in the environment (American Thoracic Society, 2000).

CLINICAL TIP

Children with tuberculosis should receive "directly observed drug therapy" by a nurse or other health care provider to ensure that the drug is being taken. Direct observation should be done daily for at least 2 weeks and then decreased to twice a week if the patient is responding to treatment (Stowe & Jacobs, 1999).

THE FOUR FS OF CYSTIC FIBROSIS

Stools of a child with cystic fibrosis have the following characteristics.

- Frothy (bulky and large quantity)
- Foul smelling
- Fat containing (greasy)
- Floaty

of cases are resistant to certain drugs (Brashers & Davey, 1998). Tuberculosis is a major public health problem and must be promptly reported to local health departments.

Nursing Management

Nursing care centers on administering medications and providing supportive care. Parents need to be taught about the disease process, medications, possible side effects, and the importance of long-term therapy (e.g., that drug therapy may last for 6 to 12 months). Most children with TB are able to lead essentially normal lives. Emphasize the importance of taking medications as prescribed on an empty stomach, and ensuring proper nutrition and rest to promote normal growth and development.

The discussion of pneumonia earlier in this chapter and the discussion of tubercular meningitis in Chapter 20 give other nursing care measures appropriate for the child with TB.

CYSTIC FIBROSIS

Cystic fibrosis is a common inherited autosomal recessive disorder of the exocrine glands that results in physiologic alterations in the respiratory, gastrointestinal, integumentary, musculoskeletal, and reproductive systems. The disorder occurs predominantly in white children, but other populations are also affected. Gender is not a factor in incidence (Figure 13-14 ◆). The median life span for individuals with cystic fibrosis is 30 years.

Etiology and Pathophysiology

A gene isolated on the long arm of chromosome 7 directs the function of the cystic fibrosis transmembrane conductance regulator (CFTR). With a defective CFTR, there is defective chloride-ion transport across the exocrine and epithelial cells. This results in an abnormal accumulation of viscous, dehydrated mucus that affects the respiratory, gastrointestinal and genitourinary systems. Inflammation and lung changes are present as early as 4 weeks of age. Ultimately, all body organs with mucous ducts become obstructed and damaged (McMullen, 2000).

Because of the blocked pancreatic ducts and resulting pancreatic damage, the natural enzymes necessary to digest fats and proteins are not secreted and thus essential nutrients are excreted in the stool.

The classic cough occurs because the lungs are always filled with mucus, which the respiratory cilia cannot clear. This causes air to become trapped in the small airways, resulting in atelectasis (pulmonary collapse). Secondary respiratory infections occur because secretions provide an environment conducive to bacterial growth. This is a major cause of morbidity and mortality.

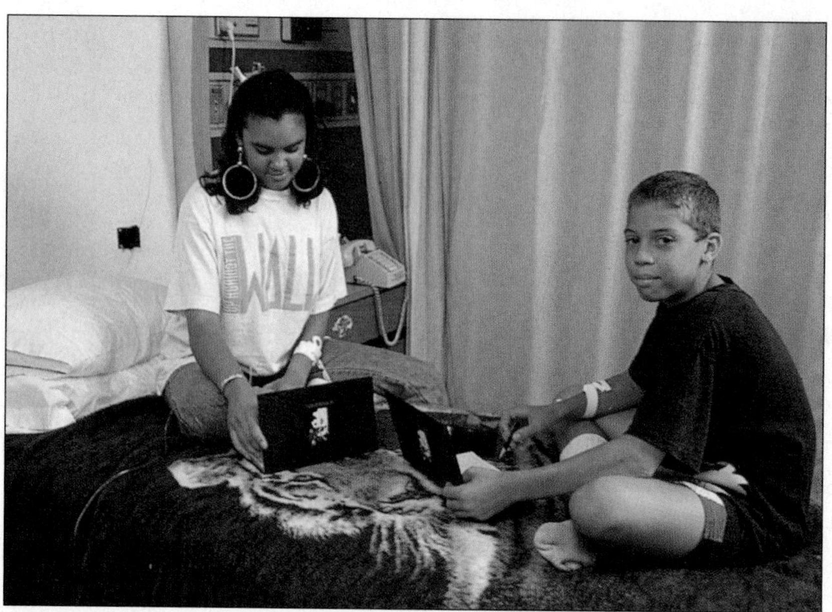

FIGURE 13-14 ◆ Cystic fibrosis is an inherited autosomal recessive disorder of the exocrine glands, so it is not uncommon to see siblings with it such as this brother and sister.

Nearly all males who have cystic fibrosis are sterile because of blockage or absence of the vas deferens. Females have difficulty conceiving because increased mucous secretions in the reproductive tract interfere with the passage of sperm (McMullen, 2000).

Metabolic function is altered as a result of the imbalances created by excessive electrolyte loss through perspiration, saliva, and mucous secretion. The "salty taste" of the skin is the result of sodium chloride that makes its way through skin pores to the skin surface.

DIAGNOSTIC CLUE

"I kissed my baby's cheek and tasted salt! Nothing would be the same after that." —The mother of a 1-week-old infant with cystic fibrosis

Clinical Manifestations

The primary symptom of cystic fibrosis is the production of thick, sticky mucus. One of the earliest signs in the newborn is meconium ileus, a small bowel obstruction that occurs during the first few days of life. In infants and toddlers, fecal impaction and intussusception ("telescoping" of the bowel) may be the first signs of the disorder (See Chapter 17). Steatorrhea (fatty stool) is another characteristic sign of cystic fibrosis. The sticky, thick stool is thought to create the initial obstruction. Intestinal peristalsis (controlled by the autonomic nervous system) is also adversely affected. Rectal prolapse, resulting from the large, bulky, difficult-to-pass stools, may occur (Figure 13-15 ◆).

Other signs and symptoms include a chronic moist, productive cough and frequent respiratory infections. Most children have difficulty maintaining and gaining weight despite a voracious appetite. Infants and children may have a delayed bone age, short stature, and delayed onset of puberty. Clubbing of the tips of the fingers and toes occurs as the disease progresses (Figure 13-16 ◆).

GENETIC CONSIDERATIONS

Recent advances in localization of the cystic fibrosis gene have led to successful techniques for prenatal diagnosis and carrier testing. There are 600 mutations of the cystic fibrosis gene with the most common being ΔF508 (Varlotta, 1998). The 1997 NIH consensus statement on genetic testing for cystic fibrosis recommended that genetic testing be offered to adults with a positive family history, partners of people with cystic fibrosis, couples planning a pregnancy in a high-risk population, and couples seeking prenatal testing (Merelle, Lees, & Nagelkerke, et al., 2000). Prenatal tests of Caucasians identify 80% of carriers (Rubin, 2001). Research is now focused on genetic treatment of the disease.

Clinical Therapy

Cystic fibrosis is usually diagnosed in infancy or early childhood with one of three major presentations: newborn meconium ileus, malabsorption or failure to thrive, or chronic recurrent respiratory infections. Some children with a milder form of the disease, however, may reach the teen or young adult years before symptoms appear. The mean age at diagnosis is 4.8 years (Farrell, Kosorok, & Rock, et al., 2001).

Cystic fibrosis is diagnosed definitively by a positive sweat test and the presence of classic symptoms or a positive family history (McMullen, 2000) (Table 13-14). Genetic testing of the child's DNA and blood immunoreactive trypsinogen can be used for newborn screening (Farrell et al., 2001). The sweat test may be performed at the child's bedside or on an outpatient basis. The parents should be present to hold and reassure the infant or small child (Figure 13-17 ◆). They should be informed that the test will indicate whether the child has cystic fibrosis and that a second test may be ordered to confirm the diagnosis. Pulmonary function tests are performed on children older than 6 years.

CULTURE

The incidence of cystic fibrosis varies by race—1:3,200 in Caucasians; 1:15,000 in African Americans; and 1:31,000 in Asian Americans (Rosenstein & Cutting, 1998).

Clinical therapy focuses on maintaining respiratory function, managing infection, promoting optimal nutrition and exercise, and preventing gastrointestinal blockage (Table 13-15). Newly diagnosed children will have no or minimal symptoms and near normal lung function if aggressively treated. Pulmonary function declines 2% to 4% per year even with aggressive treatment (Varlotta, 1998).

Improvements in medical management and optimal nutrition now enable many children with cystic fibrosis to survive well into adulthood. Lung transplantation is occasionally performed, and approximately 50% of cases survive for the first 5 years (Stubblefield & Murray, 2000). The disease is ultimately terminal, however, because of the progressive multisystem changes and the difficulty of long-term infection management.

TABLE 13-14 Diagnostic Test for Cystic Fibrosis (Sweat Test)

TEST	PURPOSE	NORMAL VALUES	DIAGNOSTIC VALUES
Sweat test (pilocarpine iontophoresis)	Analysis of sodium and chloride content in sweat	Sodium: 10–30 mEq/L; Chloride: 10–35 mEq/L	Chloride: 50–60 mEq/L—suspicious; >60 mEq/L—diagnostic with other clinical signs

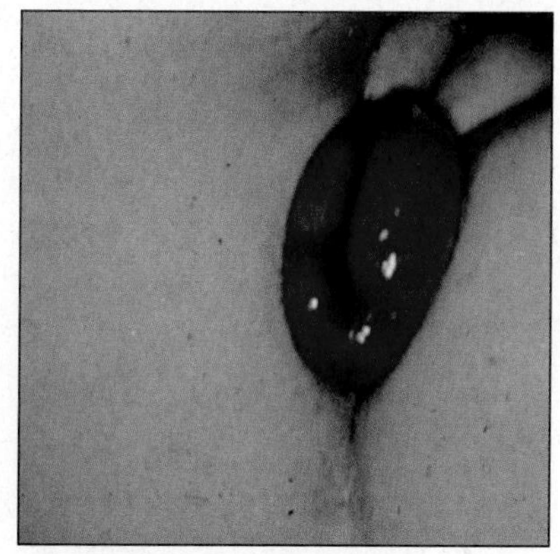

FIGURE 13-15 ◆
Rectal prolapse.

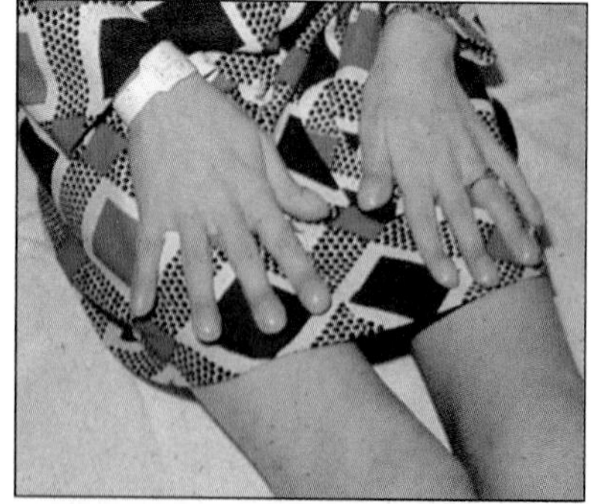

FIGURE 13-16 ◆
Digital clubbing.

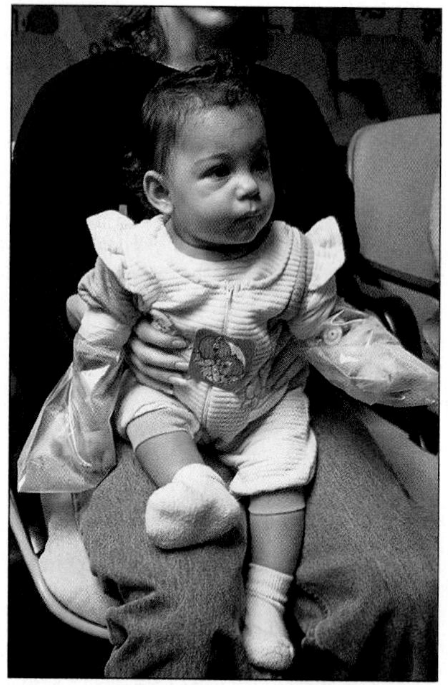

FIGURE 13-17 ◆
This 6-month-old girl is being evaluated for cystic fibrosis using the sweat test.

TABLE 13-15 Clinical Therapy for Cystic Fibrosis

CLINICAL THERAPY	RATIONALE
Respiratory Therapy	
Aerosol bronchodilators	Opens large and small airways; use before chest physiotherapy; and with symptoms
Aerosol DNAse	Loosens, liquefies, and thins pulmonary secretions; decreases risk of developing pulmonary infections requiring parenteral treatment in some patients (McMullen, 2000)
Anti-inflammatory agents: steroids, high-dose ibuprofen	Reduces inflammatory response to chronic infection; short courses to decrease side effects of steroids; decreases progression of lung damage in preadolescents with mild disease
Chest physiotherapy for all lung segments (bilateral percussion-vibration and forceful coughing)	Mobilizes secretions to bronchi for expectoration; performed twice a day
Infection Management (most susceptible to H. influenzae, S. aureus, and Pseudomonas aeruginosa bacteria, Burkholderia cepacia, and viral agents)	
Antibiotics (oral, IV, aerosol routes)	Treatment based on sputum-culture results; may need higher than normal doses to be effective
Nutritional Needs	
Pancreatic enzyme supplements (Cotazym-S, Pancrease, Viokase) taken with meals and snacks	Assists in digestion of nutrients and nutritious decreasing fat and bulk; given prior to food ingestion
Diet supplies well-balanced, food with 120%–150% of recommended (RDA) calories and 200% of RDA protein, and moderate fat; nutritional counseling necessary	Promotes essential nutrient balance for health, growth, and weight maintenance; considers child, food, and cultural-socioeconomic issues
Multivitamins and vitamin E in water-soluble form; vitamins A, D, and K given when deficient; iron	Cystic fibrosis interferes with vitamin production; supplements are required in water-soluble form for better absorption supplementation (vitamins A, D, E, and K are naturally fat soluble); iron deficiency results from malabsorption syndrome

Care of the child with previously diagnosed cystic fibrosis is the focus of the following discussion.

NURSING MANAGEMENT

Nursing Assessment and Diagnosis

Physiologic Assessment

Physical assessment of the child focuses on adequacy of respiratory function. The child with cystic fibrosis usually is admitted with symptoms of an upper respiratory infection. A set of baseline vital signs, including temperature, pulse, respirations, and blood pressure, along with a weight measurement, should be obtained on admission. Observe the child's physical appearance, noting overall body proportions and any changes characteristic of long-term cystic fibrosis.

Psychosocial Assessment

The emotional stress of this chronic disease may not be readily apparent on admission, particularly if the child's symptoms are mild and not imminently life threatening. Ongoing observation of the child's and parents' behavior helps direct nursing interventions throughout hospitalization (see Table 13-10). Parents may feel guilt as carriers of the disease. Siblings may also show signs of difficulty in dealing with the illness. Link the family to support groups.

The nurse should ask parents how the child's illness has affected day-to-day functioning and how they have adapted to the child's plan of care. What have parents told the child and siblings about the disease? What kind of questions have the child and siblings asked about cystic fibrosis, and how have parents answered them? Has the child ever asked about his or her life expectancy? If not, what would parents say if asked?

Developmental Assessment

Growth and development may be altered by the chronic nature of the disease. Children with cystic fibrosis may be growth retarded. Compare the child's height and weight to age norms and observe the adolescent for the appearance of secondary sex characteristics, which are often delayed. School-age children and adolescents often are embarrassed at being viewed as different from playmates and peers. Ask how the child or adolescent feels about the need for a special diet, medications, and limitations.

Common nursing diagnoses for the child with cystic fibrosis include the following:

- *Ineffective airway clearance,* related to thick mucus in lungs
- *Ineffective breathing pattern,* related to thick tracheobronchial secretions and airway obstruction
- *Risk for infection,* related to the presence of mucous secretions conducive to bacterial growth
- *Altered nutrition: Less than body requirements,* related to inability to digest nutrients
- *Parental role conflict,* related to interruptions in family life due to the home care regimen

Planning and Implementation

Nursing management involves supporting the child and family initially, when the diagnosis is made, during subsequent hospitalizations, and during visits to specialty and primary health care providers. The nurse's role begins with implementing specific medical therapies and providing nursing care to meet the child's physiologic and psychosocial needs. Respiratory therapy, medications, and diet must be coordinated to promote optimal body function. Psychosocial support and reinforcement of the child's daily care needs are important in preparation for home care.

Children with cystic fibrosis require periodic hospitalization when a severe infection occurs or for a pulmonary and nutritional "tune-up." Respect the parents' experiences as the child's primary care provider and include them in the child's routine care as much as possible. However, parents may view the hospital stay as a break from the rigorous daily pulmonary routine at home and need support in taking advantage of some downtime. The family often becomes proficient at providing physical care to the child, but the nurse should take the opportunity provided during rehospitalization to review basic and new information about respiratory care, medications, and nutrition. Keeping lines of communication open and validating parents' understanding of their child's disease and care needs are important steps in preparing the family to cope with this chronic health challenge.

Provide Respiratory Therapy

Chest physiotherapy is usually performed one to three times per day before meals to clear secretions from the lungs (Figure 13-18 ◆). Parents and other family members can learn to help with these necessary treatments. Pulmonary care may involve aerosol treatments and antibiotics when indicated (see Table 13-15).

Skill 10-20: Performing Chest Physiotherapy/Postural Drainage

Administer Medications and Meet Nutritional Needs

Digestive problems can be eased with special medications and dietary modification (see Table 13-15). Pancreatic enzyme supplements come in powder sprinkles and capsule form and are taken orally with all meals and large snacks. The amount needed is individualized based on the child's nutritional needs and digestive response to these supplements. The goal is to achieve near-normal, well-formed stools and adequate weight gain.

Some fat-soluble vitamins (A, D, E, and K) are not completely absorbed from food; therefore, they must be taken in water-soluble form. Multivitamins taken twice daily usually are

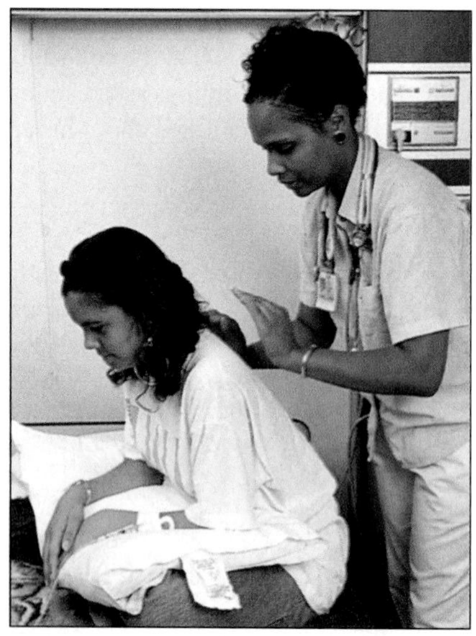

A

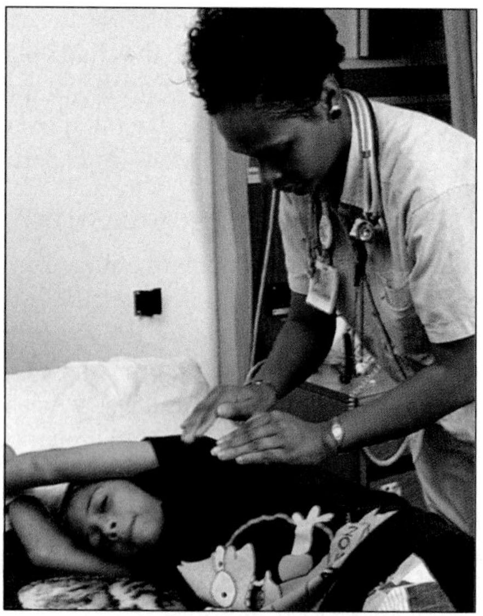

B

FIGURE 13-18 ◆
Postural drainage can be achieved by clapping with a cupped hand on the chest wall over the segment to be drained to create vibrations that are transmitted to the bronchi to dislodge secretions. A, If the obstruction is in the posterior apical segment of the lung, the nurse can do this with the child sitting up. B, If the obstruction is in the left posterior segment, the child should be lying on the right side. Several other positions can be used depending on the location of the obstruction.

sufficient to prevent deficiency. The diet should be well balanced, with an emphasis on high caloric value. Respiratory complications necessitate additional energy expenditure, and some children require special nutritional supplements, and sometimes supplemental nasogastric or gastrostomy feedings, to gain and maintain weight.

Fats and salt are both necessary in the diet. Balanced with pancreatic enzyme supplements, moderate fat intake adds an important source of extra fuel.

Provide Anticipatory Guidance

The nurse should assist the parents and child to learn what they must do to maintain health after discharge. Emotional support is essential because the diagnosis of this disorder creates anxiety and fear in both the parents and the child. They need assistance with emotional and psychosocial issues relating to discipline, body image (stooling and odor), frequent rehospitalization, the potential fatal nature of the illness, the child's feeling of being different from friends, and overall financial, social, and family concerns. Because the disorder is inherited, families may have more than one child with cystic fibrosis. Parents may have unspoken feelings of anger and guilt, blaming themselves for their children's condition.

COMMUNITY CARE

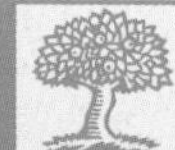

Parents often have a difficult time getting the child with cystic fibrosis to eat the extra calories needed for optimal nutrition, setting the stage for a potential mealtime battleground. To be successful, parents need guidance about managing mealtime behaviors in addition to guidelines for preparing nutritional calorie-dense foods. Increase calorie intake by adding fats and high calorie snacks between meals and before bed. Extra intervention may be needed when the child's weight is 85% to 90% of ideal weight for height (Wilson & Pencharz, 1998).

Discharge Planning and Home Care Teaching

The financial burden of medications, supplies, and medical follow-up may not be recognized immediately by a family already overwhelmed by the diagnosis. Because of the chronicity of cystic fibrosis, home care is as important as care of the child in the hospital. Initially, parents need assistance in obtaining necessary equipment. If the family requires financial assistance, they should be referred to the appropriate social services. Home care of the child with cystic fibrosis is expensive and can be draining on the family's finances.

Parents need to learn chest physiotherapy, which the child will need as often as three or four times a day. Arranging for a visiting nurse and a respiratory therapist to visit the family frequently can provide reassurance and relief to the family. Managing the child's nutritional needs is important and takes time and energy.

Parents need to learn how to mix enzymes for young children, what vitamins need to be given daily, and what foods should be avoided or eliminated because of the child's digestive problems. Referral should be made to a nutritionist either before or at the time of discharge.

Cystic fibrosis affects all family members and disrupts activities of daily living for everyone. It is important to refer families to counseling and group therapy with families of other children with cystic fibrosis if indicated. The Cystic Fibrosis Foundation is a source for information on current advances in the disorder. Local chapter activities also provide emotional support for parents and children.

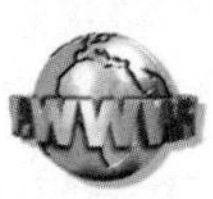

Cystic Fibrosis Family Support

Care in the Community

Nurses may encounter the child with cystic fibrosis in any of the following settings: clinics specializing in the disease, pediatricians' offices, and schools. The primary goal is to keep the disease under control by promoting optimal nutrition and assisting the family in reducing the incidence of infection. Nurses may also provide home care to the child with cystic fibrosis following hospitalization for an acute exacerbation or provide hospice care.

Assessment Assess the child's respiratory status. Inquire about the frequency and character of the child's cough and characteristics of the sputum. Compare this information with the child's baseline. Changes in the cough may be more important than its presence or absence. Auscultate the chest for breath sounds, crackles, and wheezes. Note any cyanosis or clubbing of the extremities. Oxygen saturation and spirometry readings should be obtained if changes in respiratory status are suspected.

Evaluate the child's growth, plotting the weight and height on a growth curve. Determine whether the child is maintaining an appropriate growth pattern. Inquire about the child's appetite and dietary intake. How are nutritional supplements, pancreatic enzymes, and vitamins used?

Assess the child's stooling pattern. Identify whether the child has problems with abdominal pain or bloating, and whether these problems can be related to eating, stooling, or other activities. Palpate the abdomen for liver size, fecal masses, and evidence of pain.

Inquire about the family's and child's emotional and psychosocial responses to managing the illness. These issues are important when the child is going through major developmental stages.

Management Review the child's use of bronchodilators and airway clearance techniques. To prevent a change in pulmonary status from progressing, short-term changes in care may be recommended. These may include intravenous and aerosol medications and antibiotics, an increase in the number of times chest physiotherapy is performed daily, and changes in dietary management. Help the family select the best time to fit the additional treatment into the schedule.

Malnutrition is a major problem for children with cystic fibrosis. Parents often need to plan meals and snacks for the young child to ensure that adequate calories are consumed. Nutritional supplements may be suggested when growth is not adequate. Arrange for a consultation with a nutritionist if the family would benefit from new strategies to help meet the child's nutritional needs. Children with adequate nutrition have a longer life expectancy.

Children with cystic fibrosis lose more than normal amounts of salt in their sweat. This loss can become intensified during hot weather, strenuous exercise, and fever. Parents should allow the child to add extra salt to food and should permit some salty snacks (pretzels with salt, pickles, carbonated soda). During periods of increased sweating, the child should be encouraged to drink more fluids and increase salt intake. Teach parents to recognize early symptoms of salt depletion, including fatigue, weakness, abdominal pain, and vomiting, and to contact the child's health care provider if these symptoms occur.

Talk with the child and family to identify any assistance needed with emotional and psychosocial issues. Depending on the child's developmental stage, issues related to discipline, body image (stooling and odor), or the child's feeling of being different from friends may be major concerns. The family may also have overall financial, social, and family management concerns that can be discussed.

Growth & Development

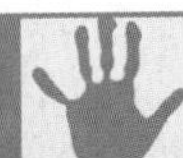

Adolescents with cystic fibrosis need special assistance in coping with their disorder. Help them identify normal adolescent changes versus those related to cystic fibrosis. Plan transitional care as they take on more responsibility for self-care and decision making, as well as preparing for a job that fits their energy level. Adolescents should also have a supportive grief process as they recognize how their remaining life will be different from their peers (Muscari, 1998).

Evaluation

Expected outcomes of nursing care include the following:

- The child and family develop proficiency in providing the daily pulmonary care and reducing the incidence of respiratory infections.
- The child and family develop a schedule and routine for daily pulmonary care that fits into family and school activities.
- The child consumes adequate calories and pancreatic enzymes to support growth and to stay within desirable weight ranges.

INJURIES OF THE RESPIRATORY SYSTEM

Airway compromise after an unintentional injury can cause death if not managed quickly and effectively. Why are children so vulnerable to changes in respiratory function after accidental injury?

The small size of the child's airway makes it vulnerable to obstruction. The tongue, small amounts of blood, mucus, or foreign debris or swelling in the respiratory tract or adjacent neck tissue may block the airway and lead to hypoxia and respiratory failure. If the child's neck is flexed or hyperextended, the soft laryngeal cartilage may compress and obstruct the airway.

Infants and young children rely on the diaphragm for air movement. They are abdominal (or "belly") breathers. Excessive crying and anxiety deplete metabolic reserves. External ventilatory support and vigorous crying may impede diaphragm function if the stomach becomes distended with air. Because the child's metabolic rate is about double that of an adult, the child has a greater need for oxygen. Respiratory distress, anxiety, and even fever can dramatically add to the child's oxygen demand.

NURSING ALERT

Never allow a child's neck to hyperextend (bend completely backward) or hyperflex (bend completely forward). Hyperextension flattens the trachea because there is no firm cartilage to provide structural support. Hyperflexion can kink and compress the trachea. Both maneuvers obstruct rather than open the airway.

AIRWAY OBSTRUCTION

Airway obstruction exists when air passage in the respiratory tract and lungs is slowed or blocked. If the blockage occurs above the trachea, inspiration is more affected. If the blockage occurs below the trachea, expiration is more affected. Earlier sections dealt with structural and functional problems that may lead to airway obstruction. This section addresses two common conditions of airway obstruction in children that result from unintentional injury: foreign body aspiration and near-drowning.

Foreign-Body Aspiration

Foreign-body aspiration is the inhalation of any object (solid or liquid, food or nonfood) into the respiratory tract. Aspiration occurs most often during feeding and reaching activities, while crawling, or during playtime in children 6 months to 4 years of age. However, aspiration may occur in children of any age.

GROWTH & DEVELOPMENT

Foreign-body aspiration is a major health problem for infants and young toddlers because of their increasing mobility and tendency to place small objects in the mouth.

ETIOLOGY AND PATHOPHYSIOLOGY In infants over 6 months of age and in children, aspiration may be caused by any number of small objects that make their way into the child's mouth. Foods such as nuts, popcorn, or small pieces of raw vegetables or hot dog; small, loose toy parts such as small wheels and bells; or household objects and substances such as beads, safety pins, coins, buttons, latex balloon pieces, colorful liquids (mouthwash, perfume) in enticing packages (screw top bottles) are frequent causes of airway obstruction.

The severity of the obstruction depends on the size and composition of the object or substance and its location within the respiratory tract. The majority of aspirated foreign bodies (AFBs) usually cause bronchial, not tracheal, obstruction. An object lodged high in the airway above the vocal cords is frequently coughed out easily or with some assistance (such as use of chest thrusts and back blows or the abdominal thrust). An object lodged in the trachea is a life-threatening situation.

Skill 10-14: Removing a Foreign Body Airway Obstruction

Coughing, choking, gagging, dysphonia, and wheezing may be brief or may persist for several hours if the object drops below the trachea into one of the mainstem bronchi. The right lung is the most common site of lower airway aspiration because of the sloped angle of its bronchus (see Figure 13-2). Objects may migrate from higher to lower airway locations. An object may also move back up to the trachea, creating extreme respiratory difficulty. If oxygen is depleted for an extended time, brain damage may occur.

CLINICAL MANIFESTATIONS Children are usually brought to the hospital after a sudden episode of coughing. Discovery of an open container with small objects may prompt parents to seek medical assistance for the child. The child may have spasmodic coughing, respiratory distress, or gagging. Sudden respiratory distress in the absence of fever or other symptoms of illness strongly suggests foreign-body aspiration (Hazinski, 1999).

CLINICAL THERAPY Clinical therapy focuses on taking a careful history to determine whether aspiration has indeed occurred. Choking associated with feeding or crawling on the floor is usually a confirming event. The physical examination often reveals decreased breath sounds, stridor, and respiratory distress in the child without a witnessed aspiration. A special radiograph, called a forced expiratory film, may be ordered. This shows local hyperinflation (air trapping) and a mediastinal shift away from the affected side (Hazinski, 1999). Sometimes, when the object aspirated is radiopaque, it can be seen on an x-ray film (Figure 13-19 ◆). Fluoroscopy and fiber-optic bronchoscopy may be used to identify, locate, and extract the AFB.

The child with an AFB that is removed is usually stabilized in the emergency department and observed for a few hours. Depending on the type of object and degree of obstruction, surgical removal of the object and hospitalization may be required.

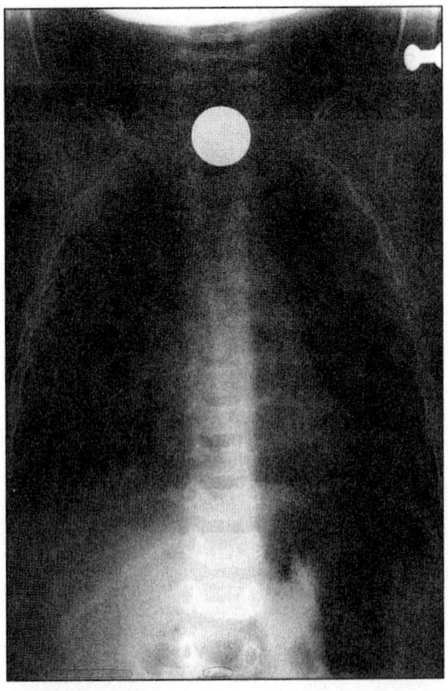

FIGURE 13-19 ◆
An aspirated foreign body (coin) is clearly visible in the child's trachea on this chest x-ray.
Courtesy of Rockwood Clinic, Spokane, WA.

NURSING MANAGEMENT

Nursing Assessment and Diagnosis

Physiologic Assessment

If the object remains lodged, the child is observed for increasing signs of respiratory distress, especially vital signs and audible wheezing on auscultation. Changes in breath sounds, from noisy to decreasing to absent, on the affected side are noted. This can indicate that the object is moving and blocking a mainstem bronchus.

Psychosocial Assessment

The unexpected and acute nature of the event creates anxiety for parents and child. They also may be experiencing a variety of other emotions—fear, anger, or guilt. The nurse should assess coping and level of stress. Providing a quiet environment and encouraging the presence of the parents can help to reduce the child's fear and anxiety.

Developmental Assessment

As the child's condition stabilizes, the nurse observes how well the child's abilities match the parents' understanding of age-appropriate behaviors. Providing anticipatory teaching or reinforcing information about developmental characteristics (see Chapter 2) helps parents to anticipate safety hazards in the future.

CLINICAL TIP

If the child cannot say "P" in words like Pluto or Peter Pan, the expiratory effort is noticeably diminished as a result of the foreign body.

Common nursing diagnoses for a child with an AFB include the following:

- *Ineffective airway clearance,* related to foreign object trauma (previously removed or coughed out object)
- *Inability to sustain spontaneous ventilations,* related to foreign object and respiratory muscle fatigue
- *Fear/anxiety (parent or child),* related to uncertainty of prognosis, unfamiliar surroundings, and procedures

Planning and Implementation

The first 12 hours after aspiration are critical, and subtle changes in the child's respiratory status during this period must be documented and reported promptly. The child and family should be apprised of procedures and provided with emotional support.

Discharge Planning and Home Care Teaching

Discharge planning centers on anticipatory guidance about childproofing the home (see Chapter 2) and encouraging the parents to learn CPR, choking-prevention techniques, and back blows, chest thrusts, or abdominal thrusts.

Skill 10-13: Performing Cardiopulmonary Resuscitation

Evaluation

Expected outcomes of nursing care include the following:

- The child regains the ability to ventilate spontaneously after removal of the foreign body.
- No future incidents of aspiration of a foreign body occur because of the parent's prevention efforts.

NEAR-DROWNING

Near-drowning incidents and death by drowning are most prevalent in children under 5 years of age. In this age group, drowning is a leading cause of death resulting from injury (Murphy, 2000). Groups at high risk include toddlers, teenage boys, and children with seizure disorders. Children with seizure disorders may experience sudden and uncontrollable loss of body position that places them at risk without warning.

Near-drowning is defined as resuscitation and survival for 24 hours following a submersion injury. Near-drowning may result in complete recovery, severe brain injury, or variable neurologic deficits. A key feature influencing survival is initiation of immediate resuscitation, followed, it is hoped, by spontaneous respiratory effort by the child within 5 minutes after removal from the water. The mouth is cleaned of foreign matter, but time should not be wasted trying to remove water from the lungs. The sooner the child is ventilated, the better the chance of survival with normal neurologic potential. Emergency transport to a hospital should occur as soon as possible, even if spontaneous breathing is initiated.

> **GROWTH & DEVELOPMENT**
>
> Toddlers have large heads, which makes them top-heavy, and an unsteady gait that compromises body control and speed of movement. When propelled into a body of water, they may be unable to escape. Teenage boys may engage in risky behavior around or in a body of water, placing themselves or others at risk.

Most drownings occur in the child's home pool or at the residence of a neighbor, friend, or relative. Usually the child is playing, is not wearing a swimsuit, and is briefly unsupervised before the immersion. Other common drowning sites for young children include bathtubs, hot tubs, toilets, and even large water-filled buckets. A child can drown in as little water as it takes to cover the nose and mouth. In most immersion cases, hypoxemia begins within seconds and irreversible nervous system cell changes begin within 4 to 6 minutes (refer to Chapter 20). Hypoxemia is the most important consequence of near-drowning. Supportive care for any progression of pathology related to cerebral edema and aspiration of water is key. Damage to the airways from loss of surface-active material can lead to capillary leakage, pulmonary edema, and acute respiratory distress syndrome (Hazinski, 1999).

Nursing Management

Nursing management focuses on observation and support of cardiopulmonary and central nervous system function. Oxygen and mechanical ventilation with positive end expiratory pressure will be needed if acute respiratory distress develops. Frequent neurologic monitoring with the Glasgow Coma Scale and assessment of vital signs provide valuable baseline information (see Chapter 20). A chest x-ray may be ordered to establish baseline information about lung expansion and pulmonary integrity. Pulse oximetry will be ordered to provide ongoing data about the child's oxygenation status. The nurse should document any change in respiratory status and notify the physician promptly.

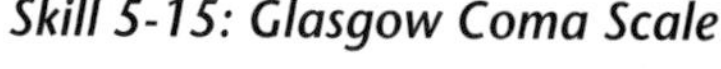

Skill 5-15: Glasgow Coma Scale

The child and family need support to work through the feelings surrounding the near-drowning incident, the unexpected hospitalization, and an uncertain prognosis that may mean the child will not return to normal functioning. Prevention is the key to avoiding a similar mishap in the future.

SMOKE-INHALATION INJURY

Exposure to fire conditions sets up dramatic responses in the respiratory tract of children. In every age group, inhalation injury significantly increases the child's chance of death (Allshouse & Eichelberger, 1993).

The severity of the smoke-inhalation injury is influenced by the type of material burned and whether the child was found in an open or closed space. The composition of materials determines how easily they ignite, how fast they burn, and how much heat they release. These factors influence the production of smoke and toxic gases. Smoke, a product of the burning process that is composed of gases and particles, is generated in varying volumes and density. The type and concentration of toxic gases, which are usually invisible, affect the severity of pulmonary damage. The duration of exposure to the smoke produced and any toxic gases contribute significantly to the child's prognosis.

Exposure to extreme heat, common in house fires, leads to surface injury and upper airway damage. The upper airway normally removes heat from inhaled gases, sparing the lower airway from thermal damage. However, this action results in marked edema, placing the small child at particular risk for airway obstruction. Edema develops rapidly over a few hours and may lead to acute respiratory distress syndrome. Burns of the face and neck, singed nasal hairs, soot around the mouth or nose, and hoarseness with stridor or voice change all indicate inhalation injury.

Carbon monoxide (CO) is a clear, colorless, odorless gas that is present in all fire conditions as the fire consumes oxygen. The CO molecule binds more firmly to hemoglobin than does oxygen. As a result, it replaces oxygen in circulation and rapidly produces hypoxia in the child. The longer the exposure to CO, the greater the hypoxia. The brain receives inadequate oxygen, resulting in confusion. This accounts for the inability of fire victims to escape as confusion progresses to loss of consciousness. The process can be rapidly reversed, however, by timely administration of 100% oxygen (Schweich & Zempsky, 1999).

Damage to the lower airway most often results from chemicals or toxic gas inhalation. Soot is carried deep into the lungs, where it combines with water in the lungs to deposit acid-producing chemicals on the lung tissue. These acids burn the tissue, causing loss of cilia, loss of surfactant, and edema. Tissue destruction, edema, and disruption of gas exchange produce the initial insult to the lungs and potential airway obstruction. Days later, the damaged tissue sloughs off, obstructing the airways. Because the cilia that normally help in removing debris have been destroyed, the lungs become a breeding ground for microorganisms. Pneumonia becomes a major health concern. The damaged alveoli heal by scar tissue formation. This can greatly reduce the future functioning of the lungs.

Nursing Management

Most children who survive smoke-inhalation injury are admitted for close observation, airway management, and ventilatory support, if indicated. Respiratory assessment and pulmonary therapy are usually required to reestablish adequate oxygenation and respiratory function.

BLUNT CHEST TRAUMA

Blunt trauma is a common injury in children, especially associated with motor vehicle crashes (Pieper, 2000). Chest injuries may not be obvious and can be extremely difficult to evaluate.

After sustaining severe blunt trauma, most children die from lack of oxygen caused by poor airway and ventilatory control. A child's elastic, pliable chest wall and thin abdominal muscles provide minimal protection to underlying organs. This elasticity often spares bone but not the underlying organs. The presence of a rib fracture in children under 12 years old indicates trauma of significant force. The energy from blunt trauma is transferred directly from an external force to the internal organs, often causing a pulmonary contusion or pneumothorax.

PULMONARY CONTUSION

A pulmonary contusion is defined as bruising damage to the tissues of the lung. This causes bleeding into the alveoli, which may lead to capillary rupture in the air sacs. Pulmonary edema develops in the lower airways as blood and fluid from damaged tissues accumulate. Lower airway obstruction and atelectasis may result in impaired gas exchange, acute respiratory distress, and respiratory failure (Hazinski, 1999).

Pulmonary contusion occurs in up to 76% of children with nonpenetrating chest trauma. Initially the child may appear asymptomatic. Respiratory distress often develops over several hours, so careful observation is required during the first 12 hours after the injury to detect decreased perfusion related to ventilatory impairment.

Nursing Management

Nursing care centers on providing necessary physiologic support, such as oxygen therapy, positioning, positive pressure ventilation, oxygen, and comfort measures. The child's level of consciousness is an excellent indicator of respiratory function. Agitation and lethargy can signal increasing hypoxia. The thorax should be inspected for symmetric chest wall movement and equal presence of breath sounds in both lungs. The child may initially appear well but requires careful and thorough monitoring to detect signs of deterioration. Children with significant injuries are cared for in the intensive care unit. Some children require ventilator support as the pulmonary tissues heal.

CLINICAL TIP 

When monitoring the status of a child who has a pulmonary contusion, do not rely on the child's color as an indicator of adequate oxygenation. Cyanosis in children is often a late indicator of respiratory distress. Observe for hemoptysis (fresh blood in the emesis), dyspnea, decreased breath sounds, wheezes, crackles, and a transient temperature elevation.

PNEUMOTHORAX

A pneumothorax occurs when air collects between the pleural layers, causing the lung to collapse. If blood collects in the pleural space, it is called a *hemothorax,* and if blood and air collect, it is called a *pneumohemothorax.* A pneumothorax is one of the more common thoracic injuries in pediatric trauma patients.

The three types of pneumothorax are open, closed, and tension. An open pneumothorax, sometimes referred to as a sucking chest wound, results from any penetrating injury that exposes the pleural space to atmospheric pressure, thereby collapsing the lung.

A closed pneumothorax is sometimes caused by blunt chest trauma with no evidence of rib fracture (Figure 13-20 ◆). The chest may be compressed against a closed glottis, causing a sudden increase in pressure within the thoracic cavity. The child spontaneously holds his or her breath when the thorax is struck, accounting for the involuntary closing of the glottis. The pressure increase is transferred to the alveoli, causing them to burst. A single burst alveolus may be able to seal itself off, but with the destruction of many alveoli the lung collapses. Breath sounds are decreased or absent on the injured side, and the child is in respiratory distress. A thoracostomy is performed and a chest tube inserted. A closed drainage system is attached to help remove the air and reinflate the lung by reestablishing negative pressure.

A tension pneumothorax is a life-threatening emergency that results when the internal pressure from a closed pneumothorax is not vented and continues to build, compressing the chest contents and collapsing the lung. Air leaks into the chest cavity during inhalation but is trapped from escape during exhalation. Venous return to the heart is impaired as the trachea, heart, vena cava, and esophagus are compressed toward the unaffected lung when the mediastinum shifts, leading to decreased cardiac output. Signs of tension pneumothorax include increasing respiratory distress, decreased breath sounds, and paradoxic breathing.

Nursing Management

Nursing management focuses on airway management and maintaining lung inflation. The child arrives on the nursing unit with a chest tube and drainage system in place. Continued

PATHOPHYSIOLOGY ILLUSTRATED

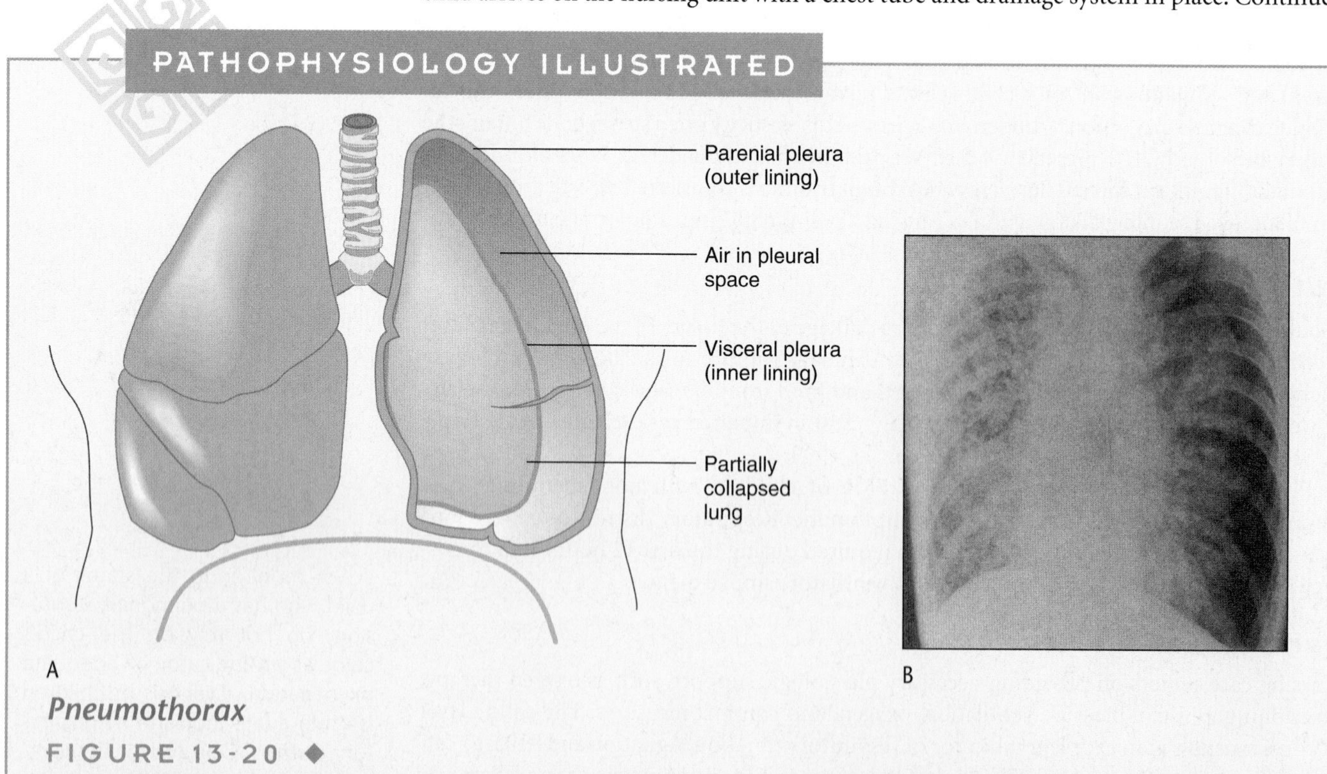

Pneumothorax

FIGURE 13-20 ◆

A, A pneumothorax is air in the pleural space that causes a lung to collapse. Whether the air results from an open injury or from bursting of alveoli due to a blunt injury, it is important to focus on airway management and maintain lung inflation. B, Pneumothorax. From: Fleisher, G.R., Ludwig, S. (1993). *Textbook of Pediatric Emergency Medicine,* 3rd ed., Fig. 89.10A, p. 398. Philadelphia: LW & W.

close observation for respiratory distress is essential. Vital signs are carefully monitored. Complications include hemothorax (if the thoracostomy and chest tube are improperly placed), lung tissue injury, and scarring from poor tube placement (especially if the tube is placed too near the breast in girls).

Chapter Highlights

- Acute respiratory problems are the most common cause of illness requiring hospitalization in infants and children less than 15 years of age.
- The child's airway is shorter and narrower than an adult's. These differences create a greater potential for obstruction. The lungs have no muscles of their own, so respiration is powered by the diaphragm and intercostal muscles.
- Apnea, by definition, is cessation of respiration lasting longer than 20 seconds, or any pause in respiration associated with cyanosis, marked pallor, hypotonia, or bradycardia.
- Sudden infant death syndrome (SIDS), a leading cause of death in infants, is the sudden death of an infant under 1 year of age that remains unexplained after a complete autopsy, a death scene investigation, and review of the history.
- Signs of impending respiratory failure in infants and children include irritability, lethargy, cyanosis, and increased respiratory effort such as dyspnea (difficulty breathing), tachypnea (increased respiratory rate), nasal flaring, and intercostal retractions.
- Laryngotracheobronchitis (LTB) is a croup syndrome viral illness with signs of a upper respiratory illness, hoarseness, tachypnea, inspiratory stridor, and a seal-like barking cough. Fever may or may not be present.
- Epiglottitis is caused by bacterial invasion of the soft tissue of the larynx causing inflammation and edema of the tissues and the epiglottis that can result in life-threatening airway obstruction. Fortunately, the number of cases of epiglottitis has decreased significantly because of the Hib vaccine.
- Asthma affects about 5 million children in the United States and, for those children, results in about 10 days of school absenteeism and 20 days of restricted activity per year.
- Bronchopulmonary dysplasia (BPD) is often a consequence of neonatal respiratory distress syndrome, congenital heart disease, meconium aspiration, and fluid overload and edema in the newborn. It is associated with respiratory infections requiring frequent hospitalization.
- Although many bacterial and mycoplasmal organisms may cause bronchiolitis, infection with respiratory syncytial virus (RSV) is the most common cause.
- Symptoms of pneumonia in infants and children include elevated temperature, rhonchi, crackles, wheezes, cough, dyspnea, tachypnea, restlessness, and if consolidation exists, decreased breath sounds.
- Clinical manifestations of tuberculosis in infants include a persistent cough, weight loss or failure to gain weight, and fever. Wheezing and decreased breath sounds may be present. Older children may be asymptomatic.
- In cystic fibrosis, defective chloride-ion transport across the exocrine and epithelial cells results in an abnormal accumulation of viscous, dehydrated mucus that affects the respiratory, gastrointestinal, and genitourinary systems.
- Foreign-body aspiration is most often caused by small objects that make their way into the child's mouth, such as foods, small toy parts, or household objects like beads, safety pins, coins, or buttons.
- A child can drown in as little water as it takes to cover the nose and mouth. Most drownings occur in the child's home pool or at the residence of a neighbor, friend, or relative. Other common drowning sites for young children include bathtubs, hot tubs, toilets, and even large water-filled buckets.
- Signs of smoke-inhalation injury in children include burns of the face and neck, singed nasal hairs, soot around the mouth or nose, and hoarseness with stridor or voice change.
- Pulmonary contusion occurs in the majority of children with nonpenetrating chest trauma. Although the child may appear initially asymptomatic, respiratory distress often develops in a few hours.
- A pneumothorax may become life threatening if internal pressure from a closed pneumothorax is not vented. Air leaking into the chest cavity during inspiration cannot escape during expiration, increasing compression. Venous blood return to the heart is impaired as the mediastinum shifts toward the unaffected lung.

EXPLORE MediaLink

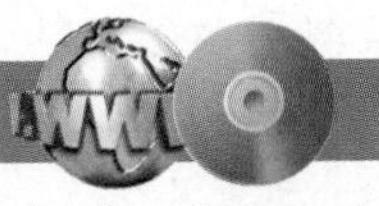

- NCLEX review, case studies, and other interactive resources for this chapter can be found on the Companion Website at **http://www.prenhall.com/ball.** Click on Chapter 13 to select the activities for this chapter.
- For animations, more NCLEX review questions, and an audio glossary, access the accompanying CD-ROM in this textbook.

References

1. Allshouse, M. J., & Eichelberger, M. R. (1993). Patterns of thoracic injury. In M. R. Eichelberger (Ed.), *Pediatric trauma: Prevention, acute care, rehabilitation* (pp. 437–448). St. Louis: Mosby.
2. American Academy of Pediatrics Committee on Child Abuse and Neglect. (2001). Distinguishing sudden infant death syndrome from child abuse fatalities. *Pediatrics, 107*(2), 437–441.
3. American Thoracic Society and Centers for Disease Control and Prevention. (2000). Diagnostic standards and classification of tuberculosis in adults and children. *American Journal of Respiratory and Critical Care Medicine, 161,* 1376–1395.
4. Bank, D. E., & Krug, S. E. (1995). New approaches to upper airway disease. *Emergency Medical Clinics of North America, 13*(2), 473–487.
5. Brashers, V. L., & Davey, S. S. (1998). Alterations in pulmonary function. In K. L. McCance & S. E. Huether, *Pathophysiology: The biologic basis for disease in adults and children* (3rd ed., pp. 1158–1200). St. Louis: Mosby.
6. Cote, A., Gerez, T., Brouillette, R. T., & Laplante, S. (2000). Circumstances leading to a change to prone sleeping in sudden infant death syndrome victims. *Pediatrics, 106*(6), 1–5.
7. Daigle, K. L., & Cloutier, M. M. (1997). Office management of bronchopulmonary dysplasia. *Comprehensive Therapy, 23*(10), 656–663.
8. D'Auria, J. P. (1997). Respiratory system. In J. A. Fox (Ed.), *Primary health care of children* (pp. 415–418). St. Louis: Mosby.
9. Eichelberger, M. R., Ball, J. W., Pratsch, G. S., & Clark, J. R. (1998). *Pediatric emergencies* (2nd ed.). Englewood Cliffs, NJ: Brady.
10. Farrell, P. M., Kosorok, M. R., Rock, M. J., Laxova, A., & Zeng, L., et al. (2001). Early diagnosis of cystic fibrosis through neonatal screening prevents severe malnutrition and improves long-term growth. *Pediatrics, 107*(1), 1–13.
11. Gilliland, F. D., Yu-Fen, L., & Peters, J. M. (2001). Effects of maternal smoking during pregnancy and environmental tobacco smoke on asthmatic and wheezing in children. *American Journal of Respiratory and Critical Care Medicine, 163,* 429–436.
12. Gross, I. (1999). Respiratory distress syndrome. In J. A. McMillan, C. D. DeAngelis, R. D. Feigin, & J. B. Warshaw, *Oski's pediatrics: Principles and practice* (3rd ed., pp. 254–258). Philadelphia: Lippincott, Williams & Wilkins.
13. Harvey, K. (2000). Bronchopulmonary dysplasia. In P. L. Jackson & J. A. Vessey (Eds.), *Primary care of the child with a chronic condition* (3rd ed., pp. 242–265). St. Louis: Mosby.
14. Hazinski, M. F. (1999). *Manual of pediatric critical care.* St. Louis: Mosby.
15. Health Resources and Services Administration's Maternal and Child Health Bureau. (2000). *Child health USA 2000.* Washington, DC: Government Printing Office.
16. Kaditis, A. G., & Wald, E. R. (1998). Viral croup: Current diagnosis and treatment. *Pediatric Infectious Disease Journal, 17*(9), 827–834.
17. Kieckhefer, G., & Ratcliffe, M. (2000). Asthma. In P. L. Jackson & J. A. Vessey (Eds.), *Primary care of the child with a chronic condition* (3rd ed., pp. 164–190). St. Louis: Mosby.
18. Loughlin, G. M., & Carroll, J. L. (1999). Apparent life-threatening events. In J. A. McMillan, C. D. DeAngelis, R. D. Feigin, & J. B. Warshaw, *Oski's pediatrics: Principles and practice* (3rd ed., pp. 589–596). Philadelphia: Lippincott, Williams & Wilkins.
19. Margo, K., & Shaughnessy, A. (1998). Antiviral drugs in healthy children. *American Family Physician, 57*(5), 1073–1077.
20. Margolis, P., & Gadomski, A. (1998). Does this infant have pneumonia? *Journal of the American Medical Association, 279*(4), 308–313.
21. McMullen, A. H. (2000). Cystic fibrosis. In P. L. Jackson & J. A. Vessey (Eds.), *Primary care of the child with a chronic condition* (3rd ed., pp. 401–425). St. Louis: Mosby.
22. Merelle, M. E., Lees, C. M., Nagelkerke, A. F., & Dezateux, C. (2000). Newborn screening for cystic fibrosis. *The Cochrane Library, 4,* 1–19.
23. Moon, R. Y., Patel, K. M., & Shaefer, S. J. M. (2000). Sudden infant death syndrome in child care settings. *Pediatrics, 106*(2), 295–300.
24. Murphy, S. A. (2000). Deaths: Final data for 1998. National Vital Statistics Reports, 48(11). Hyattsville, MD: National Center for Health Statistics.
25. Muscari, M. E. (1998). Coping with chronic illness. *American Journal of Nursing, 98*(9), 20–22.
26. National Education and Prevention Program. (1997). *Expert panel report II: Guidelines for diagnosis and management of asthma* (NIH Publication No. 97-4051). Bethesda, MD: National Institutes of Health.
27. National Respiratory and Enteric Virus Surveillance System. (2000). Respiratory syncytial virus activity—US, 1999–2000 season. *MMWR Weekly, 49*(48), 1091–1093.
28. Ozuah, P. O., Ozuah, T. P., Stein, R. E. K., Burton, W., & Mulvihill, M. (2001). Evaluation of risk assessment questionnaire used to target tuberculin skin testing in children. *JAMA, 285*(4), 451–453.
29. Parnigrahy, A., Filiano, J. J., & Sleeper, L. A., et al. (1997). Decreased kainite binding in the arcuate nucleus of the sudden infant death syndrome. *Journal of Neuropathology and Experimental Neurology, 56,* 1253–1261.
30. Pieper, P. (2000). Pediatric trauma. In B. V. Wise, C. McKenna, G. Garvin, & B. J. Harmon (Eds.), *Nursing care of the general pediatric surgical patient* (pp. 459–479). Gaithersburg, MD: Aspen.
31. Akintorin, S. M., Bez, M. L., Morales, P., & Pildes, R. S. (1996). A controlled trial of dexamethasone to prevent bronchopulmonary dysplasia in surfactant-treated infants. *Pediatrics, 98*(2), 204–210.
32. Richman, E. (1997). Asthma diagnosis and management: New severity classifications and therapy alternatives. *Clinician Reviews, 7*(8), 76–112.
33. Rosenstein, B. J., & Cutting, G. R. (1998). The diagnosis of cystic fibrosis: A consensus statement. *Journal of Pediatrics, 132*(4), 589–595.
34. Rubin, R. (2001, April 2). Cystic fibrosis carrier-testing gains support. *USA Today,* p. 5D.
35. Schweich, P. J., & Zempsky, W. T. (1999). Emergent issues. In J. A. McMillan, C. D. DeAngelis, R. D. Feigin, & J. B. Warshaw, *Oski's pediatrics: Principles and practice* (3rd ed., pp. 584–585.). Philadelphia: Lippincott, Williams & Wilkins.
36. Steinbach, S. F. (2000). Four controversies in pediatric asthma care. *Contemporary Pediatrics, 17*(10), 150–172.
37. Stowe, C. D., & Jacobs, R. F. (1999). Treatment of tuberculosis infection and disease in children: The North American perspective. *Pediatric Drugs, 1*(4), 299–312.
38. Stubblefield, C., & Murray, R. . (2000). Making the transition: Pediatric lung transplantation. *Journal of Pediatric Health Care, 14*(6), 280–287.
39. Sydnor-Greenberg, N., & Dokken, D. (2000). Communicating information at diagnosis: Helping families and children manage asthma. *Journal of Child and Family Nursing, 3*(4), 290–295.
40. Theobald, K., Botwinski, C., Albanna, S., & McWilliam, P. (2000). Apnea of prematurity: Diagnosis, implications for care, and pharmacologic management. *Neonatal Network, 19*(6), 17–24.
41. Tooley, W. H. (1996). Hyaline membrane disease. In A. M. Rudolph, J. I. E. Hoffman, & C. D. Rudolph (Eds.), *Rudolph's pediatrics* (20th ed., pp. 1598–1605). Stamford, CT: Appleton & Lange.

42. Varlotta, L. (1998). Management and care of the newly diagnosed patient with cystic fibrosis. *Current Opinion in Pulmonary Medicine, 4,* 311–318.

43. Webster, H., & Huether, S. E. (1998). Alterations in pulmonary function in children. In K. L. McCance & S. E. Huether (Eds.), *Pathophysiology: The biologic basis for disease in adults and children* (3rd ed., pp. 1201–1220). St. Louis: Mosby.

44. Wilson, D. C. & Pencharz, P. P. (1998). Nutrition and cystic fibrosis. *Nutrition, 14*(10), 792–795.

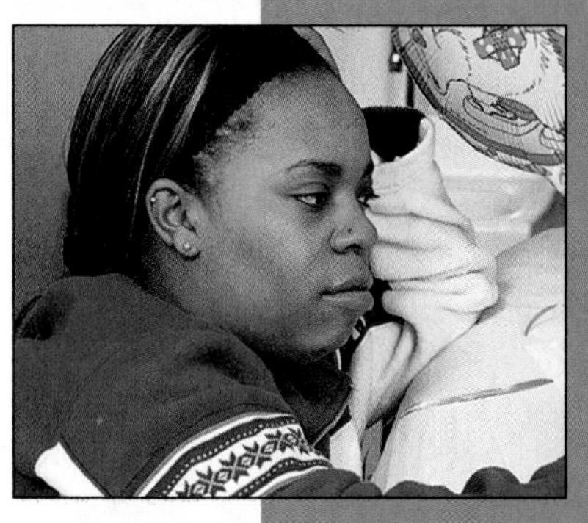

"Brandy got so sick so fast. We didn't expect her to have to have surgery when she was still so small. I just want her to get stronger and have the chance to grow up to be like other kids."

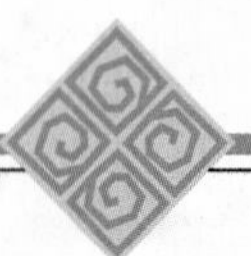

Brandy, who is 1 month old, was diagnosed with a ventricular septal defect (VSD) at birth. Her parents were just beginning to accept that she had a heart defect that might require surgical repair when signs of respiratory distress and difficulty in feeding developed.

Brandy's mother had been alerted to watch for these signs as a possible indication of congestive heart failure. Brandy was quickly hospitalized so her condition could be treated with digoxin, furosemide (Lasix), and potassium. Over the next 2 days she lost the weight she had gained due to fluid retention.

Because Brandy developed problems so soon after birth, it was decided that she should undergo surgical correction of her heart defect. Corrective surgery was performed to place a patch over the septal opening. Brandy was cared for in the intensive care unit before being transferred to another unit.

What are the causes of congestive heart failure? How is this condition treated? Is Brandy at risk to develop congestive heart failure again despite having had corrective surgery? What teaching and support do Brandy's parents need to care for her at home after the heart surgery? Answers to these and other questions can be found throughout this chapter.

CHAPTER

14

ALTERATIONS IN CARDIOVASCULAR FUNCTION

KEY TERMS

compliance Amount of distention or expansion the ventricles can achieve to increase stroke volume.

desaturated blood Blood with a lower than normal oxygen level resulting when a heart defect causes oxygenated and unoxygenated blood to mix.

digitalization Process of giving a higher than normal dose of digoxin initially to speed response to the drug.

hemodynamics Pressures generated by blood and passage of blood through the heart and pulmonary system.

palliative procedure Intervention used to preserve life in children with a potentially fatal or lethal condition.

polycythemia Above-normal increase in the number of red cells in the blood to increase the amount of hemoglobin available to carry oxygen.

preload Volume of blood in the ventricle at the end of diastole that stretches the heart muscle before contraction.

shunt Movement of blood between heart chambers through an abnormal anatomic or surgically created opening.

syncope Transient loss of consciousness and muscle tone.

MediaLink 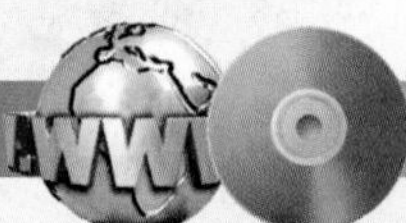 http://www.prenhall.com/ball

Resources for this chapter can be found on the CD-ROM accompanying this textbook, and on the Companion Website at http://www.prenhall.com/ball. Click on Chapter 14 to select the activities for this chapter.

CD-ROM

Animations
- Normal Heart Hemodynamics
- Congenital Heart Defects

Audio Glossary

NCLEX Review

COMPANION WEBSITE

Web Links

NCLEX Review

MediaLink Applications
- Nursing Care Plan: Pediatric Heart Transplant
- Teaching Plan: Infective Endocarditis Prophylaxis

Alterations in cardiovascular function may be the result of a congenital defect, acquired infection, or injury. Congenital heart disease is the leading cause of death, excluding prematurity, during the first year of life (Kohr & Sims, 1998). At least 35 types of heart defects are recognized (American Heart Association, 2001). Congenital heart defects, like Brandy's ventricular septal defect, occur in approximately 1% of all live births and often require surgical correction (Hoffman, 1995). Rapid advances in the treatment of congenital heart defects allow children to have surgery at younger ages. As a result, nursing care required to identify and manage responses of infants and children with heart disease has become more challenging.

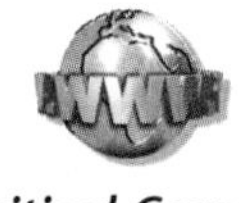

Critical Care Professional Resources

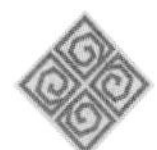

ANATOMY AND PHYSIOLOGY OF PEDIATRIC DIFFERENCES

TRANSITION FROM FETAL TO PULMONARY CIRCULATION

After the umbilical cord has been cut, the newborn must quickly adapt to receiving oxygen from the lungs. The transition from fetal to pulmonary circulation occurs in just a few hours. During fetal circulation, the constricted pulmonary vessels limit blood flow to the lungs (high pulmonary vascular resistance). Blood, however, flows easily to the extremities because systemic vascular resistance is low. The foramen ovale, an opening between the atria in the fetal heart, allows blood to flow from the right to the left atrium. Systemic vascular resistance increases after the umbilical cord is cut, causing a backup of blood flow. The pressure in the left side of the heart increases, stimulating closure of the foramen ovale. Once breathing has been initiated, the lungs expand and pulmonary vascular resistance falls. Blood that was previously shunted through the ductus arteriosus to the aorta flows to the lungs. Figure 14-1 ◆ compares fetal and postnatal pulmonary circulation.

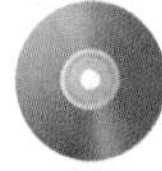

Normal Heart Hemodynamics

The ductus arteriosus, responding to higher oxygen saturation, normally constricts and closes within 10 to 15 hours after birth. Permanent closure occurs by 10 to 21 days after birth, unless oxygen saturation remains low. Fetal tissues are accustomed to low oxygen saturation. This may explain why newborns with cyanotic heart disease appear relatively comfortable even when the arterial partial pressure of oxygen (PaO_2) is 20 to 25 mm Hg. Older children and adults would rapidly develop acidosis and cerebral anoxia with such a low PaO_2.

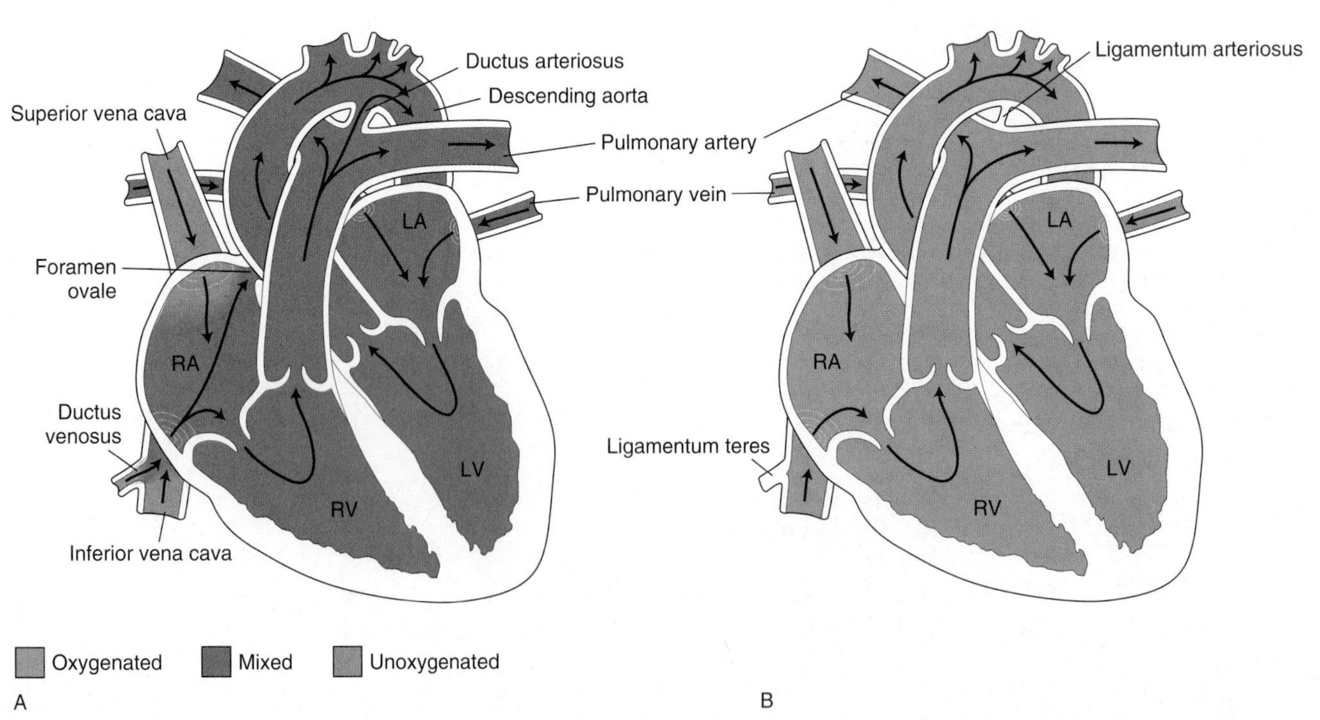

FIGURE 14-1 ◆

Normal circulation of the heart. A, Fetal (prenatal) circulation. B, Pulmonary (postnatal) circulation. *LA,* left atrium; *LV,* left ventricle; *RA,* right atrium; *RV,* right ventricle.

The ventricles are equal in size at birth, but by 2 months of age the left ventricle is twice as large as the right ventricle. The higher systemic vascular pressures force the left ventricle to develop quickly.

Infants have a greater risk of heart failure than older children because the immature heart is more sensitive to volume or pressure overload. During infancy the muscle fibers of the heart are less developed and less organized, resulting in limited functional capacity. Less **compliance** (amount of distention or expansion the ventricles can achieve to increase stroke volume) of the heart muscle means that stroke volume cannot increase substantially. The heart muscle fibers develop during early childhood and by 9 years of age, the weight of the heart has increased by 6 times (Kohr & Sims, 1998).

OXYGENATION

Oxygen bound to hemoglobin is transported to the tissues by the systemic circulation. Hematocrit and hemoglobin concentrations appropriate for the child's age are necessary for adequate oxygen transport (see Chapter 15). The oxygen arterial saturation is the amount of oxygen that can potentially be delivered to the tissues. **Desaturated blood** results when oxygenated and unoxygenated blood mix because of a congenital heart defect. Cyanosis, which indicates hypoxemia (lower than normal amounts of oxygen in the blood), results from the presence of 5 or more grams of unoxygenated hemoglobin per 100 mL of blood (Park, 1996).

The child's bone marrow responds to chronic hypoxemia by producing more red blood cells to increase the amount of hemoglobin available for oxygenation. This increase is known as **polycythemia**. A hematocrit value of 50% or higher is common in children with cyanotic heart defects.

CLINICAL TIP 

Pulse oximetry can be used to measure arterial oxygen saturation. A reading of 95%–98% is normal in children. The following values indicate hypoxemia:

- Mild hypoxemia: 90%–95%
- Moderate hypoxemia: 85%–90%
- Severe hypoxemia: <85%

CARDIAC FUNCTIONING

Oxygen requirements are high for the first 8 weeks of life. Normally the newborn's heart rate increases to provide adequate oxygen transport. The infant has little cardiac output reserve capacity until oxygen requirements begin to decrease. Cardiac output depends almost completely on heart rate until the heart muscle is fully developed at 5 years of age. Weight-specific cardiac output decreases during childhood. During stress, exercise, fever, or respiratory distress, infants and children have tachycardia, which increases their cardiac output.

Children respond to severe hypoxemia with bradycardia. Cardiac arrest in children generally results from prolonged hypoxemia related to respiratory failure or shock rather than from a primary cardiac insult as in adults. Bradycardia is therefore a significant warning sign of cardiac arrest. Appropriate management of hypoxemia reverses bradycardia and prevents cardiac arrest.

NURSING ALERT 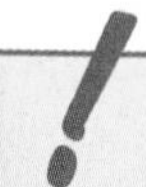

Extreme polycythemia as determined by a hemoglobin concentration greater than 20 g/dL and a hematocrit greater than 55%–60% is dangerous. Blood viscosity is increased, and the child is at risk for a thromboembolism (Park, 1996).

CONGESTIVE HEART FAILURE

Congestive heart failure is a disorder of circulation in which cardiac output is inadequate to support the body's circulatory and metabolic needs. It may result from a congenital heart defect that causes increased pulmonary blood flow or obstruction to the blood outflow tract, from problems with heart contractility, or from pathologic conditions that require high cardiac output, such as severe anemia, acidosis, or respiratory disease.

ETIOLOGY AND PATHOPHYSIOLOGY

Congenital heart defects are the most common cause of congestive heart failure in children (Wolfe, Boucek, & Schaffer, et al., 1997). Brandy, shown at the beginning of this chapter, developed congestive heart failure as a result of one such defect. Some defects allow blood to flow from the left side of the heart to the right so that extra blood must be pumped to the pulmonary system rather than through the aorta when the left ventricle contracts. This overloads the pulmonary system, and if prolonged can lead to pulmonary artery hypertension, an often irreversible condition leading to life-threatening pulmonary vascular resistance (see p. 495). Obstructive congenital defects (i.e., abnormally small pulmonary vessels) restrict the flow of blood so the heart hypertrophies to work harder to force blood through these structures. This increases cardiac output initially, but eventually the hypertrophied

CLINICAL MANIFESTATIONS OF CONGESTIVE HEART FAILURE

CAUSE	CLINICAL MANIFESTATIONS
Pulmonary venous congestion	Tachypnea, wheezing, crackles, retractions, cough, grunting, nasal flaring, feeding difficulties, irritability, tiring with play
Systemic venous congestion	Hepatomegaly, ascites, peripheral edema
Impaired cardiac output	Tachycardia, diminished pulses, hypotension, capillary refill time >2 sec, pallor, cool extremities, oliguria
High metabolic rate	Failure to thrive or slow weight gain

muscle becomes ineffective (Balaguru, Artman, & Auslender, 2000). Initially the right or left side of the heart may fail, but eventually failure is bilateral.

When cardiac output remains insufficient, the body's organs and tissues do not receive adequate oxygen. The kidneys respond to the lowered circulating volume by activating the renin–angiotensin mechanism to retain salt and water. A sympathetic response increases the heart rate and heart muscle contractility. Both responses increase cardiac output to the vital organs. Without intervention, the compensatory mechanisms increase their intensity, demanding more effort from the compromised heart. This results in progressive systemic edema and pulmonary congestion.

CLINICAL MANIFESTATIONS

Congestive heart failure often develops subtly, and symptoms may not be recognized at first. The infant tires easily, especially during feeding. Weight loss or lack of normal weight gain, diaphoresis, irritability, and frequent infections may be evident. Older children may have exercise intolerance, dyspnea, abdominal pain or distention, and peripheral edema.

As the disease progresses, symptoms such as tachypnea, tachycardia, pallor or cyanosis, nasal flaring, grunting, retractions, cough, or crackles may occur. Generalized fluid volume overload is seen more commonly in toddlers and older children. Periorbital and facial edema, jugular vein distention, and hepatomegaly are signs of fluid volume excess. See the clinical manifestation table for more detail.

Cardiomegaly occurs as the heart attempts to maintain cardiac output. Cyanosis, weak peripheral pulses, cool extremities, hypotension, and heart murmur are precursors of cardiogenic shock, which can occur if congestive heart failure is not adequately treated. (Cardiogenic shock is discussed on p. 508.)

CLINICAL THERAPY

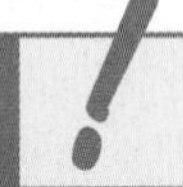

Skill 10-4: Placement of ECG Electrodes

Diagnosis is based primarily on clinical manifestations such as tachycardia, respiratory distress, and crackles. A chest x-ray study reveals cardiac enlargement and venous congestion or signs of pulmonary edema. Echocardiography may be performed to diagnose specific cardiac defects or dysfunction. An electrocardiogram may show tachycardia, bradycardia, or ventricular hypertrophy.

> **NURSING ALERT**
>
> Digoxin and digitoxin are both digitalis preparations but are not the same drug. Digoxin is the drug of choice in pediatrics. Digitoxin is 10 times more powerful than digoxin, and is rarely used in children. Read labels carefully and double-check doses to ensure that the child receives the right dose of the right drug.

The goals of medical management are to make the heart work more efficiently and to remove excess fluid, thus improving systemic circulation without flooding the pulmonary system. Inotropic medicines and afterload-reducing agents (angiotensin-converting enzyme inhibitors) are sometimes used to lessen the workload of the heart and help it to work more efficiently (Balaguru et al., 2000). Digoxin is the drug most commonly used to improve the heart's ability to contract and therefore increase its output. Occasionally a higher than normal dose is given initially, followed by a lower maintenance dose. This process, called **digitalization,** speeds the child's response to the drug. B-blockers are used in some cases to reduce the effects of catecholamines on heart rate and contractility (O'Laughlin, 1999).

Diuretics, such as furosemide, chlorothiazide, and spironolactone, are given to promote fluid excretion. Furosemide is the most commonly used medication during hospitalization; thiazides are commonly used to maintain diuresis at home. Because most diuretics (except for spironolactone) cause potassium loss, serum potassium levels are monitored and potas-

MEDICATIONS USED IN TREATMENT OF CONGESTIVE HEART FAILURE

Drug	Action
Digoxin	Increases myocardial contractility
Furosemide	Rapid diuresis
Thiazides Chlorothiazide (suspension) Hydrochlorothiazide (tablets)	Maintenance diuresis
Spironolactone	Maintenance diuresis (potassium sparing)
ACEi (angiotensin-converting enzyme inhibitor)	Promotes vascular relaxation and reduced peripheral vascular resistance
Propranolol	Increases contractility

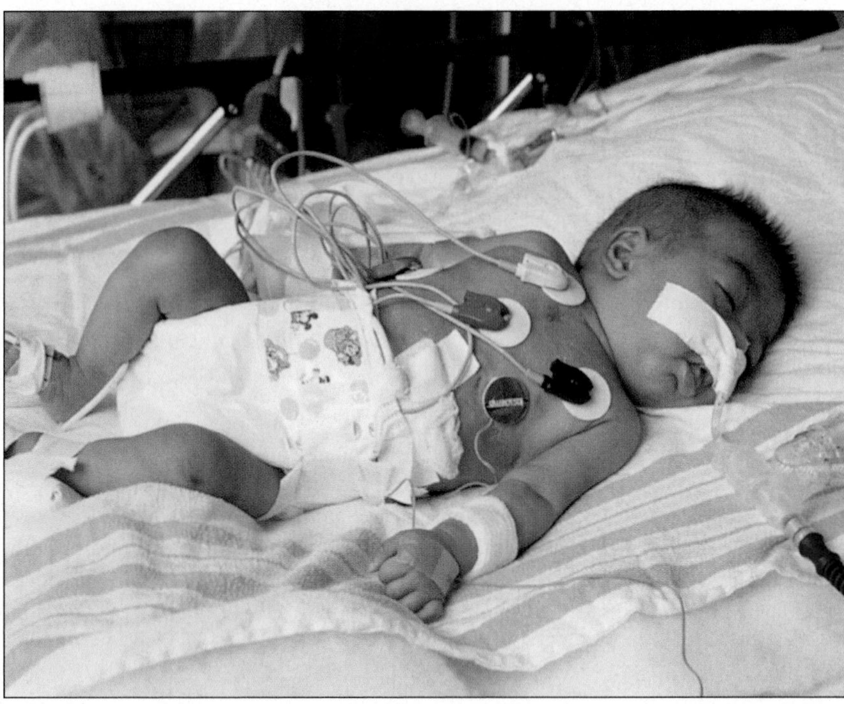

FIGURE 14-2 ◆ Jooti is receiving intravenous fluids and oxygen. Her condition is being continuously monitored for congestive heart failure.

sium supplements may be ordered. Vasodilating drugs may be given to reduce pulmonary and systemic vasoconstriction and to decrease the work of the heart.

Surgery or interventional catheterization to correct a congenital heart defect may become the treatment of choice, as occurred with Brandy. Cardiac transplantation may be performed for children with end-stage cardiomyopathy or complex congenital heart defects such as hypoplastic left heart syndrome.

Other medical therapy is supportive. Airway management, ventilatory support, rest, and fluid and dietary management are also part of the treatment plan. Oxygen may be ordered (Figure 14-2 ◆). Most children improve rapidly after medication is administered.

NURSING MANAGEMENT

Nursing Assessment and Diagnosis

Physiologic Assessment

As diagnosis of congestive heart failure depends primarily on physical symptoms, nursing observations are important. Assess the child's behavioral patterns, cardiac function, respiratory function, and fluid status. Obtain a detailed history of the onset of symptoms from the parents, as congestive heart failure often develops slowly.

Psychosocial Assessment

Take a history of the child's previous hospitalizations and assess the family's knowledge about the child's condition. Families of children with congestive heart failure are anxious and fear the potential serious outcome of the problem and the need to provide ongoing care. Assess the family's anxiety level and coping strategies. Evaluate the family's economic status. Medication is crucial to treatment, and a family's inability to afford or obtain the necessary medications jeopardizes the child's ability to survive.

The family is often overprotective and reluctant to leave the child with other caregivers. Find out if a knowledgeable person who can safely administer medications and watch the child is available for respite care.

Developmental Assessment

Because fatigue limits the activities of the child with congestive heart failure, he or she does not have the opportunity to practice the skills needed to attain normal developmental milestones. Perform developmental assessment with a tool such as the Denver II (see Chapter 6). In addition, parents can provide information about the attainment of expected developmental milestones such as sitting, manipulating objects, standing, or walking. When congestive heart failure is well controlled, the child's energy level increases and developmental skills often improve. In infants and toddlers, assessments every 2 to 3 months are useful to observe development and evaluate disease management.

Parents may limit the child's contact with other children because of frequent infections and exercise intolerance. Ask parents about contact and play with other children and a typical day's activity schedule.

Several nursing diagnoses that may apply to the child with congestive heart failure are given in the accompanying nursing care plans. The primary nursing diagnosis is *decreased cardiac output,* related to cardiac anomaly.

Planning and Implementation

Nursing care for the child with congestive heart failure focuses on administering and monitoring effects of medications, maintaining adequate oxygenation and myocardial function, promoting rest, fostering development, providing adequate nutrition, and providing emotional support to the child and family. The first of the two accompanying nursing care plans summarizes nursing care for the child who is hospitalized with congestive heart failure.

Administer and Monitor Prescribed Medications

Children with congestive heart failure usually receive digoxin and furosemide. These medications are potent and must be administered correctly.

Skill 5-22: Measuring Intake and Output

Measure intake and output carefully. Weigh the infant's diapers before and after changing (1 g = 1 mL urine). Observe for changes in peripheral edema and circulation. Weigh the child at the same time each day because fluid volume varies throughout the day. If ascites is present, take serial abdominal measurements to monitor changes (see Figure 10-11). Turn the child frequently, and provide skin care when edema is present (see Figure 10-12).

Skill 5-3: Measuring Weight

Skill 5-7: Measuring Abdominal Girth

Maintain Oxygenation and Myocardial Function

Oxygen therapy may be ordered. Make sure that tubing is patent, the oxygen flow rate is correct, the oxygen delivery device is working properly, and humidification is provided. Keep the child calm and quiet. Position the child in a semi-Fowler's or 45° angle position to promote maximum oxygenation.

Promote Rest

Group assessments and interventions together to ensure that the child has some uninterrupted rest each hour. Feedings should last no more than 20 to 30 minutes. Frequent small feedings generally work best, with burping after every half ounce of intake to minimize vomiting. Rocking is restful for infants. Encourage older children to engage in quiet activities such as playing board games or watching television.

NURSING CARE PLAN The Child Hospitalized with Congestive Heart Failure

GOAL	INTERVENTION	RATIONALE	EXPECTED OUTCOME
1. Decreased Cardiac Output related to cardiac anomaly (VSD)			
	NIC Priority Intervention: **Hemodynamic Regulation**: Optimization of heart rate, preload, afterload, and contractility.		NOC Suggested Outcome: **Cardiac Pump Effectiveness**: Extent to which blood is ejected from the left ventricle per minute to support systemic perfusion pressure.
The child's cardiac output will be sufficient to meet the body's metabolic demands.	■ Administer digoxin as ordered. ■ Take apical pulse and listen to heart sounds regularly, especially before each dose of digoxin. Record apical pulse with each recorded dose of digoxin. ■ Use cardiac monitor if ordered. ■ Prevent injury by monitoring for digoxin side effects and serum potassium level. ■ Provide for rest periods each hour.	■ Digoxin increases contractility of the heart and force of contraction. ■ Digoxin may cause bradycardia. Pulse and heart sounds provide information about heart functioning. ■ Monitor notes tachycardia and arrhythmias. ■ Digoxin is a potent drug with serious side effects. Hypokalemia increases risk of digoxin toxicity. ■ Rest increases need for high cardiac output.	The child's cardiac output is sufficient as indicated by increased energy, adequate feeding intake, and decreased edema. The child maintains normal serum levels of potassium and therapeutic levels of digoxin. The child rests hourly and has adequate energy to eat and play.
The child will manifest adequate oxygenation.	■ Place child in semi-Fowler's position. ■ Evaluate respiratory rate and sounds. Take pulse oximetry readings to determine oxygen saturation. ■ Provide oxygen and humidification if ordered. Observe for diaphoresis, a sign of increased respiratory effort.	■ Position facilitates lung expansion. ■ Absence of tachypnea and adventitious sounds and oxygen saturation above 95% indicate ease of respiration. ■ Supplemental oxygen decreases tachypnea, and humidification moistens secretions to keep airway clear.	The child has normal respiratory rate for age with no evidence of adventitious sounds or diaphoresis.
2. Fluid Volume Excess related to heart failure			
	NIC Priority Intervention: **Fluid Management**: Promotion of fluid balance and prevention of complications resulting from abnormal or undesired fluid levels.		NOC Suggested Outcome: **Fluid Balance**: Balance of water in the intracellular and extracellular compartments of the body.
The child's urinary output will remain within normal levels. Intake and output will be balanced.	■ Measure intake and output carefully. Weigh diapers to obtain output of young child. ■ Maintain fluid-restricted diet if ordered. ■ Administer diuretics as ordered. ■ Monitor electrolytes. ■ Weigh daily. ■ Measure abdominal girth daily if present. Observe for peripheral edema.	■ Adequate output is a good indicator of renal perfusion. ■ Fluid restriction is sometimes used to decrease cardiac load. ■ Diuretics mobilize fluids and facilitate excretion. ■ Electrolyte imbalance is common when fluids are restricted and diuretics are given. ■ Evaluations demonstrate effectiveness of treatment.	The child's intake and output are proportional, and electrolyte levels remain within normal ranges.

(continued)

NURSING CARE PLAN The Child Hospitalized with Congestive Heart Failure (continued)

GOAL	INTERVENTION	RATIONALE	EXPECTED OUTCOME
3. Risk for Impaired Skin Integrity related to altered fluid status			
	NIC Priority Intervention: **Pressure Management**: Minimizing pressure to body parts.		NOC Suggested Outcome: **Risk Control**: Actions to eliminate or reduce actual, personal, and modifiable health threats.
The child's peripheral and central edema will decrease.	■ Provide skin care for edematous body parts and elevate extremities. ■ Change child's position frequently. ■ Inspect skin frequently for redness and skin breakdown over pressure points.	■ Edematous skin injures easily. Elevation promotes return of fluid from extremities. ■ Position change promotes circulation to skin over pressure points. ■ Inspection identifies earliest stages of skin breakdown.	The child has no skin breakdown after edema resolves.
4. Altered Nutrition: Less Than Body Requirements related to high metabolic needs and rapid tiring while feeding			
	NIC Priority Intervention: **Nutrition Management**: Assistance with or provision of a balanced dietary intake of food and fluids.		NOC Suggested Outcome: **Nutrition Status**: Extent to which nutrients are available to meet metabolic needs.
The infant or child will demonstrate normal weight gain for age.	■ Hold infant at 45° angle for feeding. ■ Record intake carefully. ■ Weigh child daily. ■ Give frequent small meals with rest periods inbetween. Give high-calorie snacks. ■ Use soothing approaches such as holding infants for feeding and having parents eat with older child.	■ Position facilitates breathing while eating. ■ Evaluation of intake indicates whether caloric and other nutritional needs are met. ■ Weight indicates growth (in absence of edematous symptoms of congestive heart failure). ■ Digesting small meals requires less energy. High-calorie snacks provide calories efficiently. ■ Restful approach facilitates intake with minimum cardiac work.	The infant or child gains recommended weight according to growth grids. All dietary requirements are met, and mealtimes are pleasant.
5. Ineffective Family Coping, Compromised, related to unknown nature of child's disease			
	NIC Priority Intervention: **Family Involvement**: Facilitating family participation in the emotional and physical care of the patient.		NOC Suggested Outcome: Not yet developed
Parents will express lessened anxiety as hospitalization proceeds.	■ Encourage parents to room in or stay with child. Explain procedures and treatment. Involve parents in care as much as possible. Have parents plan child's play periods. ■ At discharge, provide clear instructions and information about what to do in an emergency, and whom and where to call with questions. ■ Allow parents to verbalize questions, concerns, and feelings. Refer parents to support groups or other resources as needed.	■ Involvement in child's care lessens parental anxiety and fear of unknown. ■ Having resources available provides feelings of security. ■ Emotional support is needed to lessen anxiety.	Parents participate in developing and implementing the treatment plan and providing care to the child.

Foster Development

Encourage parents to play with the child, using toys to stimulate eye–hand coordination and fine motor movements. Such toys include rattles, blocks, and stuffed animals for infants and books, paper and pencil, and dolls for older children. Encourage sitting, standing, or walking for short periods with adequate rest afterward to promote the development of large muscles. Singing, talking, and playing music facilitate cognitive and language skills.

Provide Adequate Nutrition

Teach parents about feeding techniques. The mother who chooses to breast-feed the infant should not be discouraged. The antibodies contained in breast milk reduce infections, and the milk is naturally low in sodium. However, the sucking involved in feeding may cause dyspnea and force the infant to rest frequently during feeding.

Infants should be burped frequently to permit rest and prevent vomiting. They may need small frequent feedings and longer feeding periods. Positioning the baby in an infant seat at a 45° angle decreases venous return to the heart as well as its metabolic demand. This is a favorable position for feeding and other activities (Kohr & Sims, 1998).

Make sure that parents understand that changes in feeding habits (decreased intake, vomiting, sleeping through feedings, increased perspiration with feedings) may indicate deteriorating cardiac status. The American Heart Association publishes a helpful booklet, *Feeding Infants with Congenital Heart Disease,* for parents.

Adequate nutrition is needed to support the infant's growth. It is not unusual for infants with heart problems to develop failure to thrive as the result of feeding difficulties (see Chapter 3). When infants have significant dyspnea with feeding, special feeding techniques are needed. Some infants need a higher caloric formula (24 to 30 calories per ounce) to obtain adequate nutrition. Other infants require nutritional supplementation by nasogastric or gastrostomy tube (Figure 14-3 ◆). Parents are often advised to give the infant a chance to feed normally for a specific period. The remainder of the formula is then given by nasogastric or gastrostomy tube.

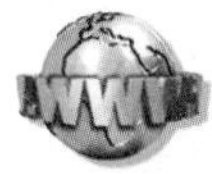

Congestive Heart Failure Support and Resources

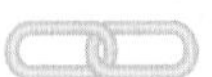

Skill 11-2: Inserting and Removing a Nasogastric Tube

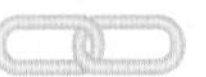

Skill 11-3: Administering a Gavage Feeding

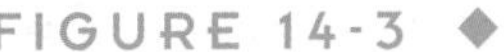

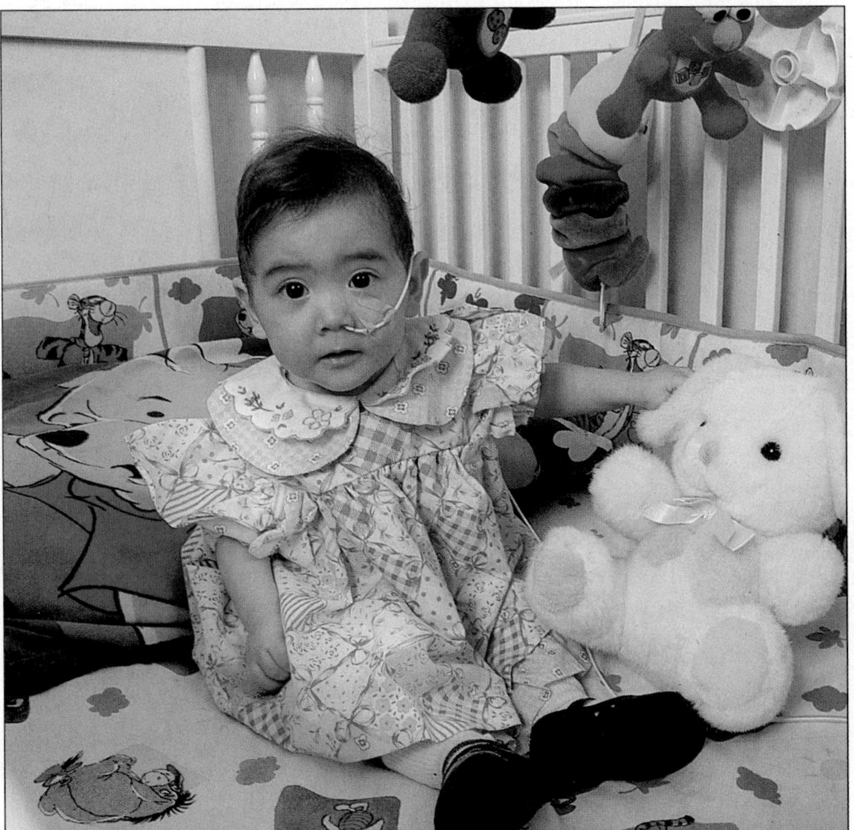

FIGURE 14-3 ◆
Infants with cardiac conditions often require supplemental feedings to provide sufficient nutrients for growth and development. The parents of this infant girl have been taught how to give her nasogastric feedings at home.

PROVIDE EMOTIONAL SUPPORT

When a child is hospitalized with congestive heart failure, the family is often anxious about his or her condition. Give parents an opportunity to express concerns about their child's condition. Explain the child's treatment regimen, and make sure family members understand the child's need for nutrition and rest. Answering questions about the child's prognosis and the ultimate outcome can be reassuring. Provide family members with information, and relay questions to the physician. Talking to other parents of children with cardiac conditions may be a source of emotional support. Refer parents to the appropriate support groups.

DISCHARGE PLANNING AND HOME CARE TEACHING

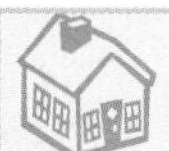

HOME CARE

Digitalis is a very dangerous drug. Encourage parents to keep it locked up at home and away from children. In case of accidental ingestion, immediate medical care is needed. Make sure the poison control number is on the parents' phones.

Home care needs should be identified and addressed well in advance of discharge. While the child is hospitalized, teach the family about the administration of medications and signs of a worsening condition.

Demonstrate administration of drugs, and then supervise while the parents measure and administer medications. Teach parents about the toxic effects of digoxin and other drugs. Advise them to notify the physician immediately if any of these side effects occur.

Show parents how to feed the child to maximize nutritional intake. Tell them to watch for symptoms such as increased feeding difficulty, irritability, lethargy, breathing difficulty, and puffiness around the eyes or extremities, which indicate that congestive heart failure is worsening. Parents are frequently taught to take the child's pulse and to report any significant change to the physician. An increase in pulse rate can signal congestive heart failure, and a decrease in pulse rate can indicate digoxin toxicity.

CARE IN THE COMMUNITY

The second of the two accompanying nursing care plans outlines home care of the child with congestive heart failure. Parents play a critical role in the care of the child with heart disease by facilitating normal development and limiting the incidence of congestive heart failure.

Evaluate family resources so that adequate child or respite care can be arranged if needed. Demonstrate to the family how to assess the child's energy level, and how to observe for feeding problems and edema. Observe medication administration and correct any errors. Watch the child feeding and provide suggestions as necessary.

Evaluation

Expected outcomes of nursing care can be found on the nursing care plans.

CONGENITAL HEART DISEASE

Congenital heart disease refers to a defect in the heart or great vessels, or persistence of a fetal structure after birth. Congenital heart defects are estimated to occur in 1% of live births (American Heart Association, 2001). In spontaneously aborted and stillborn fetuses, the incidence is much higher. Individuals with congenital heart disease are living longer than those born in past decades. Between 1979 and 1997, deaths from heart defects declined by 39.4% (Boneva, Botto, & Moore, et. al., 2001). This is attributed to diagnostic advances, surgical technique refinements, and intensive care.

CLINICAL TIP

Evidence shows that the use of multivitamins by women at the time of conception may reduce the risk of certain defects (transposition of the great vessels, tetralogy of Fallot, and truncus arteriosus) (Botto, Khoury, & Mulinare, et al., 1996).

Most congenital heart defects develop during the first 8 weeks of gestation. They are usually the result of a combined or interactive effect of genetic and environmental factors, as follows:

- Fetal exposure to drugs such as phenytoin and lithium
- Maternal viral infections such as rubella
- Maternal metabolic disorders such as phenylketonuria and diabetes mellitus
- Maternal complications of pregnancy such as increased age and antepartal bleeding
- Genetic factors (family recurrence patterns)
- Chromosomal abnormalities such as Turner syndrome, Noonan syndrome, Marfan syndrome, DiGeorge syndrome, cri du chat syndrome, Down syndrome, and trisomy syndromes 13, 15, 18, and 21 (Kohr & Sims, 1998). The prevalence of heart defects in children with Down syndrome is about 40% (Lewin, 2000).

NURSING CARE PLAN The Child with Congestive Heart Failure Being Cared for at Home

GOAL	INTERVENTION	RATIONALE	EXPECTED OUTCOME
1. Altered Growth and Development related to effects of physical disability			
	NIC Priority Intervention: **Developmental Enhancement:** Teaching parents to facilitate optimal gross motor, fine motor, language, cognitive, social, and emotional growth of preschool children.		NOC Suggested Outcome: **Child Development** (2 years): Milestones of physical, cognitive, and psychosocial progression by 2 years of age.
The child will meet developmental milestones for age group.	■ Perform baseline developmental assessment. ■ Plan for short play periods after rest. ■ Introduce age-appropriate toys and activities such as rattles and blocks for infants and art projects for older children. ■ Plan for interactions with healthy children.	■ Assessment provides comparison for later assessments and basis for planning specific games, toys, and activities. ■ Short play periods maintain energy and facilitate play. ■ Play activities facilitate learning and mastery of developmental tasks. ■ Social skills are learned through contact with others.	The child displays normal language, fine motor, and gross motor activity.
2. Ineffective Management of Therapeutic Regimen (Family) related to complexity of therapeutic regimen			
	NIC Priority Intervention: **Family Involvement**: Facilitating family participation in the emotional and physical care of the patient.		NOC Suggested Outcome: Not yet developed.
Parents will demonstrate correct administration of medications. Parents will state side effects of medications and symptoms of congestive heart failure.	■ Demonstrate administration of digoxin, diuretics, and other medications. Have parents administer them under supervision of nurse. ■ Describe side effects of medications. Give parents handouts with telephone number to call to ask questions or report side effects. ■ Describe subtle onset of congestive heart failure and its symptoms (increasing weakness, exhaustion, irritability, difficulty feeding, cough, or difficult respirations, edema).	■ Demonstration with return demonstration is an excellent method of learning psychomotor skills. ■ If side effects are understood, serious complications can be avoided. ■ Parents can evaluate child regularly and note subtle changes requiring medical management.	Parents report that child continues to demonstrate improvement and adequate cardiac output with absence of congestive heart failure.
3. Altered Nutrition: Less Than Body Requirements related to chronic illness and tiring while feeding			
	NIC Priority Intervention: **Weight Gain Assistance**: Facilitation of body weight gain.		NOC Suggested Outcome: **Nutritional Status: Food and Fluid Intake**: Amount of flood and fluid taken into the body over a 24-hour period.
The infant or child will demonstrate normal weight gain for age.	■ Teach parents methods to promote food intake related to positioning, size of feedings, food choices. ■ Observe feeding during home visit.	■ Positioning, frequency of feedings, size of feedings, and use of high-calorie foods can enhance nutritional intake. ■ Feedback can assist parents in integrating positive feeding techniques.	The infant or child shows normal weight gain. Parents report and demonstrate successful feedings of child.

(continued)

NURSING CARE PLAN The Child with Congestive Heart Failure Being Cared for at Home (continued)

GOAL	INTERVENTION	RATIONALE	EXPECTED OUTCOME
4. Activity Intolerance (Child) related to poor cardiac output			
	NIC Priority Intervention: **Energy Management**: Regulating energy use to treat or prevent fatigue and optimize function.		NOC Suggested Outcome: **Energy Conservation**: Extent of active management of energy to initiate or sustain activity.
The child will perform all necessary activities of daily living without undue tiring.	■ Help parents alternate activities and rest throughout the child's day. ■ Have parents limit child's exposure to persons with contagious disease. ■ Help family plan quiet surroundings to provide for child's rest.	■ Activities to promote development must be alternated with rest due to decreased cardiac output. ■ When the child is ill and tired, the immune system can be compromised. ■ Home setting may need to be altered to promote rest.	The child performs necessary activities and rests frequently each day.
5. Caregiver Role Strain (Parent) related to 24-hour responsibility for child's care			
	NIC Priority Intervention: **Caregiver Support**: Provision of the necessary information, advocacy, and support to facilitate primary patient care by someone other than a health care professional.		NOC Suggested Outcome: **Caregiver Endurance Potential**: Factors that promote family care provider continuance over an extended period of time.
Parents will express ability to meet own needs.	■ Assess family and community supports. Provide information related to respite care. ■ Encourage parents to seek activities to meet personal needs.	■ Variable family and community supports are available. ■ Parents need time to meet own personal needs in order to successfully care for child.	Parents report some time away from the child and report renewal in caring for the child.

Chromosome 22q11 is one of the most frequent genetic sites associated with development of cardiovascular defects such as truncus arteriosus, tetralogy of Fallot, and pulmonary atresia (Lewin, 2000). Because of this genetic component, the incidence of congenital heart defects is expected to slowly rise as persons with some of these defects survive and have children of their own.

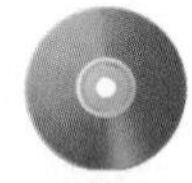

Congenital Heart Defects

A child often has more than one defect at the same time. Depending on the type of defect, signs and symptoms may be present at birth or develop later.

Congenital heart defects are generally divided into two categories, cyanotic and acyanotic, based on the hallmark sign of cyanosis. However, a child with an acyanotic defect may show clinical signs of cyanosis. The pathophysiology of a heart defect is related to **hemodynamics,** which refers to the pressures generated by blood and the pathways blood takes through the heart and pulmonary system.

ACYANOTIC DEFECTS

The majority of children with congenital heart defects have acyanotic conditions. There are two types of acyanotic defects: nonobstructive lesions, which do not interfere with the flow of blood, and obstructive lesions, which block the outflow of blood from the heart. Nonobstructive defects include patent ductus arteriosus (PDA), atrial septal defect (ASD), atrioventricular (AV) canal (endocardial cushion defect), and ventricular septal defect (VSD). Obstructive defects include pulmonic stenosis (PS), aortic stenosis (AS), and coarctation of the aorta. Tables 14-1 and 14-2 summarize the pathophysiology, clinical manifestations, and clinical therapy for these defects.

TABLE 14-1 Pathophysiology, Clinical Manifestations, and Clinical Therapy for Acyanotic Heart Defects—Nonobstructive Lesions

PATENT DUCTUS ARTERIOSUS (PDA)

Common congenital defect caused by persistent fetal circulation that accounts for 9%–12% of all congenital heart defects (Driscoll, 1999). When pulmonary circulation is established and systemic vascular resistance increases at birth, pressures in the aorta become greater than in the pulmonary arteries. Blood is then shunted from the aorta to the pulmonary arteries, increasing circulation to the pulmonary system.

Clinical Manifestations

Dyspnea; tachypnea; full, bounding pulses; and poor development occur. Infant is at risk for frequent respiratory infections and infective endocarditis. When a large PDA exists, congestive heart failure, intercostal retractions, hepatomegaly, and growth failure are also seen. A continuous systolic murmur is auscultated, and a thrill may be palpated in the pulmonic area.

Clinical Therapy

When murmur is detected, diagnosis is confirmed by chest x-ray study, electrocardiogram (ECG), and echocardiogram. Chest x-ray film and ECG show left ventricular hypertrophy. PDA can be visualized, and left-to-right shunt can be measured on echocardiogram.

Surgical ligation of PDA is the treatment of choice. Intravenous indomethacin often stimulates closure of the ductus arteriosus in premature infants. Transcatheter closure by obstructive device is sometimes attempted in children over 18 months of age.

PROGNOSIS: If PDA is not treated, child's life span is shortened because pulmonary hypertension and vascular obstructive disease develop.

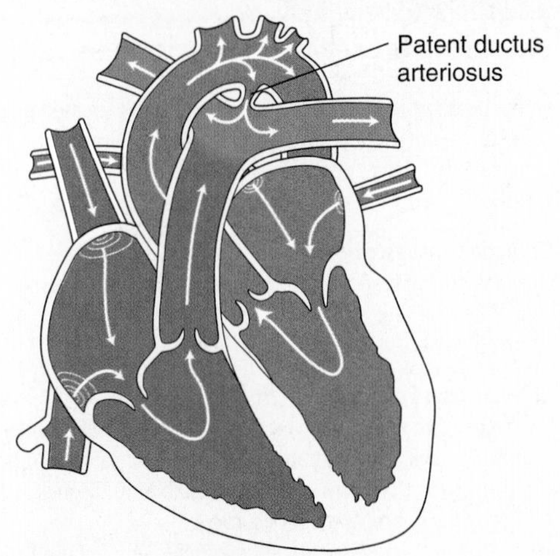

ATRIAL SEPTAL DEFECT (ASD)

An opening at any point in the atrial septum that permits left-to-right shunting of blood. The opening may be small, as when the foramen ovale fails to close, or large, as when the septum may be completely absent. Of children with congenital heart defects, 6%–10% have an ASD (Driscoll, 1999).

Clinical Manifestations

Infants and young children usually have no symptoms. Small and moderate-size ASDs are usually not diagnosed until preschool years or later. Congestive heart failure, easy tiring, and poor growth occur with a large ASD. A soft systolic murmur is usually heard in the pulmonic area with wide splitting of S_2.

Clinical Therapy

Diagnosis is made by echocardiogram that identifies right ventricular overload and shunt size. Chest x-ray film and ECG reveal little information unless ASD is large and excessive shunting is present.

Surgery to close or patch ASD is performed to prevent pulmonary vascular obstructive disease. Some ASDs may be closed by transcatheter device (septal occluder) during cardiac catheterization.

PROGNOSIS: Many persons with uncorrected small and moderate-size ASDs have lived to middle age without symptoms. Atrial arrhythmias are common late complications.

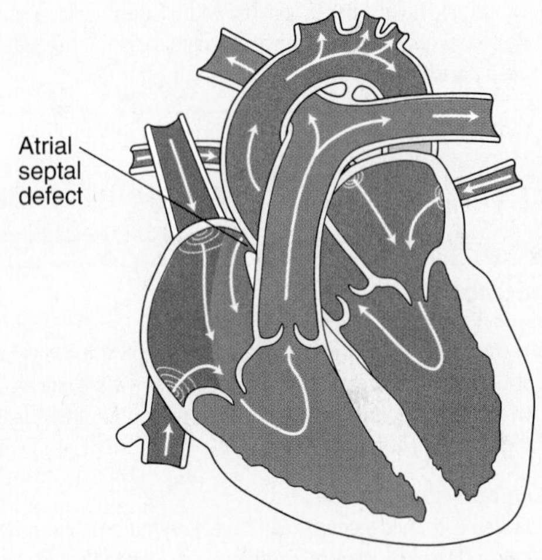

ATRIOVENTRICULAR CANAL (ENDOCARDIAL CUSHION DEFECT)

Atrioventricular (AV) canal refers to a combination of defects in the atrial and ventricular septa and portions of tricuspid and mitral valves. Of children with congenital heart defects, 4%–5% have a total or partial AV canal (Driscoll, 1999). This defect is associated with Down syndrome. Endocardial cushions are fetal growth centers for mitral and tricuspid valves and AV septum. The most complex AV canal malformation results in one AV valve and large septal defects between both atria and ventricles.

Clinical Manifestations

Severity of symptoms depends on amount of mitral regurgitation. Infants have congestive heart failure, tachypnea, tachycardia, poor growth, and repeated respiratory failure, as well as systolic murmur, which is loudest at left lower sternal border.

Clinical Therapy

On chest x-ray film, heart appears large and pulmonary vascular markings are present. Echocardiogram reveals presence of septal defects and details of valvular malformation. Cardiac catheterization is performed to evaluate pulmonary hypertension and pulmonary resistance.

Surgery is performed during infancy to prevent pulmonary vascular disease. Patches are placed over septal defects, and valve tissue is used to form functioning valves. Occasionally the mitral valve is replaced. Oxygen may be required until surgery.

PROGNOSIS: Information on long-term survival following successful surgery is lacking. Arrhythmias and mitral valve insufficiency occur postoperatively. There is no difference in short-term survival rates between infants with and without Down syndrome.

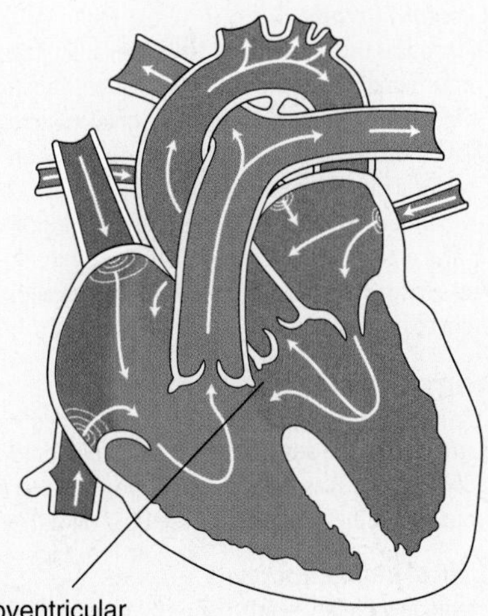

(continued)

TABLE 14-1 Pathophysiology, Clinical Manifestations, and Clinical Therapy for Acyanotic Heart Defects—Nonobstructive Lesions (continued)

VENTRICULAR SEPTAL DEFECT (VSD)

An opening in the ventricular septum results in increased pulmonary blood flow. Blood is shunted from the left ventricle directly across the open septum into the pulmonary artery. This most common congenital heart defect occurs in approximately 20% of all children with congenital heart disease (Driscoll, 1999).

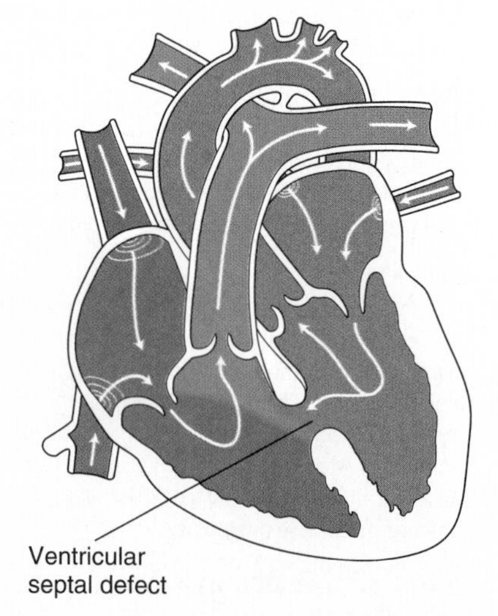

Clinical Manifestations

Only 15% of VSDs are large enough to cause symptoms, such as tachypnea, dyspnea, poor growth, reduced fluid intake, congestive heart failure, and pulmonary hypertension. Systolic murmur is auscultated in lower left sternal border.

Clinical Therapy

Chest x-ray film and ECG reveal few findings in cases of small VSDs. Larger VSDs with shunting are associated with enlarged heart and pulmonary vascular markings on chest x-ray film and left ventricular hypertrophy on ECG. Echocardiogram establishes diagnosis if shunting is present. Cardiac catheterization is used only in preparation for surgery.

Most small VSDs close spontaneously. Treatment is conservative when no signs of congestive heart failure or pulmonary hypertension are present. Surgical patching of VSD during infancy is performed when poor growth is evident. Closure of VSD by transcatheter device (i.e., Rashkind device) during cardiac catheterization may be attempted for some defects. Prophylaxis for infective endocarditis is required.

PROGNOSIS: Highest risk associated with surgical repair is in the first few months of life. Children respond well to surgery and experience substantial catch-up growth. Malignant tachyarrhythmias and heart block are a possible complication.

TABLE 14-2 Pathophysiology, Clinical Manifestations, and Clinical Therapy for Acyanotic Heart Defects—Obstructive Lesions

PULMONIC STENOSIS

Stenosis (narrowing of valve or valve area) can be above valve, below valve, or at valve. Stenosis obstructs blood flow into the pulmonary artery, which increases preload and results in right ventricular hypertrophy. Pulmonic stenosis is the second most frequent congenital heart defect, accounting for 8%–12% of all cases.

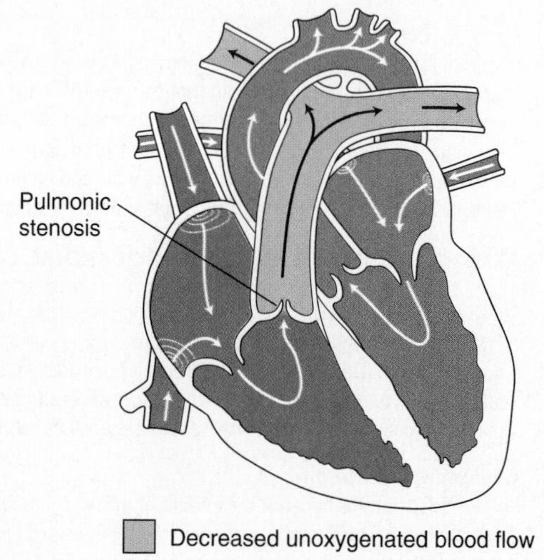

Clinical Manifestation

Children with mild stenosis may have no symptoms and grow normally. In moderate stenosis, dyspnea and fatigue occur on exertion. Signs of heart failure are rare but may result from chronic pressure overload. A systolic murmur with a fixed split S_2 and thrill may be found in the pulmonic listening area. Heart failure and chest pain on exertion may occur in severe cases.

Clinical Therapy

Diagnosis is usually made at birth after auscultation of murmur. The chest x-ray film may show heart enlargement, and the ECG may demonstrate right ventricular hypertrophy. Echocardiogram provides information about pressure gradient across valve and size of valve ring.

Dilation by balloon valvuloplasty, performed during cardiac catheterization, has been widely successful for treatment of simple pulmonic stenosis. Surgical valvotomy may still be used, especially when other defects such as VSD are present. Surgical resection may be needed for narrowing above the valve area. Pulmonary regurgitation may result, but is not a significant problem.

PROGNOSIS: Pulmonic stenosis does not typically increase in severity. Lifelong infective endocarditis prophylaxis is necessary.

AORTIC STENOSIS

Narrowing of the aortic valve obstructs blood flow to systemic circulation. Aortic stenosis accounts for 3%–6% of all cases of congenital heart defects (Fedderly, 1999). This defect is often associated with bicuspid rather than normal tricuspid valve. Stenosis is usually progressive during childhood.

Clinical Manifestations

A majority of infants and young children are asymptomatic and grow and develop normally. The blood pressure is normal, but there is often a narrow pulse pressure. Occasionally the child complains of chest pain after exercise, but exercise intolerance is uncommon. Peripheral pulses may be weak. Fainting and dizziness are serious signs that require intervention. Congestive heart failure develops in symptomatic infants. A systolic heart murmur and thrill in the aortic listening area are usually detected in routine physical examination in the school-age child or adolescent.

(continued)

TABLE 14-2 Pathophysiology, Clinical Manifestations, and Clinical Therapy for Acyanotic Heart Defects—Obstructive Lesions (continued)

Clinical Therapy

Chest x-ray film and ECG are usually normal in mild cases. An echocardiogram reveals the number of the valve cusps, pressure gradient across valve, and size of aorta. Stress testing may be used in asymptomatic children to determine amount of obstruction present with exercise.

The aortic valve may be successfully dilated by balloon valvuloplasty during cardiac catheterization. Surgical valvuloplasty may also be performed. Aortic valve replacement is performed when stenosis is severe or if significant regurgitation results from other interventions. Surgical treatment is palliative rather than curative.

PROGNOSIS: Chest pain, syncope, and sudden death can occur in symptomatic children, particularly during vigorous exercise. Stenosis is usually progressive during childhood as the valve calcifies. Valve replacement may ultimately be necessary. Lifelong infective endocarditis prophylaxis is required.

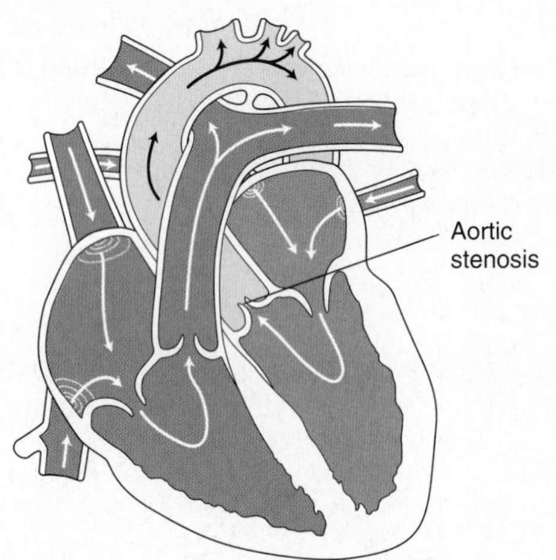

COARCTATION OF THE AORTA

Narrowing or constriction in the descending aorta, often near the ductus arteriosus, obstructs systemic blood outflow. This defect is common, occurring in 5%–8% of all children with congenital heart disease (Fedderly, 1999).

Clinical Manifestations

Many children are asymptomatic and grow normally, but constriction is progressive; 20%–30% of children develop congestive heart failure by 3 months of age. Reduction in blood flow through the descending aorta causes lower blood pressure in legs and higher blood pressure in arms, neck, and head. Brachial and radial pulses are full, but femoral pulses are weak or absent. Older children may complain of weakness and pain in the legs after exercise.

Clinical Therapy

ECG shows left ventricular hypertrophy. Chest x-ray film may reveal enlargement and pulmonary venous congestion, and indentation of descending aorta. Rib notching (change in the smooth contour of the rib apparent on x-ray) is rarely seen before 10 years of age. Magnetic resonance imaging shows coarctation.

Balloon dilation during cardiac catheterization for both initial relief and recoarctation. Surgical resection and anastomosis are palliative, as coarctation may recur. The subclavian artery can be used as a patch in the infant. Repair in the first year of life is preferred to decrease exposure to hypertension.

PROGNOSIS: Post-coarctectomy syndrome (abdominal pain and distention) occurs in 20% of patients (Walters, 2000). Persistent hypertension in adulthood is common. Infective endocarditis prophylaxis is needed.

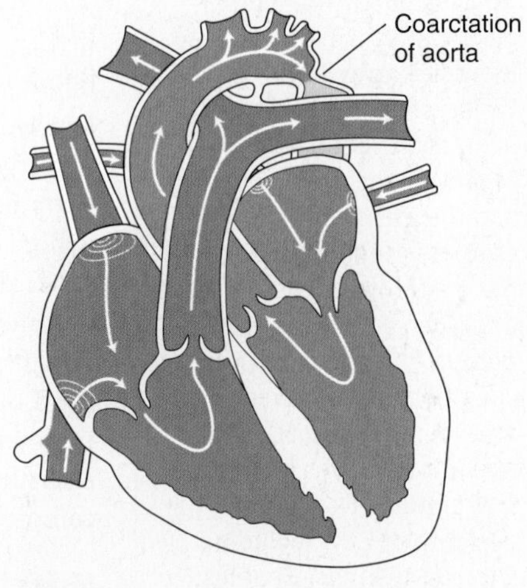

Etiology and Pathophysiology

Beginning at birth, the left side of the heart normally generates higher pressures than the right side in response to increasing systemic vascular resistance and decreasing pulmonary vascular resistance. In children who have nonobstructive defects such as openings in the septal wall, a left-to-right **shunt** (movement of blood between heart chambers through an abnormal opening) occurs. Oxygenated blood mixes with unoxygenated blood, and the extra blood volume overloads the pulmonary system, causing congestive heart failure. Pulmonary artery hypertension occurs if chronic volume overload of the pulmonary arteries is not corrected.

Clinical Manifestations

The child with a nonobstructive acyanotic heart defect may be asymptomatic except for a heart murmur. The most important consequence of these defects is volume overload. Congestive heart failure may develop if the amount of blood passing from the left to the right

CLINICAL TIP

Signs and symptoms of congenital heart disease in older children include:

- Exercise intolerance
- Chest pain
- Arrhythmias
- Syncope
- Sudden death

DIAGNOSTIC TESTS

The following tests are used in the diagnosis of congenital heart disease.

- Chest x-ray study—Reveals size and contour of the heart and characteristics of pulmonary vascular markings.
- Electrocardiogram (ECG)—Records quality of major electrical activity in the heart, identifies arrhythmias.
- Echocardiogram—Identifies heart structures, the pattern of movement, hemodynamics, and the presence of defects.
- Cardiac catheterization—Allows precise measurement of oxygen saturation, cardiac output, and pressures in each chamber and heart vessel; also identifies anatomic alterations.
- Holter monitor—Allows 24–48-hour ECG recording.
- Exercise testing—Enables ECG recording with controlled increase in activity to identify significant cardiac compensation or inadequate cardiac output.
- Hyperoxia test—Measures differences in arterial blood gas level when child is on room air and on 100% oxygen.

side of the heart overloads the pulmonary system (Nouri, 1997). If this occurs, the child has hepatomegaly, dyspnea, tachypnea, intercostal retractions, poor growth, and frequent respiratory infections. The more severe and complex the heart defect, the earlier symptoms of congestive heart failure appear.

The child with an obstructive acyanotic heart defect also has a heart murmur. See Chapter 4 for assessment of murmurs. Obstructive defects cause pressure overload and hypertrophy of the closest ventricle. Although some children experience fatigue and exercise intolerance because of their inability to increase cardiac output, many children are asymptomatic and grow normally.

Older children with a diagnosis of congenital heart disease may have additional symptoms. Exercise-induced dizziness and **syncope** (transient loss of consciousness and muscle tone) are serious signs indicating a need for medical evaluation.

Clinical Therapy

The presence of a heart murmur is often the first indication of an acyanotic defect. A loud murmur indicates higher pressures of blood flowing across the shunt or through the narrowed valve or vessel. Once the heart murmur is discovered, a chest x-ray study, electrocardiography, and echocardiography are performed. The echocardiogram usually clearly shows the defect, shunt, and heart pressures.

The selection of treatment for acyanotic defects depends on the severity of symptoms and whether the condition is imminently life threatening. Surgical correction is the treatment of choice for most acyanotic defects. Table 14-3 lists the types of surgical procedures performed on children with congenital heart defects. Conservative treatment, such as waiting until the child is symptomatic or older, may be selected initially. For example, a ventricular septal defect may close spontaneously or growth of the child may increase the probability of success of surgery. Surgical correction of defects that cause pulmonary hypertension is performed in infancy to prevent irreversible pulmonary vascular disease.

Surgery often results in complete repair of the acyanotic defect. Unless complications develop before surgery, the child should make a complete recovery without limitations. The major complication of acyanotic heart defects is pulmonary hypertension.

Cardiac catheterization, an invasive procedure previously used exclusively for diagnosis of some congenital heart defects, is now more often performed as a therapeutic procedure. Recently developed techniques using balloons and other transcatheter devices permit treatment of many acyanotic heart defects during cardiac catheterization.

Potential complications of cardiac catheterization include perforation of the pulmonary artery, allergic reaction to the contrast media, arrhythmias, hypotension, stroke, vascular compromise in the leg, and bleeding.

Nursing Care of the Child Undergoing a Cardiac Catheterization

Prepare the child for cardiac catheterization with age-appropriate information. A tour of the catheterization laboratory may reduce the child's fears about the large equipment. Because the child will be sedated but arousable for the procedure, explain the sensations that he or she will experience.

Cardiac catheterization is often an outpatient procedure, but some children will be admitted for observation. The child is NPO for several hours, except for medications, and arrives at the catheterization laboratory 1 to 2 hours before the procedure. Before entering the laboratory, the child is asked to void and is given an oral sedative.

NURSING MANAGEMENT

Nursing Assessment and Diagnosis

Before the procedure, assess the child's vital signs, hematocrit and hemoglobin concentrations, and strength of pedal pulses for comparison with postcatheterization assessments.

For several hours after the procedure, monitor the child for potential complications such as arrhythmia, bleeding, hematoma development, thrombus formation, and infection. No

TABLE 14-3 Surgical Procedures for Congenital Heart Defects

PROCEDURE	PURPOSE	THERAPEUTIC USE
Angioplasty	Dilatation of coarctation of aorta during cardiac catheterization	Palliative
Fontan	Creation of conduit between right atrium (inferior vena cava) and pulmonary artery to increase pulmonary blood flow—total right heart bypass	Corrective or palliative
Glenn	Superior vena cava connected to right pulmonary artery along with closure of aortopulmonary shunt. Systemic venous blood is sent to the lungs directly without ventricular pumping.	Palliative
Jatene (arterial switch)	Aorta and pulmonary arteries are transected and reanastomosed to opposite stumps, coronary arteries are moved to new aorta area.	Corrective
Modified Blalock-Taussig Shunt	Creation of aortopulmonary conduit to increase pulmonary blood flow	Palliative
Mustard or Senning	Baffling blood in atria to reestablish a proper blood flow in transposition of great vessels	Corrective
Norwood	Creation of conduit between aorta and pulmonary artery to increase blood flow to aorta	Palliative or corrective
Patent Ductus arteriosus closure	Closure of ductus arteriosus by surgery or an umbrella device during cardiac catheterization	Corrective
Pulmonary artery banding	Placement of constricting band around pulmonary artery to reduce pulmonary blood flow	Palliative
Rashkind—Balloon atrial septostomy	Creation of larger defect between atria to increase blood mixing, performed during cardiac catheterization	Palliative
Rastelli	Pulmonary arteries removed from truncus and conduit is placed (or a connection is made) between the right ventricle and pulmonary artery	Corrective
Transcatheter closure	Closure of a septal defect by a septal occluder or Rashkind device during cardiac catheterization	Corrective
Transplant	Replacement of diseased heart with donor heart	Corrective
Valvuloplasty	Repair of valve to relieve stenosis by balloon dilatation during cardiac catheterization or surgery	Palliative or corrective

bleeding should occur at the catheterization site. Assess vital signs, neurovascular status of the lower extremities, and the pressure dressing over the catheterization site every 15 minutes for 1 hour and then every 30 minutes for 1 hour. The child's temperature, heart rate, respiratory rate, and blood pressure should remain stable. Monitor intake and output because the contrast medium may cause diuresis. The child's intake and output should be balanced. Pedal pulses, capillary refill, sensation, warmth, and color of the lower extremities should match the precatheterization assessment.

The following nursing diagnoses may apply to the child who undergoes cardiac catheterization:

- *Fear,* related to separation from support system in a stressful situation
- *Risk for fluid volume deficit,* related to inadequate fluid intake due to NPO status and diuretic effect of contrast medium

- *Altered tissue perfusion (cardiopulmonary),* related to mechanical reduction of arterial and venous blood flow
- *Risk for decreased cardiac output,* related to ventricular restriction (obstruction by balloon catheter)

Planning and Implementation

Nursing care during a cardiac catheterization focuses on monitoring the child's vital signs, reassuring the child, and providing emergency care if necessary. After the catheters and guidewires are removed at the end of the procedure, direct pressure must be applied for 15 minutes. A pressure dressing is then placed over the site for 6 hours.

The child is kept on bedrest for 6 hours. Activity is then limited for 24 hours. Provide quiet diversional activities to keep the child occupied.

Encourage the intake of small amounts of clear liquids initially, and then progress to other fluids and food as the child tolerates them. Maintaining hydration is important because the contrast medium used during the procedure has a diuretic effect. Monitor intake and output.

Discharge Planning and Home Care Teaching

Routinely children are discharged several hours after the cardiac catheterization. Teach the parents to watch the child for signs of complications and make sure they know when to notify the physician.

Children whose heart defect is corrected by cardiac catheterization have the same risks for infective endocarditis as children with surgical correction. Use the information provided in Table 14-4, later in this chapter, to teach parents about infective endocarditis prophylaxis.

Evaluation

Expected outcomes of nursing care include the following:

- Any potential complications (thrombosis or hemorrhage) following cardiac catheterization are rapidly identified and handled.
- The child maintains fluid balance.

Nursing Care of the Child Undergoing Surgery for an Acyanotic Defect

Children with acyanotic heart defects are hospitalized either because of complications, such as congestive heart failure, or for surgery. Refer to the earlier discussion of nursing management in congestive heart failure for care of children with this condition.

FAMILIES WANT TO KNOW

Home Care after Cardiac Catheterization

- Check for signs of complications several times in the first 24 hours after catheterization such as:
  - fever
  - bleeding or a bruise increasing in size at the catheterization site
  - foot on side of catheterization site is cooler than other foot
  - loss of feeling in foot on side of catheterization
- Notify physician immediately if any of these signs are noted within the first 24 hours after the catheterization.
- Encourage fluids to help flush the dye out of the body.
- Permit quiet play such as games, puzzles, and videos for 24 hours.

NURSING MANAGEMENT

Nursing Assessment and Diagnosis

Assess the ability of the parents to cope with the diagnosis of their child's congenital heart defect. Initially parents may be in shock and feel guilty and anxious. The child often looks healthy and has few symptoms.

Parents need an opportunity to express their feelings and to begin learning to cope with their child's illness. They need special support if their infant has a life-threatening heart defect. Members of the cardiology team, including nurses, must provide counseling for the family. Counseling information may include the following:

- General information about the congenital heart disease, including a description of the heart's anatomy and physiology and the defect
- Specific information about the multiple interactive factors associated with congenital heart disease; this information can often help reduce parents' guilt about the child's defect
- Sample case histories with good and poor prognoses
- Overview of the child's prognosis and timing of medical and surgical interventions

Parents may need genetic counseling if planning a future pregnancy. Fetal echocardiography can identify structural heart defects as early as 18 to 20 weeks' gestation.

Parents may need support for their anxiety regarding an uncertain outcome of surgery. Some parents may be concerned that signing a consent for surgery is like signing the child's death warrant. The American Heart Association publishes a helpful booklet, *If Your Child Has a Congenital Heart Defect*, which can be used for education.

Following surgical correction of the heart defect, the child is usually cared for in an ICU until stable. The child may be intubated and ventilated for a few hours. In the immediate postoperative period, assess the child's vital signs, level of consciousness, pain level, heart functioning, and arrhythmias. Monitor intake and output. Monitor for hemorrhage, adequate ventilation and tissue perfusion, and acid–base and electrolyte imbalances.

After the child's return to the general nursing unit, assessment focuses on signs of surgical complications such as infection, arrhythmias, and impaired tissue perfusion. Monitor the child's temperature and inspect the surgical incision site. Fever, excessive incisional pain, spreading erythema around the incision, and wound drainage beginning 3 to 4 days postoperatively may be early signs of infection. Assess the respiratory system for breath sounds, respiratory effort, and signs of distress that may indicate pneumonia or fluid in the pleural space.

Because the child may no longer be on a cardiac monitor, auscultation of the apical pulse to detect an irregular heart rate or bradycardia is essential. Either condition is an indication of reduced cardiac output that requires intervention. To assess for impaired tissue perfusion, check capillary refill, extremity warmth, pedal pulses, level of consciousness, and urine output. Reduced urine output is a sign of decreased cardiac output. Continue to assess the child's pain.

Following are examples of nursing diagnoses associated with acyanotic heart defects and their complications:

- *Fluid volume excess,* related to heart failure and pulmonary vasculature overload
- *Decreased cardiac output,* related to ventricular restriction and an obstructed outflow tract
- *Ineffective breathing pattern,* related to respiratory muscle fatigue
- *Ineffective infant feeding pattern,* related to shortness of breath and fatigue
- *Fatigue,* related to chronic pulmonary vasculature overload
- *Altered family processes,* related to crisis of child's serious illness

Planning and Implementation

Children are often managed at home until surgery is scheduled. Nursing care following surgery focuses on promoting the child's recuperation. Pain management should be provided for several days postoperatively. Follow the guidelines given in Chapter 9.

CLINICAL TIP

Parents are at higher risk of having a child with a congenital heart defect if any of the following factors are present (Stumpflen, Stumpflen, & Wimmer, et al., 1996):

- Family history of congenital heart disease
- Maternal age >35 years
- Coexisting maternal disease (diabetes mellitus, collagen vascular disease, phenylketonuria)
- Exposure to teratogens or rubella infection

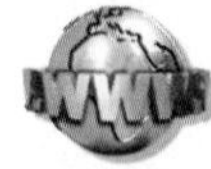

Congenital Heart Defect Support and Resources

FAMILIES WANT TO KNOW

Home Care of Children with Congenital Heart Defects Before Surgery

ROUTINE HEALTH CARE
Provide well-child care and all immunizations, including influenza vaccine.
Provide preventive dental care with fluoride treatment.

ADMINISTRATION OF MEDICATIONS
Give medications safely with a dosage schedule that fits the family's routine.

SIGNS OF ILLNESS
Notify physician if the child has the following signs: fever, vomiting, diarrhea, or is feeding poorly. Avoid dehydration.

ACTIVITY
Allow the child to set his or her own activity level. Children with congenital heart defects usually do not overexert themselves.

Note: Modified from Stinson, J., & McKeever, P. (1995). Mother's information needs related to caring for infants at home following cardiac surgery. *Journal of Pediatric Nursing*, 10(1), 48–57.

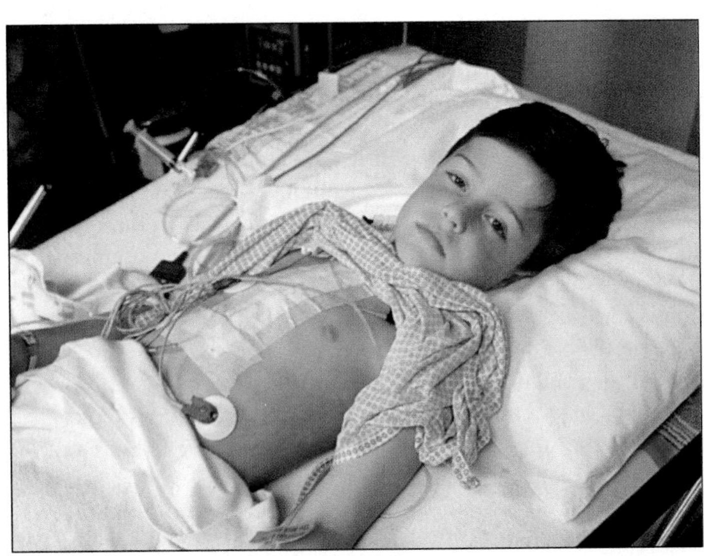

FIGURE 14-4 ◆
A child with atrial septal defect repair. Surgery is performed with this type of defect to prevent pulmonary vascular obstructive disease.

Skill 10-20: Performing Chest Physiotherapy

Skill 10-21: Using the Incentive Spirometer

Encourage the child to perform spirometry exercises regularly to promote full lung expansion. Chest physiotherapy may be performed in children under 3 years of age. Inspect the child's incision regularly and cleanse it with hydrogen peroxide if ordered (Figure 14-4 ◆).

Administer antibiotics as ordered. Intravenous lines are often converted to heparin or saline locks to continue antibiotic administration once the child's oral intake is normal. Although oral fluids are rarely limited, intake and output should be assessed carefully.

Encourage the child to increase activity gradually with longer periods out of bed every day. Provide opportunities for therapeutic play so the child can better manage the stresses associated with pain and frightening procedures.

Discharge Planning and Home Care Teaching

Infants and children may be discharged from the hospital within a few days of surgery. Parents need discharge teaching in preparation for continuing care of the child at home.

Reassure parents by telling them that the child with a repaired cardiac defect should have no further cardiovascular problems. Encourage them to allow the child to live a normal and active life.

Children are at risk for infective endocarditis, especially within the first 6 months after surgery. The child should receive prophylactic antibiotics according to the American Heart

FAMILIES WANT TO KNOW

Care of the Child After Cardiac Surgery

- Allow the child to increase activity gradually as tolerated. Report increased fatigue or decreased activity tolerance to the physician.
- Report any signs of wound infection, fever, flulike symptoms, or an increased respiratory rate or respiratory distress to the physician.
- Allow the child to return to school in approximately 3 weeks. Physical activities such as rough play, bike riding, or climbing should be postponed for 6 weeks until the incision has healed completely.
- Report any unexplained fever or illness during the first 2 months following surgery as the child is at higher risk for infective endocarditis during that time. Antibiotics should be given for dental and surgical procedures.

TABLE 14-4 Antibiotic Recommendations for Infective Endocarditis Prophylaxis in Children*

FOR DENTAL, ORAL, OR UPPER RESPIRATORY TRACT PROCEDURES Amoxicillin
FOR CHILDREN ALLERGIC TO PENICILLIN Clindamycin, cephalexin, cefadroxil, azithromycin, clarithromycin
FOR GENITOURINARY AND GASTROINTESTINAL PROCEDURES Ampicillin, gentamicin, amoxicillin
FOR CHILDREN ALLERGIC TO PENICILLIN Vancomycin, gentamicin

*One large dose is given 1 hour before the procedures. In high-risk patients, a smaller dose may be given 6 hours after the procedure.
Note: Modified from Dajani, A. S., Taubert, K. A., Wilson, W., Bolger, A. F., & Bayer, A., et al. (1997). Prevention of bacterial endocarditis: Recommendations of the American Heart Association. *Journal of the American Medical Association, 277*(22), 1794–1801.

Association recommendations (Table 14-4). Any unexplained fever or malaise seen in the 2 months following repair or after dental work may be a sign of infection. The child should be examined for petechiae and splenomegaly. Blood cultures, blood cell count, and urinalysis should be performed.

Evaluation

Examples of expected outcomes of nursing care include the following:

- The child's pain is effectively managed.
- Full lung expansion is maintained with spirometry exercises or chest physiotherapy.
- The child's incision heals without infection.

CYANOTIC DEFECTS

Cyanotic heart disease is generally caused by a valvular or vascular malformation. The most common malformations are tetralogy of Fallot and transposition of the great vessels (Figure 14-5 ◆). Table 14-5 summarizes clinical manifestations, diagnostic tests, and medical management for these defects.

Other less common congenital heart defects include hypoplastic left heart syndrome, tricuspid atresia, pulmonary atresia, truncus arteriosus, and total anomalous pulmonary venous return (Table 14-6). Not all of these defects cause cyanosis.

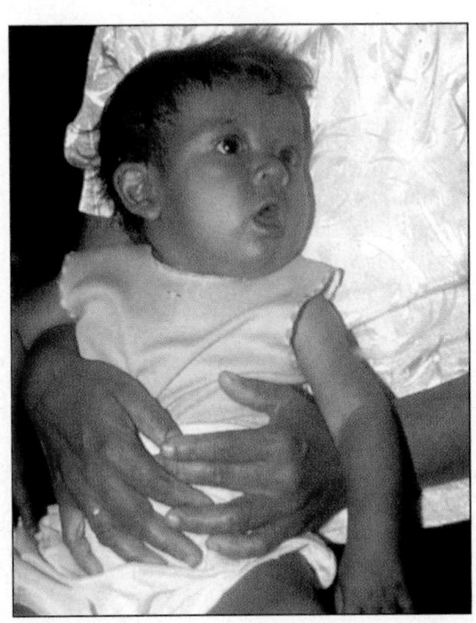

FIGURE 14-5 ◆
This infant has a cyanotic heart defect. What is the prognosis for an infant who has either of the most common malformations—tetralogy of Fallot or transposition of the great vessels?

TABLE 14-5 Cyanotic Heart Defects

TETRALOGY OF FALLOT

Combination of four defects: pulmonic stenosis, right ventricular hypertrophy, ventricular septal defect (VSD), and overriding of aorta. Some children have a fifth defect: open foramen ovale or atrial septal defect (ASD). About 10% of children with congenital heart defects have tetralogy of Fallot (Park, 1996). This defect is characterized by elevated pressures in right side of heart, causing right-to-left shunt.

Clinical Manifestations

As ductus arteriosus closes, infant becomes hypoxic and cyanotic. The degree of pulmonary stenosis determines severity of symptoms. Polycythemia, hypoxic spells, metabolic acidosis, poor growth, clubbing, and exercise intolerance may develop. Infants have a systolic murmur heard in pulmonic area that is transmitted to suprasternal notch.

Clinical Therapy

Chest x-ray film shows a boot-shaped heart due to the large right ventricle with decreased pulmonary vascular markings. Electrocardiogram (ECG) shows right ventricular hypertrophy. Echocardiogram demonstrates VSD, obstruction of pulmonary outflow, and overriding aorta. Cardiac catheterization is required before surgical correction to completely identify the location of all anatomic structures and any additional defects.

Hypercyanotic spells are managed according to guidelines given in section on nursing management of cyanotic defects. Monitoring child for metabolic acidosis or prolonged unconsciousness is critical. A total repair is performed before 6 months of age when the infant has a hypercyanotic spell. Corrective surgery may be attempted in asymptomatic children by 6 months of age.

PROGNOSIS: Not all children are cured by surgery, but most have improved quality of life and improved longevity. Arrhythmias and right ventricular dysfunction may be residual problems (Waldman & Wernly, 1999). Lifelong infective endocarditis prophylaxis is required.

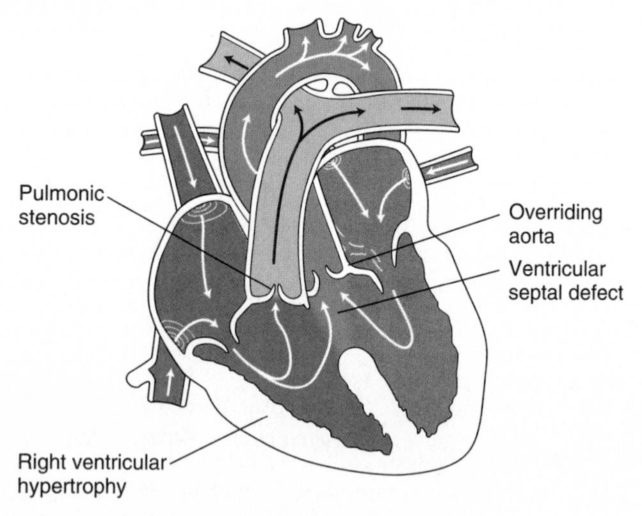

TRANSPOSITION OF THE GREAT ARTERIES (TGA)

Pulmonary artery is the outflow for left ventricle, and aorta is outflow for right ventricle. This condition is life threatening at birth, and survival initially depends on open ductus arteriosus and foramen ovale. This condition occurs in about 5% of children with congenital heart disease (Grifka, 1999). ASD or VSD may also be present with TGA.

Clinical Manifestations

Cyanosis, apparent soon after birth, progresses to hypoxia and acidosis. Cyanosis does not improve with oxygen administration. However, cyanosis may be less apparent when a large VSD is also present. Congestive heart failure may develop over days or weeks. Tachypnea (60 respirations/min) is often present without retractions or other signs of dyspnea. Infants take a long time to feed and need frequent rest periods because of rapid respiratory rate and fatigue. Growth failure may be evident as early as 2 weeks of age if corrective surgery is not performed.

Clinical Therapy

Chest x-ray study may reveal a classic egg-shaped heart on a string (narrow superior mediastinum). Diagnosis is made by echocardiogram when position of arteries arising from ventricles is visible.

Prostaglandin E_1 is initially ordered to maintain a patent ductus arteriosus until a palliative procedure can be performed. Corrective surgery (arterial switch) is usually performed before 1 week of age. Balloon atrial septostomy may be performed during cardiac catheterization in newborns as a first stage. This may also be corrected surgically.

PROGNOSIS: Survival without surgery is impossible. Arrhythmias, right ventricular failure, and sudden death are long-term complications (8–15 years) after the Mustard procedure, so the Mustard or Rastelli procedure are performed only when significant pulmonary valve stenosis is present (Grifka, 1999). Infective endocarditis prophylaxis may be necessary.

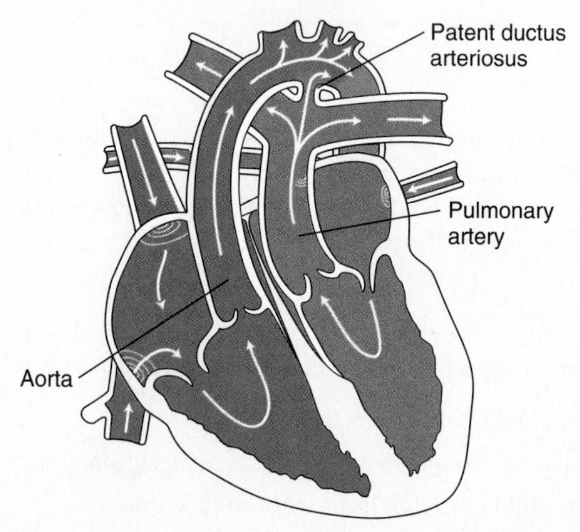

TABLE 14-6 Less Common Congenital Heart Defects

CONDITION	CLINICAL MANIFESTATIONS	CLINICAL THERAPY
Hypoplastic Left Heart Syndrome Absence or stenosis of mitral and aortic valves associated with an abnormally small left ventricle and aortic arch. Signs are initiated with closure of ductus arteriosus. Largest contributor of infant deaths due to congenital heart disease (Petrini, Damus, & Johnston, 1998). Possible genetic predisposition to the condition.	Signs include tachypnea, retractions, decreased peripheral pulses, poor peripheral perfusion, pulmonary edema, and congestive heart failure eventually leading to shock, acidosis, and death.	Echocardiogram is used for initial diagnosis. May be diagnosed in the first trimester. Prostaglandin E_1 given to maintain patent ductus arteriosus. Supplemental oxygen avoided. Surgery is done in three stages—Norwood procedure first, Glenn procedure next, and Fontan last. A heart transplant may also be performed. The survival rate is improving. May have failure of single ventricle over time.
Tricuspid Atresia/Pulmonary Atresia Absence of tricuspid or pulmonary valve. A ventricular septal defect (VSD) or transposition of the great arteries (TGA) is also often present.	Early cyanosis, dyspnea, congestive heart failure, pulmonary edema, hepatomegaly, acidosis, hypoxic spells, clubbing, polycythemia, and growth delays occur. Continuous murmur is heard in aortic area.	Chest x-ray study and echocardiogram are used for initial diagnosis. Prostaglandin E_1 is given to maintain patent ductus arteriosus. Digoxin and diuretics are also used. Palliative surgery increases pulmonary blood flow. The Rashkind procedure is used. The modified Fontan procedure results in improved survival.
Truncus Arteriosus A single large vessel empties both ventricles. VSD is usually present.	Cyanosis develops soon after birth. Severe congestive heart failure, dyspnea, retractions, fatigue, poor feeding, polycythemia, clubbing, increased pulse pressure, bounding peripheral pulses, increased respiratory infections, and cardiomegaly also occur.	Chest x-ray study and echocardiogram give initial diagnosis. Cardiac catheterization is done before surgery. Rastelli procedure is performed to close VSD and create a passage to pulmonary arteries. Digoxin and diuretics are given. Repeated surgery is necessary to enlarge pulmonary artery conduit. Survival is improved, but truncal valve stenosis and regurgitation result. Long-term prognosis is unknown.
Total Anomalous Pulmonary Venous Return Pulmonary veins empty into right atrium or veins leading to the right atrium.	Increased right ventricular impulse may occur. With severe pulmonary overload, tachycardia, dyspnea, pulmonary edema, retractions, cyanosis, hepatomegaly, poor feedings, irritability, and failure to thrive are seen.	Chest x-ray study, echocardiogram, and cardiac catheterization are used for diagnosis. Prostaglandin E_1 is given to maintain patent ductus arteriosus. Surgery to reconnect or baffle the pulmonary veins to the left atrium is performed. Survivors have lived more than 20 years after correction.

Etiology and Pathophysiology

Cyanotic defects are generally caused by a malformation or combination of defects that prevents adequate oxygenation of the blood. When the defect is associated with decreased pulmonary blood flow, pressures from obstructed blood in the right side of the heart exceed those in the left. Unoxygenated blood is shunted to the left side of the heart. Oxygenated blood destined for the systemic circulation is diluted, resulting in chronic hypoxemia and cyanosis.

When children with cyanosis rise in the morning, they may experience an abrupt decrease in systemic resistance and pulmonary blood flow. A hypercyanotic spell may be triggered by this decrease when combined with a sudden increase in cardiac output and venous return caused by crying, feeding, exercise, warm bath, and straining with defecation. The partial pressure of oxygen (PO_2) is lowered, and the partial pressure of carbon dioxide (PCO_2) rises. The hypoxemia becomes progressively worse as the respiratory center in the brain overreacts, increasing the respiratory effort. The additional respiratory effort further increases the cardiac output and contributes to a life-threatening decline unless rapid intervention is successful.

CLINICAL TIP

Cyanosis is seen at a higher oxygen saturation level when the child's hemoglobin level is normal or polycythemia exists (Park, 1996).

Hemoglobin Level	Oxygen Saturation Level
6 g% (anemia)	45%–50%
15 g% (normal)	75%–80%
20 g% (polycythemia)	80%–85%

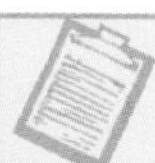

RESEARCH

Recent studies comparing cognitive performance of school-age children with heart defects revealed that most preschool and school-age children have normal IQ scores. Some children with complex lesions (transposition of great arteries and hypoplastic left heart syndrome) seem to have an increased risk for neurodevelopmental problems (Mahle & Wernovsky, 2001).

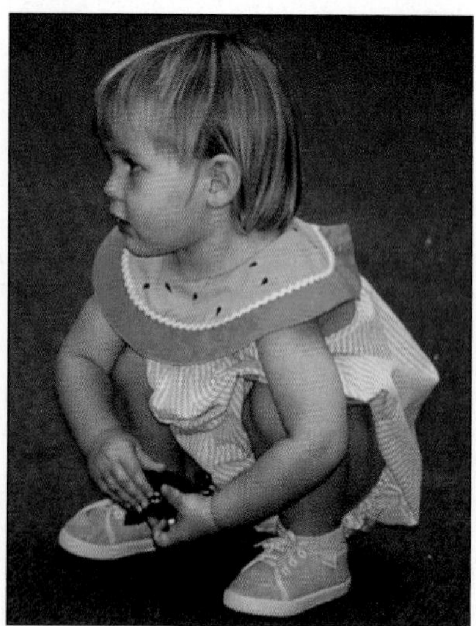

FIGURE 14-6 ◆
A child with a cyanotic heart defect squats (assumes a knee–chest position) to relieve cyanotic spells.

Children with cyanotic defects are at increased risk for thromboembolism. The chronic hypoxemia leads to polycythemia in an attempt to increase the hemoglobin available to carry oxygen. Brain abscesses are more common in children with cyanotic heart defects. Bacteria in the blood returning from the systemic circulation are usually filtered out by the capillaries in the lungs. However, when unoxygenated blood enters the systemic circulation through the right-to-left shunt, bacteria can travel directly to the brain.

Clinical Manifestations

Cyanosis often occurs when the ductus arteriosus closes, causing hypoxemia. Signs and symptoms of chronic hypoxemia include fatigue, clubbing of the fingers and toes, exertional dyspnea, and delayed developmental milestones. Because infants tire easily with feeding, they receive fewer calories, and do not grow normally. Congestive heart failure develops in some children.

The skin may have a ruddy or mottled appearance before cyanosis is observed. When pulmonary circulation is impaired, hemoglobin may not become reoxygenated. The appearance of cyanosis is related to the hemoglobin level and the oxygen saturation level.

Hypercyanotic (hypoxic) spells, the most significant problem to develop in infants and toddlers with heart defects, usually appear between 2 months and 2 years of age. Hypercyanotic spells can develop suddenly. Signs include:

- Increased rate and depth of respirations
- Increased cyanosis
- Increased heart rate
- Pallor and poor tissue perfusion
- Agitation or irritability

Children with uncorrected cyanotic heart disease often squat to relieve dyspnea (Figure 14-6 ◆). The knee–chest position reduces the cardiac output by decreasing the venous return from the lower extremities and by increasing the systemic vascular resistance.

Clinical Therapy

A systolic heart murmur may be apparent after cyanosis develops. A chest x-ray study, electrocardiogram, and echocardiogram are obtained. Usually the echocardiogram clearly shows the defect, shunt, and heart pressures. Cardiac catheterization is often used to obtain detailed anatomic information before surgery.

Early management of cyanotic heart defects is important to prevent secondary damage to the heart, lungs, and brain, including the adverse effects of hypoxemia on the child's cognitive and psychomotor development. For this reason, corrective surgery is being performed at younger ages, often in infancy. A **palliative procedure** may be performed first to preserve life in children with potentially lethal heart defects and complications (see Table 14-3). With some defects, corrective surgery can be postponed with a palliative procedure. This gives the infant an opportunity to grow and improve the success of corrective surgery.

If closure of the ductus arteriosus causes life-threatening cyanosis in newborns, prostaglandin E_1 (PGE_1) is prescribed to reopen the ductus arteriosus. These infants depend on a patent ductus arteriosus for survival or improvement in pulmonary or systemic blood flow. Treatment with PGE_1 provides time for the newborn to be transferred to a cardiac center for diagnostic evaluation and surgical intervention. Response time to PGE_1 varies depending on the type of defect.

The child's hemoglobin level and hematocrit values must be monitored to ensure that the blood does not become too viscous. Polycythemia may be managed by red blood cell pheresis if the blood viscosity becomes too high. Also monitor the child for anemia, as these children do not tolerate the lower hemoglobin and oxygen-carrying capacity.

Hypercyanotic spells are treated aggressively. To decrease the pulmonary vascular resistance, the initial treatment involves calming the child, giving oxygen, and administering morphine and propranolol intravenously. Packed red blood cells may be administered to improve oxygen delivery to the tissues when the child is anemic. Postpone all unpleasant procedures. To increase the systemic vascular resistance, the child is placed in knee–chest position and given intravenous fluids to expand circulatory volume. Dopamine or phenylephrine (Neosynephrine) are also given. Once a cyanotic spell has occurred, immediate palliative or corrective surgery is often scheduled. Oral propranolol is administered to decrease the frequency of hypercyanotic spells because of its action to minimize spasms of the pulmonary outflow tract (DeBoer, 1996).

Antibiotic prophylaxis for infective endocarditis is needed before and after surgical correction for all cyanotic conditions. See Table 14-4 for a list of recommended antibiotics.

CLINICAL TIP

Crying may improve cyanosis caused by lung disease or disorders of the central nervous system. In children with cyanotic heart disease, crying usually makes cyanosis worse.

NURSING MANAGEMENT

Nursing Assessment and Diagnosis

The cardiovascular status of infants receiving PGE_1 therapy needs to be closely monitored. Assess vital signs, heart rhythm, skin color, peripheral pulses, and capillary refill time. Observe for signs of improvement in vital signs and color as the oxygen saturation increases and acidosis decreases following the initial treatment. In addition, watch for tachycardia, tachypnea, crackles, frothy secretions, low urine output, and edema, because these infants are at risk for congestive heart failure.

The child needs careful observation for signs of increased cyanosis in the morning or at other high-risk times. Observe for neurologic signs of thromboembolitic complications from polycythemia such as headache, dizziness, excessive irritability, and paralysis. Older children with cyanotic defects may have clubbing of the fingers (Figure 14-7 ◆).

Following are nursing diagnoses that may apply to a child with cyanotic heart disease:

- *Risk for infection,* related to unfiltered bacteria in the blood and sites of blood shunting that promote bacterial growth
- *Pain,* related to palliative or corrective surgery
- *Risk for caregiver role strain,* related to care of a child with chronic illness
- *Activity intolerance,* related to cyanosis and dyspnea on exertion
- *Altered growth and development,* related to congenital anomaly and hypoxemia
- *Risk for ineffective management of therapeutic regimen,* related to complexity of therapeutic regimen: assessment and management of cyanotic spells, which are unpredictable events

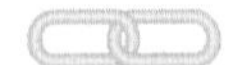

Skills 5-8 to 5-14: Assessing Vital Signs

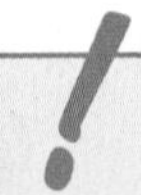

NURSING ALERT

Cyanotic spells become life threatening if not treated immediately. The child becomes progressively more hypoxic and limp, loses consciousness, is likely to have a seizure or cerebrovascular accident, and may die.

Planning and Implementation

Children with tetralogy of Fallot are often managed at home until surgery is scheduled. Home care involves reducing parental anxiety, providing adequate nutrition, helping parents recognize signs of illness, and formulating a plan for emergency treatment. Nursing care of the hospitalized child focuses on monitoring PGE_1 therapy (for newborns only; used until palliative surgery is performed), treating hypercyanotic spells, and providing postsurgical care.

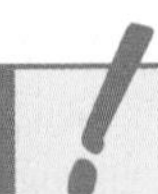

NURSING ALERT

Common side effects of PGE_1 therapy include cutaneous vasodilation, bradycardia, tachycardia, hypotension, seizure activity, fever, and apnea.

Home Care of the Child Before Surgery

Parents are usually anxious because of the need to wait before surgery can be performed. They often fear that the infant will not survive until surgery or that they will be unable to manage any problems the infant may have. Provide parents with information and teach them how to care for the child at home. Some infants have such special home care needs that home health nursing and other community services are required. Many of these children require supplemental oxygen and nutrition, either for emergencies or for regular use (Figure 14-8 ◆).

Cyanosis with or without congestive heart failure often results in delayed gross motor skills. Developmental specialists can help parents set realistic developmental goals for the child. Make referrals to community-based early-intervention programs to promote the child's development.

Encourage parents to treat the infant as normally as possible. Children with mild cyanotic lesions do not need to adjust activity. The child with moderate to severe disease should be able to tolerate crying for a few minutes without difficulty. Prolonged crying should not be permitted because it causes fatigue and further hypoxia.

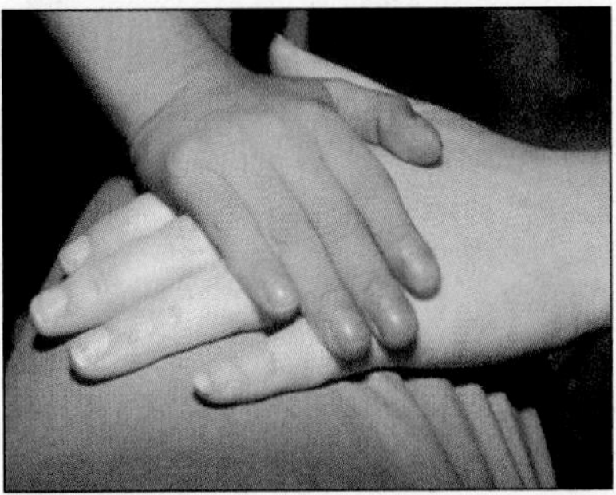

FIGURE 14-7 ◆
Clubbing of the fingers is one manifestation of a cyanotic defect in an older child. What neurologic signs may be associated with such a defect?

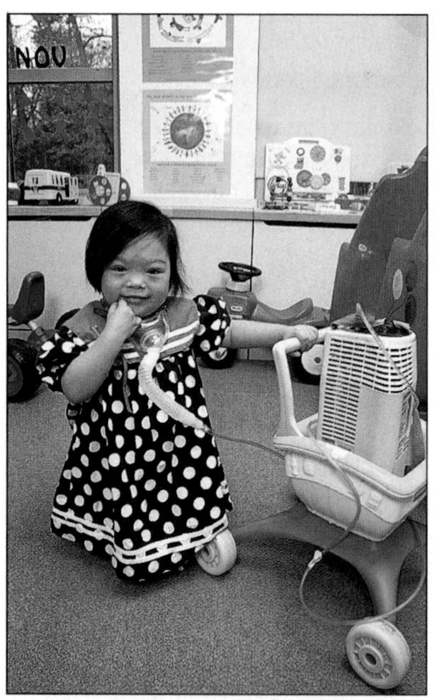

FIGURE 14-8◆
By pushing her oxygen cannister in a toy shopping cart, this toddler is able to move around in her environment. This strategy meets both her physiologic need for supplemental oxygen and her developmental need for independence.

Vomiting and diarrhea may lead to dehydration, and parents must notify the physician when the infant or child has these symptoms. Dehydration is a particular risk in children with polycythemia because the blood can become even more viscous. Fever and dehydration may increase cyanosis. The systemic vascular resistance is decreased, resulting in a further decrease in blood flow to the pulmonary system. Aggressive management with antipyretic medication and fluid volume replacement is necessary (DeBoer, 1996).

Teach parents to observe the child for signs of infective endocarditis, including low-grade fever, fatigue, and malaise. They need to notify the physician if these symptoms occur within 2 months of surgery or a high-risk procedure. Parents must learn to request antibiotic prophylaxis for the child (see Table 14-4). Children also need preventive dental care to reduce the risk of endocarditis.

Parents may want to formulate an emergency plan in case the infant develops acute problems such as a hypercyanotic spell or respiratory distress. Cardiopulmonary resuscitation should be taught to the parents. Ask parents to notify the local rescue squad about the infant's problem. Prepare a card or brief history form with information about the child's condition, medications, and necessary emergency care and the physician's name for parents to keep at home (American Academy of Pediatrics Committee on Pediatric Emergency Medicine, 1999). When an acute problem occurs, this form gives important information to the emergency medical technicians and emergency department staff.

Although parents may travel with cyanotic children, they should not take them to areas of high altitude without first consulting with the physician. Supplemental oxygen when traveling on an airplane may be necessary.

Care of the Infant and Child Undergoing Surgery

Monitor and carefully maintain the central, umbilical, or peripheral intravenous lines in the infant receiving continuous infusion of PGE_1. Observe the infant for side effects of prostaglandin treatment. Have intubation equipment and a bag and mask at bedside in case of apnea. Have intravenous fluids available to control hypotension.

If a hypercyanotic spell occurs, immediately place the child in the knee–chest position and administer oxygen. Administer morphine as ordered. Immediately notify the physician for further orders if these procedures are ineffective and the spell continues. Avoid any unpleasant or anxiety-provoking procedures.

Children are admitted to the ICU following surgery. Refer to the section on nursing assessment in the discussion of nursing care of the child undergoing surgery on page 487. Postoperative bleeding is a potential risk in children with polycythemia, because bleeding times are prolonged and platelet counts are low. Chest tube output is monitored carefully for bright red blood or excessive volume. Bright red blood in the chest tube is a significant sign of hemorrhage. Fluids and diuretics are used to maintain **preload** (the volume of blood in the ventricle at the end of diastole that stretches the heart muscle before contraction) in the right ventricle whereas inotropic drugs are used to support cardiac output. Children are transferred to the general nursing unit once heart function has stabilized.

Monitor the heart functioning of children following surgery. Assess vital signs, skin color, perfusion of the skin by capillary refill, and distal pulses. A sudden sustained increase in pulse and respirations and a decrease in peripheral perfusion may be early signs of hemorrhage. Monitoring fluid intake and output following surgery is critical. Note any signs of respiratory distress that may indicate the development of a pneumothorax or congestive heart failure.

CLINICAL TIP

To calm and reassure the infant while simultaneously positioning him or her in knee–chest position, hold the infant facing your chest. Place one arm under the knees and fold the legs upward toward the infant's chest. Use the other arm to support the infant's back.

Evaluation

Examples of expected nursing care outcomes include the following:

- The parents recognize a hypercyanotic spell, initiate emergency treatment, and seek emergency care for the child.
- The parents manage fever and medical illnesses to prevent dehydration and potential hypercyanotic spells.
- The child attains expected developmental progress in gross motor, fine motor, and language skills.

HEART TRANSPLANTATION

In 1999, 307 pediatric heart transplantations were performed. Conditions associated with transplantation include the following by age group (Odim, Laks, & Burch, et al., 2000):

- Infants—primarily congenital heart disease, such as hypoplastic left heart syndrome and other complex defects
- Children 1 to 10 years—cardiomyopathy (>50%), congenital heart disease (40%)
- Adolescents—cardiomyopathy (65%), congenital heart disease (25%)

With improved immunosuppressive protocols and surgical techniques, patient survival rates are increasing (75% at 1 year and 65% at 5 years) (Boucek, 2000).

Infection and rejection are the major causes of mortality and morbidity. The immunosuppression regimen usually includes cyclosporin A, azathioprine, and corticosteroids. Signs of organ rejection include the following (Duitsman, Suddaby, & Masterson, 1999):

- Increasing resting heart rate, arrhythmias, bradycardia
- Presence of a third heart sound
- Cool and mottled extremities
- Inspiratory crackles, diaphoresis, tachypnea, pulmonary edema
- Hepatosplenomegaly
- Oliguria

Bacterial, fungal, and viral (i.e., cytomegalovirus) infections cause the most problems; however, some common childhood illnesses (acute otitis, colds) may be well tolerated.

After recovery from surgery, children may have near-normal exercise capabilities, normal heart function, and return to school and other activities. Immunosuppressive medications will be continued long term and can cause a variety of physical side effects such as the following: hair growth, gum hyperplasia, weight gain, moon facies, acne, and rashes. Children and adolescents may need support to develop positive self-esteem due to their appearance.

Depending upon the age at time of transplant, the child may not have had all immunizations. Live virus vaccines are often not given to immunosuppressed children (see Chapter 12). Help parents arrange for schools and child care centers to provide early notification of cases of measles, mumps, rubella, and chicken pox. Preventive treatment for the child can be provided as necessary. Handwashing and other methods to reduce the spread of infection should be encouraged both at home and at school.

Organ rejection is a major concern of families. Provide education for the parents and child to recognize the signs and to seek treatment promptly.

MEDICATIONS

Immunosuppressive protocol medications commonly used include:

- Cyclosporine
- Azathioprine
- Prednisone

PULMONARY ARTERY HYPERTENSION

Pulmonary artery hypertension is a complication of many congenital heart defects, as well as pulmonary conditions. In some children with congenital heart defects, excessive pulmonary blood flow over time causes pulmonary vascular changes to decrease the blood flow. Inflammation, hypertrophy of pulmonary vessels, and fibrosis develop. Pulmonary venous hypertension develops. The increased pressure leads to a right-to-left shunt, and right heart function is impaired. The condition may become life threatening (Barst, 1999).

Hypoxemia results from pulmonary hypertension, and the infant displays tachypnea, cyanosis, retractions, and fatigue. Feeding is difficult, and weight loss with fluid and electrolyte imbalance is likely. Older children will have exertional dypsnea, chest pain, and syncope.

Clinical therapy involves surgery to correct an obstructive lesion or close a defect. Therapy for pulmonary artery hypertension related to noncardiac conditions involves bronchodilators, antibiotics, corticosteroids, and low flow oxygen. No cure is available, but life can be prolonged with these measures (Barst, 1999).

Nursing care focuses on promoting rest for oxygen conservation, monitoring fluid intake and output carefully, and administering medications and oxygen. Airplane travel may be possible with supplemental oxygen. Exercise should be tailored to avoid dyspnea. Give parents needed support and information about their child.

ACQUIRED HEART DISEASES

RHEUMATIC FEVER

Rheumatic fever is an inflammatory connective tissue disorder that follows an initial infection by some strains of group A beta-hemolytic streptococci. This disorder causes changes in the heart, joints, brain, and skin tissues. Although not common, the disorder has occurred more frequently since the 1980s, probably because of a virulent strain of group A streptococcal infections (Steeg, Walsh, & Glickstein, 2000). The exact cause of the disorder is unknown, but one possible cause is an autoimmune response in a genetically predisposed child (Steeg, 2000).

One to 3 weeks after an untreated streptococcal infection, the hallmark signs of rheumatic fever may occur. Aschoff bodies (hemorrhagic bullous lesions) develop in the connective tissue of the heart. Endocarditis may lead to permanent mitral or aortic heart valve damage. The child's joints become inflamed and painful (migratory polyarthritis), although this condition improves in several weeks. Subcutaneous nodules may be palpable near joints. A skin rash called erythema marginatum, with pink macules and blanching in the middle of the lesions, is frequently seen. Spiking fever often occurs. A condition known as Sydenham chorea (St. Vitus dance), which is characterized by aimless movements of the extremities and facial grimacing, may be seen if the central nervous system is involved. Mild anemia may also occur.

Diagnosis is based on clinical signs (Jones criteria; Table 14-7) and laboratory testing for antistreptolysin-O (ASO). An elevated ASO antibody titer indicates a recent streptococcal infection.

Clinical therapy includes antibiotics (penicillin, sufadiazine, or erythromycin) to eradicate the streptococcal infection. Aspirin may be given to control joint inflammation and reduce fever. Children should be monitored carefully for potential heart involvement by echocardiogram. Steroids may be used for severe carditis with congestive heart failure. Most children recover fully.

Nursing Management

Skill 6-12: Obtaining a Sample for Throat Culture

The most important role of the nurse is prevention of rheumatic fever. Nurses in clinics, offices, and schools need to ensure that all children with possible streptococcal infections have a throat culture taken. Even if the sore throat is mild, a culture is needed if family members

TABLE 14-7 Guidelines for Diagnosis of Initial Attack of Rheumatic Fever (Jones Criteria, updated 1992)*

MAJOR MANIFESTATIONS	MINOR MANIFESTATIONS
Carditis	**Clinical findings**
Polyarthritis	Arthralgia
Chorea	Fever
Erythema marginatum	**Laboratory findings**
Subcutaneous nodules	Elevated acute-phase reactants
	Erythrocyte sedimentation rate
	C-reactive protein
	Prolonged PR interval

Supporting evidence of antecedent group A streptococcal infection: (1) positive throat culture or rapid streptococcal antigen test; (2) elevated or rising streptococcal antibody titer.

*If supported by evidence of preceding group A streptococcal infection, the presence of two major manifestations or one major and two minor manifestations indicates a high probability of acute rheumatic fever.

Note: Data from the Special Writing Group of the Committee on Rheumatic Fever, Endocarditis, and Kawasaki Disease of the Council on Cardiovascular Disease in the Young of the American Heart Association. (1992). Guidelines for the diagnosis of rheumatic fever. Jones Criteria, 1992 update. *Journal of the American Medical Association, 268*(15), 2069–2073.

or other contacts have had a streptococcal infection. Emphasize to the family the importance of giving the entire 10-day course of antibiotics when a culture is positive.

In a case of severe rheumatic fever, the child will be hospitalized for a period of time. Nursing care focuses on assessing the child's condition, promoting recovery, and ensuring compliance with the treatment regimen.

During the acute inflammatory phase, take the child's temperature at least every 4 hours and monitor vital signs. The child is on bedrest while monitoring for the onset of carditis, and for 4 weeks if carditis develops. Auscultate the child's heart and note any unusual sounds. Observe the child for changes in skin, joints, or behavior. Family members should have throat cultures done to identify possible asymptomatic streptococcal carriers.

Administer antibiotic and aspirin as ordered. The child is usually lethargic and often has joint pain. Aspirin often relieves pain dramatically after a few doses. Position the child's joints and handle them carefully. Provide quiet activities, as the child is often confined to bed. Encourage visits or telephone calls from family members and friends. For the child with chorea, provide emotional support because the purposeless involuntary movements that can last for 5 to 15 weeks can be disturbing. Encourage the family to participate in the child's hospital care.

During the recovery phase, the child will generally be cared for at home. Activities may be limited, especially if heart damage is suspected. Help parents plan quiet activities, such as playing board games, working with computers, or reading, and arrange rest periods after the child returns to school. Reassure the child and parents that the effects of chorea will eventually subside.

On discharge, a daily oral low-dose antibiotic is prescribed or monthly long-acting antibiotic injection is given. Make sure the child and parents understand the importance of taking prescribed medication until adulthood to prevent future infection and possible heart damage from recurrent rheumatic fever. Stress the importance of telling future health care providers, including dentists and surgeons, about the child's rheumatic fever history so prophylactic antibiotics can be given to prevent infective endocarditis during invasive procedures.

Make sure the parents understand that the child's future sore throats may be streptococcal and that a throat culture should be taken even when the child is taking daily antibiotics. The child may need additional antibiotics for the infection. Emphasize the importance of follow-up care to prevent new infections and to monitor heart function.

COMMUNITY CARE

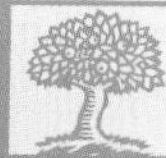

Often the sore throat that precedes the child's illness is mild and goes untreated. Nurses must carefully evaluate pharyngitis, especially when cases of group A streptococcal infection have been identified in the family or community.

INFECTIVE ENDOCARDITIS

Infective endocarditis is an inflammation of the lining, valves, and arterial vessels of the heart caused by bacterial, enterococci, and fungal infections. Children who have a congenital heart defect, rheumatic heart disease, or a central venous catheter or who have had heart surgery are at risk for infective endocarditis. Infections may occur after the causal organism enters the bloodstream during dental work or surgery and lodge on damaged or abnormal endocardial tissue. It is a significant cause of morbidity and mortality in children with complex heart defects treated with prosthetic aortopulmonary shunts and in immunocompromised children with long-term central venous catheter use (Brook, 1999).

Symptoms can be mild and develop slowly, or they can be severe and develop rapidly. Common symptoms are fever (often with elevations in the afternoon), fatigue, joint and muscle aches, headache, and nausea and vomiting. Signs may include a new or changing murmur, congestive heart failure, dyspnea, hematuria, petechia, and splenomegaly (Brook, 1999).

Infective endocarditis is diagnosed primarily by blood culture; however, urine and cerebrospinal fluid also may be cultured. Elevated erythrocyte sedimentation rate, anemia, elevated C-reactive protein level, increased white blood cell count, alterations in the electrocardiogram, and changes in heart sounds and murmurs are indicators of the condition. Echocardiography may be used to identify the presence of vegetation or infective lesions in the heart.

Clinical therapy consists of administering antibiotics such as penicillin G, ampicillin, vancomycin, nafcillin, or gentamicin. Intravenous administration is preferred, with therapy continuing for 2 to 8 weeks until the infective organism is eradicated. Serum levels of antibiotics are monitored to maintain a therapeutic range. Occasionally surgery is necessary to drain an abscess or because of heart valve failure. If congestive heart failure occurs, bedrest and medications such as digoxin and furosemide are prescribed.

Nursing Management

Nursing care focuses on assessing the child's condition, administering medications, and teaching the parents about the child's care. Take the child's vital signs and assess gastrointestinal discomfort. Administer medications as ordered and monitor serum antibiotic levels. Monitor for side effects of antibiotics and for infiltration or extravasation at the infusion site. Keep invasive procedures to a minimum. Use careful aseptic technique in performing venipunctures, urinary catheterizations, and other procedures.

The child is often lethargic and on bedrest. Encourage parents to assist with the child's care and plan quiet age-appropriate activities. Home infusion antibiotic therapy may be ordered so that care can be provided on an outpatient basis. At discharge, arrange home health nursing and instruct parents about care needed for the child's recuperation. Reinforce the need for follow-up visits. Explain the importance of informing physicians and dentists about the child's history of endocarditis so that care is taken to prevent infection before invasive procedures.

CARDIAC ARRHYTHMIAS

Cardiac arrhythmias (abnormal rhythms) are not uncommon in children. These include tachyarrhythmias (sinus tachycardia) and bradyarrhythmias (sinus bradycardia) that occur with acute conditions and resolve once the condition is treated. Less common arrhythmias are often associated with congenital heart disease, and include atrial fibrillation, atrial flutter, ventricular fibrillation, and heart block.

Supraventricular Tachycardia

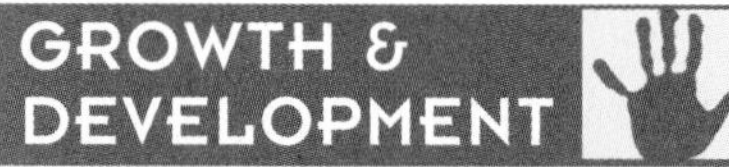

The presenting heart rate in infants with supraventricular tachycardia (SVT) may be up to 260 beats/min. In older children, a heart rate between 150 and 240 beats/min may be seen. A heart rate of 230 beats/min is seen in 60% of children under 18 years of age (Robinson, Anisman, & Eshaghpour, 1996).

Supraventricular tachycardia (SVT), the most common pathologic tachycardia, is the abrupt onset of a rapid, regular heart rate, often too fast to count. Neonates and young children may be predisposed to the condition because of a congenital heart defect or Wolff–Parkinson–White syndrome. Short periods of arrhythmia (several seconds), which may be caused by paroxysmal atrial tachycardia, are rarely dangerous; however, prolonged episodes (>24 hours) of continuous SVT may lead to congestive heart failure. Cardiac output is affected because diastolic filling cannot occur with such a rapid heart rate.

Recurrent attacks are common. Prolonged episodes of SVT are life threatening and can progress to congestive heart failure or cardiogenic shock if untreated.

Early signs in infants include poor feeding, irritability, and pallor. Older children may have episodes of altered consciousness (dizziness or syncope).

Electrocardiography, including a 24-hour rhythm recording, is used to confirm the diagnosis. Vagal stimulation such as application of ice or iced saline solution to the face may reduce the heart rate. An older child can perform the Valsalva maneuver (holding the breath and straining, or blowing forcefully on the thumb) to increase intrathoracic and venous pressures and thus slow the heart rate. Adenosine or amiodarone is the recommended emergency medication when vagal stimulation does not work. Cardioversion may be used for life-threatening episodes if other treatments are not effective. Digoxin and propranolol may be given to reduce the frequency of episodes (Starr & Freitas-Nichols, 2000). Radio-frequency catheter ablation is used in chronic cyclic tachycardia, used to obliterate the accessory pathway with much success (Case, 1999).

Long QT Syndrome

Long QT syndrome is a rhythm disturbance of autosomal dominant and autosomal recessive inheritance that places children at risk for ventricular fibrillation and sudden death. It may also result from electrolyte abnormalities, malnutrition associated with anorexia and bulimia, myocarditis, and central nervous system trauma (Berul, 2000). It is thought to be associated with some cases of sudden infant death syndrome.

The arrhythmia commonly occurs without warning and often results in death. It may be triggered by exercise or emotional stress, but in some cases has occurred during rest. Early signs include a fast heart rate (too fast to count), irritability, lethargy, poor feeding, poor perfusion (cool pale skin, increased capillary refill time), decreased responsiveness, and decreased blood pressure.

If the child is resuscitated or evaluated because of early signs, the arrhythmia is commonly detected by electrocardiogram. The disorder is treated by beta-adrenergic blockade, antiarrhythmic agents, and often a pacemaker (Lewin, 2000).

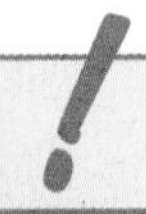

NURSING ALERT

The child with supraventricular tachycardia (SVT) should avoid subsequent use of cardiac stimulant drugs such as decongestants. These drugs might trigger another episode of SVT.

NURSING MANAGEMENT Nursing care focuses on assessing the child's condition, administering medications, and providing emotional support to the child and parents. Children are treated in the emergency department or intensive care unit. The child is placed on a cardiac monitor, and frequent assessment is critical. Report continued abnormal rates or rhythms to the physician. Carefully observe and record changes in level of consciousness, color, weakness, irritability, and feeding pattern. Administer medications as ordered. Have emergency drugs and resuscitation equipment available at bedside. Provide for rest and adequate nutrition.

Episodes of arrhythmia are frightening for both the child and parents. Carefully explain the treatment plan and home care. Teach parents to take the child's apical pulse. Make sure parents are trained in cardiopulmonary resuscitation. Provide telephone numbers of emergency medical facilities and help parents plan how to seek emergency care. Emphasize that medications help prevent or reduce episode frequency.

VASCULAR DISEASES

KAWASAKI DISEASE

Kawasaki disease, also known as mucocutaneous lymph node syndrome, is an acute systemic inflammatory illness. Although this disorder is most commonly found in Asian children, it is seen in all races. The disorder occurs primarily in children under 5 years of age. In the United States, Kawasaki disease is the most common cause of acquired heart disease in children. The etiology of Kawasaki disease is unknown, but the primary cause is theorized to be infectious in genetically predisposed children. It does not appear to be spread by person-to-person contact, but frequently is preceded by an upper respiratory tract infection.

The three stages of the disease are acute, subacute, and convalescent. The acute stage of Kawasaki disease is characterized by fever, conjunctival hyperemia, red throat, swollen hands and feet, rash on the trunk, enlargement of the cervical lymph nodes, diarrhea, and hepatic dysfunction (Figure 14-9 ◆). The subacute stage is characterized by cracking lips and fissures, desquamation of the skin on the tips of the fingers and toes, joint pain, cardiac disease, and thrombocytosis. In the convalescent stage, 6 to 8 weeks after disease onset, the child appears normal but lingering signs of inflammation may be present.

Diagnosis is based on clinical signs using the criteria given in Table 14-8. Blood studies show some abnormalities such as elevated erythrocyte sedimentation rate, elevated white blood cell count, mild anemia, thrombocytosis, elevated platelet count, and elevated C-reactive protein level. An echocardiogram may reveal some heart changes.

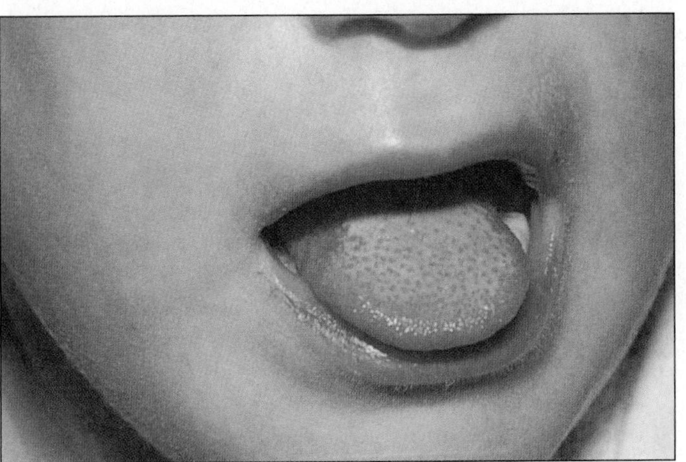

FIGURE 14-9 ◆
This child shows many of the signs of the acute stage of Kawasaki disease.

TABLE 14-8 Diagnostic Criteria for Kawasaki Disease

Kawasaki disease is diagnosed when a high spiking fever over 39°C (102.2°F) for 5 days or longer is present along with four of the following five criteria:

- Bilateral conjunctivitis without exudate, typically with distinctly visible vessels early in the disease
- Intense erythema of the buccal and pharyngeal surfaces with dry, swollen, cracked, and fissuring lips and a strawberry tongue
- Dermatitis of the extremities, intense palmar and plantar erythema, induration of the hands and feet, and then desquamation after 2 or more weeks of symptoms
- Dermatitis of the trunk with an erythematous maculopapular rash
- Acute cervical lymphadenopathy, frequently unilateral, with a node over 1.5 cm in diameter found early in the disease
- An illness not explained by another disease process

Note: Modified from Rowley, A. H., & Shulman, S. T. (1999). Kawasaki syndrome. *Pediatric Clinics of North America, 46*(2), 313–329.

Clinical therapy of Kawasaki disease involves the use of aspirin and immune globulin. High doses of aspirin (80 to 100 mg/kg/day) are given while the fever is high. The dose is decreased to 10 mg/kg/day or less once the fever has dropped. Aspirin is taken until the platelet count is normal and may be continued on a long-term basis if cardiac abnormalities occur. High doses of immune globulin and of aspirin given early in the disease have been shown to reduce the incidence of coronary artery lesions and aneurysms, and to decrease fever and inflammatory signs (Rowley & Shulman, 1999).

Children are usually hospitalized as long as fever persists. Most children recover fully. Careful monitoring for cardiac disease continues for several weeks or months. Cardiac involvement is the most serious complication. Aneurysms and early atherosclerosis lead to arrhythmias, congestive heart failure, coronary stenosis, myocardial infarction, and, potentially, death.

Nursing Management

Nursing care focuses on promoting comfort, monitoring for early signs of complications or disease progression, and supporting the family.

Assessment is important in identifying signs of Kawasaki disease, as the acute phase of this disorder is commonly confused with other diseases. The nurse in the community must be alert to early signs and symptoms. When the child is hospitalized, take the temperature every 4 hours and before each dose of aspirin. Carefully assess the extremities for edema, redness, and desquamation every 8 hours. Examine the eyes for conjunctivitis and the mucous membranes for inflammation. Monitor the child's dietary and fluid intake and weigh the child daily. Carefully assess heart sounds and rhythm.

Administer aspirin and immune globulin as ordered. Monitor for side effects of aspirin such as bleeding and gastrointestinal upset. Administer intravenous immune globulin as a blood product, carefully regulating the infusion rate to run slowly according to the physician's orders, and watching for any reactions to the infusion. The infusion rate should not be over 1 mL/min. If symptoms of reaction are noted, stop the infusion immediately (see Chapter 11).

Promote the child's comfort. Keep the child's skin clean and dry, and lubricate the lips. Use cool compresses and tepid sponges to make the feverish child more comfortable. Change the child's clothes and bed linens frequently. Give frequent small feedings of soft foods and liquids that are neither too hot nor too cold.

Use passive range-of-motion exercises to facilitate joint movement. Because the child with Kawasaki disease is frequently lethargic and irritable, plan rest periods and quiet age-appropriate activities. Encourage the parents to participate in their child's care to promote comfort and reassurance for the child. Provide the parents with information about the disease and the child's treatment.

Before the child is discharged, teach the parents to administer aspirin as ordered and to watch for side effects. Advise the parents that the child may need to avoid contact sports or

NURSING ALERT

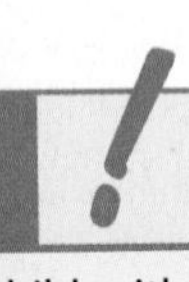

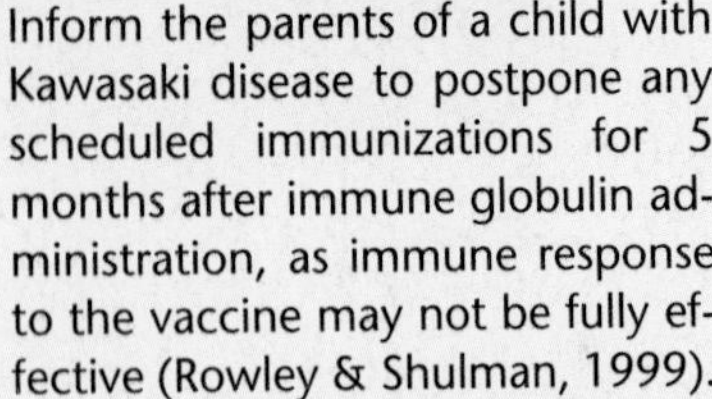

Inform the parents of a child with Kawasaki disease to postpone any scheduled immunizations for 5 months after immune globulin administration, as immune response to the vaccine may not be fully effective (Rowley & Shulman, 1999).

TABLE 14-9 Risk Factors for Hyperlipidemia

Family history of coronary heart disease before age 55	Diabetes
Cigarette smoking	Lack of exercise
Hypertension	High total and saturated fat intake
	Overweight

other activities that could cause bleeding. Have them take the child's temperature daily and report any fever above 37.8°C (100°F) to the physician. Emphasize the need for follow-up care to monitor for cardiac complications.

HYPERLIPIDEMIA

Hyperlipidemia is a condition of excessive fat in the blood that may eventually lead to atherosclerosis. Although children do not usually die of atherosclerotic heart disease, coronary heart disease, the major cause of death in the United States, begins in childhood and progresses through the adult years (Giddings, 1999). It is important to identify children who have a genetic history or lifestyle that makes them more susceptible to future coronary heart disease (Table 14-9).

Some children have hereditary disorders of lipid metabolism characterized by high levels of total cholesterol, low-density lipoprotein, or triglycerides, or by low levels of high-density lipoprotein (Winter, House, & Schatz, 1999). Children with familial hypercholesterolemia, for example, have cholesterol levels as high as 600 to 1,000 mg/dL, resulting in lipid deposits in their corneas and tendons. As the excessive fat circulates, it causes changes in blood vessels. Most commonly, children have milder lipid abnormalities that arise from a combination of heredity and lifestyle factors. The fatty streaks that appear in childhood become fibrous plaques in adolescence. These atherosclerotic plaques continue to grow in adulthood and may cause hemorrhage, thrombi, and occlusion of vessels (Williams & Bollella, 1995).

Hyperlipidemia is identified by a blood test. Cholesterol, including total cholesterol (TC), high-density lipoprotein cholesterol (HDL-C), and triglycerides are measured. The low-density lipoprotein cholesterol (LDL-C) level is calculated using an equation based on the triglyceride, HDL, and total cholesterol levels. It is recommended that all children who have a family history of cardiovascular disease before age 55 years (parents or grandparents) or who have a parent with elevated total serum cholesterol (240 mg/dL) be screened (Winter et al., 1999). Some clinicians choose to screen all children, especially those with an unknown family history, during childhood or sometime after the age of 2 years. This helps to identify children who have no risk factors but demonstrate hyperlipidemia (Purath, Lansinger, & Ragheb, 1995). Based on total cholesterol value, children are placed in a low-, moderate-, or high-risk category. The LDL cholesterol level is examined carefully in children with elevated total cholesterol (200 mg/dL). LDL cholesterol should be less than 110 mg/dL. High HDL and low LDL cholesterol levels provide protection against heart disease.

Hyperlipidemia in most children can be managed by dietary modifications, exercise, and other changes in lifestyle. The child's diet is carefully analyzed and changes are made to satisfy the dietary guidelines given in Table 14-10. If the child continues to have high serum lipid levels, a lipid specialist should be consulted. Cholestyramine or colestipol, which bind bile acid in the intestine, niacin, or some of the statin drugs are occasionally prescribed for children over 10 years of age.

Long-term studies of the effect of childhood lipid levels on life span have not yet been concluded. It is hoped that careful monitoring and management of lipid levels in childhood will decrease the incidence of cardiovascular disease.

Nursing Management

Nursing care focuses on identifying children at risk for hyperlipidemia, providing education about diet and exercise, and monitoring eating patterns. Identification and management of hyperlipidemia takes place in a variety of community agencies. Office and clinic nurses identify children who need to have serum lipid measured. Nurses in schools provide education

RECOMMENDED LIPID/LIPOPROTEIN LEVELS FOR CHILDREN

Total cholesterol
Recommended: <170 mg/dL
Borderline high: 170–200 mg/dL
High: >200 mg/dL

LDL-C
Recommended: <110 mg/dL
Borderline high: 110–130 mg/dL
High: >130 mg/dL

Triglyceride
Recommended: <100 mg/dL
Borderline: 100–130 mg/dL
High: >130 mg/dL

HDL-C
Recommended: >35 mg/dL

RESEARCH

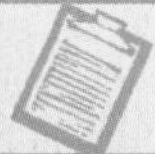

A long-term study evaluating the safety and efficacy of a cholesterol-lowering diet in children with elevated LDL-C revealed that dietary fat modification can be achieved and sustained in actively growing children. Improvements in LDL-C levels can be made without adverse effects on the child's growth and maturational development (Obarzanek, Kimm, & Barton, et al., 2001).

TABLE 14-10 Recommended Nutrient Intake in Children and Adolescents With Hyperlipidemia

NUTRIENT	RECOMMENDED INTAKE
Saturated fatty acid	Less than 10% of calories
Total fat	No more than 30% of calories
Polyunsaturated fat	Up to 10% of calories
Monounsaturated fat	10%–15% of calories
Cholesterol	Less than 300 mg/day

Note: Modified from the National Cholesterol Education Program Coordinating Committee. (1991). *Report of the expert panel on blood cholesterol levels in children and adolescents.* Washington, DC: U.S. Department of Health and Human Services; and Krauss, R. M., Eckel, R. H., Howard, B., et al. (2001). AHA scientific statement: AHA dietary guidelines, *Journal of Nutrition, 131,* 132–146.

AEROBIC ACTIVITIES

Running	Aerobic dancing
Jogging	Swimming
Fast walking	Hiking
Biking	Rollerblading
Soccer	

on ways to reduce risk factors (Howard, Bindler, & Synoground, et al., 1996). The child's history of exercise patterns, weight percentile, and dietary intake provides important information. Obtain data on familial heart disease, hypertension, diabetes, and smoking to determine risk factors. Total cholesterol level screening does not require fasting, but the child will need to fast for 12 hours before blood is drawn for a complete lipid evaluation.

Work with nutritionists to provide dietary teaching and monitor family eating patterns. Emphasize the importance of exercise in keeping the heart and blood vessels free from atherosclerotic changes. Help the child select an aerobic activity and encourage participation at least five times weekly for 30 minutes each time.

Smoking by the child or the parents should be discouraged. Secondhand smoke may affect blood pressure and plaque formation, and thus increase the risk for the development of cardiovascular disease (Giddings, 1999).

Include the entire family in the treatment plan, as changing eating and exercise patterns is difficult for a single family member. The family of a child with hyperlipidemia requires continual teaching and reinforcement. Nutrition assessments and evaluation of family diet should be performed periodically.

HYPERTENSION

Hypertension is present in 1% to 3% of the pediatric population (Porto, 2000). Most cases have unknown cause, labeled as primary or essential hypertension (Hohn, 1997). Some underlying conditions such as kidney disease or heart defects may cause secondary hypertension. A genetic predisposition to hypertension may be manifested in some children by high normal or slightly elevated blood pressures. Mildly elevated blood pressure in children and adolescents may precede adult hypertension (National High Blood Pressure Education Program, 1996). High blood pressure in adolescents is correlated with obesity and high serum lipid level (Bartosh & Aronson, 1999). All children with blood pressures in the 90th percentile for age are significantly more likely to develop hypertension as adults (Bartosh & Aronson, 1999).

The child with an elevated blood pressure should have blood chemistry (BUN, creatinine, glucose, and electrolytes), urinalysis, and culture tested to detect secondary causes of hypertension. Serum lipid studies should be performed to determine whether hyperlipidemia exists. Nonpharmacologic measures for reduction of blood pressure include dietary counseling for obesity, low-sodium and high-potassium diet, increased physical exercise, adequate calcium and dietary fiber with less than 10% of calories from saturated fats, three to five fruit servings daily, discontinuation of smoking, alcohol, and drugs, and behavioral modification (Hohn, 1997). Medications are used for children with persistent, severe hypertension.

CULTURE

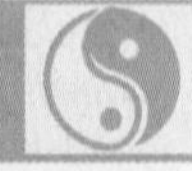

Black children may be particularly susceptible to increased blood pressure caused by dietary intake of sodium. Encouraging these children to follow a low-salt diet is important. Increasing intake of low-fat dairy products and fruits can contribute to blood pressure control.

Nursing Management

Take a complete history for the child with borderline hypertension and no other associated diseases. Are parents or siblings hypertensive? Is the child obese? How many servings of fruit does the child eat daily? What are the number of servings of dairy products? What is the child's daily salt intake? What are the child's daily exercise routines? Take the child's blood pressure regularly to monitor changes. Compare readings to normal blood pressure for age and gender (see Table 4-17).

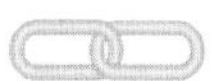

Skill 5-10: Taking Blood Pressure

Teach the child and parents how to improve the diet and develop exercise routines. Emphasize the importance of avoiding smoking. Teaching that involves the entire family is usually the most effective. Instruct the family on correct administration of prescribed medications when used.

INJURIES OF THE CARDIOVASCULAR SYSTEM

SHOCK

Shock is an acute, complex state of circulatory dysfunction resulting in failure to deliver sufficient oxygen and other nutrients to meet cell and tissue demands. It can be caused by a variety of conditions such as hemorrhage, dehydration, sepsis, obstruction of blood flow, and cardiac pump failure.

Hypovolemic Shock

Hypovolemic shock is a clinical state of inadequate tissue and organ perfusion resulting from the movement of blood or plasma out of the intravascular compartment (Figure 14-10 ◆). The blood or plasma in the vascular space may be decreased because of hemorrhage or fluid movement into the interstitial spaces.

ETIOLOGY AND PATHOPHYSIOLOGY Major causes of decreased intravascular blood volume include the following:

- Hemorrhage from significant injury
- Plasma loss from burns, nephrotic syndrome, and sepsis
- Fluid and electrolyte loss associated with dehydration, diabetic ketoacidosis, and diabetes insipidus
- Vasodilating drugs

Shock results in inadequate delivery of oxygen and nutrients to cells and accumulation of toxic wastes in the capillaries. This reduction in circulating blood volume causes a decrease in cardiac output and mean arterial pressure. Cellular hypoxia and acidosis develop simultaneously. The accumulation of toxins and inadequate tissue oxygenation cause cellular damage.

The child's body attempts to compensate by the following measures:

- The heart rate and myocardial contractility increase to improve cardiac output.
- The respiratory rate increases to improve oxygenation and decrease waste accumulation in the cells.
- The hydrostatic pressure falls, permitting fluid to shift into the vascular space and increasing the circulating blood volume.
- The peripheral vasculature constricts to maintain the systemic vascular resistance as long as possible.

The child is able to compensate until 20% to 25% of volume loss occurs, and then life-threatening hypotension results.

CLINICAL MANIFESTATIONS Signs of early hypovolemic shock in children are nonspecific, but need to be recognized before hypotension occurs. Signs indicating that the child is compensating for a decreased blood volume are tachycardia, usually sustained at a rate greater than 130 beats/min, increased respiratory effort, delayed capillary refill (>2 sec), weak peripheral pulses, pallor, and cold extremities (signs of decreased perfusion). Although the child's body attempts to compensate by preserving circulation to vital organs, urine output decreases when renal blood flow drops. In cases of dehydration, dry mucous membranes and poor skin turgor are also present.

PATHOPHYSIOLOGY ILLUSTRATED

Hypovolemic Shock

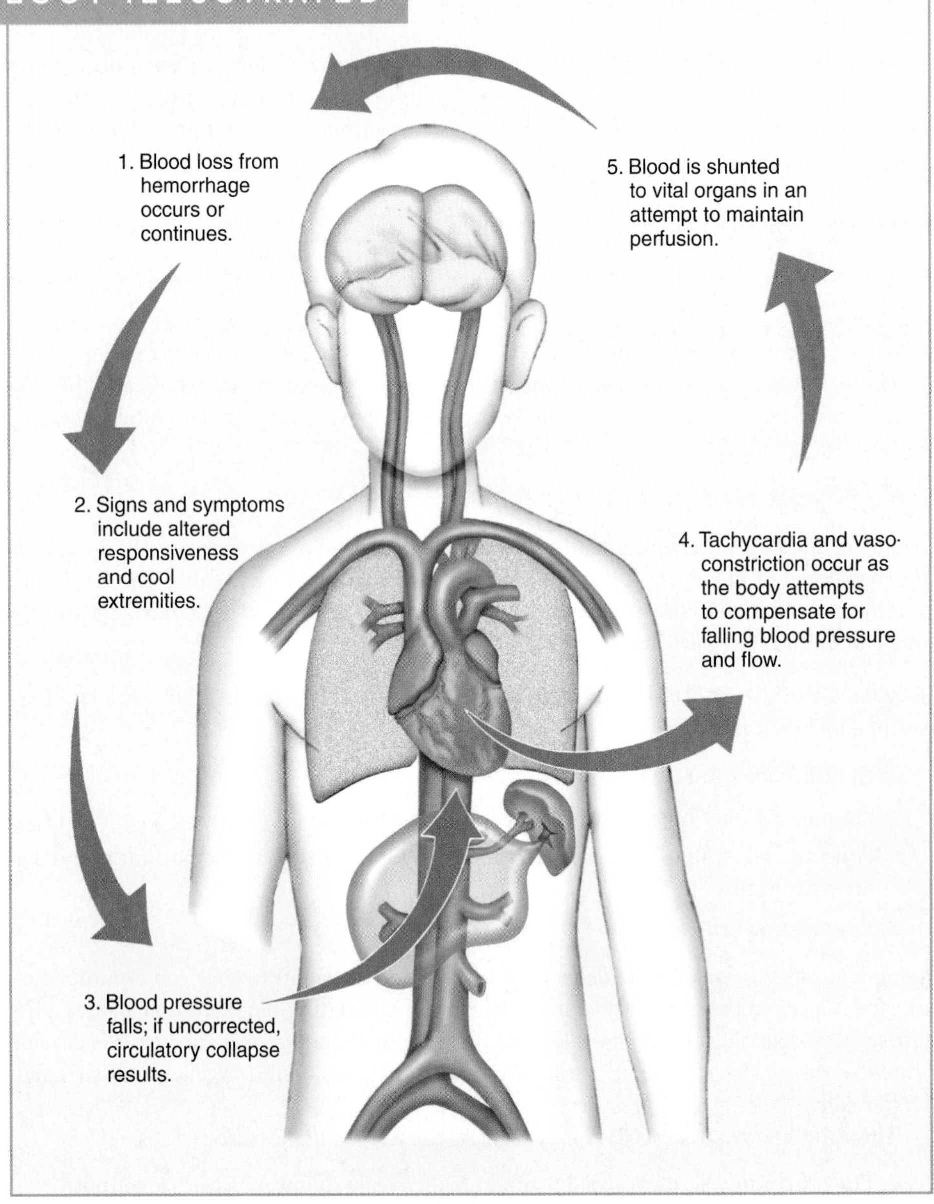

FIGURE 14-10 ◆ If hemorrhage reduces the circulating blood volume sufficiently vasocontriction occurs, shifting blood to maintain the perfusion of vital organs. When the blood loss exceeds 20%-25%, the child's body can no longer compensate and hypovolemic shock ensues.

NURSING ALERT

When the heart rate reaches 180 beats/min in a child (220 beats/min in an infant), the time needed for blood to fill the ventricles during diastole is too short. As a result, the cardiac output and stroke volume fall. Life-threatening shock may develop if corrective action is not taken to reduce the heart rate (Eichelberger, Ball, & Pratsch, et al., 1998).

If treatment is not initiated in the early stages of hypovolemic shock, the condition progresses until the child can no longer compensate. At that time, the systolic blood pressure drops and the pulse pressure decreases. A decreased level of consciousness ultimately results from reduced cerebral blood flow. If shock is not reversed, the condition progresses to cardiopulmonary failure. The clinical manifestations table compares the signs associated with early, uncompensated, and profound shock.

CLINICAL THERAPY No laboratory values can be used to evaluate the volume deficit rapidly enough to diagnose hypovolemic shock. The child is examined for characteristic signs to confirm the diagnosis. Laboratory tests commonly performed after hypovolemic shock is diagnosed include hematocrit and hemoglobin, arterial blood gases, serum electrolytes, glucose, osmolality, blood urea nitrogen, and urinalysis.

Emergency care focuses on improving tissue perfusion. An open airway is established, oxygen is administered, and ventilation is assisted if necessary. Bleeding is controlled, and an intravenous or intraosseous line is started to provide large volumes of crystalloid fluids (Ringer's lactate).

CLINICAL MANIFESTATIONS OF HYPOVOLEMIC SHOCK

SYSTEM	EARLY SHOCK	UNCOMPENSATED SHOCK	PROFOUND SHOCK
Cardiac	Tachycardia, weak distal pulses	Tachycardia, absent distal pulses, decreasing systolic blood pressure	Frank hypotension, bradycardia, weak central pulses
Neurologic	Normal, anxious, irritable, or combative behavior	Confusion, lethargy, decreased pain response	Comatose state
Skin	Mottled appearance; capillary refill time >2 sec; cool, clammy extremities	Cyanosis, capillary refill time >3 sec, cold extremities	Pale, cold skin
Renal	Decreased urine output, increased specific gravity	Oliguria, increased specific gravity	No urine output

Note: Modified from Waisman, H., & Eichelberger, M. R. (1993). Hypovolemic shock. In M. R. Eichelberger (Ed.), *Pediatric trauma: Prevention, acute care, rehabilitation* (p. 182). St. Louis: Mosby-Yearbook.

Ringer's lactate solution is the preferred fluid for initial resuscitation. A fluid volume of 20 mL/kg is administered rapidly over 5 minutes. The same amount of fluid is given in 5 minutes if the child's physiologic condition does not improve after fluid is first administered. If no improvement is seen after the second fluid bolus, blood or albumin is usually ordered.

Once the child's physiologic condition is stabilized, the cause of the hypovolemic shock becomes the focus of examination and treatment.

CLINICAL TIP

Clinical signs indicating that a child is responding to fluid resuscitation include:

- Improved color
- Improved responsiveness
- Lower heart rate
- Faster capillary refill time

NURSING MANAGEMENT

Nursing Assessment and Diagnosis

Ask the parent (or child, if appropriate) about possible injuries or the duration and severity of acute illnesses. If no external bleeding is evident, determine whether an injury may be causing internal bleeding. For example, the liver and spleen are highly vascular organs that have little protection from direct blunt forces. Significant bleeding from injury to one of these organs can cause hypovolemic shock without evidence of bleeding. An acute illness such as gastroenteritis with prolonged vomiting and diarrhea can also result in dehydration and hypovolemic shock.

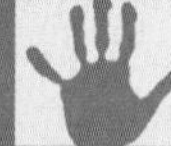

GROWTH & DEVELOPMENT

The child's total blood volume varies by weight. The child has approximately 80 mL of blood for every kilogram of body weight.

- Newborn: 3 kg × 80 mL = 240 mL (1 cup)
- 5-year-old child: 25 kg × 80 mL = 2,000 mL (2 quarts)
- 13-year-old child: 50 kg × 80 mL = 4,000 mL (1 gallon)

If external bleeding is apparent, determine the amount of blood lost. Although children lose the same amount of blood from a laceration as adults, the total volume of blood lost is proportional to their weight.

When an injured child is admitted to the hospital for a problem such as a liver or spleen laceration, assess the child's circulatory status frequently. Current medical treatment for these injuries is conservative. Surgeons give the liver or spleen a chance to heal spontaneously rather than perform immediate surgery to control bleeding and repair the laceration. Even if the child's circulatory condition was stabilized during emergency care, shock can develop again if bleeding continues.

Frequently assess the child's heart rate, respiratory rate, blood pressure, capillary refill time, level of consciousness with the Glasgow Coma Scale (see Chapter 20), color, and skin temperature to identify any changes that indicate improvement or deterioration in the child's condition. Monitor urine output and specific gravity hourly. Signs of the child's improved status include the following:

- A decrease in heart rate, respiratory rate, and capillary refill time
- An increase in systolic blood pressure and urine output
- Improved color, level of consciousness, and skin temperature
- Regaining of lost weight

The following nursing diagnoses may apply to the child with hypovolemic shock:

- *Decreased cardiac output,* related to hypovolemia
- *Fluid volume deficit,* related to active fluid volume loss
- *Altered tissue perfusion (cardiopulmonary, renal, and cerebral),* related to impaired transport of oxygen across alveolar and capillary membrane
- *Ineffective airway clearance,* related to altered level of consciousness
- *Ineffective family coping: Compromised,* related to life-threatening condition of the child

Planning and Implementation

Nurses in the emergency department and intensive care unit participate in the resuscitation of the child in hypovolemic shock. Assist with the child's assessment and the establishment of intravenous access. Calculate and prepare the amount of intravenous fluid needed for administration according to the child's weight (20 mL/kg). Ensure rapid fluid administration by intravenous push or pressure bag. Monitor the child's physiologic response to the fluid bolus within 5 minutes. Prepare a second and third fluid bolus.

Use warmed intravenous fluids for resuscitation because hypothermia may interfere with the child's response to treatment. Keep the child covered or use heat lamps to reduce body-heat loss.

When packed red blood cells are administered, verify that the correct blood has been obtained for the child. Change the intravenous fluid to normal saline solution to prevent clotting during blood administration. Assess the child carefully for a transfusion reaction (see Chapter 15). Monitor the child's physiologic circulatory responses for improvement or deterioration in status. Notify the physician of any deterioration.

Provide support to the child and family during the acute phase of treatment. Parents and children with hypovolemic shock resulting from injury are usually apprehensive. The child may be fearful because of the sudden hospitalization or agitated because of an altered level of consciousness. Determine the causes of the child's anxiety. The parents often fear for the child's life in cases of injury. Update the parents about the child's condition frequently. Explain the care being provided and how it helps the child. Listen to their concerns and correct any misconceptions.

Evaluation

Examples of expected nursing care outcomes include the following:

- The child receives adequate fluid resuscitation to prevent progression to uncompensated shock.
- The family copes with the stress of the child's injury.

Distributive Shock

Distributive (septic) shock is an abnormal pooling of blood in the extremities that may be caused by anaphylaxis, sepsis, or spinal cord injury. Immunodeficient children are at high risk for septic shock. The blood accumulates in the extremities because of vasodilation and capillary permeability. Less blood is returned to the heart, so preload drops and cardiac output falls.

Septic shock begins as an infection and progresses to sepsis. Once a bacterial toxin enters the circulatory system, the body's inflammatory processes go out of control. White blood cells multiply throughout the body and macrophages produce cytokines, which dilate the blood vessels and increase permeability. Congestion occurs in some tissue beds, and bacteria may be trapped and multiply unchecked. Systemic and pulmonary edema develop as organ ischemia occurs (Hazinski, 1999) (Figure 14-11 ◆).

Septic shock has two phases: hyperdynamic and hypodynamic. During the hyperdynamic phase, the child has a fever, tachycardia, tachypnea, warm extremities, bounding

PATHOPHYSIOLOGY ILLUSTRATED

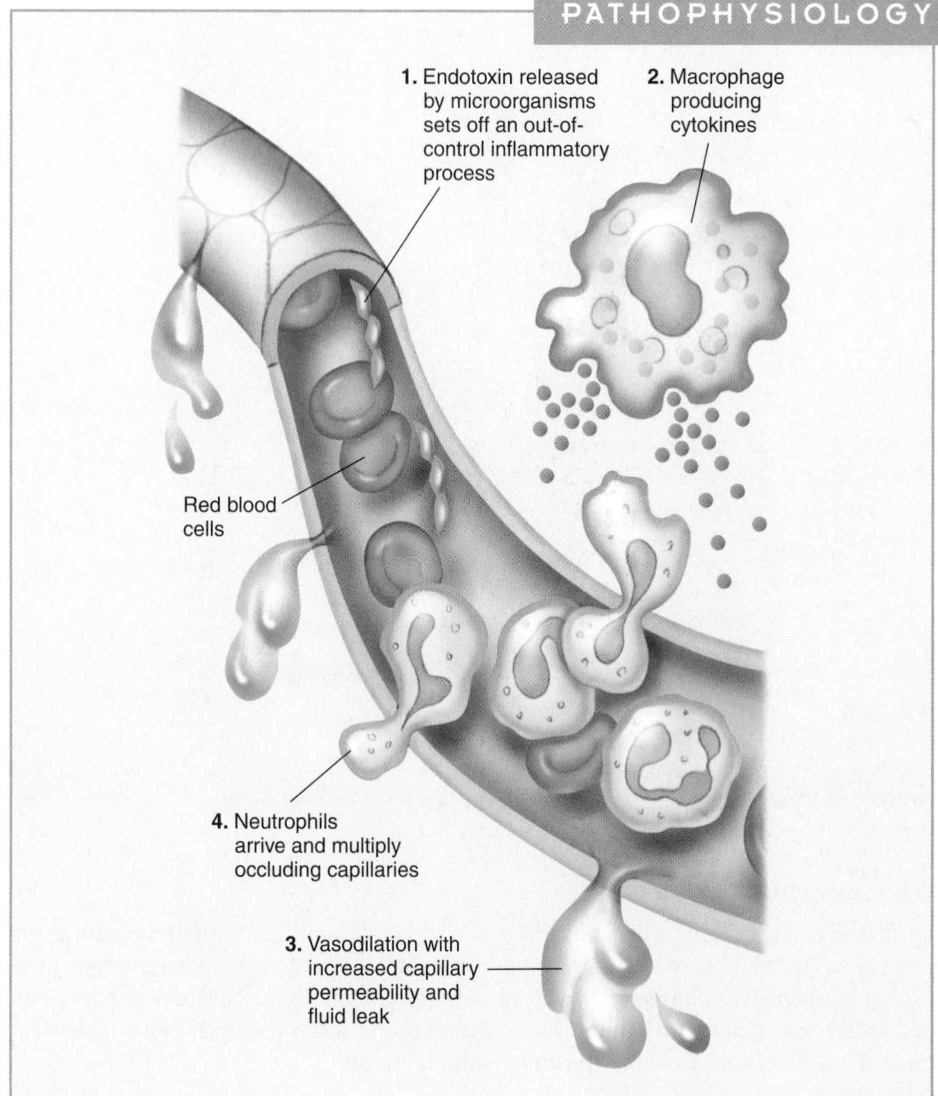

Septic Shock

FIGURE 14-11 ◆

In septic shock, blood pools in the extremities. Blood flow is sluggish and amounts of oxygen inadequate for cell metabolism are received by the tissues.

pulses, and brisk capillary refill. Perfusion appears adequate; however, because of infection and fever, oxygen demand in the tissues is much higher and perfusion is actually inadequate.

Cardiac output is high, but systemic vascular resistance is low, leading to an uneven flow and pooling in the extremities. Blood moves sluggishly, and anaerobic metabolism and lactic acidosis occur in tissue beds where oxygen no longer circulates. As the syndrome progresses, the hypodynamic phase develops. Cardiac output is low, and systemic vascular resistance is high. Blood has already pooled in the extremities. During the hypodynamic phase the child is cool, hypotensive, pale, and oliguric. Blood is shunted away from the kidneys, muscles, and skin to the heart and brain. Multisystem organ failure occurs if treatment does not improve regional perfusion.

Treatment for septic shock is initiated even before the diagnosis is confirmed. Fluid resuscitation is used in early septic shock to stabilize the circulation and ensure adequate tissue perfusion. Antibiotics effective against the suspected organism are given. Vasopressors are given during the hypodynamic phase. Morbidity and mortality are high even when treatment is initiated early. Complications include disseminated intravascular coagulation and adult respiratory distress syndrome.

PATHOPHYSIOLOGY ILLUSTRATED

Obstructive Shock

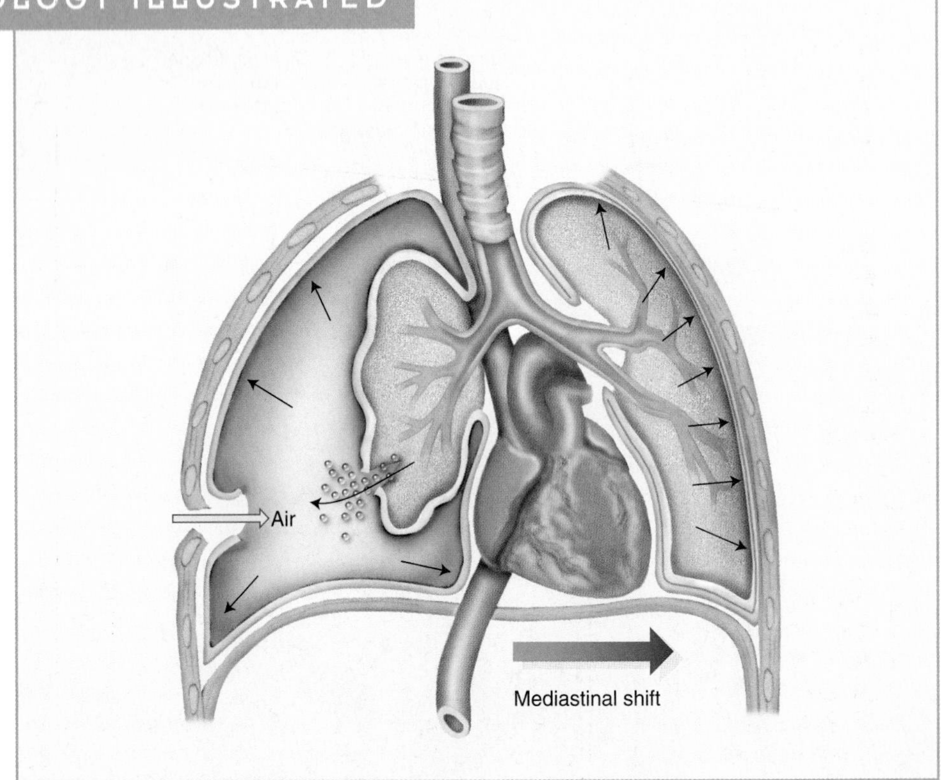

FIGURE 14-12 ◆
Mediastinal shift can occur when a tension pneumothorax obstructs blood flow to and from the heart. Here, the great vessels are compressed during the mediastinal shift leading to obstructive shock

Obstructive Shock

Obstructive shock occurs when a blockage of the main bloodstream interferes with tissue perfusion (Figure 14-12 ◆). Causes in children include compression of the vena cava, pericardial tamponade, pulmonary embolism, tension pneumothorax, pleural effusion, and congenital heart defects with outflow obstruction (e.g., coarctation of the aorta). Management is focused on treatment of the underlying condition.

Cardiogenic Shock

Cardiogenic shock is an abnormality of myocardial function in which the heart fails to maintain adequate cardiac output and tissue perfusion (Figure 14-13 ◆). Causes of cardiogenic shock in children may include congestive heart failure, congenital heart disease, cardiomyopathy, and arrhythmias such as bradycardia and supraventricular tachycardia. Cardiogenic shock may also be an end stage for other acute and chronic conditions such as sepsis, prolonged shock, asphyxia, hypoglycemia, and muscular dystrophy. Heart failure may result from obstructed outflow in congenital heart defects such as severe coarctation of the aorta and hypoplastic left heart syndrome.

Clinically, cardiogenic shock resembles hypovolemic shock with low cardiac output. Tachycardia, tachypnea, decreased oxygen saturation, hypotension, dimished peripheral pulses, and cool, pale extremities are common signs. Disorientation and restlessness occur as the compensatory mechanisms fail. Increased systemic vascular resistance puts more stress on the failing heart. Each contraction causes more blood to accumulate in the heart and pulmonary vessels, eventually leading to congestive heart failure, metabolic acidosis, and circulatory collapse.

The goal of medical treatment is rapid restoration of myocardial function with adequate ventilation, resolution of the initial metabolic insult, correction of arrhythmias, fluid management, and administration of diuretics and inotropic drugs.

PATHOPHYSIOLOGY ILLUSTRATED

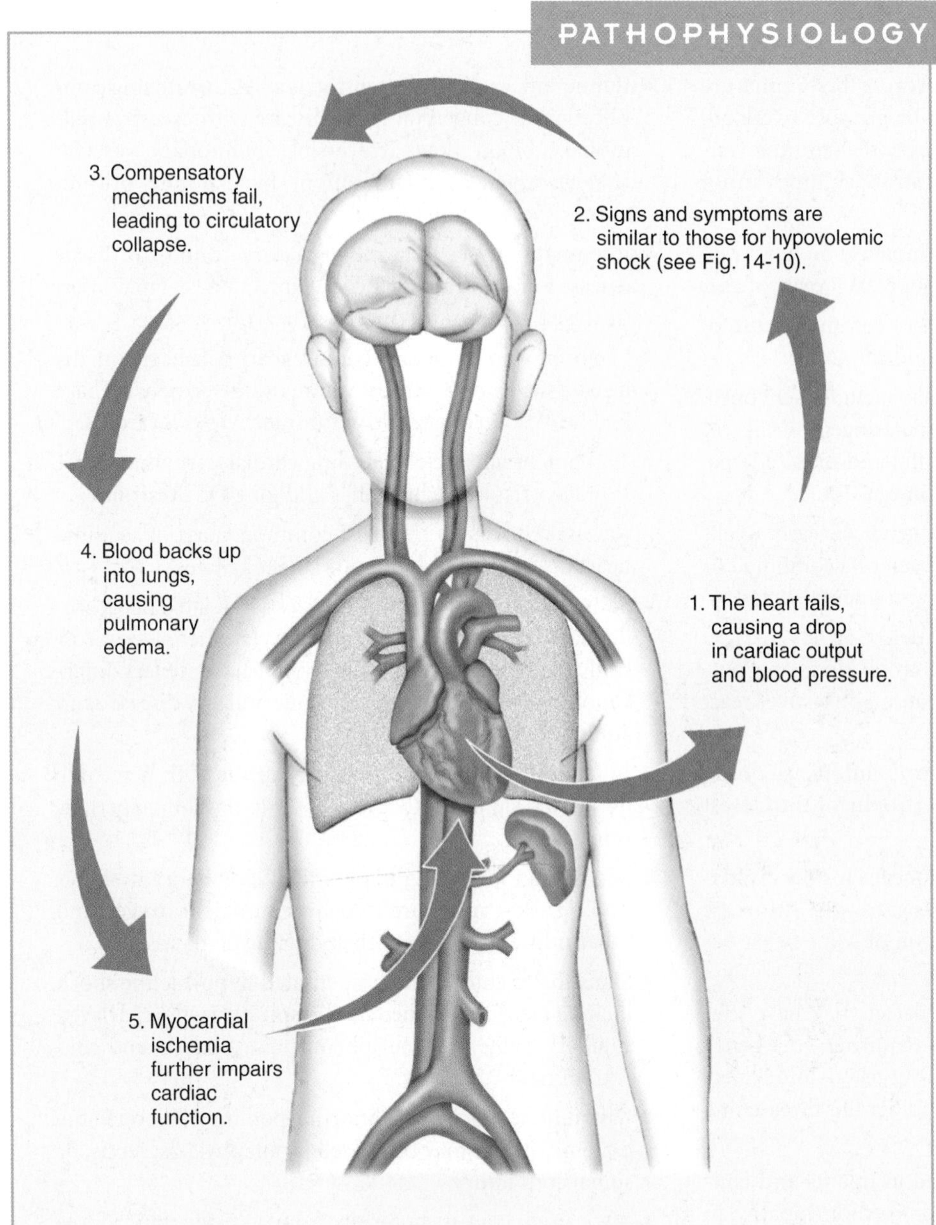

Cardiogenic Shock

FIGURE 14-13 ◆

When the heart fails, cardiac output and blood pressure decrease. Blood backs up into the lungs, causing pulmonary edema. Inadequate amounts of oxygen reach the myocardium, further impairing the heart's pumping action. The result is cardiogenic shock.

MYOCARDIAL CONTUSION

Myocardial contusion, a rare injury in children, results from a strong, blunt force against the chest wall that injures the heart muscle. Blood flow to areas of the heart muscle is disrupted, or myocardial cells are directly destroyed. This potentially life-threatening condition is often associated with a motor vehicle–related injury. It most often occurs in adolescents who have struck the steering wheel of a motor vehicle during a crash or children who have been struck in the chest with a baseball.

A myocardial contusion should be suspected in cases of injury to the anterior chest. The child has chest discomfort because of fractured ribs or chest wall contusion. An electrocardiogram reveals arrhythmias or signs of myocardial infarct. An echocardiogram may show an abnormality in heart wall movement. Cardiac isoenzyme concentrations are elevated. Because of the risk of sudden arrhythmias, the child is admitted to the intensive care unit for cardiac monitoring.

Chapter Highlights

- Infants are at risk of heart failure because their immature heart is more sensitive to volume or pressure overload. The heart muscle fibers are less developed and the ventricles have less compliance so that stroke volume cannot increase substantially.
- Cardiac output depends almost completely on heart rate until the heart muscle is fully developed at 5 years of age.
- Congenital heart defects are the most common cause of congestive heart failure in infants and children.
- Signs of congestive heart failure may include tachypnea, tachycardia, pallor or cyanosis, nasal flaring, grunting, retractions, cough, crackles, periorbital and facial edema, jugular vein distention, and hepatomegaly.
- Congenital heart defects develop during the early weeks of pregnancy and are usually the result of a combined or interactive effect of genetic and environmental factors.
- In nonobstructive acyanotic heart defects, a left-to-right shunt allows extra blood volume to overload the pulmonary system and potentially cause congestive heart failure.
- An obstructive defect (i.e., aortic or pulmonic stenosis) causes pressure overload and hypertrophy of the closest ventricle.
- Cardiac catheterization provides a means for the evaluation of hemodynamics and pressure gradients within the heart, and for noninvasive correction of some heart defects.
- The child with a cyanotic heart defect may have life-threatening hypercyanotic spells requiring emergency treatment. Palliative or corrective surgery is often performed soon afterwards to prevent other life-threatening attacks.
- Heart transplantation is performed in infants and children for complex heart defects or cardiomyopathy in children.
- Pulmonary artery hypertension is a life-threatening complication of congenital heart disease with excessive pulmonary blood flow. Irreversible pulmonary vascular changes include inflammation, hypertrophy of pulmonary vessels, and fibrosis.
- Rheumatic fever is an inflammatory connective tissue disease following a streptococcal infection that may affect the heart, joints, skin, or central nervous system.
- Children who have a congenital heart defect, rheumatic heart disease, or a central venous catheter or who have had heart surgery are at risk for infective endocarditis.
- Two potentially life-threatening cardiac arrhythmias are supraventricular tachycardias and long QT syndrome.
- Kawasaki disease is the most common cause of acquired heart disease in children in the United States.
- Some children have familial or lifestyle-related hyperlipidemia that causes undesirable levels of cholesterol or triglycerides. These children should have dietary intervention to reduce the risk of coronary artery disease as an adult.
- All children with blood pressures in the 90th percentile for age are significantly more likely to develop hypertension as adults.
- Shock is an acute, complex state of circulatory dysfunction resulting in failure to deliver sufficient oxygen and other nutrients to meet cell and tissue demands.
- Signs that a child is in compensated hypovolemic shock include tachycardia, increased respiratory effort, delayed capillary refill, weak peripheral pulses, pallor, and cold extremities.
- Distributive shock is an abnormal pooling of blood in the extremities that may be caused by anaphylaxis, sepsis, or spinal cord injury.
- Myocardial contusion results from a strong, blunt force against the chest wall that injures the heart muscle, and may cause an arrhythmia.

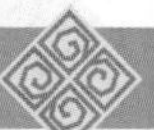

EXPLORE MediaLink

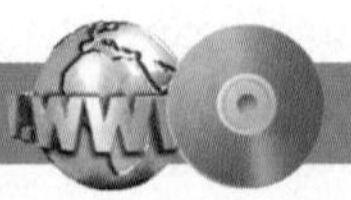

- NCLEX review, case studies, and other interactive resources for this chapter can be found on the Companion Website at **http://www.prenhall.com/ball.** Click on Chapter 14 to select the activities for this chapter.
- For animations, more NCLEX review questions, and an audio glossary, access the accompanying CD-ROM in this textbook.

References

1. American Academy of Pediatrics Committee on Pediatric Emergency Medicine. (1999). Emergency preparedness of children with special health care needs. *Pediatrics, 104*(4), e53.
2. American Heart Association. (2001). Incidence of congenital heart defects. *www.americanheart.org/children/hworks.html.*
3. Balaguru, D., Artman, M., & Auslender, M. (2000). Management of heart failure in children. *Current Problems in Pediatrics, 30*(1), 1–36.
4. Barst, R. J. (1999). Recent advances in the treatment of pediatric pulmonary artery hypertension. *Pediatric Clinics of North America, 46*(2), 331–345.
5. Bartosh, S. M., & Aronson, A. J. (1999). Childhood hypertension: An update on etiology, diagnosis, and treatment. *Pediatric Clinics of North America, 46*(2), 235–252.
6. Berul, C. I. (2000). Cardiac evaluation in the young athlete. *Pediatric Annals, 29*(3), 162–165.
7. Boneva, R. S., Botto, L. D., Moore, C. A., Yang, O., Correa, A., & Erickson, J. D. (2001). Mortality associated with congenital heart defects in the United States: Trends and racial disparities, 1979–1997, *Circulation, 103*(19), 2376–2381.
8. Botto, L. D., Khoury, M. J., Mulinare, J., & Erickson, J. D. (1996). Periconceptional multivitamin use and the occurrence of contruncal heart defects: Results from a population-based, case-control study. *Pediatrics, 98*(5), 911–917.
9. Boucek, M. M. (2000). Issues in pediatric heart transplantation. *http://transplantation.medscape.com/Medscape/transplantation/Clinical Mgmt/CM.v08/index-CM.v08.html*
10. Brook, M. M. (1999). Pediatric bacterial endocarditis: Treatment and prophylaxis. *Pediatric Clinics of North America, 46*(2), 275–287.
11. Case, C. L. (1999). Diagnosis and treatment of pediatric arrhythmias. *Pediatric Clinics of North America,* 46(2), 347–354.
12. Dajani, A. S., Taubert, K. A., Wilson, W., Bolger, A. F., & Bayer, A., et al. (1997). Prevention of bacterial endocarditis: Recommendations of the American Heart Association. *Journal of the American Medical Association, 277*(22), 1794–1801.
13. DeBoer, S. (1996). The care of the blue baby: Emergency department management of tetralogy of Fallot. *Journal of Emergency Nursing,* 22(2), 73–76.
14. Driscoll, D. J. (1999). Left-to-right shunt lesions. *Pediatric Clinics of North America, 46*(2), 355–368.
15. Duitsman, D. M., Suddaby, E. C., & Masterson, G. (1999). Unique considerations for the pediatric heart transplant recipient: The role of the school nurse. *Journal of School Nursing, 15*(3), 10–13.
16. Eichelberger, M. R., Ball, J. W., Pratsch, G. S., & Clark, J. R. (1998). *Pediatric emergencies* (2nd ed.). Englewood Cliffs, NJ: Brady.
17. Fedderly, R. T. (1999). Left ventricular outflow obstruction. *Pediatric Clinics of North America, 46*(2), 369–384.
18. Giddings, S. (1999). Preventive pediatric cardiology: Tobacco, cholesterol, obesity, and physical activity. *Pediatric Clinics of North America, 46*(2), 253–262.
19. Grifka, R. G. (1999). Cyanotic congenital heart disease with increased pulmonary blood flow. *Pediatric Clinics of North America, 46*(2), 405–425.
20. Hazinski, M. F. (1999). *Manual of pediatric critical care* (pp. 130–160). St. Louis: Mosby.
21. Hoffman, J. I. E. (1995). Incidence of congenital heart disease: I. Postnatal incidence. *Pediatric Cardiology, 16*(3), 103–113.
22. Hohn, A. R. (1997). Diagnosis and management of hypertension in childhood. *Pediatric Annals, 26*(2), 105–110.
23. Howard, J. K., Bindler, R. M., Synoground, G., & Van Gemert, F. C. (1996). A cardiovascular risk reduction program for the classroom. *Journal of School Nursing, 12*(4), 5–11.
24. Kohr, L. M., & Sims, S. L. (1998). Alterations in cardiovascular function in children. In K. L. McCance, & S. E. Huether, *Pathophysiology: The biologic basis for disease in adults and children,* (3rd ed., pp. 1093–1130). St. Louis: Mosby.
25. Krauss, R. M., Eckel, R. H., Howard, B., Appel, L. J., & Daniels, S. R., et al. (2001). AHA scientific statement: AHA dietary guidelines. *Journal of Nutrition, 131,* 132–146.
26. Lewin, M. B. (2000). The genetic basis of congenital heart disease. *Pediatric Annals, 29*(8), 469–480.
27. Mahle, W. T., & Wernovsky, G. (2001). Long-term developmental outcome of children with complex congenital heart disease. *Clinics in Perinatology, 28*(1), 235–247.
28. National High Blood Pressure Education Program, Working Group on Hypertension Control in Children and Adolescents. (1996). Update on the 1987 task force report on high blood pressure in children and adolescents: A working group report from the National High Blood Pressure Education Program. *Pediatrics, 98*(4), 649–658.
29. Nouri, S. (1997). Congenital heart defects: Cyanotic and acyanotic. *Pediatric Annals, 26*(2), 94–98.
30. Obarzanek, E., Kimm, S. Y. S., Barton, B. A., Van Horn, L., Kwiterovich, P. O., & Simons-Morton, D. G., et al. (2001). Long-term safety and efficacy of a cholesterol-lowering diet in children with elevated low-density lipoprotein cholesterol: Seven-year results of the dietary intervention study in children (DISC). *Pediatrics, 107*(2), 256–264.
31. Odim, J., Laks, H., Burch, C., Komanapalli, C., & Alejos, J. C. (2000). Transplantation for congenital heart disease. *Advances in Cardiac Surgery, 12,* 59–76.
32. O'Laughlin, M. P. (1999). Congestive heart failure in children. *Pediatric Clinics of North America, 46*(2), 263–273.
33. Park, M. K. (1996). *Pediatric cardiology for practitioners* (3rd ed.). St. Louis: Mosby Yearbook.
34. Petrini, J., Damus, K., & Johnston, R. B. Jr. (1998, September 25). Trends in infant mortality attributable to birth defects—United States, 1980–1995. *Morbidity and Mortality Weekly Report, 47,* 773–778.
35. Porto, I. (2000). Hypertensive emergencies in children. *Journal of Pediatric Health Care, 14*(6), 312–317.
36. Purath, J., Lansinger, T., & Ragheb, C. (1995). Cardiac risk evaluation for elementary school children. *Public Health Nursing, 12*(3), 189–195.
37. Robinson, B., Anisman, P., & Eshaghpour, E. (1996). Is that fast heart beat dangerous (and what should you do about it)? *Contemporary Pediatrics, 13*(9), 52–85.
38. Rowley, A. H., & Shulman, S. T. (1999). Kawasaki syndrome. *Pediatric Clinics of North America, 46*(2), 313–329.
39. Starr, N. B., & Freitas-Nichols, J. (2000). Cardiac arrythmias in children. *Journal of Pediatric Health Care, 14*(3), 127–129.
40. Steeg, C. N., Walsh, C. A., & Glickstein, J. S. (2000). Rheumatic fever: No cause for complaisance. *Contemporary Pediatrics,* 17(1), 128–141.
41. Stinson, J., & McKeever, P. (1995). Mother's information needs related to caring for infants at home following cardiac surgery. *Journal of Pediatric Nursing, 10*(1), 48–57.
42. Stumpflen, I., Stumpflen, A., Wimmer, M., & Bernaschek, G. (1996, September 28). Effects of detailed fetal echocardiography as part of routine prenatal ultrasonographic screening on detection of congenital heart disease. *Lancet, 348,* 854–857.
43. Waldman, J. D., & Wernly, J. A. (1999). Cyanotic congenital heart disease with decreased pulmonary blood flow in children. *Pediatric Clinics of North America, 46*(2), 385–404.
44. Walters, H. L. (2000). Congenital cardiac surgical strategies and outcomes: HEARTS. *Pediatric Annals, 29*(8), 489–498.
45. Williams, C. L., & Bollella, M. (1995). Guideline for screening, evaluating, and treating children with hypercholesterolemia. *Journal of Pediatric Health Care, 9*(4), 153–161.
46. Winter, W. E., House, D. V., & Schatz, D. (1999). Measuring and managing lipid levels. *Contemporary Pediatrics, 16*(5), 96–105.
47. Wolfe, R. R., Boucek, M., Schaffer, M. S., & Wiggins, J. W. (1997). Cardiovascular diseases. In W. W. Hay, J. R. Groothius, A. R. Hayward, & M. J. Levin (Eds.), *Current pediatric diagnosis and treatment* (13th ed., pp. 474–536). Stamford, CT: Appleton & Lange.

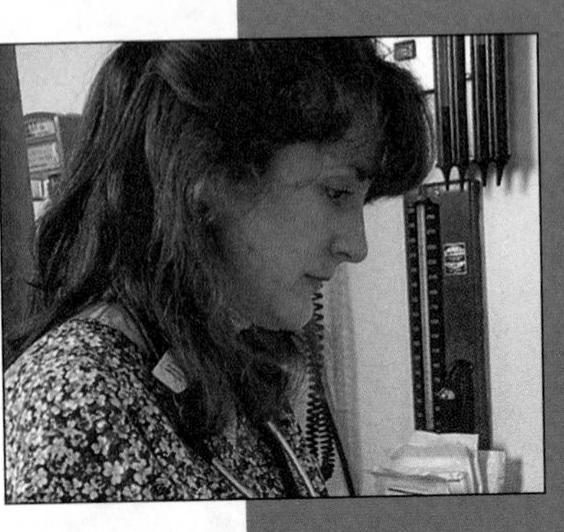

"My major concern is helping Michael to be comfortable. His pain was intense when he was admitted, and he was anxious and breathing rapidly. Once his pain is controlled, and the results of testing show what treatment he needs, we will manage the specific complications of his condition."

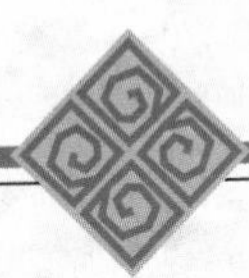

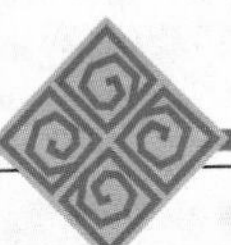

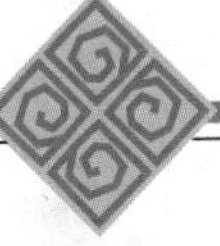

Michael is a 12-year-old black boy who is admitted to the hospital with severe abdominal pain. He was diagnosed with sickle-cell anemia at 1 year of age and has been in fairly good health. He has, however, been hospitalized on two previous occasions with complications of the disease. Recently, Michael has had several viral illnesses, leading his physician to suspect that his spleen is filled with abnormal cells, which are impairing his immune function.

Michael is small for his age and has several bruises on his lower legs. His respirations are rapid and he appears anxious. Michael's parents are knowledgeable about sickle-cell anemia, as his uncle also has the disease. They know that Michael is experiencing an episode of sickle-cell crisis.

An intravenous infusion is started, and Michael is medicated for pain. The nurse attempts to perform multiple tests and procedures together to allow Michael time to rest in between. Michael is receiving oxygen by nasal cannula to increase his oxygen saturation to normal levels.

What immediate and long-term care does Michael require? What do Michael and his parents need to know about this crisis? How could you help them manage the challenges of this condition? This chapter will assist you in planning care for children like Michael who have disorders of the hematologic system.

CHAPTER 15

ALTERATIONS IN HEMATOLOGIC FUNCTION

KEY TERMS

anemia Reduction in the number of red blood cells, the quantity of hemoglobin, and the volume of packed red cells per 100 mL of blood to below-normal levels.

ecchymosis A bruise.

erythropoiesis Formation of red blood cells.

hemarthrosis Bleeding into joint spaces.

hematopoiesis Blood cell production.

hemoglobinopathy Disease characterized by abnormal hemoglobin.

hemosiderosis Increased storage of iron in body tissues; associated with diseases involving the destruction of red blood cells.

leukopenia A lower than normal white blood cell count.

menorrhagia Increased menstrual bleeding.

pancytopenia A decreased number of blood cell components.

petechiae Pinpoint red lesions.

polycythemia Above-normal increase in the number of red cells in the blood to increase the amount of hemoglobin available to carry oxygen.

purpura Bleeding into the tissues, particularly beneath the skin and mucous membranes, causing lesions that vary from red to purple.

thrombocytopenia A low platelet count.

vaso-occlusion Blockage of a blood vessel.

MediaLink WWW http://www.prenhall.com/ball

Resources for this chapter can be found on the CD-ROM accompanying this textbook, and on the Companion Website at http://www.prenhall.com/ball. Click on Chapter 15 to select the activities for this chapter.

CD-ROM

Audio Glossary

NCLEX Review

COMPANION WEBSITE

Web Links

NCLEX Review

MediaLink Applications

- Ethical Considerations: Hemophilia
- Growth and Development Considerations: Bone Marrow Transplantation

The hematologic system is one of a few body systems that regulate, directly or indirectly, all other body functions. Because blood is involved in the function of all tissues and organs, changes in the blood may result in altered functioning of many body organs and structures. A tendency toward easy bruising is a characteristic sign of many bleeding disorders. Other signs include nosebleeds, pallor, frequent infections, and lethargy. This chapter discusses the most common disorders of the blood and blood-forming organs in children. (See Chapter 16 for a discussion of leukemia.)

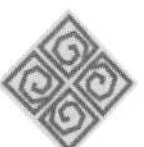

ANATOMY AND PHYSIOLOGY OF PEDIATRIC DIFFERENCES

Blood has two components: a fluid portion called plasma and a cellular portion known as the formed elements of the blood. The cellular elements are red blood cells (erythrocytes), white blood cells (leukocytes), and platelets (thrombocytes) (Figure 15-1 ◆). Table 15-1 gives normal values for these blood components in children.

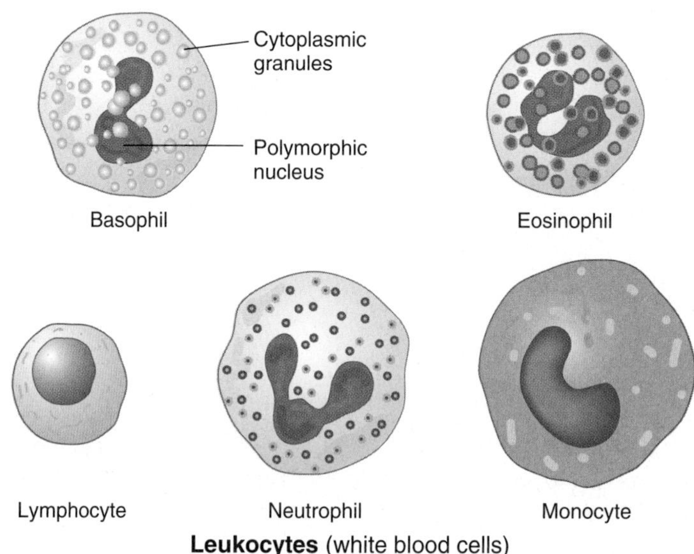

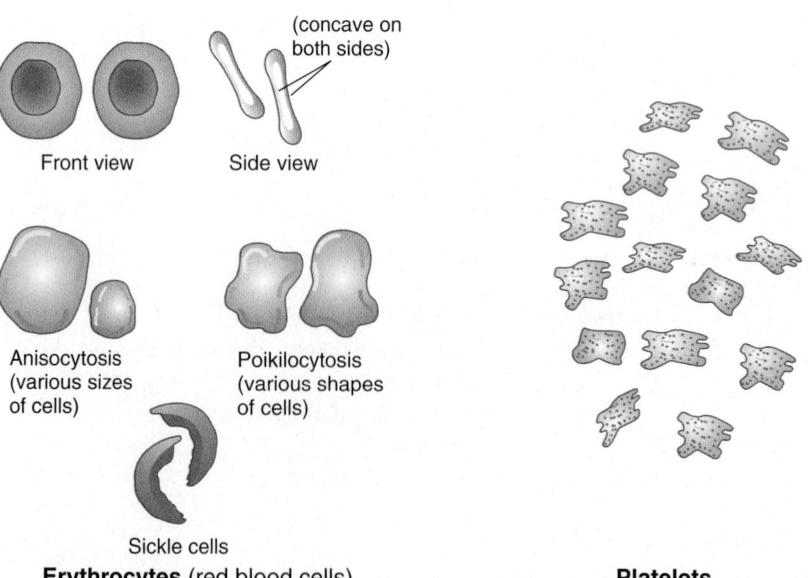

FIGURE 15-1 ◆
Types of blood cells.

TABLE 15-1 Normal Blood Values in Children

	NEWBORN	2 YEARS	12 YEARS	18 YEARS
Red blood cells (RBCs) (values × $10^6/\mu L$)	3.4–5.5	4.0–4.9	4.0–5.3	3.8–5.4
Hematocrit (Hct) (%)	37.4–56.1	31.7–37.7	34.0–43.9	33.0–46.2
Hemoglobin (Hgb) (g/dL)	12.7–18.6	10.5–12.7	11.2–14.8	10.7–15.7
White blood cells (WBCs) (values × $10^3/\mu L$)	6.8–14.3	5.3–11.5	4.5–10.1	4.4–10.2
Platelets (values × $10^3/\mu L$)	164–351	204–405	165–335	143–326

Note: Modified from Soldin, S. J., Brugnara, C., & Hicks, J. M. (1999). *Pediatric reference ranges* (3rd ed.). Washington, DC: AACC Press.

Production of red blood cells occurs in the fetus by the second week of gestation, with white blood cell and platelet production beginning at 8 weeks. Most of this early production occurs in the liver; however, by 20 to 24 week's gestation, liver production decreases as bone marrow production begins to predominate (Ohls & Christensen, 2000).

At birth, **hematopoiesis,** or blood cell production, occurs in the marrow of almost every bone. The flat bones, such as the sternum, ribs, pelvic and shoulder girdles, vertebrae, and hips, retain most of their hematopoietic activity throughout life.

RED BLOOD CELLS

Red blood cells, or erythrocytes, are the most abundant of the cellular elements of blood. They are formed through a process called **erythropoiesis.** The primary function of red blood cells is to transport oxygen from the lungs to the tissues. These cells also help to carry carbon dioxide back to the lungs. Hemoglobin, a red pigment composed of protein and iron, is essential to this function.

Polycythemia is an above-average increase in the number of red cells in the blood. Any condition that causes the quantity of oxygen transported to the tissues to decrease ordinarily increases the rate of red blood cell production. When a child becomes anemic secondary to hemorrhage, for instance, the bone marrow immediately begins to produce large quantities of red cells. **Anemia** is a reduction in the number of red blood cells; the various types of anemia will be discussed in the following section.

At birth, the newborn has a naturally occurring elevation in red blood cells (RBCs) due to a high level of erythropoietin, which stimulates red cell production (see Table 15-1). Once the newborn begins breathing air and the oxygen level in the blood increases, this production slows. Levels of RBCs fall until about 2 to 3 months of age, and then begin increasing. Adult levels are reached during adolescence. Teenage males have red blood cell levels slightly higher than teenage females (see Appendix C) (Lane, Nuss, & Ambruso, 1999).

WHITE BLOOD CELLS

White blood cells, or leukocytes, are the mobile units of the body's protective system. They are formed in bone marrow and lymph tissue. The white blood cell count is highest at birth, although levels vary greatly among infants. By 1 week of age, white blood cell values stabilize. Throughout childhood, there is a very slow decrease in white blood cell count (Boxer, 2000).

There are five types of white blood cells, each with a distinct function (Table 15-2). A differential blood count indicates the percentages of the different types of white cells present in the blood and is sometimes useful in identifying the cause of an illness. For example, infections cause an increase in neutrophils; and allergies are related to an increase in eosinophils. The role of lymphocytes is discussed with acquired immunodeficiency syndrome in Chapter 11. A decrease in the number of white blood cells is called **leukopenia,** and can be caused by immune or bone marrow disorders.

TABLE 15-2 White Blood Cells and Their Functions

TYPE	FUNCTION
Neutrophils	Phagocytosis
Eosinophils	Allergic reactions
Basophils	Inflammatory reactions
Monocytes (macrophages)	Phagocytosis, antigen processing
Lymphocytes	Humoral immunity (B cell), cellular immunity (T cell)

PLATELETS

Platelets, or thrombocytes, are cell fragments that can form hemostatic plugs to stop bleeding. They are synthesized from components in the red bone marrow and are stored in the spleen. Platelet levels in newborns are lower than in older children and adults. Levels of many clotting factors, particularly those requiring vitamin K for activation, are also lower in infants. For this reason, all newborns receive a prophylactic injection of vitamin K at birth. Values of platelets and other coagulation products soon reach normal childhood levels (Montgomery & Scott, 2000). A deficiency of platelets can lead to bleeding disorder and is termed **thrombocytopenia.**

ANEMIAS

TYPES OF ANEMIA IN CHILDREN

- Iron deficiency
- β-Thalassemia
- Aplastic
- Normocytic
- Sickle cell

Anemia is defined as a reduction in the number of red blood cells, the quantity of hemoglobin, and the volume of packed red cells to below-normal levels. This condition can be caused by loss or destruction of existing red blood cells or by an impaired or decreased rate of red cell production. Anemia also can be a clinical manifestation of an underlying disorder, such as lead poisoning or hypersplenism (a syndrome characterized by splenomegaly and blood cell deficiencies).

IRON DEFICIENCY ANEMIA

CULTURE

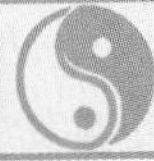

A number of genetic abnormalities of red blood cells that are rare in the United States are found among Southeast Asian immigrants. Many of these conditions can be confused with iron deficiency; however, most do not cause serious illness. Nurses who work with these cultural groups should seek out more specific information about such conditions (Glader & Look, 1996).

Iron deficiency anemia is the most common type of anemia and the most common nutritional deficiency in children. It can occur secondary to blood loss, or as a result of increased internal demands (rapid growth) for blood production, or due to poor nutritional intake. See Chapter 3 for a discussion of iron deficiency anemia due to deficits in nutritional intake.

Rapidly growing adolescents whose diets are high in fat and low in vitamins and minerals are particularly susceptible to iron deficiency anemia. Infants who do not take in adequate solid foods after 6 months of age and are fed only breast milk or formula that is not fortified with iron are also at risk because neonatal iron stores have been depleted by this time and their iron needs are not being met. Similarly, among mothers whose nutritional status during pregnancy was inadequate, and infants who were born prematurely or are products of multiple births, insufficient iron may have been stored in the latter part of pregnancy, placing the infant at higher risk for anemia in the first months of life.

Chronic blood loss is always a potential cause of iron deficiency anemia. The infant who has had bleeding in the neonatal period, the child who loses blood as a result of conditions such as hemophilia or parasitic gastrointestinal illness, and the adolescent girl who has **menorrhagia** (heavy menstrual bleeding), may all be at risk of anemia.

Clinical manifestations depend on the severity of the anemia. Pallor, fatigue, and irritability are characteristic findings. With prolonged anemia, nailbed deformities, growth retardation, developmental delay, tachycardia, and systolic heart murmur can occur.

Diagnosis is made on the basis of laboratory studies, including hemoglobin level, mean corpuscular volume, microscopic analysis (Figure 15-2 ◆), and serum iron-binding capacity. The red blood cells are microcytic (small) in size and hypochromic (pale) in appearance

(Cook, 2000). A diet history and analysis can provide information related to food intake; see Chapter 3 for guidelines about diet history.

Treatment involves correction of the iron deficiency with oral elemental iron preparations and a diet high in iron. Because oral iron preparations cause several side effects such as constipation and gastrointestinal discomfort, the child may receive iron supplements (to restore blood levels of iron) while the iron content of the diet is increased above the recommended dietary allowances (RDAs). Oral supplements can then be tapered off once the child's food intake can supply the needed iron. If the anemia is a result of bleeding, the cause is identified and treated to prevent future excess blood loss.

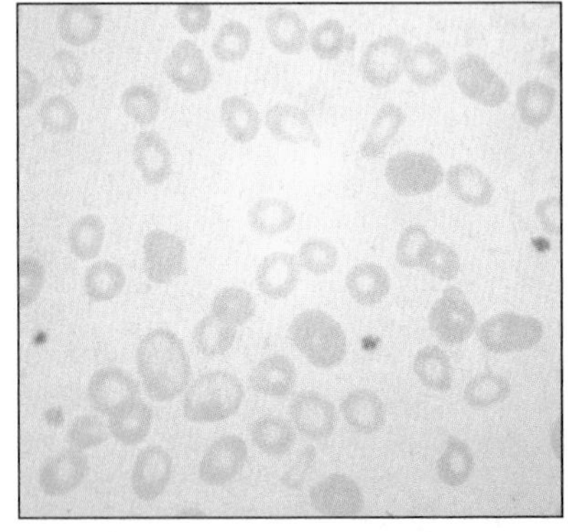

FIGURE 15-2 ◆ In iron deficiency anemia, red blood cells appear hypochromic as a result of decreased hemoglobin synthesis. Courtesy of Dr. Ed Wong, Laboratory Medicine, Children's National Medical Center, Washington, DC.

Nursing Management

Children with iron deficiency anemia are usually not hospitalized unless they have another serious illness. Nursing care focuses on screening for the disorder and educating the parents and children about the causes of iron deficiency anemia, dietary management, and the importance of complying with the medication regimen.

Screening for anemia is recommended at 9 months of age and again at adolescence (see Chapter 6) (American Academy of Pediatrics, 2000). A hematocrit or hemoglobin level is obtained. More detailed tests are performed if the blood test is abnormal. Children at high risk for nutritional deficiencies, such as those in low-income groups and WIC programs, may require additional tests. Most children in Head Start are screened annually by nurses. In addition, children showing signs of anemia should be screened. Height and weight measurements should be obtained at each health care visit, plotted on growth charts, and compared with percentiles obtained at previous visits. Slow downward trends in percentiles are of concern and require further nutritional analysis (see Chapter 3). Developmental screening tests should be performed to assess for developmental delays (see Chapter 6).

Dietary management is the preferred long-term treatment for iron deficiency anemia. Teach the family and child about foods that are rich in iron. Iron-fortified formula and baby cereals should be used in the diet of the infant. Older infants and toddlers can be provided with finger foods such as thinly sliced meats. Adolescents can be encouraged to eat foods with a high iron content, such as hamburgers and dried fruits.

Oral iron preparations are given to correct anemia. Teach the child and family that the liquid iron preparation should be taken through a straw because it stains the teeth. Instruct about side effects such as black stools, constipation, and a foul aftertaste. Emphasize the importance of drinking fluids and eating foods high in dietary fiber to minimize these side effects. Expected outcomes of nursing care are intake of recommended levels of iron and return to normal hematocrit level.

CULTURE 

According to traditional Chinese beliefs, a person who does not feel well is lacking in chi (inner energy) and blood. Chinese-Americans who follow traditional practices may be hesitant to have blood drawn for laboratory studies for fear of causing bodily weakness.

NORMOCYTIC ANEMIA

In normocytic anemia, the red blood cells, although decreased in number, are of normal size with a pale center (Cook, 2000). This type of anemia may occur as a result of hemorrhage, disease-induced inflammation, disseminated intravascular coagulation (DIC; see the discussion later in this chapter), G6PD deficiency, hemolytic–uremic syndrome (see Chapter 18), or several other conditions. When one of these conditions exists in a child diagnosed with anemia, the infectious or inflammatory condition should be suspected as the cause of the identified anemia and treated first. The anemia will often then correct itself if ample time is provided (Abshire, 1996). Some of the infectious and inflammatory causes of anemia are listed in Table 15-3.

Clinical manifestations are similar to those seen in iron deficiency anemia, with the possible occurrence of hepatomegaly and splenomegaly, as well. The etiology of normocytic anemia associated with chronic inflammation or infection is related to increased red blood cell destruction, decreased iron release from storage sites, and ineffective bone marrow response (Lane, Nuss, & Ambruso, 1999). In hemorrhage, anemia is a direct result of loss of blood.

Treatment of normocytic anemia depends on the underlying cause. When the anemia is associated with inflammation or infection, the underlying condition is treated. For anemia caused by renal failure, recombinant human erythropoietin is administered. When

TABLE 15-3 Infectious and Inflammatory Causes of Anemia

INFECTIONS	INFLAMMATIONS
Haemophilus influenzae type b	Arthritis
HIV/AIDS	Cancers
Orbital cellulites	Chronic heart or liver disease
Meningitis	
Septic arthritis	

hemorrhage is the underlying cause, the source of the bleeding is identified and treated. In acute emergencies, blood products are infused to make up for some of the losses.

Nursing management of normocytic anemia depends on the cause of the decreased red blood cells. Children with inflammatory or infectious diseases require careful assessment and management of medication and other treatment regimens. Administer blood products and other intravenous fluids as ordered to restore blood volume. Follow-up and home visits are used to assess hematocrit, hemoglobin, and dietary intake. (Refer to the discussion later in this chapter for management of DIC; to Chapter 17 for management of intestinal infections; and to Chapter 18 for management of hemolytic–uremic syndrome.)

SICKLE-CELL ANEMIA

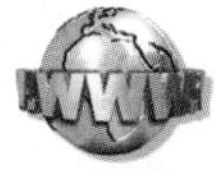

Sickle Cell Anemia Resources for Professionals

Sickle-cell anemia is a hereditary **hemoglobinopathy,** characterized by the partial or complete replacement of normal hemoglobin with abnormal hemoglobin S (Hgb S) (Table 15-4). Sickle-cell anemia occurs primarily in blacks, although occasionally it affects people of Mediterranean descent. Sickle-cell anemia occurs in about 1 in 375 black infants born in the United States, and 1 in 12 blacks have sickle-cell trait (i.e., they carry one gene for the disease) (Jakubik & Thompson, 2000).

Etiology and Pathophysiology

Sickle-cell anemia is an autosomal recessive disorder. If both parents have the trait, with each pregnancy the risk of having a child with the disease is 25%. (See Chapter 2 for a discussion of recessive gene transmission.)

In sickle-cell anemia, the hemoglobin in the red blood cell acquires an elongated crescent or sickle shape (Figure 15-3 ◆). The sickled cells are rigid and obstruct capillary blood flow. Microscopic obstructions lead to engorgement and tissue ischemia. This local tissue hypoxia causes further sickling and ultimately large infarctions. Damaged tissues in organs

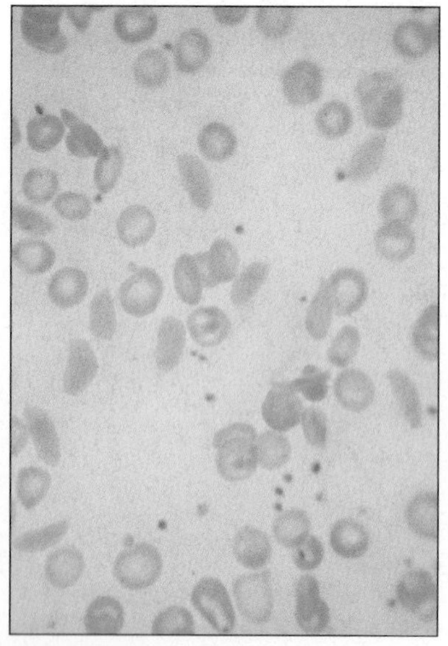

FIGURE 15-3 ◆
Many of these red blood cells show an elongated crescent shape characteristic of sickle cell anemia.
Courtesy of Dr. Ed Wong, Laboratory Medicine, Children's National Medical Center, Washington, DC.

TABLE 15-4 Sickle-Cell Disorders

Sickle-Cell Trait (Hgb SA) Most common form of sickle-cell disease in the United States Heterozygous condition (child has one sickle-cell hemoglobin gene and one normal hemoglobin gene) Child is carrier of sickle-cell anemia and rarely has symptoms of the disease
Sickle-Cell Anemia (Hgb SS) Homozygous condition (child has two sickle hemoglobin genes) Child is subject to sickle-cell crises
Sickle-Cell Syndromes *Sickle-cell–Hgb C disease (Hgb SC)* Second most frequent form of sickle-cell disease in blacks Different from sickle-cell anemia only in that the sickle-cell assumes a **C** shape instead of an **S** shape **Rarely occurs** Combination of sickle-cell trait and thalassemia trait most often seen in people of Mediterranean descent *Sickle-Cell–β-Thalassemia Disease (Hgb SB)*

throughout the body become scarred, resulting in impaired function. For example, children with sickle-cell anemia can suffer from splenic sequestration when blood is trapped in the spleen, a life-threatening complication. Many children must undergo splenectomy in early childhood, leading to severely compromised immunity. Infection rate is high due to impaired immunity, and bacterial infections are the leading cause of death in young children with sickle-cell disease. Strokes occur in 5% to 10% of children with sickle-cell disease and can lead to developmental delay, mental retardation, and other neurologic outcomes (Hendricks-Ferguson & Nelson, 1999).

Sickling may be triggered by fever and emotional or physical stress. Precipitating factors for sickle-cell crisis include increased blood viscosity (such as from a low fluid intake or fever) and hypoxia or low oxygen tension. Potential causes of hypoxia or low oxygen tension include high altitudes, poorly pressurized airplanes, hypoventilation, vasoconstriction when cold, or an emotionally stressful event. Any condition that increases the body's need for oxygen or alters the transport of oxygen (such as infection, trauma, or dehydration) may result in sickle-cell crisis.

Sickled cells can resume a normal shape when rehydrated and reoxygenated. The membrane of these cells becomes more fragile, however, and cell life is shortened to 10 to 20 days rather than the usual 120 days. In response, bone marrow spaces enlarge to produce more red blood cells. Continuous formation and destruction of the child's red blood cells contributes to the severe hemolytic anemia that is characteristic of sickle-cell anemia (Lane, Nuss, & Ambruso, 1999).

Clinical Manifestations

Affected children are usually asymptomatic until 4 to 6 months of age because sickling is inhibited by high levels of fetal hemoglobin. Clinical manifestations are directly related to the shortened life span of blood cells (hemolytic anemia) and tissue destruction resulting from **vaso-occlusion** (blockage of a blood vessel). Pathologic changes occur in most body systems and result in multiple signs and symptoms (Figure 15-4 ◆).

Illness results from recurrent vaso-occlusive events that involve painful crises and chronic organ damage (Odesina, 2001). Sickle-cell crises are acute exacerbations of the disease that vary markedly in severity and frequency. Table 15-5 outlines the most common types of crises affecting children with sickle-cell disease. These crises may occur individually or in combination. Michael, the boy described at the beginning of this chapter, was in sickle-cell crisis.

Children with sickle-cell trait rarely have such crises. However, because they have some abnormal hemoglobin, they may develop symptoms of the disease under conditions of abnormally low oxygen such as flying in an unpressurized airplane over 7,000 feet or during anesthesia. The most common symptoms experienced by those with sickle-cell trait are splenic infarction and hematuria. However, most persons who carry the trait never have symptoms, even with low oxygen concentrations.

TABLE 15-5 Types of Sickle-Cell Crises

Vaso-occlusive Crises (Thrombotic) Most common type of crisis; painful Caused by stasis of blood with clumping of cells in the microcirculation, ischemia, and infarction Signs include fever, pain, tissue engorgement
Splenic Sequestration Life-threatening crisis; death can occur within hours Caused by pooling of blood in the spleen Signs include profound anemia, hypovolemia, and shock
Aplastic Crises Diminished production and increased destruction of red blood cells Triggered by viral infection or depletion of folic acid Signs include profound anemia, pallor

PATHOPHYSIOLOGY ILLUSTRATED

Sickle Cell Anemia

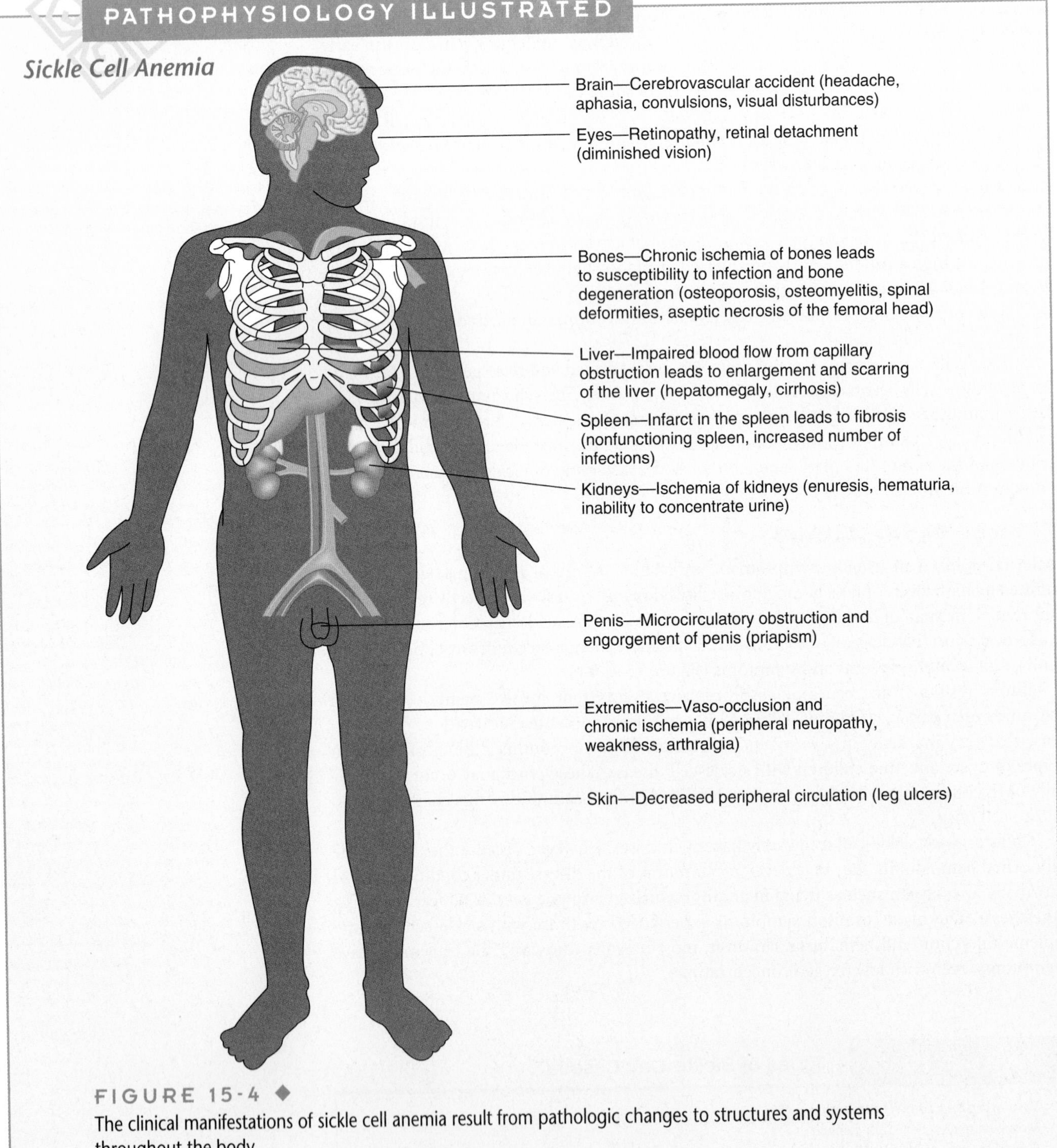

FIGURE 15-4 ◆
The clinical manifestations of sickle cell anemia result from pathologic changes to structures and systems throughout the body.

Clinical Therapy

The initial diagnosis of sickle-cell anemia in newborns is often made by testing cord blood using hemoglobin electrophoresis. The sickle-turbidity test (Sickledex) may be used for quick screening purposes in children over 6 months of age, once the fetal hemoglobin levels have fallen. Hemoglobin electrophoresis is performed to verify positive Sickledex test results. Newborn screening of infants for hemoglobinopathies occurs in forty-three states (Zimmerman, Ware, & Kinney, 1997). It is recommended that all newborns be screened, as sickle-cell disease can occur in several groups in addition to African Americans, such as those of Mediterranean, South American, Arabian, and East Indian descent. A child's heritage cannot be predicted from appearance or name alone.

No cure for sickle-cell anemia exists. Supportive care is aimed at the prevention and treatment of sickling episodes. Preventing exposure to infections and maintaining normal hydration are important steps in avoiding crises. Aggressive treatment of infection with antibiotics and use of daily prophylactic penicillin in children from 2 months to 5 years of age is effective (Davis, Schoendorf, & Gergen, et al., 1997). The reticulocyte count is monitored regularly to ensure that the bone marrow is still functioning.

Treatment of crises involves hydration, oxygen, pain management, and bedrest to reduce energy expenditure. Cultures (blood, urine, and throat) are taken to identify sources of infection. Other therapeutic measures include blood transfusions to treat the anemia and to make the sickled blood less viscous. In children who have had strokes from the disease, periodic transfusions (about every 3 to 4 weeks) can reduce the incidence of future strokes (National Heart, Lung, and Blood Institute, 1997). If given early in the crisis, blood transfusions may sometimes relieve the ischemia in major organs and body parts (spleen, lung, kidney, brain, and penis) caused by the vaso-occlusion. Antibiotics are administered for infection control, during acute infection, and sometimes as a prophylactic measure. Treatment with hydroxyurea has been helpful in adults, and is now sometimes used in children. This cytotoxic drug decreases production of abnormal blood cells and leads to a lesser amount of pain being experienced (Day & Wynn, 2000).

Children who have suffered a cerebrovascular accident (stroke) as a complication of the disease may be treated with blood transfusions on a regular basis. However, frequent transfusions may result in an overload of iron in the body. The iron is stored in tissues and organs (**hemosiderosis**), because the body has no way of excreting it. For this reason, an iron-chelating drug such as deferoxamine may be given with vitamin C to promote iron excretion.

Neonatal screening, early intervention, prophylactic antibiotics, and parent education have allowed children with sickle-cell disease to live into adulthood. Prognosis depends on the severity of the child's disease; children with more frequent exacerbations and hospitalization have poorer prognosis.

NURSING MANAGEMENT

Nursing Assessment and Diagnosis

The nurse may be involved in sickle-cell gene testing to identify carriers and children who have the disease. Once a child is diagnosed with the disease, a comprehensive physical assessment is essential because sickle-cell anemia can affect any body system.

Physiologic Assessment

In children who are known to have sickle-cell anemia, obtain a detailed history from the parents or child about past crises, precipitating events, medical treatment, and home management. Measure the child's height and weight accurately and compare with past measurements, since failure to thrive is common. Ask about chronic or acute pain that the child is experiencing. Pain may occur in nearly any body part, but most commonly manifests as headache, extremity pain, or abdominal discomfort.

The ill child with sickle-cell disease should receive a careful multisystem assessment. Fever is an emergency that necessitates prompt treatment (Zimmerman et al., 1997).

When the child is in crisis, assess pain and note the presence of any signs of inflammation or infection. Carefully monitor the child for signs of shock (see Chapter 14).

Psychosocial Assessment

The family of a child with sickle-cell disease requires a thorough psychosocial assessment. If the child is newly diagnosed with the disorder, the family will need assistance to deal with feelings related to the serious, life-threatening nature of the disease. Assess parents' understanding of the disease transmission and ask whether genetic counseling has been obtained. Determine whether the family has adequate health care coverage to pay for the

LAW & ETHICS

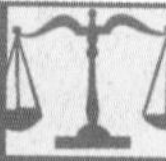

Information about genetic testing is confidential and must not be shared with persons other than those tested. In the 1970s, when genetic testing for sickle-cell disease and trait first became available, discrimination in jobs and insurance occurred against blacks who had the trait for sickle-cell disease.

Skill 8-6: Administering Blood or Blood Products

SAFETY PRECAUTIONS

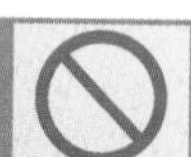

It is important for all health facilities to have current guidelines for transfusion protocols. Become familiar with the policies and procedures where you work. For example, does the child's blood type and patient identification need to be checked by two nurses before starting the infusion? See the Skills Manual for further discussion of blood transfusions.

NURSING CARE PLAN The Child with Sickle-Cell Anemia

GOAL	INTERVENTION	RATIONALE	EXPECTED OUTCOME
1. Risk for Altered Peripheral Tissue Perfusion related to affinity of hemoglobin for oxygen			
	NIC Priority Intervention: **Circulatory Care:** Promotion of arterial and venous circulation		NOC Outcome: **Tissue Perfusion, Peripheral:** Extent to which blood flows through the small vessels of the extremities and maintains tissue function.
The child will show few signs and symptoms of tissue hypoxia.	■ Instruct child to avoid physical exertion, emotional stress, low oxygen environments (e.g., airplanes, high altitudes), and known sources of infection. ■ Administer blood transfusions as ordered. ■ Perform several caregiving activities together when possible. ■ Give oxygen as ordered.	■ Decreased activity and exposure reduce body's need for oxygen. ■ Packed cells increase number of red blood cells available to carry oxygen to tissue cells. Transfusions promote circulation. ■ Grouping activities allows for optimum rest. ■ High concentration of oxygen in alveoli increases diffusion of gas across membranes.	The child has no shortness of breath and shows no signs of hypoxia.
Repeated cerebrovascular accidents will be avoided.	■ Administer and teach the family to administer prophylactic transfusions for the child who has had a cerebrovascular accident.	■ Lowers potential for a future cerebrovascular accident.	The child does not suffer a cerebrovascular accident.
2. Risk for Fluid Volume Deficit related to inadequate fluid intake			
	NIC Priority Intervention: **Fluid Management:** Promotion of electrolyte balance and prevention of complications resulting from abnormal or undesired fluid levels.		NOC Suggested Outcome: **Hydration:** Amount of water in the intracellular and extracellular compartments of the body.
The child will maintain or be restored to adequate hydration.	■ Calculate the child's daily fluid requirements. Moniter the child's usual fluid consumption and make necessary adjustments. Encourage the child to take fluids. Observe for signs dehydration. ■ Record intake and output.	■ Optimizing fluid intake ensures that the child gets needed fluid. Dehydration exacerbates crises. ■ Recording enables you to monitor daily fluid intake and spacing throughout the day.	The child shows signs of adequate hydration.

(continued)

child's medical expenses. Ask older children about their knowledge of the disease, and explore their feelings related to the management of a chronic condition. When siblings or other family members are carriers, counseling is needed periodically during the life span so that implications for dating, marriage, and having children can be understood.

Several nursing diagnoses that may apply to the child with sickle-cell anemia are presented in the accompanying nursing care plan. Other nursing diagnoses may include the following:

- *Caregiver role strain,* related to illness chronicity
- *Risk for altered parenting,* related to having a child with a physical illness

NURSING CARE PLAN The Child with Sickle-Cell Anemia (continued)

GOAL	INTERVENTION	RATIONALE	EXPECTED OUTCOME
3. Pain related to chronic physical disability			
	NIC Priority Intervention: **Pain Management:** Alleviation of pain or a reduction in pain to a level of comfort acceptable to the patient.		NOC Suggested Outcome: **Comfort Level:** Feelings of physical and psychological ease.
The child will verbalize that pain is controlled.	■ Administer analgesics, such as morphine or hydromorphine (Dilaudid), as ordered. Continuous intravenous infusion is used for the duration of a painful crisis. ■ Position carefully.	■ Pain of sickle-cell crises is excruciating. ■ Joints and extremities can be extremely painful.	The child is pain-free or pain control is significantly improved.
4. Risk for Infection related to chronic disease and splenic malfunction			
	NIC Intervention: **Infection Control:** Minimizing the acquisition and transmission of infections agents		NOC Suggested Outcome: **Risk Control:** Actions to eliminate or reduce actual, personal, and modifiable health threats.
The child will not develop infection.	■ Ensure adequate nutrition by providing high-calorie high-protein diet. Ensure that the child's immunizations are up to date. Report any signs of infection to physician immediately. ■ Isolate the child from possible sources of infection. Instruct parents about signs of infection and encourage them to seek prompt health care.	■ Chronically ill children are at greater risk of infection. ■ Restriction of persons with infection decreases the child's contact with infectious agents. Prompt care for infection reduces the chance of sickle-cell crisis.	The child is free of infection.
5. Knowledge Deficit (Child and Parents) related to lack of exposure about cause and treatment of sickle-cell anemia			
	NIC Intervention: **Teaching Disease Process:** Assisting the patient to understand information related to a specific disease process.		NOC Suggested Outcome: **Knowledge:** Extent of understanding conveyed about sickle-cell disease.
The child and family will verbalize understanding of risk factors for sickle-cell crises and how to minimize them.	■ Review basics of sickle-cell disease. Teach the child and family about signs and symptoms of crises. ■ Arrange for genetic counseling and testing for sickle-cell trait for family members if desired.	■ Knowledge of disease helps ensure compliance with treatment regimen and adherence to preventive measures. ■ Questions and concerns regarding future pregnancies can be allayed through knowledge of disease and transmission.	The child and parent can verbalize precipitating events of crises.

- *Altered growth and development,* related to effects of physical disability
- *Impaired physical mobility,* related to pain

Planning and Implementation

The accompanying nursing care plan summarizes nursing care for the child with sickle-cell anemia. Nursing management for the child in crisis focuses on increasing tissue perfusion, promoting hydration, controlling pain, preventing infection, ensuring adequate nutrition, preventing complications, and providing emotional support to the child and family.

CLINICAL TIP

When giving a transfusion, never infuse cold blood because it may increase sickling. Use a blood-warming coil to bring blood to room temperature.

NURSING ALERT

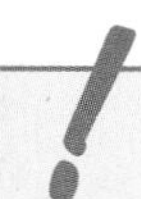

Blood reactions can occur as soon as the blood transfusion begins. Administer the first 20 mL of blood slowly and observe the child carefully for a reaction. Repeatedly assess the child according to hospital policy.

GROWTH & DEVELOPMENT

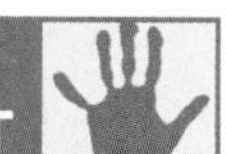

To encourage fluid intake in a small child:

- Use a favorite cup or glass.
- Use straws.
- Take advantage of times the child is thirsty, such as on awakening or after play.
- Leave a cup within easy reach of the child.
- Offer frozen juice pops, crushed ice drinks, and flavored ice chips.

NURSING ALERT

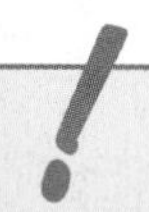

Neither hot nor cold compresses should be used for pain management in the child who has sickle-cell anemia. Ischemic tissue is fragile and has reduced sensation, increasing the risk of burn injury. Cold compresses promote sickling.

TABLE 15-6 Nursing Considerations for Blood Transfusion Reactions

TYPE OF REACTION	CAUSE	CLINICAL MANIFESTATIONS	NURSING INTERVENTIONS
Allergic reaction	Immune response	Urticaria, itching, respiratory distress	Stop the transfusion; call physician; give antihistamines as ordered; monitor vital signs; maintain intravenous infusion of normal saline; keep intravenous line open; check urine for hematuria
Hemolytic reaction	Mismatched blood, history of multiple transfusions	Fever, chills, hematuria, headache, chest pain; can progress to shock	

Increase Tissue Perfusion

Administer blood transfusions and oxygen as ordered. To prevent hemolysis, the intravenous fluid used before and after a blood transfusion must be saline rather than D5W. In small children, the blood is usually infused without saline because the child cannot manage the extra volume. Monitor for transfusion reactions (Table 15-6). Encourage the child to rest. Work with the child and family to avoid emotional stress. Any activities that increase cellular metabolism also result in tissue hypoxia. Schedule caregiving activities and play to allow for optimal rest.

Promote Hydration

The child with sickle-cell anemia is adversely affected by dehydration. Calculate the child's fluid maintenance requirements (minimum daily fluid intake) (see Chapter 10) and monitor the child's oral fluid intake. Administer intravenous fluids as ordered. Adjust oral intake as necessary to keep the child well hydrated.

Control Pain

Give prescribed analgesics around the clock during crises. If patient-controlled analgesia is used, be sure that the constant infusions run as ordered and that the parent or child understands the use of bolus infusions, when needed (see Chapter 9). Assist the child to assume a comfortable position. Avoid putting stress on painful joints.

Prevent Infection

Infection makes the child more susceptible to a crisis, and the crisis, in turn, increases susceptibility to infection. Teach the parents how to administer antibiotics for prophylaxis or treatment of infection. Be sure they have the finances and other resources to obtain and give daily antibiotics. Because infections can be particularly virulent and can cause death in these children, parents should be instructed to obtain immediate care when the child is ill. Encourage the use of the pneumococcal vaccine for all infants and children with the disease. The *Haemophilus influenzae* type b (Hib) vaccine series should be started at 2 months of age and continued at recommended ages to prevent another common source of infection.

Ensure Adequate Nutrition

Emphasize the importance of adequate nutrition to promote growth. Encourage the child to eat a high-protein, high-calorie diet. Emphasize the importance of folic acid supplements as ordered.

Prevent Complications of Crises

Observe the child for signs of increasing anemia and shock (mental status change, pallor, vital sign changes). Assess the child's neurologic status for evidence of altered cerebral function. If ordered, assess for an enlarged spleen by gentle palpation. Administer blood transfusions and watch the child for any adverse reaction.

Provide Emotional Support

Sickle-cell anemia is a chronic disease that is accompanied by life-threatening episodic crises. Family members often need support to help them deal with their feelings about the diagnosis and its implications. Explore resources in the home and community to see if parents will be able to administer medications and fluids and to provide adequate nutrition. Assess their knowledge of signs of infection and of sickle-cell crisis and when to seek medical care for the child. Refer the parents for genetic counseling, particularly if they plan to have more children. Encourage adolescents and young adults in the family to receive genetic counseling and testing, as well. Referrals to support groups and contact with others with the disease can be helpful.

COMPLICATIONS OF SICKLE-CELL ANEMIA

- Poor growth
- Delayed maturation
- Nonfunctional spleen
- Infection
- Crisis

Discharge Planning and Home Care Teaching

Home care needs should be identified and addressed well in advance of discharge. Provide parents with information about sickle-cell disease and the child's treatment. Even parents of a child previously diagnosed with the disorder may benefit from information about the disease process and its management. Explain the basic effect of tissue hypoxia and the effects of sickling on circulation. Refer parents to support groups such as the National Association of Sickle Cell Disease for further information.

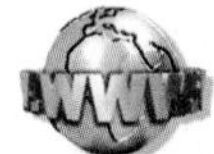

Sickle Cell Anemia Resources for Parents

Teach parents to look for signs of dehydration, such as dry mucous membranes, weight loss, and sunken fontanels in infants. Give specific instructions about how many ounces of liquid the child needs to drink each day. Emphasize that increased fluid intake is needed to replace the fluids lost from overheating or exposure to hot weather. Make sure both the child and family understand the triggers and precipitating factors for sickle-cell crises. Encourage them to avoid situations that cause crises. Instruct the child and parents about signs and symptoms of crises that should be reported to their health care provider (see Table 15-5).

Provide the family with careful instructions about infusion therapy. When regular blood infusions are used, the resulting iron overload is damaging to body organs. These children will need infusion of deferoxamine (Desferal) for iron overload. The medication is usually given by subcutaneous or intravenous routes over 8 to 10 hours. Prompt recognition of side effects and careful management of the lengthy infusion process are important. The child needs to be monitored for skin reactions and allergic responses. Have parents demonstrate the infusion technique and state what to do in case of reactions. Pain management is needed during infusion as the site may be tender and uncomfortable (Odesina, 2001).

Tell parents that it is important to inform all treating physicians and dentists of the child's medical condition. The child should also wear a medical identification tag. Special precautions are necessary when the child undergoes surgery of any kind, as hypoxia resulting from anesthesia is a major surgical risk.

FAMILIES WANT TO KNOW

Home Care Considerations for the Child with Sickle-Cell Anemia

Follow recommended schedules for well-child care visits.

Be sure the child is up to date with immunizations, including hepatitis B, annual influenza, pneumococcal vaccine, and tuberculosis skin test.

Special testing, such as heart and eye examinations, may be needed periodically to check for any sequelae of the disease.

Special medications, such as antibiotics, may be needed; pain relief medicine and blood transfusions may be administered.

Dehydration is dangerous. Be sure the child gets extra fluids in hot weather, when ill, during physical activity, and during travel.

As the child develops, provide information about the disease and encourage self-care. Be sure the school personnel understand the child's diagnosis and any care required during school hours.

Contact your health care provider if the child has a high fever, a common illness that lasts more than a day, seizures, change in behavior, severe pain, abnormal skin color or breathing pattern, or any other symptoms of concern.

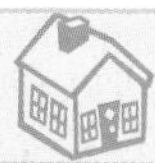

HOME CARE

Sickle-cell disease and some other hematologic disorders of childhood require that parents provide ongoing monitoring and care for their children with chronic conditions. Nurse researchers have found that parents describe a sense of chronic sorrow and eventual adjustment to the uncertainty of the condition. Nurses should realize that parents are constantly changing in their understanding and coping mechanisms. Periodic evaluations of their coping skills and needs are helpful in adapting teaching and resource recommendations to them (Northington, 2000).

Family members need ongoing support to deal with the stress of having a child with a chronic condition. Provide resources, respite care for parents, and information as needed for siblings.

Encourage older children with sickle-cell anemia to participate in activities with other children between crises, but to avoid strenuous physical exertion and contact sports. Play and social interactions that promote learning and development are important.

Evaluation

Expected outcomes of nursing care for the child with sickle-cell anemia include the following:

- Management of pain to facilitate comfort level
- Maintenance of adequate hydration state to prevent cell sickling
- Absence of side effects of disease in respiratory system, central nervous system and body organs
- Maintenance of normal immune status and prevention of infection
- Prompt recognition and treatment of complications of the disease
- Maintenance of normal growth and development for the child
- Provision of necessary services and resources for the parents and other family members
- Knowledge of disease and treatment by family

β-THALASSEMIA

The thalassemias are a group of inherited blood disorders of hemoglobin synthesis characterized by anemia that can be mild or severe. β-Thalassemia, also known as Cooley anemia, is the most common type. These disorders most often occur in people of Mediterranean descent but are also found among Middle Eastern, Asian, and African populations (Cook, 2000; Lane et al., 1999). If both parents carry the abnormal gene, with each pregnancy there is a 25% chance of passing the disorder on to the child.

There are three types of β-thalassemia: thalassemia minor, or thalassemia trait (produces mild anemia); thalassemia intermedia (produces severe anemia); and thalassemia major (produces anemia requiring transfusion). Clinical manifestations of β-thalassemia are caused by the defective synthesis of hemoglobin, structurally impaired red blood cells (Figure 15-5 ◆), and the shortened life span of the red blood cells. β-Thalassemia can be detected early in infancy. The infant with β-thalassemia manifests pallor, failure to thrive, hepatosplenomegaly, and severe anemia (hemoglobin < 6 g/dL). Diagnosis is made by hemoglobin electrophoresis, which shows a decreased production of one of the globin chains in hemoglobin. Characteristic erythrocyte cell changes often can be recognized in infants by 6 weeks of age.

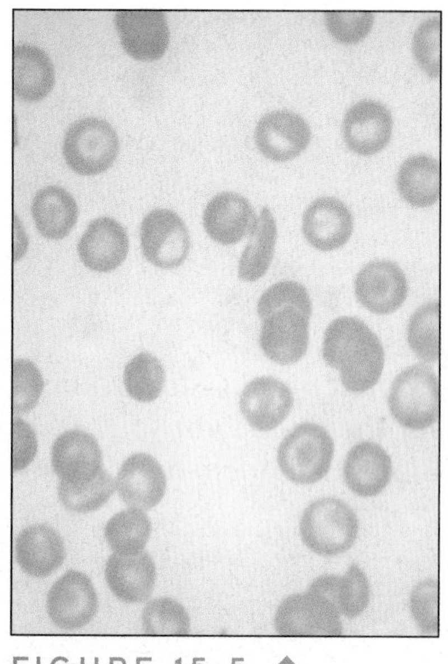

FIGURE 15-5 ◆
Red blood cell appearance in β-thalassemia. What characteristic abnormalities can be seen on this microscopic view?
Courtesy of Dr. Ed Wong, Laboratory Medicine, Children's National Medical Center, Washington, DC.

Treatment is supportive. The goal of medical management is to maintain normal hemoglobin levels. Blood transfusion is the conventional therapy used to treat children with severe disease. Since iron overload is a side effect of this treatment, children may need to receive an iron-chelating drug such as deferoxamine, which binds excess iron so it can be excreted by the kidneys. Other potential complications of long-term transfusion therapy are transfusion reactions and alloimmunization (antibody formation). Bone marrow transplantation may be offered as an alternative therapy for children newly diagnosed with the disorder.

Nursing Management

Nursing care focuses on observing for complications of transfusion therapy, providing emotional support, and referring the family for genetic counseling. Transfusions of packed cells are often given (see Table 15-6). Teach parents the technique for subcutaneous infusion of deferoxamine (to prevent iron overload) if that route is to be used for therapy at home. Give parents information about thalassemia and its treatment, and encourage them to obtain genetic counseling. Provide emotional support and encourage parents to take an active role in the child's treatment regimen.

Compliance with transfusion therapy often becomes an issue as children reach adolescence. Offering the adolescent treatment options, such as when to undergo transfusion, can

CLINICAL MANIFESTATIONS OF OF β-THALASSEMIA

BODY ORGANS	CLINICAL MANIFESTATIONS
Red Blood Cells (Anemia)	Hypochromic and microcytic changes Folic acid deficiency Frequent epistaxis
Skeletal Changes	Osteoporosis Delayed growth Susceptibility to pathologic fractures Facial deformities: enlarged head, prominent forehead due to frontal and parietal bossing, prominent cheek bones, broadened and depressed bridge of nose, enlarged maxilla with protruding front teeth, eyes with mongolian slant and epicanthal fold
Heart	Chronic congestive heart failure Myocardial fibrosis Murmurs
Liver/Gallbladder	Hepatomegaly Hepatic insufficiency
Spleen	Splenomegaly
Endocrine System	Delayed sexual maturation Fibrotic pancreas, resulting in diabetes mellitus
Skin	Darkening of skin

help to improve compliance. Adolescents with β-thalassemia and parents of newly diagnosed children can be referred to the Thalassemia Action Group, a national organization for patients, or to the Cooley's Anemia Foundation. Expected outcomes of nursing care include maintenance of normal hemoglobin and hematocrit, safe transfusion of blood products, maintenance of recommended body iron levels, and family understanding about the genetic transmission of the disease.

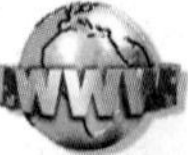

β-Thalassemia Online Support

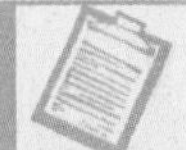

RESEARCH

The results of treating children with β-thalassemia by transplantation with bone marrow stem cells from family members have been successful. In a study at the University of California, San Francisco, overall survival with this treatment was 94%, those surviving without complications was 71% (Mentzer & Cowan, 2000). It is expected that collection of cord blood from siblings of affected children will also be a treatment of choice in the future (Reed, Walters, & Lubin, 2000).

APLASTIC ANEMIA

Aplastic anemia is a deficiency of the blood cells that results from failure of the bone marrow to produce adequate numbers of circulating blood cells. The condition may be congenital or acquired.

Congenital aplastic anemia (Fanconi anemia) is a rare autosomal recessive syndrome consisting of multiple congenital anomalies. Symptoms can include **purpura** (bleeding into the tissues) (Figure 15-6 ◆), **petechiae** (pinpoint lesions), bleeding, fatigue, and pallor. Laboratory findings include neutropenia or anemia and thrombocytopenia (low platelet count) that progresses to **pancytopenia** (decreased number of blood cell components).

Children with congenital aplastic anemia are at risk for developing malignancies such as acute nonlymphocytic leukemia (Pizzo & D'Andrea, 2000). The treatment of choice is bone marrow transplantation; however, the prognosis is poor, and death usually results from overwhelming infection, hemorrhage, or malignancy.

Acquired aplastic anemia in children is either idiopathic or occurs from a drug reaction. It can develop after exposure to ionizing radiation or insecticides or after ingestion of drugs such as sulfonamides, chloramphenicol, quinacrine, benzene solvents in model airplane glue, or lead. This type of anemia can also be a result of an infectious process such as viral hepatitis or mononucleosis.

Symptoms are related to the degree of bone marrow failure and can include petechiae, purpura, bleeding, pallor, weakness, tachycardia, and fatigue. Diagnosis is made by blood studies, which reveal leukopenia (low white blood cell count) with marked neutropenia, thrombocytopenia, and pancytopenia; and by bone marrow aspiration, which reveals yellow, fatty bone marrow instead of red bone marrow.

FIGURE 15-6 ◆
Nonpalpable purpura with bleeding into the tissues below the skin.
Courtesy of the Department of Hematology/Oncology, Children's National Medical Center, Washington, DC.

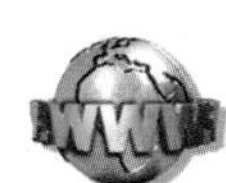

Aplastic Anemia Support

Supportive treatment includes transfusions of packed cells and/or platelets. Immunosuppressive drug therapy is effective for many children. The treatment of choice is bone marrow transplantation from a compatible sibling or family member donor.

Nursing Management

Nursing care is similar to care provided for the child with leukemia (see Chapter 16). Nursing actions focus on preventing bleeding, administering and monitoring blood transfusions, preventing infection, encouraging mobility as tolerated, educating the parents and child about the disorder, and providing emotional support. Families need support in dealing with a child who has a life-threatening disease. Refer them to support groups for counseling, if indicated, and to social services. Expected outcomes of nursing care include maintenance of normal levels of white and red blood cells and platelets to support body functions.

CLOTTING DISORDERS

HEMOPHILIA

Hemophilia refers to a group of hereditary bleeding disorders that result from a deficiency in specific clotting factors. Hemophilia A, or classic hemophilia, is caused by a deficiency of factor VIII in the blood and accounts for 80% of persons with hemophilia. About 1 in 5,000 male births result in hemophilia A (DiMichele, 1996). Hemophilia B, known as Christmas disease, is caused by a deficiency of factor IX. Of persons with hemophilia, 15% have hemophilia B.

Etiology and Pathophysiology

Hemophilia is an X-linked recessive trait, which manifests almost exclusively as affected males and carrier females. A daughter who inherits the trait from her father has a 50% chance at each pregnancy of transmitting it to her sons (see Chapter 2 for a description of genetic transmission). However, as many as one-third of hemophiliacs have no family members with a history of clotting disorders. In these cases, the disorder is caused by a new mutation. The degree of bleeding is related to the amount of clotting factor and the severity of the injury.

Clinical Manifestations

Hemophilia is manifested in different children by bleeding tendencies that range from mild to moderate or severe. Children with hemophilia often do not manifest symptoms until after 6 months of age as they become more mobile and incur injuries and bleeding from falls or from tooth eruption. Spontaneous bleeding, **hemarthrosis** (bleeding into a joint space), and deep tissue hemorrhage occur. Affected children frequently experience bleeding into the joint spaces of the knees, ankles, and elbows. Bleeding into joint spaces or bursae causes the child to have limited motion because of pain, tenderness, and swelling. Bone changes, contractures, and disabling deformities can result from immobility and from the effects of blood in the joint structures.

Children may have bleeding after circumcision, easy bruising (**ecchymosis**), nosebleeds, hematuria, and bleeding after tooth extraction, minor trauma, or minor surgical procedures. Large subcutaneous and intramuscular hemorrhages sometimes occur. Bleeding into the tissues of the neck, mouth, or chest is particularly serious because of the potential for airway obstruction. Retroperitoneal and intracranial bleeding may also occur and can be life threatening (Stover, 2000).

Females who carry the trait for hemophilia do not usually manifest symptoms of the disease. However, they may have prolonged bleeding during dental work, surgery, or trauma.

Clinical Therapy

Diagnosis of affected individuals and carriers can be done before birth through chorionic villus sampling or amniocentesis. Genes for clotting factors VIII and IX are located near the terminal long arm of the X chromosome (Montgomery & Scott, 2000). Genetic testing of family members is increasingly being used to identify carriers. Diagnosis can also be made on the basis of the history, physical examination, and laboratory data. Laboratory tests will show low levels of factor VIII or IX, and prolonged activated partial prothrombin time (APPT). Prothrombin time (PT), thrombin time (TT), fibrinogen, and platelet count are normal.

The goal of medical management is to control bleeding by replacing the missing clotting factor. Replacement therapy is indicated when the child experiences a mild or major hemorrhage or faces a life-threatening situation. Prompt and adequate treatment is needed to prevent serious bleeding episodes and their sequelae (Stover, 2000). A synthetic drug that is effective against mild hemophilia is desmopressin acetate (DDAVP). An analog of vasopressin, DDAVP is administered intravenously and causes a two- to fourfold increase in factor VIII activity. The outlook for children with hemophilia has been greatly improved by the availability of transfusion therapy. Transfusions started at home and early interventions prevent many disease complications. In the past, many children with factor VIII deficiency died in the first 5 years of life. Today, children with moderate or mild hemophilia can lead normal lives. Gene therapy is being explored for treatment of hemophilia. One approach is to infuse carrier organisms into the body where they would act on target cells to promote manufacture of deficient clotting factor. These research approaches offer the promise of new treatment options in the future (White, 2001).

NURSING MANAGEMENT

Nursing Assessment and Diagnosis

Physiologic Assessment

Obtain a complete medical history from the parents or child. In particular, ask about previous episodes of bleeding and the occurrence of hemophilia or any other bleeding disorders in family members. The history of bleeding will vary, depending on the severity of the disease.

Assess the child for any joint pain, swelling, or permanent deformity, particularly around the knees, elbows, ankles, and shoulders. Note the presence of hematuria and mild flank pain. A neurologic assessment should be conducted, as the risk for intracranial hemorrhage and bleeding can lead to peripheral neuropathies.

The adolescent with hemophilia should be screened for human immunodeficiency virus (HIV). Present testing methods make transmission of HIV to individuals with hemophilia very unusual. However, before universal testing of the blood supply began in 1985, significant numbers of hemophiliacs acquired HIV from infusions (see Chapter 11).

Psychologic Assessment

It is difficult for families to manage care of the hemophiliac child, especially if the disease is severe. Assess the family's coping mechanisms and support systems. Ask whether the family's health insurance covers the child's medical expenses; the factor concentrates and infusion equipment are costly. Find out if the parents have respite care that enables them to take time for themselves while knowing that the child is cared for safely. Assess older children's understanding of the disease and their adaptation to it.

Developmental Assessment

Because the child with hemophilia may have physical activity restrictions, physical skills may be delayed. Perform frequent developmental assessments, being particularly attentive to fine and gross motor skills.

The most important nursing diagnosis for the child with hemophilia is *risk for injury,* related to bleeding disorder. Following are other nursing diagnoses that may apply:

- *Pain,* related to bleeding episodes
- *Impaired physical mobility,* related to joint stiffness or contractures
- *Knowledge deficit (child and parent),* related to lack of exposure to illness

- *Altered family processes,* related to family role shift required to care for a child with a chronic illness
- *Altered growth and development,* related to effects of physical disability

Planning and Implementation

Nursing care focuses on preventing and controlling bleeding episodes, limiting joint involvement and managing pain, and providing emotional support. Both short-term interventions and long-term management are necessary.

Prevent and Control Bleeding Episodes

Bleeding problems are rare in infants with hemophilia. As children learn to walk and develop other motor skills, however, they often fall and suffer cuts and bruises. The risk of injury can be reduced by emphasizing to parents the need for close supervision and a safe environment. Parents should encourage children to play with toys that are safe and age appropriate.

If dental surgery or tooth extraction is necessary, it is performed in a controlled environment by experienced staff. Use of a dental irrigation device is often recommended if the child has excess bleeding from gums. Advise adolescents to shave only with an electric razor.

Control any superficial bleeding by applying pressure to the area for at least 15 minutes. Immobilize and elevate the affected area, and apply ice packs to promote vasoconstriction.

If significant bleeding does occur, offer supportive measures and assist with factor replacement therapy. Carefully monitor the child's condition for any side effects when factor replacement therapy is administered.

CLINICAL TIP

Take the following precautions when caring for children with bleeding disorders.

- Avoid taking temperatures rectally or giving suppositories.
- Check blood pressure by cuff as infrequently as possible.
- Avoid intramuscular or subcutaneous injections.
- Use only paper or silk tape for dressings.
- When indicated, perform mouth care every 3 hours with a glycerin swab.
- Except for factor replacement therapy, avoid all venipunctures.
- Use a peripheral fingerstick to obtain blood samples.
- Do not give aspirin.

Limit Joint Involvement and Manage Pain

During bleeding episodes, hemarthrosis is managed by elevating and immobilizing the joint and applying ice packs. Administer analgesics as ordered. Once bleeding has been controlled, range-of-motion exercises are performed to strengthen muscles and joints and to prevent flexion contractures. Physical therapy may be needed. Because excessive weight can place an added stress on joints, encourage the child to maintain an appropriate weight.

Provide Emotional Support

The needs of families with hemophiliac children are best met through a comprehensive team approach. Refer the parents for genetic counseling as soon as possible after diagnosis. It is important to identify family members who carry the trait, as they may suffer excessive bleeding during surgery.

Encourage the parents to verbalize their feelings. Be understanding and sensitive to their needs. Teach the parents about hemophilia and explain how the disorder affects both the child and other family members. Refer the parents and child to organizations such as the National Hemophilia Foundation for further information.

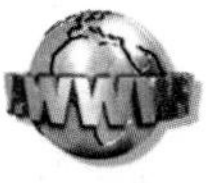

Hemophilia Family Resources

Discharge Planning and Home Care Teaching

The child may be hospitalized briefly during the first manifestation of bleeding or diagnosis and management. Most care will subsequently take place in the home. Home care needs should be identified and addressed well in advance of discharge. Advise parents to have the child wear a medical identification tag. Explain the cause of bleeding so both the child and parents understand the disease process. Teach the child and family how to identify internal bleeding. Signs and symptoms such as joint pain, abdominal pain, and obvious bleeding are indicators for immediate factor infusion. Make sure the child and parents know what situations could cause bleeding to occur. Teach parents to give acetaminophen instead of aspirin to relieve pain.

Instruct the parents and the child, when appropriate, in the preparation and administration of factor concentrate. If infusion of the missing factor is scheduled on a regular basis, bleeding episodes can be controlled or avoided. Have the parents demonstrate the procedure and make sure they can administer the product correctly. The parents need to be familiar with properties of the factor concentrate to prepare the mixture correctly.

COMMUNITY CARE

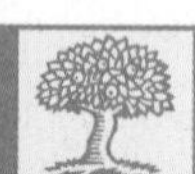

School personnel must be able to care for the hemophiliac child when bleeding occurs. Prompt care is essential. The nurse can identify key staff members in the school and teach them the actions that need to be taken.

The child will need an individual school health plan (see Chapter 6). Members of the school staff should be instructed in management of emergencies, and infusion equipment should be readily available. Dentists and other health care providers should be aware of the diagnosis.

Help the family and school to plan an appropriate schedule of activities without overprotecting the child. Children with hemophilia should not engage in contact sports such as football and soccer, which may result in injury and trauma. Instead, sports such as swimming, hiking, and bicycling should be encouraged.

Explain how the parents can coordinate their child's care with a number of health professionals. Provide ongoing case management, assisting the family to take on this task if able.

Hemophilia is not only a debilitating disorder for the child. It also can be financially draining for the family. Frequent outpatient visits, emergency department visits, hospital admissions, and the cost of factor concentrate can exhaust a family's resources. If indicated, referral should be made to appropriate social services (e.g., the state's maternal and child health program for children with special health care needs) and organizations such as the National Hemophilia Foundation. Sharing experiences with other families of children with hemophilia can provide support.

GROWTH & DEVELOPMENT

Encourage adolescents with hemophilia to participate in leisure activities such as computer games, reading clubs, and crafts. Knee pads, elbow pads, and helmets should be used when participating in any physical sports. Activities important to development can be encouraged when coaches, teachers, and others know how to treat bleeding episodes.

Evaluation

Expected outcomes of nursing care include the following:

- Prevention of injury to the child
- Maintenance of normal joint mobility
- Management of pain to promote comfort level
- Provision of safe and timely infusions as needed to treat the disease and prevent complications
- Promotion of normal growth and development
- Adequate knowledge of child and family for disease management, including recognition of bleeding and prompt initiation of infusions
- Support for family members in providing care for a chronic illness and in dealing with genetic implications of the disease

VON WILLEBRAND DISEASE

Like hemophilia, von Willebrand disease is a hereditary bleeding disorder. There are about 20 different disorders involving a deficiency of von Willebrand factor, which is a plasma protein and the carrier for clotting factor VIII, thereby playing a necessary role in platelet adhesion (McDaniel, 2000). The most common form of the disorder is transmitted as an autosomal dominant trait, and it can occur in both males and females. The gene for the disease is located on chromosome 12.

The characteristic manifestations are easy bruising and epistaxis. Children with von Willebrand disease frequently have gingival bleeding and increased bleeding with lacerations or during surgery. Affected teenage girls may have menorrhagia (increased menstrual bleeding).

Diagnosis of von Willebrand disease is made after laboratory studies reveal decreased von Willebrand factor levels, von Willebrand factor antigen levels, and factor VIII activity; reduced platelet agglutination; prolonged bleeding time; and prolonged or normal activated partial thromboplastin time (APPT). Treatment is similar to that for the child with hemophilia and involves infusion of von Willebrand protein concentrate. For bleeding episodes or prior to surgery, DDAVP is infused. Locally administered medications such as aminocaproic acid are sometimes used to manage bleeding in the mucous membranes.

Nursing Management

Teach parents about the disorder and instruct them not to give the child any aspirin or other drugs that can cause bleeding or inhibit platelet function. Teach management of bleeding episodes and intravenous infusion techniques, as for hemophilia. The prognosis is good, and children with von Willebrand disease usually have a normal life expectancy. Expected outcomes of nursing care include prompt management of bleeding and prevention of disease complications.

DISSEMINATED INTRAVASCULAR COAGULATION

Disseminated intravascular coagulation (DIC) is a life-threatening, acquired pathologic process in which the clotting system is abnormally activated, resulting in widespread clot formation in the small vessels throughout the body. Excess thrombin is generated, followed by deposition of fibrin strands in body tissues. These changes cause tissue hypoxia, resulting in eventual tissue necrosis. The circulating fibrin fragments later begin to interfere with platelet aggregation and other aspects of the clotting mechanism, resulting in bleeding or hemorrhage.

DIC is a complication of other serious illnesses in infants and children, such as hypoxia, shock, cancer, and viruses. Symptoms can include diffuse bleeding manifested by hematuria, petechiae, or purpura; an injection site that continues to ooze; circulatory collapse; and major vessel thrombosis (Lane et al., 1999). The prothrombin time and partial thromboplastin time are prolonged, platelet count and fibrinogen levels are increased, and levels of fibrin–fibrinogen split products are high.

Medical management is supportive and includes identification and treatment of the underlying disorder; replacement of depleted coagulation factors, fibrinogen, and platelets; and anticoagulant therapy (heparin).

Nursing Management

DIC is a complex disorder that is managed by a critical care team. Nursing care focuses on assessing the bleeding, preventing further injury, and administering prescribed therapies. Observe for petechiae, ecchymoses, and oozing every 1 to 2 hours. Be sure to check dependent areas, as blood will pool there. Intravenous sites are particularly prone to oozing and should be assessed every 15 minutes. Examine stool for the presence of blood, and measure blood loss as accurately as possible. Measure intake and output.

Because all body systems can be involved, careful assessment of all systems is needed on a continual basis. Institute bleeding control precautions, monitor prescribed therapy (transfusion, anticoagulant therapy), and report any signs of complications. Expected outcomes of nursing care are management of bleeding and adequate functioning of all body systems. Adequate family support in this life-threatening situation is a focus of nursing care.

IDIOPATHIC THROMBOCYTOPENIC PURPURA

Idiopathic thrombocytopenic purpura (ITP), also known as autoimmune thrombocytopenic purpura, is a disorder characterized by increased destruction of platelets, even though platelet production in the bone marrow is normal. When the rate of platelet destruction exceeds the rate of platelet production, the number of circulating platelets decreases and blood clotting slows.

ITP is the most common bleeding disorder in children. It occurs most frequently in children 2 to 10 years of age and usually follows a viral infection such as measles, chickenpox, or rubella, as part of an inappropriate immune response (Bolton-Maggs, 2000). Symptoms include multiple ecchymoses and petechiae. Diagnosis is made by history and through physical and laboratory findings, which show a decreased platelet count and antiplatelet antibodies in the peripheral blood. Treatment includes administering corticosteroids and intravenous immunoglobulins. For those children who do not respond to drug therapy over a period of 6 months to 1 year, splenectomy may be the treatment of choice. Spontaneous remission is seen in 90% of children with ITP.

Nursing Management

Nursing care focuses on controlling and reducing the number of bleeding episodes. Preventive measures are similar to those for the child with hemophilia. Teach parents to use acetaminophen, rather than aspirin, to control pain. Provide emotional support. Expected outcomes of nursing care are prevention of bleeding and restoration of normal coagulation patterns.

MENINGOCOCCEMIA

Meningococcemia is the most severe disease process that follows infection with *Neisseria meningitidis* or, occasionally, other microorganisms such as *H. influenzae* or *Streptococcus pneumoniae.* The disorder is thought to be an immune response to the endotoxins of the organism.

Onset is sudden: A respiratory infection is followed by high fever, petechial rash, massive skin and mucosal hemorrhage, hypotension, disseminated intravascular coagulation, and shock (Herf, Nichols, & Fruh, et al., 1998). The child, usually under 2 years of age, is critically ill and demonstrates multisystem disease. Symptoms can progress to a critical level within 12 to 48 hours of onset. Commonly the skin turns pink and then black as the tissues are damaged from reduced oxygen delivery. Limbs may need to be amputated as a result of impaired circulation.

Treatment consists of antibiotics, removal from sources of infection, and multisystem shock management. (See to Chapter 14 for a description of distributive shock.) Prompt administration of antibiotics to the child who manifests fever with purpura can decrease the severity of outcome. Depending on the child's condition, total parenteral nutrition, sedation and pain relief, dialysis, or amputation may be required. Close contacts of the child should receive prophylactic antibiotics.

Nursing Management

Nursing care of the child with meningococcemia is complex. Treatment must begin quickly and the child generally has a lengthy hospitalization in a pediatric intensive care unit (Hoag-Apel, 1997). Thorough assessments of all body systems are performed. Intravenous infusions must be administered when ordered to ensure correct and timely administration of antibiotics and other therapies. Urinary output is measured to evaluate kidney function. Meticulous skin care is necessary to preserve the integrity of tissues. Care is taken to prevent further infections. Nutritional support in the form of total parenteral nutrition is common. The family needs support to deal with the changing critical nature of the child's illness and the possibility that death or permanent, severe deformities will result. When the child improves, continuing comprehensive care in the hospital and then in the community is needed to manage complex issues related growth, development, nutrition, amputations, and prosthetics. Expected outcomes of nursing care include prevention of further infection, maintenance of body systems during the acute phase of illness, and positive adjustment to amputations and deformities resulting from the disease.

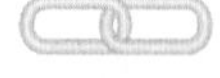

Skill 8-7: Administering Total Parenteral Nutrition

> **NATIONAL BONE MARROW REGISTRY**
>
> With the development of the National Bone Marrow Registry, bone marrow transplantation from HLA-matched unrelated donors has become possible for some children. Nurses may be typed and registered if they wish, or can assist in bone marrow registry drives.

BONE MARROW TRANSPLANTATION

Bone marrow transplantation is a treatment used for diseases such as severe combined immunodeficiency disease, severe and unresponsive aplastic anemia, and leukemia (see Chapter 16).

There are three types of bone marrow transplant: autologous, isogeneic (or syngeneic), and allogeneic. In autologous transplantation, the child's own marrow is taken, stored, and reinfused after the child has received chemotherapy. In isogeneic transplantation, the marrow is taken from an identical twin. In allogeneic transplantation, the donor, usually a sibling, has a compatible human leukocyte antigen (HLA). When no relative is found to match the child, a histocompatible donor may be sought from the National Bone Marrow Registry.

The transplantation procedure begins with chemotherapy and, sometimes, total body irradiation directed at destroying circulating blood cells and the diseased bone marrow in the ill child. Following this treatment, the child is transfused with the donor marrow. If the transplantation is successful, the donor marrow implants itself in the bone and begins to grow. Healthy bone marrow, capable of making blood cells, is the result.

The chemotherapy program for destruction of bone marrow takes 4 to 12 days. During this time, the child is cared for in strict isolation in a special unit that provides a germ-free environment (Figure 15-7 ◆). Side effects of chemotherapy provide challenges for care in addition to those of preventing infection (see Chapter 16). The child is without any immunity for a minimum of 10 days after transplantation. It takes 2 to 4 weeks for the donor cells

> **GROWTH & DEVELOPMENT**
>
> 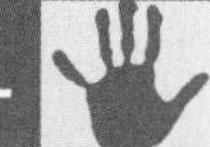
>
> Hospitalizations of children undergoing bone marrow transplantation are usually lengthy. Evaluate the child's age and developmental stage and establish developmental goals to be met during the hospitalization. Implement nursing plans to meet the child's developmental needs and encourage further growth.

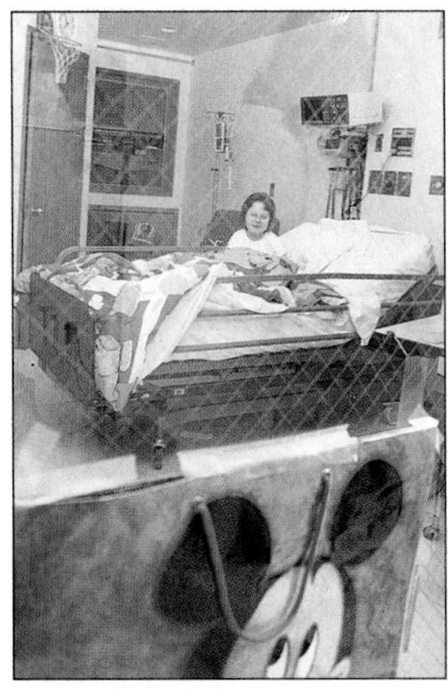

FIGURE 15-7 ◆
The child undergoing bone marrow transplantation is hospitalized in a special sterile unit while receiving chemotherapy before the transfusion. The child remains in the unit for several weeks afterward until the new marrow produces enough cells to maintain health.

to begin proliferation and maturation. Medications to stimulate the production of red and white blood cells are administered during this period.

Once the bone marrow begins to produce new cells, graft-versus-host disease (rejection) is the major threat. Refer to Chapter 11 for a discussion of this disease.

Monitor for this multisystem disorder by assessing the skin, mucous membranes, gastrointestinal function, respiratory function, cardiac function, and hydration status. Because graft-versus-host disease may occur at any time, even after the child returns home, frequent thorough assessments are necessary after discharge.

Supportive care after the transplantation procedure focuses on preventing infection, controlling bleeding, maintaining adequate nutrition and hydration, monitoring for signs of rejection, and providing psychosocial support. The treatment is lengthy, the child is often critically ill, and parents may have traveled to a medical center many miles from home for the procedure. Ask parents about other family members and how they are managing. Provide information about inexpensive housing available near the medical center, such as in a Ronald McDonald house. Encourage parents to discuss their feelings with other parents of children receiving bone marrow transplantation. Organizations such as the Bone Marrow Transplant Family Support Network can serve as resources for families.

When the child is ready for discharge, be sure the family is prepared to administer medications, recognize signs of graft-versus-host disease, provide adequate nutrition for the child, and perform other necessary care. Arrange for follow-up visits and provide the names of local health care contact persons who can offer support and provide information. The child may need tutors or other educational assistance to promote integration back into the school setting. The major expected outcome of nursing care is the proper activity of bone marrow in the child with resulting normal levels and function of blood cells. Other outcomes are provision of family support, ongoing care and education for the child, adequate nutrition, and prevention of infection.

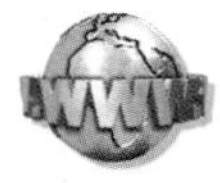

Bone Marrow Transplant Resources for the Family

Chapter Highlights

- Erythrocytes (red cells) are a major component of the blood and transport oxygen from the lungs to body tissues.
- Polycythemia is an increase in the number of red blood cells and anemia characterized by a decrease in red blood cell number. Leukocytes (white cells) are important in the cell's defenses against disease.
- Thrombocytes (platelets) are necessary for normal clotting of blood.
- The major anemias of childhood include iron deficiency anemia, thalassemia, aplastic anemia, normocytic anemia, and sickle-cell anemia.
- Sickle-cell anemia is a genetic disease in which an abnormal shape, or sickling of red blood cells, prevents the normal flow of blood.
- Major complications of sickle-cell anemia include pain, strokes, retinopathy, enlarged liver and spleen, urinary complications, poor peripheral blood flow, and osteoporosis.
- Nurses assist families in dealing with chronic diseases such as sickle-cell anemia by providing information about the disorder and resources that can provide assistance, monitoring child growth and development, instituting preventive care, and managing exacerbations of the disease.
- β-Thalassemia is also a genetic disease of red blood cells, and causes defective synthesis of hemoglobin.
- Treatment of thalassemia frequently involves regular blood transfusions; bone marrow transplantation is used in severe cases.
- Aplastic anemia is a deficiency of all blood cells related to poor bone marrow function; it can be congenital or acquired after exposure to certain drugs or harmful environmental toxins.
- Hemophilia is a bleeding disorder transmitted by genes; hemophilia A is most common and causes a decrease in clotting factor VIII.
- The goal of treatment for hemophilia is to control bleeding by preventive care and replacement of the missing factor.
- Major nursing concerns for the child with hemophilia include managing bleeding episodes, controlling pain during bleeds, minimizing physical immobility, supporting the family in learning management of this chronic disease, and explaining genetic implications of the disease.
- Disseminated intravascular coagulation is a serious condition in which clotting mechanisms are disturbed, leading to extensive clotting and tissue damage.

- Idiopathic thrombocytopenic purpura causes destruction of platelets and most frequently follows a childhood viral disease.
- Management of idiopathic thrombocytopenic purpura includes corticosteroids and immunoglobulins since the disease is considered to be autoimmune in nature.
- Occasionally, infection with organisms such as *Neisseria meningitidis* or *Streptococcus pneumoniae* is followed by a severe systemic disease known as meningococcemia.
- Meningococcemia is manifested by sudden high fever, rash, skin and mucosal hemorrhage, and shock; prompt treatment with antibiotics is needed.
- Bone marrow transplantation is a useful treatment in some diseases of the hematologic system and some cancers; it involves infusion of bone marrow from a donor into the blood where it circulates, implants into the bone marrow, and begins making new blood cells.
- Nursing care before and after bone marrow transfusions includes infection prevention, careful physical assessment, administration of medications, and support for the family.

EXPLORE MediaLink

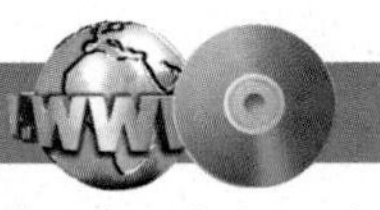

- NCLEX review, case studies, and other interactive resources for this chapter can be found on the Companion Website at **http://www.prenhall.com/ball.** Click on Chapter 15 to select the activities for this chapter.
- For animations, mor NCLEX review questions, and an audio glossary, access the accompanying CD-ROM in this textbook.

References

1. Abshire, T. C. (1996). The anemia of inflammation: A common cause of childhood anemia. *Pediatric Clinics of North America, 43*(3), 623–638.
2. American Academy of Pediatrics. (2000). *Guidelines for health supervision III.* Elk Grove Village, IL: American Academy of Pediatrics.
3. Bolton-Maggs, P. H. B. (2000). Idiopathic thrombocytopenic purpura. *Archives of Disease in Childhood, 83,* 220–223.
4. Boxer, L. A. (2000). Leukopenia. In R. E Behrman, R. M. Kliegman, & H. B. Jenson (Eds.), *Nelson textbook of pediatrics* (16th ed., pp. 621–626). Philadelphia: WB Saunders.
5. Cook, L. S. (2000). A simple case of anemia: Pathophysiology of a common symptom. *Journal of Intravenous Nursing, 23,* 271–281.
6. Davis, H., Schoendorf, K. C., Gergen, P. J., & Moore, R. M. (1997). National trends in the mortality of children with sickle cell disease, 1968 through 1992. *American Journal of Public Health, 87*(8), 1317–1322.
7. Day, S. W., & Wynn, L. W. (2000). Sickle cell pain & hydroxyurea. *American Journal of Nursing AJN, 100,* 32–38.
8. DiMichele, D. (1996). Hemophilia 1996: New approach to an old disease. *Pediatric Clinics of North America, 43*(3), 709–736.
9. Glader, B. E., & Look, K. A. (1996). Hematologic disorders in children from Southeast Asia. *Pediatric Clinics of North America, 43*(3), 665–682.
10. Hendricks-Ferguson, V. L., & Nelson, M. (1999). Update of the health care management needs of infants with sickle cell disease. *Journal of Pediatric Health Care, 13,* 217–222.
11. Herf, C., Nichols, J., Fruh, S., Holloway, B., & Anderson, C. U. (1998). Meningococcal disease: Recognition, treatment, and prevention. *Nurse Practitioner, 23*(8), 33–6, 39–40.
12. Hoag-Apel, C. (1997). Meningococcal disease. *American Journal of Nursing AJN, 97,* 33.
13. Jakubik, L. D., & Thompson, M. (2000). Care of the child with sickle cell disease: Acute complications. *Pediatric Nursing, 26,* 373–380.
14. Lane, P. A., Nuss, R., & Ambruso, D. R. (1999). Hematologic disorders. In W. W. Hay, A. R. Hayward, M. J., Levin, & J. M. Sondheimer, (Eds.), *Current pediatric diagnosis and treatment* (14th ed., pp. 723–773). Stamford, CT: Appleton & Lange.
15. McDaniel, P. (2000). Focus on factors. *Journal of Intravenous Nursing, 23,* 282–289.
16. Mentzer, W. C., & Cowan, M. J. (2000). Bone marrow transplantation for beta-thalassemia: The University of California San Francisco experience. *Journal of Pediatric Hematology and Oncology, 22,* 598–601.
17. Montgomery, R. R., & Scott, J. P. (2000). Hemorrhagic and thrombotic diseases. In R. E Behrman, R. M. Kliegman, & H. B. Jenson (Eds.), *Nelson textbook of pediatrics* (16th ed., pp. 1504–1515). Philadelphia: WB Saunders.
18. National Heart, Lung, and Blood Institute. (1997). *Periodic transfusions lower stroke risk in children with sickle cell anemia.* Washington, DC: U.S. National Library of Medicine.
19. Northington, L. (2000). Chronic sorrow in caregivers of school age children with sickle cell disease: A grounded theory approach. *Issues in Comprehensive Pediatric Nursing, 23,* 141–154.
20. Odesina, V. (2001). Intravenous support for the patient in sickle cell crisis. *Journal of Intravenous Nursing, 24,* 32–37.
21. Ohls, R. K., & Christensen, R. D. (2000). The hematopoietic system. In R. E. Behrman, R. M. Kliegman, & H. B. Jenson (Eds.), *Nelson textbook of pediatrics* (16th ed., pp. 1456–1460). Philadelphia: WB Saunders.
22. Pizzo, P. A. & D'Andrea, A. D. (2000). The pancytopenias. In R. E Behrman, R. M. Kliegman, & H. B. Jenson (Eds.), *Nelson textbook of pediatrics* (16th ed., pp. 1495–1498). Philadelphia: WB Saunders.
23. Reed, W., Walters, M., & Lubin, B. H. (2000). Collection of sibling donor cord blood for children with thalassemia. *Journal of Pediatric Hematology and Oncology, 22,* 602–604.
24. Stover, B. (2000). Training the client in self-management of hemophilia. *Journal of Intravenous Nursing, 23,* 304–309.
25. White, G. C. (2001). Gene therapy in hemophilia: Clinical trials update. *Thrombosis and Haemostasis, 86,* 172–177.
26. Zimmerman, S., Ware, R., & Kinney, T. (1997). Gaining ground in the fight against sickle cell disease. *Contemporary Pediatrics, 14*(10), 154–177.

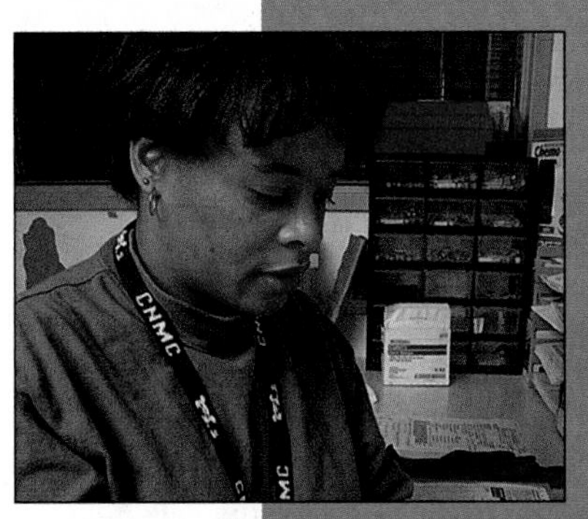

"THE NEWS THAT RASHEED HAD ENTEROCOLITIS WAS A BLOW TO HIM AND HIS FAMILY, BUT THAT SETBACK SEEMED TO MAKE RASHEED EVEN MORE DETERMINED TO FIGHT HIS DISEASE."

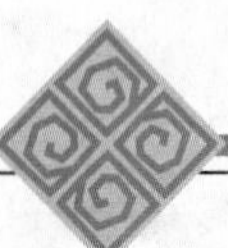

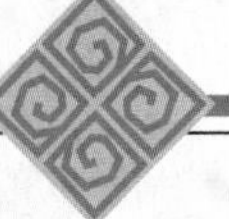

Twelve-year-old Rasheed is admitted to the hospital with fever and explosive diarrhea. He is diagnosed with enterocolitis, an invasive infection of the small intestine and colon that has occurred several months into his therapy for acute myelogenous leukemia. As Rasheed's condition worsens day by day, his anxiety grows. His mother, who took a 3-month leave from work during the early phases of his treatment, is unable to take additional time off from work to be with him. At last, with aggressive antibiotic therapy and supportive nursing care, Rasheed conquers the complication and returns home.

Rasheed and his parents feel they have met another challenge in his treatment for leukemia. When he was first diagnosed, 7 months earlier, Rasheed was severely anemic and bruised easily. He was hospitalized for a short time after diagnosis for implantation of a medication port and the first chemotherapy treatments. Soon, however, he was discharged home, returning for outpatient visits to receive chemotherapy and monitor his condition.

Rasheed has maintained a positive attitude throughout his treatment. He studied at home for a short time but has now returned to school. Keeping up with his school work has been made easier by the gift of a computer from the Make-a-Wish Foundation.

CHAPTER

16

ALTERATIONS IN CELLULAR GROWTH

KEY TERMS

benign A growth that does not endanger life or health.

biotherapy Use of biologic response modifiers to treat cancer.

carcinogens Chemicals or processes that, when combined with genetic traits and in interaction with one another, cause cancer.

chemotherapy Treatment to combat cancer that involves drugs taken orally, intravenously, intrathecally, or by injection, which kill both normal and cancerous cells.

complementary therapy Approaches to health care that are usually not part of conventional western medicine; sometimes called "alternative therapy."

extravasation Damage that occurs when a chemotherapeutic drug leaks into the soft tissue surrounding the infusion site.

leukocytosis A higher than normal leukocyte count.

leukopenia A lower than normal white cell count.

malignant The progressive growth of a tumor that will, if not checked by treatment, result in death.

metastasis The spread of cancer cells to other sites in the body.

myelosuppression A decreased production of blood cells in the bone marrow.

neoplasms Cancerous growths.

oncogene A portion of the DNA that is altered and, when duplicated, causes uncontrolled cellular division.

polypharmacy The use of many drugs at one time to treat multiple health conditions.

protocol A plan of action for chemotherapy that is based on the type of cancer, its stage, and the particular cell type.

protooncogene A gene that regulates cellular growth and development but can become an oncogene, capable of causing cancerous growth.

radiation Cancer treatment using unstable isotopes that release varying levels of energy to cause breaks in the DNA molecule and thereby destroy cells.

thrombocytopenia A low platelet count.

tumor suppressor genes Genetic material that controls the growth of cells, decreasing the effects of oncogenes.

MediaLink 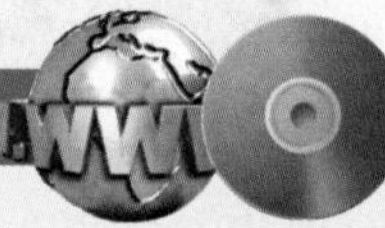 http://www.prenhall.com/ball

Resources for this chapter can be found on the CD-ROM accompanying this textbook, and on the Companion Website at http://www.prenhall.com/ball. Click on Chapter 16 to select the activities for this chapter.

CD-ROM

Audio Glossary

NCLEX Review

COMPANION WEBSITE

Web Links

NCLEX Review

MediaLink Applications

Exploring the Controversy: Stem Cell Transplantation

Life with Leukemia: A Teen in Transition

Why do children like Rasheed develop different types of cancers than adults? Cancer in adults is often the result of dietary practices or habits such as smoking. Some adult-onset cancers are the result of oncogenic responses to stimuli, that is, responses that stimulate cancerous changes in cells. Other cancers that occur in adults result from prolonged exposure to toxins such as coal dust and asbestos. Some cancers are known to be related to genetic causes. In adults, prevention through general lifestyle changes is a major focus of interventions. In children, however, cancer is usually embryonic (occurring during development of the fetus) or oncogenic in origin. Thus, lifestyle changes that begin in childhood have little effect on the incidence of childhood cancer, although they may have a positive influence on the incidence of later cancer or other diseases. Occasionally, an environmental exposure is linked to the incidence of cancer in children.

Abnormal cellular growth can occur in any area of the body. Why are some growths called cancer and others not? Changes in cellular growth within the body are called **neoplasms** (meaning new growth). A neoplasm is further classified as benign or malignant. **Benign** means that a growth does not endanger life or health. **Malignant** means that progressive growth of the tumor will, if not checked by treatment, result in spread to other sites in the body (**metastasis**), ending in death. The common term for this type of cellular growth is cancer.

ANATOMY AND PHYSIOLOGY OF PEDIATRIC DIFFERENCES

The major physiologic difference between adults and children that affects cellular growth involves the immune system and how well it functions in the defense of the body. The rate of cell growth in children also can play a role in the rapidity with which some childhood cancers progress. The continuing presence of fetal cells in small children is related to some cancers.

The immune system defends the body against foreign organisms and substances through two responses: nonspecific and specific. In a nonspecific response, the components of the immune system attack a variety of targets. Nonspecific components include phagocytic (cell destroying) cells such as mononuclear leukocytes, polymorphonuclear (PMN) leukocytes, natural killer (NK) cells, and complements (noncellular proteins) that work together to destroy invading cells and substances. During the first month of a child's life, the nonspecific response is immature, so phagocytic cells have little ability to move toward cancer cells and fulfill their function. The nonspecific response is also impaired in premature and small-for-gestational-age (SGA) infants.

In a specific response, T lymphocytes and immunoglobulin (Ig) attack only one type of invader. The specific response capability also is immature in infants. B-cell production of various proteins called immunoglobins (IgM, IgG, and IgA) is below adult levels, so that the infant is vulnerable to bacterial and viral infections. (For a discussion of immune function, see Chapter 11.)

In children, many cells are growing quickly; this fast growth can lead to the proliferation of both cancerous and normal cells.

CHILDHOOD CANCER

The care of children who have cancer is a challenging specialty in pediatric nursing. For several years, the child undergoes aggressive treatments that may be life threatening and cause temporary illness. Often the prognosis is quite hopeful; at other times, a terminal result may be expected. The child is cared for at home with outpatient visits for treatment and occasional hospitalization when needed. The periods of hospitalization are times of intense physical vulnerability for the child and intense emotional vulnerability for both the child and the family. To monitor the child closely, nurses need a sound knowledge of physiologic and psychologic responses, medical interventions, and nursing care. Effective communication skills are necessary to support the child and family and promote realistic hope.

INCIDENCE

During 2001, in the United States, cancer was diagnosed in approximately 8,600 children. In children under 15 years of age, cancer is the leading cause of disease-related death. In 2001, about 1,500 U.S. children died of cancer, one-third of these from leukemia (American Cancer

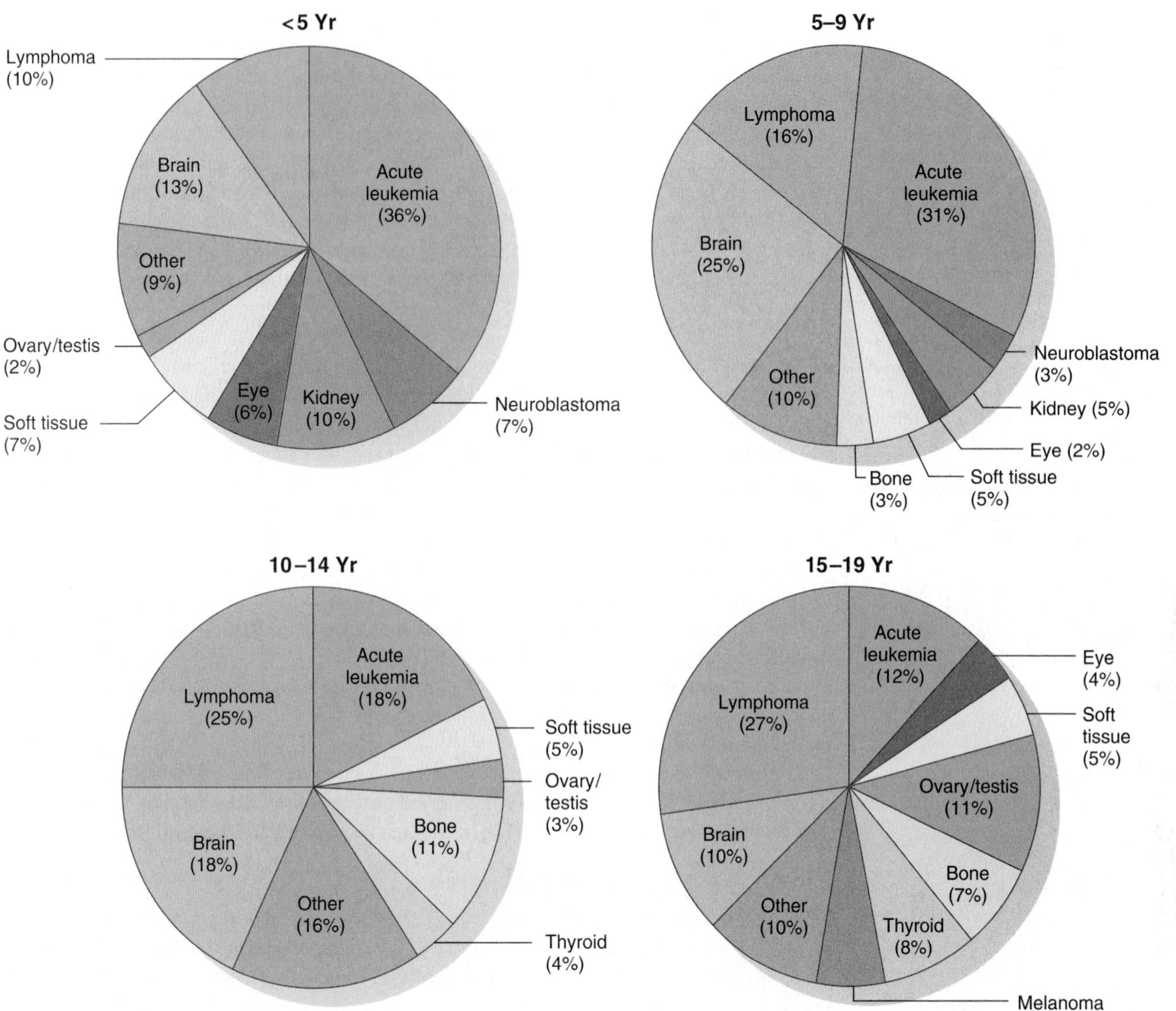

FIGURE 16-1 ◆

Percentage of primary tumors by site of origin for different age groups.

From Crist, W. M. (2000). *Neoplastic disease and tumors.* In R. E. Behrman, R. M. Kliegman, & H. B. Jenson (Eds.), *Nelson textbook of pediatrics* (16th ed., p. 1531). Philadelphia: Saunders.

Society, 2001). Mortality rates have declined by over 60% since 1960, and the rates continue to improve. Children treated in the 1980s and 1990s have had significantly lower mortality rates than those treated in the 1960s and 1970s. Mortality rates are higher for females than males, for those diagnosed before 5 years of age, and for children with a central nervous system tumor or leukemia. The cause of death for most children is recurrence of the primary cancer (Moller, Garwicz, & Barlow, et al., 2001). The most common forms of childhood cancers among children in different age groups are shown in Figure 16-1 ◆ (Behrman, Kliegman, & Jenson, 2000).

ETIOLOGY AND PATHOPHYSIOLOGY

Alterations in cellular growth occur in response to external and internal stimuli. Neoplasms are caused by one or a combination of three factors: (1) external stimuli that cause genetic mutations, (2) immune system and gene abnormalities, and (3) chromosomal abnormalities.

External Stimuli

External stimuli may affect the child's general health and cause mutations in body cells. **Carcinogens** are chemicals or industrial processes that, when combined with genetic traits and

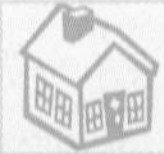

HOME CARE

Many parents ask what they can do to decrease the incidence of cancer in children as they grow into adulthood. The three major teaching areas to address are as follows:

1. Have children increase intake of fruits and vegetables. Most children do not eat enough of these foods and increased intake is associated with lower rates of many cancers.
2. Protect skin with sunscreen. Early excessive exposure to sun and having been sunburned increase chance of skin cancers in adulthood.
3. Discourage smoking among children and be sure children are not exposed to environmental tobacco smoke. This will decrease future chance of developing lung cancer.

in interaction with one another, result in cancer. Several carcinogens cause cancers that are diagnosed during childhood. Others cause cancers that begin in childhood but are not identified until adulthood. Some chemicals suspected of causing childhood cancer include diethylstilbestrol (maternal use of therapeutic estrogen hormones), anabolic androgenic steroids, alkylating chemotherapy agents, and immunosuppressants used for organ transplantation. Radiation exposure has been known to cause cancers such as leukemia and thyroid tumors in children exposed to atomic bombs and excessive radiation during diagnostic medical procedures. Secondary cancers can result when the child is treated for a primary cancer with high doses of radiation. Excessive exposure to ultraviolet radiation from the sun predisposes children to development of skin cancer in adulthood.

Immune System and Gene Abnormalities

One critical function of a normal immune system is immune surveillance, in which phagocytic cells circulate throughout the body, detecting and destroying abnormal and cancerous cells. Children with congenital immune deficiencies, such as Wiskott–Aldrich syndrome, in which immune surveillance may fail, are at high risk for cancer. A form of non-Hodgkin's lymphoma develops in some children treated with immune system–suppressing drugs. Children with acquired immunodeficiency syndrome (AIDS) may be at higher risk of certain types of cancer.

Viruses and other substances may act in the body to alter the immune system, thereby allowing cancer to occur (Figure 16-2 ◆). Their action is based on changing certain genes that normally regulate cellular growth and development (called **protooncogenes**) to related genes that allow unregulated cell division and cancerous growth (called **oncogenes**). Among the cancers thought to be linked to virus action and the change of protooncogenes to oncogenes are certain leukemias, rhabdomyosarcoma, Burkitt's lymphoma, and some forms of Hodgkin's disease.

Tumor suppressor genes counteract the effect of oncogenes, keeping cellular growth within normal limits. When tumor suppressor genes are missing, unstemmed cellular growth can occur. These genes are commonly missing in children with retinoblastoma and Wilms' tumor.

Chromosomal Abnormalities

Normal chromosomes undergo change as a part of the genetic process. Most of the changes are not harmful. However, some changes result in chromosomal abnormalities such as hyperploidy (more than the normal number of chromosomes), deletion, translocation, and breakage.

PATHOPHYSIOLOGY ILLUSTRATED

Protooncogene Alteration

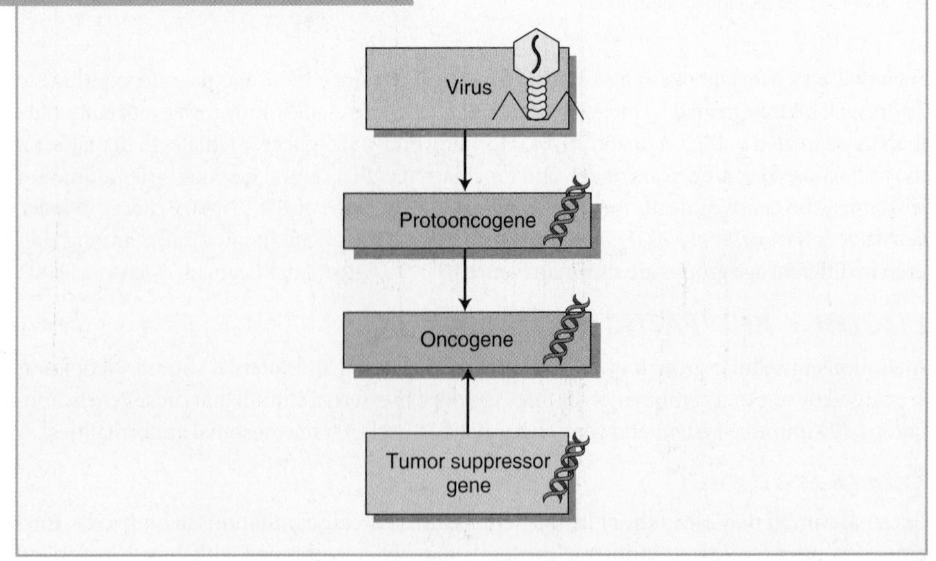

FIGURE 16-2 ◆
A protooncogene normally regulates cellular growth and development. When altered by a virus or other external cause, it can change to an oncogene, which allows unregulated genetic activity and tumor growth. Tumor-suppressor genes regulate the effects of oncogenes to decrease wildly proliferating cellular growth.

Some of these chromosomal abnormalities have been linked to an increased incidence of cancer. Children with Down syndrome have a 200 times higher incidence of leukemia than nonaffected children. Children who are missing a band of genetic material on chromosome 13 often have retinoblastoma. Similarly, a Wilms' tumor often develops in children missing part of the genetic material from chromosome 11. Regardless of the location of abnormal cellular growth, the pathophysiologic process is similar. The altered cell begins to multiply as directed by the altered genetic structure of its DNA and the absence or inactivation of tumor suppressor genes. Each new cell transmits the new or altered pattern to the next generation. As the abnormal cells replicate, the neoplastic mass grows. Normal cells usually die as the increased metabolic rate of the neoplastic cells depletes available nutrition. The altered DNA in the tumor cells may also cause the abnormal cells to invade adjoining tissue. Through continued growth, the mass expands until it enters and disrupts a major vessel or a vital organ.

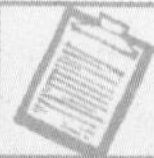

RESEARCH

In an analysis of cancer reports in children infected with acquired immune deficiency syndrome (AIDS), higher than expected numbers of cancers were reported. The most common cancers in AIDS-infected children were non-Hodgkin's lymphoma, Kaposi sarcoma, leiomyosarcoma (smooth-muscle sarcoma), and Hodgkin's disease (Biggar, Frisch, & Goedert, 2000).

CLINICAL MANIFESTATIONS

Each type of childhood cancer signals its presence differently. Because many of the presenting signs and symptoms of cancer are typical of common childhood illnesses, a delay in diagnosis can occur. In some cases, no symptoms are noted until the cancer is advanced. Some of the common presenting symptoms of cancer follow:

- *Pain* may be the result of a neoplasm either directly or indirectly affecting nerve receptors through obstruction, inflammation, tissue damage, stretching of visceral tissue, or invasion of susceptible tissue.
- *Cachexia* is a syndrome characterized by anorexia, weight loss, anemia, asthenia (weakness), and early satiety (feeling of being full).
- *Anemia* may be experienced during times of chronic bleeding or iron deficiency. In chronic illness the body uses iron poorly. Anemia is also present in cancers of the bone marrow when the number of red blood cells (RBCs) is reduced, in part because of the presence of large numbers of other bone marrow products. Treatment of cancer often promotes further anemia.
- *Infection* is usually a result of an altered or immature immune system. In addition, infection occurs when bone marrow cancers inhibit maturation of normal immune system cells. Infection may also occur in children who are treated with corticosteroids. Because their immune response is altered, the normal signs of infection may not appear.
- *Bruising* can occur if the bone marrow cannot produce enough platelets and bleeding occurs after minor trauma.

NURSING ALERT

The American Academy of Pediatrics Subcommittee on Cancer Pain in Children recommends that children be given some type of sedation before lumbar puncture is performed.

CLINICAL THERAPY

The most common diagnostic tests performed on children with cancer are complete blood counts, bone marrow aspiration, lumbar puncture (Table 16-1), peripheral blood studies, radiographic examination, magnetic resonance imaging (MRI), computed tomography (CT; Figure 16-3 ◆), ultrasound, and biopsy.

Cancer is treated with one or a combination of therapies: surgery, chemotherapy, radiation, biotherapy, and bone marrow transplantation. Many families also choose some type of complementary therapy, in addition to traditional medical approaches. The choice of treatment is determined by the type of cancer, its location, and the degree of metastasis (spread to other sites in the body).

The goal of treatment may be curative, supportive, or palliative. Curative treatment rids the child's body of the cancer. Supportive treatment includes transfusions, pain management, antibiotics, and other interventions to assist the body's defenses and increase the child's comfort. Palliative treatment is designed to make the child as comfortable as possible when no curative treatment is possible (see Chapter 8 for a detailed discussion of palliative care for children). Whatever combination of treatment is used, families have many questions and need resources for information.

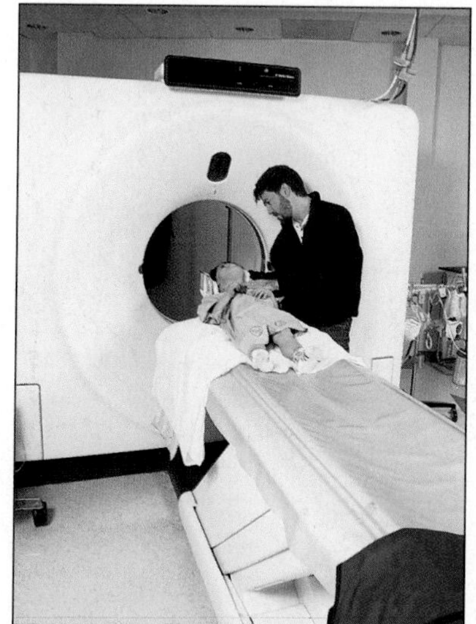

FIGURE 16-3 ◆ Computed tomography (CT) can be a frightening procedure for children. This 2-year-old boy is comforted by his father before the procedure.

NURSING ALERT

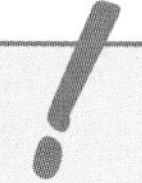

Any child who has an implanted metallic object in the body should not undergo MRI scanning because of the strong magnetic field generated. Metallic objects include orthodontic braces, metal dental bridgework, surgical clips or plates, and orthopedic rods. Remove all jewelry and clothes with metal snaps from the child before the test.

TABLE 16-1 Selected Diagnostic Tests for Childhood Cancer

TEST	PURPOSE	NORMAL LABORATORY VALUES	DIAGNOSTIC VALUES
Bone marrow aspiration	Examines bone marrow	<5% blast cells (immature)	>25% blast cells in acute lymphoblastic leukemia, most with hypercellular marrow
Lumbar puncture	Examines cerebrospinal fluid	Cell count (μL) Polymorphonuclear leukocytes 0 Monocytes 0–5 RBCs 0–5	Presence of malignant cells indicates central nervous system involvement
Complete blood count and differential	Examines cellular components of blood	WBC <10,000/μL Platelets 150,000–400,000/μL Hemoglobin 12–16 g/dL	WBC >10,000/μL Platelets 20,000–100,000/μL Hemoglobin 7–10 g/dL

FAMILIES WANT TO KNOW

Cancer Therapy

Most parents are not aware of the effects of cancer treatment and how they can help children through this experience. Depending on the stage and type of treatment, there are several ways to help:

- Children in radiation and chemotherapy are fatigued. Provide extra rest periods with shorter activity periods between them.
- Have a bag ready in case the child develops a complication and needs to be taken to stay in the hospital for a few days. Several hospital stays of a few days are normal during treatment.
- When concerned about a symptom in the child, ask the care provider. Parents are often key in identifying problems early.
- Parents are usually concerned about central line care, but feel more comfortable after a few days of caring for the line.
- Children may not feel hungry and so nutritional intake is needed when they are ready to eat.
- Remember that the child is still at the normal developmental age. Treat them like their ages, not as if they are older or younger.
- Try to maintain contact with the child's peer group and family members.
- Seek information from other parents and resources on cancer care.

Remind parents to get time away and relax so that parental energy remains high and they are better able to deal with the child's therapy.

Surgery

Surgery is used to remove or debulk (reduce the size of) a solid tumor. An example of a cancer that is commonly treated with surgery is a Wilms' tumor. Surgery is also used to determine the stage and type of cancer.

Chemotherapy

Chemotherapy is the administration of specific drugs that kill both normal and cancerous cells. The administration of various chemotherapeutic drugs is timed to achieve the greatest cellular destruction. The schedule is determined by the cell's cycle of replication (Figure 16-4 ◆). Several chemotherapeutic drugs are administered simultaneously to maximize their lethal impact on cells at all stages of activity. Table 16-2 provides examples of common chemotherapy drug combinations.

Whereas DNA in a normal cell can repair itself after chemotherapy, the DNA in a neoplastic cell cannot. The particular chemotherapy treatment protocol used is based on re-

PATHOPHYSIOLOGY ILLUSTRATED

Chemotherapy Drug Action

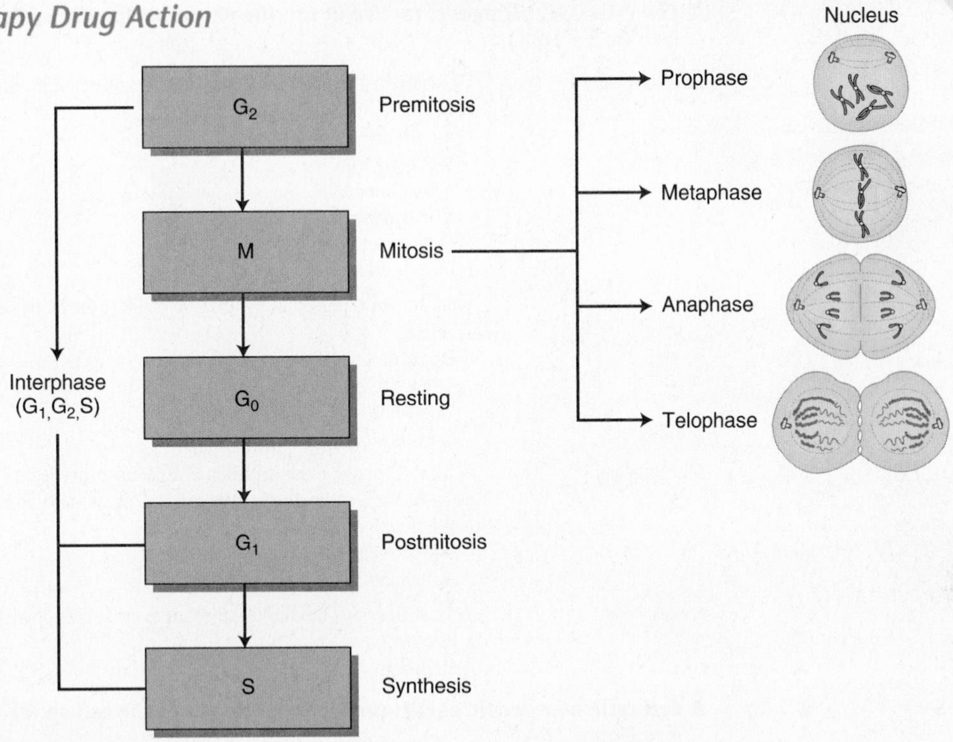

G_2 — Premitosis
M — Mitosis
G_0 — Resting
G_1 — Postmitosis
S — Synthesis
Interphase (G_1, G_2, S)
Nucleus
Prophase
Metaphase
Anaphase
Telophase

FIGURE 16-4 ◆
Chemotherapy drugs either act at specific parts of the cell cycle or are non-specific for action (act throughout all cell phases).

search into different types of cancer cells. A **protocol** is a plan of action for chemotherapy that is based on the type of cancer, its stage, and the particular cell type (Figure 16-5 ◆).

Other drugs used in the treatment of children with cancer include colony-stimulating factors, antiemetics, and nutritional supplements. Colony-stimulating factors are hormonelike glycoproteins that enhance blood cell production and counteract the myelosuppressive effects of chemotherapy drugs. For example, erythropoietin is produced in the kidney, and a recombinant form (epoetin) is available which can be used to treat anemia of cancer, thereby decreasing the number of transfusions needed (Agency for Healthcare Research and Quality, 2001a). Antiemetics can be used to treat the nausea and vomiting that are common side effects of therapy. Nutritional supplements can be given to maintain nutritional status.

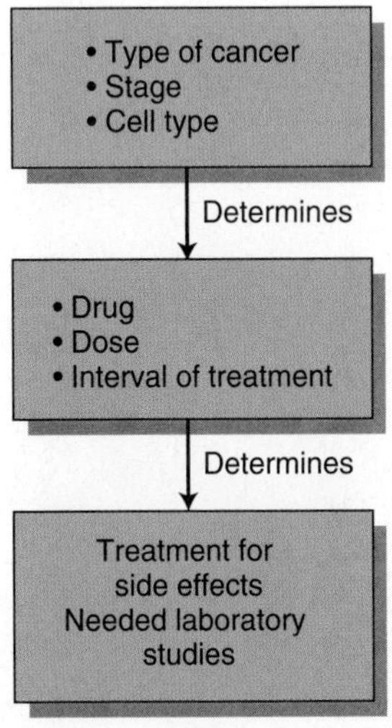

FIGURE 16-5 ◆
Chemotherapy protocol. A protocol is a map or plan of action that directs therapy by identifying the drug and its accompanying treatment.

Radiation

Radiation therapy involves the use of unstable isotopes that release varying levels of energy to cause breaks in the DNA molecule and thereby destroy cells. Radiation has been used as a treatment method since the early 1900s, shortly after its discovery. It is often used for the local and regional control of cancer, and in combination with surgery and chemotherapy.

The area to be irradiated (treatment field) includes the tumor site and sometimes other involved areas, such as lymph glands. The goal is to irradiate the tumor but not healthy adjacent tissue. The total dose of radiation is divided (or fractionated) and given over several weeks. A common course of radiation treatment might be once daily 4 or 5 days per week for a period of 2 to 6 weeks.

Tumors that are highly sensitive to radiation include Hodgkin's disease, Wilms' tumor, retinoblastoma, and rhabdomyosarcoma. Tumors that have a low sensitivity to radiation, such as osteosarcoma and soft-tissue sarcomas, require higher doses of radiation.

MEDICATIONS USED FOR CHEMOTHERAPY AND THEIR ACTIONS

■ *Cell cycle specific agents (active in specific phases of the cell cycle) (see Figure 16-4)*

Antimetabolites	Work at synthesis phase; interfere with function of nucleic acid, inhibiting DNA or RNA synthesis 5-Azacytidine 5-Fluorouracil 6-Mercaptopurine 6-Thioguanine Cytosine arabinoside Methotrexate
Vinca alkaloids	Work at mitosis phase; bind with cell proteins to inhibit nucleic acid and protein synthesis Etoposide Teniposide Vinblastine Vincristine
Miscellaneous	Work at G_1 phase; cause depletion of asparagine, needed by cancer cells and cause lysis of lymphoid cells; make cell in G phase vulnerable to other agents; interfere with prosynthesis 1-Asparaginase Prednisone
Miscellaneous	Work at G_2 phase; bind cellular proteins to cause metaphase arrest Bleomycin Etoposide

■ *Cell cycle nonspecific agents (active in all stages of the cell cycle) (see Figure 16-4)*

Alkylating agents	Substitute an alkyl group for a hydrogen atom, leading to DNA replication Cyclophosphamide Cisplatin Busulfan Chlorambucil Thiotepa Mechlorethamine
Antibiotics	Interfere with nucleic acid, inhibiting DNA or RNA synthesis Doxorubicin Mitomycin-C Dactinomycin Bleomycin Daunorubicin
Nitrosureas	Cause breakage in DNA; cross blood-brain barrier Carmustine Lomustine
Miscellaneous	Affect DNA and RNA synthesis Dacarbazine Procarbazine

Biotherapy

Biotherapy is the use of biologic response modifiers, such as interleukins, interferons, or radiolabeled monoclonal antibodies, to treat cancer (Bertolone, 1997). The three major classes of biologic response modifiers are (1) agents that restore, augment, or modulate the host's immunologic mechanisms; (2) agents that have direct antitumor activity; and (3) agents that have other biologic effects. The actions of many of these agents are not completely understood, and some agents have more than one effect. For example, interferon has both antiviral and antiproliferative effects on some malignant cells. Interferon and tumor necrosis factor are undergoing clinical trials to study their effectiveness and to develop protocols for their safe use against selected cancers.

TABLE 16-2 Commonly Used Chemotherapy Drug Combinations

ACRONYM	DRUG COMBINATION
A-COPP	doxorubicin + cyclophosphamide + vincristine (oncovin) + procarbazine + prednisone
ABVD	doxorubicin + bleomycin + vinblastine + dacarbazine
ACE	doxorubicin + cyclophosphamide + etoposide
APE	doxorubicin + procarbazine + etoposide
CAF	cyclophosphamide + doxorubicin + fluorouracil
CAMP	cyclophosphamide + doxorubicin + methotrexate + procarbazine
CAVe	lomustine + doxorubicin + vinblastine
CAVE or ECHO or CAPO or EVAC or VOCA	etoposide + cyclophosphamide + doxorubicin + vincristine
CHOP	cyclophosphamide + doxorubicin + vincristine + prednisone
CHOR	cyclophosphamide + doxorubicin + vincristine
CISCA	cisplatin + cyclophosphamide
CMF	cyclophosphamide + methotrexate + fluorouracil
COPP	cyclophosphamide + vincristine + procarbazine + prednisone
CY-VA-DIC	cyclophosphamide + vincristine + doxorubicin + dacarbazine
FAC	fluorouracil + doxorubicin + cyclophosphamide
MACC	methotrexate + doxorubicin + cyclophosphamide + lomustine
MOPP	mechlorethamine + vincristine + procarbazine + prednisone
MTX + MP + CTX	methotrexate + mercaptopurine + cyclophosphamide
PVB or VBP	vinblastine + bleomycin + cisplatin
T-2	dactinomycin + doxorubicin + vincristine + cyclophosphamide
VAP	vincristine + dactinomycin + cyclophosphamide
VP-*L*-asparaginase	vincristine + prednisone + *L*-asparaginase

Note: From Bindler, R.M., & Howry, L.B. (1997). *Pediatric drugs and nursing implications* (2nd ed., pp. 579–580). Stamford, CT: Appleton & Lange.

COLONY-STIMULATING FACTORS

Filgrastin (neupogen): Stimulates neutrophil production
Erythropoietin (epoetin): Stimulates red blood cell production

SAFETY PRECAUTIONS

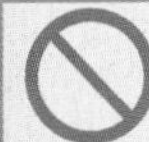

Nurses who care for a child receiving implant radiation or who work in a radiation department must wear a dosimeter film badge at all times.

LAW & ETHICS

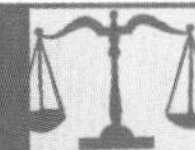

Consent by parents is mandatory if a child is to be started on a medication that is considered a clinical trial drug. Children who are cognitively able should give assent verbally or in writing. This consent can usually be obtained from children by the age of 7–9 years, depending on the child's level of understanding.

Bone Marrow and Blood Stem Cell Transplantation

Bone marrow transplantation is used to treat leukemia, neuroblastoma, and some non-cancerous conditions such as aplastic anemia. The goal of therapy is to administer a lethal dose of chemotherapy and radiation that will kill the cancer, and then to resupply the body with bone marrow stem cells either from the child's own marrow previously removed and stored or from a compatible donor.

Bone marrow transplantation has become the treatment of choice when a relapse occurs while the child is receiving another form of cancer therapy. First, a histocompatible donor must be located. The child then receives intensive chemotherapy, often followed by total

TYPES OF BONE MARROW TRANSPLANT

Allogenic: Donor and recipient are of same species
Autologous: Donor and recipient are the same person
Isogenic or syngeneic: Donor and recipient are genetically the same (twins)

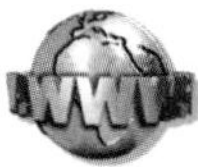

Cord Blood Registry and Resources

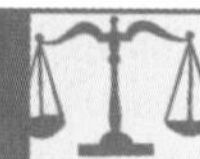

LAW & ETHICS

A child advocate whose role is to objectively safeguard the rights and needs of a minor child scheduled to receive a bone marrow transplant is frequently a part of the bone marrow transplant team.

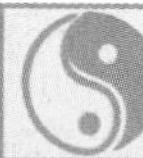

CULTURE

Traditional Chinese view cancer as a result of weak or toxic blood, which allows pollutants to accumulate and become toxic. A variety of plant products and acupuncture are used to detoxify the blood, and good nutrition helps it to rebuild (Swerdlow, 2000).

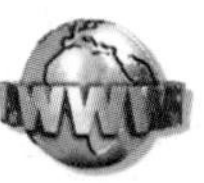

Complementary Cancer Therapies

FOODS USED FOR CANCER PREVENTION AND TREATMENT

Carrots
Garlic
Green tea
Cabbage
Citrus fruits
Ginger root
Willow bark
(Swerdlow, 2000)

body irradiation. Beginning 7 to 10 days before the transplant, this treatment kills all circulating blood cells and bone marrow contents (Alcoser & Burchett, 1999). Following this treatment, the child is intravenously transfused with the donor bone marrow. New blood cells usually form within 6 to 8 weeks. (See Chapter 15 for a description of care for the child undergoing bone marrow transplantation.)

Stem cells that become established in the host child's bone marrow can also be obtained from newborn cord blood. For some children this has become a better option than waiting for a matching bone marrow donor. Cord blood can be easily collected at birth from a sibling of the ill child, as histocompatible matches often occur in siblings, or cord blood banks may offer a match. The cord blood is then infused into the child undergoing treatment and the same mechanism occurs as in bone marrow transplantation—implantation of the stem cells into the child's bone marrow and production of normal blood cells over about 2 to 6 weeks. Advantages of cord blood are that, unlike bone marrow collection, it is not painful for the donor and does not require anesthesia; there is an opportunity to easily collect samples from many ethnic groups that are underrepresented in bone marrow donor registries; graft-versus-host disease after treatment is less prevalent; and storage of cord blood for use later in life is possible (Chang, 1998; Crooks, Lill, & Feig, et al., 1997). A variety of federally funded and private blood banks are available to store and provide cord blood.

Complementary Therapies

Many families use **complementary therapies** in treatment of a child's cancer. These approaches to care are also referred to as alternative or unconventional, and may involve nutritional supplements, herbal ingestion, touch therapy, and mind/body interventions. Little research has been done on complementary therapies, although up to 80% of children have used at least one such therapeutic approach (Kelly, Jacobsen, & Kennedy, et al., 2000). Health care providers should be aware of these practices, inquire in a nonjudgmental manner about what therapies are used, and attempt to learn about specific therapies and practices. Although some herbs and nutritional products such as St. John's Wort may decrease serum concentration of chemotherapeutic agents, or some may act as hormones in the body, most are not known to negatively impact contemporary medical treatment, and the families should be assisted in seeking information and supported in use of their chosen therapies (Dean, 2000; Chase, 2000). Intake of fruits and vegetables is associated with lower cancer incidence in adults, and some foods such as garlic and oranges may slow cancer growth or enhance medical chemotherapy (Swerdlow, 2000). Some herbal supplements are used to treat cancer by some individuals; these include cat's claw (bark of a tree root), mistletoe, and shark cartilage. The Food and Drug Administration has allowed testing of the efficacy of some herbal treatments for cancer (Kemper & Longwood Herbal Task Force, 1999). Several cancer drugs such as vincristine and paclitaxel are obtained from plant products. Some herbs are useful in treatment of nausea and vomiting, and others can boost the immune system's function (Kemper & Longwood Herbal Task Force, 1999).

Palliative Care

In spite of modern medicinal practices and complementary therapies, some children do not survive childhood cancer. In these cases, the focus of health care is to provide comfort and emotional support for the child and family. Too often, health care providers feel uncomfortable when a child is expected to die and may withdraw from close contact with the child or family, fail to provide adequate comfort measures, and leave the family without access to needed resources. When delay in the recognition of prognosis occurs, children experience greater suffering and less integration of palliative care (Wolfe, Klar, & Grier, et al., 2000). Some of the symptoms for which children are commonly undertreated include pain, dyspnea, nutrition, elimination, and fatigue (Wolfe, Grier, & Klar, 2000). See Chapter 8 for a detailed description of palliative care for children with terminal disease.

Oncologic Emergencies

Oncologic emergencies can be organized into three groups: metabolic, hematologic, and those involving space-occupying lesions.

TABLE 16-3 Tumor Lysis Syndrome

Laboratory Evaluation CBC Serum sodium, potassium, chloride, bicarbonate, calcium, phosphorus, uric acid, BUN, creatinine, magnesium Urinalysis ECG if potassium is >7 mEq/L
Management Hydration to maintain urine specific gravity <1.010 Alkalinization with drugs and intravenous fluids to keep urine pH between 7 and 7.5 Diuretics Phosphate reduction with aluminum hydroxide

METABOLIC EMERGENCIES Metabolic emergencies result from the lysis (dissolving or decomposing) of tumor cells, a process called tumor lysis syndrome. This cell destruction releases high levels of uric acid, potassium, phosphates, and calcium into the blood and can lower serum sodium levels. This syndrome is seen most commonly in children with Burkitt's lymphoma and acute lymphocytic leukemia (Kelly & Lange, 1997). Table 16-3 presents laboratory tests and managment of tumor lysis syndrome.

A second type of metabolic emergency is septic shock. During periods of immune suppression the child is vulnerable to overwhelming infection, resulting in circulatory failure, inadequate tissue perfusion, and hypotension. Septic shock can be fatal (see Chapter 14 for a description of septic shock). Factors contributing to massive infection include inadequate neutrophil production, abnormal granulocytes (not able to be actively phagocytic), erosions through normal barriers such as blood vessels and mucous membranes, and altered bone marrow production caused by chemotherapy and some forms of radiation. Such infections must be vigorously treated with antimicrobial therapy and hydration management.

A third type of metabolic emergency occurs when large amounts of bone are destroyed by treatment, resulting in hypercalcemia (elevated calcium in the serum). Hypercalcemia is most common in children with acute lymphocytic leukemia and rhabdomyosarcoma. Treatment includes hydration and adequate intake of phosphate by oral supplement.

HEMATOLOGIC EMERGENCIES Hematologic emergencies result from bone marrow suppression or infiltration of brain and respiratory tissue with high numbers of leukemic blast cells (hyperleukocytosis). Bone marrow suppression results in anemia and **thrombocytopenia** (decreased platelets) with resultant hemorrhage. Gastrointestinal and central nervous system bleeding (strokes) are common.

Treatment involves infusion of packed red blood cells for anemia; and platelet transfusion, vitamin K, and fresh frozen plasma for thrombocytopenia and hemorrhage. Hyperleukocytosis is treated by hydration, bicarbonate infusion, and allopurinol (Kelly & Lange, 1997).

SPACE-OCCUPYING LESIONS Extensive tumor growth may result in spinal cord compression, increased intracranial pressure, brain herniation, seizures, massive hepatomegaly, and superior vena cava syndrome (obstruction of the superior vena cava by tumor). These emergencies are often caused by neuroblastoma, medulloblastoma, astrocytoma, Hodgkin's disease, or lymphoma. After biopsy of the mass, treatment involves radiation therapy, chemotherapy, and corticosteroids.

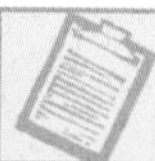

RESEARCH

Health care providers often feel uncomfortable in treating children who are dying of cancer, and may not be adequately prepared for the task by their educational programs. The presence of a palliative care team; an integrated plan of care; collaboration between families, primary care provider, and other practitioners; and focus on the child's developmental level and the needs of the family can enhance the care provided for the dying child (Chaffee, 2001; Hilden, Emanuel, & Fairclough, et al., 2001).

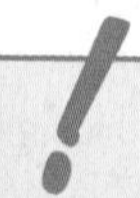

NURSING ALERT

Watch for signs of septic shock: hyperthermia or hypothermia, tachycardia, tachypnea, hypotension, mental changes, and peripheral cyanosis or coolness.

NURSING MANAGEMENT

Nursing Assessment and Diagnosis

PHYSIOLOGIC ASSESSMENT

Physiologic assessment focuses on identifying the signs and symptoms of cancer and ongoing assessment of the side effects of treatment (see the discussion of side effects following under "Planning and Implementation"). Assessment of children with the most significant types of childhood cancers is presented later in the chapter.

Skills 5-1 to 5-21: Performing a Physical Assessment

GROWTH & DEVELOPMENT

Children of different ages experience differing threats to body image as a result of cancer treatment. A preschool girl may be most upset at hair loss, since she now looks like a boy. A school-age child has the most difficult time with changes that interfere with the developmental task of industry. Amputation, which decreases the child's ability to participate in activities such as sports, dancing, and school work, can be a major challenge during the school-age years. Teenagers are often most worried about such changes as hair loss and cushingoid features, which cause them to look different from peers.

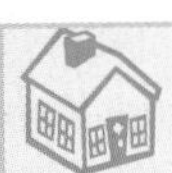

HOME CARE

For many parents, especially of daughters, the loss of the child's hair can be devastating. Ask the parents and the child what this issue is like for them. Prepare them for the fact that it can be rapid or slow. Find out how they will plan to cope. Some children want the hair cut very short so its loss will not be as traumatic. Offer resources for wigs, hats, or other ideas. Put them in touch with children who have lost hair and with those who have now regrown it.

A thorough physical assessment of all systems is needed to help in identifying the presence and extent of cancer (see Chapter 4). Height and weight should be carefully measured, and compared with prior findings for the child. Observe gait and coordination, as well as any changes in mental status. Evaluate pain, nutritional intake, fatigue, infections, bruising, shortness of breath, and elimination problems. Periodic laboratory studies will be performed.

Psychosocial Assessment

Assessment of body image, stress and coping abilities, knowledge of the condition and cognitive level, support systems, and developmental level provides data that help determine the appropriate nursing interventions for the child with cancer and the family.

Body Image Hair loss, surgical scars, and cushingoid changes are three common treatment-induced threats to body image. Most children being treated for cancer experience hair loss (Figure 16-6 ◆). Children who have cranial surgery lose hair as part of the surgical preparation. Chemotherapy frequently results in some degree of hair loss. The speed of hair loss is unique to the child and can be as rapid as overnight or slower, evidenced by hair left on the pillow and in the hairbrush.

A second challenge to the child's body image is surgery. The scars of cranial and neck surgery are obvious, as are amputation and limb salvaging. Abdominal surgery for lymphoma is more easily concealed but is still a threat to the child's body image.

A third source of altered body image is the cushingoid features such as round and flushed face, prominent cheeks, double chin, and generalized obesity (Figure 16-7 ◆) that result from the use of corticosteroids. As the child's weight increases, stretch marks similar to those of pregnancy may occur. These stretch marks often remain after the corticosteroids are decreased.

Body image disturbances occur when a child cannot integrate changes and continues to cling to old images despite their inconsistency with reality. Common means for assessing body image are drawings, colored pictures cut out by the child to form a collage, discussion, and observation. See Chapter 5 for further discussion of these and other assessment techniques that can be used with children.

Stress and Coping The diagnosis of cancer is a major stressor for both the child and the family. Although each child's prognosis and each family's coping mechanisms are unique, most families deal with the diagnosis in a manner similar to that of other families who have a child with a life-threatening illness (see Chapter 8). Assess the family (and child if old enough) for their understanding and acceptance of the diagnosis. Evaluate if the family has told the child about the diagnosis and whether the family needs assistance in deciding how

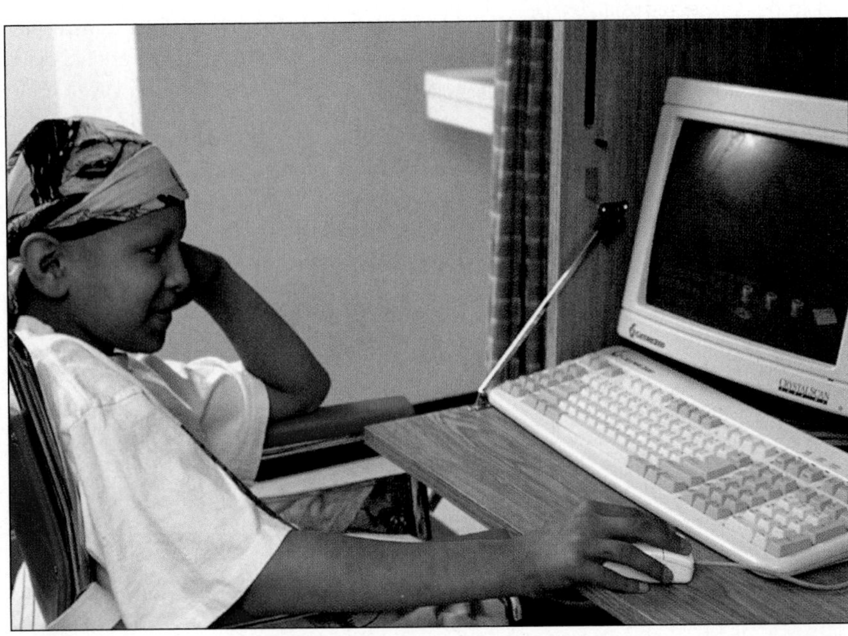

FIGURE 16-6 ◆
One of the most common threats to a child's body image at any age is hair loss induced by chemotherapy. Use of hats can improve self concept.

to do this (Ishibashi, 2001). Assess the level of anxiety during health care visits and scheduled treatments (Figure 16-8 ◆). Evaluate the family's methods of coping, such as the ability to integrate relaxing and meaningful activities into family life, the use of support systems in the community and extended family, and the ability to alter expectations to take into account the child's health status. Concurrent stressors increase the family's difficulty in coping with childhood cancer. Evaluate the family for stressors such as illness or death of another family member, occupational changes, financial problems, relocation, and change in vacation plans.

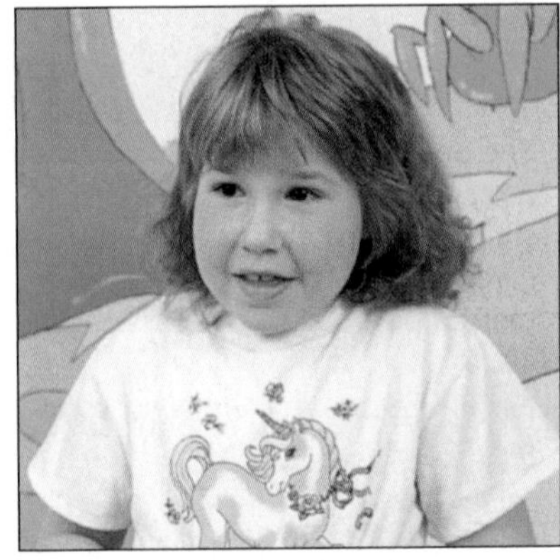

FIGURE 16-7 ◆
The child with cushingoid changes frequently has a rounded face and prominent cheeks

Knowledge People who are anxious tend to narrow their scope of attention and may read unintended messages into the behaviors of health care personnel. Anxiety also limits a person's ability to retain information.

The child's knowledge of cancer and its treatment should be assessed throughout the treatment period. As the child matures cognitively, new evaluations of knowledge are needed. Cancer and its treatment are complex topics and parents are exposed to information in various forms, including written material, news reports, and internet websites and resources. Evaluate their knowledge and provide an opportunity for them to ask questions.

Support Systems Cancer treatment generally occurs over a long period of time. The extended family is crucial in providing necessary support to the child, parents, and siblings. Identify key persons in the family. They may be the parents, grandparents, or aunts and uncles. Thoroughly assess the coping strategies used by the family to meet the various challenges posed by the child's illness. This information helps to predict the success of interventions, such as home care with intravenous medications, and to decide when referrals for other supportive therapies are needed.

Assess family resources to identify support systems available to help the family during crises and if a child is expected to die. Extended supports include friends, jobs, insurance coverage, religious affiliations, cultural support systems, and the school system. Parents commonly lose contact with close friends following the diagnosis of cancer in a child. This is an additional stressor for the family. Jobs are often a source of support because co-workers may have gone through the same experience. It may also be comforting for parents to return to a job where they can feel a sense of security in tangible accomplishments. However, jobs can also be a source of stress if employers are unsympathetic to the demands of the child's hospitalization and clinic or office visits.

Religious affiliations can be an important source of support. Evaluate whether such affiliations are meaningful for the family and, if so, plan for visits from the appropriate clergy. In some cultures, spiritual leaders are an important part of the family's support.

The return to school may pose difficulties for the child with cancer or it may be a source of support to be connected again to peers. The child is encouraged to go to school, even if

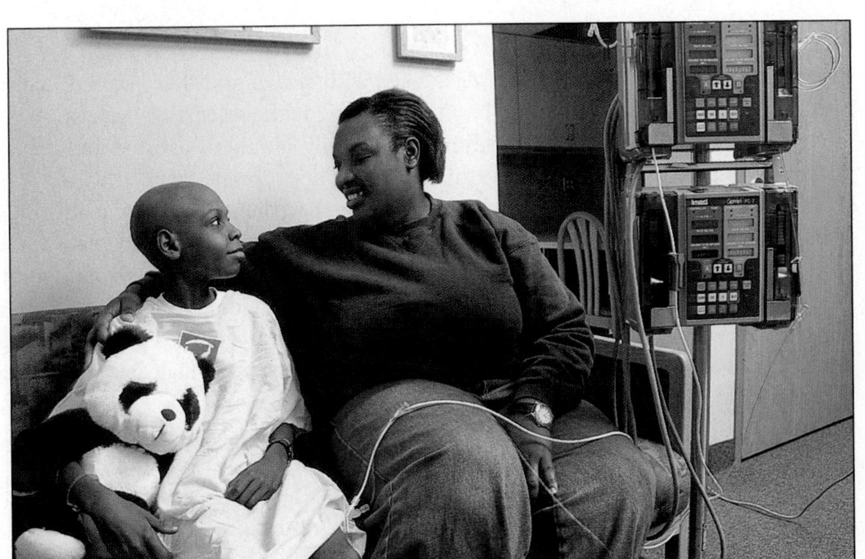

FIGURE 16-8 ◆
The child with cancer depends on parents and family members to provide support. Nurses can assist families to draw upon their strengths to help the child.

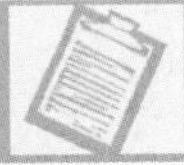

RESEARCH

The death of a child from cancer is a major traumatic event. Research shows that during the palliative care phase, when no further treatment is possible, the family's needs are to:

- Have the child recognized as special
- Experience care and connectedness with health care professionals
- Retain responsibility for the dying child

(James & Johnson, 1997)

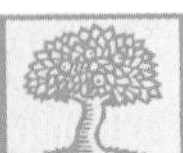

COMMUNITY CARE

The child who is returning to school with a changed appearance from cancer treatment needs support and assistance. Discuss and role-play how the child can tell friends about the changes. A nurse or child life specialist can visit the child's class to explain what the child is experiencing. Offer to talk with the teacher to devise a plan for preparing classmates.

only for half a day per week, to stay connected to peers. Evaluate the ability of the school to accept a medically vulnerable child into the classroom. Assess whether the other children and teachers have been prepared for the appearance and needs of the child with cancer. Arrangements can be made for tutors to help the child keep up with school work if he or she cannot attend school.

Developmental Assessment

Developmental assessment of children should be performed regularly during treatment for cancer. Assessment of the child's physical and neurologic development helps in determining the progress made during treatment and provides a baseline for evaluating the long-term effects of treatment. Children under 6 years of age who have cancer should receive regular developmental assessment with a standardized tool such as the Denver II Developmental Screening Test (see Chapter 6). Performance in school and social activities with friends provides important information about expected developmental milestones in older children.

Children who have received cranial radiation and intrathecal chemotherapy need regular scholastic evaluations. Impaired neurocognitive performance may occur as long-term effects of treatment and appropriate interventions should be planned in these cases (Challinor, Miaskowski, & Moore, et al., 2000).

Children with cancer have a variety of common psychologic and physiologic problems, regardless of their specific type of cancer. They and their families are dealing with a complex illness that influences their lives for years. The impact of this experience extends into all areas of function.

The accompanying nursing care plans include several diagnoses that may be appropriate for the child with cancer who is receiving care in the hospital or at home. Among the many other diagnoses that may be appropriate for a child with cancer are the following:

- *Diarrhea,* related to radiation therapy and toxins
- *Altered urinary elimination,* related to chemotherapy
- *Altered oral mucous membrane,* related to chemotherapy and radiation therapy
- *Impaired skin integrity,* related to altered nutritional state, effects of medication, radiation, and immobilization
- *Ineffective individual coping,* related to situational crises of chronic and acute illness
- *Sleep pattern disturbance,* related to biochemical agents, anxiety, and unfamiliar surroundings
- *Diversional activity deficit,* related to frequent lengthy treatments
- *Body image disturbance,* related to chronic illness and treatments
- *Knowledge deficit (child or parents),* related to lack of exposure to disease or treatments
- *Anticipatory grieving,* related to actual or potential loss of significant other

Planning and Implementation

The nursing care of children newly diagnosed with cancer and their families includes immediate physiologic and psychologic support, along with anticipatory guidance about imminent and future medical interventions. The family should be assisted and supported in making decisions about types of treatment that are appropriate for their child.

Nursing care of the hospitalized child with cancer and the child receiving ongoing therapy at home is summarized in the accompanying nursing care plans. These care plans are designed for the child who is beyond the cancer diagnosis phase and is receiving chemotherapy.

Physiologic care of the hospitalized child focuses on providing support during treatment. This includes ensuring optimal nutritional intake, administering medications, managing the multiple side effects of chemotherapy and radiation, ensuring adequate hydration, preventing infection, and managing pain.

Ensure Optimal Nutritional Intake

The high metabolic rate of cancer growth depletes the child's nutritional stores. Added to this is the catabolic effect of chemotherapy and radiation on normal cells, necessitating additional cellular replacement. The child needs increased nutritional intake at a

NURSING CARE PLAN Hospital Care of the Child with Cancer

GOAL	INTERVENTION	RATIONALE	EXPECTED OUTCOME
1. Pain related to tissue injury			
	NIC Priority Intervention: **Pain Management:** Alleviation or reduction in pain to a level of comfort acceptable to patient.		NOC Suggested Outcome: **Comfort Level:** Feelings of physical and psychologic ease.
The child will report reduced pain that is manageable.	■ Give analgesics as ordered. ■ Teach relaxation techniques, deep breathing and distraction.	■ Adequate medications can reduce pain. ■ Nonpharmacologic methods work with the medication to reduce pain.	The child experiences pain reduced to the level that allows child to interact appropriately and gain rest.
2. Sleep Pattern Disturbance related to lack of sleep privacy/control			
	NIC Priority Intervention: **Sleep Enhancement:** Facilitation of regular sleep/wake cycles.		NOC Suggested Outcome: **Rest:** Extent and pattern of diminished activity for mental and physical rejuvenation.
The child will sleep for hours appropriate to age. The child will report feeling rested.	■ Alter the environment to allow designated rest periods. ■ Plan care to reduce frequency of interruptions during normal rest and sleep times.	■ A quiet environment encourages relaxation needed for resting. ■ Reduced interruptions allow continuous sleep and rest.	The child rests and sleeps for an age-appropriate amount of time per day.
3. Altered Nutrition: Less Than Body Requirements related to inability to ingest or digest food or absorb nutrients			
	NIC Priority Intervention: **Nutrition Management:** Assistance with and provision of a balanced dietary intake.		NOC Suggested Outcome: **Nutritional Status:** Extent to which nutrients are available to meet metabolic needs.
The child will maintain adequate nutritional intake.	■ Offer small feedings. Encourage favorite foods. Refer to dietitian for special meals: Weigh daily.	■ Measures can increase caloric intake. Taste changes and mouth sores alter desire for food.	The child maintains admission weight.
The child will experience reduced effects of chemotherapy (i.e., nausea and vomiting).	■ Teach the child distraction and relaxation techniques. Give antiemetics according to orders.	■ Pharmacologic and nonpharmacologic methods are effective in helping to reduce nausea.	The child has minimal side effects of nausea and vomiting.
4. Constipation related to change in usual foods and eating patterns			
	NIC Priority Intervention: **Constipation Management:** Prevention and alleviation of constipation.		NOC Suggested Outcome: **Bowel Elimination:** The ability of the gastrointestinal tract to form and evacuate stool effectively.
The child will reestablish normal bowel pattern.	■ Record all output by size and description. Administer stool softeners. Test stool for guaiac. Report changes in stool to physician. Encourage adequate fluid intake.	■ Chemotherapy or tumor may create constipation, diarrhea, or blood in stool.	The child has normal bowel pattern.
5. Fluid Volume Excess or Deficit related to medications			
	NIC Priority Intervention: **Fluid Management:** Promotion of fluid balance and prevention of complications resulting from abnormal fluid levels.		NOC Suggested Outcome: **Fluid Balance:** Balance of water in the intracellular and extracellular compartments of the body.

(continued)

NURSING CARE PLAN Hospital Care of the Child with Cancer (continued)

GOAL	INTERVENTION	RATIONALE	EXPECTED OUTCOME
5. Fluid Volume Excess or Deficit related to medications (continued)			
The child will be adequately hydrated.	■ Record all intake. Monitor intravenous rate and solution as appropriate. ■ Test specific gravity of urine daily.	■ Some drugs (e.g., cyclophosphamide) necessitate a high level of fluid intake to prevent complications. ■ Renal function may be affected by chemotherapy.	The child demonstrates adequate hydration. Mucous membranes are hydrated. Specific gravity remains within normal range.
6. Risk for Infection related to immunosuppression, invasive procedures, malnutrition, or pharmaceutical agents			
	NIC Priority Intervention: **Infection Protection:** Prevention and early detection of infection in patient at risk.		NOC Suggested Outcome: **Risk Control:** Actions to eliminate or reduce health threats.
The child will remain free of infection.	■ Wash hands often. Maintain in isolation if needed. ■ Monitor temperature. Report elevation to physician. ■ Administer intravenous antibiotics as ordered. Monitor temperature. Use cooling mattress as ordered. Report elevations over 38° C (101° F) to physician.	■ Handwashing is effective in killing organisms. ■ Elevated temperature is a sign of infection. ■ Multiple antibiotics are needed to deal with bacterial and fungal infections during neutropenia. Blood cultures may be taken to identify organism.	The child remains infection free. The child with an infection is effectively treated.
7. Ineffective Individual Coping related to situational crisis			
	NIC Priority Intervention: **Coping Enhancement:** Assisting a patient to adapt to stressors which interfere with meeting life demands and roles.		NOC Suggested Outcome: **Coping:** Actions to manage stressors that tax an individual's resources.
The child will demonstrate normal adaptive coping methods.	■ Encourage drawings and other therapeutic play for expression of feelings. Allow for expression of angry feelings, such as hitting dolls and throwing sponge balls. Discuss how to behave during treatments.	■ Expression of feelings helps identify avoidance coping for further intervention. Play is a normal way for child to express self and ideas. Misinterpretations can be corrected. Knowledge of appropriate and helpful behaviors supports self-esteem.	The child continues to use usual coping-strategies expected for developmental stage.
8. Altered Health Maintenance related to complex treatment, and lack of resources			
	NIC Priority Intervention: **Health System Guidance:** Facilitating use of health services		NOC Suggested Outcome: **Knowledge: Health Behaviors:** Extent of understanding conveyed about promotion and protection of health.
The child will state understanding of treatments and procedures.	■ Use age-appropriate teaching methods. Content areas include child's cancer, medications (actions and side effects), how to deal with body changes, and how to deal with response of others to those changes. Correct misinterpretations. Anticipate upcoming events and teach the child and family about them.	■ Education helps by increasing understanding, removing fantasy, and clarifying fears. Education promotes the use of new learning in all areas of life.	The child demonstrates age-appropriate knowledge of the cancer, its treatments, and medications. The child has age-appropriate understanding of how to deal with changes in the body.

FAMILIES WANT TO KNOW

Nutrition and the Child with Cancer

Because of the effects of cancer and chemotherapy or other treatment, the child often has a poor appetite. Mucosal sores lead to difficulty chewing and swallowing. Parents can enhance the nutritional intake of the child in the following ways.

- Provide frequent small feedings rather than three meals daily.
- Integrate the child's favorite foods into daily menus.
- Have nutritious snacks available for times when the child feels like eating.
- Sprinkle dried milk on top of cereals and other foods.
- Serve smooth, soft foods. Milkshakes with added peanut butter, puddings, and soft casseroles may be well tolerated and preferred. Try a variety of liquid protein–calorie supplements to find those the child likes.
- Avoid making food an area for disagreement. Do not force foods, but make them readily available.
- If the child is vomiting due to therapy, do not encourage food at that time. Food aversions may develop to foods that are vomited.
- Administer antiemetics as ordered during therapy because they can prevent nausea and vomiting.
- Report weight loss and increased fatigue.
- Bring the child in for scheduled health visits so growth, development, and effects of therapy can be monitored.
- Request a temporary feeding tube to ensure adequate nutrition. Feedings at night can often increase intake and promote health. Occasionally a central line is inserted to provide total parenteral nutrition.
- Know that supplements and tube feedings will usually be covered by insurance if the provider writes an order for them.

time when nausea and vomiting are occurring as drug side effects, and when decreased activity and general health status result in diminished appetite. This often leads to extreme concern on the part of parents, and they may focus excessive attention on the child's intake.

Administer antiemetic drugs to lessen nausea from chemotherapy. Offer frequent, small meals. It may be helpful to offer the child's favorite foods at times when nausea and vomiting are decreased. Ask the family what treatments they use to decrease the child's nausea and vomiting. Perform 24-hour dietary recalls to assess the child's intake, and evaluate height and weight regularly. Special nutritional products may be given orally, nasogastric or nasoduodenal tube feedings may be given, or total parenteral nutrition may be necessary.

Administer Medications

One important intervention of the oncology nurse is administering medications safely. Most chemotherapeutic drugs are prescribed and calculated as dose per meter squared (dose/m^2), with m^2 calculated from the child's height and weight. (Refer to the section on administering medications in the Skills Manual.)

Several chemotherapeutic drugs are often used in combinations (see Table 16-2). These drugs are prepared with special techniques under laminar flow devices to minimize potential toxic effects on health care providers. Gloves and other hazardous drug protocols are used. Care must be taken to avoid **extravasation** of intravenous drugs (leakage into the soft tissue around the infusion site), as permanent tissue damage can result.

In addition to chemotherapy drugs, the nurse administers other medications, such as antiemetics to control nausea, vitamin supplements, and antibiotics. Parents are asked about complementary therapy and medications they are obtaining from other sources and using at home. All medications must be safely administered and the child should be monitored for side effects. **Polypharmacy** (the use of several drugs at one time to treat multiple health conditions) can lead to multiple side effects and can challenge the body's ability to metabolize and excrete drugs.

SAFETY PRECAUTIONS

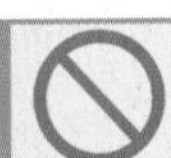

Health care professionals who have contact with chemotherapy drugs must follow careful guidelines. The Occupational Safety and Health Administration (OSHA) publishes an instruction manual, entitled "Controlling Occupational Exposure to Hazardous Drugs," which outlines general guidelines, protective equipment, and procedures (OSHA Instruction TED 1–0.15, Office of Science and Technology Assessment, Washington, DC, 1999).

Skills 7-1 to 7-13: Administration of Medication

NURSING ALERT

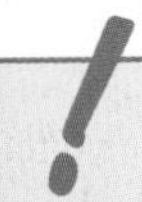

Chemotherapeutic drugs are given through intravenous infusion. Care should be taken to prevent leakage at the infusion site, because many drugs can cause tissue damage due to extravasation.

CLINICAL MANIFESTATIONS OF COMMON SIDE EFFECTS OF CHEMOTHERAPY

SIDE EFFECT	CLINICAL MANIFESTATIONS	CLINICAL THERAPY
Bone marrow suppression	Evidence of suppression usually appears 7–10 days after administration of chemotherapy; recovery is usually complete within 3–4 weeks	Blood transfusions are administered when anemia is severe (Hgb <7 g/dL) or platelets are very low Some institutions use a low-microbial diet to decrease the possibility that infectious organisms will colonize the intestine Septra is used for *Pneumocystis carinii* pneumonia prophylaxis; nystatin and oral vancomycin for antifungal and antibacterial prophylaxis Instruct the family and child about the importance of protecting the body from bruising during periods of mild to moderate thrombocytopenia (platelet count $< 5{,}000/mm^3$) Careful handwashing is essential Encourage use of masks if family or staff have nasopharyngeal infections
Nausea and vomiting	Symptoms may occur immediately or 5–6 hours after administration of chemotherapy and may last 48 hours	Antiemetics, such as andansetron, Kytril, Reglan, and Benadryl are used to treat this side effect Teach relaxation techniques, hypnosis, and systematic desensitization (a hypnotic process that progressively reduces reactions to objects that cause strong emotional or physical responses) to help to decrease the child's symptoms Encourage mild exercise and change of diet (eating only easily digestible foods) 12 hours before chemotherapy
Anorexia and weight loss	May occur at any time	Hyperalimentation is necessary if dietary changes are unsuccessful in halting the child's weight loss. Pay careful attention to changes in taste that affect food preferences Referral to a dietician may be helpful to achieve successful modification of the child's diet
Mouth sores	The oral mucositis resulting from chemotherapy usually occurs within 3–4 days and is often a contributing factor in anorexia	Antifungal agents, such as nystatin or clotrimazole, lessen the possibility of candidal infection Promote good oral hygiene, use soft foam wand or water irrigation to clean teeth; commercial mouthwashes are not recommended because they contain alcohol and increase drying of the oral cavity
Constipation	Can occur at any time in treatment but becomes more common as therapy progresses and dietary intake and physical activity decrease	Stool softeners and laxatives are used to treat this side effect Advise parents to increase fluids and fibrous foods in the child's diet
Pain	Pain can occur at any time and is best understood by subjective explanations of the child.	Acetaminophen, morphine, steroids, nonsteroidal anti-inflammatory drugs, and antidepressants may be used to manage pain Careful pain assessment is important; the location of the pain may provide a clue to its cause, for example, metastasis to the skull, infiltration of joints, or damage to soft tissue; pain associated with chemotherapy may also be related to oral mucositis, myalgia, or tumor embolization; painful polyneuropathy can follow treatment with vincristine or cisplatin Acetaminophen for pain can mask the presence of fever, which signals infection; careful and complete physical assessment is needed to identify infection Pharmacologic, nonhypnotic (deep breathing, self-control), and hypnotic methods of pain control may be used; the nonpharmacologic methods often prove helpful to children with pain from multiple etiologies

Manage Treatment Side Effects

All cancer treatments affect some normal body cells as well as cancer cells, causing a wide variety of side effects. A frequent occurrence is **myelosuppression,** or suppression of blood cell production in the bone marrow. Be alert for signs of a decreased white blood cell count, such as infections. Take the child's temperature, isolate the child from others with infections, and perform serum laboratory studies as ordered. A colony-stimulating factor for white cell production may be administered, if necessary.

Protect the child from bruises and be alert for signs of bleeding such as petechiae, an effect of decreased platelets. When thrombocytopenia occurs, minimize needle sticks and other intrusive procedures. Be ready to deal with nosebleeds and watch for bleeding gums. Report any bleeding episodes to the physician.

Inadequate red blood cell production can result in anemia. Encourage the child to eat iron-rich foods and administer nutritional supplements, as needed.

Chemotherapy affects all rapidly growing cells in the body, but especially those of the mucous membranes. Provide good oral hygiene with a soft toothbrush, foam wand, or water irrigation device. Report oral breakdown promptly. Be alert for blood in vomitus and stool, which can be indicators of bleeding in the gastrointestinal tract. Evaluate the effects of hair loss on the child.

Radiation can cause burns to the skin. Examine the skin daily during hospitalization or weekly when making home visits. Leave the marks on the skin that outline the radiation target area. Avoid use of lotions, powders, and soaps on the target skin area. Some children may need to be anesthetized to ensure correct positioning for radiation; postanesthesia care will then be needed.

COMMUNITY CARE

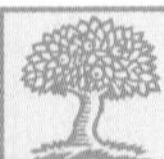

Children being treated for cancer usually have low immune response to disease, and thus need to avoid places where they might come in contact with many antimicrobials, such as child care centers, church schools, play areas at fast-food restaurants, and community fairs. Help parents find alternative activities that do not involve contact with multiple children at one time. They can often attend church services with the parent, spend special time with an older sibling, or have a video night at home with popcorn and a favorite friend.

Ensure Adequate Hydration

Hydration management can be a challenge as the child may not be thirsty but is excreting large numbers of cell fragments and other substances as a result of treatment. Offer frequent small amounts of fluid. Include frozen ice pops or other fluid-containing foods such as Jell-O. Measure intake and output. To ensure adequate excretion, a number of chemotherapy drugs are given with intravenous fluids. It is important to administer fluids as ordered and ensure that the recommended urinary output excretion rate is maintained after drug administration.

NURSING ALERT

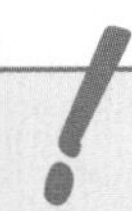

A treatment known as leucovorin rescue is used in conjunction with high-dose methotrexate chemotherapy. Leucovorin (citrovorum factor) is a form of folic acid that helps to protect normal cells from the destructive action of methotrexate. It is started within 24 hours of methotrexate administration and is given along with hydration therapy. Usual administration is q 6 hours X 72 hours or until serum methotrexate is at the desired level.

Prevent Infection

Children with cancer have an altered immune system, both from the disease and from the effects of immunosuppressant drugs, and must be kept away from persons with known infections. Teach parents to avoid taking the child to places that attract large gatherings of people, such as department stores, once the child returns home. Emphasize the need to report any exposure to contagious diseases, especially chickenpox. Signs of infection may be masked by some drugs, so be alert for any signs of mild infection. Fever, malaise, and mild respiratory infection must be reported promptly. Follow recommendations for the immunization of children with cancer as published by the Centers for Disease Control and Prevention and the American Academy of Pediatrics. Usually no immunizations are given to the child until 6 months after receiving chemotherapy.

Manage Pain

The child with cancer may experience pain from the disease itself and from the medical interventions, such as lumbar puncture, bone marrow aspiration, and frequent intravenous infusions and blood draws. Use all possible pain management techniques to keep the child comfortable, as this will assist with comfort and encourage cooperation throughout the long treatment period. (See Chapter 9 for suggestions on methods of pain management.)

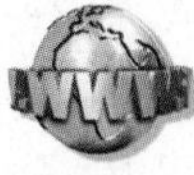

Professional Resources Online

Management of cancer pain has been the subject of an evidence-based practice report by the Agency for Healthcare Research and Quality. The agency found a lack of adequate studies on pain management and a limited application of existing work. These factors limit effective pain management in many patients with cancer (Agency for Healthcare Research and

Skills 9-1 to 9-4: Pain Assessment and Management Techniques

CLINICAL TIP

EMLA (eutectic mixture of local anesthetics) cream is a combination of lidocaine 2.5% and prilocaine 2.5% in an emulsion. Apply a thick layer of the cream to intact skin and cover with an occlusive dressing. Leave in place 1 hour for minor procedures and 2 hours for major procedures.

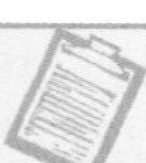

RESEARCH

The most common unmet needs for parents when their child has cancer are:

- Financial assistance
- Time
- Rest

These needs were identified in a survey of parents of children with cancer who were receiving treatment both at a medical center and at home. (Mercer & Ritchie, 1997).

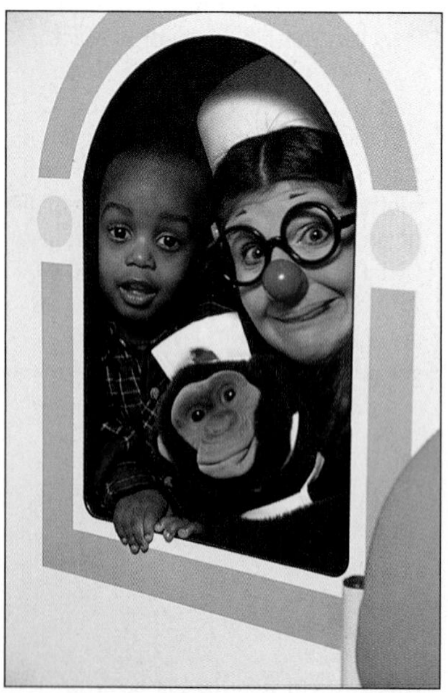

FIGURE 16-9 ◆
Clowns from the Big Apple Clown Care Unit can help to ease the stress of hospitalization for seriously ill children and their families. Here, a clown doctor and her puppet distract a toddler who is waiting for his clinic appointment.

Quality, 2001b). Nurses must examine research on effective pain management for children and integrated findings into practice.

Conscious sedation (see Chapter 9) may be used for some procedures. Administer sedation as ordered for young children who are undergoing radiation. Coordinate other painful or intrusive tests so they can be done while the child is sedated for radiation.

Topical anesthetics such as EMLA cream may be used to numb the skin before an intravenous start, lumbar puncture, or bone marrow aspiration. When possible, include the parents in comforting the child after painful procedures.

PROVIDE PSYCHOSOCIAL SUPPORT

A diagnosis of cancer brings with it many emotions for the family. Initially parents experience shock and anger. They need basic information about the disease and the purpose of the tests that will be performed. Instructions often need to be repeated as parents may not process information the first time it is presented due to their increased stress levels. Assist the parents to plan how and when to tell the child the diagnosis. What the child needs to know is based on his or her developmental level and understanding.

After progressing from the initial state of shock about the diagnosis, the family needs to learn more about the disease, including the pathophysiology, treatment, and expected outcome or the prognosis. Clarify the family's understanding of these areas and be ready to answer questions. Provide verbal explanations and written material. Parents may talk with friends, purchase books, or search the internet for information. Find out where they are getting information and provide additional resources when appropriate. Correct misconceptions and misinformation.

The family needs many strategies to deal with the challenge of long-term treatment for cancer. As the child experiences remissions and exacerbations or complications, the family feels alternately hopeful and discouraged. This was the case with Rasheed's family at the beginning of the chapter. Identify the family's support systems and intervene as needed to enhance these systems. Facilitate contact with extended family members who might be of help, religious or spiritual connections, social service agencies, and other resources such as internet and parent support groups. Assist parents who are concerned about job obligations and financial concerns.

The child undergoing treatment for cancer needs support appropriate to his or her developmental stage and cognitive level (Figure 16-9 ◆). (See Chapters 2 and 5 for developmental levels and effective support strategies for children of different ages.) Younger children primarily need support during painful procedures and separation from parents. Older children need intervention strategies to assist in working through feelings related to treatments (Figure 16-10 ◆). A major developmental task of adolescence is to attain independence and control, but cancer often interferes with adolescents' ability to achieve this task. Therefore, plan nursing strategies that empower adolescents as much as possible.

Talk with the child's teachers before the return to school after treatment to explain the child's condition. Arrange for tutors if necessary to assist the child with school work during hospitalization and home care. Explore the option of summer camp for children with cancer. The Make-a-Wish Foundation strives to make dreams come true for ill children by sponsoring them for a desired activity or outing. Refer the child to this foundation if appropriate.

The siblings of a child who has cancer can be stressed by the changes in the family. They may grieve over the ill brother or sister and may feel sad and depressed. They also can experience anger, guilt, or resentment and may have a lack of knowledge about the disease and treatment. Inquire about siblings and ask what they know about the child's condition. Find out who is caring for siblings and whether their teachers have been informed about the family situation. Include siblings in care when possible. Invite them to visit and to participate both during hospitalization and at home care visits. They can be involved in play therapy sessions and recreational activities with the ill child. Ask the parents if the siblings are demonstrating symptoms such as depression, behavioral changes, or decrease in school performance and suggest interventions as appropriate. They may benefit from speaking with a school counselor or can be referred to a support group for siblings of children with cancer. Some cancer summer camps welcome siblings as well as children with cancer.

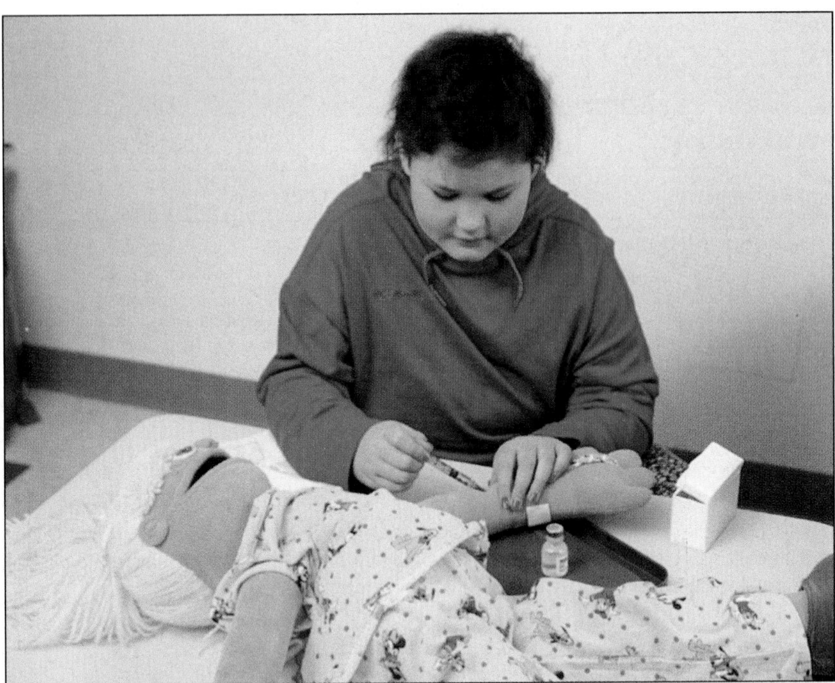

FIGURE 16-10 ◆
A child in a pediatric oncology clinic giving injections to a doll. This type of play therapy helps the child deal with fear, thus lowering his or her stress level.

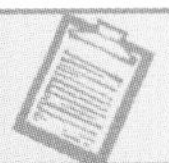

RESEARCH

Research has shown that two of the worst stressors for adolescents with cancer are (1) waiting for care and (2) dependence on parents. Nurses can devise interventions to minimize waiting for chemotherapy and other treatments or provide options such as meetings with other teens and computer use while waiting. When possible, enable the adolescent to make choices independently of parents (Enskar, Carlsson, & Golsater, et al., 1997).

The family of a child with cancer is faced with a life-threatening illness. Refer to Chapter 8 for strategies to assist the family in coping with this stressor. For some types of cancer, the child may experience a remission with treatment, but then a recurrence of disease later as cancer cells grow again. The family may become angry or depressed about the relapse. Repeated treatments challenge the family's support systems. Waiting for the outcome of diagnostic tests can be an especially challenging time. Provide information as soon as possible. If the child's illness progresses, refer the family to hospice to assist them in caring for the terminally ill child and in working through the grieving process. Explore support groups and information related to cancer in order to share this information with families.

Discharge Planning and Home Care Teaching

Preparation for home care centers on creating a normal environment while supporting the child's physiologic and psychosocial responses to the cancer and treatments. Education is

FAMILIES WANT TO KNOW

Reportable Events for Children Receiving Chemotherapy

Report the following events to your child's oncologist if they occur while the child is receiving chemotherapy:

- Temperature above 38°C (101°F)
- Any bleeding, such as nosebleeds, blood in stool or urine, petechiae, bruising
- Pain or discomfort with urination or defecation
- Sores in the mouth
- Vomiting or diarrhea
- Persistent pain anywhere, including headache
- Signs of infection, such as cough, fever, runny nose, tugging at ears
- Signs of infection in central lines, such as redness, drainage, or tenderness
- Exposure to communicable diseases, especially varicella (chickenpox)

Inform dentists and other health care providers that the child is receiving chemotherapy prior to procedures. Prophylactic antibiotics should be given before and after dental care.

Note: Adapted from Bindler, R. M., & Howry, L. B. (1997). *Pediatric drugs and nursing implications* (2nd ed., p. 587). Stamford, CT: Appleton & Lange.

NURSING CARE PLAN Home Care of the Child with Cancer

GOAL	INTERVENTION	RATIONALE	EXPECTED OUTCOME
1. Risk for Infection related to immunosuppression, chemotherapy, and presence of invasive lines			
	NIC Priority Intervention: **Infection Protection:** Prevention and early detection of infection in child at risk.		NOC Suggested Outcome: **Risk Control:** Actions to eliminate or reduce health risks.
The child will remain infection free.	■ Educate the child and parents about meaning of blood counts. ■ Encourage parents/family members to use masks when they are ill. ■ Encourage good handwashing at all times. ■ Advise the child's teacher to tell parents if the child is exposed to communicable illness at school. ■ Clean vascular access site and inject heparin per protocol. Observe for signs of infection. Report infection to physician.	■ Knowledgeable parents and child can protect themselves. ■ Masks help decrease airborne infection if used properly. ■ Handwashing is best prevention. ■ Exposure can be reported to physician for possible use of acyclovir or admission for treatment. ■ Use of heparin maintains an open access route by preventing clotting.	The child remains infection free. All exposures are reported to physician immediately.
2. Altered Nutrition: Less Than Body Requirements related to inability to ingest or digest adequate quantities of food or absorb adequate nutrients			
	NIC Priority Intervention: **Nutrition Management:** Assistance with and provision of a balanced dietary intake.		NOC Suggested Outcome: **Nutritional Status:** Extent to which nutrients are available to meet metabolic needs.
The child will maintain adequate nutritional intake.	■ Encourage small and frequent high-calorie meals. Encourage small bites of a variety foods ■ Promote good oral hygiene and use of nonalcohol mouthwashes. ■ Teach home parenteral nutrition if ordered.	■ Measures to increase caloric intake. Taste changes and favorite foods may no longer be preferred. ■ Mouth sores interrupt eating. Alcohol stings open sores. ■ Parenteral nutritional support may be used to enhance intake.	The child maintains normal weight for height.
3. Ineffective Management of Therapeutic Regimen related to complex therapy			
	NIC Intervention: **Family Involvement:** Facilitating family participation in the emotional and physical care of the child.		NOC Suggested Outcome: **Care Management:** Family ability to manage complex therapy.
The child will comply with oral medication regimen.	■ Educate parents and child about the importance of taking medication as prescribed. ■ Set up calendar with dates, times, and medications clearly labeled. ■ Reward the child for taking medications.	■ Understanding can assist parents and child in placing importance on medication intake. ■ Visual reminders can help them recall instructions. ■ Reinforcing desired behaviors, through rewards is effective with children.	The child takes all medications according to prescription.

(continued)

NURSING CARE PLAN Home Care of the Child with Cancer (continued)

GOAL	INTERVENTION	RATIONALE	EXPECTED OUTCOME
4. Altered Growth and Development related to serious illness			
	NIC Priority Intervention: **Developmental Enhancement:** Facilitating parents/caregivers to promote optimal growth and development of child.		NOC Suggested Outcome: **Child Growth and Development:** Normal increase in body size and developmental skills.
The child will demonstrate normal physical, emotional, and cognitive development.	■ Encourage play appropriate to age. ■ Encourage the child to attend school. ■ Encourage seeing peers when unable to attend school. ■ Work with teachers to support reentry to school. Use puppets, videotape, and discussion with classmates.	■ Normal activities support self-esteem and self-knowledge. ■ School is the work of the child and promotes cognitive and social growth. ■ Peer contacts help the child in normal developmental tasks. ■ Classmates need to understand what has happened to their friend without asking the child directly.	The child continues to develop physically, emotionally, and cognitively at a normal pace.
5. Fatigue related to disease state			
	NIC Priority Intervention: **Energy Management:** Regulating energy use to prevent fatigue and optimize function.		NOC suggested Outcome: **Energy Conservation:** Extent of management of energy to initiate and sustain activity.
The child will maintain energy levels necessary for normal activities.	■ Problem solve ways to save energy for play and school. ■ Plan with child for quiet activities during low-energy times.	■ The child and parents are assisted to see school and play as important. ■ Child is empowered to select and plan own activities.	The child plans use of time effectively to maintain energy for school and play. The child conserves energy during times of increased fatigue.
6. Altered Family Processes related to situational crisis			
	NIC Priority Intervention: **Family Process Maintenance:** Minimization of family process disruption events.		NOC Suggested Outcome: **Family Process:** Extent of maintenance of family support system.
The child and family will demonstrate healthy adaptation.	■ Encourage open communication. ■ Suggest that all family members develop support networks. ■ Parents should be proactive with siblings about their feelings and needs. ■ Encourage attendance of all family members at oncology camps.	■ Open discussion allows problem solving and ego support. ■ Networks expand support systems. ■ Siblings feel valued and problems are confronted early. ■ Oncology camps promote open discussion between peers for further support and fun.	Parents report better communication between themselves and the children. Family members report an increase in friends with whom they can share feelings. Family reports attending oncology camp and describes benefit of sharing with other families in same situation.

the primary focus of discharge planning. Teach the parents how to ensure adequate nutritional intake, to be alert for signs of infection, to protect the child from exposure to communicable diseases during times of neutropenia, to administer medications at home, and to handle vomiting and pain. Assist the parents and child to deal with any obstacles to normal development and functioning. Teach the parents and family about symptoms that need to be treated immediately.

Skills 8-8 to 8-10: Managing Central Venous Catheters

Home management of a vascular access device or central line, such as a Broviac catheter (refer to the Skills Manual), is an initial challenge for parents (Figure 16-11 ◆). An implanted port may be used and allows the child freedom to swim and engage in other activities. Parents will need information about whatever device the child has received. Details about cleaning the site, instilling heparin in the line or reservoir, and other needed care are demonstrated. After teaching the parents, observe them performing the procedure before the child is discharged.

Emphasize the need for the child and family to have fun and be as normal as possible. Play distracts the child and is essential in reducing fears. Children, parents, and siblings often benefit from participation in cancer support groups and cancer summer camps. These activities create additional support systems, build the child's self-esteem, and enhance coping skills through role modeling.

Make home visits to evaluate the family's strengths and needs. Be sure that the family has adequate support from a hospice and other end-of-life services when the child's condition is terminal.

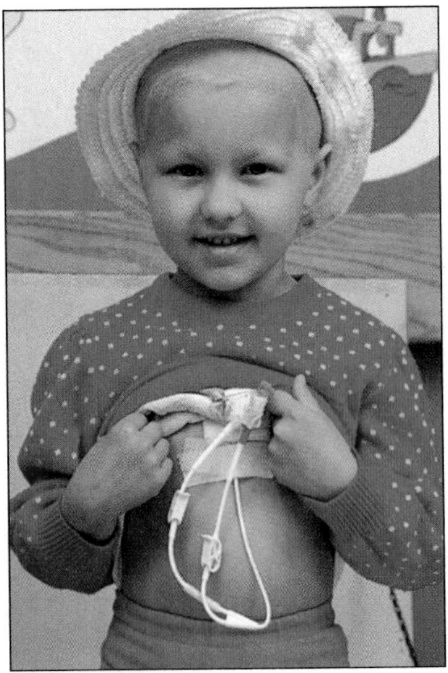

FIGURE 16-11 ◆
A vascular access device allows chemotherapeutic agents to be administered without the need for repeated "sticks" to the child.

GROWTH & DEVELOPMENT

An adolescent can decide which type of medication port would be best (e.g., an implantable port under the skin or a venous access device with tubing outside the body). This enables the teen to feel more in control of the disease and treatment.

Evaluation

The following expected outcomes of nursing care for the child with cancer relate to the specific disease, treatments, and responses:

- Adequate intake to promote normal growth
- Hydration that supports body processes and ensures drug and cancer cell product elimination
- Prompt identification and treatment to minimize treatment side effects
- Management of pain to a level of comfort satisfactory to child and family
- Family use of resources to provide necessary support during hospitalizations and treatments
- Knowledge of management of treatment regimens
- Acceptance of prognosis and support of all family members

BRAIN TUMORS

Central nervous system or brain tumors are the most commonly occurring solid tumors in children and the second most common malignancy, after leukemia (Baker, 1998; Smith, Freidlin, & Ries, et al., 1998). Each year approximately 1,500 children under the age of 15 are diagnosed with tumors of the brain and central nervous system, accounting for one in five childhood cancers (Conway, Asuncion, & DaRosso, 1999).

ETIOLOGY AND PATHOPHYSIOLOGY

Brain tumors in children usually occur below the roof of the cerebellum and involve the cerebellum, midbrain, and brainstem (Figure 16-12 ◆). In contrast, brain tumors in adults are usually located above the areas between the cerebrum and cerebellum.

The most common brain tumors in children are medulloblastoma, cerebral and cerebellar astrocytoma, ependymoma, and gliomas of the cerebrum or brainstem. Less common are supratentorial embryonal tumors and craniopharyngioma.

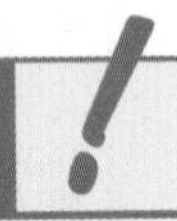

NURSING ALERT

Some children with brain tumors have nonspecific signs. They may have a slight behavior change, perform poorly at school, or show some incoordination. Be alert to such signs and to the parents' statement that they notice a change in the child. Report such findings so appropriate assessments can be made.

CLINICAL MANIFESTATIONS

Brain tumors in children can be manifested by behavioral and nervous system changes that occur either rapidly or more slowly and subtly. Some common symptoms include headache, nausea, vomiting, dizziness, change in vision or hearing, fatigue, and nonspecific signs. See the clinical manifestations table for common manifestations of certain types of tumors.

Medulloblastomas are brain tumors in the external layer of the cerebellum. They account for 20% of childhood brain tumors, and commonly occur in children aged 5 to 6 years. Astrocytomas arise from glial cells and can be either above or below the area between the cerebrum and cerebellum. They comprise 40% of childhood brain tumors (Kun, 1997).

PATHOPHYSIOLOGY ILLUSTRATED

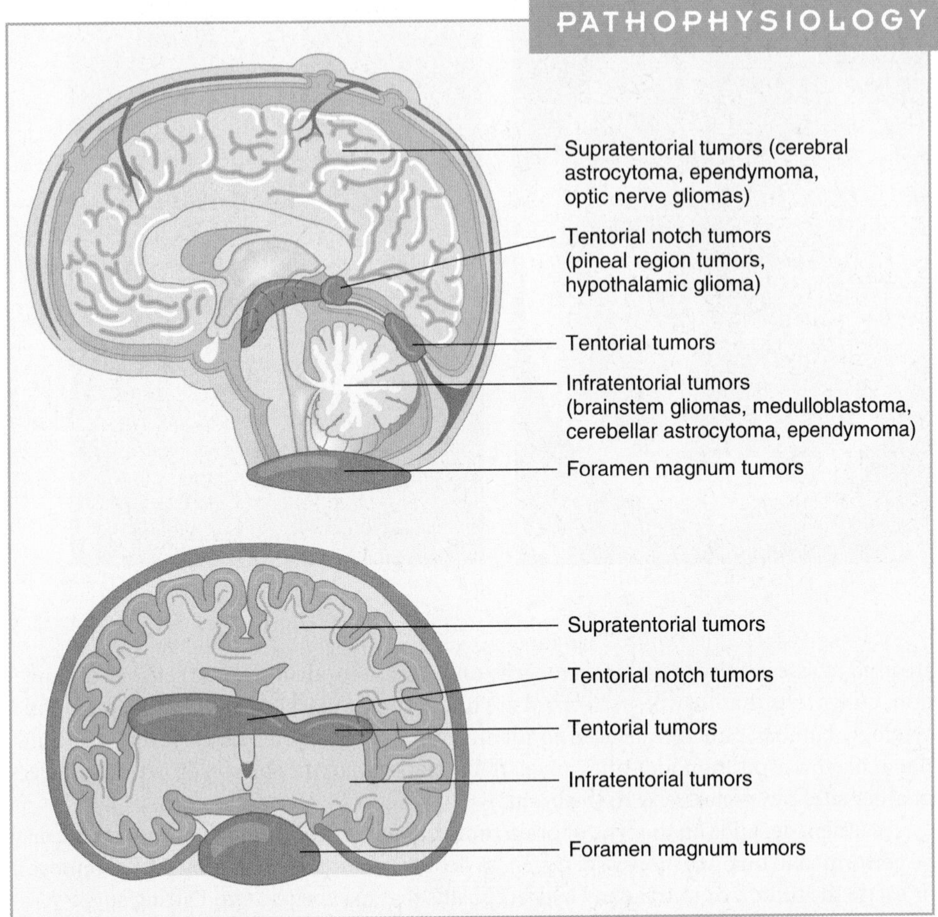

Brain Tumors

FIGURE 16-12 ◆
Sites of brain tumors in children. Approximately 1500 children under the age of 15 years are diagnosed annually as having tumors of the brain and central nervous system. The four most common brain tumors in children are medulloblastoma, cerebral astrocytoma, ependymoma, and brainstem glioma.

CLINICAL MANIFESTATIONS OF BRAIN TUMORS

TUMOR	ETIOLOGY	CLINICAL MANIFESTATIONS	CLINICAL THERAPY
Medulloblastoma	External layer of cerebellum	Headache, vomiting, ataxia	Surgery; chemotherapy with lomustine, vincristine, prednisone, cisplatin, radiation
Astrocytomas	Glial cells, supratentorial or infratentorial	Seizures, visual disturbances, increased intracranial pressure, vomiting	Surgery; chemotherapy with vincristine, dactinomycin; radiation
Ependymoma	Fourth ventricle, posterior fossa	Hydrocephalus	Surgery, radiation
Brainstem gliomas	Pons	Cranial nerve (VI + VII) tract signs, nystagmus, ataxia, motor symptoms	Surgery, radiation

Ependymomas commonly occur in the fourth ventricle of the posterior fossa and comprise 8% of childhood brain tumors. Brainstem gliomas are located in the pons and typically spread into the surrounding tissue. They account for 15% of childhood brain tumors (Conway, et al., 1999). Cerebral gliomas are another common cancer type in children.

CLINICAL THERAPY

Brain tumors are commonly diagnosed by means of computed tomography (CT; Figure 16-13A ◆), magnetic resonance imaging (MRI; Figure 16-13B ◆), myelography, and angiography. Neurophysiologic tests (electroencephalography and brainstem evoked potentials)

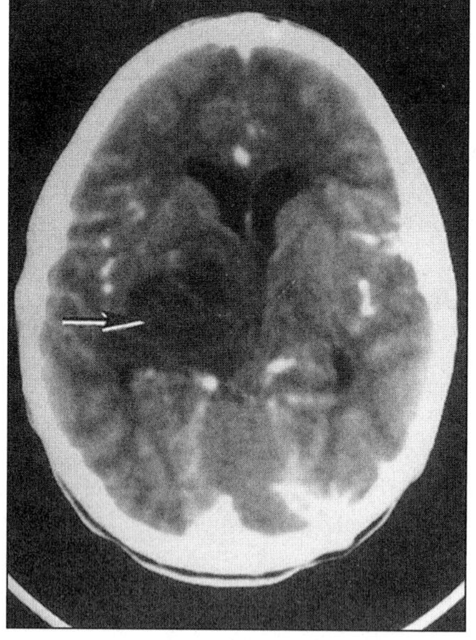
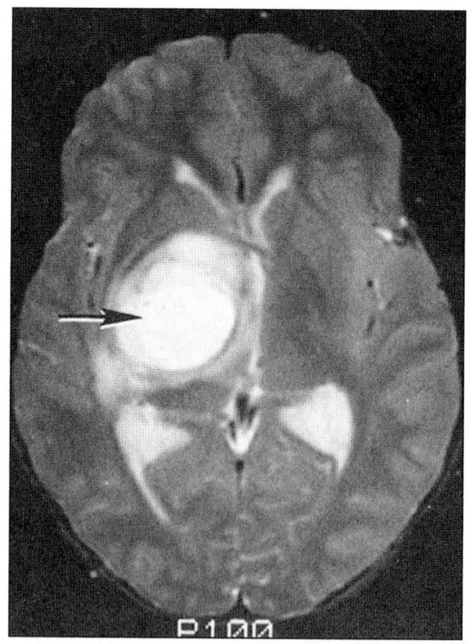

A B

FIGURE 16-13 ◆
Radiologic imaging of a child with a brain tumor. A, CT scan. B, MRI.
Courtesy of Carlos Sivit, M. D., Children's National Medical Center, Washington, DC.

are used to assess sensory pathway integrity and disease- or drug-related sensory dysfunction. Other tests that may be performed are use of tumor markers and cerebrospinal fluid cytology. Lumbar puncture is used to identify abnormal cells in the cerebrospinal fluid. Bone marrow aspiration identifies any extracranial primary neoplastic growth, as cancers in other sites can metastasize to the brain.

Treatment depends on the type of brain tumor. Surgery is a common treatment, and may be performed to obtain a biopsy specimen, to debulk (reduce the tumor by partial removal) or excise the tumor, or to treat any hydrocephalus that may be present. During surgery, radiology images allow the neurosurgeon to see computerized images of the brain while at the same time stimulating nerves to determine their functioning. These techniques provide rapid feedback to the neurosurgeon. Laser surgery, which has delicate precise control and accuracy, is used when tumors are close to sensitive neural or vascular structures.

DRUGS USED TO TREAT BRAIN TUMORS

- Cyclophosphamide
- Ifosfamide
- Lomustine
- Vincristin
- VP-16
- Cisplatin
- Carboplatin

Use of radiation following surgery and chemotherapy has improved the survival of children with medulloblastoma and ependymoma. High-dose chemotherapy is often used, and this modality has improved the survival of children with central nervous system tumors (Conway et al., 1999). Low-dose chemotherapy can shrink and help manage some tumors. Intrathecal administration of chemotherapy is useful in some cases. However, the blood-brain barrier is a factor in the effectiveness of chemotherapy for children with brain tumors. For example, when methotrexate is administered intrathecally (in the spinal canal), only a small amount crosses normal brain capillaries. Radiation is not used in children under 3 years because of resultant damage to brain cells. Bone marrow and stem cell transplantation is an increasingly used treatment option.

Complications of treatment for children with brain tumors are significant. They include severe infections (associated with high-dose chemotherapy), seizure activity, sensorimotor defects, hydrocephalus, and growth problems. Care is taken to treat infections early and aggressively. If a cerebrospinal shunt is used, infection or blockage can occur (see Chapter 20 for further discussion of cerebrospinal shunts in children). Anticonvulsants are commonly given prophylactically following surgery. Endocrine problems, such as growth hormone changes, hypothyroidism, and panhypopituitarism, may occur when the tumor is in the hypothalamic-pituitary area (Vernon-Levett & Geller, 1997). Treatment may also lead to impaired cognitive function and emotional or behavioral problems in some children. Memory deficits and selective attention deficits are the most common problems.

Diabetes insipidus is a special consideration in children with midline brain tumors, such as those that compress the hypothalamus, pituitary stalk, or posterior pituitary gland. Manifestations of diabetes insipidus include voiding of large amounts of dilute urine with a specific gravity of less than 1.005 (see Chapter 18).

NURSING MANAGEMENT

Nursing Assessment and Diagnosis

The focus of physiologic assessment of the child with a brain tumor is determined by its presentation (Table 16-4). Presenting signs can be categorized as follows:

- Nonspecific signs related to increasing intracranial pressure
- Secondary signs related to displacement of intracranial structures
- Focal signs suggesting direct involvement of the brain and cranial nerves

Thorough neurologic examination before surgery is essential to provide a record of baseline functioning and allow the evaluation of the child's changing physiologic status before surgery. Ask if the child has manifested slow changes over time or has had quickly developing symptoms. Measurement of head circumference and assessment of the anterior fontanel are necessary in children under the age of 18 months.

Perform developmental screening on young children using the Denver II or other developmental test (see Chapter 6). Ask about the child's social interactions, school performance, and any behavior changes that have occurred.

The following nursing diagnoses can be identified for the child with a brain tumor, depending on the type and location of the tumor:

- *Altered nutrition: Less than body requirements,* related to loss of appetite
- *Impaired physical mobility,* related to tumor pressure on coordination centers
- *Altered growth and development,* related to effects of disability
- *Impaired memory,* related to neurologic disturbance
- *Pain,* related to physical injury

Planning and Implementation

The child with a brain tumor requires multidisciplinary care by a neurologist, neurosurgeon, pediatrician, dietician, social worker, and other specialists. The nurse can act as a case manager to coordinate the complex care needed by the child.

For the nursing care of children immediately following surgery, refer to Chapter 5. In addition, close monitoring of neurologic status is needed postoperatively (refer to Chapter 20). Be especially alert for signs of increased intracranial pressure and infection. Observe for seizure activity. Administer drugs such as antibiotics and anticonvulsants as ordered.

Signs and symptoms of diabetes insipidus may occur following brain surgery (see Chapter 18 for a description of diabetes insipidus). Nursing care includes hourly measurement of intake and output, measurement of serum sodium levels every 4 to 6 hours, accurate fluid replacement, and frequent assessment of neurologic status. An indwelling urinary catheter is useful for accurate measurement of urinary output.

NURSING ALERT

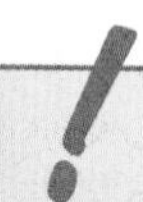

Report abnormally high or low urinary output in the child after brain surgery. Either amount can be indicative of problems with management of urinary output.

TABLE 16-4 Physiologic Assessment of Brain Tumors

CLINICAL MANIFESTATIONS	ASSESSMENT
Nonspecific signs: headache, morning vomiting, somnolence, irritability	Level of consciousness, pupil response, pupil shape and size
Secondary signs: disturbances of cranial nerves; other signs depend on site of tumor	All cranial nerves
Focal signs: truncal ataxia (midline brain tumors), general nystagmus, head tilting	Motor ability, head positions when watching television or looking at people (double vision, sixth cranial nerve involvement)

Discharge Planning and Home Care Teaching

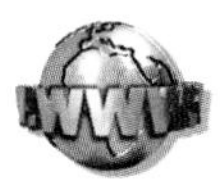

Cancer Resources Online

Teach the parents to watch for an increase in voiding of dilute urine. Be sure they can recognize the signs of infection and changes in the child's neurologic status. Once the child is ready for discharge, chemotherapy or radiation may begin; inform parents of the reason and potential side effects of these treatments. Assist the family in obtaining any special equipment they may need to care for the child at home, such as a wheelchair, bed rails, or dressings. The American Cancer Society is a potential resource for assistance with these needs.

Children with brain tumors, especially those who have received radiation, often have some permanent sequelae. They may have slowed development, incoordination, learning disabilities, or other effects. These sequelae are most common in children who are 3 years of age or younger at the time of radiation therapy. Perform accurate height and weight measures at each health care visit. Assess developmental milestones. Ask about progress in school and any special services that might be needed. Perform thorough neurologic assessments. Support the family as they learn to deal with unknown or changed expectations for the child's performance (Freeman, O'Dell, & Meola, 2000).

Evaluation

Expected outcomes of nursing care for the child with a brain tumor depend on the site of tumor, clinical therapy, and medical outcome. Possible outcomes include the following:

- Adequate nutritional intake to support growth and prevent malnutrition
- Maintenance of a safe environment
- Physical mobility allowed by developmental level and alterations of disease
- Provision of an environment to meet normal developmental milestones within capability of the child
- Management of pain to comfort level
- Parental understanding of diagnosis and treatment plan

NEUROBLASTOMA

Neuroblastoma is the solid tumor most commonly occurring outside the cranium of children. It is responsible for 8% of childhood cancers and 15% of cancer deaths in children. The average age at onset is 22 months. Prognosis varies, depending on the staging of the tumor (Table 16-5) and the age of the child, with more favorable outcomes in infants under 1 year of age (Castleberry, 1997).

TABLE 16-5 International Neuroblastoma Staging System

STAGE	DESCRIPTION
1	Localized tumor confined to the area of origin; complete gross excision, with or without microscopic residual disease; identifiable ipsilateral and contralateral lymph nodes negative microscopically
2A	Unilateral tumor with incomplete gross excision; identifiable ipsilateral and contralateral lymph nodes negative microscopically
2B	Unilateral tumor with complete or incomplete gross excision; with positive ipsilateral regional lymph nodes; identifiable contralateral lymph nodes negative microscopically
3	Tumor infiltrating across the midline with or without regional lymph node involvement; or unilateral tumor with contralateral regional lymph node involvement; or midline tumor with bilateral regional lymph node involvement
4	Dissemination of tumor to distant lymph nodes, bone, bone marrow, liver, and/or other organs (except as defined in stage 4S)
4S	Localized primary tumor as defined for stage 1 or 2 with dissemination limited to liver, skin, and/or bone marrow

Note: Adapted from Castleberry, R.P. (1997). Biology and treatment of neuroblastoma. *Pediatric Clinics of North America, 44*, 919–938.

Neuroblastoma is commonly a smooth, hard, nontender mass that can occur anywhere along the sympathetic nervous system chain. A frequent location is the abdomen, although other sites are the adrenal, thoracic, and cervical areas. It is usually diagnosed in children under 5 years of age, with the median age at diagnosis being 2 years (McManus & Gilchrist, 2000).

ETIOLOGY AND PATHOPHYSIOLOGY

Neuroblastoma originates in primitive neurocrest cells that form the adrenal medulla, paraganglia, and sympathetic nervous system of the cervical sympathetic chain and the thoracic chain. Fifty percent of neuroblastomas develop in the adrenal medulla, 20% develop in the thorax, and the remaining 30% are elsewhere along the sympathetic chain (McManus & Gilchrist, 2000). Lymph node metastasis is common.

The cause of neuroblastoma is unknown. Theories that have been proposed center on the possible effects of environmental factors such as prenatal drug exposure from the mother and disturbed cellular nerve growth factors. Oncogenes are present in neuroblastoma cells in a DNA sequence known as N-myc. High levels of the N-myc oncogene are associated with rapid disease progression and a poorer prognosis.

CLINICAL MANIFESTATIONS

The location of the mass determines the symptoms. Altered bowel and bladder function occur when the mass is retroperitoneal; characteristic signs are weight loss, abdominal fullness, irritability, fatigue, and fever. Dyspnea or infection may occur when the tumor is mediastinal. Neck and facial edema may result from vena cava syndrome if the tumor is mediastinal and large. Malaise, fever, and a limp can occur if there has been metastasis to the bone (Castleberry, 1997).

CLINICAL THERAPY

The International Neuroblastoma Staging System (INSS) recommends different diagnostic and laboratory evaluations for diagnosis of the primary disease and of metastases (Table 16-6).

Vanillylmandelic acid (VMA) and homovanillic acid (HVA) are byproducts of adrenal hormones and their levels are usually elevated in the urine and blood (see Appendix C for normal values). They are used initially to diagnose the disease and later to follow its progress. Areas of necrosis and calcification are readily identifiable with radiologic tests. These tests also help in the staging of the disease by identifying metastases.

Routine blood cell counts may reveal anemia and thrombocytopenia. There is no classic WBC response, although thrombocytopenia may occur in association with disseminated intravascular coagulation. **Leukocytosis** (higher than normal leukocyte count) and **leukopenia** (lower than normal leukocyte count) have been observed with bone marrow involvement.

The stage of the tumor (see Table 16-5) determines the treatment protocol. Surgical excision of the mass is performed, followed by chemotherapy with a combination of drugs. Ra-

TABLE 16-6 Diagnostic Tests for Neuroblastoma

Tests for initial diagnosis Tumor tissue diagnosis by light microscopy, or Biopsy of tumor cells plus laboratory evaluation showing increased urine or serum catecholamines (two separate measures each more than 3 standard deviations above the norm for age)
Tests for metastases Bone marrow biopsy Radiolabeled scanning with metaiodobenzylguanidine (MIBG) Skeletal x-ray CT or MRI of abdomen and liver Chest x-ray, with added CT or MRI if x-ray shows lesions

DRUGS USED TO TREAT NEUROBLASTOMA

Cyclophosphamide
Doxorubicin
Cisplatin
Ifosfamide
Teniposide
Etoposide
Carboplatin

diation is occasionally used. Bone marrow transplantation may be performed for advanced disease. Neuroblastoma is most responsive to treatment in children under 1 year of age.

NURSING MANAGEMENT

Nursing Assessment and Diagnosis

The presenting site of the tumor, such as the neck or abdomen, is assessed by observation and inspection. Palpation is contraindicated. Carefully document related functioning, such as bowel and bladder function. Take vital signs to watch for elevated temperature and vital sign changes caused by a thoracic mass. Observe gait and coordination. Take weight and height and compare with earlier percentiles for the child. Specific assessments during treatment will depend on the treatment methods used (refer to the earlier discussions of chemotherapy and radiation treatment). Psychosocial assessment and emotional assessment of the family are needed.

The following nursing diagnoses may be appropriate for the child with neuroblastoma, depending on the location and extent of the presenting disease:

- *Impaired gas exchange,* related to ventilation-perfusion imbalance
- *Impaired physical mobility,* related to neuromuscular impairment
- *Sensory/perceptual alteration (visual),* related to altered sensory perception
- *Pain,* related to tumor pressure and injury
- *Anticipatory grieving (family),* related to potential loss of significant person

Planning and Implementation

The nursing management of the child with neuroblastoma can encompass the three phases of medical treatment: chemotherapy, surgery, and radiation. Specific postsurgical care depends on the size and site of the tumor. Normal postoperative care includes providing fluid support and respiratory care and preventing infection.

Nursing care during the chemotherapy phase includes minimizing side effects, preventing infection, teaching parents about the medications their child is receiving, and monitoring physical and emotional growth and development of the young child. When radiation is part of the treatment, use common nursing measures described earlier in the chapter.

FAMILIES WANT TO KNOW

The Child with a Neuroblastoma

SURGERY PHASE

- Teach the parents to observe for signs of infection at the wound site and to take the child's temperature, if necessary.
- Advise parents to note bowel movements and report a lack of one for 3 days to the physician.
- Continue with progression to a regular diet.

CHEMOTHERAPY PHASE

- The child frequently has a central line placed early in the chemotherapy phase. The central line greatly reduces the emotional trauma associated with chemotherapy and blood tests.
  - Teach the child how to help the parents with cleaning of the central line.
  - Teach the child how to protect the central line.
  - Teach the parents how to clean and dress the site of the central line.
  - Have the parents practice central line care with a model and then on the child before discharge to increase the parents' confidence.
  - Give the parents written and illustrated information about care of a central line.
  - Arrange for home care dressing supplies before discharge.
- Give the parents detailed chemotherapy information.
- Refer the family to the American Cancer Society for coloring books for children receiving chemotherapy.

Topics for parent and family teaching and discharge planning are presented in the Families Want to Know feature on page 566. Ongoing support and connection to resources to assist in management of the child's treatment at home will be needed. When the prognosis is poor, parents may appreciate referrals to hospice, to other parents who have experienced similar child illnesses, and to other community resources. See Chapter 8 for additional nursing care for end of life.

CLINICAL TIP

Many centers give notebooks with information on chemotherapy and other relevant treatment methods to families shortly after diagnosis. Information that is pertinent to the child is highlighted during the teaching sessions. Blank pages are included to encourage parents to use the notebook for recording information, tests and results, personal thoughts, and questions.

Evaluation

Expected outcomes of nursing care for the child with neuroblastoma include the following:

- Respiratory exchange to support daily activities
- Physical mobility to level possible considering developmental age
- Management of sensory/perceptual alterations to provide for safety and sensory input
- Management of pain to level of comfort
- Acceptance and integration of diagnosis into lives of family members

WILMS' TUMOR (NEPHROBLASTOMA)

Nephroblastoma, an intrarenal tumor that is called Wilms' tumor, is a common abdominal tumor of childhood and accounts for 6% to 7% of all childhood tumors (Anderson, 2000). Each year the incidence is 8.1 cases per million children. Wilms' tumor occurs most frequently between 2 and 5 years of age, but may also occur in adolescents and adults.

ETIOLOGY AND PATHOPHYSIOLOGY

Wilms' tumor is associated with several congenital anomalies: aniridia (absence of the iris), hemihypertrophy (abnormal growth of half of the body or a body structure), genitourinary anomalies, nevi, and hamartomas (benign, nodulelike growths). This connection suggests a genetic link; however, most children with Wilms' tumor have no other abnormalities. A tumor suppressor gene has been identified that acts to promote normal kidney development. This gene and others may be missing in children with Wilms' tumor (Anderson, 2000).

CLINICAL MANIFESTATIONS

Wilms' tumor is usually an asymptomatic, firm, lobulated mass located to one side of the midline in the abdomen. Often a parent discovers the mass during the child's bath. Hypertension caused by increased renin activity related to renal damage is reported in 25% of cases. Hematuria is sometimes present. Bilateral Wilms' tumors occur in 5% to 10% of cases (Anderson, 2000).

CLINICAL THERAPY

The diagnosis of Wilms' tumor is based on an ultrasound study of the abdomen and an intravenous pyelogram. CT scanning or MRI of the lungs, liver, spleen, and brain may be performed to identify any metastasis. This information is used in staging the tumor (Table 16-7). A complete blood count is obtained, as well as BUN and creatinine levels. Liver function tests are performed.

Treatment is multifaceted. Surgery is performed to remove the affected kidney, to examine the opposite kidney, and to look for other sites of metastasis. Chemotherapy or radiation therapy, alone or in combination, is sometimes used before surgery to reduce the size of the tumor. Radiation and/or chemotherapy may also follow surgery. Children whose tumors are almost completely excised and who have a favorable prognosis do not require irradiation of the tumor bed.

Long-term complications of treatment include liver damage, portal hypertension, and mild cirrhosis, which may occur in children treated for right-sided Wilms' tumor. Radiation damage (such as thinning or weakening) of the skeleton, pelvis, and thorax has been reported. Kyphosis and scoliosis may occur from irradiation of vertebral bodies and the

TABLE 16-7 National Wilms' Tumor Study Staging System

STAGE	DESCRIPTION
I	The tumor is limited to the kidney and completely excised. The surface of the renal capsule is intact. The tumor is not ruptured before or during removal. No residual tumor is apparent beyond the margins of the excision.
II	The tumor extends beyond the kidney but is completely excised. Regional extension of the tumor is present, i.e., penetration through the outer surface of the renal capsule into the perirenal soft tissues. Vessels outside the kidney substance are infiltrated or contain tumor thrombus. Biopsy may have been performed on the tumor, or local spillage of tumor confined to the flank has occurred. No residual tumor is apparent at or beyond the margin of excision.
III	Residual nonhematogenous tumor is confined to the abdomen. Any of the following may occur: Lymph nodes on biopsy are found to be involved in the hilus, the periaortic chains, or beyond. Diffuse peritoneal contamination by the tumor has occurred, such as by spillage of tumor beyond the flank before or during surgery, or by tumor growth that has penetrated through the peritoneal surface. Implants are found on peritoneal surfaces. The tumor extends beyond the surgical margins either microscopically or grossly. The tumor is not completely resectable because of local infiltration into vital structures.
IV	Hematogenous metastasis: deposits are present beyond stage III, e.g., lung, liver, bone, and/or brain.
V	Bilateral renal involvement is present at diagnosis. An attempt should be made to stage each side according to the above criteria on the basis of extent of disease before biopsy.

Note: Adapted from Green, D. M., Grigoriev, Y. A., Nan, B., Takashima, J. R., Norkool, P. A., D'Angio, G. J., & Breslow, N. E. (2001). Congestive heart failure after treatment for Wilms' tumor: A report from the National Wilms' Tumor study group. *Journal of Clinical Oncology, 19,* 1926–1934.

DRUGS USED TO TREAT WILMS' TUMOR

Vincristine
Actinomycin D
Doxorubicin
Cyclophosphamide

pelvis. Glomerular damage to the remaining kidney may also occur. Second malignancies in the original radiation field have occurred with orthovoltage radiation, but recent changes in radiation therapy have reduced this risk.

NURSING MANAGEMENT

Nursing Assessment and Diagnosis

Perform a thorough baseline assessment of the child. Do not palpate the abdomen because of the potential for spreading the cancerous cells. Monitor the child's blood pressure carefully as hypertension is a common finding that may require treatment.

Nursing diagnoses for a child with Wilms' tumor will differ depending on the phase of treatment. Common nursing diagnoses may include the following:

- *Risk for infection,* related to inadequate defenses
- *Altered urinary elimination,* related to anatomic obstruction
- *Altered cardiopulmonary tissue perfusion,* related to hypertension caused by mechanical reduction of blood flow
- *Risk for caregiver role strain,* related to child's illness severity
- *Risk for impaired home maintenance management,* related to child's disease

NURSING ALERT

If a mass is felt during palpation of a child's abdomen, stop palpating immediately and report the finding to the physician. Never palpate the liver or abdomen of a child with Wilms' tumor as this could cause a piece of the tumor to dislodge. Place a sign on the child's bed and in the chart alerting health providers not to palpate the abdomen.

Planning and Implementation

Nursing management can be divided into two phases: the postrenal surgery phase and the chemotherapy phase. (See Chapter 5 for general care of the child after surgery.) Drawings and special teaching dolls with removable kidneys can be used to teach young children about the surgery. Although chemotherapy may occur at two different times, before and after surgery, nursing management considerations remain the same.

Nursing care during the postrenal surgery phase focuses on pain management and close monitoring of fluid levels. A large incision is necessary to remove the kidney, and the resultant postoperative shift of organs and fluid in the abdominal cavity may create discomfort for the child. Frequently reposition the child and use noninvasive and pharmacologic pain interventions to improve the child's comfort. Gentle handling is important. Monitor fluids closely following surgery to prevent hypovolemia and to assess the shift of fluids out of the third space and out of the body. Assess daily weight, intake and output (I& O), and urine specific gravity. Monitor the function of the remaining kidney. Take blood pressure measurements frequently to watch for signs of shock and to assess the functioning of the remaining kidney.

During the chemotherapy phase, monitor the child for side effects of drugs, the potential for infection from the central line site, and the function of the remaining kidney. Advise parents about home care needs, administration of medications, and monitoring for drug side effects and ongoing needs for health monitoring.

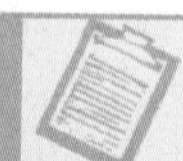

RESEARCH

Children treated for Wilm's tumor with doxorubicin are at risk of developing congestive heart failure later in life, and need to be followed indefinitely for signs of this secondary treatment effect (Green, Grigoriev, & Nan, et al., 2001).

Evaluation

Desired outcomes for nursing care of the child with nephroblastoma include balanced intake and output, normal vital signs, recovery from surgery, and successful family management of postsurgical care and ongoing treatments.

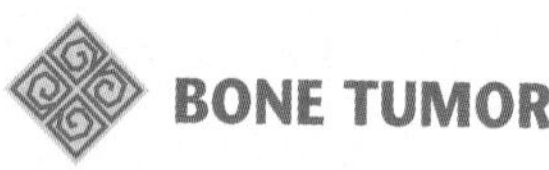

BONE TUMORS

OSTEOSARCOMA

Osteosarcoma is a rare, malignant bone tumor that occurs predominantly in adolescent boys. Its peak incidence is during the rapid growth years. The tumor is usually located at the metaphysis of the distal femur, proximal tibia, or proximal humerus (Meyers & Gorlick, 1997).

Etiology and Pathophysiology

Bone tissue produced by osteosarcoma never matures into compact bone. Although the cause of osteosarcoma is unknown, radiation exposure (either environmental or treatment related) is associated with its development. Survivors of retinoblastoma have a greatly increased incidence of osteosarcoma. An abnormality of gene p53 has been noted in some cases of this cancer, leading to oncogene malformations and possibly to an absence of tumor suppressor genes (Meyers & Gorlick, 1997).

Clinical Manifestations

The common initial symptoms of osteosarcoma are pain and swelling. The pain can be referred to the hip or back, which can delay diagnosis. Pulmonary metastasis occurs in 20% of cases.

DRUGS USED TO TREAT OSTEOSARCOMA

Methotrexate
Doxorubicin
Cisplatin
Cyclophosphamide
Bleomycin
Dactinomycin
Ifosfamide

Clinical Therapy

Diagnosis of osteosarcoma is made through radiographic tests (radiographic studies of the affected area, bone scan, CT or MRI scans of involved bone), blood test for serum alkaline phosphatase (level may be elevated), and tumor biopsy (to confirm the diagnosis). Arteriography may be performed if limb-sparing surgery is contemplated.

Treatment involves both surgery and chemotherapy. The surgery is either a limb-sparing procedure or limb amputation. In limb-sparing procedures the tumor is removed and an internal prosthesis is inserted. A limb-sparing procedure is possible if bone growth has taken place and a neurobundle (area where several nerves converge) is not involved in the tumor. If these two criteria are not met, limb amputation is necessary. Aggressive chemotherapy following surgery has improved the survival rate. At the time of diagnosis, most children have metastases (even though they may not be identifiable), so chemotherapy is needed. Chemotherapy may be started before surgery, especially in cases where limb-sparing surgery is performed.

Research is being carried out to test the benefit of drugs to stimulate the immune system in the treatment for osteosarcoma. In addition, muramyl-tripeptide (MTP), a derivative of the tuberculosis vaccine BCG, is showing promise in reducing the risk of recurrence (Meyers & Gorlick, 1997).

EWING'S SARCOMA

Ewing's sarcoma is a malignant, small, round cell tumor usually involving the diaphyseal (shaft) portion of the long bones. The most common sites are the femur, pelvis, tibia, fibula, ribs, humerus, scapula, and clavicle, but any bone may be involved. Ewing's sarcoma occurs in two children per million, is most common in whites and Hispanics, and is rare in black and Asian children. The incidence is highest in children between the ages of 10 and 20 years (Grier, 1997).

DRUGS USED TO TREAT EWING'S SARCOMA

Vincristine
Cyclophosphamide
Dactinomycin
Doxorubicin
Ifosfamide
Etoposide
Adriamycin

Although full mechanisms have not been described, abnormalities on chromosomes 11 and 22 have been identified in children with Ewing's sarcoma. A translocation of genetic material is apparent. In addition, these tumors express a protooncogene, c-myc.

The symptoms are similar to those of osteosarcoma and may include pain, swelling, fever, an elevated WBC count, and elevated erythrocyte sedimentation rate. A tumor biopsy is necessary for diagnosis. Diagnostic tests are the same as those for osteosarcoma.

Initial treatment for Ewing's sarcoma is chemotherapy to reduce the tumor, followed by surgical removal of the entire bone or intensive high-dose irradiation of the entire bone. Surgery is preferred because of the possibility of a secondary cancer from radiation. Chemotherapy is always used following initial treatment, as nondetectable metastases are nearly always present (Grier, 1997).

NURSING MANAGEMENT

Nursing Assessment and Diagnosis

Physiologic assessment of the child with a bone tumor includes assessment of the site before surgery. Assess the child's pain or discomfort, mobility, and gait. Take careful vital signs, especially noting temperature and respirations. Psychologic assessment of the child and family are needed, especially if amputation is planned. Body image disturbances occur when a limb is lost, particularly with school-age children and adolescents. Assess the child's understanding of the treatment and of care after surgery. Find out what support systems are available for assistance.

Observe the wound postoperatively for infection and hemorrhage. Assess circulation above and below the operative site. If edema is found, elevate the limb. If a limb salvage procedure is performed, the child's extremity will be intact but it will not function as before, because muscle insertion sites and mass have been removed with the tumor during surgery. Detailed charting of the condition of the surgical site and limb function is important.

If the limb has been amputated, assess the child for the following signs indicating a disturbed body image:

- Refusal to look at or touch the altered or missing body part
- Preoccupation with loss or change
- Feelings of shame or embarrassment, either verbalized or demonstrated
- Distorted perception of normal body (easily seen in the child's drawings of the body)
- Fears of rejection or unwanted attention from others
- Overexposure or hiding of the affected body part
- Actual or perceived change in the structure and function of the body or body parts

Psychosocial assessment of the child and family is discussed in more detail earlier in the general section on Childhood Cancer (see p. 556).

Appropriate nursing diagnoses for the child with a bone tumor are based on the treatment and needs of each child:

- *Risk for infection,* related to amputation
- *Impaired skin integrity,* related to mechanical forces of prosthesis

- *Impaired physical mobility,* related to musculoskeletal impairment
- *Impaired adjustment,* related to disability and lifestyle change
- *Body image disturbance,* related to treatment and injury
- *Pain,* related to physical injury of tissues

Planning and Implementation

Care of the child after surgery involves general postoperative care (see Chapter 5). The child who has had an amputation has special needs regarding skin care and rehabilitation. Inspect the tissue at the surgical site, using sterile technique, and turn the child at least every 2 hours. The site needs to heal completely before chemotherapy can begin and a prosthesis can be made.

Discuss insurance and other financial arrangements with the parents, as prosthetics can be costly. Referral to a Shriners Hospital is an option for some families.

Implement plans to help the child deal with body image disturbance. Plan for a visit from another child who is well adjusted to a prosthesis. Help the child to gradually learn how to care for the stump. Slow progress may be made as the child first looks briefly, then for longer periods, and finally is willing to touch the stump. Show the child how it is possible to continue with sports such as baseball, skiing, or biking with a prosthesis. A discussion group with others can be very useful for adolescents. Plan with the child how to tell friends about the surgery and what issues he or she may face upon return to school. Make plans for elevator access if needed and emergency evacuation procedures. Some children or adolescents may need referral for counseling to assist in dealing with body image disturbance.

The child will be receiving physical rehabilitation while hospitalized and after discharge. When the child is discharged, explain to the family the importance of bringing the child for outpatient chemotherapy and physical rehabilitation visits. Special arrangements may be needed at the child's school to facilitate a wheelchair, crutches, or ambulation with a new prosthesis. Call or visit the school to evaluate the presence of buttons to open doors, wide doorways to facilitate passage, and any limitations of the building. Contact school personnel to plan the child's return.

Evaluation

The following expected outcomes of nursing care for the child with a bone tumor focus on the treatments required and adaptation to changes in lifestyle:

- Healed surgical site with no signs of infection
- Adaptation to changes in mobility status
- Successful adjustment to changes required in school settings
- Maintenance of healthy skin
- Positive body image
- Management of pain to comfort level
- Successful integration of continuing medical therapy

LEUKEMIA

Leukemia is among the most commonly diagnosed pediatric malignancies; an increase of acute leukemia in children has occurred in the last decade, perhaps due to enhanced early diagnosis (Friebert & Shurin, 1998). A cancer of the blood-forming organs, leukemia is characterized by a proliferation of abnormal white blood cells in the body. Several types of leukemia are differentiated, depending on the blood cells affected. The main types are acute lymphoblastic leukemia, acute myelogenous leukemia, and the rare chronic leukemias of childhood.

The most common type of childhood leukemia is acute lymphoblastic leukemia (ALL), which accounts for 25% of all childhood cancer and 75% of leukemias in children. The peak age at onset is 2 to 4 years (Landier, 2001). ALL is more common in whites and in boys (Figure 16-14 ◆) (Friebert & Shurin, 1998).

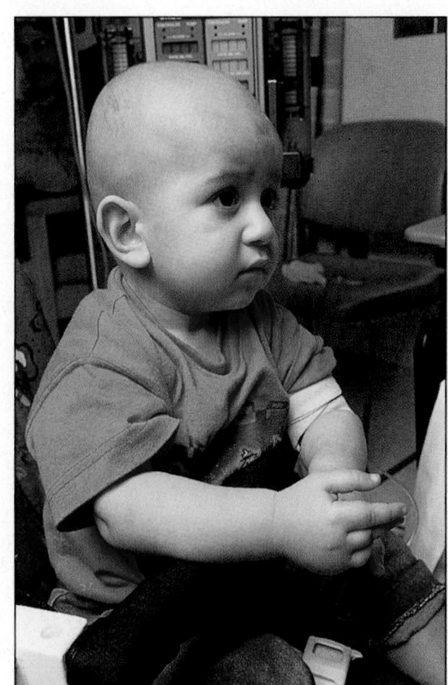

FIGURE 16-14 ◆
Acute lymphoblastic leukemia is the most common type of leukemia in children and the most common cancer affecting children under 5 years of age.

Acute myelogeous leukemia (AML) affects all ethnic groups equally, and there is no peak age at onset (Golub, Weinstein, & Grier, 1997). Rasheed, the boy described at the beginning of the chapter, has AML.

Because chronic leukemias such as chronic myelocytic, chronic myelomonocytic, and chronic lymphocytic leukemia are rare in children, the following discussion will focus on ALL and AML.

ETIOLOGY AND PATHOPHYSIOLOGY

The causes of leukemia are not well understood. Genetic factors are believed to play a role in some types of the disease. For instance, children with chromosomal defects such as Down syndrome have an increased incidence of ALL, and chromosomal abnormalities are present in most children with ALL (Friebert & Shurin, 1998). Ionizing radiation and chemical agents such as treatment with chemotherapy for other cancers are thought to play some role in the development of AML. Children with immune deficiency states, such as ataxia-telangiectasia, congenital hypogammaglobulinemia, and Wiskott–Aldrich syndrome, have an increased risk of ALL. Some investigators theorize that exposure to infectious agents can predispose children to leukemia (Kinlen & Balkwill, 2001).

Leukemia occurs when the stem cells in the bone marrow produce immature WBCs that cannot function normally. These cells proliferate rapidly by cloning instead of normal mitosis, causing the bone marrow to fill with abnormal WBCs. The abnormal cells then spill out into the circulatory system where they steadily replace the normally functioning WBCs. As this occurs, the protective lymphocytic functions such as cellular and humeral immunity are reduced, leaving the body vulnerable to infections.

The malignant WBCs rapidly fill the bone marrow, replacing stem cells that produce erythrocytes (red blood cells) and other blood products such as platelets, thereby decreasing the amount of these products in circulation. The stem cells are replaced by leukemic clones, eventually resulting in anemia. Children with leukemia commonly experience abnormal bleeding because of the reduced platelet amounts.

CLINICAL MANIFESTATIONS

Children with ALL and AML usually have fever, pallor, overt signs of bleeding, lethargy, malaise, anorexia, and large joint or bone pain. Petechiae, frank bleeding, and joint pain are cardinal signs of bone marrow failure. Enlargement of the liver and spleen (hepatosplenomegaly) and changes in the lymph nodes (lymphadenopathy) are common. If the leukemia has infiltrated the central nervous system (entered it by means of the circulatory or lymphoid system), the child will have signs such as headache, vomiting, papilledema, and sixth cranial nerve palsy (inability to move the eye laterally). These findings are caused by the leukemic cells massing and putting pressure on nerves. The testicles, spinal cord, and bone marrow are common sites for infiltration. The leukemic cells in the testicle become a mass that causes the testicle to enlarge, often painlessly.

LABORATORY VALUES IN LEUKEMIA

	Usual	Common values in leukemia
Leukocytes	<10,000/μL	>10,000/μL
Platelets	150,000–400,000/μL	20,000–100,000/μL
Hemoglobin	12–16 g/dL	7–11 g/dL

CLINICAL THERAPY

Diagnosis is based initially on blood counts and bone marrow aspiration. Blood counts reveal anemia, thrombocytopenia, and neutropenia. Bone marrow aspiration reveals immature and abnormal lymphoblasts and hypercellular marrow. Bone marrow aspiration is the differential test. Neutropenia, thrombocytopenia, and anemia are commonly noted. Other abnormal laboratory findings include elevated serum uric acid and elevated calcium, potassium, and phosphorus levels. New laboratory studies such as rapid flow cytometric assay are making the presence of even very small numbers of leukemic cells possible, so that treatment can be used to improve prognosis in children with minimal residual disease (Coustan-Smith, Sancho, Hancock et al., 2000).

Treatment of ALL involves radiation and chemotherapy. Radiation is used for central nervous system prophylaxis and involvement and for testicular involvement. Chemotherapy is organized into four phases: (1) induction, (2) consolidation, (3) delayed intensification, and (4) maintenance of remission. Additional drugs may be used for treatment of central nervous system involvement. Maintenance therapy may continue for 2 to 3 years, causing decreased resistance to infection for this prolonged period of time (Kanarek, 1998).

Treatment of AML involves use of a wide variety of drugs during the induction and consolidation phases.

Maximum cell death occurs during the induction phase. The cells that remain after this period are more resistant to treatment. After 3 to 4 weeks, when a remission has occurred, central nervous system prophylaxis begins. Drugs are used in combination with cranial irradiation. During the consolidation phase, chemotherapy with l-asparaginase and doxorubicin is administered. Delayed intensification uses additional drugs to target the leukemic cells that have survived. Treatment during the maintenance phase is aimed at destroying the remaining leukemic cells. Combinations of active drugs are used to prevent resistance. Occasionally other drugs are added to the regimen, such as vincristine, prednisone, cyclophosphamide, intravenous methotrexate, cytosine arabinoside, or anthracyclines.

The prognosis for children with leukemia is much improved with current therapy. However, several risk factors affect the long-term outcome. The most favorable findings are as follows:

- Age at onset between 2 and 10 years
- Initial hemoglobin level less than 10 g/dL
- Low initial WBC count
- Lack of B- or T-cell antigens
- Absence of extramedullary (outside bone marrow or spinal cord) involvement
- Rapid response to chemotherapy

The most important factor is the initial leukocyte count. The higher the leukocyte count (over 50,000/mm^3) at diagnosis, the worse the prognosis. For children in the low-risk group, the probability of prolonged survival is as high as 90%. Infants under 12 months of age have a poor prognosis. Treatment methods and duration are adjusted for each child, depending on that child's risk factors. More aggressive treatment is undertaken for those in the higher risk groups.

Approximately 10% of children have a relapse within a year after completing treatment. Treatment for relapse consists of additional chemotherapy drugs. The prognosis is best if the relapse occurs late after the initial diagnosis and after the initial treatment is completed. Bone marrow transplantation is a treatment option for the child who has a relapse with ALL or who is in remission from AML. Chemotherapy itself can create numerous complications, affecting all body organs. Secondary malignancies sometimes occur later in life.

DRUGS USED TO TREAT ACUTE LYMPHOBLASTIC LEUKEMIA

Induction phase
Prednisone
Vincristine
l-Asparaginase
Daunorubicin

Central nervous system prophylaxis
Intrathecal methotrexate

Consolidation phase
l-Asparaginase
Doxorubicin

Delayed intensification
Vincristine
ARA-C
Cyclophosphamide

Maintenance phase
6-Mercaptopurine or 6-Thioguanine
Methotrexate

DRUGS USED TO TREAT ACUTE MYELOGENOUS LEUKEMIA

Induction phase
Daunorubicin
Doxorubicin
Mitoxantrone
Cytarabin

Consolidation phase
Etoposide
Teniposide

NURSING MANAGEMENT

Nursing Assessment and Diagnosis

A thorough physical assessment is important to ensure prompt identification of problems without injuring the child who has deficient coagulation and immune function. Perform assessments every 8 hours or more often depending on the chemotherapy regimen. Observe carefully for bruising and other new sites of bleeding. Once chemotherapy has begun, closely monitor renal functioning through specific gravity, intake and output (I& O), and daily weight measurement. Monitor dietary intake, nausea, vomiting, and constipation. Observe for mucosal sores in the mouth. A central line is usually in place for intravenous infusion of medications, so careful assessment of the line for proper functioning and for signs of infection is needed. Ask the parents about any behavioral changes. Central nervous system infiltration can affect the child's level of consciousness, causing irritability, vomiting, and lethargy. However, these nonspecific signs can also be induced by chemotherapeutic drugs and antiemetics. Frequent venipunctures, bone marrow aspirations, and spinal taps require pain assessment, and an evaluation of the level of knowledge and coping skills of child and family.

Leukemia causes many changes in the body and confirmation of the disease is difficult for families to face. Among the many nursing diagnoses that might be appropriate for the child with leukemia are the following:

- *Altered nutrition: Less than body requirements,* related to inability to ingest food
- *Risk for infection,* related to altered immune system functioning

COMPLICATIONS OF LEUKEMIA THERAPY

- Central nervous system toxicity or damage
- Potential damage to the pituitary, liver, kidneys, gastrointestinal tract, heart, lungs, gonads, and hematopoietic and immune systems
- Secondary malignancies

Skill 8-8: Managing a Central Venous Catheter Site

- *Risk for injury,* related to bleeding
- *Activity intolerance,* related to generalized weakness
- *Pain,* related to chemotherapy and disease process
- *Anxiety (child and parent),* related to change in health status

Planning and Implementation

Infection Control Methods

Bone marrow suppression may necessitate transmission-based precautions (refer to the Skills Manual). Instruct parents in the prevention of infection. Care of mouth sores and other side effects of chemotherapy is presented in the Nursing Care Plan for Hospital Care of the Child with Cancer, earlier in this chapter.

Special attention to renal function is needed when the child receives cyclophosphamide. Gross hematuria is a side effect of this drug. Hydration with intravenous fluids to attain a specific gravity of less than 1.010 prevents or reduces the severity of hematuria. To achieve this specific gravity, the child receives intravenous fluids at 1.5 times maintenance volume for at least 6 to 8 hours before and at least 1.5 hours after administration of the drug. Careful monitoring of I&O is required to record the intravenous fluids and assess kidney functioning. Monitor specific gravity every 8 hours, as well as before and during administration of the drug, and when the intravenous fluids are reduced to maintenance volume levels. Daily weight measurements are important to assist in planning adequate hydration during chemotherapy, as well as to measure nutritional status.

Many children are treated in an oncology clinic, staying in the hospital only on the day of intravenous drug administration, and receiving oral medications at home. Careful teaching for the family is needed to ensure safe drug administration and identification of symptoms requiring care.

Nurses play a key role in the long-term multidisciplinary treatment of children with leukemia. The impact of a diagnosis of leukemia and the long-term nature of treatment can severely stress the coping abilities of both the child and the family. Ongoing psychosocial assessment and emotional support are essential (see the general discussion of Psychosocial Assessment in the section on Childhood Cancer, p. 556). Referral to support groups and social services may be beneficial. Assist the family in exploration of alternative therapies such as relaxation, imagery, and nutritional support that may aid the child. Be alert for any interactions that could occur between alternative therapies and the medical regimen.

FAMILIES WANT TO KNOW

Chemotherapy for Leukemia

PHYSICAL CARE

- Have rest periods each day.
- Avoid areas of exposure to people with illnesses.
- Drink generous amounts of water.
- Eat a healthy diet, using frequent, small, and nutritious meals to obtain enough nutrients.
- Take medicines prescribed to decrease nausea.
- Maintain good oral hygiene with soft toothbrush and water pik.
- Avoid sun exposure and check skin each day for any signs of bruises, pressure areas, cuts, or scratches.
- Allow time and eat foods to promote bowel elimination.
- Report any signs of infection, changes in condition, or other concerns.

EMOTIONAL CARE

- Be prepared for loss of hair with plans for hats, wigs, or other alternatives.
- Continue contact with friends via phone, internet, and in person when possible.
- Try relaxation techniques to aid in sleep and management of treatments.
- Talk with clergy, teachers, parents, counselors, friends, or other supportive people about the experience of having leukemia.
- Keep a journal to record feelings and experiences.

Evaluation

Following are expected outcomes for nursing care of the child with leukemia:

- Prevention of infection
- Adequate hydration
- Normal urinary output
- Blood values within normal limits
- Successful family adaptation to parenting a child with chronic illness
- Adequate parental knowledge related to disease process

SOFT TISSUE TUMORS

HODGKIN'S DISEASE

Hodgkin's disease is a disorder of the lymphoid system. It usually arises in a single lymph node or an anatomic group of lymph nodes (Figure 16-15 ◆). There are approximately 3 cases per 100,000 people, with the peak occurrence in adolescent boys. Hodgkin's disease has a childhood form but is rare in those under 14 years. Most cases involve a young adult form that affects those between 15 and 35, and an older adult form, usually seen in persons over 55 years (Thompson, 1999).

Etiology and Pathophysiology

Hodgkin's disease occurs in clusters and has been reported in families. This suggests a possible genetic link as well as an infectious agent or environmental hazard.

Clinical Manifestations

The main symptom of Hodgkin's disease is nontender, firm lymphadenopathy, usually in the supraclavicular and cervical nodes but occasionally in the mediastinal area. A mediastinal growth can cause respiratory difficulty because of pressure on the trachea or bronchi. Fever, night sweats, and weight loss occur in one-third of children with Hodgkin's disease

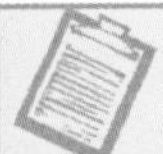

RESEARCH

The role of an infectious agent in Hodgkin's disease is being investigated. Infectious agents that may be associated with Hodgkin's disease include a herpesvirus, cytomegalovirus, and Epstein-Barr virus (EBV). High EBV titers and EBV-associated antigens are commonly found in individuals with Hodgkin's disease.

PATHOPHYSIOLOGY ILLUSTRATED

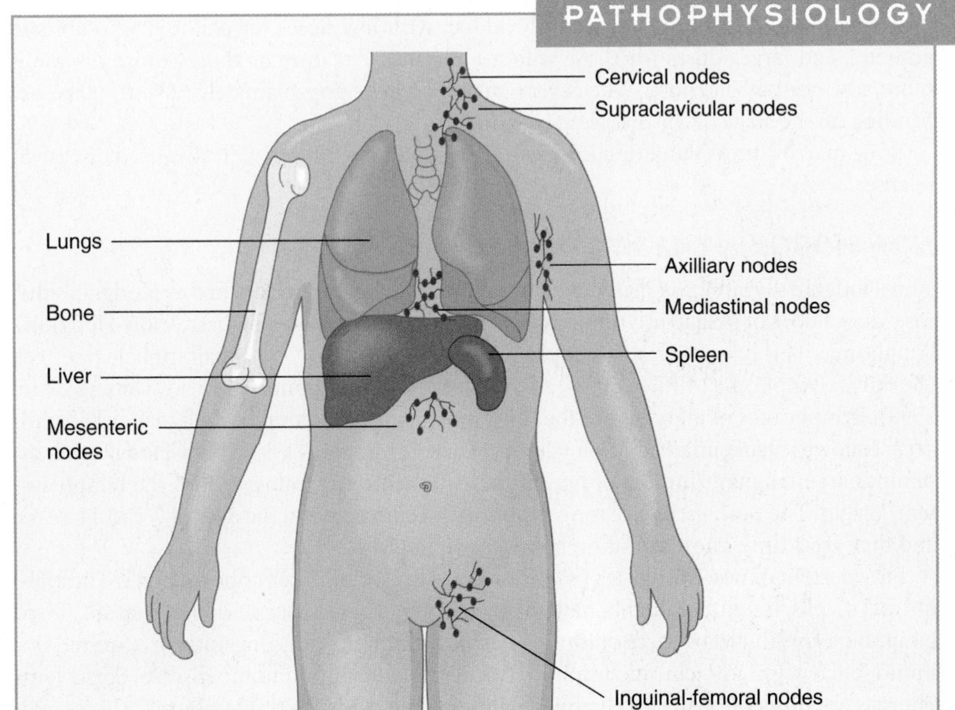

Hodgkin's Disease

FIGURE 16-15 ◆ Lymph nodes and organs affected in Hodgkin's disease in children.

CLINICAL TIP

An oral contrast medium is often given to children having CT scanning of the abdomen and pelvis. Mixing this contrast medium with fruit juice or punch makes it more palatable. Mix it in a small amount so the child can easily drink it all.

TABLE 16-8 Staging System for Hodgkin's Disease

STAGE	DESCRIPTION
I	Disease within a single lymph node region
IE	Disease within a single extralymphatic organ
II	Disease within two or more lymph node regions on same side of diaphragm
IIE	Disease within extralymphatic organ, and of one or more lymph node regions on same side of diaphragm
III	Disease of lymph node regions on both sides of diaphragm
IIIE	Disease of lymph node regions on both sides of the diaphragm with involvement of extralymphatic organ
IIIS	As in III, plus disease within spleen
IIISE	As in III, plus disease in extralymphatic organs and spleen
IV	Disseminated disease within one or more lymphatic organs with or without lymph node involvement

DRUGS USED TO TREAT HODGKIN'S DISEASE

MOPP (mechlorethamine, Oncovin [vincristine], procarbazine, prednisone)
COPP (cyclophosphamide, Oncovin, procarbazine, prednisone)
COMP (cyclophosphamide, Oncovin, methotrexate, prednisone)
OPPA (Oncovin, procarbazine, prednisone, adriamycin)
ABVD (adriamycin, bleomycin, vinblastine, dacarbazine)

and are associated with a more aggressive form of the disease. The leukocyte count and erythrocyte sedimentation rate (ESR) may be elevated.

Clinical Therapy

Diagnosis is based on lymph node biopsy; Reed-Sternberg cells (large cells with two nucleoli) are present. A staging classification is used to determine disease severity. (Table 16-8). The basis for staging is data obtained from the history, physical examination, chest x-ray study (for metastasis), chest CT scan, CT or MRI scans of the retroperitoneal nodes, lymphangiogram, laboratory studies (complete blood count, erythrocyte sedimentation rate, serum copper level, liver function tests), and a radionuclide scan with gallium. Bone marrow biopsy, bone scan, or a staging laparotomy may be performed in certain situations when advanced disease is suspected. Increasingly, minimally invasive surgery can be used to biopsy or remove the spleen for diagnosis, avoiding the potential complications of major surgery (Kleinhaus & Boley, 1999).

Chemotherapy using a four-drug combination has been found to be the most effective drug treatment. Radiation is commonly added, with low doses for children who are still growing, and larger doses for those who are physically mature or those whose disease is more advanced at diagnosis. The 5-year survival rate is approximately 80% to 90%, depending on the stage of the disease at diagnosis.

Bone marrow transplantation is a treatment option in children with advanced disease or relapse.

NON-HODGKIN'S LYMPHOMA

Non-Hodgkin's lymphoma includes all lymphomas that are not classified as Hodgkin's disease (about 60% of pediatric lymphomas). There are three types of pediatric non-Hodgkin's lymphoma: (1) lymphoblastic lymphoma (30% to 40%), (2) small noncleaved cell (Burkitt's) lymphoma (40% to 50%), and (3) large cell lymphoma ($\leq$ 15%) (Derengowski, 1999). Lymphomas of all types are the third most common group of malignancies in children, following leukemia and brain tumors (Shad & Magrath, 1997). Non-Hodgkin's lymphomas are malignant tumors of lymphoreticular (internal framework of the lymph system) origin. The peak incidence for lymphomas occurs between the ages of 7 and 11 years, and they are 3 times more common in boys than in girls.

Fifty percent of non-Hodgkin's lymphomas are caused by T-cell abnormalities. These abnormal T cells are diffuse, highly malignant, and very aggressive and do not mature. T-cell lymphomas produced by these cells often occur in children with congenital or acquired immunodeficiency states, chronic immune stimulation, or autoimmune disease. Some lymphomas are observed with B-cell abnormalities. The incidence of lymphomas shows geographic variability. For example, a high incidence of Burkitt's lymphoma is found in equatorial Africa, where it causes 50% of childhood cancer. Incidence in Hispanic children is higher than in whites, and blacks have the lowest incidence (Wilkinson, Fleming, & MacKinnon, et al., 2001).

Children with non-Hodgkin's lymphoma frequently present with fever and weight loss. The lymph glands are usually enlarged or nodular, with the most frequent sites being the cervical, axillary, inguinal, and femoral nodes. However, the disease may be diffuse, without nodular glands. The anterior mediastinum is the primary site for T-cell lymphomas. Tumors that occur in this area may compress the airway (causing breathing difficulty) or superior vena cava (leading to swelling of the face, neck, or arms), and can cause pain. Jaw involvement is common in Burkitt's lymphoma.

Diagnosis is confirmed by tissue biopsy. Several staging systems relate to the tumor mass and extension to other body areas. Because systemic disease is present in 80% of children with non-Hodgkin's lymphoma, the treatment is aggressive chemotherapy similar to that used for ALL. The induction phase of chemotherapy results in a 90% remission rate. Treatment also includes localized radiation and surgery to remove the tumor mass. Between 50% and 75% of children with non-Hodgkin's lymphoma have a good outcome. Children with localized diseases have a more favorable prognosis.

DRUGS USED TO TREAT NON-HODGKIN'S LYMPHOMA

- Cyclophosphamide
- Ifosfamide
- Prednisone
- Methotrexate
- ARA-C
- VM-26
- Adriamycin
- Vincristine

RHABDOMYOSARCOMA

Rhabdomyosarcoma is a soft tissue cancer that is common in children. It occurs most often in the muscles around the eyes (extraorbital), in the neck, and less commonly in the abdomen and genitourinary tract. Among children under 15 years of age, rhabdomyosarcoma occurs more often in whites than in blacks or Asians (Wexler & Helman, 1997). Most cases are diagnosed in children under 5 years of age.

Tumors occurring close to the eye produce swelling, ptosis, visual disturbances, and eye movement abnormalities (Figure 16-16 ◆). When the tumor occurs in the genitourinary tract, the result can be obstruction, hematuria, dysuria, vaginal discharge, and a protruding vaginal mass. Rhabdomyosarcoma occurring in the abdomen may be asymptomatic. There is rapid metastasis to the lungs, bones, bone marrow, and distant lymph nodes.

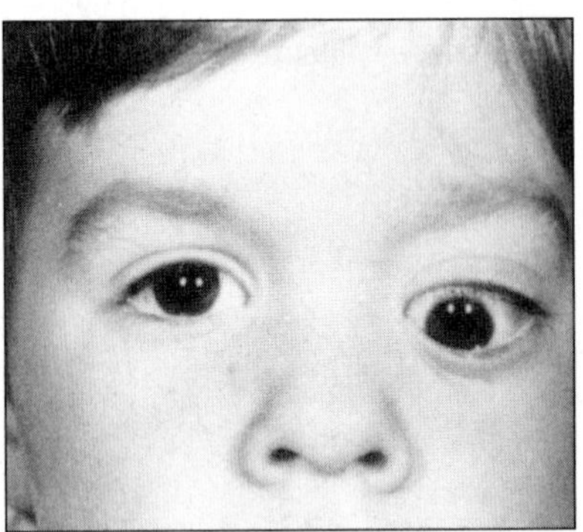

FIGURE 16-16 ◆
Rhabdomyosarcoma is characterized by ptosis and swelling.
From Vaughn, D., Asbury, T., & Riordan-Eva, P. (1995). *General opthalmology* (14th ed.). Norwalk, CT: Appleton & Lange.

Diagnosis is confirmed by CT, MRI, bone marrow aspiration, and biopsy. A useful biologic marker, Desmin, allows differentiation of rhabdomyosarcoma from other round cell tumors. Because 20% of children have metastatic disease at the time of diagnosis, chest and lung CT scans are performed.

Treatment includes surgical removal of the tumor followed by wide-field radiation and chemotherapy with a combination of drugs. Prognosis depends on the site, staging (Table 16-9), and histologic findings. Children with stage II or IV disease or abdominal tumors have a poor prognosis.

DRUGS USED TO TREAT RHABDOMYOSARCOMA

- Dactinomycin
- Cyclophosphamide
- Vincristine
- Doxorubicin
- Cisplatin
- Etoposide

RETINOBLASTOMA

Retinoblastoma is an intraocular malignancy of the retina. It may be bilateral (20% to 30%) or unilateral. In 40% of children, the disease is inherited by an autosomal dominant gene (Donaldson, Egbert, & Newsham, et al., 1997).

TABLE 16-9 Classification of Rhabdomyosarcoma

GROUP	DESCRIPTION
I	Localized, completely resected disease
II	Total gross resection with regional microscopic spread
III	Incomplete gross resection of biopsy
IV	Distant metastatic disease present

Note: From Wexler, L. H., & Helman, L. J. (1997). Rhabdomyosarcoma and the undifferentiated sarcomas. In P. A. Pizzo & D. G. Poplack (eds.), *Principles and practices of pediatric oncology* (3rd ed., p. 808). Philadelphia: Lippincott-Raven.

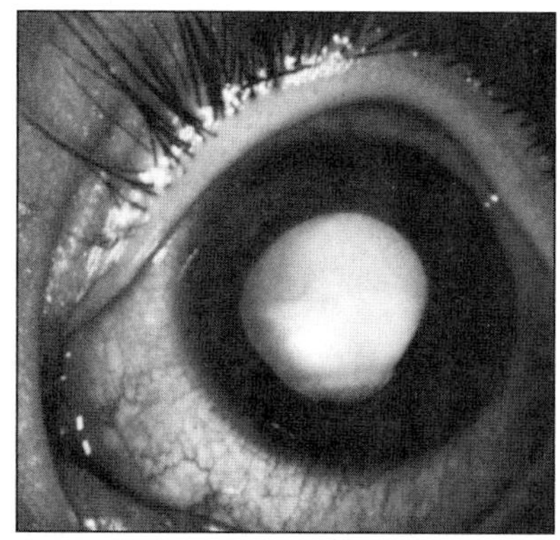

FIGURE 16-17 ◆
Retinoblastoma is characterized by leukocoria, a white reflection in the pupil.
From Hathaway, W. E., Hay, W. W., Jr., Groothuis, J. R., & Paisley, J. W. (1993). *Current pediatric diagnosis and treatment* (11thed.) Norwalk, CT: Appleton & Lange.

The first sign of retinoblastoma is a white pupil, termed leukokoria or cat's-eye reflex (Figure 16-17 ◆). Other symptoms may include a fixed strabismus (a constant deviation of one eye from the other), orbital inflammation, glaucoma, and heterochromia (irises of different colors).

Retinoblastoma is usually diagnosed when the child is between 1 and 2 years of age. The overall tumor-free survival rate is 90%, 5 to 10 years after diagnosis. Diagnostic tests include full ocular examination and CT or MRI scans of the eye orbit. All children with a history of retinoblastoma in the family should be examined by an ophthalmologist after birth and on a regular basis to aid in early diagnosis. Tumors are classified according to a staging system, from a very small localized tumor (group I) to tumors involving more than half the retina and with seeding into the vitreous (group V).

Treatment for retinblastoma may include removal of the eye. Other surgical treatments involve cryotherapy or photocoagulation (argon laser therapy). Radiation is nearly always used, either as the sole treatment or before surgery to shrink the tumor. Chemotherapy is occasionally used but is generally ineffective as the drugs often fail to penetrate sufficiently into the eye. Multiple therapies are more commonly used in children with bilateral retinoblastoma. Children with retinoblastoma are at increased risk of developing a secondary tumor, including another retinoblastoma or a sarcoma, most commonly osteogenic sarcoma. However, most young children who have been treated for the disease have good health and normal mental abilities several years after treatment. Over 90% of children with small unilateral tumors survive. Increased size and invasion by a tumor decrease success of treatment. The most common sequella of retinoblastoma is decrease in visual acuity (Ross, Lipper, & Abramson, et al., 2001).

NURSING MANAGEMENT

Nursing Assessment and Diagnosis

PHYSIOLOGIC ASSESSMENT

Physiologic assessment of the child with a soft tissue tumor, such as Hodgkin's disease, non-Hodgkin's lymphoma, rhabdomyosarcoma, and other lymphomas, focuses on the child's general condition. Accurate height and weight measurements are essential to provide a baseline against which to measure the child's growth during treatment, as well as for calculation of chemotherapeutic drug dosages.

Observe the area of the tumor, such as the face, neck, and abdomen, and describe any changes. Monitor respiratory status if the tumor is on the face or neck. Report any changes in respiratory pattern to the physician. Avoid palpation of any tumor site or enlarged area; metastasis can be influenced by injudicious palpation and manipulation of a tumor site. Notify the physician of a change in any lymph node or any other area of the body.

Gastrointestinal and genitourinary function can be altered by the presence of a tumor and by treatment such as chemotherapy and radiation. Careful monitoring of the child's intake and output measurement is essential. Abdominal tumors may affect defecation, so charting of all bowel movements is important. Explain to the family and child why keeping accurate records is necessary.

Observe wounds closely for lack of healing as a result of chemotherapy or radiation. Examine the mouth and extremities for wounds or ulcers. Nutritional changes caused by treatment will affect the body's ability to support healthy cells and heal wounds.

A thorough eye examination is warranted for any child who has a family history of retinoblastoma or has undergone treatment for a prior tumor. Assess color and position of the iris, eye movements, cover–uncover test, and other eye tests described in Chapter 4. Ask whether the child has been evaluated by an ophthalmologist.

PSYCHOSOCIAL ASSESSMENT

Assessment of the family's psychosocial status and coping mechanisms is an essential component of nursing care. Refer to the general discussion of Psychosocial Assessment under

Childhood Cancer, earlier in this chapter. Assessment of body image is needed when the child has a soft tissue tumor affecting appearance of the head and neck.

The location and type of soft tissue tumor determine the specific nursing diagnoses for a particular child. Common nursing diagnoses may include the following:

- *Altered tissue perfusion (peripheral),* related to interruption of blood flow
- *Ineffective breathing pattern,* related to effect of tumor deformity on neck or chest wall
- *Impaired swallowing,* related to acquired anatomic defect
- *Altered Growth and Development,* related to effects of treatment
- *Body image disturbance,* related to illness and treatment
- *Sensory/perceptual alteration (visual),* related to illness

Planning and Implementation

Nursing management of children with soft tissue tumors varies depending on the specific tumor. Children with lymphoma affecting the mediastinum may need respiratory support. Position the child so that the head is elevated. Administer chemotherapy drugs as ordered, maintaining adequate fluids to facilitate excretion of the resultant breakdown products. Monitor the central line used for chemotherapy administration, and teach parents care of the central line when the child is at home.

For the child with a rhabdomyosarcoma involving the bladder, monitor urinary output carefully. Report hematuria and painful urination. Monitor the changes that occur during therapy. For example, in children with eye tumors, observe for a decrease in ptosis, which may indicate successful treatment. Administer pain medications as needed and use distraction and other techniques to decrease the child's discomfort. Emphasize to parents the need for follow-up CT and MRI scans after completion of treatment.

When the child with retinoblastoma undergoes removal of the eye, the parents and child will need detailed instructions on postsurgical care. Demonstrate to the parents care of the socket and use of a conformer to maintain the eye socket shape. When healing is complete and the child receives a prosthetic eye, instruct parents about its insertion and care. The child can gradually be taught to take over this care when old enough. Encourage periodic health care visits to monitor for signs of a tumor in the other eye. Interventions to encourage normal developmental milestones are adapted if sensory alteration has resulted.

Attention is directed at the body changes of the cancer and its treatment. Children and adolescents may need suggestions to deal with hair loss, disfigurement, and living with serious illness. Referral to other children and teens with similar concerns may be helpful. Parents of all children need help to encourage normal development in the child with cancer.

The child with a soft tissue tumor often receives chemotherapy or radiation, or sometimes both modalities. Nursing management during chemotherapy and radiation is discussed earlier in this chapter in the general sections on these treatment measures (see pp. 542–543) and in the Nursing Care Plan for Hospital Care of the Child with Cancer. Generally, the family will need help to adjust to the diagnosis of a life-threatening disease and to the care of the ill child. Refer to Chapter 5 for a description of postsurgical care. Consult Chapter 19 for strategies to assist the child and family if the child has a visual impairment resulting from a retinoblastoma. Topics for parent and family teaching

FAMILIES WANT TO KNOW

The Child with a Soft Tissue Tumor

- Teach the family about the chemotherapy drugs and their side effects.
- Teach about the care of venous access devices surgically placed.
- Provide written and illustrated information about the chemotherapy protocol(s).
- Provide radiation and surgery education specific to the tumor treatment.
- Refer the family to nutrition resources such as dietitians to improve the child's nutritional status.

and discharge planning are similar to those previously presented. Referral resources to support the families of children with these types of cancer can be found at our companion website.

Evaluation

The following expected outcomes of nursing care for the child with a soft tissue tumor are examples that illustrate the varied tumor presentations:

- Successful management of treatment side effects
- Healed surgical site with no signs of infection
- Adaptation to sensory loss
- Growth and development to maximum potential
- Anticipatory grieving by parents in cases of terminal disease.

IMPACT OF CANCER SURVIVAL

Over the past 20 to 30 years, treatment for childhood cancers has been increasingly successful. About 1 in 1,000 young adults is a survivor of childhood cancer. The success of new modalities and treatment combinations has, however, created special health care needs for many survivors (see Figures 16-18A, B, and C).

Surgery can have many results. Body organs may be removed and manipulated, leading to adhesions, intestinal obstruction, visual impairment, neurologic disruption, and even sterility. Removal of the spleen can lead to serious infections. Amputation necessitates the need for prosthetic devices and physical rehabilitation.

Radiation has several long-term effects. It can impair the growth of bones and teeth, leading to conditions such as scoliosis, leg length discrepancy, or poor dental health. Cardiotoxicity and pulmonary toxicity can result from mediastinal radiation. Delayed puberty and

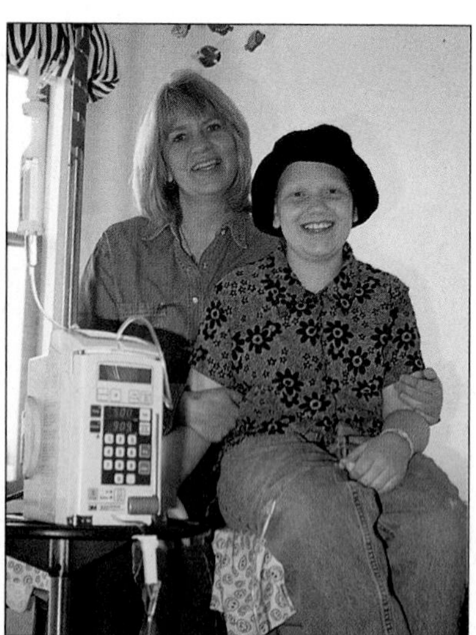

A

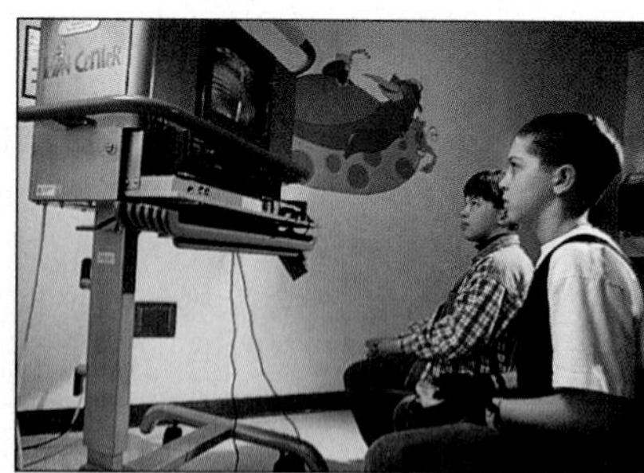

B

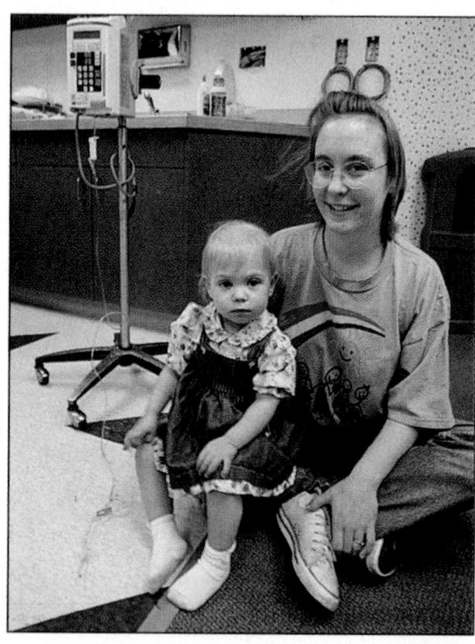

C

FIGURE 16-18 ◆

Survivors of Childhood Cancer A, Nicole, 11 years old, is undergoing chemotherapy for Ewing's sarcoma. Her mother emphasizes, "It's our faith that has gotten us through this. The hardest part is how busy you are coming to treatments all the time. Nicole's younger brother sometimes feels neglected." B, According to Jesse, who is 10 years old and waiting for a bone marrow transplant, "The thing that has helped me the most [in dealing with acute lymphoblastic leukemia] is all the mail I got from my friends." His mother adds, "We're just really positive and think that everything will turn out all right." C, Cassie, 19 months old, has been diagnosed with neuroblastoma. At this age, it is hard for her to understand what is happening. Her mother has stayed with her each time she has come to the hospital, which has helped Cassie adjust to therapy. Her caregivers are confident that she will respond well to her treatment.

sterility can result from radiation effects to the cranium and spinal regions. Neural damage can occur. Secondary cancers, most commonly solid tumors, occur in some survivors.

Chemotherapy can cause a wide variety of effects, both during its administration and for years afterward. Cardiomyopathy can occur with some drugs, especially the anthracyclines. Pulmonary toxicity and renal complications can develop. Neurologic effects of some drugs can lead to hearing loss (e.g., cisplatin and ifosfamide), cataracts, and paraplegia (e.g., intrathecal methotrexate for leukemia). Learning disabilities and change in intelligence quotient (IQ) occur in some children (Blatt, Copeland, & Bleyer, 1997). Although radiation is responsible for most secondary tumors, some chemotherapy drugs have also been implicated.

The diagnosis and stress of treatment, along with the risk of recurrence, are significant stressors for the child with cancer. See Chapter 8 for a discussion on types of family stress when a child has a life-threatening illness. Families may find it difficult to obtain full insurance coverage for the child who has had a prior cancer. Employment can be a potential problem for cancer survivors if employers have concerns about the earlier cancer diagnosis (Monaco, Fiduccia, & Smith, 1997). Most people with cancer report fear of recurrence of the disease, which is a stressor. On the other hand, hopefulness and the sense of having an added purpose in life can be positive outcomes for many cancer survivors.

Nurses are involved with families when a diagnosis of cancer is made, during the therapy process, and in the years that follow. For a child who survives cancer, ongoing care is essential. Evaluate the child regularly with thorough physical, psychosocial, developmental, and cognitive assessments. Carefully monitor all body systems (e.g., cardiovascular; respiratory; musculoskeletal; eye, ear, nose, and throat; genitourinary). Record height and weight and general growth patterns. Ask about the child's interactions with peers and performance at school. Be alert for signs and symptoms that could indicate a secondary tumor. Ask the parents about insurance coverage and other financial difficulties with ongoing care.

Plan care to assist the family to manage any long-term effects of cancer treatment. This may involve physical rehabilitation, support related to visual impairment, or treatment for cardiac or musculoskeletal abnormalities. Provide resources for information and support. Facilitate periodic evaluations in a health care agency so that serious outcomes of treatment can be identified early.

Chapter Highlights

- Cancer is a leading cause of illness and death among children.
- In spite of improvement in mortality and prevalence rates from childhood cancer, the incidence of some types of cancer, such as brain tumors and leukemia, continues to rise.
- Cancer may be caused by chromosomal alterations or genetic messages, environmental carcinogens, or infectious processes. Often a combination of factors seems to be present.
- Cancer treatments include surgery, chemotherapy, radiation, biotherapy, and alternative therapies. Palliative care is needed when the prognosis is poor.
- Oncologic emergencies are life-threatening conditions caused by cancer or its treatment.
- Main types of oncologic emergencies are metabolic, hematologic, or space occupying.
- Key signs of childhood cancer are pain, cachexia, anemia, infection, and bruising.
- A protocol is a plan of action for chemotherapy that is based on the type of cancer, its stage, and the particular cell type.
- Nursing assessment for children with cancer involves detailed physical data, as well as psychological factors and developmental achievements.
- Common physical nursing interventions for children with cancer involve nutrition, medication administration, hydration, infection prevention, pain management, and measures to decrease side effects of treatment. Families require ongoing psychosocial support, information, and referral to diverse resources when caring for a child with cancer.
- Common brain tumors in children include medulloblastoma, astrocytoma, ependymoma, and gliomas.
- Headache, vomiting, ataxia, seizures, increased intracranial pressure, hydrocephalus, and sensory disturbances are the major clinical manifestations of brain tumors.
- Neuroblastoma is a tumor that is located along the sympathetic nervous system chain.

- Nephroblastoma (Wilms' tumor) is an intrarenal tumor; when suspected, the abdomen should not be palpated.
- Common bone tumors in childhood are osteosarcoma and Ewing's sarcoma; both are most common among adolescents.
- Leukemia is a common childhood malignancy, with the major types being acute lymphoblastic leukemia and acute myelogenous leukemia.
- A variety of soft tissue tumors are seen in children and adolescents; they include Hodgkin's disease, non-Hodgkin's lymphoma, rhabdomyosarcoma, and retinoblastoma.
- While the number of children who are long-term survivors continues to grow, it is known that some of these children experience lasting effects such as cognitive or behavioral problems, recurrent or secondary cancers, or discrimination.
- Nurses are in a key position to assist families during a diagnosis for cancer, while therapy is carried out, in adjustment to school and other life tasks, and in providing palliative care for children who do not survive.

EXPLORE MediaLink

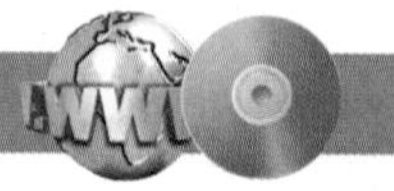

- NCLEX review, case studies, and other interactive resources for this chapter can be found on the Companion Website at **http://www.prenhall.com/ball.** Click on Chapter 16 to select the activities for this chapter.
- For animations, more NCLEX review questions, and an audio glossary, access the accompanying CD-ROM in this textbook.

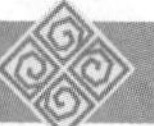

References

1. Agency for Healthcare Research and Quality. (2001a). *Uses of epoetin for anemia in oncology*. Washington, DC: U.S. Department of Health and Human Services (Evidence Report/Technology Assessment #30).
2. Agency for Healthcare Research and Quality. (2001b). *Management of cancer pain*. Washington, DC: U.S. Department of Health and Human Services (Evidence Report/Technology Assessment #35).
3. Alcoser, P. W., & Burchett, S. (1999). Bone marrow transplantation. *American Journal of Nursing 99,* 26–31.
4. American Cancer Society. (2001). Statistics. *www.cancer.org.*
5. Anderson, P. M. (2000). Neoplasms of the kidney. In R. E. Behrman, R. M. Kliegman, & H. B. Jenson, Eds. *Nelson textbook of pediatrics* (16th ed., pp. 1554–1556). Philadelphia: WB Saunders.
6. Baker, B. (1998). CNS tumors now most common cancer in children. *Pediatric News, 32* (7), 12.
7. Behrman, R. E., Kliegman, R. M. & Jenson H. B. (2000). Nelson Textbook of Pediatrics 16th ed. Philadelphia: Saunders.
8. Bertolone, K. (1997). Pediatric oncology: Past, present, and new modalities of treatment. *Journal of Intravenous Nursing, 20,* 136–140.
9. Biggar, R. J., Frisch, M., & Goedert, J. J. (2000). Risk of cancer in children with AIDS. *Journal of the American Medical Association, 284,* 205–209.
10. Bindler, R. M., & Howry, L. B. (1997). *Pediatric drugs and nursing implications* (2nd ed., pp. 579–580, 587). Stamford CT: Appleton & Lange.
11. Blatt, J., Copeland, D. R., & Bleyer, W. A. (1997). Late effects of childhood cancer and its treatment. In P. A. Pizzo & D. G. Poplack (eds.), *Principles and practice of pediatric oncology* (3rd ed., pp. 1301–1330). Philadelphia: Lippincott–Raven.
12. Castleberry, R. P. (1997). Biology and treatment of neuroblastoma. *Pediatric Clinics of North America, 44,* 919–938.
13. Chaffee, S. (2001). Pediatric palliative care. *Primary Care, 28,* 365–370.
14. Challinor, J., Miaskowski, C., Moore, I., Slaughter, R., & Franck, L. (2000). Review of research studies that evaluated the impact of treatment for childhood cancers on neurorecognition and behavioral and social competence: Nursing implications. *Journal of the Society for Pediatric Nurses, 5,* 57–74.
15. Chang, C. C. (1998). Cord blood stem cell transplantation. *Clinician Reviews, 8,* 67–83.
16. Chase, S. (2000). St. John's Wort: Not so safe. *RN, 63,* 114.
17. Conway, E. E., Asuncion, A., & DaRosso, R. (1999). Diagnosing and managing brain tumors: The pediatrician's role. *Contemporary Pediatrics, 16,* 84–97.
18. Coustan-Smith, E., Sancho, J., Hancock, M. L., Boyett, J. M., Behm, F. G., Raimondi, S. C., Sandlund, J. T., Rivera, G. K., Rubnitz, J. E., Ribeiro, R. C., Piu, C. H., & Campana, D. (2000). Clinical importance of minimal residual disease in childhood acute lymphoblastic leukemia. *Blood, 96,* 2691–2696.
19. Crooks, G. M., Lill, J., Feig, S., & Parkman, R. (1997). Cord blood—New source of stem cells for transplants. *Contemporary Pediatrics, 14,* 25–26, 30, 34–36, 41.
20. Dean, R. (2000, September). Alternative therapies may cause interactions in oncology patients. American College of Clinical Pharmacology meeting. Reported by Reuters. http://pediatrics.medscape.com/reuters/prof/2000/09/09.19/20000919prof003.html. Retrieved 9/25/2000 www.
21. Derengowski, S. (1999, June 14). Pediatric non-Hodgkin's lymphoma. *Advance for Nurses,* 26–28.
22. Donaldson, S. S., Egbert, P. R., Newsham, I., & Cavenee, W. K. (1997). Retinoblastoma. In P. A. Pizzo & D. G. Poplack (eds.), *Principles and practice of pediatric oncology* (3rd ed., pp. 699–716). Philadelphia: Lippincott–Raven.
23. Enskar, K., Carlsson, M., Golsater, M., & Hamrin, E. (1997). Symptom distress and life situation in adolescents with cancer. *Cancer Nursing, 20,* 23–33.
24. Freeman, K., O'Dell, C., & Meola, C. (2000). Issues in families of children with brain tumors. *Oncology Nursing Forum, 27,* 843–848.
25. Friebert, S. E., & Shurin, S. B. (1998). ALL: Diagnosis and outlook. *Contemporary Pe-*

diatrics, 15, 118–119, 123–124, 127–128, 131–132, 134, 136.

26. Golub, T. R., Weinstein, H. J., & Grier, H. E. (1997). Acute myelogenous leukemia. In P. A. Pizzo & D. G. Poplack (eds.), *Principles and practice of pediatric oncology* (3rd ed., pp. 463–482). Philadelphia: Lippincott–Raven.
27. Green, D. M., Grigoriev, Y. A., Nan, B., Takashima, J. R., Norkool, P. A., D'Angio, G. J., & Breslow, N. E. (2001). Congestive heart failure after treatment for Wilms' tumor: A report from the National Wilms' Tumor study group. *Journal of Clinical Oncology, 19,* 1926–1934.
28. Grier, H. E. (1997). The Ewing family of tumors: Ewing's sarcoma and primitive neuroectodermal tumors. *Pediatric Clinics of North America, 44,* 991–1004.
29. Hilden, J. M., Emanuel, E. J., Fairclough, D. L., Link, M. P., Foley, K. M., Clarridge, B. C., Schnipper, L. E., & Mayer, R. J. (2001). Attitudes and practices among pediatric oncologists regarding end-of-life care: Results of the 1998 American Society of Clinical Oncology Survey. *Journal of Clinical Oncology, 19,* 205–212.
30. Ishibashi, A. (2001). The needs of children and adolescents with cancer for information and social support. *Cancer Nursing, 24,* 61–67.
31. James, L., & Johnson, B. (1997). The needs of parents of pediatric oncology patients during the palliative care phase. *Journal of Pediatric Oncology Nursing, 14,* 83–95.
32. Kanarek, R. C. (1998). Facing the challenge of childhood leukemia. *American Journal of Nursing, 98,* 42–50.
33. Kelly, K. M., & Lange, B. (1997). Oncologic emergencies. *Pediatric Clinics of North America, 44,* 809–830.
34. Kelly, K. M., Jacobsen, J. S., Kennedy, D. D., Braudt, S. M., Mallick, M., & Weiner, M. A. (2000). Use of unconventional therapies by children at an urban medical center. *Journal of Pediatric Hematology/Oncology, 22,* 412–416.
35. Kemper, K. J., & Longwood Herbal Task Force. (1999). Shark cartilage, cat's claw, and other complementary cancer therapies. *Contemporary Pediatrics, 16,* 101–102, 105–106, 112, 115, 117–118, 121, 125–126.
36. Kinlen, L. J., & Balkwill, A. (2001). Infective cause of childhood leukemia and wartime population mixing in Orkney and Shetland, UK. *Lancet, 357,* 858.
37. Kleinhaus, S., & Boley, S. J. (1999). The latest news about minimally invasive surgery. *Contemporary Pediatrics, 16,* 125–134.
38. Kun, L. E. (1997). Brain tumors: Challenges and directions. *Pediatric Clinics of North America, 44,* 907–918.
39. Landier, W. (2001). Childhood acute lymphoblastic leukemia: Current perspectives. *Oncology Nursing Forum, 28,* 823–833.
40. McManus, J., & Gilchrist, G. S. (2000). Neuroblastoma. In R. E. Behrman, R. M. Kliegman, & H. B. Jenson, Eds. *Nelson textbook of pediatrics* (16th ed., pp. 1552–1554). Philadelphia: WB Saunders.
41. Mercer, M., & Ritchie, J. A. (1997). Home community care: Parents' perspectives. *Journal of Pediatric Nursing, 12,* 133–141.
42. Meyers, P. A., & Gorlick, R. (1997). Osteosarcoma. *Pediatric Clinics of North America, 44,* 973–990.
43. Moller, T. R., Garwicz, S., Barlow, L., Falck Winther, J., Glattre, E., Olafsdotti, G., Olsen, J. H., Perfekt, R., Ritvanen, A., Sankila, R., & Tulinius, H. (2001). Decreasing late mortality among five-year survivors of cancer in childhood and adolescence: A population-based study in the Nordic countries. *Journal of Clinical Oncology, 19,* 3161–3181.
44. Monaco, G. P., Fiduccia, D., & Smith, G. (1997). Legal and societal issues facing survivors of childhood cancer. *Pediatric Clinics of North America, 44,* 1043–1058.
45. Ross, G., Lipper, E. G., Abramson, D., & Preiser, L. (2001). The development of young children with retinoblastoma. *Archives of Pediatric and Adolescent Medicine, 155,* 80–83.
46. Shad, A., & Magrath, L. J. (1997). Non-Hodgkin's lymphoma. *Pediatric Clinics of North America, 44,* 863–890.
47. Smith, M. A., Freidlin, B., Ries, L. A., & Simon, R. (1998). Trends in reported incidence of primary malignant brain tumor in children in the United States. *Journal of the National Cancer Institute, 90,* 1269–1277.
48. Swerdlow, J. L. (2000). *Nature's medicine: Plants that heal.* Washington, DC. National Geographic Society.
49. Thompson, K. A. (1999). Detecting Hodgkin's disease. *American Journal of Nursing AJN, 99,* 61–64.
50. Vernon-Levett, P., & Geller, M. (1997). Posterior fossa tumors in children: A case study. *AACN Critical Issues, 8,* 214–226.
51. Wexler, L. H., & Helman, L. J. (1997). Rhabdomyosarcoma and the undifferentiated sarcomas. In P. A. Pizzo & D. G. Poplack (eds.), *Principles and practice of pediatric oncology* (3rd ed., pp. 799–830). Philadelphia: Lippincott–Raven.
52. Wilkinson, J. D., Fleming, L. E., MacKinnon, J., Voti, L., Wohler-Torres, B., Peace, S., & Trapido, E. (2001). Lymphoma and lymphoid leukemia incidence in Florida children: Ethnic and racial distribution. *Cancer, 91,* 1402–1408.
53. Wolf, J., Grier, H. E., & Klar, N. (2000). Symptoms and suffering at the end of life in children with cancer. *New England Journal of Medicine, 342,* 326–333.
54. Wolfe, J., Klar, N., Grier, H. E., Duncan, J., Salem-Schatz, S., Emanuel, E. J., & Weeks, J. C. (2000). Understanding of prognosis among parents of children who died of cancer. *Journal of the American Medical Association, 284,* 2469–2475.

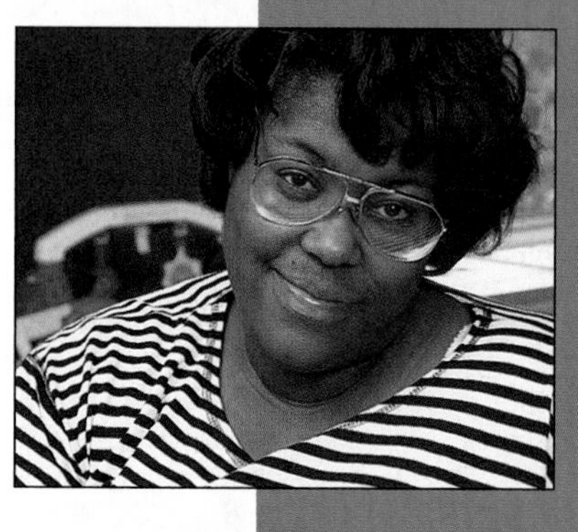

"I was so worried when Jerome was born. He had so many problems. Now he's growing and doing pretty well, and I'm so happy to see him starting to smile. I can't wait until he is able to eat on his own."

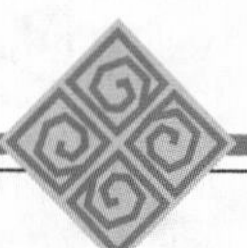

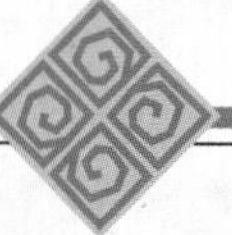

Jerome was born 2 weeks prematurely after a normal pregnancy. Soon after birth, he was diagnosed with multiple gastrointestinal anomalies, the most severe of which were an imperforate anus and esophageal atresia (an incomplete esophagus leading to a blind pouch). He underwent two major surgeries in the immediate newborn period and has been hospitalized several times since birth to treat infections and electrolyte imbalance, provide nutritional support, and evaluate his condition.

Jerome is now 8 months old and weighs 15 pounds. Although he still receives most of his nutrition through enteral feedings, he is learning to suck more vigorously and is given a bottle every few hours. The muscle development facilitated by sucking will promote his intake of foods and formation of speech later.

Jerome has a colostomy that was placed during surgery on his imperforate anus. It is hoped that this can be closed at about 2 years of age and that he will be able to develop normal bowel function. An ostomy nurse visits Jerome both at home and when he is in the hospital to evaluate his care.

Jerome's mother has been devoted to his care, providing nearly all of his tube feedings and other care at home. A home health nurse visits frequently and helps arrange occasional respite care for her. Jerome's mother has received materials and talks on the phone with members of an ostomy support group. She finds this contact very helpful in providing additional ideas about colostomy care and the opportunity to discuss her feelings and concerns about Jerome.

CHAPTER

17

ALTERATIONS IN GASTROINTESTINAL FUNCTION

KEY TERMS

cholestasis Disruption of bile flow.

chronic vomiting Low grade nearly daily emesis.

constipation Difficult and infrequent defecation with passage of hard, dry stool.

cyclic vomiting Repeated severe vomiting of an episodic nature.

deamination Removal of an amino group from an amino compound.

diarrhea Frequent passage of abnormally watery stool.

gluconeogenesis Formation of glycogen from noncarbohydrate sources such as protein or fat.

hernia Protrusion or projection of a body part or structure through the muscle wall of the cavity that normally contains it.

occult blood Blood that is present in minute quantities and can be seen only on microscopic examination or through chemical testing.

ostomy An artificial abdominal opening into the urinary or gastrointestinal canal that provides an outlet for the diversion of urine or fecal matter.

peristalsis A progressive, wavelike muscular movement that occurs involuntarily throughout the gastrointestinal tract.

projectile vomiting Vomiting in which the stomach contents are ejected with great force.

stoma An opening, commonly in the abdominal wall, to provide for drainage from the intestinal or urinary systems.

MediaLink WWW http://www.prenhall.com/ball

Resources for this chapter can be found on the CD-ROM accompanying this textbook, and on the Companion Website at http://www.prenhall.com/ball. Click on Chapter 17 to select the activities for this chapter.

CD-ROM

Animations
- Insider's View: Effects of Lead in the Body

Audio Glossary

NCLEX Review

COMPANION WEBSITE

Web Links

NCLEX Review

MediaLink Applications
- Care of the Child with Cleft Palate
- Evaluating the Home for Poisons
- Managing Emesis in Pediatric Conditions

What causes structural defects such as esophageal atresia and imperforate anus? What special care will Jerome require to promote his growth and development while he undergoes treatment for his anomalies? This chapter discusses the care of infants, like Jerome, who have structural defects and those with other common disorders of gastrointestinal functioning.

Through the gastrointestinal (GI) tract, a child ingests and absorbs the foods and fluids necessary to sustain life and promote growth. Most GI disturbances produce symptoms that are short term and interfere with nutrition and fluid balance for only a brief period. Some disorders or severe defects lead to complications that prevent optimal nutrition and adequate growth. This chapter explores some of the common GI disorders in children. (See Chapter 10 for a discussion of specific fluid imbalances that may accompany GI disorders.)

GI disorders can result from a congenital defect, acquired disease, infection, or injury. Structural problems may occur when development is altered or ceases in the first trimester of gestation. Because various parts of the gastrointestinal system are developing at this point in gestation, it is not unusual for infants to have more than one structural defect of the gastrointestinal system. This was the case with Jerome in the opening vignette. Infections can cause an increase or decrease in motility and prevent proper absorption of nutrients. Interruption or destruction of the GI system can also result from trauma or ingestion of caustic substances. As you read this chapter, remember that any interruption or alteration in the GI system will decrease the body's ability to obtain nutrients, thus impairing growth.

ANATOMY AND PHYSIOLOGY OF PEDIATRIC DIFFERENCES

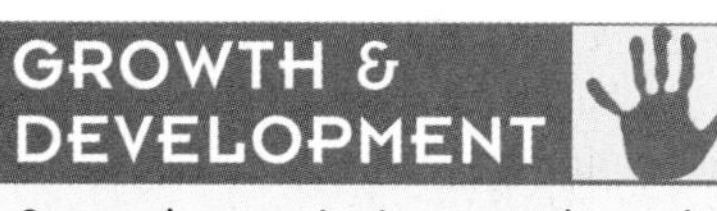

Stomach capacity increase throughout early childhood:

Age	Capacity (mL)
Newborn	10–20
1 week	30–90
2–3 weeks	75–100
1 month	90–150
3 months	150–200
1 year	210–360
2 years	500

Although the fetus makes sucking and swallowing movements in utero and ingests amniotic fluid, the GI system is immature at birth. The processes of absorption and excretion do not begin until after birth, because the placenta is responsible for providing nutrients and removing waste. Sucking is a primitive reflex that occurs when the lips or cheeks are stroked. The infant does not have voluntary control over swallowing until about 6 weeks of age.

The stomach capacity of the newborn is quite small, and intestinal motility (**peristalsis**) is greater than in older children. These characteristics explain the newborn's need for small, frequent feedings and the increased frequency and liquid consistency of bowel movements. Because of the relaxed cardiac sphincter, infants frequently regurgitate small amounts of feedings.

Digestion takes place in the duodenum. Infants have a deficiency of the following enzymes: amylase (which digests carbohydrates), lipase (which enhances fat absorption), and trypsin (which catabolizes protein into polypeptides and some amino acids). Enzymes are usually not present in sufficient quantities to aid digestion until 4 to 6 months of age. Thus, abdominal distention from gas is common.

Liver function is also immature. After the first few weeks of life, the liver is able to conjugate bilirubin and excrete bile. The processes of **gluconeogenesis** (formation of glycogen from noncarbohydrates), plasma protein and ketone formation, vitamin storage, and **deamination** (removal of amino group from amino compound) remain immature during the first year of life.

By the second year of life, digestive processes are fairly complete. Stomach capacity increases to accommodate a three-meals-per-day feeding schedule. At about the same time, myelination of the spinal cord becomes complete and voluntary control over excretory functions can be achieved.

STRUCTURAL DEFECTS

Structural defects can involve one or more areas of the GI tract. These defects occur when growth and development of fetal structures are interrupted during the first trimester. This can leave the structure incomplete, resulting in **atresia** (absence or closure of a normal body orifice), malposition, nonclosure, or other abnormalities.

CLEFT LIP AND CLEFT PALATE

Cleft lip and cleft palate are two distinct facial defects that can occur singly or in combination (Figure 17-1 ◆). Incomplete fusion of the lip occurs in approximately 1 in 700 births (Mitchell & Wood, 2000). It is more common in Native Americans and Asians than in

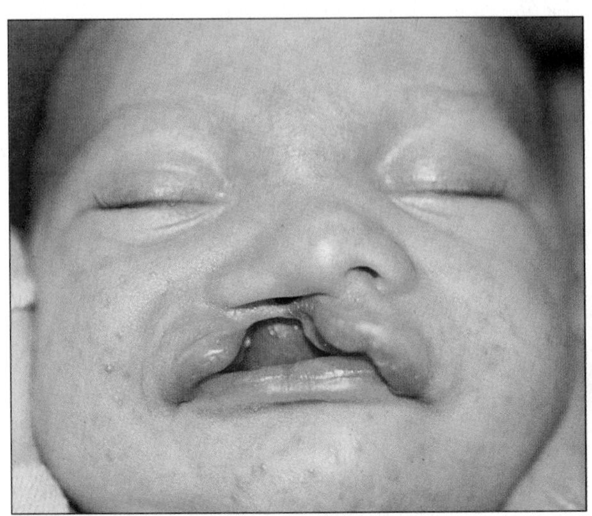

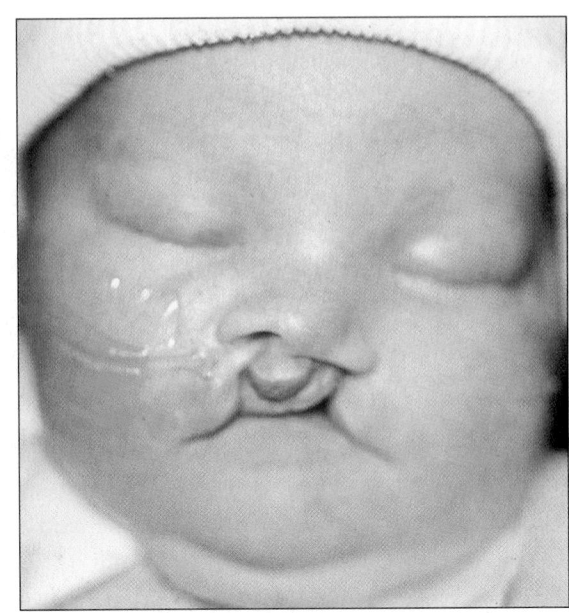

A B

FIGURE 17-1 ◆
A, Unilateral cleft lip. B, Bilateral cleft lip.
Courtesy of Dr. Elizabeth Peterson, Spokane, WA.

whites, and less common in blacks. Incomplete fusion of the palate occurs in approximately 1 in 2,000 births (Balasubrahmanyam, Scherer, & Martin, et al., 1998). Each defect involves various degrees of severity.

Etiology and Pathophysiology

Cleft lip with or without cleft palate results from a failure of the maxillary processes to fuse with the elevations on the frontal prominence during the sixth week of gestation. Normally union of the upper lip is complete by the seventh week. Fusion of the secondary palate occurs between 5 and 12 weeks of gestation. Failure of the tongue to move downward at the correct time will prevent the palatine processes from fusing.

The intrauterine development of the hard and soft palates is completed in the first trimester. It is during this time that other major organ systems develop. Congenital defects such as tracheoesophageal fistula, omphalocele, trisomy 13, and skeletal dysplasias are associated with cleft lip and palate defects in 20% to 30% of cases. There is an increased incidence in families with a prior history of cleft lip or palate. The cause is believed to be multifactorial, involving a combination of environmental and genetic influences. When fortification of cereals and breads with folate began in the United States in 1996 as a measure to decrease neural tube defects, it was found that the incidence of orofacial clefts also decreased. This may suggest a role for folate in formation of maxillary processes in the fetus (Wong, Eskes, & Kuihpers-Jagtman, et al., 1999).

Clinical Manifestations

Cleft lip may be seen during pregnancy on ultrasound by 13 to 16 weeks' gestation (Mitchell & Wood, 2000). A cleft that involves the lip is apparent at birth. It may be a simple dimple in the vermilion border of the lip or a complete separation extending to the floor of the nose. The defect may be unilateral or bilateral and may occur alone or in combination with a cleft palate defect. Varying degrees of nasal deformity may also be present.

Cleft palate defects are less obvious when they occur without a cleft lip and may not be detected at birth. Clefts of the hard palate form a continuous opening between the mouth and nasal cavity and may be unilateral or bilateral, involving just the soft palate or both the soft and hard palate.

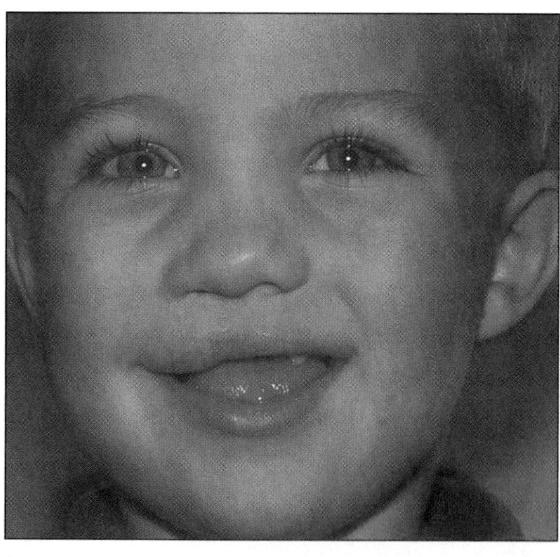

A

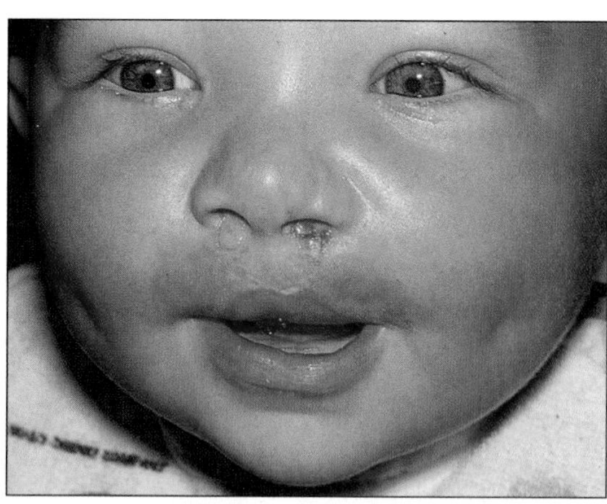

B

FIGURE 17-2 ◆

A, Repaired unilateral cleft lip (see Fig 17-1A). B, Repaired bilateral cleft lip (see Fig. 17-1B).
Courtesy of Dr. Elizabeth Peterson, Spokane, WA.

Clinical Therapy

Cleft lip and palate are usually diagnosed at birth or during the newborn assessment. Medical management requires the combined efforts of a multidisciplinary team. Because speech, hearing, and dentition may be affected, coordinated care by specialists in plastic surgery, hearing, speech, and dentistry is necessary.

The cleft lip is usually repaired by 2 to 3 months of age (Figure 17-2 ◆). The lip is sutured together, and a Logan bow or other stabilizing device or dressing is put in place to prevent tension on the suture line. After surgery, the infant's elbows are restrained to prevent flexion (refer to the Skills Manual). To prevent injury to the suture line, crying is minimized by use of medication.

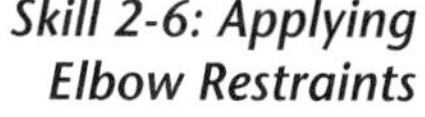

Skill 2-6: Applying Elbow Restraints

Early closure of the lip enables the infant to form a better seal around the nipple for feeding. The sucking motion strengthens the muscles necessary for speech. Special feeding devices such as longer nipples with enlarged holes are available to help meet the infant's nutritional needs before surgical correction.

Timing of the cleft palate repair is controversial and depends on the size and severity of the cleft. Most surgeons perform closure operations when the infant is about 18 months old. This protects the formation of tooth buds and allows the infant to develop more normal speech patterns.

Infants with cleft lip and cleft palate are prone to recurrent otitis media, which can lead to tympanic membrane scarring and hearing loss. Antibiotic therapy is prescribed to treat any infections that might lead to an ear infection. Because infants with chronic otitis media often have difficulty hearing, speech patterns may be altered. These infants require early and continuous intervention to prevent complications. (Refer to Chapter 19 for care of the child with chronic otitis media.) The child who has had cleft palate repair will require orthodontic care. Early visits will permit assessment of tooth eruption and the need for future orthodontic work.

CULTURE

In many developing countries, infants do not have access to surgery for correction of cleft lip and palate. They may grow into childhood and adulthood with these abnormalities. Medical teams from the United States, Canada, and other countries sometimes travel to developing nations for short medical missions, performing surgery on the children and teaching local doctors surgical techniques.

NURSING MANAGEMENT

Nursing Assessment and Diagnosis

Physiologic Assessment

A cleft lip defect is observable at birth. A cleft palate defect is usually noted during the newborn assessment by palpation of the hard palate with the finger. A description of the location and extent of the defect will assist the nurse in determining the correct method of feeding. Thorough and complete physical assessment is needed because additional defects are sometimes present.

Psychosocial Assessment

Assessment of the family's reactions is an integral part of the overall nursing assessment. Physical deformities, especially of the face, can be devastating to parents. A poorly corrected defect can lead to the development of low self-esteem in the older child. Assess the child's developmental level and social interactions with peers.

The accompanying nursing care plan lists common nursing diagnoses for the infant with a cleft lip and/or palate. Other diagnoses that may be appropriate include the following:

- *Anxiety (parent),* related to situational crisis and threat to self-concept
- *Ineffective infant feeding pattern,* related to anatomical abnormality
- *Risk for caregiver role strain,* related to complexity of caregiving tasks
- *Risk for impaired home maintenance management,* related to infant's defect(s) and inadequate family support

Planning and Implementation

Nursing care involves providing emotional support, performing postsurgical care, helping parents to coordinate care and maintain a healthy home environment, and making appropriate referrals. The accompanying nursing care plan summarizes nursing care for the infant with a cleft lip and/or cleft palate.

Provide Emotional Support

Parents may need assistance to view their infant as a whole person, rather than focusing solely on the physical defect. Nurses can promote parent–infant bonding by explaining the nature of the structural defect and the procedure for correction. Interact and speak to the infant in the parents' presence and point out positive attributes such as alertness, soft skin, or active movements. Self-blame is common among parents. Parents can also be referred to the American Cleft Palate Association for information about the disorder. Some plastic surgeons have photos of children before and after correction to reassure parents that their child can have a "normal" appearance (Uhrich & Mackin, 2001).

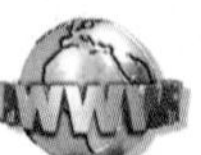

Cleft Palate Resources Online

Parental anxiety is usual when children undergo surgery. This anxiety is heightened when the surgery involves an infant. To minimize anxiety, explanations to parents should be clear and concise. Allow sufficient time for parents to ask questions. Encourage parents to hold and cuddle the infant before surgery.

Provide Postoperative Care

Provide general postoperative care for the infant. (See the accompanying nursing care plan for the infant with a cleft lip and/or palate and also the nursing care plan for the child undergoing surgery in Chapter 5.) Assess vital signs frequently and maintain the infant's airway. Measure intake and output. When oral fluids with clear liquids are started, they are usually given through a dropper or an Asepto syringe. Position the infant in a sitting position for the feedings to avoid aspiration. The infant then progresses to half-strength formula or breast milk. After each feeding, clean the suture line with water or normal saline to avoid accumulation of feedings.

It is important to maintain the suture line to ensure healing. Place the infant in a supine or a side-lying position to avoid rubbing the suture line on the bedding. Keep elbows in soft restraints. Maintain the metal device or Steri-Strips placed over the incision. Place antibiotic cream on the incision site as ordered. Medicate the infant regularly to control pain and to minimize crying and stress on the suture line. After cleft palate surgery, avoid the use of metal utensils or straws, which may disrupt the surgical site.

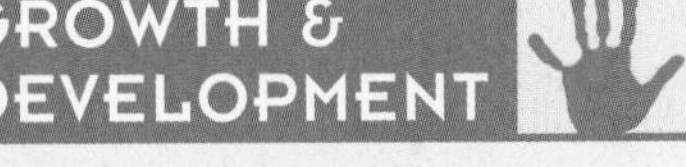

An infant who has had a cleft lip repair needs stimulation to provide distraction. This approach will minimize crying, which can damage the suture line. Soft colorful toys, mobiles, and other visual objects are helpful. Music also can be used to soothe the infant.

Care in the Community

Home care needs should be identified and addressed well in advance of discharge. Discuss all aspects of the infant's care with the parents throughout hospitalization and after surgery. Involve parents in the infant's care to increase their comfort level before discharge and to promote bonding. Teach them feeding techniques, how to recognize signs of infection, how

NURSING CARE PLAN — The Infant with a Cleft Lip and/or Palate

GOAL	INTERVENTION	RATIONALE	EXPECTED OUTCOME
Preoperative Care			
1. Risk for Aspiration (Breast Milk, Formula, or Mucus) related to anatomic defect			
	NIC Priority Intervention: **Aspiration Precautions:** Prevention or minimization of risk factors in the patient at risk of aspiration.		NOC Suggested Outcome: **Airway Maintenance:** Toleration of enteral feedings without aspiration.
The infant will have no episodes of gagging or aspiration.	■ Assess respiratory status and monitor vital signs at least every 2 hours. ■ Position on side after feedings. ■ Feed slowly and use adaptive equipment as needed. ■ Burp frequently (after every 15–30 mL of fluid). ■ Position upright for feedings. ■ Keep suction equipment and bulb syringe at bedside.	■ Allows for early identification of problems. ■ Prevents aspiration of feedings. ■ Facilitates intake while minimizing risk of aspiration. ■ Helps to prevent regurgitation and aspiration. ■ Minimizes passage of feedings through cleft. ■ Suctioning may be necessary to remove milk or mucus.	The infant exhibits no signs of respiratory distress.
2. Ineffective Family Coping related to situational crisis of birth of a child with a defect			
	NIC Priority Intervention: **Family Involvement:** Facilitating family participation in the emotional and physical care of the child.		NOC Suggested Outcome: **Positive Coping:** Extent of coping mechanisms and ability to perform child's physical and emotional care.
Parents will begin bonding process with the infant.	■ Help parents to hold the infant and facilitate feeding process. ■ Point out positive attributes of infant (hair, eyes, alertness, etc). ■ Explain surgical procedure and expected outcome. Show pictures of other children's cleft lip repair.	■ Contact is essential for bonding. ■ Helps parents see the child as a whole, rather than concentrating on the defect. ■ Eliminating unknown factors helps to decrease anxiety.	Parents hold, comfort, and show concern for the infant.
The family's coping ability will be maximized. Parents will verbalize the nature and sequelae of the defect.	■ Assess parents knowledge of the defect, their degree of anxiety and level of discomfort, and the interpersonal relationships among family members. ■ Explore the reactions of extended family members. ■ Support open visitation. ■ Encourage parents to participate in caretaking activities (holding, diapering, feeding).	■ Helps to determine the appropriate timing and amount of information to be given regarding the child's defect. ■ Extended family is an important source of support for most parents of a newborn. Family members can often help promote acceptance and compliance with the treatment plan. ■ Allows parents to continue the bonding process. ■ Participation in infant care decreases anxiety and provides parents with a sense of purpose.	The family demonstrates improved coping ability before discharge. Parents receive necessary support to care for their infant.

(continued)

NURSING CARE PLAN The Infant with a Cleft Lip and/or Palate (continued)

GOAL	INTERVENTION	RATIONALE	EXPECTED OUTCOME
2. Ineffective Family Coping related to situational crisis of birth of a child with a defect (continued)			
	■ Provide information about the etiology of cleft lip and palate defects and the special needs of these infants. Encourage questions. ■ Refer to parent support groups.	■ Concrete information allows parents time to understand the defect and reduces guilt. ■ Support groups allow parents to express their feelings and concerns, to find people with concerns similar to their own, and to seek additional information.	
3. Altered Nutrition: Less Than Body Requirements related to the infant's inability to ingest nutrients			
	NIC Priority Intervention: **Nutrition Management:** Provision of a balanced dietary intake of foods and fluids.		NOC Suggested Outcome: **Nutrition Status:** Amount of food and fluid taken into the body over a 24-hour period.
The infant will gain weight steadily.	■ Assess fluid and calorie intake daily. Assess weight daily (same scale, same time, with infant completely undressed).	■ Provides an objective measurement of whether the infant is receiving sufficient caloric intake to promote growth. Using the same scale and procedure when weighing the infant provides for comparability between daily weights.	The infant maintains adequate nutritional intake and gains weight appropriately.
	■ Observe for any respiratory impairment.	■ Any symptoms of respiratory compromise will interfere with the infant's ability to suck. Feedings should be initiated only if there are no signs of respiratory distress.	
	■ Provide 100–150 cal/kg/day and 100–130 mL/kg/day of feedings and fluid. If the infant needs an increased number of calories to grow, referral to a nutritionist should be made. Formulas with higher calorie concentrations per ounce are available without increasing total fluids.	■ Provides optimal calories and fluids for growth and hydration.	
	■ Facilitate breastfeeding.	■ Breast milk is recommended as the best food for an infant. The process of breastfeeding helps to promote bonding between mother and infant.	Successful breastfeeding is achieved if desired.
	■ Hold the infant in a semisitting position.	■ Makes swallowing easier and reduces the amount of fluid return from the nose.	
	■ Give the mother information on breastfeeding the infant with a cleft lip and/or palate such as plugging the cleft lip and eliciting a let-down reflex before nursing.	■ Information and specific suggestions may encourage the mother to persist with breastfeeding.	
	■ Contact the LaLeche League for the name of a support person.	■ The LaLeche League promotes breastfeeding for all infants. It can provide support people with experience who will aid the mother.	

(continued)

NURSING CARE PLAN The Infant with a Cleft Lip and/or Palate (continued)

GOAL	INTERVENTION	RATIONALE	EXPECTED OUTCOME
3. Altered Nutrition: Less Than Body Requirements related to the infant's inability to ingest nutrients (continued)			
	■ If the mother is unable to breast-feed (or prefers not to), initiate bottle feeding:		
	■ Hold infant in an upright or semisitting position for feeding.	■ Facilitates swallowing and minimizes the amount of fluid return from the nose.	Feeding provides necessary nutrients and is a positive experience for parents and infant.
	■ Place nipple against the inside cheek toward the back of the tongue. May need to use a premature nipple (slightly longer and softer than regular nipple with a larger opening) or a Brecht feeder (an oval bottle with a long, soft nipple).	■ Use of longer, softer nipples makes it easier for the infant to suck. A Brecht feeder decreases the amount of pressure in the bottle and makes the formula flow more easily.	
	■ Feed small amounts slowly.	■ Small amounts and slow feeding do not tire the infant as quickly as do larger amounts given at a faster rate. They also decrease the energy used during feeding.	
	■ Burp frequently, after 15–30 mL of formula has been given.	■ Frequent burping prevents the accumulation of air in stomach, which can cause regurgitation or vomiting.	
	■ Initiate nasogastric feedings if the infant is unable to ingest sufficient calories by mouth.	■ Adequate nutrition must be maintained. Use of a feeding tube allows the infant who has difficulty with oral feeding to receive adequate nutrition for growth.	
Postoperative Care			
1. Risk for Infection related to location of surgical procedure			
	NIC Priority Intervention: **Infection Control:** Minimizing the acquisition and transmission of infectious agents.		NOC Suggested Outcome: **Risk Control:** Actions to eliminate or reduce actual, personal, or modifiable health risks.
The infant's mucosal tissue will heal without infection.	■ Assess vital signs every 2 hours.	■ Elevated temperature may indicate infection.	The infant remains free of infection in the oral cavity. Tissues remain intact and pink.
	■ Assess oral cavity every 2 hours or as needed for tenderness, reddened areas, lesions, or presence of secretions.	■ Aids in identifying infection.	
	■ Cleanse suture line with normal saline or sterile water if ordered.	■ Helps decrease the presence of bacteria.	Healing process progresses without adverse events in postoperative period.
	■ Cleanse the cleft areas by giving 5–15 mL of water after each feeding.	■ Prevents accumulation of carbohydrates, which encourage bacterial growth.	
	■ If a crust has formed, use a cotton swab to apply a half-strength peroxide solution.	■ Helps loosen the crust, aiding in removal.	
	■ Apply antibiotic cream to suture line as ordered.	■ Counteracts the growth of bacteria.	

(continued)

NURSING CARE PLAN The Infant with a Cleft Lip and/or Palate (continued)

GOAL	INTERVENTION	RATIONALE	EXPECTED OUTCOME
1. Risk for Infection related to location of surgical procedure (continued)			
	■ Use careful handwashing and sterile technique when working with suture line.	■ Prevents the spread of microorganisms from other sources.	
2. Ineffective Breathing Pattern related to surgical correction of defect			
	NIC Priority Intervention: **Airway Management:** Facilitation of patency of air passages.		NOC Suggested Outcome: **Vital Signs Status:** Temperature, pulse, respiration, and blood pressure within expected range for the infant/child.
The infant will maintain an effective breathing pattern.	■ Assess respiratory status and monitor vital signs at least every 2 hours.	■ Allows for early identification of problems.	The infant shows no signs of respiratory infection or compromise.
	■ Apply a cardiorespiratory monitor.	■ Enables early detection of abnormal respirations, facilitating prompt intervention.	
	■ Keep suction equipment and bulb syringe at bedside. Gently suction oropharynx and nasopharynx as needed.	■ Gentle suctioning will keep the airway clear. Suctioning that is too vigorous can irritate the mucosa.	
	■ Provide cool mist for first 24 hours postoperatively if ordered.	■ Moisturizes secretions to reduce pooling in lungs. Moisturizes oral cavity.	
	■ Reposition every 2 hours.	■ Ensures expansion of all lung fields.	
	■ Allows for early identification of problems.		
3. Impaired Tissue Integrity related to mechanical factors			
	NIC Priority Intervention: **Wound Care:** Prevention of wound complications and promotion of wound healing.		NOC Suggested Outcome: **Wound Healing:** The extent to which cells and tissues have regenerated following intentional closure.
Lip and/or palate will heal with minimal scarring or disruption.	■ Position the infant with cleft lip repair on side or back only.	■ Prone position could cause rubbing on suture line.	Lip/palate heals without complications.
	■ Use soft elbow restraints. Remove every 2 hours and replace. Do not leave the infant unattended when restraints are removed.	■ Prevents the infant's hands from rubbing surgical site. Regular removal allows for skin and neurovascular checks.	
	■ Maintain metal bar (Logan bow) or Steri-Strips placed over cleft lip repair.	■ Maintaining suture line will minimize scarring.	
	■ Avoid metal utensils or straws after cleft palate repair.	■ These devices may disrupt suture line.	
	■ Keep the infant well medicated for pain in initial postoperative period. Have parents hold and comfort the infant.	■ Good pain management minimizes crying, which can cause stress on suture line. Increases bonding and soothes the child to decrease crying.	
	■ Provide developmentally appropriate activities (e.g., mobiles, music).	■ Soothes and keeps the infant calm.	

(continued)

NURSING CARE PLAN The Infant with a Cleft Lip and/or Palate (continued)

GOAL	INTERVENTION	RATIONALE	EXPECTED OUTCOME
4. Knowledge Deficit (Parent) related to lack of exposure and unfamiliarity with resources			
	NIC Priority Intervention: **Teaching, Disease Process:** Assisting the patient to understand information related to cleft lip/palate.		NOC Suggested Outcome: **Knowledge:** Extent of understanding conveyed about cleft lip/palate treatment.
Before discharge, parents will verbalize home care methods for care of the infant with cleft lip and palate defect.	■ Explain care and treatment (both short term and long term). Discuss potential complications. ■ Demonstrate feeding techniques and alternatives. Allow parents to demonstrate before discharge. ■ Provide written instructions for follow-up care arrangements. ■ Introduce the parents (if possible) to a primary care provider in the setting where the infant will receive follow-up care after discharge.	■ Assists the family to deal with the physical and psychosocial aspects of a child with a congenital defect. ■ Provides visual instructions. Redemonstration confirms learning. ■ Written instructions reinforce verbal instruction and provide a reference after discharge. ■ Continuity of care is important. Since the infant will require long-term follow-up, a contact with the new provider is helpful.	Parents accurately describe and demonstrate feeding techniques to facilitate optimal growth of the infant; describe interventions if respiratory distress occurs; and take the written instructions home with them on discharge.
5. Altered Nutrition: Less Than Body Requirements related to inability to ingest nutrients			
	NIC Priority Intervention: **Nutrition Management:** Promotion of a balanced dietary intake of foods and fluids.		NOC Suggested Outcome: **Nutritional Status:** Extent to which nutrients are available to meet metabolic needs.
The infant will receive adequate nutritional intake.	■ Maintain intravenous infusion as ordered. ■ Begin with clear liquids, then give half-strength formula or breast milk as ordered. ■ Use Asepto syringe or dropper in side of mouth. ■ Do not allow pacifiers. ■ Give high-calorie soft foods after cleft palate repair.	■ Provides fluid when NPO. ■ Ensures adequate fluids and nutrients. ■ Avoids suture line and resultant accumulation of formula in that area. ■ Sucking can disrupt suture line. ■ Rough foods, utensils, and straws could disrupt the surgical site.	The infant receives adequate nutritional intake. Infant resumes usual feeding patterns and gains weight appropriately.

to position the infant, and how to care for the suture line. Breastfeeding is usually possible with some assistance from a lactation specialist, even if the mother pumps her breasts and milk is fed by a special nurser. Some infants may need a device placed in the mouth to enable them to establish suction. Several companies provide special nursers that may be helpful for children with cleft lip or palate.

Management, especially in the first few months of life, involves many different health care professionals. In addition to hospital, clinic, and home health nurses, members of the health care team often include specialists such as the surgeon, speech therapist, geneticist, dentist, prosthodontist, audiologist, social worker, and pediatrician (Balasubrahmanyam et al., 1998). The parents are the best coordinators of the child's care. Encourage them to keep a diary listing the professionals with whom they talk and the content of the discussions.

Discuss with the parents the financial implications of long-term care. Private insurance does not always cover all the costs of care necessary for the child. Refer parents to social services familiar with programs and financial aid for which the parents and child may be eligible. Relief of financial worries enables parents to concentrate on caring for the child.

Teach parents how to care for the child after discharge. If the child has siblings, emphasize that they will need preparation to accept the child. Sibling rivalry can be heightened when one child receives more attention within the home. Remind parents of the importance of setting limits and of spending time with each child. Determine whether additional family supports are necessary. Provide parents with information on support groups, physicians, social workers, internet resources, and local services that can help maintain family continuity.

Discuss ways to prevent the infant from touching the suture line. Teach parents how to bundle an infant in a blanket with arms tucked inside the blanket. A front-sling baby carrier may also be used to immobilize the arms. Front-sling carriers provide the additional benefits of comforting the infant through contact with the parent and of holding the infant upright, which aids in optimal positioning after feedings.

After surgical repair, parents need to be taught how to feed the infant and identify signs of complications (fever, vomiting, respiratory distress). Referral to a home health care agency for support may be helpful. Encourage follow-up visits with health care professionals. The child may need further evaluation of speech development, ear infections, or a recommendation for plastic surgery.

Evaluation

Following are expected outcomes of nursing care in the preoperative period:

- Absence of respiratory distress and maintenance of normal respirations
- Positive parent–infant bonding
- Parental expression of support and comfort by family and community
- Maintenance of normal weight by infant
- Parental knowledge of defect, its correction, and infant needs

Following are expected outcomes of postoperative nursing care:

- Absence of infection
- Clean healing of surgical area
- Absence of respiratory distress
- Effective pain management
- Fluid and electrolyte balance and adequate weight gain
- Parental description of infant care and feeding

ESOPHAGEAL ATRESIA AND TRACHEOESOPHAGEAL FISTULA

Esophageal atresia is a malformation that results from failure of the esophagus to develop as a continuous tube during the fourth and fifth weeks of gestation. Esophageal atresia with tracheoesophageal fistula occurs in 1 in 3,000 to 4,500 births. About 30% of the infants are premature (Herbst, 2000)

In esophageal atresia, the foregut fails to lengthen, separate, and fuse into two parallel tubes (the esophagus and trachea) during fetal development. Instead the esophagus may end in a blind pouch or develop as a pouch connected to the trachea by a fistula (tracheoesophageal fistula) (Figure 17-3 ◆). Esophageal atresia is often associated with a maternal history of polyhydramnios. Associated anomalies may occur, including congenital heart defects, gastrointestinal or urinary tract anomalies, and musculoskeletal abnormalities. Jerome, described at the beginning of the chapter, had esophageal atresia as well as an imperforate anus.

Symptoms in the newborn include excessive salivation and drooling, often accompanied by cyanosis, choking, coughing, and sneezing. During feeding, the infant returns fluid through the nose and mouth. Aspiration places the infant at risk for pneumonia. Depending on the type of defect, the abdomen may become distended because of air trapping.

Diagnosis is usually confirmed by attempting to pass a 5 or 8 French nasogastric tube into the stomach. In most cases, the tube meets resistance and can be advanced only minimally. Specific defects and associated anomalies are determined by x-ray examination.

PATHOPHYSIOLOGY ILLUSTRATED

Esophageal Atresia and Tracheoesophageal Fistula

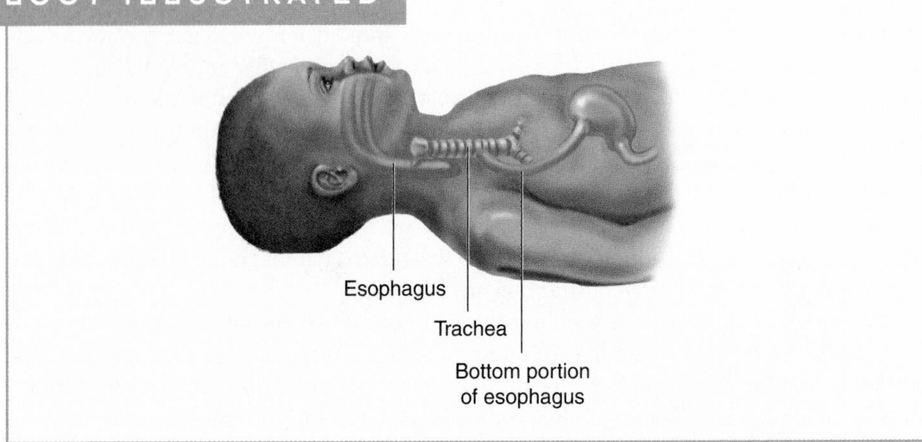

FIGURE 17-3 ◆
In the most common type of esophageal atresia and tracheoesophageal fistula, the upper segment of the esophagus ends in a blind pouch connected to the trachea; a fistula connects the lower segment to the trachea.

CLINICAL TIP

When using a small-bore nasogastric tube, gurgling can occur when the tube is in the esophagus or lung. To confirm placement, aspiration of stomach contents and pH testing are required.

Echocardiogram and abdominal ultrasound are performed. Careful examination of the lungs is needed. A delay in diagnosis can be fatal because ingested fluid or secretions may enter the lungs.

A tube is inserted to suction the upper pouch. Intravenous antibiotics and fluids are begun. Surgery is performed as soon as possible. Surgical correction may be accomplished in several stages. The first stage usually involves ligation of the fistula and insertion of a gastrostomy tube. In the second stage, the two ends of the esophagus are reconnected, if possible. When surgical closure (anastomosis) is not possible, a gastrostomy tube must remain in place for use in feeding. Potential postoperative complications include gastroesophageal reflux, aspiration, and stricture formation. The prognosis is usually good with surgery.

Nursing Management

Esophageal atresia is a surgical emergency. Preoperatively the infant requires close observation and intervention to maintain a patent airway. Suction should be readily available to remove any secretions that accumulate in the nasopharyngeal airway. Place the infant with the head of the bed slightly lowered to minimize aspiration of secretions into the trachea. Continuous or low intermittent suction is used to remove secretions from the blind pouch. Oral fluids are withheld, and the infant is maintained with intravenous fluids administered through an umbilical artery catheter.

After surgery, gastrostomy drainage is maintained, and intravenous fluids and antibiotics are administered. Total parenteral nutrition may be needed until gastrostomy or oral feedings are tolerated.

The parents require emotional support throughout the infant's hospitalization. All procedures should be clearly explained. Encourage parents to bond with the infant by stroking and talking to the child. Eliciting questions and allowing parents to participate in the infant's care, especially feeding (when permitted), can facilitate bonding and help to prepare parents for care of the infant after discharge.

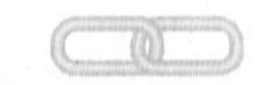

Skill 11-3: Administering a Gavage Feeding

Once enteral feedings have been established, the infant may be discharged from the hospital with a gastrostomy tube in place (Figure 17-4 ◆). (Refer to the Skills Manual for care of the child with a gastrostomy tube.) Teach the parents about gastrostomy tube care and feeding, signs of infection, and how to prevent postoperative complications.

The outcomes of nursing care will depend on the extent of the defect and correction. Examples include the following:

- Adequate intake of fluids to promote hydration and growth
- Absence of respiratory distress
- Positive parent–infant bonding
- Absence of infection
- Parental use of support and information resources regarding the condition

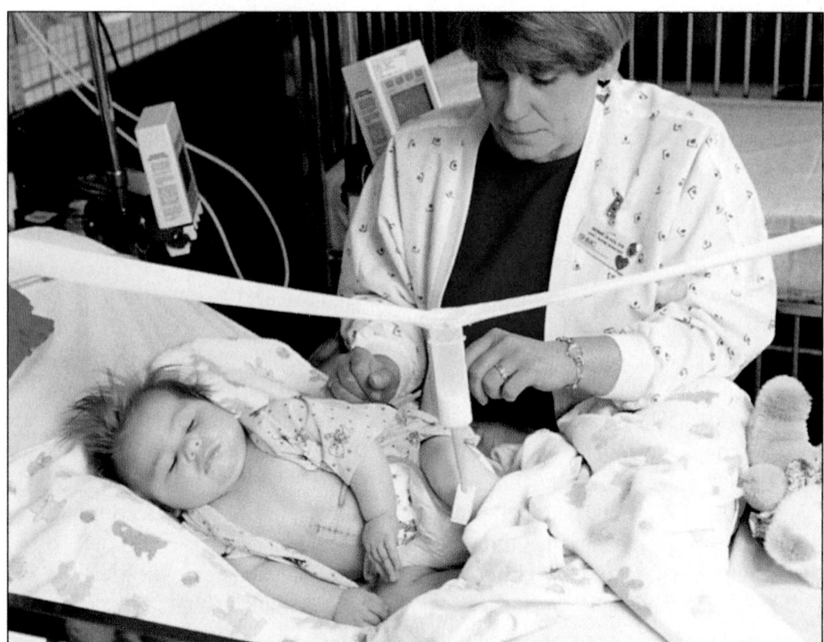

FIGURE 17-4 ◆
Children with esophageal atresia and other gastrointestinal disorders often require a gastrostomy tube for feedings.

PYLORIC STENOSIS

Pyloric stenosis is a hypertrophic obstruction of the circular muscle of the pyloric canal. It is a common problem that most often affects first-born male infants.

Etiology and Pathophysiology

The exact cause of pyloric stenosis is unknown, although frequently there is a family history of the disorder. It is relatively common, with about three cases in 100 births (Irish, Pearl, & Caty, et al., 1998). Hypertrophy of the circular pylorus muscle results in stenosis of the passage between the stomach and the duodenum, partially obstructing the lumen of the stomach (Figure 17-5 ◆). The lumen becomes inflamed and edematous, which narrows the opening until the obstruction becomes complete. At this time, vomiting becomes more forceful. As the obstruction progresses, the infant becomes dehydrated and electrolytes are depleted, resulting in metabolic imbalances.

Clinical Manifestations

Symptoms usually become evident 2 to 4 weeks after birth, although onset may vary. Initially the infant appears well or regurgitates slightly after feedings. The parents may describe the infant as a "good eater" who vomits occasionally. As the obstruction progresses, the vomiting becomes projectile. In **projectile vomiting,** the contents of the stomach may be ejected up to 3 feet from the infant. The vomitus is nonbilious and may become blood tinged because of repeated irritation to the esophagus. The infant is always hungry, appears irritable, fails to gain weight, and has fewer and smaller stools. Dehydration, alkalosis, and hyperbilirubinemia can occur.

Clinical Therapy

On physical examination, visible peristaltic waves across the abdomen and an olive-sized mass in the left upper quadrant are often found. A sonogram is usually performed to confirm the diagnosis, and an upper GI series may be performed as well. Blood tests are used to determine the degree of dehydration, electrolyte imbalance, and anemia (see Chapter 10).

Surgical correction is the treatment of choice. Preoperatively the infant's condition is stabilized with intravenous fluids and electrolytes. A nasogastric tube is inserted to decompress the stomach. Surgery is performed as soon as possible after the infant's condition is stabilized. During surgery, the circular muscle fibers are released to allow the passage of food and fluid (pyloromyotomy). The prognosis is good. The infant is usually taking fluids in 12 to 24 hours, and discharged on a regular diet by 36 to 48 hours after surgery.

FAMILIES WANT TO KNOW

Home Care Instructions for the Child Requiring Gastrostomy Tube Feedings and Care

EQUIPMENT

Prepared, prescribed feeding; enteral feeding pump; long-nosed syringe

PROCEDURE

1. Wash hands.
2. Warm prescribed formula to room temperature.
3. Pour formula to run through the feeding bag.
4. Allow formula to run through the tubing to remove air. Close clamp.
5. Attach syringe to the end of the gastrostomy tube. Unclamp the gastrostomy tube.
6. Pull plunger back until resistance is felt. Check amount of formula in syringe. If more than half of the prescribed amount is withdrawn, refer to the section on problem solving (below). If less than the prescribed amount is withdrawn, push the formula gently back through the syringe.
7. Instill water through the tube.
8. Attach the feeding bag to the gastrostomy tube. Infuse at the prescribed rate.
9. Burp or bubble the infant throughout the feeding.
10. After feeding, flush the gastrostomy tube with water and clamp the tube.
11. Position the infant prone or side lying for 30 to 60 minutes after feedings.

PSYCHOSOCIAL NEEDS

Hold and rock the infant or child during feedings.
Give a pacifier to an infant or a bottle or cup to a child to meet developmental needs.

MEDICATION ADMINISTRATION

Use liquid medication when possible.
Crush only uncoated tablets.
Crush tablets to a fine powder and mix with water or juice.
Flush tubing before and after medication administration.

STOMA CARE

Wash the area around the stoma twice a day with soap and water.
Use half-strength hydrogen peroxide to remove any crusting.
Look for signs of infection, such as redness, swelling, and discharge.
Notify the physician if any signs of infection or leakage are present.

PROBLEM SOLVING

Problem	Cause	Action
Formula will not flow	Blocked tube (clamped, foreign material, viscous formula)	Check clamp. Reposition. Pull back on syringe. Instill water. Milk tube. Notify physician.
	Pump malfunction	Check pump. Call company. Give feeding by gravity.
Large volume of undigested formula removed before feeding	Delayed absorption	Reinfuse remaining formula. If more than half of feeding, subtract from the next feeding. Do not discard the residual.
	Constipation	Check for last bowel movement. Notify physician.
Constipation	Decreased free fluids	Give water and juice between feedings as tolerated. Report bowel problems or hard stools to physician.
Diarrhea	Hyperosmolar formula	Dilute formula.
	Rapid rate of flow	Feed at a slower rate.
	Cold formula	Warm formula to room temperature before feeding.
	Bacterial contamination	Treat with antibiotics.
Dislodged tube	Inadequate stabilization	Bring child for emergency care.
Skin irritation	Formula leakage	Provide skin care; barrier if needed.

Note: Data from Borkowski, S. (1998). Pediatric stomas, tubes, and appliances. *Pediatric Clinics of North America, 45,* 1419–1435; Young, C., & White, S. (1992). Preparing patients for tube feeding at home. *AJN, 92,* 46–53.

PATHOPHYSIOLOGY ILLUSTRATED

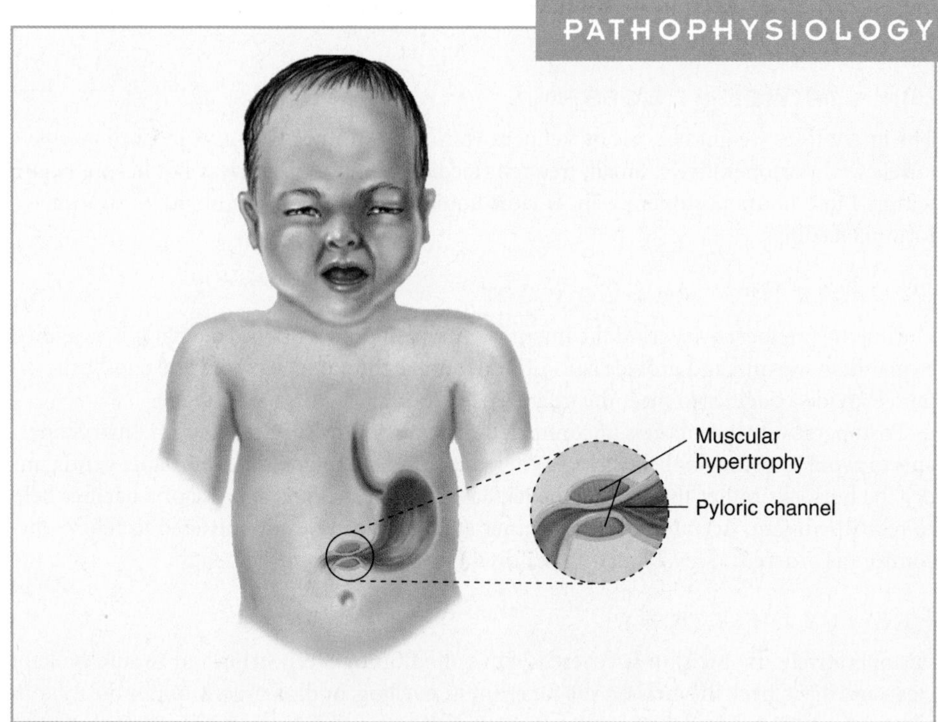

Pyloric Stenosis

FIGURE 17-5 ◆
In pyloric stenosis, the hypertrophied pyloric muscle causes symptoms of projectile vomiting and visible peristalsis.

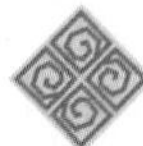

NURSING MANAGEMENT

Nursing Assessment and Diagnosis

Observe the infant's abdomen for the presence of peristaltic waves. Bowel sounds are hyperactive on auscultation. Palpation reveals an olive-shaped mass in the right upper quadrant of the abdomen.

Assess skin turgor, fontanels, urinary output, and mucous membranes to determine whether hydration is adequate. Measure vomitus and describe vomiting episodes. Be alert for signs of an electrolyte imbalance, particularly low levels of serum chloride, sodium, and potassium, and an elevated pH. (See Chapter 10 for a discussion of these electrolyte imbalances.) Assess the parents' level of anxiety related to the child's condition.

CLINICAL TIP

Auscultate for bowel sounds before palpating the abdomen because bowel patterns may change in response to the examiner's touch.

Following are nursing diagnoses that may be appropriate for the child with pyloric stenosis:

- *Fluid volume deficit,* related to active fluid volume loss
- *Altered nutrition: Less than body requirements,* related to vomiting and inability to ingest nutrients
- *Sleep pattern disturbance,* related to discomfort
- *Altered family processes,* related to health status of family member

Planning and Implementation

Nursing care centers on meeting the infant's fluid and electrolyte needs, minimizing weight loss, promoting rest and comfort, preventing infection, and providing supportive care for parents.

MEET FLUID AND ELECTROLYTE NEEDS

Because projectile vomiting will continue until the obstruction is relieved surgically, oral feedings are withheld. Intravenous fluid therapy is administered to correct fluid and electrolyte imbalances and to maintain adequate hydration. Because gastric fluid is high in potassium, hypokalemia can result (see Chapter 10 for a discussion of this electrolyte imbalance and the signs of its occurrence). Monitor intake and output (including vomitus) and urine specific gravity. Inform parents that all diapers will be weighed to measure the infant's output of urine and stool.

MINIMIZE WEIGHT LOSS

The infant loses weight because of frequent vomiting. Monitor weight daily both preoperatively and postoperatively. Small, frequent feedings consisting of clear liquids are begun within 4 to 6 hours postoperatively. If clear liquids are tolerated, the infant is advanced to formula feedings.

PROMOTE REST AND COMFORT

During the preoperative period the infant is hungry and cries often. The infant is swaddled to maintain warmth and provide comfort. Encourage the parents to hold and cuddle the infant. Provide a pacifier to meet the infant's need to suck.

Postoperatively the infant is uncomfortable because of the surgical incision. Instruct parents to avoid pressure on the incision. When diapering the infant, slide the diaper gently under the buttocks rather than lifting the legs. Swaddling, rocking, and use of a pacifier help to relax the infant. Acetaminophen or other analgesics can be administered to relieve discomfort as ordered. (See Chapter 9 for a discussion of pain management.)

PREVENT INFECTION

Postoperatively the incision is covered with collodion or Steri-Strips and should be kept clean and dry. Check the incision site for redness, swelling, or discharge. Monitor the infant's temperature every 4 hours. Auscultate lungs to listen for clear respiratory sounds.

PROVIDE SUPPORTIVE CARE

The need for hospitalization and surgery creates anxiety for parents. Encourage them to participate in the infant's care and to discuss their fears and concerns. Provide simple and clear explanations about the infant's condition and care. Advise parents that occasional vomiting after surgery may occur.

DISCHARGE PLANNING AND HOME CARE TEACHING

Instruct parents to observe the incision for redness, swelling, or discharge and to notify the physician immediately if these occur or if the infant's temperature is higher than 38.5°C (101°F). To reduce the possibility of infection, advise parents to fold the infant's diaper so that it does not touch the incision.

Evaluation

Expected outcomes of care include pain control, intake of recommended fluid and food with absence of vomiting, and manifestation of normal growth patterns.

CLINICAL TIP 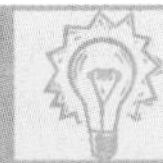

Vomiting and feeding disorders can occur throughout childhood as well as in infancy. In older children, a pattern of **chronic vomiting** (low-grade nearly daily emesis) or **cyclic vomiting** (repeated severe vomiting of an episodic nature) can occur. These patterns differ from vomiting seen in colic or gastroesophageal reflux. Chronic vomiting is most often associated with peptic ulcer or irritable bowel, and cyclic vomiting is indicative of a syndrome known as abdominal migraine. Continuous vomiting of any nature should be evaluated (Li, 1996).

GASTROESOPHAGEAL REFLUX

Gastroesophageal reflux, the return of gastric contents into the esophagus, is the result of relaxation of the lower esophageal sphincter. It may occur at any time and is not necessarily related to having a full stomach.

Some "spitting up" after feedings is considered normal in newborn infants, because of the weak cardiac sphincter of the stomach. However, regurgitation that continues and increases in frequency, resulting in delayed growth, may be called reflux disease, and requires further investigation. Gastroesophageal reflux is more common in premature infants and in children with neurologic impairments. It often resolves without surgical intervention by 12 to 18 months of age (Berube, 1997).

Children with gastroesophageal reflux are frequently hungry and irritable. They eat often but still lose weight. They have a history of vomiting and frequent upper respiratory infections. Reflux of stomach contents can lead to aspiration, resulting in frequent bouts of pneumonia, reactive airway disease, color changes during feeding, apnea, or *hematemesis* (vomiting blood) (Levy, 2001).

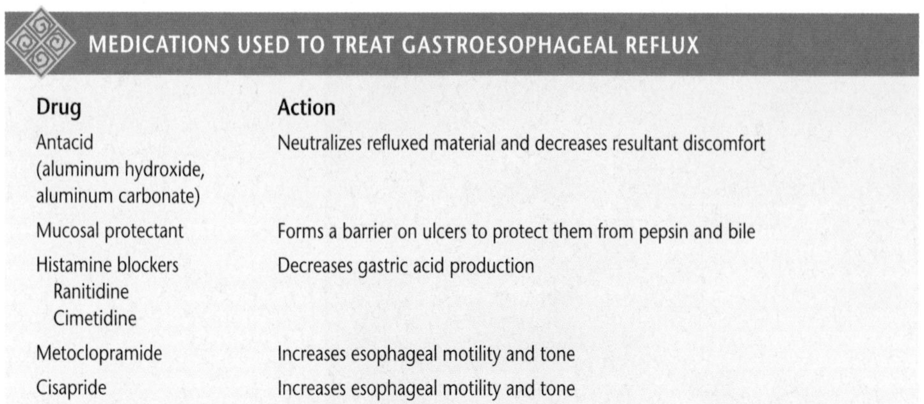

MEDICATIONS USED TO TREAT GASTROESOPHAGEAL REFLUX

Drug	Action
Antacid (aluminum hydroxide, aluminum carbonate)	Neutralizes refluxed material and decreases resultant discomfort
Mucosal protectant	Forms a barrier on ulcers to protect them from pepsin and bile
Histamine blockers Ranitidine Cimetidine	Decreases gastric acid production
Metoclopramide	Increases esophageal motility and tone
Cisapride	Increases esophageal motility and tone
Acetaminophen	Controls pain

Diagnosis is confirmed by a thorough history of the child's feeding patterns and by diagnostic evaluation using contrast upper gastrointestinal series, upper gastrointestinal endoscopy, pH probe monitoring (insertion of a small catheter into the esophagus through the nose that is left in place for 18 to 24 hours to measure pH and thus determine number of reflux episodes), or gastroesophageal scintigraphy (radionuclide scanning to evaluate gastric emptying) (Murray & Christie, 2000).

Treatment depends on the severity of the condition. Mild cases may require only a modification of feeding habits, and usually resolve by 12 to 18 months (Murray & Christie, 2000). Rice cereal is often placed in the infant's bottle to thicken feedings. Fatty foods and citrus juices are avoided. Medications (cholinergics, antacids, and histamine antagonists) may be prescribed to reduce the amount of stomach acid and lessen the child's discomfort. The child should be positioned with the upper body raised 30 degrees after feedings.

Treatment for severe cases may include surgery to create a valve mechanism by wrapping the greater curvature of the stomach (fundus) around the distal esophagus (Nissen fundoplication). A gastrostomy tube is usually inserted during surgery and left in place for 6 weeks. Infants with mild conditions and those undergoing surgical correction usually have decreased incidence of reflux. They may have episodes of mild reflux throughout life and may occasionally require medication for treatment.

Nursing Management

Nursing management focuses on obtaining a thorough history of the child's feeding patterns. Observe vomiting episodes and document amount, color, and consistency of emesis.

Monitor the infant's weight daily and plot progress on a growth chart. Observe for any signs of respiratory distress and keep the infant's nose and mouth clear of vomitus.

Adequate nutrition must be maintained. Infants receiving oral feedings should be given small, frequent feedings. Elevate the head of the bed to prevent aspiration if vomiting should occur. If the child has difficulty maintaining this position, a Tracy harness or reflux board may be used. The harness, which is pinned to the mattress, supports the infant in an upright position. If the child has a gastrostomy tube, it is important to maintain skin integrity around the stoma site. Secure the tube so the infant cannot dislodge or pull on it.

Discharge planning focuses on instructing parents in how to feed and position the infant, as well as providing comfort and emotional support. Encourage parents to hold and cuddle the infant during all feedings. Providing the infant with a pacifier helps to meet nonnutritive sucking needs. Teach parents how to suction the nose and mouth if vomiting occurs.

OMPHALOCELE

Omphaloceles are congenital malformations in which intra-abdominal contents herniate through the umbilical cord (Figure 17-6 ◆). They result from failure of the abdominal contents, such as intestines and liver, to return to the abdomen when the abdominal wall begins to close by the tenth week of gestation. The protrusion is covered by a translucent sac (peritoneum) into which the umbilical cord inserts. Omphalocele is often associated with other

CLINICAL TIP

To thicken formula, add 1 teaspoon to 2 tablespoons of rice cereal to each ounce of formula. Cut a slightly larger hole in the infant's nipple to accommodate the thicker feeding. This may not be recommended for all children, because they may not eat enough formula to meet their nutritional needs. Breast milk will not readily thicken when mixed with rice cereal.

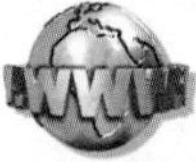

Reflux Resources

CLINICAL TIP

Measure and record the length of the gastrostomy tube daily to be sure it remains properly placed. Coil the tube that is outside the body, tape in place, and put a shirt on the infant to cover it. Frequently clean any drainage around the tube as the acidic gastric contents are harmful to the skin.

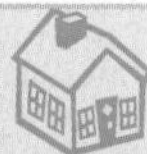

HOME CARE

Be sure that parents know not to place an infant with gastroesophageal reflux in an infant seat. The infant's position in this type of seat increases intra-abdominal pressure and will actually worsen the condition.

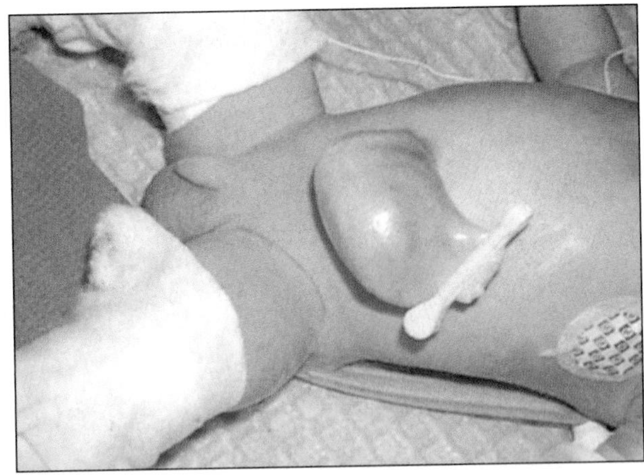

FIGURE 17-6 ◆
In omphalocele, the size of the sack depends on the extent of the protrusion of abdominal contents through the umbilical cord.
From Rudolph, A.M., Hoffman, J.I.E., & Rudolph, C.D. (Eds.). (1991). *Rudolph's pediatrics.* (19th ed., p. 1040) Stamford, CT: Appleton & Lange.

congenital anomalies such as cardiac defects; genitourinary anomalies; trisomy 13, 18, or 21; craniofacial abnormalities; and diaphragmatic abnormalities (Brown, Irish, & Rice, et al., 1998). Omphalocele with intestinal contents in the sac occurs in 1 in 5,000 births, while those involving liver and intestines occur in 1 in 10,000 births (Stoll & Kliegman, 2000).

The size of the sac varies depending on the extent of the protrusion. Rupture of the sac results in evisceration of the abdominal contents. Treatment involves protecting the sac from injury, providing fluids and warmth, and surgical repair to replace the abdominal contents and close the abdominal wall. For smaller defects, primary closure is accomplished with one surgery. If the defect is severe, surgical correction may be performed in several steps. If an omphalocele occurs without associated defects, the child usually recovers from the surgery without incident and leads a normal life.

Nursing Management

Be alert for signs of associated congenital anomalies. (Refer to the discussions of tracheoesophageal fistula earlier in this chapter, to genitourinary anomalies in Chapter 18, and to congenital heart defects in Chapter 14.)

Immediately after birth, the sac is covered with sterile gauze soaked in normal saline solution to prevent drying of the abdominal contents. A layer of plastic wrap is placed over the gauze to provide additional protection against heat and moisture loss. Monitor vital signs every 2 to 4 hours, paying close attention to temperature, as the infant can lose heat through the sac. The child should be in a warmer or isolette for maintenance of temperature control. Inspect the area for signs of infection.

Because the infant is NPO preoperatively, fluid and electrolyte balance is maintained by administering intravenous fluids. Postoperative care includes measures to control pain, prevent infection, maintain fluid and electrolyte balance, and ensure adequate nutritional intake.

Throughout the infant's hospitalization, parents need clear, accurate explanations about the infant's condition. To help the parents deal with the crisis of an acutely ill newborn, provide emotional support and encourage parents to express their feelings. When the child has multiple anomalies, parents need ongoing support for the lengthy treatment, numerous hospitalizations, and management of nutritional intake.

Expected outcomes of nursing care depend on the severity of defect and its correction. Some examples include maintenance of normal vital signs, prompt identification of additional problems, healing of surgical site without signs of infection, pain control, proper intake of fluids, and establishment of an intake to support growth patterns.

INTUSSUSCEPTION

Intussusception occurs when one portion of the intestine prolapses and then invaginates or telescopes into another. It is one of the most frequent causes of intestinal obstruction during infancy, with an incidence of 1 to 4 in 1,000 births. Most cases occur in boys between the ages of 3 months and 6 years (Wylie, 2000).

The most common site of intussusception is the ileocecal valve (Figure 17-7 ◆). Telescoping of the intestine obstructs the passage of stool. The walls of the intestine rub to-

PATHOPHYSIOLOGY ILLUSTRATED

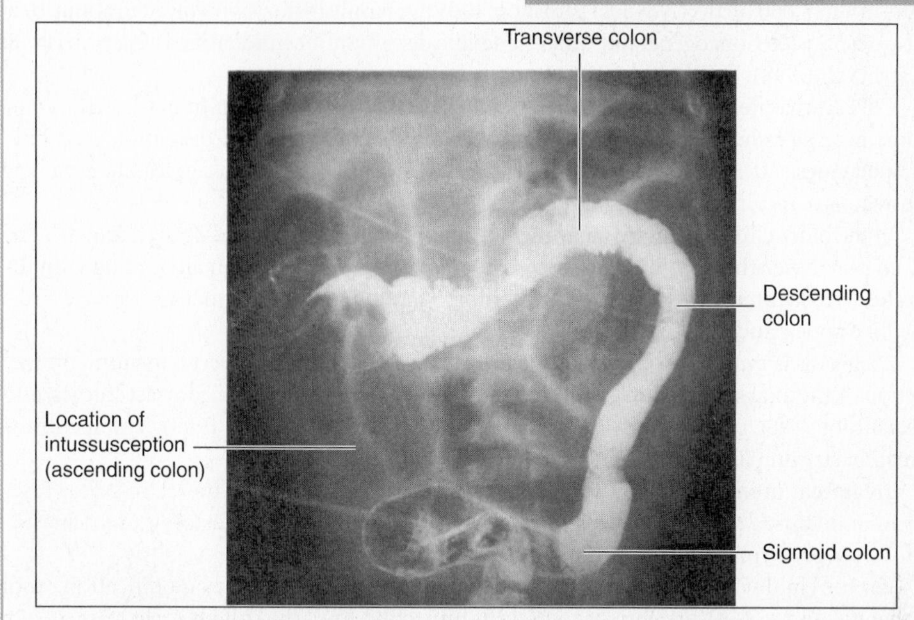

Intussusception

FIGURE 17-7 ◆

In infants, intussusception is commonly associated with measles, viral disease, and gastroenteritis syndromes.

From Fleisher, G.R., Ludwig S. (1993). *Textbook of Pediatric Emergency Medicine*, 3rd ed., Fig. 112.5, p. 1315. Philadelphia: LW&W.

gether, causing inflammation, edema, and decreased blood flow. This can lead to necrosis, perforation, hemorrhage, and peritonitis.

The onset is usually abrupt. A previously healthy infant or child suddenly experiences acute abdominal pain with vomiting and passage of brown stool. There may be periods of comfort between acute episodes of pain. As the condition worsens, painful episodes increase. The stools become red and resemble currant jelly because of the mix of blood and mucus. A palpable mass may be present in the upper right quadrant or mid-upper abdomen.

Diagnosis is made on the basis of the history and confirmed by radiographs and ultrasound of the abdomen; barium enema may be used (Orenstein, 2000). In some cases, the hydrostatic pressure from the barium moves the bowel back into place. Oxygen, saline, and aqueous contrast material may also be used to reduce the intussusception. If this does not occur, surgical intervention to reduce the invaginated bowel and remove any necrotic tissue is necessary. Surgery is usually successful in correcting the problem.

Nursing Management

Nursing management focuses on maintaining or restoring fluid and electrolyte balance. Intravenous fluids are started immediately. Serum electrolyte monitoring is essential to correct imbalances.

Postoperative care focuses on monitoring for early signs of infection, managing the child's pain, and maintaining nasogastric tube patency. Assess vital signs, check for abdominal distention, and listen for bowel sounds every 4 hours. After normal bowel function returns, clear liquid feedings are begun. Feedings are advanced to half-strength milk and other foods as the infant or child tolerates it.

Discharge usually occurs shortly after the infant or child begins taking full feedings. Instruct parents to watch for infection and to call the physician if symptoms recur, a fever develops, or appetite decreases.

HIRSCHSPRUNG'S DISEASE

Hirschsprung's disease, also known as congenital aganglionic megacolon, is a congenital anomaly in which inadequate motility causes mechanical obstruction of the intestine. The absence of autonomic parasympathetic ganglion cells in the colon prevents peristalsis at that portion of the intestine, resulting in the accumulation of intestinal contents and abdominal distention. Hirschsprung's disease is more common in boys (4:1 ratio) and can

CLINICAL TIP

Chronic intestinal pseudo-obstruction (pseudo-Hirschprung's disease) is a rare condition of small bowel dysmotility, and should be differentiated from the presence of Hirschsprung's disease. It results from disorders of the smooth muscle of the bowel (myopathic type) or of the neurological network of the bowel (neuropathic type). Treatment includes drugs to increase intestinal motility and generally total parenteral nutrition (Barr, 2000).

occur in combination with congenital heart defects, Down syndrome, and such syndromes as Smith-Lemli-Opitz and Waarendenburg's syndromes. It can be acute or chronic and occurs in 1 in 5,000 births (Nowicki & Bishop, 1999). A family history is involved in about 10% of cases; a proto-oncogene and other genetic causes have been identified (Pearl, Irish, & Caty, et al., 1998).

Clinical manifestations vary depending on the child's age at onset. In newborns, symptoms include failure to pass meconium, refusal to suck, abdominal distention, and bile-stained emesis. If Hirschsprung's disease is not treated, the condition can lead to complete obstruction, respiratory distress, and shock.

In the older child, symptoms may include failure to gain weight and delayed growth. The child may have a history of abdominal distention, severe constipation alternating with **diarrhea** (frequent, watery stools), and vomiting. The stool may be normal size or have a ribbonlike appearance.

Diagnosis is made on the basis of the history, bowel patterns, anorectal manometry (reaction of the anal sphincter to distention of the rectum), radiographic contrast studies, and rectal biopsy for presence or absence of ganglion cells (Pearl et al., 1998). The rectum is small in size on palpation and does not contain stool.

Treatment in infancy involves surgical removal of the aganglionic bowel. In severe cases or in ill infants, a temporary colostomy is created. Closure of the colostomy and reanastomosis are performed at a later point (Pearl et al., 1998).

For the child with a milder defect, management may involve dietary modification, stool softeners, and isotonic irrigations to prevent impaction until the child is toilet trained.

The return of normal bowel function depends on the amount of bowel involved. Some fecal incontinence and constipation may persist following surgery. A serious complication is enterocolitis (inflammation of the intestines), which occurs in 20% to 60% of children after surgery (Pearl et al., 1998). Symptoms of enterocolitis include gastrointestinal bleeding and diarrhea. Enterocolitis can occur before or after surgery, resulting in ischemia and ulceration of the bowel wall. Treatment may include total parenteral nutrition and a lactose-free diet.

Nursing Management

Nursing assessment in the newborn period includes careful observation for the passage of meconium. When the disease is diagnosed later in infancy or in childhood, obtain a thorough history of weight gain, nutritional intake, and bowel habits.

Nursing management consists of carefully monitoring fluid and electrolyte balance and maintaining nutrition. Teach parents how to ensure regular bowel movements. Daily rectal irrigations with normal saline solution are necessary to promote adequate elimination and prevent obstruction. Teach parents how to prevent skin breakdown in the rectal area by changing diapers frequently, cleansing the area carefully, and applying protective ointment at each diaper change.

If surgical correction is necessary, nursing care will include monitoring for infection, managing pain, maintaining hydration, measuring abdominal circumference to detect any distention, and providing support to the child and family. Parents will need instruction in ostomy care in those cases when the child has a colostomy (refer to the discussion later in this chapter). Provide appropriate referrals to an ostomy support group and enterostomal nurse specialist when indicated. Teach parents to be alert for and immediately report signs of complications. These include diarrhea and pelvic abscess from leakage of intestinal contents at the surgical site (characterized by fever and pain). Children occasionally develop constipation, and parents may need guidance to adapt the diet and fluid intake to manage this complication. Because some children develop malabsorption, be alert for signs of poor growth or malnutrition.

Expected outcomes of nursing care include prompt identification of obstruction, maintenance of normal bowel patterns, adequate hydration, and maintenance of clear skin.

HOME CARE

Because newborns are often discharged within 24 hours of birth, it is important to describe to parents the characteristics of infants' first bowel movements. Parents should be instructed to notify the physician if no stool is passed or if the abdomen becomes distended.

ANORECTAL MALFORMATIONS

Malformations of the anus and rectum are common congenital anomalies. Minor anomalies occur in 1 in 4,000 to 5,000 births. They are often associated with anomalies of the uri-

TABLE 17-1 Management of Anorectal Malformations

CONDITION	MANAGEMENT
Males	
Cutaneous fistula Anal stenosis Anal membrane	No colostomy required
Rectourethral fistula Bulbar Prostatic Rectovesical fistula Anorectal agenesis without fistula Rectal atresia	Colostomy required
Females	
Cutaneous perineal fistula	No colostomy required
Vestibular fistula Vaginal fistula Anorectal agenesis without fistula Rectal atresia Persistent cloaca	Colostomy required

Note: From Warner, B. W. (1996). Classification of congenital disorders of the anorectum. In A. M. Rudolph, J.I.E. Hoffman & C.D. Rudolph. *Rudolph's pediatrics (29th ed.).* Stamford, CT: Appleton & Lange, pg, 1112.

nary tract, esophagus, and duodenum (Brown et al., 1998). Table 17-1 describes the most common anorectal anomalies.

Diagnosis is usually made at birth or during the newborn assessment of anorectal structures and rectal patency. Failure to pass meconium may indicate a malformation high in the colon. Stool in the urine is indicative of a fistula between the colon and urinary tract. Ribbonlike stools may occur with some malformations. Ultrasound and lower GI radiographic studies are used to confirm the diagnosis and demonstrate the extent of the anomaly. Higher defects are often less apparent at birth and involve more complicated treatment (Hendren, 1998).

Medical management depends on the extent of the malformation. Some stenosed anal openings can be treated with dilation alone. An imperforate anal membrane (Figure 17-8 ◆) is excised surgically, followed by daily manual dilations. More severe defects require reconstructive surgery. A temporary colostomy is sometimes performed to rest the bowel after reconstruction. Closure of the colostomy is generally performed between the age of 6 months and 1 year.

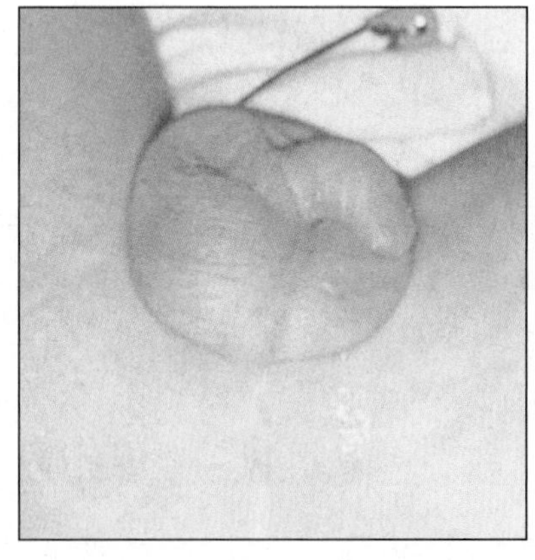

FIGURE 17-8 ◆ Imperforate anus, which is often obvious at birth, can range from mild stenosis to a complex syndrome that includes associated congenital anomalies.

Nursing Management

During the initial newborn assessment, the perineal area is inspected for a poorly developed anal dimple or sacral anomalies. A rectal thermometer is lubricated and inserted a short distance into the rectum to determine patency. Observation and recording of passage of meconium are essential.

Once the diagnosis has been made, intravenous fluids are initiated and a nasogastric tube is inserted to decompress the stomach. Monitor the child's intake and output and cardiorespiratory functioning. Provide emotional support to the parents and give them information about the upcoming surgery.

Postoperative care centers on preventing infection and respiratory complications from surgery, as well as maintaining hydration. Observe the incision for signs of infection, and provide careful wound care. Assess vital signs at least every 4 hours. Once the child's condition is stable, clear fluid oral intake is allowed, advancing to half- and full-strength formula or breast milk as tolerated. The infant will have a colostomy after surgery, and careful skin care around the stoma is essential to prevent breakdown of the fragile area. Colostomy care was a particular focus of nursing management for Jerome, who was described at the beginning of this chapter.

DISCHARGE PLANNING AND HOME CARE TEACHING Infants are increasingly discharged shortly after birth, so parents need clear instructions about normal newborn stools and what abnormalities to report.

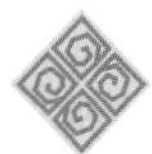

Skill 5-13: Taking an Axillary Temperature

After surgery, teach parents how to take the infant's temperature using the axillary route (see the Skills Manual). Have them demonstrate the proper technique before discharge. Explain the signs and symptoms of infection. Discuss feeding regimens and bowel habits necessary to maintain adequate nutrition for growth and development. Advise parents that children with anorectal malformations may have difficulty achieving bowel control. Patience in toilet training is important. When the child reaches an age that is appropriate for toilet training, encourage the family to speak with a health care provider to discuss the child's progress.

If a colostomy is performed, teach parents how to care for the ostomy site (see discussion of ostomies later in this chapter). Reassure parents that the colostomy will be closed in the future, and assist them in planning for that hospitalization. Discuss follow-up care and long-term management. Arrange follow-up visits and home care visits to evaluate the child's ostomy site and monitor growth.

Expected outcomes of nursing care include adequate fluid intake, normal bowel patterns, parental knowledge of ostomy or other treatment protocols, and eventual success with toilet training.

HERNIAS

A **hernia** is the protrusion or projection of an organ or a part of an organ through the muscle wall of the cavity that normally contains it. This protrusion may result from the failure of normal openings to close during fetal development or from weakness in the supporting musculature. When intra-abdominal pressure increases (as when the infant cries or strains to pass stool), the weakened area separates, causing a protrusion of underlying organs. Inguinal hernias are the most common type of hernia occurring in children (see Chapter 18). Other hernias that occur frequently in children are diaphragmatic and umbilical.

DIAPHRAGMATIC HERNIA

In a diaphragmatic hernia, abdominal contents protrude into the thoracic cavity through an opening in the diaphragm. Sites of herniation include the substernal space, posterolateral region, and the esophageal hiatus. The posterolateral site (foramen of Bochdalek) is the most common location. The cause is a delay or failure in closure of the pleuroperitoneal musculature. The overall incidence of diaphragmatic hernia is 1 in 5,000 live births, and 1 in 2,000 stillbirths (Hartman, 2000). Associated anomalies, particularly cardiac defects, occur in some infants.

A diaphragmatic hernia is a life-threatening condition. Severe respiratory distress occurs shortly after birth. As the infant cries, abdominal organs extend into the thorax, decreasing the size of the thoracic cavity. The infant becomes dyspneic and cyanotic. Characteristic findings include a barrel-shaped chest and sunken abdomen.

Some cases of congenital diaphragmatic hernia are diagnosed in utero by ultrasound. Postnatal diagnosis is confirmed by chest x-ray examination. Immediate respiratory support is essential. The infant is positioned with the head and thorax higher than the abdomen to facilitate downward movement of abdominal organs. A nasogastric tube is inserted to decompress the stomach. Ventilator support is necessary to manage respiratory compromise. Intravenous fluids are administered through an umbilical artery catheter.

Once the infant's condition is stabilized, surgery is performed to correct the defect. Extracorporeal membrane oxygenation (ECMO) may be used to provide cardiopulmonary bypass to rest the lungs. The prognosis is poor. Only 50% of infants survive, with death usually resulting from pulmonary hypoplasia. Even after surgery, the infant may do well initially and then manifest severe respiratory decompensation.

Nursing Management

The infant with a diaphragmatic hernia is admitted to the NICU and requires continuous monitoring. Preoperative management centers on providing supportive care to the infant and parents. Note the infant's vital signs every 30 minutes on the cardiorespiratory monitor. Observe for worsening of respiratory compromise. Maintain intravenous fluid administration. Promote decreased stimulation to keep the infant calm and thus maintain low abdominal pressure. Keep parents informed about the infant's condition and provide emotional support both before and after surgery.

Postoperative care includes positioning the infant on the affected side to facilitate expansion of the lung on the unaffected side, observing closely for signs of infection, maintaining respiratory support, and carefully monitoring fluid and electrolyte balance.

Before discharge, instruct parents in wound care, prevention of infection, and feeding techniques.

UMBILICAL HERNIA

An umbilical hernia results from imperfect closure or weakness of the umbilical ring (Figure 17-9 ◆). The condition is often associated with diastasis recti (lateral separation of the abdominal muscles). It is more common in black children, girls, and infants with low birth weight (O'Donnell, Glick, & Caty, 1998).

The hernia appears as a soft swelling covered by skin. The herniated area protrudes with coughing, crying, or straining during a bowel movement. It is easily reduced by pushing the bowel back through the fibrous ring. The size of the defect may vary among individuals. Contents of the hernia include omentum or portions of the small intestine.

Most defects resolve spontaneously by 3 to 4 years of age. Surgery is indicated in cases of strangulation (closure of the umbilical ring around a portion of the bowel, preventing it from moving back into the abdomen), increased protrusion of the hernia after the age of 2 years, or little or no improvement in a large defect after the age of 4 years.

Nursing management is generally supportive. Instruct parents not to apply tape, straps, or coins to reduce the hernia. This can cause strangulation of the hernia, necessitating immediate surgery. If surgery is required, it is usually performed in a short-stay unit. Postoperatively, teach parents how to care for the surgical site, to watch for bleeding, and to recognize signs of infection. Reinforce the importance of returning for follow-up evaluation.

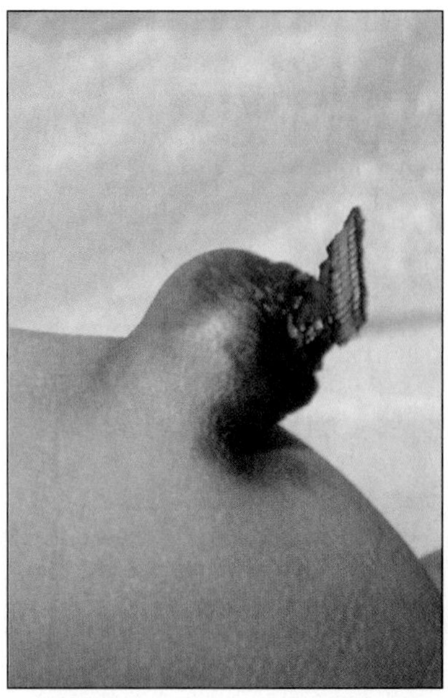

FIGURE 17-9 ◆
The umbilical hernia of the newborn usually closes as the muscles strengthen in later infancy and childhood.
From Zitelli, B., & Davis, H. (Eds.) (1994). *Atlas of pediatric physical diagnosis.* (2nd ed.). London: Mosby-Wolfe Publishing.

OSTOMIES

An intestinal **ostomy** is an opening, or **stoma,** into the small or large intestine that diverts fecal matter to provide an outlet when a distal surgical anastomosis, obstruction, or nonfunctioning structures prevent normal elimination. Depending on the integrity and function of anatomic structures, the ostomy may be temporary or permanent. Infants and small children with necrotizing enterocolitis, Hirschsprung's disease, volvulus, or intussusception may require a temporary colostomy or ileostomy. Ostomies may also be indicated for children with inflammatory bowel disease, intestinal tumors, or abdominal trauma.

An ostomy may be elective or a surgical emergency. In all cases it affects a child's lifestyle, alters body image, causes anxiety, and increases the risk for alterations in physiologic processes (electrolyte imbalance, increased nutritional requirements). For adolescents, it may also result in dependence at a time when autonomy is a major developmental need (Figure 17-10 ◆).

In assessing the family and child approaching ostomy surgery, it is important to determine their ability to understand and accept the physical changes that will occur. Parents may feel guilt and anger about the ostomy surgery when the child has a genetically transmitted disease, has sustained an injury, or has developed an obstruction from necrosis of the bowel. Encourage the parents and child to express their feelings, and correct any misunderstandings. Parents and older children may be referred for counseling and to support groups to help them deal with their feelings. Adolescents often benefit from a visit with an adolescent ostomate (someone who has an ostomy) who can answer questions about living with an ostomy.

PREOPERATIVE CARE

Preoperative education focuses on educating the child and family and preparing them for postoperative management. Discuss how the appliance will look, and explain the purpose of the pouch in developmentally appropriate terms. Encourage the parents and

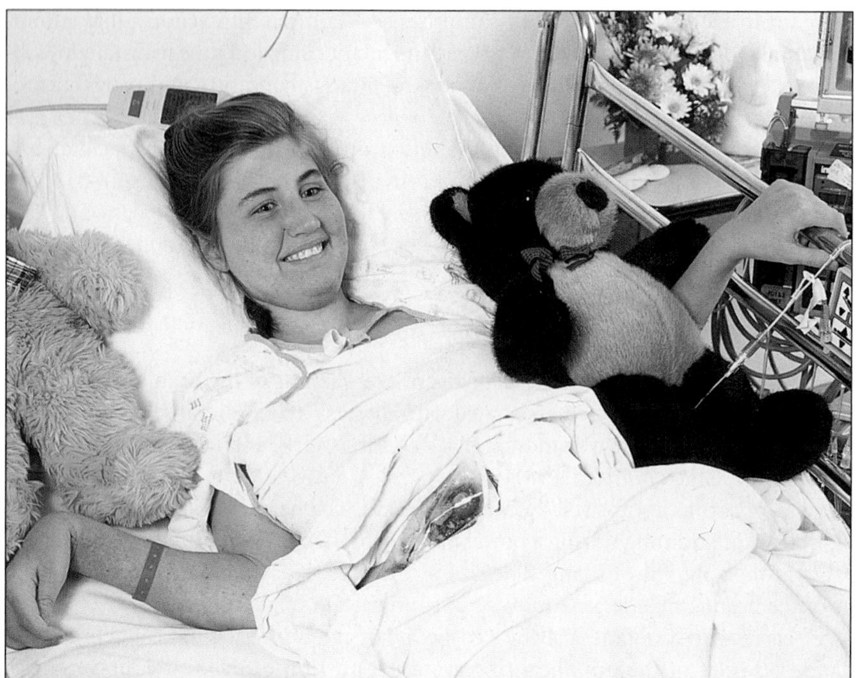

FIGURE 17-10 ◆ Nursing strategies to address altered perceptions of body image and increased feelings of dependence are important when working with adolescents who have ostomies. Support groups or a visit from another teenager who has had an ostomy can facilitate positive coping, as demonstrated by this teenage girl.

GROWTH & DEVELOPMENT

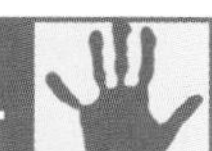

The preschooler has some manual dexterity and can help with some parts of the procedure for changing an ostomy appliance and cleaning the stoma. Teach the child using a doll or stuffed animal. Many school-age children are able to care for their ostomy independently. Teach them how to avoid leakage around the bag, which could be embarrassing. Adolescents are generally totally independent in their self-care of ostomies; however, they may need support to deal with the fact that they are different from their peers.

CLINICAL TIP

The nurse should be aware of the most common complications in children with stomas. These include:

- Prolapse
- Retraction
- Stenosis
- Skin breakdown
  - Dermatitis
  - Allergy (latex or adhesive)
  - Infections
  - Mechanical trauma

(Borkowski, 1998)

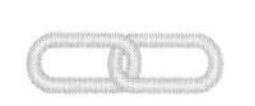

Skills 12-3, 12-4: Changing the Ostomy Dressing and Pouch

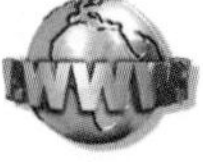

Ostomy Resources and Support

child to touch and manipulate all equipment. A younger child can be shown how to place a pouch on a doll. Older children can practice placing a pouch on their skin. These measures help relieve anxiety by providing information and increasing familiarity with the appliance.

In addition to discussion of the appliance, preoperative education should include discussion of pain control and measures that will be used to prevent postoperative complications (turning, coughing, and breathing deeply). Instructions should be geared to the child's developmental level. Encourage parental participation to promote compliance.

POSTOPERATIVE CARE

Postoperative care of a child with an ostomy is similar to that for any child who undergoes abdominal surgery. (See the earlier discussion of nursing management for appendicitis and the nursing care plan for the child undergoing surgery in Chapter 5.) Management of the stoma may be done by an ostomy nurse or other nurses. Major interventions involve ensuring proper function of the stoma, identifying complications, and instituting daily stoma care. Assess the stoma, quality and amount of fecal matter, skin condition, and adherence of the pouch (Borkowski, 1998). Evaluate the understanding and ability of the family to care for the ostomy.

Home care needs should be identified and addressed well in advance of discharge. Instructions include skin care, care of the stoma, appliance removal and application, and frequency of appliance changes. Teaching should begin immediately after surgery with responsibility for care transferred gradually to the parents and child as they are ready. (For information on caring for an ostomy, refer to the Skills Manual.) Discuss diet, activity level, hygiene, clothing, equipment, and financial considerations. Arrange for home visits to check periodically on the home management program.

Parents and children can be referred to the United Ostomy Association or a local ostomy group for information and support. Referrals should be made to social service, counseling, and a home health agency, if appropriate.

Expected outcomes of nursing care include successful adjustment to the ostomy, thorough evacuation of the bowel, absence of infection and other complications, intact skin, and formation of a positive self-image in the child.

INFLAMMATORY DISORDERS

Inflammatory disorders are reactions of specific tissues of the GI tract to trauma caused by injuries, foreign bodies, chemicals, microorganisms, or surgery. These disorders may be acute or chronic and may involve various segments of the GI tract.

APPENDICITIS

Appendicitis is an inflammation of the vermiform appendix, the small sac near the end of the cecum. The condition occurs most often in adolescent boys (10 to 19 years of age) (Hamilton, Rao, & Wagner, et al., 1998). It is rarely seen before 2 years of age.

Etiology and Pathophysiology

Appendicitis almost always results from an obstruction in the appendiceal lumen. It can be caused by a fecalith (hard fecal mass), parasitic infestations, stenosis, hyperplasia of lymphoid tissue, or a tumor. Continued secretion of mucus following acute obstruction of the lumen increases pressure, causing ischemia, cellular death, and ulceration.

Perforation or rupture of the appendix may occur, resulting in fecal and bacterial contamination of the peritoneum. Peritonitis spreads quickly and if untreated can result in small bowel obstruction, electrolyte imbalances, septicemia, and hypovolemic shock.

Clinical Manifestations

At onset, symptoms include periumbilical cramps, abdominal tenderness, and fever (Pena, Taylor, & Lund, 1999). In adolescent and young adult females, symptoms must be differentiated from those associated with ovulation (mittelschmerz), ruptured ectopic pregnancy, and pelvic inflammatory disease. As the inflammation progresses, pain in the right lower abdomen becomes constant. Pain is often most intense halfway between the anterior superior iliac crest and the umbilicus (Figure 17-11 ◆). In 30% of children, however, the appendix

CLINICAL TIP

Avoid adhesive enhancers on the skin of newborns and premature infants. Their skin layers are so thin that removal of the appliance can strip off the skin. Remember also that adhesive contains latex and its constant use is not advised due to risk of latex allergy development (see Chapter 11).

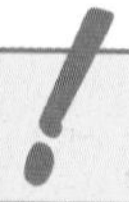

NURSING ALERT

Signs and symptoms of a ruptured appendix include:

- Fever
- Sudden relief from abdominal pain
- Guarding
- Abdominal distention
- Rapid shallow breathing
- Pallor
- Chills
- Irritability or restlessness

PATHOPHYSIOLOGY ILLUSTRATED

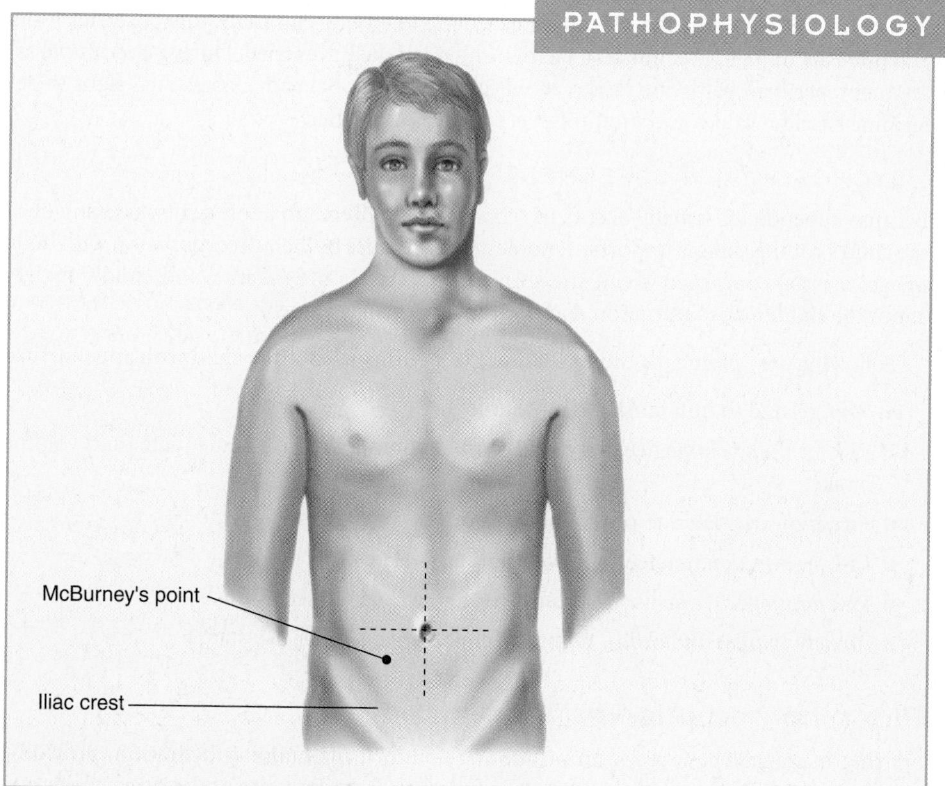

Appendicitis

FIGURE 17-11 ◆
Common location of pain in children and adolescents with appendicitis.

is in a different location, so the pain may occur elsewhere. Symptoms progress to include guarding, rigidity, and rebound tenderness following palpation over the right lower quadrant (Hamilton et al., 1998).

Vomiting, diarrhea, or constipation may be present. As appendicitis progresses, the child remains motionless, usually in a side-lying position with knees flexed. Sudden relief of pain usually means that the appendix has ruptured.

Clinical Therapy

Diagnosis of appendicitis in young children can be difficult because their pain may be less localized and their symptoms more diffuse than in the older child. Continuing evaluations over several hours are often needed to establish the diagnosis.

An elevated white blood cell count (above 15,000/mm^3) may occur. This leukocytosis occurs less often in young children than in teenagers. A history of abdominal pain, presence of a fecalith in the right lower abdomen on x-ray, and abdominal ultrasound help to confirm the diagnosis. Focused appendiceal computerized tomography (FACT) is a relatively new technique that shows success in diagnosing the condition (Rao, Rhea, & Novelline, et al., 1998).

Treatment involves immediate surgical removal (appendectomy). Preoperatively the child is kept NPO. Intravenous fluids, electrolytes, and antibiotics are administered. A nasogastric tube may be inserted before or after surgery. Postoperatively the child has an abdominal incision, and intravenous antibiotics are administered to prevent infection. If the appendix has ruptured before surgery, a Penrose drain is inserted and the wound may not be completely sutured. Wound irrigations may be needed to assist with cleansing of the peritoneum. Recovery is usually complete following uncomplicated removal of the appendix.

NURSING MANAGEMENT

Nursing Assessment and Diagnosis

PHYSIOLOGIC ASSESSMENT

A detailed assessment of the child's pain is necessary to differentiate appendicitis from other illnesses (see Chapter 9). Ask the child to point to the painful area and describe the pain. Recognize that localizing the pain may be difficult for young children. Note onset, location, and intensity of pain; precipitating factors; and relief measures tried. During abdominal assessment, perform palpation last to avoid causing additional pain. Assess vital signs to determine baseline values and monitor every 4 hours thereafter.

PSYCHOSOCIAL ASSESSMENT

Because appendicitis usually occurs in school-age children and adolescents, assessment of the child's coping skills is important. Adolescents, because of their preoccupation with body image, may be concerned about the surgical scar. Assess the parents' and child's anxiety about the sudden hospitalization and need for emergency surgery.

Following are nursing diagnoses that may be appropriate for the child with appendicitis.

- *Pain,* related to inflammation and surgery
- *Risk for fluid volume deficit,* related to fluid volume loss and inadequate fluid volume intake
- *Anxiety/fear,* related to physical condition
- *Risk for infection,* related to bowel trauma
- *Risk for ineffective airway clearance,* related to retained secretions
- *Anxiety (parent and child),* related to child's change in health status

Planning and Intervention

Nursing management focuses on promoting comfort, maintaining hydration, providing emotional support, supporting respiratory function, providing care of the surgical site, and monitoring for symptoms of infection.

Promote Comfort

A side-lying position with knees bent is usually the most comfortable. Administer analgesics as ordered, and note relief from pain. Postoperative pain is managed in a similar manner. The child should be placed in a semi-Fowler or side-lying position on the right side. If the appendix has ruptured, lying on the right side facilitates drainage from the peritoneal cavity. Administer pain medication as ordered.

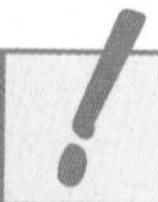

NURSING ALERT

Use of a heating pad is contraindicated in children with appendicitis. Heat will only increase the inflammation and may contribute to rupture of the appendix.

Skill 9-1: Selected Pediatric Pain Scales

Maintain Hydration

Assess fluid volume status every 2 hours. Assess skin turgor, eyes, and mucous membranes for signs of dehydration. Monitor intake and output and assess vital signs. An intravenous infusion is initiated preoperatively and continued until bowel function returns after surgery. Once bowel sounds return, offer water in small amounts and then other clear fluids.

Provide Emotional Support

For many children, this may be their first hospitalization and their first experience with health care personnel beyond their usual provider. The nurse must elicit a history, perform a physical examination, coordinate diagnostic tests, and prepare the child for surgery in a short period of time. Emotional support is essential for both child and parents. Good preoperative education can reduce anxiety. Answer any questions the child or parents may have. In the postoperative period, phone calls from friends or family members may be helpful.

Support Respiratory Function

General anesthesia during surgery compromises respiratory function. It is important for the child to turn, cough, and breathe deeply to prevent atelectasis. Encourage the child to splint the incision area with a pillow during coughing to decrease pain.

Recognize Symptoms of Infection

Assess vital signs and observe the abdominal incision every 4 hours for redness, edema, or drainage. If a drain is present, assess drainage for color, consistency, and amount. After the initial dressing has been changed, perform dressing changes frequently and keep the incision area clean and dry. Administer antibiotics as prescribed.

Discharge Planning and Home Care Teaching

The child is discharged once bowel function returns and he or she has a bowel movement. Give parents instructions on reestablishing a nutritious diet slowly and as tolerated. Teach parents to recognize the signs and symptoms of infection and to seek early treatment.

Normal activities can be resumed fairly quickly, but strenuous activities and contact sports should be avoided in the immediate postoperative period. Parents should check with the child's physician before allowing the child to resume sports activities. Home tutoring may be needed for a short time so the child can keep up with school work.

Evaluation

Expected outcomes of nursing care include the following:

- Successful management of pain
- Absence of bodily infection
- Expressed knowledge and understanding by parent and child of the condition and treatment
- Clear respiratory sounds
- Adequate hydration
- Restoration of normal nutritional intake

CLINICAL TRIAD OF NECROTIZING ENTEROCOLITIS

- Abdominal distention
- Bilious vomiting
- Bloody stools

NURSING ALERT

Signs of sepsis include:

- Hypothermia or hyperthermia
- Jaundice
- Respiratory distress
- Hepatomegaly
- Abdominal distention
- Anorexia
- Vomiting
- Lethargy

CHOLESTASIS

Cholestasis is a disruption of bile flow, the most common problem in survivors of necrotizing enterocolitis. It is a complication of total parenteral nutrition (TPN) and commonly occurs 2 weeks after TPN therapy has been initiated. It is characterized by an elevated bilirubin (>2 mg/dL), hepatomegaly, and elevated serum transaminase.

NECROTIZING ENTEROCOLITIS

Necrotizing enterocolitis is a potentially life-threatening inflammatory disease of the intestinal tract that occurs primarily in premature infants. It affects from 1% to 8% of infants in the NICU, and has up to a 40% mortality rate (Pearl et al., 1998). It can be caused by several factors, among them intestinal ischemia, bacterial or viral infection (a result of the premature infant's decreased immune response and greater risk for infection), and immaturity of the gut (a result of the premature infant's decreased amount of gastric acid and proteolytic enzymes and underdeveloped protective intestinal mucin layer). The disease occurs most often in the terminal ileum and colon.

The infant may initially show signs of feeding intolerance (increased gastric residuals, vomiting, irritability, and abdominal distention). These signs are caused by inflammation and dilation of the bowel and accumulation of gas in the intestine. Bloody diarrhea may be present because of the hemorrhagic bowel. Signs of sepsis usually follow, and the infant's condition rapidly deteriorates.

Diagnosis is made on the basis of characteristic clinical findings and the presence of free peritoneal gas, dilated bowel loops, bowel distention, and bowel wall thickening on abdominal x-rays. Necrotizing enterocolitis requires prompt intervention. Management begins with discontinuation of all enteral feedings. An orogastric tube is inserted to prevent gastric distention, and intravenous fluids are started. Total parenteral nutrition may be initiated through a central line. Antibiotics are administered prophylactically or to treat sepsis. Perforation or necrosis of the bowel necessitates surgical resection of the bowel. An ileostomy or colostomy may be performed in some cases.

All cases of necrotizing enterocolitis are treated with strict enteric precautions to prevent the spread of infection to other premature infants on the unit. Early aggressive enteral formula feedings of premature infants is avoided because of the increased incidence of the disease in these cases. Human milk has been shown to be protective against the disease; thus, breastfeeding or feeding the mother's expressed milk is the feeding method of choice for premature infants.

Long-term complications of necrotizing enterocolitis include short bowel syndrome, strictures, **cholestasis,** impaired nutrition and growth, and delayed developmental performance.

Nursing Management

Nursing care centers on prevention and early detection of necrotizing enterocolitis to minimize bowel loss and providing postoperative care. Watch for feeding intolerance by aspirating gastric residual (if the infant is receiving enteral feedings). Enteral feedings should slowly progress, by no more than 20 mL/kg/day (Committee on Nutrition, American Academy of Pediatrics, 1998). Measure abdominal circumference in the premature or high-risk infant every 4 to 8 hours (see Figure 10-11). Even minimal changes in circumference can indicate necrotizing enterocolitis and should be reported to the physician.

Maintaining fluid and electrolyte balance is essential. Provide comfort by holding and cuddling an infant who is NPO, and offer a pacifier to meet nonnutritive sucking needs. Careful assessment for infection and maintenance of skin integrity are essential. Feedings are gradually reestablished once bowel function returns.

Parents need emotional support and reassurance and help in bonding with their infant. They are coping with the birth of an infant who is critically ill. Because the symptoms of necrotizing enterocolitis do not appear until approximately 5 to 7 days after feedings are begun, parents may not be prepared for the infant's decline. The recovery of a premature infant is slow and can be complicated. Give clear explanations and encourage parents to ask questions and express their fears and concerns. If the infant's condition worsens, support for the parents of a dying child should be offered (see Chapter 8).

Once the child is discharged, frequent follow-up is needed. Encourage regular health care visits. Schedule home visits to help the family manage health care and normal developmental issues. If TPN is administered at home, the parents will need to know how to administer it correctly and how to care for the central line. Oral and enteral nutritional intake is carefully assessed. Growth of the child is monitored and compared with previous findings. Several medications are likely to be used, and correct administration techniques must be reinforced. The infant requires regular and thorough physical assessments to identify any complications. Parents need to learn care of the ostomy if the child has one in place. Developmental progress is assessed by regular administration of a developmental test such as the Denver II (see Chapter 6).

Expected outcomes of nursing care for the child with necrotizing enterocolitis include successful treatment of infection, absence of signs of sepsis, management of fluid and electrolyte status, and provision of adequate nutrition. If surgery is performed, complete healing without infection or other complication is desired. If the infant is not successfully treated, support and comfort for the parents is a necessary outcome. When the child survives, long-term outcomes include normal developmental progression and nutrition to support growth.

MECKEL'S DIVERTICULUM

Meckel's diverticulum results when the omphalomesenteric duct, which connects the midgut to the yolk sac during embryonic development, fails to atrophy. Instead, an outpouching of the ileum remains, usually located near the ileocecal valve. The pouch contains gastric or pancreatic tissue, which secretes acid, causing irritation and ulceration. Meckel's diverticulum is the most common gastrointestinal malformation and cause of lower gastrointestinal bleeding in children; it occurs in 2% of the population, although many individuals are asymptomatic and do not know they have the disorder (Pearl et al., 1998). Clinical manifestations usually appear by 2 years of age. The most common sign is painless dark or bright red rectal bleeding, which results from the obstruction or ulceration. Often blood is passed without stool. Abdominal pain is uncommon, but when it occurs, it may resemble the pain of appendicitis. The child may have symptoms of intussusception, incarcerated hernia, volvulus, or intestinal obstruction. If untreated, diverticulitis may progress to perforation and peritonitis.

Diagnosis is based on the history. Contrast studies are usually not helpful, because the diverticulum is often too small to visualize and may not fill with barium. Radionuclide imaging and scanning can usually detect the gastric tissue, confirming the diagnosis.

Treatment is surgical excision of the diverticulum and removal of any involved bowel. The prognosis is good following surgical excision.

Nursing Management

Preoperatively an intravenous infusion is initiated to correct fluid and electrolyte imbalances. Monitor intake and output. Observe for rectal bleeding and test stools for **occult blood** (blood that is present in small quantities and measurable only by laboratory testing). The child should be kept on bedrest. Assess vital signs every 2 hours, and monitor for signs of shock.

Postoperative care is similar to that for an infant or child undergoing abdominal surgery. (See the earlier discussion of postsurgical nursing management of appendicitis and the nursing care plan for the child undergoing surgery in Chapter 5.)

At the time of discharge, parents need instructions on caring for the surgical site, preventing infection, providing an adequate diet, and administering prescribed medications.

INFLAMMATORY BOWEL DISEASE

Crohn's Disease and Ulcerative Colitis

Inflammatory bowel disease encompasses two distinct chronic disorders, Crohn's disease and ulcerative colitis, which have similar symptoms and treatment. Both diseases involve faulty regulation of the immune response of the intestinal mucosa in individuals who are genetically predisposed and have a genetic trigger (Gokhale, 2001). Inflammatory bowel disease differs from irritable bowel syndrome, which is discussed in the section on feeding and elimination disorders in Chapter 7.

Crohn's disease is a chronic, inflammatory process. It can occur randomly throughout the GI tract, with the ileum, colon, and rectum the most common sites. A distinct feature of Crohn's disease is the development of enteric fistulas between loops of bowel or nearby

CLINICAL MANIFESTATIONS OF ULCERATIVE COLITIS AND CROHN'S DISEASE

	ULCERATIVE COLITIS	CROHN'S DISEASE
Type of lesions	Continuous, superficial involvement	Segmental, transmural (through the wall) involvement
Clinical manifestations		
Anal or perianal lesions	Rare	Common
Anorexia	Mild to moderate	Can be severe
Diarrhea	Often severe	Moderate
Growth retardation	Mild	Significant
Pain	Present	Common
Rectal bleeding	Present	Absent
Weight loss	Moderate	Severe
Risk of cancer	Slightly increased	Greatly increased

organs. Mucosal ulcers begin in small locations, and then grow in size and depth into the mucosal wall. Submucosal inflammation can be severe. The etiology is unknown. There is strong evidence to support a genetic association. Crohn's disease is more common in whites and three to six times more prevalent in individuals of Jewish descent. It most often develops between 15 and 25 years of age, and has been increasing in incidence (Gokhale, 2001).

The onset of Crohn's disease is subtle. Crampy abdominal pain is usually reported first, followed by diarrhea. Other symptoms include fever, anorexia, growth failure or weight loss, general malaise, and joint pain. Diagnosis is based on laboratory evaluation (anemia is common; an elevated erythrocyte sedimentation rate, hypoalbuminemia, and thrombocytosis are other possible findings), diffuse abdominal tenderness, and radiologic and biopsy examinations.

Ulcerative colitis is a chronic recurrent disease of the colon and rectal mucosa of unknown etiology. Inflammation is limited to the mucosa and can involve the entire length of the bowel with varying degrees of inflammation, ulceration, hemorrhage, and edema. Emotional and other psychosocial factors may influence the presentation and course of the disease. It is more prevalent among persons of Jewish heritage. The disease develops before 20 years of age with peak onset at about 12 years.

The first symptom of ulcerative colitis is usually diarrhea. Lower abdominal pain and cramping are present before and during a bowel movement and are relieved by the passage of stool and flatus. The stool is often mixed with blood and mucus. Weight loss or delayed growth, nutritional deficiencies, and arthralgias often occur as effects of the disease.

Diagnosis centers on evaluating the cause and identifying the extent of involved bowel and differentiating an infectious process (organisms such as *Shigella* and *Salmonella*) from ulcerative colitis. Endoscopy with biopsy is helpful to determine the extent and severity of the inflammatory process. Laboratory and bone age studies help to identify related nutritional, growth, and blood abnormalities.

Crohn's disease and ulcerative colitis have periods of remission and exacerbation. Treatment for both diseases includes pharmacologic interventions (administration of antibiotic, anti-inflammatory, immunosuppressive, and antidiarrheal medications), nutrition therapy, and in severe cases, surgery. Corticosteroids are given orally and in the form of enemas to children with more severe disease. For children with milder disease, sulfasalazine has been shown to decrease the number of relapses.

A nutritionist is part of the team treating the child. The goal of nutrition therapy is to provide adequate caloric intake and nutrients necessary for growth. Vitamin, iron, zinc, and folic acid supplementation is frequently required. Total parenteral nutrition is often given to treat nutritional deficiencies and malnutrition, which accompany inflammatory bowel disease. A high-protein, high-carbohydrate, low-fiber diet with normal amounts of fat is recommended.

If other treatment measures fail to reduce inflammation, surgery is generally indicated. A temporary colostomy or ileostomy is performed to allow the bowel to rest. In Crohn's dis-

DRUGS USED IN TREATMENT OF INFLAMMATORY BOWEL DISEASE

Aminosalicylates
Sulfasalazine
Mesalamine
Olsalazine
Balsalazide

Corticosteroids
Prednisone
Methylprednisone
Hydrocortisone enema

Immunosuppressants
6-Mercaptopurine (6-MP)
Azathioprine
Cyclosporine
Methotrexate
Tacrolimus (FK-506)

Antibacterial
Metronidazole
Ciprofloxacil

ease, however, ulcerations tend to recur elsewhere in the GI tract. In ulcerative colitis, removal of the diseased bowel provides a permanent cure.

NURSING MANAGEMENT Nursing management occurs mainly in the community and home and focuses on helping the child and family adjust to the emotional impact of a chronic disease, administering medications and diet therapy, monitoring nutritional status, and providing appropriate referrals. Provide emotional support and counseling to help the child adjust to feeling "different" from peers. Inability to compete with peers and frequent absences from school can affect the child's self-esteem. Have the parents contact the school district to arrange for tutoring in case extended absences from school become necessary. Encourage the child who is not attending school regularly to maintain contact with friends through telephone calls, cards, and visits.

If the child is unable to eat or the intake of calories is insufficient to meet basic nutritional and metabolic needs, TPN will be ordered. If the child is able to eat, parents need instructions about dietary needs. Frequent growth measurements and nutritional evaluations must be carried out.

Body image is a major concern for children and adolescents with inflammatory bowel disease. Corticosteroid therapy causes growth retardation and delayed sexual maturation. Encourage the child to discuss feelings about these side effects. If a permanent colostomy or ileostomy is required, the nurse can assist the child and family to understand the need for surgical treatment. (See the discussion of ostomies earlier in this chapter.) Introduce the child and family to other children who have stomas.

Teach parents about medication administration and diet therapy. Reinforce to both the parents and child the importance of adhering to a strict medication regimen. Emphasize that medications should be continued even when the child is asymptomatic. Discuss the side effects of the drugs and what to do if any of these symptoms occur.

Parents also will need instructions for TPN and care of a central venous catheter, including dressing changes, sterile and nonsterile techniques, signs of infection, how to handle infusion pumps and tubing, and how to measure the child's intake and output. Assist parents in obtaining equipment and supplies necessary for the child's care. Have parents demonstrate their mastery of care for the central venous catheter and their understanding of TPN techniques during home visits and appointments for health care.

Refer parents to social services, the visiting nurse association, and home health care agencies if they are not receiving any of these services. For information about inflammatory bowel disease, refer families to the Crohn's Colitis Foundation.

Expected outcomes of nursing care for the child with inflammatory bowel disease include the following:

- Normal growth and development
- Absence of gastrointestinal distress
- Successful management of medications without demonstration of side effects
- Freedom from infection due to TPN line

RESEARCH

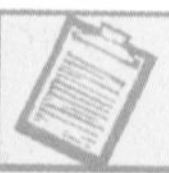

Increased production of inflammatory cytokines in the intestine has been observed in patients with Crohn's disease. The intravenous infusion of antitumor necrosis factor antibody has therefore shown promise of treatment for the disorder, decreasing the symptoms and incidence of surgery (Gokhale, 2001).

Skill 8-7: Administering Total Parenteral Nutrition

GROWTH & DEVELOPMENT

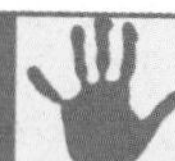

Providing adequate stress reduction may be helpful in control of inflammatory bowel disease. Teach young children relaxation techniques, such as deep breathing, progressive tensing and relaxing of muscles, and visualization of favorite places. Encourage busy school-age children and teens to have quiet and restful times each day, in addition to physical activity periods.

NURSING ALERT

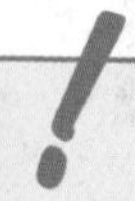

Corticosteroids can decrease a child's immune response and alter growth. Immunizations (especially for live vaccines such as varicella) are contraindicated when systemic steroids are being administered.

FAMILIES WANT TO KNOW

Diet Instructions for Inflammatory Bowel Disease

- Several small feedings are usually better tolerated than three meals daily.
- Limiting fiber intake can help to decrease intestine motility and inflammation. Peel fruits and avoid large quantities of whole grains and nuts.
- If the child is not eating well, offer high-calorie meals. If lactose intolerance is not a problem for the particular child, then cream soups, milkshakes, puddings, and custards can be offered.
- Liquid dietary supplements may be helpful to ensure that protein and caloric requirements are met.
- Watch for foods that cause intestinal problems for the individual child, and avoid them in the future.
- Avoid having mealtime become a reason for family strife. Seek help of nurses and dietitians if needed.

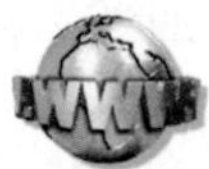

Crohn's and Colitis Resources and Support

- Establishment of positive body image
- Integration of stress-lowering practices into daily life

PEPTIC ULCER

A peptic ulcer is an erosion of the mucosal tissue in the lower end of the esophagus, in the stomach (usually along the lesser curvature), or in the duodenum. Boys are more likely to have peptic ulcers than girls; however, peptic ulcers are much less common in children than in adults.

Ulcers are classified as primary or secondary, depending on their etiology. Primary peptic ulcers occur in healthy children. Secondary (stress) ulcers occur in children with a preexisting illness or injury (often a burn) and in children receiving medications such as salicylates, corticosteroids, and nonsteroidal anti-inflammatory drugs. Diet usually is not a major factor in the development of peptic ulcers in children, although caffeine and alcohol consumption in adolescents may exacerbate the disease. It is now known that many cases of ulcer, in both adults and children, are caused by *Helicobacter pylori,* a gram-negative rod (Herbst, 2000). This organism is transmitted by the fecal–oral or oral–oral route. Infections often occur in several members of a family, especially when the family's water supply is contaminated.

Clinical manifestations vary according to the age of the child and location of the ulcer. The most common symptom is abdominal pain (burning) associated with an empty stomach, which may awaken the child at night. Vomiting and pain after meals, anemia, occult blood in stools, and abdominal distention may also be present.

Diagnosis is based on the history and radiologic studies. *H. pylori* can be diagnosed by culture of the organism taken via gastroscopy, and by measuring urea in the urine and on the breath, since the organism hydrolyzes urea. The goals of medical management are to relieve discomfort and promote healing. When *H. pylori* is the causative agent, antimicrobial agents such as bismuth salts, tetracycline, and metronidazole combination are given. Other drug combinations such as antacids in liquid form (Maalox, Mylanta) and histamine antagonists (ranitidine, cimetidine, and famotidine) are also used. Antibody titers are measured several times over 6 months to evaluate the effectiveness of therapy. The prognosis is usually good with early intervention.

Nursing Management

Nurses may identify children with peptic ulcer disease by looking for the symptoms and noting family history of *H. pylori* infection. Nursing care centers on interventions to promote adequate nutritional intake, promote healing, and prevent recurrences. A nutritionally sound, age-appropriate diet is provided. Foods should be omitted only if they exacerbate the disorder.

Antibiotics must be given as scheduled. Emphasize the importance of continuing drug therapy. The family needs encouragement to continue the medications as ordered and to return for follow-up visits. Children who attend school may prefer to take antacids in the form of tablets, which are easier to carry than liquid preparations. A permission form to take medications at school will need to be filled out by the prescriber. Parents should check with the child's physician before giving any additional medication. Caution parents to avoid aspirin products, which irritate the gastric mucosa. If an antipyretic or pain medication is needed, acetaminophen should be given. Advise parents to read medication labels if they are unsure of product contents.

Because psychologic stress can contribute to peptic ulcer disease, the parents and child should be assisted to identify sources of stress in the child's life. Assess coping mechanisms and provide referral for psychologic counseling, if appropriate. Teach relaxation techniques and recommend community classes on yoga or other stress reduction.

DISORDERS OF MOTILITY

Fluids are produced in large quantities as part of normal GI functioning. As food passes through the intestines, fluids are reabsorbed and moderately soft stool is formed and evacuated. In disorders such as diarrhea and constipation, fluid production is altered, causing either more or less fluid to be reabsorbed. This can severely alter the characteristics of the stool. Reabsorption of too little water produces diarrhea and can lead to fluid and electrolyte alterations. Reabsorption of too much fluid can cause constipation, which if untreated can lead to bowel obstruction.

GASTROENTERITIS

Gastroenteritis (acute diarrhea) is an inflammation of the stomach and intestines that may be accompanied by vomiting and diarrhea. It can affect any part of the GI tract. Diarrhea is a common problem in children. It may be an acute problem, caused by viral, bacterial, or parasitic infections, or a chronic problem. Children under age 5 years average approximately two episodes of gastroenteritis each year (Burkhart, 1999). Infants and small children with gastroenteritis or diarrhea can quickly become dehydrated and are at risk for hypovolemic shock if fluid and electrolyte losses are not replaced (see Chapter 10).

Etiology and Pathophysiology

Diarrhea in children can have many different causes (Table 17-2). The specific etiology is not always identified. The common mechanism is a decrease in the absorptive capacity of the bowel through inflammation, decrease in surface area for absorption, or alteration of parasympathetic innervation. Children in child care centers and those living in substandard housing with improper sanitation are at increased risk.

Clinical Manifestations

Diarrhea may be mild, moderate, or severe. In mild diarrhea, stools are slightly increased in number and have a more liquid consistency. In moderate diarrhea, the child has several loose or watery stools. Other symptoms include irritability, anorexia, nausea, and vomiting. Moderate diarrhea is usually self-limiting, resolving without treatment within 1 or 2 days. In severe diarrhea, watery stools are continuous. The child exhibits symptoms of fluid and electrolyte imbalance (see Chapter 10), has cramping, and is extremely irritable and difficult to console.

Clinical Therapy

Diagnosis is based on the history, physical examination, and laboratory findings. A thorough history may help in identifying the causative factor. Ask parents about recent exposure to illnesses, use of antibiotics, travel, food and formula preparation, food sensitivities or allergies, and whether the child attends daycare. Physical examination provides a guide to the severity of dehydration (see Chapter 10). The stool can be examined for the presence of ova,

TABLE 17-2 Causes of Diarrhea in Children

ETIOLOGY	BOWEL MANIFESTATIONS
Emotional stress (anxiety, fatigue)	Increased motility
Intestinal infection (bacteria [*E. coli, Salmonella, Shigella*], viral [human rotavirus, enteric adenovirus], fungal overgrowth)	Inflammation of mucosa; increased mucous secretion in colon
Food sensitivity (gluten, cow's milk)	Decreased digestion of food
Food intolerance (lactose, introduction of new foods, overfeeding)	Increased motility; increased mucous secretion in colon
Medications (iron, antibiotics)	Irritation and suprainfection
Colon disease (colitis, necrotizing enterocolitis, enterocolitis)	Inflammation and ulceration of intestinal walls; reduced absorption of fluid; increased intestinal motility
Surgical alterations (short bowel syndrome)	Reduced size of colon; decreased absorption surface

CLINICAL MANIFESTATIONS AND TREATMENT OF DEHYDRATION IN DIARRHEA

DEHYDRATION	CLINICAL MANIFESTATIONS
None	Feed age-appropriate diet of breast milk or regular formula, complex carbohydrates, and meats (especially chicken) Oral rehydration of 10 mL/kg/stool for ongoing losses
Mild (3%–5%)	Oral rehydration with 50 mL/kg for 4–6 hours or until rehydrated 10 mL/kg/stool for ongoing losses and replacement of estimated emesis volume After rehydration, feed age-appropriate diet
Moderate (6%–9%)	100 mL/kg plus replacement of continuing losses during a 4-hour period Reassess ongoing losses every hour and replace volume for volume After rehydration, feed age-appropriate diet
Severe (≥10%)	True emergency which causes shock or near-shock condition Bolus intravenous therapy with normal saline or Ringer's lactate, 20–40 mL/kg/hr Begin oral rehydration solution when level of consciousness improves After rehydration, feed age-appropriate diet

Note: From Snyder, J. (1997). Feeding during diarrhea: New AAP guidelines and innovations in oral rehydration solutions. *Contemporary Pediatrics Meeting Reporter, July 1997*, pg. 6. Adapted.

parasites, infectious organisms, viruses, fat, and undigested sugars. Laboratory evaluation of serum and urine helps in identification of electrolyte imbalances and other deficiencies (Murphy, 1998).

Medical management depends on the severity of the diarrhea and fluid and electrolyte imbalances. The goal of treatment is to correct the fluid and electrolyte imbalances. For mild to moderate dehydration, the child is rehydrated by means of oral rehydration therapy (see Chapter 10). This may be accomplished at home or in the short-stay observation unit in a hospital with solutions such as Pedialyte, Ricelyte, or Lytren. Carbonated beverages and those containing high amounts of sugar should not be given. Fermentation of sugar in the GI tract causes increased gas, abdominal distention, and an increased frequency of diarrhea.

For severe dehydration, rehydration is accomplished by intravenous infusion with a solution chosen to correct the specific imbalances. Isotonic fluid such as normal saline with glucose or Ringer's lactate are commonly used solutions (see Chapter 10 for further information about solutions to correct dehydration). As soon as possible, clear liquids are introduced and then the child progresses to a regular diet. Foods generally are not withheld for more than 1 or 2 days (Eliason & Lewan, 1998).

If the diarrhea is caused by bacteria or parasites, antimicrobial therapy may be prescribed.

NURSING MANAGEMENT

Nursing Assessment and Diagnosis

The nurse may encounter the child and family in the emergency department, urgent care center, clinic, or office. The child may be cared for over several hours at a clinic or urgent care center so that dehydration is treated with intravenous infusion and/or oral rehydration, and then sent home with instructions for parents to care for the child. If the child is hospitalized, it is important to assess onset, frequency, color, amount, and consistency of stools. If the child is also vomiting, monitor the amount and type of vomitus. Initial and ongoing physical assessment of the child focuses on observing for signs and symptoms of dehydration, which reflect underlying fluid and electrolyte status. Evaluate urinary output and specific gravity. Weigh the infant or child on admission and daily thereafter. Monitor vital signs every 2 to 4 hours. If the child is febrile, water loss will be increased, contributing to the dehydration. Assess skin integrity, especially in the perineal and rectal areas, and note any breakdown or rashes.

NURSING ALERT

Antiemetics and antidiarrheals (e.g., Donnagel and Kaopectate) should generally not be used in infants and young children, as they do not reduce actual fluid loss, and can mask the signs and symptoms of more serious illnesses.

The accompanying nursing care plan lists common nursing diagnoses for a child with gastroenteritis. The following diagnoses may also be appropriate:

- *Anxiety (child and parent),* related to change in health status
- *Sleep pattern disturbance,* related to pain
- *Altered nutrition: Less than body requirements,* related to inability to ingest sufficient nutrients

CLINICAL TIP

Avoid using commercial baby wipes when changing the diaper of an infant with diarrhea. Chemicals in the wipes may cause additional irritation and skin breakdown.

Planning and Implementation

Nursing care focuses on providing emotional support, promoting rest and comfort, and ensuring adequate nutrition. The accompanying nursing care plan summarizes nursing care for the child with gastroenteritis.

Provide Emotional Support

The child may have been ill for several days or become suddenly ill a short time before seeking health care. The child and parents are usually anxious, so it is important to allow them to talk and ask questions. The child may require blood tests to help direct rehydration therapy. Using therapeutic play techniques, such as allowing the child to manipulate equipment, can reduce anxiety (see Chapter 5). To promote a trusting relationship, be honest if a procedure will hurt. Encourage the child to express anger, fear, and pain.

Promote Rest and Comfort

Most children with gastroenteritis are quite ill and awaken frequently with periods of vomiting and diarrhea. Provide a quiet, restful environment. Darken the room and keep interruptions to a minimum. To reduce the child's anxiety, encourage parents to room-in. Place the child's favorite toys and comfort objects within reach. Keep the child's mouth moistened with a glycerine swab, a wet washcloth, or an occasional ice chip.

Ensure Adequate Nutrition

Liquids are offered throughout the illness, even if an intravenous infusion is in place. Follow guidelines for oral rehydration therapy in Chapter 10. If tolerated, the CRAM diet can be started. Infants are breast fed or given formula. After about 1 week, the child should be consuming a normal diet for age.

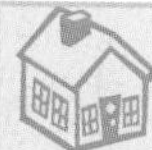

HOME CARE

An effective way to treat diarrhea is the CRAM diet. Teach its components to parents and give them ideas of how to include the following foods in the child's diet.

Complex carbohydrates (e.g., cereals, toast, pasta)
Rice
and
Milk

Discharge Planning and Care in the Community

Discharge teaching should begin on arrival at the health care facility. Instruct parents on what to expect as the child's GI system returns to normal function. Teach the parents about the symptoms of dehydration and what to do if diarrhea recurs. Be sure that parents understand the recommended diet progression. Emphasize the necessity of good hygiene practices to prevent the spread of microorganisms that can cause gastroenteritis. If the child attends child care, then ask the parent to alert the care center about the gastroenteritis so the staff can watch for other cases and take steps to prevent the spread of infection.

Evaluation

Expected outcomes of nursing care for the child with gastroenteritis include the following:

- Correction of dehydration
- Adequate nutritional intake
- Return to normal bowel function
- Parental description of signs of dehydration
- Parental knowledge of importance of handwashing in decreasing transmission of infectious agents
- Maintenance of intact skin

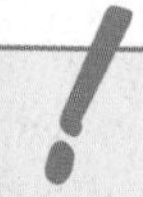

NURSING ALERT

Handwashing is the most important measure that can be taken to prevent the spread of gastroenteritis.

NURSING CARE PLAN The Child with Gastroenteritis

GOAL	INTERVENTION	RATIONALE	EXPECTED OUTCOME
1. Diarrhea related to infectious process			
	NIC Priority Intervention: **Diarrhea Management:** Prevention and alleviation of diarrhea.		NOC Suggested Outcome: **Fluid and Electrolyte Balance:** Balance of water and electrolytes in the intracellular and extracellular compartments of the body.
The child's bowel function will be restored to normal.	■ Obtain baseline vital signs and monitor every 2–4 hours. ■ Observe stools for amount, color, consistency, odor, and frequency. ■ Test stools for occult blood. ■ Monitor results of stool culture and sample for ova and parasites. ■ Wash hands well before and after contact with the child. ■ Isolate the child until the cause of the diarrhea is determined. ■ Assist the child with toileting and hygiene. ■ Administer prescribed oral rehydration and intravenous solutions. ■ Notify the physician if diarrhea persists, stool characteristics change, or other symptoms of dehydration/electolyte imbalance occur.	■ Fluid and electrolyte imbalances can alter vital body functions. ■ Aids in the diagnosis and in monitoring the child's status. ■ Frequent defecation and some infectious organisms can cause bleeding. ■ Rapid notification of the physician will facilitate treatment. ■ Helps prevent transmission of microorganisms. ■ Prevents exposure of other patients and staff. ■ The child may be weak, incontinent, physically impaired, or anxious and require assistance to use the bathroom. ■ Provides necessary fluids and nutrients. ■ Ensures early intervention.	The child's bowel function returns to normal.
2. Fluid Volume Deficit related to active fluid volume loss			
	NIC Priority Intervention: **Fluid Monitoring:** Collection and analysis of patient data to regulate fluid balance.		NOC Suggested Outcome: **Fluid and Electrolyte Balance:** Balance of water and electrolytes in the intracellular and extracellular compartments of the body.
The child will remain hydrated and will begin to drink fluids within 24 hours of admission.	■ Monitor intake and output. Be sure to document time of each voiding. ■ Compare admission weight to preadmission weight. Assess weight daily. ■ Assess level of consciousness, skin turgor, mucous membranes, skin color and temperature, capillary refill, eyes, and fontanels every 4 hours.	■ Will determine if output exceeds input. Long periods of time without urine output can be an early indicator of poor renal function. A child should produce 1 mL of urine/kg/hr. ■ The degree of dehydration can be determined by the percentage of weight loss. Daily weights aid in determining progress toward rehydration. ■ Will determine degree of hydration and adequacy of interventions.	The child has normal fluid and electrolyte balance as indicated by laboratory evaluation and physical examination.

(continued)

NURSING CARE PLAN The Child with Gastroenteritis (continued)

GOAL	INTERVENTION	RATIONALE	EXPECTED OUTCOME
2. Fluid Volume Deficit related to active fluid volume loss (continued)			
	■ Assess for vomiting. ■ Provide oral fluid and electrolyte replacement solution if able to tolerate. ■ Provide and maintain IV replacement therapy, as ordered.	■ Vomiting frequently accompanies diarrhea and contributes to the child's fluid loss. ■ Less invasive than IV fluids. Provides for replacement of essential fluids and electrolytes. ■ Use of IV replacement is based on the degree of dehydration, ongoing losses, insensible water losses and electrolyte results.	
3. Risk for Impaired Skin Integrity related to altered fluid status			
	NIC Suggested Intervention: **Skin Surveillance:** Collection and analysis of patient data to maintain skin integrity		NOC Priority Outcome: **Tissue Integrity:** Structural intactness and normal physiologic function of skin.
The child will remain free of skin breakdown and rashes.	■ Assess skin of perineum and rectum for signs of skin breakdown or irritation. ■ Provide prevention or restorative care for infants as follows:	■ Early assessment and intervention can prevent worsening of the condition.	The child's perianal and rectal tissue remains pink and intact.
Preventive care:			
	■ Change diapers every 2 hours or as needed. ■ Use cloth diapers rather than disposable. ■ Wash diaper area after each soiling. ■ Apply A & D ointment.	■ Minimizes skin contact with chemical irritants from stool and urine. ■ Minimizes the mechanical and chemical irritation from disposables. ■ Removes traces of stool if present. ■ Provides a barrier and protects intact or reddened skin from becoming excoriated.	
Restorative care:			
	■ Place the infant prone and leave the buttocks open to air. ■ Notify the physician if the skin is severely broken or peeling or if a rash is present. ■ For toddlers and older children: ■ Tub bathe at least daily (if condition allows) in tepid water. Pat the area dry. ■ Discourage the wearing of underwear if possible. ■ Apply A & D ointment at least four times daily.	■ Promotes air circulation to the area. ■ Helps loosen any fecal matter without scrubbing, which can cause additional irritation to the skin. ■ Allows air to circulate and prevents accumulation of moisture. ■ Provides a barrier and protects intact or reddened skin from becoming excoriated.	

CONSTIPATION

Constipation is characterized by a decrease in the frequency or passage of stools; the formation of hard, dry stools; or the oozing of liquid stool past a collection of hard, dry stool. Because stooling patterns vary among children, identification of an abnormal pattern is sometimes difficult. Infants usually have several bowel movements a day. For a young child, one bowel movement a day may be normal. As the child grows, however, three to four bowel movements a week may be a normal pattern.

Constipation may be caused by an underlying disease, diet, or psychologic factor. It may result from defects in filling, or more commonly emptying, of the rectum. Pathologic causes of defective filling include ineffective colonic propulsive activity, caused by hypothyroidism or use of medication, and obstruction, caused by a structural anomaly (stricture or stenosis) or by an aganglionic segment (Hirschsprung's disease). If the rectum fails to fill, stasis leads to excessive drying of the stools. Emptying of the rectum depends on the defecation reflex. Lesions of the spinal cord, weakness of the abdominal muscles, and local lesions blocking sphincter relaxation all may impede attempts to defecate.

Constipation during infancy is rare and is most often caused by mismanagement of diet. The transition from formula to cow's milk may cause a transient constipation, because the bowel must adjust to the increased protein content of cow's milk. Constipation in young infants can usually be corrected by increasing the amount of fluids or adding 2 oz of pear or apple juice to daily intake. In older infants, increasing the intake of fluids, cereals, fruits, and vegetables in the diet should correct the problem.

Constipation occurs most frequently in the toddler and preschool age groups. This increased incidence is often associated with learning to control bodily functions. Many children do not like the sensations of a bowel movement and may begin withholding stool, which accumulates in and dilates the rectum until the next urge to defecate. The increasingly hard and painful bowel movement reinforces the child's behavior, and a pattern develops (Castiglia, 2001). See Chapter 7 for a discussion of encopresis.

Removing constipating foods (bananas, rice, and cheese) from the child's diet often decreases the constipation. Increasing the child's intake of high-fiber foods (whole grain breads, raw fruits and vegetables) and fluids also promotes defecation.

In the school-age child, constipation may occur because time for toileting is limited. Busy school-age children may delay going to the bathroom. Children may also be hesitant to use an unfamiliar bathroom. Encouragement from parents and relaxation of bathroom privileges at school promote regularity and return of usual bowel patterns within a short time.

Diagnosis is based on a thorough history and physical examination. When constipation occurs along with growth failure, vomiting, or abdominal pain, further investigation is necessary to rule out other disorders. Dietary management is the treatment of choice for constipation that has no underlying pathologic cause. A single glycerin suppository or enema may be needed to remove hard stool, followed by dietary and fluid management.

Constipation may follow surgery, especially in children who are immobilized, such as by traction or a body cast. Stool softeners and a diet high in roughage and fluids are given to prevent and treat constipation. Many families use herbal or other plant remedies to treat constipation.

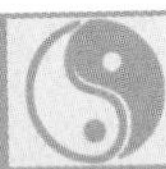

CULTURE

Herbal stimulant laxatives are used by some families as complementary therapies. The following are not recommended for use in children under 12 years:

- Aloe
- Buckthorn bark
- Cascara sagrada bark
- Senna leaf or pod
- Coffee
- Tea
- Cola nut
- Mate
- Ma huang

Nursing Management

Take a diet history and obtain a description of bowel patterns from parents. Ask what the family does to treat constipation. Assessment of the child's food likes and dislikes may provide a clue to the cause of constipation. Nursing care focuses on teaching parents what constitutes normal bowel patterns in children and the importance of diet in maintaining such patterns. Regular bowel habits are encouraged by placing the child on the toilet 30 minutes after a meal or around the time defecation usually occurs. Providing positive reinforcement during toilet training helps to prevent a withholding pattern.

Teach parents dietary measures to promote regularity of bowel movements. Children can be given a high-fiber diet that includes fruits and vegetables. Cut-up fresh fruits, dried fruits, and fruit juice can be offered as snacks. A glycerine suppository can be used periodically. This is a natural stimulant and lubricant of the bowel. Caution parents to avoid frequent use of laxatives, stool softeners, and enemas, because overuse can cause bowel dependency. Herbal stimulant laxatives are discouraged for children less than 12 years, although other intestinal motility aids are not generally harmful. Find out more about any herbs your patients commonly use.

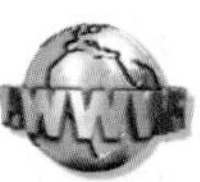

Complementary Therapy for Motility

INTESTINAL PARASITIC DISORDERS

Intestinal parasitic disorders occur most frequently in tropical regions. Outbreaks take place in areas where water is not treated, food is incorrectly prepared, or people live in crowded conditions with poor sanitation. In the United States, outbreaks of diseases caused by protozoa or helminths (worms) are increasing. Young children, especially those in childcare, are most at risk of infection. They often lack good hygiene practices and are more likely to put objects and their hands into their mouths. The most common intestinal parasitic disorders are summarized in the clinical manifestations table on the following pages.

In addition, parasites are emerging in the United States that previously were not commonly seen. The possibility of enteric infection should always be considered in children with continuing diarrhea or other intestinal symptoms (Cowden & Hotez, 2001).

Another common cause of young childhood infection is exposure to pets and wildlife. Pets should be checked for parasites and dewormed regularly. Public policies for cleanup of pet fecal material in parks can also decrease contamination. Sand and play boxes should be kept covered when not in use and children should be taught good handwashing after exposure to their pets and not to approach or touch unfamiliar or wild animals (Kazacos, 2000).

Laboratory examination of stool specimens identifies the causative organism (protozoa, worms, larvae, or ova). Treatment usually involves an anthelmintic. Nursing care centers on preventive teaching. Emphasize the importance of good hygiene practices, especially careful handwashing, after toileting and when handling food. Instruct parents to give prescribed medications as directed even if the child's condition seems to be improved.

RESEARCH

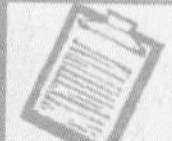

Following are newly emerging enteric protozoa seen in U.S. children:

- *Cryptosporidium parvum*
- *Dientamoeba fragilis*
- *Blastocystis hominis*
- *Entamoeba coli*

DRUGS USED TO TREAT INTESTINAL PROTOZOAN INFECTIONS

Diloxanide furoate
Furazoladine
Iodoquinol
Mebendazole
Metronadazole
Paromomycin
Piperazine citrate
Pyrantel pamoate
Tetracycline
Thiabendazole
Trimethoprim/sulfamethoxazole

FEEDING DISORDERS

Feeding problems that interfere with a child's ability to ingest or tolerate formulas and foods usually become apparent during the first year of life. To prevent complications of poor nutrition, feeding methods or diet may need to be altered. The following discussion focuses on the common disorders of colic and rumination. See Chapter 3 for a discussion of food allergy and sensitivity and of feeding disorder of infancy and childhood (failure to thrive). Chapter 7 has a discussion of the eating disorders anorexia nervosa and bulimia.

COLIC

Colic is a feeding disorder characterized by paroxysmal abdominal pain of intestinal origin and severe crying. It usually occurs in infants under 3 months of age. The etiology of colic is unknown. Proposed causes include feeding too rapidly and swallowing large amounts of air.

Characteristically the infant cries loudly and continuously, often for several hours. The infant's face may become flushed. The abdomen is distended and tense. Often the infant draws up the legs and clenches the hands. Episodes occur at the same time each day, usually in the late afternoon or early evening. Crying may stop only when the child is completely exhausted or after passage of flatus or stool. Carrying the child in the upright position is often helpful.

The symptoms initially may resemble intestinal obstruction or peritoneal infection. These conditions must be ruled out along with sensitivity to formula. Treatment is supportive. Usually by 3 months of age the severity and frequency of symptoms decrease.

Nursing Management

Nursing care requires a thorough history of the infant's diet and daily schedule and the events surrounding episodes of colicky behavior. Assessment of the infant's feeding patterns and diet includes type, frequency, and amount of feeding (if breast-feeding, maternal diet history) and frequency of burping. Episodes of colic are assessed for onset, duration, and characteristics of

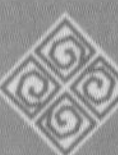

CLINICAL MANIFESTATIONS OF COMMON INTESTINAL PARASITIC DISORDERS

PARASITIC INFECTION	TRANSMISSION, LIFE CYCLE, PATHOGENESIS	CLINICAL MANIFESTATIONS	CLINICAL THERAPY	COMMENTS
Giardiasis Organism: protozoan *Giardia lamblia* *Giardia lamblia*	Transmission is through person-to-person contact, unfiltered water, improperly prepared infected food, and contact with animals. Cysts are ingested and passed into the duodenum and proximal jejunum, where they begin actively feeding. They are excreted in the stool.	May be asymptomatic. *Infants:* diarrhea, vomiting, anorexia, failure to thrive *Older children:* abdominal cramps; intermittent loose, foul-smelling, watery, pale, and greasy stools	Available medications include furazolidone and quinacrine. Furazolidone has fewer side effects than quinacrine but is more expensive. Metronidazole is also effective but is not licensed in the United States for treatment of giardiasis.	Most common intestinal parasitic organism in the United States. Infection may resolve spontaneously in 4–6 weeks without treatment. Parents or caregivers should wear gloves when handling diapers or stool of parasite-infected infant or child.
Enterobiasis (Pinworm) Organism: nematode *Enterobius vermicularis* Pinworm	Transmission is from discharged eggs inhaled or carried from hand to mouth. Eggs hatch in the upper intestine and mature in 15–28 days. Larvae then migrate to the cecum. After mating, the female migrates out of the anus and lays up to 17,000 eggs. Movement of worms causes intense itching. Scratching deposits eggs on the hands and under the nails.	Intense perianal itching, irritability, restlessness, and short attention span; in females, can migrate to the vagina and urethra to cause infection. Itching intensifies at night when the female comes to the anal opening to lay eggs.	Available medications include mebendazole, pyrantel pamoate, and piperazine citrate. The child and all household members should be treated at the same time. Treatment may be repeated in 2–3 weeks.	Most common helminthic infection in United States. Transmission is increased in crowded conditions such as housing developments, schools, and childcare centers.
Ascariasis (Roundworm) Organism: nematode *Ascaris lumbricoides* Roundworm	Transmission is from discharged eggs carried from hand to mouth. Adult lays eggs in small intestine. Eggs are excreted in stool, where they incubate for 2–3 weeks. Swallowed eggs hatch in the small intestine. Larvae may penetrate intestinal villi, entering the portal vein and liver, then moving to the lung. Larvae that ascend to upper respiratory tract are swallowed and proceed to the small intestine, where they repeat the cycle.	Mild infection may be asymptomatic. Severe infection may result in intestinal obstruction, peritonitis, obstructive jaundice, and lung involvement.	Available anthelmintic medications include mebendazole, pyrantel pamoate, or piperazine citrate. Stools should be examined 2 weeks after treatment and monthly for 3 months. Family members and contacts of the child should be treated if indicated. If the child has intestinal obstruction, treatment may include administering piperazine through a nasogastric tube and duodenal suction. Obstructing worms sometimes have to be surgically removed.	Most common in warm climates. Primarily affects children 1–4 years of age.

Note: Giardia lamblia *courtesy of the Centers for Disease Control and Prevention, Atlanta, GA;* pinworm (*p. 718*), roundworm (*p. 714*), hookworm (*p. 719*), and threadworm (p. 721) from Rudolph, A.M., Hoffman, J.I.E., Rudolph, C.D. (1996). *Rudolph's pediatrics* (20th ed.). Stamford, CT: Appleton & Lange.

(continued)

CLINICAL MANIFESTATIONS OF COMMON INTESTINAL PARASITIC DISORDERS (continued)

PARASITIC INFECTION	TRANSMISSION, LIFE CYCLE, PATHOGENESIS	CLINICAL MANIFESTATIONS	CLINICAL THERAPY	COMMENTS
Hookworm disease Organism: nematode *Necator americanus* Hookworm	Transmission is through direct contact with infected soil containing larvae. Worms live in the small intestine and feed on villi, causing bleeding. Eggs are deposited in the bowel and excreted in feces. Eggs hatch in damp shaded soil. Larvae attach to and penetrate the skin then enter the bloodstream, migrating to the lungs. Larvae then migrate to the upper respiratory passages and are swallowed.	In healthy individuals mild infection seldom causes problems. More severe infection may result in anemia and malnutrition. Presence of larvae on the skin may cause burning and itching, followed by redness and papular eruption.	Available medications include mebendazole and pyrantel pamoate. Stools should be examined 2 weeks after treatment and monthly for 3 months. Family members and contacts of the child should be treated if indicated.	Children should wear shoes when outdoors, although other unprotected areas of the skin may still come in contact with larvae.
Strongyloidiasis (Threadworm) Organism: nematode *Strongyloides stercoralis*	Transmission is from the ingestion of discharged larvae in the soil. Life cycle is similar to that of the hookworm, except the threadworm does not attach to the intestinal mucosa and feeding larvae (rather than eggs) may be deposited in the soil. Threadworm	Mild infection may be asymptomatic. Severe infection may result in abdominal pain and distention, nausea, vomiting, and diarrhea. Stools may be large and pale, with mucus. Severe infection may lead to a nutritional deficiency.	Available medications include thiabendazole or mebendazole. Treatment may need to be repeated if symptoms recur after treatment. Family members and contacts of the child should be examined and treated if indicated.	Most common in older children and adolescents.
Visceral larva migrans (Toxocariasis) Organism: nematode *Toxocara canis* or *T. catis,* commonly found in dogs and cats	Transmission is through the ingestion of eggs in the soil. Ingested eggs hatch in the intestine. Mobile larvae then migrate to the liver and eventually to all major organs (including the brain). Once migration is complete, they encapsulate in dense fibrous tissue.	Most cases are asymptomatic. Affected children may have a low-grade fever and recurrent upper airway diseases. Severe symptoms include hepatomegaly, pulmonary infiltration, and neurologic disturbances. In all cases there is a hypereosinophilia of the blood.	There is no specific treatment. Corticosteroids have been used in severe cases. Thiabendazole has been recommended but efficacy is not established (infection usually resolves spontaneously).	Most common in toddlers. Deworm household pets monthly if indicated. Keep children away from areas contaminated with animal droppings.

FAMILIES WANT TO KNOW

Suggestions for Alleviating Colic

PROVIDE RHYTHMIC MOVEMENT
Front-carrying sling carriers
Infant swing (battery-operated swing provides continuous motion)
Car ride

ALTERNATE POSITIONS
Swaddle infant in a soft, stretchy blanket with knees flexed up against abdomen or with legs straight
Place infant prone on parent's arm, supporting the body with one hand under the abdomen and cradling the head in the crook of the other arm

REDUCE ENVIRONMENTAL STIMULI
Respond to crying
Provide quiet, soothing music
Prevent sudden loud noises
Avoid smoking

PROVIDE VARIOUS TACTILE STIMULI
Offer a pacifier
Provide a warm bath
Massage abdomen

ALTER INTAKE
Feed smaller amount and burp frequently
Use a bottle with a collapsible bag to prevent sucking air
Breast-feeding mothers: eliminate milk products and spicy or gas-producing foods
Hold upright for 30 minutes after feeding

cry. What measures are used to relieve crying? How effective are they? When possible, the feeding method should be observed. Parents of infants with colic are often tired and frustrated. They require frequent reassurance that they are not to blame for the infant's condition. Suggest ways of alleviating some of the infant's symptoms and discomfort.

RUMINATION

Rumination is a rare and serious form of chronic regurgitation that may lead to malnutrition and growth failure in infancy. Chewing movements and mouthing of fingers often precede or accompany regurgitation. Close observation may reveal the infant actively initiating gagging with the tongue and fingers.

Rumination is most often associated with poor maternal–infant bonding. This kind of behavior is seen in infants who are deprived of tactile, visual, or auditory stimuli for long periods. The infant substitutes repetitive self-stimulation for the lack of appropriate external stimulation. (See the discussion of failure to thrive in Chapter 3.)

Diagnostic evaluation focuses on ruling out an organic cause and determining the degree and type of nutritional deficiencies. Treatment involves correcting the nutritional deficits and developing normal feeding patterns. Medical and nursing staff and social services are often involved in helping parents meet the infant's nutritional and psychologic needs (see Chapter 3).

Nursing Management

Nursing care focuses on establishing a warm, caring relationship with the infant and the parents. Making eye contact with the infant, providing food regularly, and stimulating the infant through all the senses are ways to break the pattern of rumination.

Parents need to be included in the infant's care. Discuss proper nutrition and demonstrate feeding techniques and interactions that promote development. Determine the parents' support needs and make a referral to social service agencies as appropriate. A parent who is preoccupied with financial or other problems is less likely to attend to an infant's needs, resulting in continuation or recurrence of the pattern of rumination.

DISORDERS OF MALABSORPTION

Malabsorption occurs when a child is unable to digest or absorb nutrients in the diet. Disorders of malabsorption include celiac disease, lactose intolerance, and short bowel syndrome. Cystic fibrosis is a common cause of malabsorption and is discussed in Chapter 13.

CELIAC DISEASE

Celiac disease, or gluten-sensitive enteropathy, is a chronic malabsorption syndrome that is more common in white European children than in black or Asian children. It is also more common among members of the same family, so a genetic factor may play a role in etiology (Connon, 1999). About 1% to 4% of children with Down syndrome have celiac disease (Nehring & Vessey, 2000). Current research is being directed at locating the potential genetic abnormalities that occur in celiac disease. The disease is characterized by an intolerance for gluten, a protein found in wheat, barley, rye, and oats. Inability to digest glutenin and gliadin (protein fractions) results in the accumulation of the amino acid glutamine, which is toxic to mucosal cells in the intestine. Damage to the villi ultimately impairs the absorptive process in the small intestine.

In the early stages, celiac disease affects fat absorption, resulting in excretion of large quantities of fat in the stools (steatorrhea). Stools are greasy, foul smelling, frothy, and excessive. As changes in the villi continue, the absorption of protein, carbohydrates, calcium, iron, folate, and vitamins A, D, E, K, and B_{12} becomes impaired.

Symptoms usually occur when solid foods containing gluten are introduced to the child's diet (in the first 2 years of life), although celiac disease is sometimes first diagnosed in adulthood (Connon, 1999). The child exhibits chronic diarrhea, vomiting, irritability, and failure to grow (Figure 17-12 ◆). If diagnosis is delayed, the child begins to show evidence of protein deficiency (wasted musculature, abdominal distention), delayed dentition, and changes in bone density.

Diagnosis is confirmed through measurement of fecal fat content, jejunal biopsy, and improvement with removal of gluten products from the diet. Blood screening tests are more often being used successfully for diagnosis. Serum antigliadin antibody (AGA) and reticulin antibody levels are elevated. Symptoms usually improve within a few days to weeks. The intestinal villi return to normal in about 6 months. Growth should improve steadily, and height and weight should reach normal range within 1 year. Vitamin supplementation may be needed for a period of time if the child has become malnourished.

Nursing Management

Nursing care focuses on supporting the parents in maintaining a gluten-free diet for the child. The parents should receive a thorough explanation of the disease process. Emphasize the necessity of following a gluten-free diet. Help parents to understand that celiac disease requires lifelong dietary modifications that should not be discontinued when the child is symptom free. Discontinuation of the diet places the child at risk for growth retardation and the development of GI cancers in adulthood. All children with celiac disease should be seen by a dietitian several times during childhood. Nutritional assessment and continued teaching to maintain a gluten-free diet take place at these visits.

The diet of an infant or toddler is easily monitored at home. When the child enters school, however, ensuring adherence to dietary restrictions becomes more difficult. In addition to easily identified gluten-based foods such as bread, cake, doughnuts, cookies, and crackers, the child must also avoid processed foods that contain gluten as a filler. School-age children and adolescents are often tempted to eat these foods, especially when among peers. Emphasize the need for compliance while meeting the child's developmental needs.

The child's special dietary needs can place a financial burden on the family. Parents will need to purchase prepared rice or corn flour products or make their own bread and bakery products. Advise parents that obtaining a dietary prescription will enable them to deduct the cost of these ingredients and commercially prepared products as a medical expense.

Because adaptation to the diet must be made by the entire family, support and management skills are needed by parents and siblings (Huff, 1997). For information and support,

RESEARCH

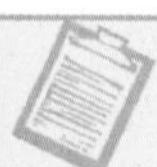

By studying children at genetic risk of celiac disease, researchers have found that a transglutaminase antibody titer level identifies 70%–85% of children who have intestinal changes on biopsy. The test may help in the future to identify and begin treatment for children with early nonsymptomatic celiac disease. The researchers also found that the consumption of 24 g of oat cereal daily did not worsen celiac disease, so once verified with further study, this may make management of the disease easier for children and families (Hoffenberg, Bao, & Eisenbarth, et al., 2000).

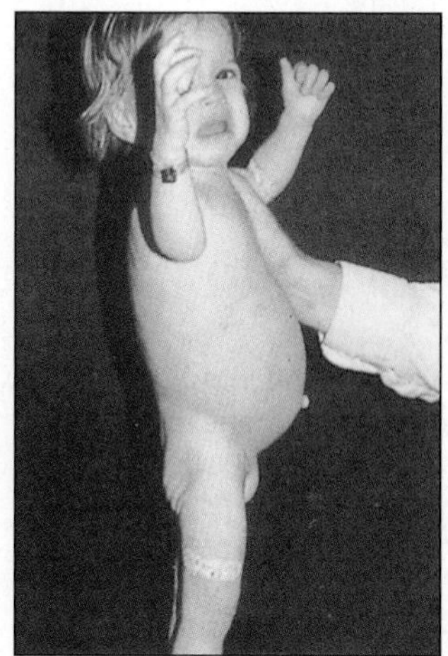

FIGURE 17-12 ◆
The child with celiac disease commonly shows failure to grow and wasting of extremities. The abdomen can appear large due to intestinal bloating and malnutrition.
From Zitelli, B. J., and Davis, H. W. (Eds.). (1997). *Atlas of Pediatric Physical Diagnosis.* St. Louis, MO: Mosby, Inc.

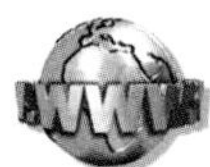

Celiac Disease Support and Resources

NURSING ALERT

Many prepared foods contain hidden gluten. Examples include certain types of chocolate candy, some prepared hamburgers, hot dogs, luncheon meats, milk preparations such as malts and processed ice cream, canned soups, mayonnaise, catsup, malt flavoring, vinegar (except apple cider vinegar), hydrolyzed vegetable protein, and modified food starch.

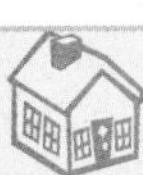

HOME CARE

Caution parents to read food labels carefully to identify hidden sources of lactose. For example, milk solids are found in breads, cakes, some candies (e.g., milk chocolate, caramels, and toffee), some salad dressings, margarine, and various processed foods.

CLINICAL TIP

The section of the intestine that is resected will determine the vitamin and nutrient deficiencies of the child with short bowel syndrome. When the ileum is resected, bile salts, fluids, and electrolyte absorption decrease so diarrhea can result. Loss of ileum also leads to steatorrhea and fat soluble vitamins. When the colon is resected, fluid and electrolyte management is impaired. Resection of the jejunum is compensated for effectively by the remaining bowel (Jakubik, Colfer, & Grossman, 2000).

parents and children can be referred to several organizations, including the American Celiac Society, the Celiac Sprue Association/United States of America, and the Gluten Intolerance Group. Written materials are also available from Children's Memorial Hospital in Chicago.

Expected outcomes of nursing care include the following:

- Maintenance of normal dietary patterns
- Adequate absorption of essential nutrients as demonstrated by normal growth patterns and absence of deficiency symptoms
- Child and family knowledge of sources of dietary gluten

LACTOSE INTOLERANCE

Lactose intolerance is the inability to digest lactose, a disaccharide found in milk and other dairy products. It results from a congenital or acquired deficiency of the enzyme lactase. Congenital lactase deficiency of infancy is a rare disorder. See Chapter 3 for a general discussion of food intolerance. Abdominal pain, flatulence, and diarrhea occur shortly after birth when the infant is unable to hydrolyze lactose. The prevalence of secondary (acquired) lactase deficiency is highest (approximately 100%) among Asian and Native American children and affects approximately 70% of blacks after the age of 3 years. Diarrhea develops rapidly after the child ingests milk and milk products. Some children are able to tolerate small ingestions of lactose but have symptoms when larger amounts are consumed. Incidence of lactose intolerance increases with advancing age throughout childhood.

Diagnosis is based on a thorough history and a hydrogen breath test, which measures the amount of hydrogen left after fermentation of unabsorbed carbohydrates. Implementing a lactose-free diet for a period of time may eliminate the symptoms, thus confirming the diagnosis. Treatment for infants includes switching to a soy-based formula. For older children, eliminating lactose-containing foods is recommended. Enzyme tablets such as LactAid can be added to milk or sprinkled on foods to aid digestion.

Nursing Management

Nursing care is primarily supportive. Carefully explain dietary modifications to parents and discuss alternate sources of calcium (see Chapter 10). Discuss the need for supplementation of calcium and vitamin D to prevent deficiencies. Suggest lactase tablets for children who want to have some dairy product intake.

SHORT BOWEL SYNDROME

Short bowel syndrome is a decreased ability to digest and absorb a regular diet because of a shortened intestine. Loss of intestine may result from extensive bowel resection for treatment of necrotizing enterocolitis or inflammatory disorders or from a congenital bowel anomaly such as intestinal malrotation, gastroschisis, or atresia.

The extent and location of the involved bowel determine the severity of the disorder. Because specific types of absorption occur primarily in certain parts of the bowel, the section lost determines the particular vitamins and other nutrients that are inadequate. During the first 3 months after bowel resection, watery diarrhea is common. In the transition period, the remaining bowel usually increases its absorptive surface area and partially compensates for the absent intestine. The infant or young child requires nutritional support initially to provide sufficient nutrients for adequate growth and development. A combination of total parenteral nutrition via central line and oral fluids may be required. Once the bowel begins to recover, enteral feedings may be started. Careful management of enteral feedings includes a high-fat, low-carbohydrate diet with added stimulants for mucosal growth hormones (gastrin, insulin, enteroglucagon, and growth hormone). Careful management of nucleotide, glutamine, polyamine, and fatty acid components in enteral feedings can also encourage growth of normal intestinal mucosa (Committee on Nutrition, American Academy of Pediatrics, 1998).

Nursing Management

Nursing care focuses on meeting the child's nutritional and fluid needs and teaching parents how to care for the child at home. Establishing an adequate nutritional intake and bowel pattern is a lengthy process. Total parenteral nutrition is provided initially until a feeding regimen can be established. Oral and enteral feedings are instituted gradually to allow the bowel time to compensate. Provide support to the family and child throughout this period. Teach parents how to prepare and administer total parenteral feedings and care for the central line (see description in the Skills Manual). Once enteral or tube feedings are begun, teach management of the feeding pump and care of the feeding tube. Ensure regular bowel function and maintain skin integrity. Arrange home visits to monitor the child's growth and development, care of the central line and tube feeding site, and any side effects such as fluid and electrolyte imbalance and diarrhea.

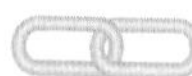

Skills 8-8 to 8-10: Managing Central Venous Catheters

HEPATIC DISORDERS

The liver is one of the most vital organs in the body. Among its essential functions are blood storage and filtration; secretion of bile and bilirubin; metabolism of fat, protein, and carbohydrates; synthesis of blood-clotting components; detoxification of hormones, drugs, and other substances; and storage of glycogen, iron, fat soluble vitamins, and vitamin B_{12}. Thus, any inflammatory, obstructive, or degenerative disorder that affects liver function can be life threatening. The following discussion focuses on three common liver disorders in children: biliary atresia, viral hepatitis, and cirrhosis.

LIVER TRANSPLANT

The most common reasons for liver transplants in children are:

- Biliary atresia
- Metabolic liver disease
- Acute idiopathic hepatic necrosis
- Cirrhosis

(Cox, 2000)

BILIARY ATRESIA

Biliary atresia is the pathologic closure or absence of bile ducts outside the liver. It is the most common pediatric liver disease necessitating transplantation and the most common cause of infant jaundice (Brown et al., 1998).

Initially the newborn is asymptomatic. Jaundice may not be detected until 2 or 3 weeks after birth. At that point, bilirubin levels increase, accompanied by abdominal distention and hepatomegaly (see Appendix C for bilirubin levels and other liver function tests). As the disease progresses, splenomegaly occurs. The infant experiences easy bruising, prolonged bleeding time, and intense itching. Stools are puttylike in consistency and white or clay colored because of the absence of bile pigments. Excretion of bilirubin and bile salts results in tea-colored urine. Failure to thrive and malnutrition occur as the destructive changes of the disease progress.

The cause of biliary atresia is unknown. Absence or blockage of the extrahepatic bile ducts results in blocked bile flow from the liver to the duodenum. This altered bile flow soon causes inflammation and fibrotic changes in the liver. In addition to blockage, the disease can also be caused by hepatocellular dysfunction (Brown et al., 1998). Lack of bile acids also interferes with digestion of fat and absorption of fat soluble vitamins A, D, E, and K, resulting in steatorrhea and nutritional deficiencies. Without treatment the disease is fatal.

Diagnosis is based on the history, physical examination, and laboratory evaluation. Laboratory findings reveal elevated bilirubin levels, elevated serum aminotransferase and alkaline phosphatase values, prolonged prothrombin time, and increased ammonia levels. Ultrasound is used to rule out other causes, and a liver biopsy is performed. Because liver damage develops rapidly in infants with biliary atresia, early diagnosis is essential.

Treatment involves surgery to attempt correction of the obstruction (hepatoportoenterostomy) and supportive care. In the hepatoportoenterostomy (Kasai procedure), a segment of the intestine is anastomosed to the porta hepatis. In most children this is a palliative treatment to promote bile drainage, maintain as much hepatic function as possible, and prevent the complications of liver failure. Supportive treatment is directed at managing the bleeding tendencies by administering oral vitamin K, preventing rickets through vitamin D supplementation, controlling itching and irritability with cholestyramine and antihistamines, and promoting adequate nutrition.

Although the hepatoportoenterostomy improves the prognosis, complications of liver disease continue to develop and eventually necessitate liver transplantation. Advances in transplantation surgery now make it possible to perform partial liver transplants from living donor resections. This enables transplantation to be performed when the child is in optimal health, rather than waiting until an appropriate-size cadaver liver is available, and allows for donations from close family members who are often good tissue matches.

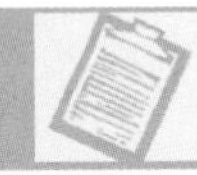

RESEARCH

The Studies of Pediatric Liver Transplantation (SPLIT) had registered 1,144 child liver transplants in the United States and Canada by June 2000. Survival rate was 85% at 1 year and 77% at 2 years. Of the survivors, 89% of the school-age children attended school full time by 18 months after transplant (SPLIT Research Group, 2001).

CLINICAL TIP

When drying the skin, pat the towel against the skin rather than rubbing and massaging. Rubbing and massaging promote vasodilation, which worsens the infant's itching and irritation.

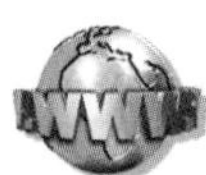

Hepatitis Statistics and National Resources

These advances, along with the development of cyclosporine and other immunosuppressants, have improved the first-year survival rate for children receiving liver transplantation to between 75% and 80%.

Nursing Management

Nursing care in the initial stages of biliary atresia is the same as that for any healthy newborn. As symptoms develop, the focus of nursing care becomes long-term management and support.

Diagnosis of this potentially fatal disorder can be devastating to parents. Provide emotional support and offer frequent explanations of tests during the initial diagnostic evaluation. As the disease progresses, the infant becomes irritable because of intense itching and the accumulation of toxins. Tepid baths may help to relieve itching and provide comfort. Promote rest by grouping nursing activities while the infant is awake. Care following a hepatoportoenterostomy is similar to that for a child undergoing abdominal surgery. (See the earlier discussion of postsurgical nursing management for appendicitis and the nursing care plan for the child undergoing surgery in Chapter 5.) Posttransplant care includes immunosuppressant drugs and close monitoring for vascular complications (see Table 17-3).

Discharge planning focuses on teaching parents how to care for the child's skin, provide for nutritional needs, administer medications, and monitor for increasing symptoms of liver disease. For the child who has received a transplant, teach parents how to identify signs of rejection (nausea, vomiting, fever, and jaundice), as well as the administration and side effects of immunosuppressant medications. Refer parents to support groups, clergy, or social services if indicated. They will need ongoing visits from a home health care nurse to help them in managing the complex care of the child. The main expected outcomes of nursing care are the parent's ability to cope with the child's health status and to provide the necessary care. The child is expected to function at maximum potential considering the extent of disease.

VIRAL HEPATITIS

Hepatitis is an inflammation of the liver caused by a viral infection. It may occur as an acute or chronic disease. Acute hepatitis is rapid in onset and if untreated may develop into chronic hepatitis. The most frequently diagnosed causative organisms are hepatitis A virus (HAV), hepatitis B virus (HBV), hepatitis C virus (HCV), hepatitis D virus (HDV), and hepatitis E virus (HEV). An estimated 136,000 cases of hepatitis occur annually in the United States, and one-third of these are in children. Most cases are types A and B (Table 17-4).

Etiology and Pathophysiology

Hepatitis A is the most common form of acute viral hepatitis. It is highly contagious and traditionally has been referred to as infectious hepatitis. Infection occurs primarily through the

TABLE 17-3 Problems Encountered in Pediatric Liver Transplant

- **Lack of donors.** This problem is being solved by increasing use of split liver transplants when partial transplants are provided by a family member, alleviating the need to wait for cadaver donations.
- **Immunosuppression.** Immunosuppressive therapies have been tested less in children than in adults and increased research is needed.
- **Morbidity and mortality of treatment.** Many of the drugs used after transplant have side effects of renal toxicity, malignancy, and other serious sequellae. The effects can be magnified in children who have decades of exposure to these drugs.
- **Recurrent and new diseases.** Diseases that may be caused by immunosuppression can occur, such as those caused by infectious agents. Other liver diseases such as cirrhosis and nonspecific hepatitis are seen in some children.
- **Influences on growth and development.** Drugs, liver disease, emotional strain, and disturbed nutritional intake and metabolism may all influence the growth, cognitive function, and developmental variation of children. Attention and consistent screening of development and family adaptation are needed.

Note: From McDiarnid, S.V. (2000). Liver transplantation. The pediatric challenge. *Clinical Liver Disease, 4,* 879–927.

TABLE 17-4 Comparison of Hepatitis Types

TYPE	INCUBATION	% ICTERIC	% WHO BECOME CHRONIC CARRIERS	CLINICAL FEATURES
Hepatitis A				
Children <5 years	4 weeks (10–50 days)	<5	0	More acute onset; frequently subclinical in young children
Adults		50–75		
Hepatitis B				
Infants	1–6 months	<5	>90	Extrahepatic manifestations more common
Adults		20–60	5–10	
Hepatitis C				
All ages	6–7 weeks	20–30	≥60	Frequently manifests without jaundice; predisposes to hepatocellular carcinoma
Hepatitis D				
Coinfection with HBV	2–8 weeks	Not known	<5	Most common viral cause of fulminant hepatitis
Superinfection of HBV carrier			>80	
Hepatitis E				
All ages	2–9 weeks	~10	0	Severe in pregnant women; high mortality and fetal loss

Note: From Holst, B., & Ritter, D. (2001). Managing viral hepatitis. *Clinician Reviews, 11,* 51–62.

fecal–oral route. Transmission is by direct person-to-person spread or through ingestion of contaminated water or food (particularly shellfish). Hepatitis A frequently occurs in children in child care settings where hygiene practices are poor. Food handlers can spread hepatitis A if not aware of their infection; it is a common cause of foodborne illness. The virus can live on surfaces for 1 month. Because the virus is transmitted in the early stages of the disease when individuals are often asymptomatic or only mildly ill, large numbers of people may be exposed before the diagnosis is confirmed (Table 17-5). Although hepatitis A is a mild disease in many people, others may experience severe liver damage (Shovein, Damazo, & Hyams, 2000).

Hepatitis B, which has been known traditionally as serum hepatitis, is a serious disease. Transmission is usually by the parenteral route through the exchange of blood or any bodily secretion or fluid. Other common transmission routes include sexual activity and transmission from mother to fetus in utero. Adolescents who use intravenous drugs and have unprotected sexual intercourse are at risk for contracting hepatitis B. Major sources for the spread of HBV are healthy chronic carriers. All body fluids of infected individuals are potentially contaminated with the virus.

The hepatitis C virus is transmitted primarily through blood and blood products, and blood banks now test for this virus. Infected children are commonly individuals who have had repeated transfusions (as in sickle-cell disease or hemophilia). Intravenous drug use , body piercing, and multiple sexual partners are also risk factors. Infected mothers may infect their children before birth or during breastfeeding (Estrada, 2000; National Institutes of Health, 2000).

Hepatitis D (delta virus) is a defective virus that can gain entry to a human only in connection with hepatitis B. This virus is suspected when someone who has been diagnosed with hepatitis B has diminishing liver function, increasing jaundice, and deteriorating mental status.

Hepatitis E infection is primarily transmitted through contaminated water and is most common in developing countries. Outbreaks may occur in flooding and rainy seasons. A related infection transferred primarily through blood transfusion is hepatitis G (Holst & Ritter, 2001).

TABLE 17-5 Transmission, Immunization, and Prophylaxis for Hepatitis

TYPE	PRIMARY TRANSMISSION	IMMUNIZATION AVAILABLE	PROPHYLAXIS
Hepatitis A	Fecal–oral	Yes	Immune serum globulin Hepatitis A vaccine
Hepatitis B	Blood products Intravenous drug use In utero Sexual activity	Yes	Hepatitis B immune globulin Hepatitis B vaccine
Hepatitis C	Blood products Sexual activity Intravenous drug use Body piercing	No	None
Hepatitis D	Blood products Intravenous drug use In utero Sexual activity	No	Hepatitis B vaccine
Hepatitis E	Fecal–oral	No	None

The liver's response to injury by the viruses that cause hepatitis is similar (Figure 17-13 ◆). Initially, invasion of the parenchymal cells by the virus results in local degeneration and necrosis. Subsequent infiltration of the parenchyma by lymphocytes, macrophages, plasma cells, eosinophils, and neutrophils causes inflammation that blocks biliary drainage into the intestine. Impaired bile excretion causes a buildup of bile in the blood, urine, and skin (jaundice). Structural changes in the parenchymal cells account for other altered liver functions. Regeneration of parenchymal cells occurs within 3 months, and most children recover completely.

In some children, however, a progressive and total destruction of the hepatic parenchyma known as acute fulminating hepatitis develops. Children with this form of the disease usu-

PATHOPHYSIOLOGY ILLUSTRATED

Viral Hepatitis

FIGURE 17-13 ◆

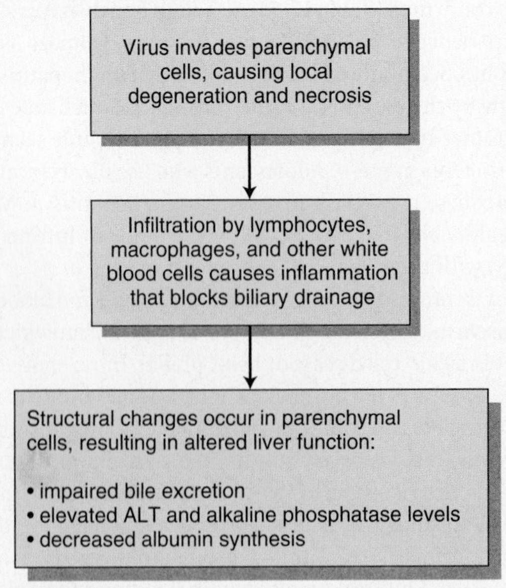

ally die of liver failure within 2 weeks of onset unless they receive a liver transplant. Another complication, chronic active hepatitis, may lead to scarring of the liver and progressive deterioration of liver function. The prognosis depends on the degree of liver involvement. In some persons, especially those who develop chronic hepatitis, liver cancers and cirrhosis can develop.

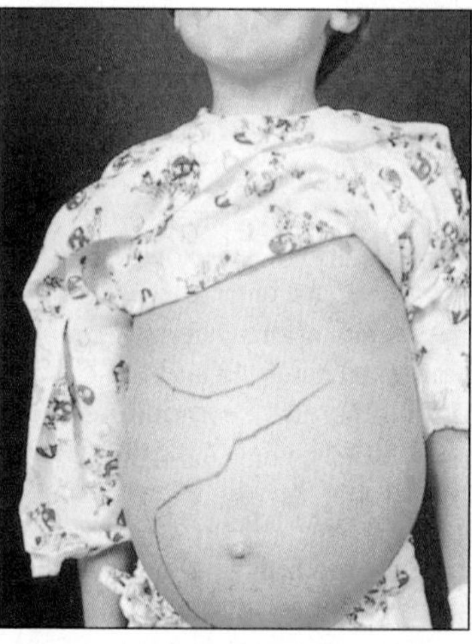

FIGURE 17-14 ◆
Hepatosplenomegaly is a common finding in the child with hepatitis. Can you tell which organs are enlarged in this photo? Review methods for finding an enlarged spleen or liver in Ch. 4.
From Zitelli, B. J., and Davis, H. W. (Eds.). (1997). *Atlas of Pediatric Physical Diagnosis.* St. Louis, MO: Mosby, Inc.

Clinical Manifestations

Acute hepatitis infection is characterized by two phases, the anicteric (absence of jaundice) phase and the icteric (jaundice) phase. The anicteric phase usually lasts 5 to 7 days. Signs and symptoms include nausea, vomiting, anorexia, malaise, fatigue, right upper quadrant pain, hepatosplenomegaly (Figure 17-14 ◆), and fever (see Table 17-4). The child becomes irritable, looks ill, and requires rest. In the icteric phase, signs and symptoms include darkening of urine, clay-colored stools, and the characteristic yellowing of the skin and sclera. In many cases of hepatitis in children, there is no jaundice, leading to difficulty in disease diagnosis and management. As the jaundice worsens, the child begins to feel better. This phase lasts approximately 4 weeks. Complete recovery with return of normal liver function and laboratory values may take 1 to 3 months.

In some cases hepatitis becomes chronic. The individual with chronic hepatitis carries the virus, can transfer it to others, and may develop serious liver disease after several years.

Clinical Therapy

Diagnosis is often made on the basis of a thorough history and physical examination. A history of exposure to persons with the disease is significant. Physical examination reveals a tender, enlarged liver, abdominal pain, and flulike symptoms. Laboratory evaluation includes serologic testing (to detect the presence of antigens and antibodies to HAV, HBV, HCV, or HDV) and liver function studies. Although a test for HEV has been developed, it is not available in developing countries, so diagnosis is usually based on the history.

The three goals of medical management are early detection to prevent complications, support and monitoring during the acute phase of the disease, and prevention of the spread of the disease. Early diagnosis is essential to follow the course of the illness and identify potential complications. Management of the illness includes bedrest during the flulike phase. If prothrombin times are increased, vitamin K is administered.

The spread of viral infections can be interrupted by elimination of the virus from the infected population, institution of proper hygiene, and passive or active immunization. To date, no antiviral agent has been developed to combat the hepatitis viruses. Prevention depends on breaking the cycle of infection. Active immunization for hepatitis A, a two-dose series, is recommended for all persons at risk of acquiring and transmitting the disease and for children and child care workers in certain states with endemic disease (see Chapter 12). Individuals at risk include child care staff and food handlers (Centers for Disease Control and Prevention, 1999). Immunization for hepatitis B, a three-dose series, is recommended for all children and at-risk adults. The first dose is given within 12 hours of birth to the infant born of an infected mother (refer to the discussion of immunization in Chapter 12).

Passive immunity to HAV can be achieved with standard pooled immune globulin. It must be administered within 2 weeks of exposure. Passive immunity to HBV can be achieved with hepatitis B immune globulin (HBIG). It is used for one-time exposure and for infants of infected mothers and is given within 12 hours of birth.

NURSING MANAGEMENT

Nursing Assessment and Diagnosis

The nurse usually encounters the child and family in an outpatient setting. In addition to being observed for characteristic signs of hepatitis (jaundiced skin and sclera), the child is assessed for the presence of abdominal pain, anorexia, nausea and vomiting, malaise, and arthralgia. A history of the child's contacts over the past 45 days for HAV and up to 180 days for HBV is also obtained. For an infant, the hepatitis history of the mother and other family members is important.

NURSING ALERT

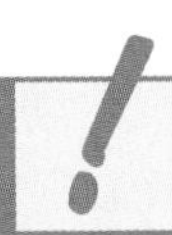

When hepatitis A is present, drug metabolism is altered and the liver's ability to detoxify drugs is decreased. As with all liver disorders, medications need to be administered carefully and the child's condition must be monitored for possible side effects. Caution parents to check with health professionals before giving any nonprescription medication. For example, acetaminophen is metabolized in the liver, and liver disease can interfere with its breakdown.

NURSING ALERT

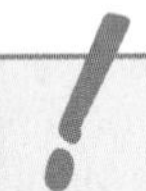

Health care workers who come in contact with blood or other body fluids of children infected with hepatitis B are at risk for contracting the virus. Standard precautions should be used at all times (see the Skills Manual). Hepatitis B immunization (3 doses) is recommended for nurses and other persons at high risk for exposure as well as all infants and adolescents (see Chapter 12).

COMMUNITY CARE

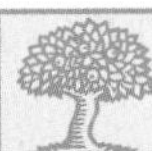

Nurses in child care centers can provide assessment of the center's procedures and teaching to prevent hepatitis A transmission. Help the center to set standards related to the following areas.

- Handwashing after each diaper change
- Disposing of diapers properly
- Cleaning diaper-changing surfaces after each diaper change
- Never having food handlers perform diaper changes
- Instructing parents to keep children at home for at least 2 weeks after a diagnosis of hepatitis A
- Informing parents of other children when there is a case of hepatitis A and teaching them the symptoms of the condition

Common nursing diagnoses for the child with acute hepatitis may include the following:

- *Risk for altered nutrition: Less than body requirements,* related to chronic illness
- *Fatigue,* related to disease state
- *Risk for diversional activity deficit,* related to forced inactivity
- *Risk for body image disturbance (older child),* related to jaundice
- *Anxiety (parent and child),* related to threat to health status
- *Pain,* related to liver injury

Planning and Implementation

Nursing care involves home and community considerations, as children with hepatitis are seldom admitted to the hospital. The hospitalized child is placed in isolation. Prevention of the diseases is integrated into all health care by discussion of immunization and universal precautions. When hepatitis cases have occurred in the family or community, parents need additional detailed information about health precautions and infection control measures. In addition, teach parents the importance of maintaining adequate nutrition, promoting rest and comfort, and providing diversional activities.

Prevent Spread of Infection

Teach the parents and the child infection control measures to help prevent transmission of the virus. Good hygiene practices, such as washing hands before and after toileting and proper disposal of soiled diapers, should be reinforced to parents. Siblings of a child with hepatitis B who have not already been immunized with the hepatitis B vaccine should be vaccinated immediately. Contacts of the child with hepatitis A should receive immune serum globulin and the first immunization in the hepatitis A series. Rifampin may be given in some cases.

Maintain Adequate Nutrition

Initially the child is encouraged to eat favorite foods. Once the anorexia and nausea have resolved, a high-protein, high-carbohydrate, low-fat diet is recommended. Increased protein helps to maintain protein stores and prevent muscle wasting. Increased carbohydrates ensure adequate caloric intake and prevent protein depletion. The use of low-fat foods lessens stomach distention. Offer the child small, frequent feedings.

Promote Rest and Comfort

Bedrest is necessary only if the child has severe fatigue and malaise. However, most children voluntarily limit their activities during the initial phase of the disease. Keep the child quiet and comfortable. Offer comfort items such as favorite toys, blankets, and pillows.

Provide Diversional Activities

Hospitalized children with hepatitis are kept in isolation. Nonhospitalized children with hepatitis do not need to be isolated, but they should be kept at home for 2 weeks following the onset of symptoms. Parents who cannot arrange to take time off from work may need to arrange home sitters to stay with the child. Offer suggestions for diversional activities during this period. Young children can be provided with a new toy or favorite activities. Older children and adolescents can be provided with board games, puzzles, books or magazines, movies, or video games. Phone calls and short visits from friends help school-age children and adolescents maintain contact with peers.

Evaluation

Expected outcomes of nursing care for hepatitis include the following:

- Prevention of new cases of the disease
- Full immunization coverage at recommended ages
- Restoration to normal liver function

- Reestablishment of nutritional intake to support growth
- Return to full energy and activity level
- Developmental progression during and after the disease
- Control of pain to level of comfort
- Absence of chronic liver disease

CIRRHOSIS

Cirrhosis is a degenerative disease process that results in fibrotic changes and fatty infiltration in the liver. It can occur in children of any age as the end stage of several disorders. The diffuse destruction and regeneration of the hepatic parenchymal cells result in an increase in fibrous connective tissue and disorganization of the liver structure. The balance between destruction and regeneration determines the specific clinical presentation.

Clinical manifestations of cirrhosis vary. When the disease process results from obstruction, as in biliary atresia, jaundice is an initial sign that intensifies with progression of the disease. In other diseases that cause cirrhosis, jaundice may be a late sign, intermittent, or absent. Steatorrhea is frequently present and can lead to rickets, hemorrhage, and failure to gain weight. Anemia can occur as a result of chronic blood loss from the GI tract. Pruritus is common, particularly in children with biliary malformations. Clubbing of the digits and cyanosis are other common findings. Severe end-stage complications signaling hepatic failure can occur at any time and with little warning

Diagnostic evaluation is based on the child's history of infection or disease with liver involvement. Physical examination may reveal jaundice, skin changes, ascites, and hemodynamic changes. Laboratory evaluation reveals abnormal liver function tests. A liver biopsy may help to determine the extent of the parenchymal damage.

Medical management focuses on treating the child's symptoms and achieving optimal nutritional status and growth. See the clinical manifestations table below for a summary of treatment for complications of cirrhosis. Liver transplantation is the most common treatment for biliary atresia and metabolic disorders and is the only treatment for end-stage liver disease.

Nursing Management

Nursing care focuses on monitoring physiologic and psychosocial changes to identify early signs of end-stage hepatic failure. Monitor vital signs every 2 to 4 hours. Daily weight measurement is performed to assess for fluid retention. Close monitoring of electrolytes and liver function test results helps determine the need for fluid replacement therapy.

Careful administration of medications and monitoring for side effects are necessary because drug metabolism is altered in liver disorders. If ascites is present, provide a low-sodium, low-protein diet and restrict fluids. Remove all water pitchers, glasses, and straws to minimize the child's desire to drink.

Parents of a child with cirrhosis are coping with a life-threatening disorder, and their anxiety and stress are high. The child may be awaiting a liver transplantation that represents

CLINICAL MANIFESTATIONS OF CIRRHOSIS COMPLICATIONS

ETIOLOGY	CLINICAL MANIFESTATIONS	CLINICAL THERAPY
Fluid and electrolyte imbalance	Ascites	Restrict sodium, protein, and fluids. Administer diuretics (e.g., furosemide [Lasix]). Administer intravenous albumin.
Liver dysfunction	Hepatic encephalopathy	Restrict protein. Administer lactulose (to control increased ammonia levels). Administer antibiotics. Correct any imbalances that can lead to coma (fluid and electrolyte imbalance).
Esophageal varices	Hemorrhage from esophageal varices	Administer blood and blood products. Replace fluid and electrolytes. Administer vitamin B complex and vitamin K. Insertion of Sengstaken-Blakemore tube in cases of severe bleeding.

the only hope for recovery. Provide support to parents and encourage them to verbalize their fears and concerns (see Chapter 8). Encourage parents to participate in the child's care. Referral to a support group or counseling may be beneficial.

INJURIES TO THE GASTROINTESTINAL SYSTEM

ABDOMINAL TRAUMA

Abdominal injuries may be caused by blunt or penetrating trauma. The kind of injury determines the extent of organ damage. Low-velocity trauma, which may occur when a child strikes the handlebars of a bicycle, usually results in single-organ injury.

High-velocity blunt trauma, which may occur in motor vehicle crashes, usually involves multiple organs. Solid organs such as the liver and spleen are more vulnerable to injury than hollow organs such as the stomach, intestines, and bladder.

Motor vehicle crashes are the most common and also the most preventable unintentional injury in children (National Safety Council, 2000). On impact, small children who are held on a parent's lap or improperly restrained in a safety seat can easily become airborne, striking objects or being thrown from the car. When older children involved in severe crashes are wearing only lap belts, injury to the hollow organs may result. Bicycles are another cause of abdominal injuries in children. Such injuries commonly occur when the child strikes the handlebars during a fall or sudden stop or is struck by a car. Child abuse is another major cause of abdominal trauma.

PERITONEAL LAVAGE

During peritoneal lavage, a dialysis catheter is inserted into the abdominal cavity and normal saline or lactated Ringer's solution is instilled. The fluid is then drained and analyzed for the presence of red blood cells, amylase, and bacteria, which could indicate organ damage.

Suspected abdominal trauma in a child necessitates a thorough history and physical examination. The description of the event should be compared with the child's signs and symptoms. Clinical manifestations of abdominal injury include pain, abdominal distention, muscle guarding, decreased or absent bowel sounds, nausea and vomiting, hypotension, and shock. See Chapter 4 for techniques of abdominal assessment.

A sonogram or a CT scan is performed to assess for internal bleeding and air in the abdomen. CT scans are also used to locate areas of internal trauma. Peritoneal lavage may be performed. Baseline laboratory studies, including blood type and cross-match, are done. A urinary catheter may be inserted to check for the presence of blood and bladder rupture.

Treatment of a liver or spleen injury takes place in the ICU and focuses on preventing or managing hemorrhage and monitoring for signs of shock. An intravenous infusion is started for fluid maintenance and to provide access for blood products. The child will be kept NPO. A nasogastric tube is inserted. Blood transfusions and pharmacologic management are used to treat blood loss. Use of analgesics is minimized to avoid masking symptoms. Serial hematocrit levels are monitored during this period. Healing of the liver and spleen usually occurs without further intervention.

Exploratory laparatomy is performed to resect hollow organ injuries or to repair liver or spleen lacerations when bleeding is not controlled. The spleen is salvaged to help maintain immune function. The child is usually discharged within 5 to 7 days. No strenuous activity is allowed for 6 to 8 weeks. The prognosis is generally good.

Nursing Management

Nursing care includes initial and ongoing assessments of the child's condition. Monitor vital signs every hour as warranted. Measurement of abdominal circumference, intake and output monitoring, serial hematocrits, and auscultation of bowel sounds are also performed hourly. Notify the physician of any changes.

The child and parents are usually fearful and anxious when the child is admitted to the hospital. If the injury was preventable, parents may have feelings of guilt or anger. Provide emotional support and avoid judgmental comments or statements that assign blame.

Once the child's condition is stabilized, the focus of nursing care shifts to preventive teaching. Parents should be taught safety measures to prevent future injuries and given written materials, when available, to use as a reference when they return home.

Discuss the use of car safety restraint devices for riding in an automobile (see Chapter 2). If the child's injury was the result of a bicycle fall or crash, discuss the importance of the proper bicycle size and teach bike safety measures such as use of a helmet and knowledge and proper use of hand signals (see Chapter 2). Have the child practice safe biking habits at a bike rodeo sponsored by a local affiliate of the National SAFE KIDS Campaign.

WWW *Injury Prevention*

POISONING

Poisoning is a common cause of death and injury in children between 1 and 4 years of age. About 1.5 million poisons occur annually in the United States (Powers, 2000). Young children are at risk for poisoning because of their characteristic behaviors, which involve exploration of the environment (see Chapter 2). Infants and toddlers commonly place objects in their mouths. Some household items are nontoxic and cause little harm; however, items that contain caustic agents or toxic chemicals can cause irreversible damage or death.

The Poison Prevention Packaging Act of 1970 mandates child protective devices for all potentially toxic substances, such as household cleansers and medications. However, many are still ingested by children; analgesics and hydrocarbons remain the two most common causes of poisoning deaths (Powers, 2000). Many other items commonly found in the home are less obvious sources of toxins. The leaves, stems, or flowers of many common household and garden plants are poisonous. Examples include Boston ivy, poinsettia, philodendron, lily-of-the-valley, daffodil (bulbs), azalea, and rhododendron. Nail care products, mothballs, weed and bug killers, and rodent killers are other potential hazards (Emery & Singer, 1998).

CLINICAL MANIFESTATIONS OF COMMONLY INGESTED TOXIC AGENTS

TYPE	SOURCES	CLINICAL MANIFESTATIONS	TREATMENT
Corrosives (strong acids and alkaline products that cause chemical burns of mucosal surfaces)	Batteries, household cleaners, Clinitest tablets, denture cleaners, bleach, toilet bowl cleaners	Severe burning pain in mouth, throat, or stomach; swelling of mucous membranes; edema of lips, tongue, and pharynx (respiratory obstruction); violent vomiting; hemoptysis; drooling; inability to clear secretions; signs of shock, anxiety, and agitation	*Do not induce vomiting!* Dilute toxin with water to prevent further damage. Give activated charcoal.
Hydrocarbons (organic compounds that contain carbon and hydrogen; most are distillates of petroleum)	Gasoline, kerosene, furniture polish, lighter fluid, paint thinners	Gagging, choking, coughing, nausea, vomiting, alteration in sensorium (lethargy), weakness, respiratory symptoms of pulmonary involvement, tachypnea, cyanosis, retractions, grunting	*Do not induce vomiting!* (Aspiration of hydrocarbons places child at high risk for pneumonia.) Use gastric lavage if severe central nervous system and respiratory impairment are present. Use of activated charcoal is controversial. Provide supportive care. Decontaminate skin by removing clothing and cleansing skin.
Acetaminophen	Many over-the-counter products	Nausea, vomiting, sweating, pallor, hepatic involvement (pain in upper right quadrant, jaundice, confusion, stupor, coagulation abnormalities)	Induce vomiting or perform gastric lavage, depending on amount ingested. Administer charcoal or NAC (concentrated form of Mucomyst), which binds with the metabolite, preventing absorption and protecting the liver.
Salicylate	Products containing aspirin	Nausea, disorientation, vomiting, dehydration, diaphoresis, hyperpnea, hyperpyrexia, bleeding tendencies, oliguria, tinnitus, convulsions, coma	Depends on amount ingested. Induce vomiting. Administer intravenous sodium bicarbonate, fluids, and vitamin K.
Mercury	Broken thermometers, chemicals, paints, pesticides, fungicides	Tremors, memory loss, insomnia, weight loss, diarrhea, anorexia, gingivitis	Similar to that for lead poisoning (see text discussion).
Iron	Multiple vitamin supplements	Vomiting, hematemesis, diarrhea, bloody stools, abdominal pain, metabolic acidosis, shock, seizures, coma	Induce vomiting. Administer intravenous fluids and sodium bicarbonate. Desferoxamine chelation therapy.

CLINICAL TIP

The acronym SIRES is a useful mnemonic device for recalling the essentials of care in cases of poisoning:

Stabilize the child's condition.
Identify the toxic substance.
Reverse its effect.
Eliminate the substance from the child's body.
Support the child physically and psychologically.

Most poisonings occur in the home (see Chapter 2). Although 75% of poisons are ingested, other routes of contamination include dermal, inhalation, and ocular (Litovitz, Klein-Schwartz, & White, et al., 2000). Parents who suspect that their child has ingested a poison should immediately call the Poison Control Center (PCC). The PCC will advise parents about treatment to begin at home, and if the child needs treatment in the emergency department. If the child has vomited, the vomitus should be brought to the emergency department. With older children, the possibility of intentional ingestion needs to be considered.

In the emergency department the child's vital signs and level of consciousness are assessed and specific information about the poison is obtained from the parent. The goal of treatment is to prevent further absorption of the poison and to reverse or eliminate its effects. Table 17-6 summarizes emergency management for poisoning.

TABLE 17-6 Emergency Management for Poisoning

1. Stabilize the child. Assess ABCs (airway, breathing, and circulation). Provide ventilatory and oxygen support.
2. Perform a rapid physical examination, start an IV infusion, draw blood for toxicology screen, and apply a cardiac monitor.
3. Obtain a history of the ingestion, including substance ingested, where child was found, by whom, position, when, how long unsupervised, history of depression or suicide, allergies, and any other medical problems.
4. Reverse or eliminate the toxic substance using the appropriate method:

Syrup of ipecac

The use of ipecac is no longer widely promoted because it may not remove all poison and can be harmful in some situations. Activated charcoal is used instead for many types of poisons (West, 1997).

- Assess level of consciousness before administering. Recommended doses are:
  6–12 months: 10 mL; do not repeat
  1–12 years: 15 mL; may repeat one time if vomiting does not occur
  Over 12 years: 30 mL; may repeat one time if vomiting does not occur
- Administer clear fluids, 10–20 mL/kg, after giving ipecac.

Apomorphine

- Assess level of consciousness before administering.
- Given IM or SQ; has rapid onset.
- Give plenty of oral fluids.

Gastric lavage

- Insert a gastric tube through the mouth (use the largest size possible for the size of the child).
- Instill and aspirate normal saline solution until the return is clear. Considered a less effective method of removing ingested substances from the stomach than vomiting. Reserved for children with central nervous system depression, diminished or absent gag reflex, or unwillingness to cooperate with other measures.
- Contraindicated in children who have ingested alkaline corrosive substances, as insertion of the tube may cause esophageal perforation. Used in children who have ingested acids to decrease continued damage and potential perforation of stomach and intestines.

Activated charcoal

- Give to absorb and remove any remaining particles of toxic substances.
- Give a commercial preparation of activated charcoal orally or through a gastric tube. It is available as a ready-to-drink solution in an opaque container. Use a covered cup and straw when giving orally, to prevent the child from seeing the black liquid and to minimize spillage. Give activated charcoal only after the child has stopped vomiting, because aspiration of charcoal is damaging to lung tissue.

Cathartics

- Hasten excretion of a toxic substance and minimize absorption. The most commonly used cathartic is magnesium sulfate.

Antidotes and antagonists

These agents are few, but the most common is Narcan, used for opiate ingestion.

5. Other measures will depend on the child's condition, the nature of the ingested substance, and the time since ingestion. May include diuresis, fluid loading, cooling or warming measures, anticonvulsive measures, antiarrhythmic therapy, hemodialysis, or exchange transfusions.
6. Remember always to treat the child first, not the poison. Maintain the ABCs.

Nursing Management

Once immediate care has been provided, the focus of nursing care shifts to providing emotional support and preventing recurrence.

PROVIDE EMOTIONAL SUPPORT Wait until the child is out of immediate danger before questioning parents in detail about the incident. Encourage parents to express feelings of anger, guilt, or fear about the incident.

PREVENT RECURRENCE Discuss with parents the need to supervise infants and young children at all times. Ask parents how medicines and cleaning agents are stored and whether the house contains any plants. Teach parents proper methods of childproofing the home. Have the PCC number readily available. Instruct parents to keep two bottles of syrup of ipecac available for each child in the home and to be familiar with its use and proper dosage. The PCC must be contacted before this medication is administered at home since it is contraindicated in some poisons (see Table 17-6). Suggest measures for preventing recurrence of poisoning.

SAFETY PRECAUTIONS

The toll-free number for the American Association of Poison Control Centers (AAPCC) is 1-800-222-1222. This number can be accessed from anywhere in the United States and Puerto Rico, and the caller will be connected to the nearest poison control center.

LEAD POISONING

Lead poisoning has been successfully prevented in many areas of the United States, with a substantial decline in lead levels from the mid-1970s. The average serum lead level for children is now 0.6 μg/dL, down from 15 μg/dL in 1976. About 7.6% of children (1.5 million) have levels above the recommended level of <10 μg/dL. Many of these children are poor and live in older houses in inner cities (Centers for Disease Control and Prevention, 2000). Even children with levels below 10 μg/dL may experience cognitive defects due to lead exposure. Lead in paint is the most common source of lead exposure for preschool children. Children are also exposed to lead when they ingest contaminated food, water, and soil or when they inhale dust contaminated with lead. Table 17-7 summarizes several sources of lead exposure.

SAFETY PRECAUTIONS

Mercury is another heavy metal that can produce similar effects in the body to those seen in lead poisoning. Recent mercury levels measured in the National Health and Nutrition Examination Survey found that about 10% of women of childbearing age have had more mercury exposure than is recommended. The major source of mercury begins with pollution from power plants, waste incinerators, and industrial processes. Mercury is emitted into the air and falls to waters where it is ingested by fish. In most states, women of childbearing age and young children are warned to limit consumption of local fish. Other sources of potential mercury contamination such as mercury thermometers should be eliminated (Centers for Disease Control and Prevention, 2001).

TABLE 17-7 Sources of Lead Exposure

Sources
Lead-based paint
Soil and dust
Drinking water from coolers with lead-soldered or lead-lined tanks, from lead-soldered teapots, or from lead pipes or lead-soldered pipes
Food grown in contaminated soil, stored in lead-soldered cans or leaded crystal, or prepared in improperly fired pottery
Parental occupations and hobbies that involve exposure to lead (e.g., plumbing, battery manufacturing, highway construction, furniture refinishing, stained glass work, pottery making)
Airborne lead in areas surrounding smelters and battery manufacturing plants

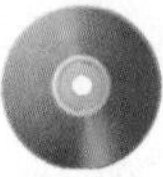

Insider's View: Effects of Lead in the Body

FAMILIES WANT TO KNOW

Avoiding Childhood Poisoning

- Put PCC phone number by every phone in the house.
- Place household cleaners, medications, vitamins, and other potentially poisonous substances out of the reach of children or in locked cabinets. Use warning stickers such as Mr. Yuk on all containers.
- Buy products with childproof caps.
- Store products in their original containers. Never place household cleansers or other products in food or beverage containers.
- Remove all house plants from the child's play areas.
- Use caution when visiting other settings that are not childproofed (e.g., grandparents' homes). Remember that visitors may have pills in their purses or pockets that are easily accessible.

CLINICAL MANIFESTATIONS OF LEAD POISONING

MILD TOXICITY (10–15 μg/dL)	MODERATE TOXICITY (25–69 μg/dL)	SEVERE TOXICITY (>70 μg/dL)
Myalgia or paresthesia	Arthralgia	Paresis or paralysis
Mild fatigue	General fatigue	Encephalopathy (may lead abruptly to seizures, changes in consciousness, coma, and death)
Irritability, Lethargy	Difficulty concentrating	Lead line (blue-black) on gingival tissue
Occasional abdominal discomfort	Muscular exhaustibility Tremor Headache Diffuse abdominal pain Vomiting Weight loss Constipation Anemia	Colic (intermittent, severe abdominal cramps)

Note: Adapted from Agency for Toxic Substances and Disease Registry. (1990). Lead toxicity. *Case studies in environmental medicine* (p. 11). Atlanta: Author.

CULTURE

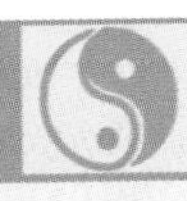

Traditional medicines and cosmetics may contain large amounts of lead. Examples include azarcon and greta, preparations that are used by Mexican-Americans to treat empacho, a coliclike illness; chifong tokuwan, pay-loo-ah, ghasard, bali goli, and kandu, used by some Asian communities; and alkohl, kohl, surma, saoott, and cebagin, used by some Middle Eastern communities.

Children are at greater risk for lead poisoning because they absorb and retain more lead in proportion to their weight than adults do. Lead is particularly harmful to children under the age of 7 years.

Lead interferes with normal cell function, primarily of the nervous system, blood cells, and kidneys, and adversely affects the metabolism of vitamin D and calcium. Clinical manifestations depend on the degree of toxicity. Neurologic effects include decreased IQ scores, cognitive deficits, impaired hearing, and growth delays. Impaired mental function can occur with blood levels even lower than 10 μg/dL. Lead ingestion by a woman during pregnancy can result in fetal malformations, reduced birth weight, and premature birth. Severe lead poisoning, which can result in encephalopathy, coma, and death, is now rare.

Once in the body, lead accumulates in the blood, soft tissues (kidney, bone marrow, liver, and brain), bones, and teeth. Lead that is absorbed by the bones and teeth is released slowly; thus, exposure to even small doses, over time, can result in dangerously high levels of lead in the body.

The Centers for Disease Control and Prevention now recommends screening children at high risk with reduced screening for those at low risk (Harvey, 1997; Centers for Disease Control and Prevention, 1997). In addition, all children enrolled in Medicaid should be tested, with follow-up management and care (Advisory Committee on Childhood Lead Poisoning Prevention, 2000). A blood lead (Pb-B) level is the most useful screening and diagnostic test for lead exposure.

A Pb-B below 10 μg/dL is considered acceptable, although may still not screen out all children with impaired development due to lead. An environmental history should be obtained for children with Pb-B levels between 10 and 19 μg/dL to identify removable sources of lead. Follow-up testing is required. Children with Pb-B levels between 20 and 69 μg/dL require a full medical evaluation, including a detailed environmental and behavioral history, physical examination, and tests for iron deficiency. Interventions to remove sources of lead from the child's environment are necessary. For levels above 25 μg/dL, chelation therapy is also administered. Children with Pb-B levels greater than 70 μg/dL are critically ill from lead poisoning and require immediate chelation therapy and interventions to provide a lead-free environment.

Chelation therapy involves the administration of an agent that binds with lead, increasing its rate of excretion from the body. Calcium disodium ethylenediamine tetraacetate ($CaNa_2$ EDTA), dimercaprol (BAL), d-penicillamine, or succimer (DMSA) may be used. Children with Pb-B levels between 25 and 69 μg/dL receive $CaNa_2$ EDTA for 5 to 7 days, followed by a rest period and then a second chelation treatment. Children with Pb-B levels greater than 70 μg/dL are given both BAL and $CaNa_2$ EDTA, followed by a rest period and a second chelation treatment using $CaNa_2$ EDTA alone. Long-term follow-up of children receiving chelation therapy is essential. The child should never be discharged unless a lead-free home environment has been ensured.

Nursing Management

Nursing care centers on screening, education, and follow-up. Nurses often work with state and local health officials to plan screening for children at high risk of lead exposure. Ask parents about the child's development and eating habits and be alert for risk of lead exposure. Educate parents about sources of lead in the environment and techniques to reduce exposure. Emphasize the importance of housekeeping interventions to reduce exposure to lead dust. These interventions include damp mopping of hard surfaces, floors, window sills, and baseboards; washing the child's hands and face before meals; and frequent washing of toys and pacifiers.

Teach parents the importance of including foods high in iron and calcium in the child's diet to counteract losses of these minerals associated with lead exposure. The child should eat meals at regular intervals, as lead is absorbed more readily on an empty stomach.

Be sure that parents understand the importance of follow-up testing of lead levels. If the child is developmentally delayed, refer the family to an infant stimulation or child development program. Referral to social services and either a visiting nurse or home health care nurse may also be appropriate.

Expected outcomes of nursing care for the child with lead or other poisoning include the following:

- Normal growth and development, including cognition
- Adequate nutritional intake
- Removal of lead or other poisons from the child's environment
- Expressed understanding by family of measures to establish a safe environment for the child

Chapter Highlights

- A variety of structural defects caused by fetal development alterations can affect the gastrointestinal system of infants.
- Cleft lip and palate are structural defects that often involve care by a team of providers such as plastic surgeon, pediatrician, nurse, audiologist, speech therapist, and orthodontist.
- A variety of defects of the esophagus can manifest as mild to life-threatening problems in the newborn period.
- Pyloric stenosis is a common cause of projectile vomiting in the newborn period.
- Children with gastroesophageal reflux are irritable due to lack of food and discomfort when feeding.
- Anatomical malformations of the intestines include omphalocele, Hirschsprung's disease, and anorectal disorders.
- Hernias can be present in the diaphragmatic area, umbilicus, or inguinal canal.
- The most common inflammatory disorder of the gastrointestinal tract is appendicitis.
- Necrotizing enterocolitis is a potentially life-threatening inflammatory disease of the intestines seen primarily in premature infants after enteral feedings are begun.
- Common inflammatory bowel diseases affecting primarily adolescent and young adult age groups are Crohn's disease and ulcerative colitis.
- Peptic ulcer may be primary (often caused by *H. pylori*) or secondary, in situations of stress, trauma, or other disease.
- Several of the intestinal problems of childhood necessitate temporary or permanent ostomy placement.
- Acute vomiting and diarrhea (gastroenteritis) is a common disease that threatens the fluid and electrolyte status of young children.
- A variety of parasitic disorders are seen in children, and preventive methods can be followed to minimize their spread.
- Feeding disorders such as colic and rumination may require teaching and other nursing interventions.
- Celiac disease is a malabsorption disorder caused by gluten sensitivity.

- Short bowel syndrome occurs when surgery is used to treat an intestinal disease and significant sections of the bowel are removed.
- Biliary atresia and hepatitis are the most common liver diseases in young children.
- Abdominal trauma most often occurs to children during motor vehicle crashes.
- Numerous medicines, plants, pesticides, and other household products are accidentally ingested by children each year. Parents must learn how to avoid these poisonings and how to contact the AAPCC in case of accidental exposure.

EXPLORE MediaLink

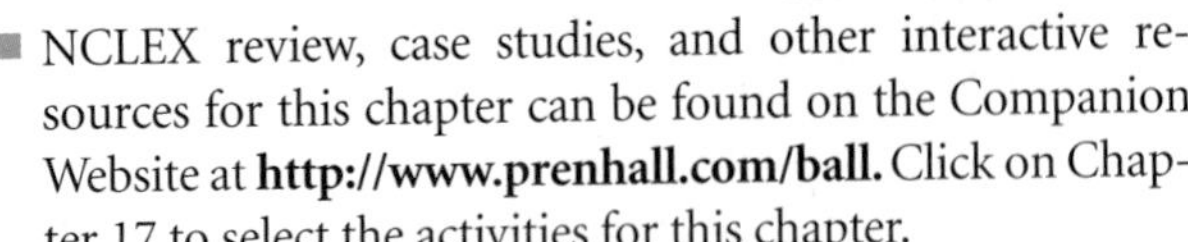

- NCLEX review, case studies, and other interactive resources for this chapter can be found on the Companion Website at **http://www.prenhall.com/ball.** Click on Chapter 17 to select the activities for this chapter.
- For animations, more NCLEX review questions, and an audio glossary, access the accompanying CD-ROM in this textbook.

References

1. Advisory Committee on Childhood Lead Poisoning Prevention. (2000). Recommendations for blood lead screening of young children enrolled in Medicaid: Targeting a group at high risk. *MMWR, Morbidity and Mortality Weekly Report, 49*(RR14), 1–13.
2. Balasubrahmanyam, G., Scherer, N. J., Martin, J. A., & Michal, M. L. (1998). Cleft lip and palate: Keys to successful management. *Contemporary Pediatrics, 15,* 133–153.
3. Barr, J. M. B. (2000). Chronic intestinal pseudo-obstruction: Pediatric case presentations and review of the literature. *Journal of the Society of Pediatric Nurses, 5,* 175–182.
4. Berube, M. (1997). Gastroesophageal reflux. *Journal of the Society of Pediatric Nurses, 2,* 43–46.
5. Borkowski, S. (1998). Pediatric stomas, tubes, and appliances. *Pediatric Clinics of North America, 45,* 1419–1436.
6. Brown, R. L., Irish, M. S., Rice, H. E., Caty, M. G., & Glick, P. L. (1998). Care of the surgical intensive care nursery graduate: The primary care pediatrician's perspective. *Pediatric Clinics of North America, 45,* 1327–1352.
7. Burkhart, D. M. (1999). Management of acute gastroenteritis in children. *American Family Physician,* 60, 2555–63, 2565–6.
8. Castiglia, P. T. (2001). Constipation in children. *Journal of Pediatric Health Care, 15,* 200–202.
9. Centers for Disease Control and Prevention. (1997). *Screening young children for lead poisoning: Guidance for state and local public health officials.* Atlanta: Author.
10. Centers for Disease Control and Prevention. (1999). Prevention of hepatitis A through active or passive immunization: Recommendations of the ACIP. *MMWR, 48*(RR12), 1–37.
11. Centers for Disease Control and Prevention. (2000). Blood lead levels in young children—United States and selected states, 1996–1999. *MMWR, 49,* 1133–1137.
12. Centers for Disease Control and Prevention. (2001). Blood and hair mercury levels in young children and women of childbearing age—United States, 1999. *MMWR, 50,* 140–143.
13. Committee on Nutrition, American Academy of Pediatrics. (1998). *Pediatric nutrition handbook.* Elk Grove Village, IL: American Academy of Pediatrics.
14. Connon, J. J. (1999). Celiac disease. In M. E. Shils, J. A. Olson, J. Shike, & A. C. Ross (eds.), *Modern nutrition in health and disease* (9th ed., pp. 1163–1168).
15. Cowden, J. D., & Hotez, P. J. (2001). A field guide to emerging enteric protozoa. *Contemporary Pediatrics, 18,* 440–447.
16. Cox, K. L. (2000). Liver transplantation. In R. E. Behrman, R. M. Kliegman, & H. B. Jenson, *Nelson textbook of pediatrics* (16th ed., pp. 1227–1229). Philadelphia: Saunders.
17. Eliason, B. C., & Lewan, R. B. (1998). Gastroenteritis in children: Principles of diagnosis and treatment. *American Family Physician, 58,* 1769–1776.
18. Emery, D., & Singer, J. I. (1998). Highly toxic ingestions for toddlers: When a pill can kill. *Emergency Medicine Reports, 3,* 111–122.
19. Estrada, B. (2000). Breast-feeding and vertical transmission of hepatitis C. *Infectious Medicine, 17,* 526–528.
20. Gokhale, R. (2001). Chronic abdominal pain: Inflammatory bowel disease and eosinophilic gastroenteropathy. *Pediatric Annals, 30,* 49–55.
21. Hamilton, J., Rao, P. M., Wagner, J. M., & Miller, D. (1998). Appendicitis: Unmasking the great masquerader. *Patient Care Nurse Practitioner, 1*(5), 11–27.
22. Hartman, G. E. (2000). Diaphragmatic hernia. In R. E. Behrman, R. M. Kliegman, & H. B. Jenson, *Nelson textbook of pediatrics* (16th ed., pp. 1231–1234). Philadelphia: Saunders.
23. Harvey, B. (1997). New lead screening guideline from the Centers for Disease Control and Prevention: How will they affect pediatricians? *Pediatrics, 100,* 384–388.
24. Hendren, W. H. (1998). Pediatric rectal and perianal problems. *Pediatric Clinics of North America, 45,* 1353–1372.
25. Herbst, J. J. (2000). The esophagus; Ulcer disease. In R. E. Behrman, R. M. Kliegman, & H. B. Jenson, *Nelson textbook of pediatrics* (16th ed., pp. 1121–1128; 1147–1150). Philadelphia: Saunders.
26. Hoffenberg, E. J., Bao, F., Eisenbarth, G. S., Uhlhom, C., Haas, J. E., Sokol, R. J., & Rewers, S. (2000). Transglutaminase antibodies in children with a genetic risk for celiac disease. *Journal of Pediatrics, 137,* 356–366.
27. Holst, B., & Ritter, D. (2001). Managing viral hepatitis. *Clinician Reviews, 11,* 51–62.
28. Huff, C. (1997). Celiac disease: Helping families adapt. *Gastroenterology Nursing, 20,* 79–81.
29. Irish, M. S., Pearl, R. H., Caty, M. G., & Glick, P. L. (1998). The approach to common abdominal diagnoses in infants and children. *Pediatric Clinics of North America, 45,* 729–773.
30. Jakubik, L. D., Colfer, A., & Grossman, M. B. (2000). Pediatric short bowel syn-

drome: Pathophysiology, nursing care, and management issues. *Journal of the Society of Pediatric Nurses, 5,* 111–121.

31. Kazacos, K. R. (2000). Protecting children from helminthic zoonoses. *Contemporary Pediatrics* (Suppl.), 1–24.

32. Levy, J. (2001). Gastroesophageal reflux and other causes of abdominal pain. *Pediatric Annals, 30,* 42–47.

33. Li, B. U. K. (1996). Cyclic vomiting: New understanding of an old disorder. *Contemporary Pediatrics, 13,* 48–62.

34. Litovitz, T. L., Klein-Schwartz, W., White, S., Cobaugh, D. J., Youniss, J., Drab, A., & Benson, B. E. (2000). 1999 annual report of the American Association of Poison Control Centers Toxic Exposure Surveillance System. *American Journal of Emergency Medicine, 18,* 517–574.

35. McDiarnid, S. V. (2000). Liver transplantation. The pediatric challenge. *Clinical Liver Disease, 4,* 879–927.

36. Mitchell, J. C., & Wood, R. J. (2000). Management of cleft lip and palate in primary care. *Journal of Pediatric Health Care, 14,* 13–19.

37. Murphy, M. S. (1998). Guidelines for managing acute gastroenteritis based on a systematic review of published research. *Archives of Disease in Childhood, 79,* 279–288.

38. Murray, K. F., & Christie, D. L. (2000). Vomiting in infancy: When should you worry? *Contemporary Pediatrics, 17,* 81–115.

39. National Institutes of Health. (2000). Hepatitis C. *Community Drug Alert Bulletin* (NIH Publication No. 00–4663). Bethesda MD: author.

40. National Safety Council. (2000). *Injury facts.* Itasca, IL: Author.

41. Nehring, W. M., & Vessey, J. A. (2000). Down syndrome. In P. L. Jackson & J. A. Vessey, *Primary care of the child with a chronic condition* (pp. 445–474). St. Louis: Mosby.

42. Nowicki, M. J., & Bishop, P. R. (1999). Organic causes of constipation in infants and children. *Pediatric Annals, 28,* 293–300.

43. O'Donnell, K. A., Glick, P. L., & Caty, M. G. (1998). Pediatric umbilical problems. *Pediatric Clinics of North America, 45,* 791–812.

44. Orenstein, J. (2000). Update on intussusception. *Contemporary Pediatrics, 17,* 180–191.

45. Pearl, R. H., Irish, M. S., Caty, M. G., & Glick, P. L. (1998). The approach to common abdominal diagnoses in infants and children: Part II. *Pediatric Clinics of North America, 45,* 1287–1326.

46. Pena, B. M. G., Taylor, G. A., & Lund, D. P. (1999). Appendicitis revisited: New insights into an age-old problem. *Contemporary Pediatrics, 16,* 122–133.

47. Powers, K. S. (2000). Diagnosis and management of common toxic ingestions and inhalations. *Pediatric Annals, 29,* 330–343.

48. Rao, P. M., Rhea, J. J., Novelline, R. A., Mostatavi, A. A., & McCabe, C. J. (1998). Effect of computed tomography of the appendix. *New England Journal of Medicine, 338,* 141–146.

49. Shovein, J. T., Damazo, R. J., & Hyams, I. (2000). Hepatitis A: How benign is it? *American Journal of Nursing, 100,* 43–48.

50. Snyder, J. (1997, July). Feeding during diarrhea: New AAP guidelines and innovations in oral rehydration solutions. *Contemporary Pediatrics Reporter,* 6.

51. SPLIT Research Group. (2001). Studies of pediatric liver transplantation (SPLIT): Year 2000 outcomes. *Transplantation, 72,* 463–476.

52. Stoll, B. J., & Kliegman, R. M. (2000). Digestive system disorders. In R. E. Behrman, R. M. Kliegman, & H. B. Jenson, *Nelson textbook of pediatrics* (16th ed., pp. 510–518). Philadelphia: Saunders.

53. Uhrich, K. S., & Mackin, A. L. (2001). Cleft lip and palate. *AJN, 101,* 24AA–FF.

54. Warner, B. W. (1996). Classification of congenital disorders of the anorectum. In A. M. Rudolph, J. I. E. Hoffman, & C. D. Rudolph, *Rudolph's pediatrics* (29th ed., pp. 1112). Stamford, CT: Appleton & Lange.

55. West, L. (1997). Innovative approaches to the administration of activated charcoal in pediatric toxic ingestions. *Pediatric Nursing, 23,* 616–619.

56. Westerdahl, J. (1999). Botanicals in pediatrics. In P. Q. Samour, K. K. Helm, & C. E. Lang, *Handbook of pediatric nutrition* (2nd ed., pp. 589–600). Gaithersburg, MD: Aspen Publishers.

57. Wong, W. Y., Eskes, T. K., Kuihpers-Jagtman, A. M., Spauwen, P. H., Steegers, E. A., Thomas, C. M., Hamel, B. C., Blom, H. J., & Steegers-Theunissen, R. P. (1999). Nonsyndromic orofacial clefts: Association with maternal hyperhomocysteinemia. *Teratology, 60,* 253–257.

58. Wylie, R. (2000). Ileus, adhesions, intussusception, and closed loop obstructions. In R. E. Behrman, R. M. Kliegman, & H. B. Jenson, *Nelson textbook of pediatrics* (16th ed., pp. 1141–1144). Philadelphia: Saunders.

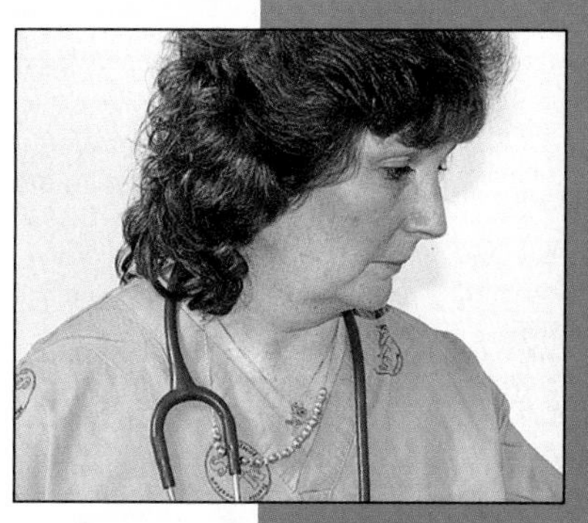

"PROVIDING CARE TO CHILDREN LIKE TERRELL IS CHALLENGING, BECAUSE THE TREATMENT OFTEN INTERFERES WITH A CHILD'S REGULAR ACTIVITIES. WE ALL HOPE THAT TERRELL RECEIVES A KIDNEY TRANSPLANT SOON SO HIS GROWTH WILL IMPROVE AND HE WILL NOT HAVE TO CONTINUE TO MISS SCHOOL DURING TREATMENT."

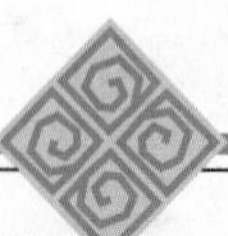

Terrell, who is now 5 years old, was born with posterior urethral valves, which caused damage to his kidneys. Despite undergoing surgery to correct the defect at 2 years of age, his kidney function continued to deteriorate. End-stage renal disease was diagnosed 2 years ago, and dialysis treatment was started 3 months later. Terrell is waiting for a kidney transplant, but no family member is able or willing to donate a kidney. As a result, Terrell has been placed on the list for a cadaver kidney.

Terrell was initially treated with peritoneal dialysis, but after having several peritoneal infections in the first year, his health care team and family decided that hemodialysis should become his recommended treatment. He comes to the dialysis center three afternoons a week for treatments that last about 3 to 4 hours. This schedule permits him to go to kindergarten classes in the morning.

What are the special concerns of the nurse in monitoring a child who is receiving hemodialysis treatment? Is Terrell at any higher risk for infection than other children? Does he need a special diet? What are the potential complications of this disease and of the hemodialysis treatments for Terrell's growth and development? If a kidney becomes available for transplant, what special teaching will the family need to receive to assure the best survival of the kidney graft? The answer to these questions and information about many other genitourinary conditions are presented in this chapter.

CHAPTER 18

ALTERATIONS IN GENITOURINARY FUNCTION

KEY TERMS

azotemia Accumulation of nitrogenous wastes in the blood.

dialysate The solution used in dialysis.

end-stage renal disease Irreversible kidney failure.

enuresis Involuntary micturition by a child who has reached the age at which bladder control is expected.

hydronephrosis Collection of urine in the renal pelvis as a result of obstructed outflow.

oliguria Diminished urine output (less than 0.5–1 mL/kg/hr).

osteodystrophy Defective mineralization of bone caused by renal failure and chronic hyperphosphatemia.

renal insufficiency Any degree of renal failure in which the kidneys' ability to conserve sodium and concentrate the urine decreases.

stent A device used to maintain patency of the urethral canal after surgery.

uremia Toxicity resulting from the buildup of urea and nitrogenous waste in the blood.

vesicoureteral reflux The backflow of urine from the bladder into the ureters during voiding.

MediaLink 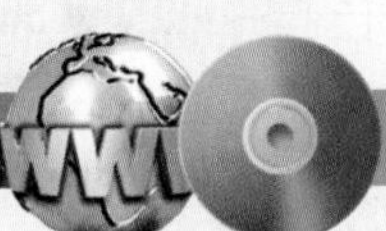 http://www.prenhall.com/ball

Resources for this chapter can be found on the CD-ROM accompanying this textbook, and on the Companion Website at http://www.prenhall.com/ball. Click on Chapter 18 to select the activities for this chapter.

CD-ROM

Animation
- Renal Function

Audio Glossary

NCLEX Review

COMPANION WEBSITE

Web Links

NCLEX Review

MediaLink Applications
- Developing an Enuresis Care Plan
- Discussing Sexual Activity with Adolescents

What are the consequences of urinary and renal disorders such as end-stage renal disease, or irreversible kidney failure, in children? What specific and nonspecific signs alert parents and health care professionals to suspect these disorders?

Many infections, structural disorders, and disease processes alter genitourinary function. Because the kidneys and other urinary system organs perform several essential body functions, including removal of waste products and maintenance of fluid and electrolyte balance, disorders that affect these organs pose a significant threat to the health of children.

Although the reproductive system is functionally immature until puberty, disorders involving these organs may also have a significant impact on the health of children. Uncorrected structural defects and sexually transmitted diseases can have both psychologic and physiologic implications on the developing child.

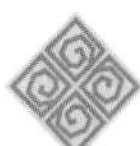

ANATOMY AND PHYSIOLOGY OF PEDIATRIC DIFFERENCES

The genitourinary system consists of the urinary and reproductive organs. The urinary system—kidneys, ureters, bladder, and urethra (Figure 18-1 ◆)—functions to excrete wastes and maintain acid–base and fluid and electrolyte balance. The reproductive system consists of internal and external organs that at maturity function to promote the conception and healthy development of a fetus.

URINARY SYSTEM

All of the nephrons that will comprise the mature kidneys are present at birth. The kidneys grow and the tubular system matures gradually during childhood, reaching full size by adolescence. Most renal growth occurs during the first 5 years of life. This increase in size is due primarily to enlargement of the nephrons. The efficiency of the kidney also increases with age. During the first 2 years of life, the kidneys are less efficient at regulating electrolyte and acid–base balance (refer to Chapter 10) and eliminating some drugs from the body. After the age of 2 years, the kidneys' efficiency increases markedly. Because the kidney is less able

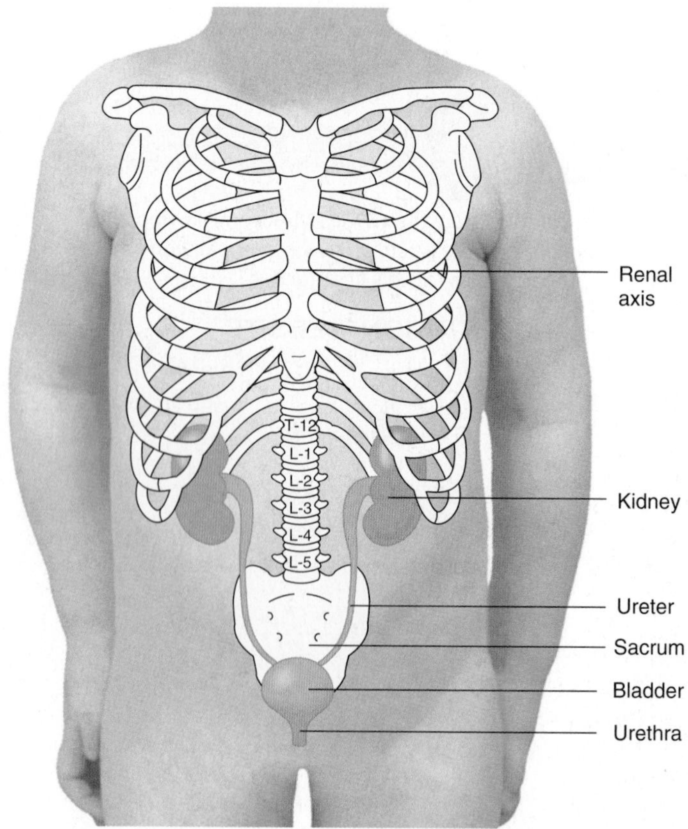

FIGURE 18-1 ◆
The kidneys are located between the twelfth thoracic (T12) and third lumbar (L3) vertebrae.

to concentrate urine in infancy, urine output per kilogram of body weight is higher in infancy than in later childhood or adolescence.

Bladder capacity increases with age from 20 to 50 mL at birth to 700 mL in adulthood. Stimulation of "stretch receptors" within the bladder wall initiates urination. Simultaneous contraction of the detrusor muscle of the bladder and relaxation of the internal and external sphincters result in emptying of the bladder. Children less than 2 years of age cannot maintain bladder control because of insufficient nerve development.

REPRODUCTIVE SYSTEM

The reproductive system in children is functionally immature until puberty. Throughout childhood the genitalia (with the exception of the clitoris in girls) enlarge gradually. Anatomic and functional development accelerates with the hormonal changes of puberty (see Chapter 4 and Figures 4-41 and 4-42). In girls, the mons pubis becomes more prominent and hair begins to grow. The vagina lengthens and the epithelial layers thicken. The uterus and ovaries enlarge, and the musculature and vascularization of the uterus also increase. In boys, downy hair begins to appear at the base of the penis, and the scrotum becomes increasingly pendulous. The penis increases in length and width.

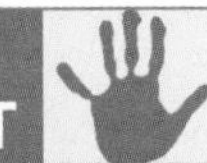

GROWTH & DEVELOPMENT

Urinary output per kilogram of body weight decreases as the child ages, because the kidney becomes more efficient at concentrating urine. Expected output:

Infants	2 mL/kg/hr
Children	0.5–1 mL/kg/hr
Adolescents	40–80 mL/hr

CLINICAL TIP

A child's bladder capacity (in ounces) can be estimated by adding 2 to the child's age. For example, the normal bladder capacity of a 4-year-old is 6 ounces.

STRUCTURAL DEFECTS OF THE URINARY SYSTEM

BLADDER EXSTROPHY

Bladder exstrophy is a rare defect in which the posterior bladder wall extrudes through the lower abdominal wall (Figure 18-2 ◆). Failure of the abdominal wall to close during fetal development results in eversion and protuberance of the bladder wall and a wide separation of the rectus muscles and the symphysis pubis. The upper urinary tract is usually normal. The defect occurs in approximately 1 in every 400,000 live births and is more common in boys than girls by a ratio of 3 to 1 (Ben-Chaim, Docimo, & Jeffs, et al., 1996). The bladder mucosa appears as a mass of bright red tissue, and urine continually leaks from an open urethra. Females have a bifid clitoris. Males have a short, stubby penis; and the glans is flattened with dorsal chordee and a ventral prepuce. Epispadias and bilateral inguinal hernias are also common.

Treatment is surgical reconstruction, which is performed in several stages. The initial stage (bladder closure) is usually completed within 24 to 48 hours after birth. Epispadias repair and closure of the symphysis pubis are often performed simultaneously. Surgery to reconstruct the bladder neck and reimplant the ureters is performed when the child is 2 to 3 years of age. The goals of surgical reconstruction are (1) bladder and abdominal wall closure; (2) urinary continence, with preservation of renal function; (3) creation of functional and normal-appearing genitalia; and (4) improvement of sexual functioning. Some children require permanent urinary diversion, because a functional bladder cannot be reconstructed. In some patients with a very small or bifid penis, gender reassignment may be considered.

Because the bladder epithelium is abnormal, it is prone to neoplasms. Periodic examination and cystoscopy after the age of 20 years are recommended to evaluate for possible malignancies.

Nursing Management

Preoperative nursing care centers on preventing infection and trauma to the exposed bladder. The bladder mucosa is covered in sterile plastic wrap to prevent trauma and irritation, and the surrounding area is cleaned daily and protected from leaking urine with a skin sealant.

Postoperatively, the wound and pelvis are immobilized to facilitate healing. Internal and external immobilization techniques are used for pelvic closure (see Chapter 21). Avoid abduction of the infant's legs. Nursing care includes maintaining proper alignment, monitoring peripheral circulation, and providing meticulous wound and skin care.

Renal function is monitored by assessing the adequacy of urine output and blood and urine chemistries. Observe for any signs of obstruction in the drainage tubes such as increased intensity of bladder spasms, decreased urine output, or urine or blood draining from the urethral meatus. Promote comfort and give antibiotics as ordered.

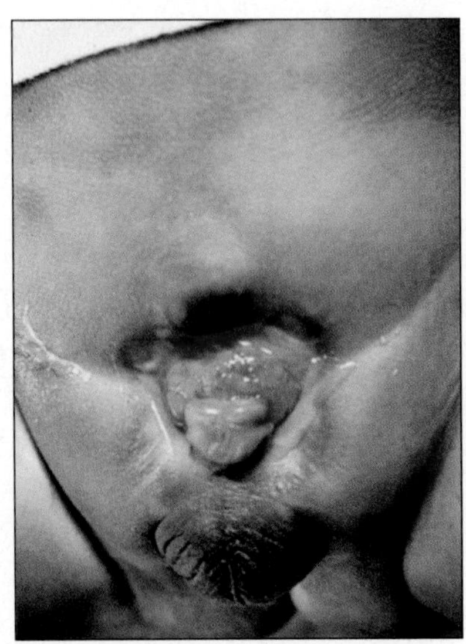

FIGURE 18-2 ◆ This child has bladder exstrophy, noted by extrusion of the posterior bladder wall through the lower abdominal wall.

Parents need emotional support to help them cope with the disfiguring nature of the infant's defect and the uncertainty of complete repair. To promote parent–infant bonding, encourage parents to participate in all aspects of the infant's care, including bathing, feeding, and wound care. Discharge teaching should include instructions about dressing changes and diapering and the need to immediately report any signs of infection or change in renal function. Emphasize the need for routine follow-up visits after surgery to assess urinary function and to ensure that the next stages of surgery for continence control are performed at the appropriate time and age in the child's development. However, continence is not always achieved by these children. Parents need help to promote the child's self-esteem and self-confidence with sexual identity and function. Psychological counseling may be beneficial to the child during adolescence.

HYPOSPADIAS AND EPISPADIAS

Hypospadias and epispadias are congenital anomalies involving the location of the urethral meatus in males (Figure 18-3 ◆). Both defects result from failure of the urethral folds to fuse completely over the urethral groove.

The reported incidence of hypospadias is 1 in every 300 male births, nearly double that of earlier rates (Paulozzi, Erickson, & Jackson, 1997). The increased incidence is thought to be associated with environmental elements or genetic factors. The urethral meatus can be located anywhere along the course of the anterior urethra on the ventral surface of the penile shaft, from the perineum to the tip of the glans. Most cases are mild, with the meatus slightly off center from the tip of the penis; in severe cases, the meatus is located on the scrotum. Hypospadias often occurs in conjunction with congenital chordee, a fibrous line of tissue that results in ventral curvature of the penile shaft and undescended testes.

In epispadias, the meatal opening is located on the dorsal surface of the penile shaft. Epispadias often occurs in conjunction with exstrophy of the bladder.

Diagnosis is made prenatally by ultrasound or by examination at birth. The infant should not be circumcised because the dorsal foreskin tissue will be used for surgical repair. The defects are corrected surgically, usually during the first year of life, to minimize psychologic effects when the child is older. Surgery is usually performed in a single operation, often as an outpatient procedure. The goals of surgical repair are (1) placement of the urethral meatus at the end of the glans penis with satisfactory caliber and configuration for a urinary stream (enabling the child to void in a standing position) and (2) release of chordee to straighten the penis (enabling future sexual function).

A caudal nerve block is often used for postoperative pain relief. Muscle relaxants may be prescribed to relieve bladder spasms.

Nursing Management

It is important for the nurse to address parents' concerns at the time of birth. Preoperative teaching can relieve some of their anxiety about the future appearance and functioning of the penis.

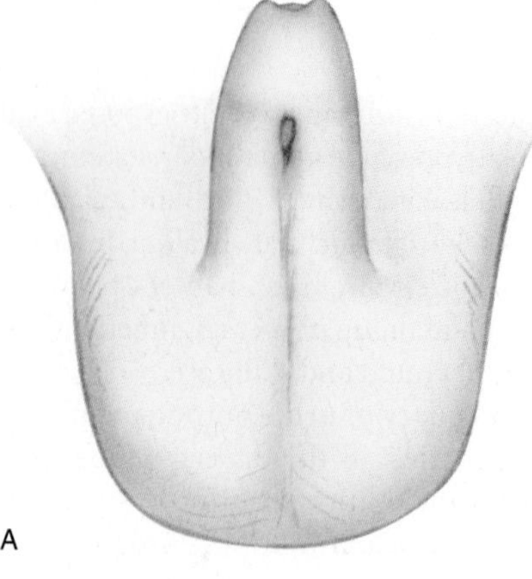

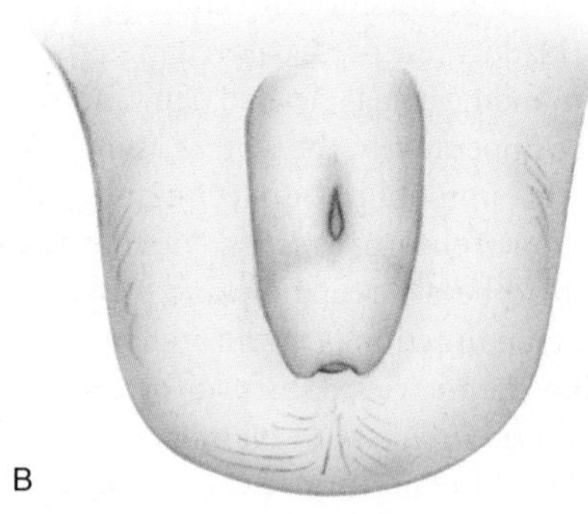

FIGURE 18-3 ◆
Hypospadias and epispadias. A, In hypospadias the urethral canal is open on the ventral surface of the penis. B, In epispadias the canal is open on the dorsal surface.

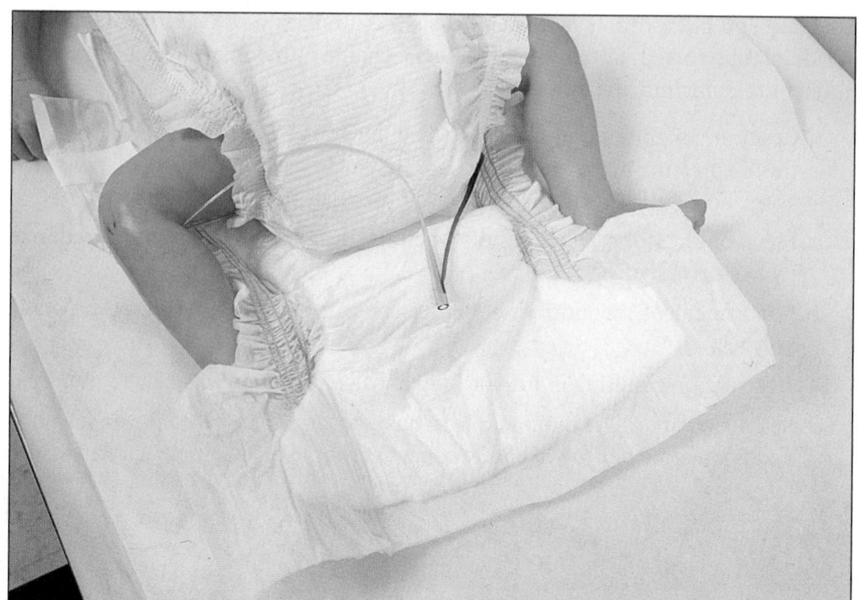

FIGURE 18-4 ◆
A double diapering technique protects the urinary stent after surgery for hypospadias or epispadias repair. The inner diaper collects stool; the outer diaper, urine.

Postoperative care focuses on protecting the surgical site from injury. The infant or child returns from surgery with the penis wrapped in a simple dressing, and sometimes a urethral **stent** (a device used to maintain patency of the urethral canal) is placed to keep the new urethral canal open. Plan care to ensure that the stent does not get removed. Refer to the hospital's policy for the appropriate use of mechanical restraints in this situation.

Skill 12-2: Double Diapering with a Stent in Place

Encourage fluid intake to maintain adequate urinary output and patency of the stent. Accurate documentation of intake and output is essential. Notify the physician if there is no urine drainage for 1 hour, as this may indicate kinks in the system or obstruction by sediment. Pain may be associated with bladder spasms. Anticholinergic medications such as oxybutynin or hyoscyamine may be prescribed. Acetaminophen may also be given for pain. Antibiotics are often prescribed until the urinary stent falls out.

Patients are often discharged the day of surgery. Discharge teaching should include instructions for parents about care of the reconstructed area, fluid intake, medication administration, and signs and symptoms of infection (Figure 18-4 ◆). Inform parents of the need to go to the physician's office for dressing removal about 4 days after surgery.

OBSTRUCTIVE UROPATHY

Obstructive uropathy refers to structural or functional abnormalities of the urinary system that interfere with urine flow. The pressure caused by urine backup compromises kidney

FAMILIES WANT TO KNOW

Caring for the Child after Hypospadias and Epispadias Repair

- Use the double-diapering technique shown to protect the stent (the small tube that drains the urine).
- Restrict the infant or toddler from activities (e.g., playing on riding toys) that put pressure on the surgical site. Avoid holding the infant or child straddled on the hip. Limit the child's activity for 2 weeks.
- Encourage the infant or toddler to drink fluids to ensure adequate hydration. Provide fluids in a pleasant environment or using a special cup. Offer fruit juice, fruit-flavored ice pops, fruit-flavored juices, flavored ice cubes, and gelatin.
- Be sure to give the complete course of prescribed antibiotics to avoid infection.
- Watch for signs of infection: fever, swelling, redness, pain, strong-smelling urine, or change in flow of the urinary stream.
- The urine will be blood tinged for several days. Call the physician if urine is seen leaking from any area other than the penis.

function and often causes **hydronephrosis** (accumulation of urine in the renal pelvis as a result of obstructed outflow). Physiologic changes that may occur as a result of hydronephrosis include the following:

- Cessation of glomerular filtration when the pressure in the kidney pelvis equals the filtration pressure in the glomerular capillaries (In response, the blood pressure increases as the body attempts to increase the glomerular filtration pressure.)
- Metabolic acidosis, which results when the distal nephrons are impaired in their ability to secrete hydrogen ions
- Impairment of the kidney's ability to concentrate urine, resulting in polydipsia and polyuria
- Obstruction resulting in urinary stasis, which promotes the growth of bacteria
- Restriction of urinary outflow, which causes progressive renal damage if left untreated (As a consequence, the growth of the kidneys may be arrested, or renal failure may occur.)

PATHOPHYSIOLOGY ILLUSTRATED

Obstruction Sites

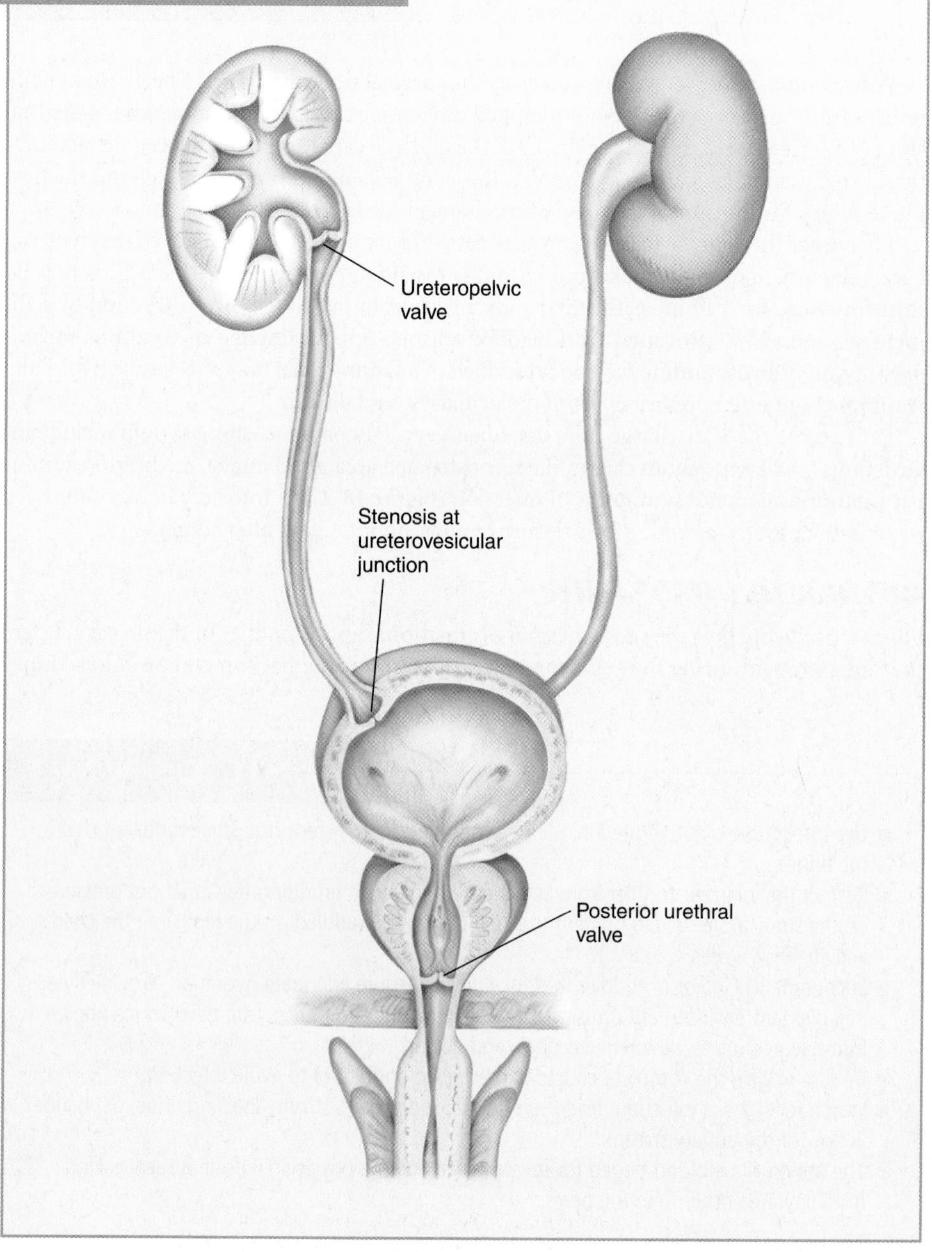

FIGURE 18-5 ◆
The common sites of obstruction in the upper and lower urinary tract. Why would damage from posterior urethral valves potentially be worse than other obstructions? Upper urinary tract infections are often unilateral. Renal failure is most likely to occur when both kidneys are affected by hydronephrosis.

Obstructive uropathy may be caused by several congenital lesions such as ureteropelvic junction (UPJ) obstruction, posterior urethral valves (PUVs), and stenosis at the ureterovesicular junction (Figure 18-5 ◆). The ureteropelvic junction is the most common site of obstruction of the upper urinary tract in infants and children. Posterior urethral valves (abnormal folds of mucosa in the male urethra) are the most common cause of anatomic bladder outlet obstruction, occurring in approximately 1 in every 5,000 to 8,000 live male births. Other conditions that can lead to hydronephrosis include myelomeningocele, neoplasms, and prune-belly syndrome. Clinical manifestations vary, depending on the cause and location of the obstruction.

Early diagnosis and treatment are necessary to prevent kidney damage and deterioration of renal function. Hydronephrosis may be detected by prenatal ultrasound, but milder obstructions may not become apparent until later in infancy or childhood. Table 18-1 lists diagnostic tests commonly used to identify urinary tract conditions.

The goals of surgical correction or diversion are to lower the pressure within the collecting system, which prevents parenchymal damage, and to prevent stasis, which decreases the risk of infection. Surgical correction may necessitate pyeloplasty (removal of an obstructed segment of the ureter and reimplantation into the renal pelvis) or valve repair or reconstruction, depending on the cause of the obstruction. Urinary incontinence resulting from sphincter weakness is a common problem after surgery.

PRUNE-BELLY SYNDROME

Prune-belly syndrome, also known as Eagle–Barrett syndrome, is a congenital defect characterized by failure of the abdominal musculature to develop. The skin covering the abdominal wall is thin and resembles a wrinkled prune. Other characteristics include urinary tract anomalies, poor ureteral peristalsis, enlarged bladder, high risk for recurrent urinary tract infection, and bilateral cryptorchidism. Prune-belly syndrome occurs predominantly in males (95%), with an incidence of 1 in 29,000–40,000 births (Becker & Avner, 1995).

Nursing Management

Preoperative nursing care focuses on preparing the parents and child for the procedure and addressing parents' concerns about the postsurgical outcome. Provide parents with an opportunity to discuss concerns about the effect of the disorder on the child's long-term renal functioning.

CLINICAL MANIFESTATIONS OF OBSTRUCTIVE LESIONS OF THE URINARY SYSTEM

OBSTRUCTIVE LESION	CLINICAL MANIFESTATIONS
Ureteropelvic junction obstruction	In infants: Abdominal mass (enlarged kidney), hypertension, urinary tract infection In children: Hematuria, pain, intermittent nausea and vomiting
Posterior urethral valves	In infants: Abdominal mass (enlarged kidney), distended bladder, poor urinary stream, urinary tract infection, sepsis, low specific gravity, polyuria, increased creatinine level, failure to thrive In children: Urinary frequency and incontinence
Ureterovesicular junction obstruction	Urinary tract infection (recurrent or chronic), hematuria, pain, abdominal mass (enlarged kidney), enuresis

TABLE 18-1 Diagnostic Tests for Urinary System Conditions

TEST	USE
Voiding cystourethrogram	Shows bladder structure and function, urethral anatomy, bladder masses. Detects vesicoureteral reflux
Renal ultrasound	Identifies large renal scars, renal anomalies, obstruction, abscesses, masses, and hydronephrosis
Diuretic renogram	Identifies lesions that become symptomatic during increased urine flow
Radionucleotide scan	Detects renal parenchymal lesions, renal atrophy, or scars. Differentiates between hydronephrosis caused by obstructive lesions, reflux, or a cyst
Renal cortical scintigraphy	Documents pyelonephritis and renal scarring
Serum creatinine	Evaluates kidney function

Postoperative care involves monitoring vital signs and intake and output and observing for signs of urine retention, such as decreased output and bladder distention. Many children are discharged with stents or catheters. Teach parents how to change dressings, care for catheters, assess pain and give analgesics, and recognize signs of possible obstruction or infection. Parents should encourage the child to participate in age-appropriate activities; however, contact sports should be avoided because of their potential to injure the bladder.

URINARY TRACT INFECTION

A urinary tract infection (UTI) is of bacterial, viral, or fungal origin, and occurs in the urinary tract. Cystitis is a lower UTI that involves the urethra or bladder. Pyelonephritis is an upper UTI that involves the ureters, renal pelvis, and renal parenchyma. UTIs can be acute or chronic (the latter either recurrent or persistent).

UTIs are the second most common infections in children. What accounts for the high incidence of these infections? Among newborns and young infants, most infections occur in boys. These infections are usually associated with structural defects having a higher incidence in males (e.g., obstructive uropathy), which predispose the infant to infection. A higher rate of UTIs also occurs among uncircumcised infants (Anderson & Anderson, 1999). Among older infants and children, the incidence of UTIs is higher in girls. This is attributed to the shorter female urethra (2 cm [1 in.] in young girls) and its proximity to the anus and vagina, which increases the risk of contamination by fecal bacteria.

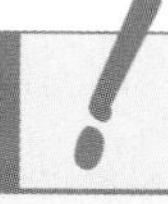

NURSING ALERT

Rule out a urinary tract infection in any child under 2 years of age with a fever of unknown origin.

ETIOLOGY AND PATHOPHYSIOLOGY

Many first UTIs are caused by *Escherichia coli,* a common gram-negative enteric bacterium. Other causative organisms include *Staphylococcus, Klebsiella, Proteus, Pseudomonas, Enterobacter,* and *Enterococcus.*

Urinary stasis enhances the risk of UTI. Stasis may be caused by abnormal anatomic structures or abnormal function (e.g., a neurogenic bladder, which is common in children with myelomeningocele). Infrequent voiding, which is common in school-age children, also increases the risk of UTI. Children normally void five to six times a day. Some children, however, develop the habit of urinating only once or twice a day, which results in incomplete emptying of the bladder and urinary stasis. Other factors associated with increased risk of UTI include an irritated perineum, constipation, masturbation, sexual abuse, and sexual activity in adolescent females.

Another cause of UTI is **vesicoureteral reflux,** the backflow of urine from the bladder into the ureters during voiding. This prevents complete emptying of the bladder and creates a reservoir for bacterial growth. Vesicoureteral reflux can also result from a structural anomaly in which the ureters insert in an abnormal position into the bladder.

Renal scarring can result from hydronephrosis or pyelonephritis due to the inflammatory and ischemic effects of the infection. Scars have been associated with hypertension, proteinuria, and kidney failure. The risk of kidney damage increases in the following instances:

- Children less than 1 year of age
- Delay in diagnosis and effective antibacterial treatment for an upper UTI
- Anatomic or neurologic obstruction
- Recurrent episodes of upper UTIs

CLINICAL MANIFESTATIONS

Symptoms depend not only on the location of the infection, but also on the age of the child. Symptoms in the newborn period tend to be nonspecific—unexplained fever, failure to thrive, poor feeding, vomiting and diarrhea, strong-smelling urine, and irritability. Not until the toddler years are the more "classic" symptoms of lower urinary tract infection listed in the clinical manifestations table. About 40% of UTIs are asymptomatic.

URINARY TRACT INFECTION CLINICAL MANIFESTATIONS AND THERAPY

TYPE OF UTI	CLINICAL MANIFESTATIONS	CLINICAL THERAPY
Lower UTI—Cystitis	Frequency, dysuria, urgency, enuresis, strong-smelling urine.	Five to 7-day course of trimethoprim or sulfamethoxazole or antibiotic matching organism sensitivity, encourage fluids, analgesic such as acetominophen or pyridium
Upper UTI—Pyelonephritis	High fever, chills, abdominal pain, flank pain, persistent vomiting, moderate to severe dehydration	Rehydration, antipyretics, IV antibiotics initially then transitioned to oral antibiotics matching organism sensitivity for a total of 7 to 10 days

CLINICAL THERAPY

A urine specimen is examined for the presence of bacteria. A dipstick leukocyte esterase test identifies white blood cells and pyuria. A nitrite dipstick detects bacteria. Using both dipsticks increases the sensitivity (88%) and specificity (93%) for diagnosing a UTI (Shaw & Gorelick, 1999). Diagnosis is confirmed with a urine culture collected by midstream clean-catch void, sterile catheterization, or suprapubic aspiration. Urine collection bags used on infants are reliable only when no pathogens are found. The diagnosis of infection is made from the number of colony-forming units (between 10^3 to 10^5), depending upon the method of urine collection (Shaw & Gorelick, 1999). Antibiotic sensitivity for the specific organisms cultured is then determined.

Skills 6-7, 6-8: Collecting Clean-Catch Urine and Catheter Specimens

Radiologic studies are often performed to detect structural abnormalities and renal scarring. A renal ultrasound is often obtained soon after the diagnosis, and a voiding cystourethrogram (VCUG) is obtained after the infection has cleared. These are the most commonly performed tests. Renal cortical scintigraphy has become the most commonly used imaging study to detect pyelonephritis and renal scarring (Hellerstein, 2000).

Antibiotic therapy is initiated as soon as urine samples have been collected. Once the culture sensitivity information is obtained, the antibiotic is changed if necessary. Follow-up cultures should be obtained 48 to 72 hours after drug therapy initiation, at which time the urine should be sterile. Follow-up urine cultures should then be obtained monthly for 3 months, every 3 months for 6 months, and then annually. Subsequent infections may be asymptomatic. For children with vesicoureteral reflux or recurrent infections, a long-term suppressive dose of an antibiotic may be ordered for prophylaxis. Children with renal scarring should have their blood pressure monitored.

Children who appear ill and cannot tolerate oral antibiotics are often hospitalized because of the need for rehydration and initiation of parenteral antibiotic treatment. Infants may develop permanent kidney damage or generalized sepsis if the UTI is not treated aggressively. If a structural defect is identified, surgical correction may be necessary to prevent recurrent infections that could lead to renal damage.

NURSING MANAGEMENT

Nursing Assessment and Diagnosis

PHYSIOLOGIC ASSESSMENT

A history of urinary symptoms is obtained. Assess the infant for toxic (very ill) appearance, fever, and oral fluid intake. Measure the child's height and weight and plot on a growth curve to identify any change in growth pattern associated with a chronic illness. Take the infant's or child's blood pressure. Palpate the abdomen and suprapubic and costovertebral areas for masses, tenderness, and distention. Observe the urinary stream if possible and perform a urinalysis, including specific gravity. Proper collection of the urine specimen is essential. A clean-catch urine specimen may be obtained if the child is able to cooperate (refer to the Skills Manual). If not, a catheterized sample is obtained. An-early morning urine specimen is preferred because the urine is more concentrated. A blood culture may be obtained to assess for sepsis.

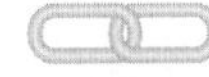

Skills 5-2, 5-3: Measuring Height and Weight

Psychosocial Assessment

Sexually active adolescents may deny having symptoms because they fear disclosure of their sexual activity to their parents. Careful questioning may be necessary to elicit these concerns. Be open and approachable and allow the patient and family the opportunity to address their concerns (see informed consent in the Skills Manual).

Following are common nursing diagnoses for the child with a UTI:

- *Altered urinary elimination,* related to recurrent urinary tract infections
- *Risk for altered growth,* related to chronic infection and renal damage
- *Urinary retention,* related to infrequent voiding habits or vesicoureteral reflux
- *Risk for ineffective management of therapeutic regimen,* related to lack of knowledge of preventive measures (adequate fluid intake, proper hygiene, signs and prophylactic antibiotics)
- *Risk for fluid volume deficit,* related to fever and inadequate intake

Planning and Implementation

Skill 5-21: Measuring Intake and Output

Skill 12-1: Performing a Urinary Catheterization

Nursing care for the hospitalized child with a complicated UTI centers on administering prescribed medications, promoting rehydration, assessing renal function, and teaching parents and older children how to minimize the risk of future infection.

Administer antibiotics and antipyretics as prescribed to maintain therapeutic drug levels and reduce fever. Encourage fluid intake to dilute the urine and flush the bladder. Document intake and output. Assess renal function by comparing the child's output with the expected measure of 1 mL/kg/hr and weigh the child daily. Frequent voiding minimizes urinary stasis. Postvoid catheterization may be needed to determine the amount of residual urine left after urinating. Palpate or percuss the bladder after voiding to evaluate bladder emptying.

Because bladder training is such an important milestone for young children, any disorder that affects voiding may have developmental implications. A toddler who has been potty trained may regress and require diapers temporarily due to incontinence related to the UTI. Reassure parents that this is normal and emphasize that they should offer the toddler support rather than disapproval. A preschooler may perceive the infection as punishment for an imagined wrong such as masturbation. Provide support and reassurance that the child is not being punished for any actions.

Care in the Community

Teach prevention through proper hygiene, especially for girls, reinforcing the importance of (1) avoiding bubble baths, (2) wearing cotton underwear, (3) avoiding tight-fitting pants, and (4) always wiping the perineum from front to back after bowel movements.

Children with UTIs are usually cared for at home. Teach parents the importance of giving antibiotics as prescribed and assist them to develop an effective schedule. Emphasize that antibiotics must be taken for the full course and that they may be continued even after the infection has cleared to prevent a recurrence.

FAMILIES WANT TO KNOW

Preventive Strategies for Urinary Tract Infections

- Teach proper perineal hygiene. Girls should always wipe the perineum from front to back after voiding.
- Encourage the child to drink plenty of fluids and avoid long periods of "holding urine."
- Caution against tight underwear; children should wear cotton rather than nylon underwear.
- Encourage the child to void more frequently and to fully empty the bladder.
- Discourage bubble baths and hot tubs, which can irritate the urethra.
- Encourage abstinence of sexual activity. However, if girls are sexually active instruct them to void before and after sexual intercourse to prevent urinary stasis and flush out bacteria introduced during intercourse.

Give parents specific guidelines for oral fluid intake. Ensure that the amount of fluids recommended for a 24-hour period equals the maintenance fluids needed plus additional fluids required because of fever and diuresis to flush out pathogens (see Chapter 10.) Suggest that the parents avoid giving the child caffeinated and carbonated beverages as these may potentially irritate the bladder mucosa (Miller, 1996).

Encourage the child to void more frequently even after the infection has cleared. A wristwatch with an alarm may be a helpful reminder. The child with a neurogenic bladder needs to have clean intermittent catheterization performed several times a day to reduce urinary stasis and the potential for UTI. See guidelines below for teaching this procedure to families and children.

Teach parents the signs and symptoms of recurrent infection and to seek care promptly.

Evaluation

Expected outcomes of nursing care include the following:

- The child increases fluid intake and number of times voiding each day.
- Future UTIs are prevented.

FAMILIES WANT TO KNOW

Clean Intermittent Catheterization

Clean intermittent catheterization (CIC) is performed to empty the bladder when nerves for bladder control are missing or damaged. This procedure must be performed every 3 to 4 hours during the day, but is usually not done when the child sleeps at night. The child is ready to learn self-catheterization when he or she really wants to be dry and is learning independence. Until that time, the parents usually perform CIC.

EQUIPMENT NEEDED

- Four or five catheters of the size and type recommended. Each catheter is used until it becomes hard and brittle (about 1 month).
- Water-soluble lubricant (not Vaseline)

HOW PERFORMED

- Usually clean technique is used. Wash hands with soap and water, then spread lubricant on the tip of the catheter. Hold the catheter like a pencil in one hand, about 8 cm (3 in.) from the tip. Position the other end of the catheter over the toilet or a container.

GIRLS

- Spread the labia with the other hand and slide the catheter 5 to 8 cm (2 to 3 in.) into the urethra until urine begins to flow, then 2.5 cm (1 in.) further, up to 8 cm (3 in.) maximum.
- Hold the catheter in place until all urine flows out, then slowly remove it. If more urine begins to flow, let it drain before removal.

BOYS

- Hold the penis outward with the other hand and slide the catheter into the penis until urine begins to flow, then 2.5 cm (1 in.) further, up to 12 to 15 cm (5 to 6 in.) maximum. A sphincter muscle is located at the opening to the bladder, and it sometimes feels very tight. If the catheter will not slide into the bladder easily, use constant but gentle pressure on the sphincter muscle with the tip of the catheter. It will soon feel the pressure and gradually open up, allowing the catheter to slip in.
- Hold the catheter in place until all urine flows out, then slowly remove it. If more urine begins to flow, let it drain before removal.

STORAGE

- Wash the catheter with soap and water and shake out excess water. Store the catheter in a plastic bag after use.
- Keep a catheter in the car, bookbag, fanny pack, or at school. (The catheter can be carried to school in a toothbrush holder to avoid embarrassment.)

Note: Adapted from Ball, J. W. (1998). Mosby's pediatric patient teaching guides. St. Louis: Mosby.

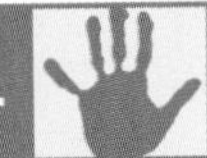

GROWTH & DEVELOPMENT

An estimated 15% to 20% of children who are partially toilet trained will continue to have wetting episodes after 5 years of age. An estimated 5% of 10-year-olds and 2% of 12- to 14-year-olds continue to have nocturnal enuresis (Issenman, Filmer, & Gorski, 1999).

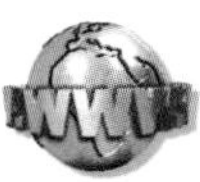

Enuresis Support and Resources

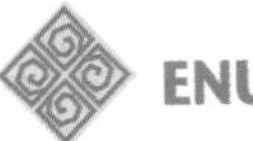

ENURESIS

Enuresis is repeated involuntary voiding by a child who has reached an age at which bladder control is expected, usually about 5 to 6 years of age (see Table 18-2 for bladder control milestones). Enuresis can occur either at night (nocturnal, 50% of cases), during the day (diurnal, 10% of cases), or both night and day (40% of cases) (Kelleher, 1997). Nocturnal enuresis occurs more often in boys than in girls, with a 3.5:1 ratio, whereas diurnal enuresis is more common in girls. Three types of enuresis are distinguished: primary, intermittent, and secondary (Table 18-3).

Enuresis may result from neurologic or congenital structural disorders, illness, or stress. Nocturnal enuresis occurs with high frequency in children whose parents have a history of bedwetting. There is a 77% risk if both parents had enuresis, a 44% risk if one parent had enuresis, and a 15% risk if neither parent had enuresis (Tobias, 2000). In most children with primary enuresis, the bladder has a smaller functional capacity, and neuromuscular maturation of the inhibitory fibers is delayed. Minor abnormalities of the bladder neck and urethra are also associated with enuresis. Some children are believed to have mild developmental delays. Often children with nocturnal enuresis are harder to arouse and may fail to respond to full bladder signals. In some children, unstable bladder contractions may occur during sleep resulting in enuresis. The majority of cases (95%) are not associated with structural or neurologic pathology.

Diabetes mellitus or renal insufficiency should be ruled out in children with both enuresis and polyuria or oliguria. Examine the child's lower spine for fistulas, sacral dimples, or tufts of hair that could be signs of occult spina bifida. Prolonged hospitalization, family stressors, and preoccupation with school concerns also have been associated with secondary enuresis. Children with diurnal enuresis may have frequency, urgency, constant dribbling, and involuntary loss of control after voiding.

TABLE 18-2 Milestones in the Development of Bladder Control

AGE	DEVELOPMENTAL MILESTONE
1 1/2 years	Child passes urine at regular intervals.
2 years	Child announces when he or she is voiding.
2 1/2 years	Child makes known need to void; can hold urine.
3 years	Child goes to the bathroom by himself or herself; holds urge if preoccupied with play.
2 1/2–3 1/2 years	Child achieves nighttime control.
4 years	Child shows great interest in going to bathrooms when away from home (shopping centers, movies).
5 years	Child voids approximately 7 times a day; prefers privacy; is able to initiate emptying of bladder at any degree of fullness.

TABLE 18-3 Types of Enuresis

Primary enuresis: Child has never had a dry night; attributed to maturational delay and small functional bladder; not associated with stress or psychiatric cause.
Intermittent enuresis: Child has occasional nights or periods of dryness.
Secondary enuresis: Bedwetting that occurs in a child who has been reliably dry for 6–12 months; associated with stress, infections, and sleep disorders.

A thorough history can help identify potential causes of enuresis (Table 18-4). Asking about the child's elimination patterns and developmental milestones and the parents' methods of toilet training can provide essential information (see Table 2–18). Laboratory evaluation includes urinalysis and urine culture. Renal studies such as ultrasound and VCUG are done in cases of secondary enuresis.

A multitreatment approach is usually most effective. Fluid restriction, bladder training, and enuresis alarms are common approaches (Table 18-5). A spontaneous cure rate occurs in 15% of children each year, regardless of intervention used or lack of intervention. Approximately one-third of children with nocturnal enuresis are treated with medications. Imipramine, a tricyclic antidepressant, is often used but requires close monitoring because of its effects on mood and sleep-arousal patterns and the associated dangers of overdoses. Desmopressin, given as a nasal spray, has an antidiuretic effect but is not used long term because of its expense. Its use is primarily reserved for times when the child is away from home for a short period (e.g., sleep-overs or camp). Relapse often occurs when medications are stopped. Avoidance of foods believed to contribute to enuresis may be recommended such as those containing caffeine, milk, chocolate, and citrus (Tobias, 2000).

CLINICAL TIP

Enuretic children often have a history of constipation. Rectal pressure on the posterior bladder wall stimulates the bladder to empty.

NURSING MANAGEMENT

Teach the child and parents about the physiologic development of bladder control and causes and treatment of enuresis. Explore feelings of guilt or blame. Make sure the parents are aware that the child cannot control the wetting. Psychosocial support is an essential part of care since stress is an important cause of secondary enuresis. Provide emotional support to the parents and child, and encourage the child's participation in the treatment plan. Refer the child for counseling or therapy if appropriate.

Assess the parents' and child's motivation and readiness for interventions. Before parents purchase an enuresis alarm, suggest they use an alarm clock in the child's room for several

TABLE 18-4 Questions to Ask When Taking an Enuresis History

Family History
Is there a family history of renal or urinary structural abnormalities?
Is there a family history of bedwetting?

Family Management
How serious is the problem for the family?
What happens when the child wets? (Who gets up and changes sheets?)
How is the child treated? Is the child punished or blamed for wetting?
What remedies have been tried?

Toilet Training
Did the child have a difficult time with toilet training?
What method of toilet training was used? When was toilet training initiated?
What are the child's current voiding and stooling patterns?
How long is the child's longest dry period, and when does it occur?
Does the child have a history of constipation or encopresis?

Stressors
How is the child doing in school?
Are any new or chronic stressors present in the child's life?
How does the problem interfere with play and other activities?

Risk Factors
Diabetes
- Does the child void often or have urgency?
- Is the child frequently thirsty?

Urinary Tract Infection
- Does the child experience burning on urination?
- Has the child had a urinary tract infection before?

TABLE 18-5 Treatment Approaches for Enuresis

APPROACH	DESCRIPTION
Fluid restriction	Fluid intake is limited in the evening and before the child goes to bed.
Bladder exercises	The child drinks a large amount and then holds urine as long as possible. The child practices stopping voiding midstream. Exercises should continue for at least 6 months.
Timed voiding	The child with diurnal enuresis is instructed to void every 2 hours and to use a double voiding pattern; this trains the bladder to empty completely and avoid overdistention.
Enuresis alarms	A detector strip is attached to the child's pants. The alarm sounds a buzzer that alerts the child when wetting occurs, so the child can get up and finish voiding in the bathroom. This works best for children over 7 years old, and takes 3–4 months for success.
Reward system	Set realistic goals for the child and reinforce dry days or nights with stars and stickers on a chart.
Medications	Imipramine is prescribed nightly for 2–4 months and then tapered over several months to reduce the rate of relapse. It is effective in 50%–70% of children. Desmopressin is prescribed for special events such as camp or sleep-overs in cases of nocturnal enuresis. Oxybutynin is used for diurnal enuresis to relieve urgency and frequency from bladder irritability.

nights to see if the child will arouse. Determine whether the child shares a room with others who will be disturbed by the alarm. Ask if the child and parents are willing to persist with an enuresis alarm, as it may take months to work. Evaluation of nursing care includes families selecting the intervention that is best suited for their lifestyle, and an increase in the number of dry nights.

RENAL DISORDERS

NEPHROTIC SYNDROME

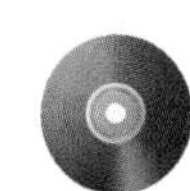

Renal Function

Nephrotic syndrome refers not to a specific disease, but to a clinical state characterized by edema, massive proteinuria, hypoalbuminemia, hypoproteinemia, hyperlipidemia, and altered immunity. Nephrotic syndrome is classified as congenital, primary, or secondary. Congenital nephrotic (CNF) syndrome, an autosomal recessive disorder, is extremely rare. The CNF gene is localized on the long arm of chromosome 19 (19q13.1) (Goodyer & Kashtan, 1998). Primary nephrotic syndrome results from a disease, such as glomerulonephritis, that affects only the kidney. Secondary nephrotic syndrome results from a disease, such as diabetes, lupus, or sickle-cell anemia, with multisystem effects.

Approximately 80% of children with nephrotic syndrome have a type of primary disease called minimal change nephrotic syndrome (MCNS). MCNS usually occurs in children between the ages of 2 and 7 years, with an incidence of 3 per 100,000 children, and is approximately twice as common in boys as in girls (Gilman & Mooney, 1998). MCNS derives its name from the fact that the glomeruli appear normal or show only minimal changes on light microscopic evaluation. Because MCNS is the most common form of nephrotic syndrome, it is the focus of the following discussion.

Etiology and Pathophysiology

What accounts for the dramatic symptoms of altered renal functioning in children with nephrotic syndrome? Why do proteinuria, hypoalbuminemia, hyperlipidemia, and altered immunity develop in these children?

The cause of primary MCNS is unknown, but an immune system role is strongly suspected. The mechanism of increased glomerular permeability is unknown as the glomeruli appear normal. Usually, a minute amount of protein is present in the urine. In MCNS, however, increased permeability of the glomerular membrane permits large, negatively charged molecules such as albumin to pass through the membrane and be excreted in the urine. Proteinuria results in decreased oncotic pressure and the development of edema, because fluid remains in the interstitial spaces instead of being pulled back into the vascular compartment. Loss of protein in the urine, as well as insufficient albumin production by the liver and a decreased albumin concentration as a result of salt and water retention by the kidney contribute to the development of hypoalbuminemia.

Because the kidney reabsorbs salt and water, edema develops. Immunoglobulins are lost, resulting in altered immunity. The liver, stimulated perhaps by hypoalbuminemia or decreased osmotic pressure, responds by increasing synthesis of lipoprotein (cholesterol), resulting in hyperlipidemia.

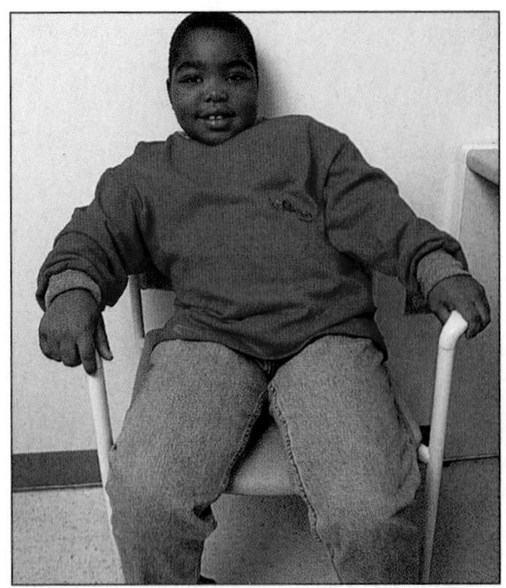

FIGURE 18-6 ◆
This boy has generalized edema, a characteristic finding in nephrotic syndrome.

Clinical Manifestations

In most children, edema develops gradually over several weeks. Children may have a history of periorbital edema on waking that resolves during the day as fluid shifts to the abdomen and lower extremities. Other signs include weight gain, hypertension, irritability, anorexia hematuria, and nonspecific malaise (Gilman & Mooney, 1998). The child's urine may be frothy or foamy. Medical treatment often is not sought until generalized edema develops on the child's extremities, abdomen, or genitals (Figure 18-6 ◆). Respiratory distress from pleural effusion may occur in some cases.

Massive edema resulting in a dramatic weight gain and abdominal pain, with or without vomiting, may occur, depending on the amount of albumin lost and the amount of sodium ingested. The child becomes malnourished as a result of protein loss in the urine. The skin is pale and shiny with prominent veins, and the hair quality becomes more brittle.

CLINICAL TIP

The following signs may indicate that a child has MCNS.

- Weight gain greater than expected in relation to previous pattern
- Snug fit of clothing, tight-fitting shoes
- Extreme skin pallor
- Irritability and fatigue
- Decreased urine output

Clinical Therapy

Diagnosis is based on the history, physical examination, presence of characteristic symptoms, and laboratory findings. Serum albumin and other blood studies may be ordered. Edema begins to develop in children when the serum albumin concentration falls below 20 g/L (Tune & Mendoza, 1997). Urinalysis reveals massive proteinuria (50 mg/kg/day), the primary indicator of nephrotic syndrome. Microscopic hematuria may also be present. The serum creatinine or BUN are increased in some cases.

Children may be hospitalized when severe edema or a major infection is present. Treatment generally occurs on an outpatient basis. Clinical therapy focuses on decreasing proteinuria, relieving edema, managing associated symptoms, improving nutrition, and preventing infection. A corticosteroid (such as prednisone), the drug of choice, is prescribed to decrease proteinuria. In most children, urine protein levels fall to trace or negative values within 2 to 3 weeks of the start of therapy. Children who respond successfully to therapy continue to take corticosteroids daily for 6 weeks and 6 weeks of alternate-day treatment. The relapse rate has been improved with this protocol (Tune & Mendoza, 1997).

LABORATORY VALUES

A protein-to-creatinine (PR/CR) ratio of the first-morning void is used to estimate protein excretion in children because of the challenges in obtaining 24-hour urines. A ratio of >0.2 is found in children over 2 years with MCNS.

Approximately 85% of children experience complete remission with corticosteroid therapy. A relapse is commonly associated with a respiratory infection or live virus immunizations; however, relapses become less frequent or stop during puberty (Gilman & Mooney, 1998). Repeat therapy is administered to children who have a relapse after drug therapy is discontinued. Alkylating agents such as chlorambucil and cyclophosphamide have been effective in children with frequently recurring nephrotic syndrome, but they have serious side effects, including carcinogenesis and 15% to 20% risk of sterility in males (Tune & Mendoza, 1997). If steroid therapy is ineffective, a renal biopsy is performed to identify other causes for the child's symptoms.

To reduce massive edema, intravenous administration of albumin or oral diuretics may be ordered. Since diuretics can precipitate hypovolemia, hyponatremia, and hypokalemia, electrolyte levels should be carefully monitored. An angiotensin-converting enzyme (ACE) inhibitor may be used to decrease protein excretion. Broad-spectrum antibiotics are prescribed to treat any infections.

NURSING ALERT

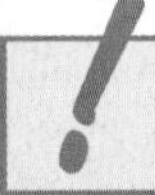

No live virus immunizations should be given to a child with nephrotic syndrome who is relapsing or receiving corticosteroid treatment.

A diet that is normal for the child's age is recommended. No attempt should be made either to restrict or to increase protein intake. A "no added salt" diet is recommended during corticosteroid treatment.

NURSING MANAGEMENT

Nursing Assessment and Diagnoses

Physiologic Assessment

Careful assessment of the child's hydration status and edema is essential. Monitor intake and output and vital signs and record these findings accurately. Perform a careful assessment for respiratory distress associated with pleural effusion (see Chapter 13). Test urine for proteinuria and specific gravity at least once each shift.

Psychosocial Assessment

Children and parents are often fearful or anxious on admission. Because edema often develops gradually, parents may feel guilty if they did not seek medical attention immediately. School-age children with generalized edema are often concerned about their appearance. Careful questioning may be necessary to elicit these concerns. The child who is hospitalized for a recurrence of nephrotic syndrome may be frustrated or depressed. Assess individual and family coping mechanisms, support systems, and level of stress.

Following are common nursing diagnoses for the child with MCNS:

- *Risk for infection,* related to immunosuppressive therapy
- *Risk for impaired skin integrity,* related to edema, lowered resistance to infection and injury, immobility, and malnutrition
- *Fluid volume excess,* related to renal dysfunction and sodium retention
- *Altered nutrition: Less than body requirements,* related to loss of appetite and protein loss in urine
- *Fatigue,* related to fluid and electrolyte imbalance, albumin loss, altered nutrition, and renal failure
- *Diversional activity deficit,* related to fatigue, immobility, and social isolation

Planning and Implementation

Nursing care is mainly supportive and focuses on administering medications, preventing infection, preventing skin breakdown, meeting nutritional and fluid needs, promoting rest, and providing emotional support to the parents and child.

Administer Medications

It is important to give prescribed medications at the scheduled times. Watch for side effects of corticosteroids such as moon face, increased appetite, increased hair growth, abdominal distention, and mood swings. If the child is receiving albumin intravenously, monitor closely for hypertension or signs of volume overload caused by fluid shifts. If diuretics are used, observe for shock. The child may need to have albumin infused simultaneously with diuretics.

Prevent Infection

Children with MCNS are at risk for infection because of the loss of immunoglobulins in the urine, other alterations of the immune system associated with renal failure, and corticosteroid therapy. Careful handwashing is important. Use standard precautions. Strict aseptic technique is essential during invasive procedures. Monitor the child's white blood cell count when cytotoxic drugs are given because of bone marrow suppression. Monitor vital signs carefully to detect early signs of infection that may be masked by corticosteroid therapy. Decrease the child's social contacts during immunosuppressive treatment, and caution parents and children to avoid exposure to individuals with respiratory infections and communicable diseases. Emphasize the importance of avoiding shopping malls, sporting arenas, grocery stores, game stores, and other public areas where the risk of exposure to such infections is increased.

Prevent Skin Breakdown

Meticulous skin care is essential to prevent skin breakdown and potential infection. Perform repeated skin assessments, turn the child frequently, and use therapeutic mattresses (e.g., egg crate, airflow) to help prevent skin breakdown. Keep the skin clean and dry.

Meet Nutritional and Fluid Needs

Keep the child's food preferences in mind when planning menus. Encourage the child to eat by presenting attractive meals with small portions. Mealtimes should center on pleasurable socialization. Encourage the child to eat meals with other children on the unit. Fluids are not usually restricted.

Carefully monitor intake and output. Weigh the child daily using the same scale, and measure abdominal girth to monitor changes in edema and ascites (see Figure 10-12). Monitor vital signs every 4 hours to watch for signs of respiratory distress, hypertension, or circulatory overload.

Promote Rest

Provide opportunities for quiet play as tolerated, such as drawing, playing board games, listening to tapes, and watching videos. Adjust the child's daily schedule to allow rest periods after activities. Signs of fatigue may include irritability, mood swings, or withdrawal. Inform the parents and child about the importance of rest. Limiting visitors during the acute phase of the illness may be necessary. Telephone contacts may be encouraged as an alternative to visitors. To provide a sense of control, encourage the child to set his or her own limits on activity.

Provide Emotional Support

Parents and children often need support to cope with this chronic disease. Provide parents with thorough explanations about the child's disease and treatment regimen. Parental anxiety in combination with the hospitalization may interfere with the child's independence. Assist parents to promote the child's independence by allowing the child to select food from the menu or to select the daily activity schedule. This gives the child some sense of control.

Children with MCNS may have a distorted body image because of sudden weight gain and edema. Behavioral manifestations may include refusal to look in the mirror, refusal to participate in care, and decreased interest in appearance. Encourage children to express their feelings. Help them maintain a normal appearance by promoting normal grooming routines. Encourage children to wear their own pajamas rather than hospital gowns. Scarves or hats may be used to lessen the child's edematous appearance.

Discharge Planning and Home Care Teaching

Provide parents and school-age children with explanations of the disease process, prognosis, and treatment plan. Ensure that parents know how to administer medications and can identify potential side effects. Inform parents about restricting fluid intake until the edema resolves. Instruct parents about the need to monitor urine daily for protein, and have them keep a diary to record results. Monitoring the child's weight each week may help identify early stages of fluid retention. This helps parents to identify signs of a relapse before edema occurs.

Tutoring may be required for a short period after discharge. However, parents should be encouraged to allow the child to return to normal activities once the acute episode has resolved. Emphasize the importance of avoiding contact with individuals who have infectious diseases, because of the child's reduced immunity. Reinforce to parents that as long as the child is receiving corticosteroid therapy or shows signs of MCNS, the no added salt diet should be followed. Warn them about the appetite stimulant effects of steroids and to control food intake and weight gain. Immunizations should be withheld until 6 months after the completion of corticosteroid therapy. Although immunizations may trigger a relapse, pneumococcal vaccine and other immunizations are important to protect the child from serious preventable infections.

Most children do well with corticosteroid therapy; however, relapses commonly occur. Even those children with frequent relapses usually have a spontaneous resolution of MCNS before 30 years of age.

NURSING ALERT

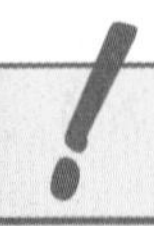

Traditionally, a high-protein, low-salt diet was recommended for children with MCNS. Current data, however, suggest that the high-protein diet increases urinary protein loss and may accelerate the development of renal failure. On the other hand, low-protein diets may lead to protein deficiency. For these reasons, a regular-protein, low-salt diet is recommended.

Skill 5-7: Measuring Abdominal Girth

Evaluation

Expected outcomes of nursing care include the following:

- The child responds to corticosteroid therapy.
- Dietary guidelines of no added salt are followed and food intake is controlled during corticosteroid therapy.
- Relapses are identified by parents before edema occurs.
- The child receives the additional recommended immunizations.

A discussion of Wilm's tumor can be found in Chapter 16.

CLINICAL TIPS

Normal renal function requires the following:

- Unimpaired renal blood flow
- Adequate glomerular ultrafiltration
- Normal tubular function
- Unobstructed urine flow

GROWTH & DEVELOPMENT

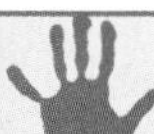

The following factors increase the risk of acute renal failure.

Infants
- Critically ill neonate
- Obstructive uropathy
- Dehydration
- Hemolytic-uremic syndrome

Toddler
- Poisoning (e.g., acetaminophen, mushrooms)

School-age Child and Adolescent
- Trauma

NURSING ALERT

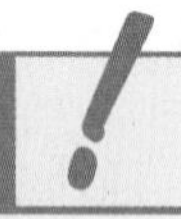

Nephrotoxic drugs include the following:

- Antimicrobials: aminoglycosides, cephalosporins, tetracycline, sulfonamides
- Radiographic contrast media with iodine
- Heavy metals: lead, barium, iron
- Nonsteroidal anti-inflammatory drugs (NSAIDS): indomethacin, aspirin

RENAL FAILURE

Renal failure occurs when the kidney is unable to excrete wastes and concentrate urine. There are two types of renal failure: acute and chronic. Acute renal failure occurs suddenly (over days or weeks) and may be reversible, whereas in chronic renal failure, kidney function diminishes gradually and permanently over months or years.

Both types of renal failure are characterized by **azotemia** (accumulation of nitrogenous wastes in the blood) and sometimes **oliguria** (urine output <0.5 to 1 mL/kg/hr), indicating the kidney's inability to excrete metabolic waste products. The degree of renal impairment is estimated by the degree of azotemia and the increase in serum creatinine level. **Uremia** occurs when there is an excess of urea and other nitrogenous waste products in the blood.

Acute Renal Failure

Acute renal failure (ARF), which occurs when kidney function abruptly diminishes, is characterized by a rapid rise in the BUN level. The kidneys are also unable to regulate extracellular fluid volume, sodium balance, and acid–base homeostasis. ARF occurs most frequently in neonates who are critically ill with asphyxia, shock, and sepsis. It can also be a postoperative complication of cardiac surgery or may result from drug toxicity.

ETIOLOGY AND PATHOPHYSIOLOGY ARF may be caused by prerenal, postrenal, or intrinsic factors. Prerenal ARF is a result of decreased perfusion to an otherwise normal kidney in association with a systemic condition. Hypovolemia (hemorrhage or dehydration), septic shock, or cardiac failure may precipitate prerenal ARF. This is the most common type of ARF in infants and young children.

Intrinsic ARF results from primary damage to the parenchymal cells of the kidneys. Damage can be caused by infection, diseases such as hemolytic-uremic syndrome or acute glomerulonephritis, cortical necrosis, nephrotoxic drugs, or accidental ingestion of drugs or poisons. The structure most susceptible to damage is the kidney tubule. Injury to the tubule resulting in acute tubular necrosis is the most frequent cause of intrinsic renal failure in children.

Postrenal ARF is caused by obstruction of the urinary flow from both kidneys, such as occurs in posterior urethral valves or a neurogenic bladder. Children may have oliguria, or normal or increased urine output. Renal failure without oliguria usually indicates a less severe renal injury. Children who recover from ARF may have residual kidney damage and compromised renal function.

CLINICAL MANIFESTATIONS Characteristically, a healthy child suddenly becomes ill with nonspecific symptoms, including nausea, vomiting, lethargy, edema, gross hematuria, oliguria, and hypertension (Vogt, 1997). These symptoms are a result of electrolyte imbalances, uremia, and fluid overload. The child appears pale and lethargic. See the clinical manifestations tables for more information.

Hyperkalemia is the most life-threatening electrolyte disorder associated with ARF. An increase in serum potassium adversely affects the electrical conductivity within the heart. Hyponatremia affects central nervous system function, resulting in symptoms that range from fatigue to seizures. Edema occurs as a result of sodium and water retention. (Refer to Chapter 10 for a discussion of these fluid and electrolyte alterations.) Children with ARF are also more susceptible to infection because of depressed immune functioning.

CLINICAL MANIFESTATIONS OF ACUTE VERSUS CHRONIC RENAL FAILURE

TYPE OF RENAL FAILURE	CLINICAL MANIFESTATIONS
Acute renal failure	Gross hematuria, headache, edema, severe hypertension, lethargy, nausea and vomiting, oliguria
Chronic renal failure	Fatigue, malaise, poor appetite, prolonged unexplained nausea and vomiting, failure to thrive, poor school performance, secondary enuresis, chronic anemia, hypertension, and unusual bone disease (fractures with minimal trauma, rickets, valgus deformity)

Note: From Vogt, B. A. (1997). Identifying kidney disease: Simple steps can make a difference. *Contemporary Pediatrics, 14*(3), 115–119.

CAUSES AND CLINICAL MANIFESTATIONS OF ELECTROLYTE IMBALANCES IN ACUTE RENAL FAILURE

ELECTROLYTE IMBALANCE AND CAUSE	CLINICAL MANIFESTATIONS
Hyperkalemia Results from inability to inadequately excrete potassium derived from diet and catabolized cells. In metabolic acidosis, there is also movement of potassium from intracellular fluid to extracellular fluid.	■ Peaked T waves, widening of QRS on ECG. ■ Dysrhythmias: ventricular dysrhythmias, heart block, ventricular fibrillation, cardiac arrest ■ Diarrhea ■ Muscle weakness
Hyponatremia In the acute oliguric phase, hyponatremia is related to the accumulation of fluid in excess of solute.	■ Change in level of consciousness ■ Muscle cramps ■ Anorexia ■ Abdominal reflexes, depressed deep tendon reflexes ■ Cheyne-Stokes respirations ■ Seizures
Hypocalcemia Phosphate retention (hyperphosphatemia) depresses the serum calcium concentration. Calcium is deposited in injured cells. Hyperkalemia and metabolic acidosis may mask the common clinical manifestations of severe hypocalcemia.	■ Muscle tingling ■ Changes in muscle tone ■ Seizures ■ Muscle cramps and twitching ■ Positive Chvostek sign (contraction of facial muscles after tapping facial nerve just anterior to parotid gland)

Note: Data from Chan, J. C. M., Alon, U., & Oken, D. E. (1992). Acute renal failure. In C. M. Edelman, Jr. (Ed.), *Pediatric kidney disease* (2nd ed., pp. 1923–1940). Boston: Little, Brown.

CLINICAL THERAPY Diagnosis of renal failure is based primarily on urinalysis and blood chemistry results, including BUN, serum creatinine, sodium, potassium, and calcium levels (Table 18-6). The kidneys are normal in size and no signs of osteodystrophy are found on x-ray. Various imaging studies to assess kidney size, renal blood flow, and renal perfusion and function may be performed to determine whether the child has ARF or chronic renal failure.

Treatment depends on the underlying cause of the renal failure. The goal of treatment is to minimize or prevent permanent renal damage while maintaining fluid and electrolyte balance and managing complications. Eliminate all potential sources of potassium intake until hyperkalemia is controlled (see Chapter 10). Initial emergency treatment of children with fluid depletion focuses on fluid replacement at 20 mL/kg of saline or lactated Ringer's solution given rapidly or over 5 to 10 minutes to ensure renal perfusion. Albumin may also be administered when blood loss is the cause of circulatory depletion. If oliguria persists after restoration of adequate fluid volume, intrinsic renal damage is suspected. Children with fluid overload, like those with pulmonary edema, need diuretic therapy, and dialysis if the response to diuretics is poor.

TABLE 18-6 Diagnostic Tests for Renal Failure

TEST	NORMAL VALUES	FINDINGS IN ARF
Urinalysis		
pH	4.5–8.0	Lowered
Osmolarity	50–1,400 mosm/L	>500 prerenal <350 intrinsic
Specific gravity	1.001–1.030	High: prerenal ARF Low: intrinsic ARF Normal: postrenal ARF
Protein	Negative	Positive
Blood Chemistry		
Potassium	3.5–5.8 mmol/L	Elevated
Sodium	135–148 mmol/L	Normal, low, or high, depends solely on the amount of water in the body
Calcium	2.2–2.7 mmol/L	Low
Phosphorus	1.23-2.0 mmol/L	High
Urea nitrogen	3.5–7.1 mmol/L	Increased
Creatinine	0.2–0.9 mmol/L	Increased
pH	7.38–7.42	Low acidic

ARF, acute renal failure.

Fluid requirements are calculated to maintain zero water balance. Intake should equal output. Nutrition must be maintained with extra carbohydrate intake during the catabolic state. Antibiotics are prescribed for infection. Nephrotoxic antibiotics such as aminoglycosides are avoided.

Some children whose ARF is unresponsive to management require dialysis to correct severe electrolyte imbalances, manage fluid overload, and cleanse the blood of waste products. The clinical situation and age of the child will determine whether hemodialysis or peritoneal dialysis will be used. Refer to "Renal Replacement Therapy" later in this chapter.

Prognosis depends on the cause of ARF. When renal failure results from drug toxicity or dehydration, the prognosis is generally good. However, ARF that results from diseases such

MEDICATIONS USED TO TREAT COMPLICATIONS OF ACUTE RENAL FAILURE

Complication	Medication	Action or Indication	Nursing Implications
Hyperkalemia (>5.8 mmol/L)	Kayexalate	Exchanges sodium for potassium.	May require up to 4 hours to take effect.
	Calcium gluconate 10%	Counteracts potassium-induced increased myocardial irritability.	Monitor for ECG changes. Intravenous infiltration may result in tissue necrosis.
	Albuterol	Shifts potassium to the cells.	Give by inhalation.
	Sodium bicarbonate	Helps correct metabolic acidosis by exchanging hydrogen for potassium.	*Do not mix with calcium.* Complications include fluid overload, hypertension, and tetany.
Hypocalcemia (<2.2 mmol/L)	Calcium gluconate 10%	Used in presence of tetany; provides ionized calcium to restore nervous tissue function to control serum phosphorus.	Administer slowly to prevent bradycardia. Monitor for ECG changes.
Malignant hypertension (blood pressure >95% for age)	Sodium nitroprusside, nitroglycerin	Relaxes smooth muscle in peripheral arterioles.	Administer by continuous intravenous infusion; fall in blood pressure is seen within 10–20 minutes.

as hemolytic-uremic syndrome or acute glomerulonephritis may be associated with residual kidney damage.

NURSING MANAGEMENT

Nursing Assessment and Diagnoses

A complete history and physical examination are necessary to identify progression of symptoms and possible causes for renal failure.

Physiologic Assessment

Assessment of vital signs, level of consciousness, and other neurologic indicators helps to identify clinical signs of electrolyte imbalance (see the clinical manifestations table on page 663). Measurement of the child's weight on admission provides a baseline for evaluating changes in fluid status. Monitor urinalysis, urine culture, and blood chemistry studies. Inspect urine for color (Figure 18-7 ◆). Cloudy urine may indicate infection; tea-colored urine suggests hematuria. Assess urine specific gravity and intake and output.

Psychosocial Assessment

The unexpected and acute nature of the child's hospitalization creates anxiety for parents and child. Assess for feelings of anger, guilt, or fear associated with the hospitalization. Such feelings are likely if ARF developed as a result of dehydration, a preventable injury, or poisoning. Assess coping mechanisms, family support systems, and level of stress.

Following are nursing diagnoses that may apply to the child with ARF.

- *Altered renal tissue perfusion,* related to hypovolemia, sepsis, or drug toxicity
- *Fluid volume excess,* related to renal dysfunction and sodium retention
- *Altered nutrition: Less than body requirements,* related to anorexia, nausea, vomiting, and catabolic state
- *Risk for infection,* related to invasive procedures and monitoring equipment, and diminished immune functioning
- *Ineffective family coping (compromised),* related to sudden hospitalization and uncertain prognosis of child

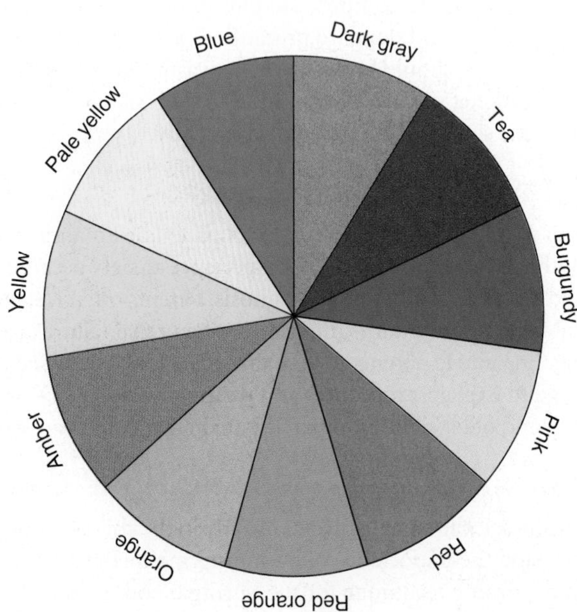

FIGURE 18-7 ◆
A color wheel, such as the one shown here, can be used as a guide in standardizing descriptions of urine color. Normal urine is pale yellow. Changes in urine color can indicate the following alterations: *yellow*—concentrated urine; *amber*—bile in urine; *orange*—alkaline or concentrated urine; *red orange*—acid pH, medications; *red*—blood, menses; *pink*—dilute blood; *burgundy*—laxatives; *tea*—melanin, hematuria; *dark gray*—medications, dyes; *blues*—dyes, medications.
From Cooper, C. (1993). What color is that urine specimen? *American Journal of Nursing, 93,* 37. Copyright © 1993 Connie Cooper, R. N., M. S. N.; graphics by Mike O'Grady, R. N. M. S. N.

CLINICAL TIP

If serum sodium concentration rises and weight falls, insufficient fluids are being administered. If the serum sodium level falls and the weight increases, excessive fluids are being administered.

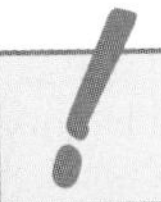

NURSING ALERT

The child with renal insufficiency has a concentrating defect. In cases of acute gastrointestinal illness, children are at greater risk for dehydration.

Planning and Implementation

Nursing care focuses on preventing complications, maintaining fluid balance, administering medications, meeting nutritional needs, preventing infection, and providing emotional support to the child and parents.

Prevent Complications

Complications are best prevented by ensuring compliance with the treatment plan. Careful monitoring of vital signs, intake and output, serum electrolytes, and level of consciousness can alert the nurse to changes that indicate potential complications.

Maintain Fluid Balance

Estimate the child's fluid status by monitoring weight (on the same scale), intake and output, and blood pressure two or three times a day. Also monitor serum chemistry values, especially for sodium. The aim of maintaining fluid balance is to achieve a stable serum sodium concentration and a decrease in body weight by 0.5% to 1.0% a day.

If the child has oliguria, fluid intake, including parenteral nutrition, is limited to replacement of insensible fluid loss from the lungs, skin, and gastrointestinal tract (about one-third the daily maintenance requirements in afebrile children). If the child is febrile, fluid administration is increased by 12% for each centigrade degree of temperature elevation.

Administer Medications

Because the kidney's ability to excrete drugs is impaired in ARF, dosages of all medications should be adjusted. The actual dosage of the drug can be reduced or the time interval between doses can be increased. Check drug levels to monitor for drug toxicity. Be aware of signs of drug toxicity for each medication the child is receiving.

Meet Nutritional Needs

Children are at risk of malnutrition because of their high metabolic rate. Parenteral or enteral feeding may be used initially to minimize protein catabolism. The diet is tailored to the individual child's need for calories, carbohydrates, fats, and amino acids or protein hydrolysates. Depending on the degree of renal failure, sodium, potassium, and phosphorus may be restricted. Oral feeding is initiated as soon as the child can tolerate it.

Prevent Infection

The child with ARF is extremely susceptible to nosocomial infections as a result of altered nutritional status, compromised immunity, and numerous invasive procedures. Thorough handwashing and standard precautions are imperative to decrease the risk of infection. Sterile technique should be used for all invasive procedures and when caring for lines. Drainage from catheter sites should be cultured to check for the presence of infectious organisms. Assess vital signs and lung sounds frequently.

Provide Emotional Support

The sudden onset of ARF presents parents with an unexpected threat to their child's life. Both the child and the parents experience anxiety because of the unexpected hospitalization and the uncertainty of the prognosis. Parents often feel guilty, regardless of the cause of renal failure. This guilt is intensified when renal failure is a result of dehydration or poisoning. Encourage parents to verbalize their fears and assist them in working through feelings of guilt. Explain procedures and treatment measures to decrease anxiety. Encouraging parents and older siblings to participate in the child's care can increase their sense of control.

Discharge Planning and Home Care Teaching

Encourage parental involvement early in the child's hospitalization. Be sure that parents understand the importance of administering medications correctly. Instruct family members in the proper technique for measuring blood pressure so they can monitor the child's hypertension, if ordered. Have them demonstrate how to take the blood pressure.

Diet counseling is a key component of discharge planning and is usually performed by a renal dietitian. Depending on the degree of renal failure, the child's diet may include restrictions on protein, water, sodium, potassium, and phosphorus. The parents should be given written guidelines listing appropriate food choices to assist in menu planning. Ethnic and cultural preferences should be considered in listing menu options.

Continued monitoring of renal function during follow-up examinations is critical as deterioration may occur over time. Referral to support groups can be helpful for parents and children alike. The National Kidney Foundation is a source of numerous publications.

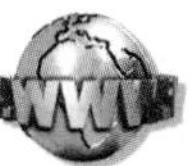

Renal Failure Support and Resources

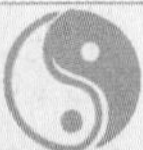

CULTURE

Special effort is often needed to reduce the sodium in the diet of an Asian child. Sauces and seasonings for foods (soy sauce, mustards, monosodium glutamate, and garlic salt) are sodium rich even though the foods seasoned (rice, vegetables, shrimp, and chicken) are low in sodium. The child may ingest up to 18 g of sodium a day with these added sauces and seasonings whereas 4 g per day is the goal. The typical Mexican diet, high in sodium and potassium (avocados, tomatoes, beans) may also require significant modification. Individualized counseling and motivation are needed to encourage families to reduce the child's sodium intake and to use spices low in sodium when preparing meals.

Evaluation

Expected outcomes of nursing care include the following:

- The child's fluid status is balanced with edema-associated weight loss.
- Nutritional needs are met.
- The child acquires no secondary infections.

Chronic Renal Failure

Chronic renal failure (CRF) is a progressive, irreversible reduction in kidney function. CRF is rare in children, occurring in 0.6 to 1.6 per million (Saborio, Hahn, & Hisano, et al., 1998). Blacks have a higher rate of the most advanced form of CRF **end-stage renal disease** (ESRD) than whites by a ratio of 2.7:1 (Balinsky, 2000).

ETIOLOGY AND PATHOPHYSIOLOGY In children, CRF usually results from developmental abnormalities of the kidney or urinary tract. Terrell, described at the beginning of the chapter, had ESRD resulting from posterior urethral valves, which caused bilateral kidney damage. CRF may also be caused by hemolytic-uremic syndrome, glomerulonephritis, or other renal diseases (see discussions later in the chapter).

The gradual, progressive loss of functioning nephrons ultimately results in ESRD, which is characterized by minimal renal function (less than 5% of normal), uremic syndrome, anemia, and abnormal blood values. In ESRD, the kidneys can no longer maintain homeostasis and the child requires dialysis.

The kidneys function to excrete excess acid in the body and to regulate the body's fluid and electrolyte balance. Renal failure upsets this fluid and electrolyte balance. As renal failure progresses, metabolic acidosis occurs because the kidneys cannot excrete the acids that build up in the body. Retention of excessive sodium and water is a common cause of the elevated blood pressure associated with CRF. Insufficient calcium loss, phosphorus retention, and elevated parathyroid hormone levels lead to uremic bone disease. Because the kidneys are also the site of production of erythropoietin (the growth factor responsible for the production and maturation of red cells), lack of erythropoietin and progressive renal disease are the underlying causes of the anemia of CRF.

SPECTRUM OF CHRONIC RENAL FAILURE

1. Early renal failure with glomerular filtration rate (GFR) of 50%–75% of normal; few or no clinical signs
2. Chronic renal insufficiency with GFR of 25% of normal; some clinical signs
3. Chronic renal failure with GFR of 10%–15% of normal; increased clinical signs
4. End-stage renal disease with GFR of less than 10% of normal; clinical signs requiring treatment with dialysis or renal transplantation (Taylor, 1996)

CLINICAL MANIFESTATIONS Children with CRF frequently have no symptoms initially. Symptoms do not appear until the child is in advanced renal failure (see the clinical manifestations table on page 663). In the early stages, the child may appear pale and complain of headache, nausea, and fatigue. Decreased mental alertness and ability to concentrate may be seen. Anemia leading to tachycardia, tachypnea, and dyspnea on exertion may occur. As the disease progresses, the child experiences a loss of appetite and complications of renal impairment, including hypertension, pulmonary edema, growth retardation, **osteodystrophy** (defective mineralization of bone caused by renal failure and chronic hyperphosphatemia), delayed fine and gross motor development, and delayed sexual maturation.

Growth retardation is caused by disturbances in the metabolism of calcium, phosphorus, and vitamin D; decreased caloric intake; and metabolic acidosis. Osteodystrophy increases the child's risk for spontaneous fractures, rickets, and valgus deformity of the legs.

In end-stage renal disease (ESRD), the most advanced form of CRF, all body systems are adversely affected by renal failure. As the severity of the clinical and biochemical disturbances resulting from progressive renal deterioration increase, uremic symptoms develop.

UREMIC SYNDROME

Signs and symptoms of uremic syndrome include nausea and vomiting, progressive anemia, anorexia, dyspnea, malaise, uremic frost (urea crystals deposited on the skin), unpleasant (uremic) breath odor, headache, progressive confusion, tremors, pulmonary edema, and congestive heart failure.

CLINICAL THERAPY Laboratory evaluation, including serum electrolyte, phosphate, BUN, and creatinine levels and pH, is used to confirm the diagnosis of CRF. A urine sample is collected for culture, and a 24-hour urine sample is obtained to quantify creatinine and protein excretion. From the 24-hour urine creatinine and serum creatinine levels, it is possible to calculate the remaining glomerular filtration rate. Laboratory values vary depending on the child's size and muscle mass. Age-specific normal ranges for laboratory values must be used. Tests to identify renal diseases that could be causing the renal failure are also performed if necessary. A renal biopsy is the best method for establishing or confirming the diagnosis, predicting the prognosis, and directing treatment (Taylor, 1996).

The goals of treatment are to slow the progression of renal disease and to prevent complications. Conservative treatment includes a combination of dietary and fluid and electrolyte management, control of hypertension, and if that fails and the child progresses to ESRD, dialysis is initiated.

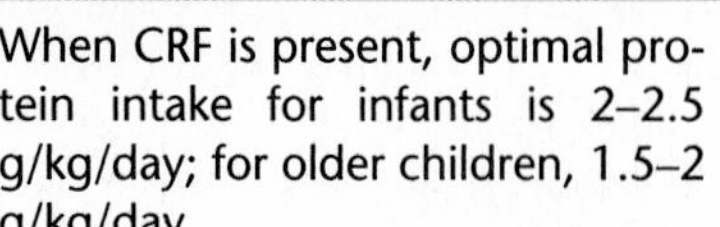

When CRF is present, optimal protein intake for infants is 2–2.5 g/kg/day; for older children, 1.5–2 g/kg/day.

Dietary management focuses on maximizing caloric intake for growth while limiting demands on the kidneys and minimizing fluid and electrolyte disturbances. Tube feedings or parenteral nutrition may be required to achieve optimal protein intake, especially in children under 1 year of age. Sodium bicarbonate (Bicitra) is used for treatment of metabolic acidosis. Restricting sodium to as little as 2 g/day may be necessary if the child is hypertensive or edematous. As renal failure progresses, potassium and phosphate restrictions become necessary. Calcium-based phosphate binders may be prescribed to remove the excess phosphate.

Diuretics are given to reduce the edema associated with renal failure. Antihypertensives (calcium channel blockers or ACE inhibitors) are prescribed to reduce blood pressure and prevent the progression of renal disease. As in ARF, medication dosages are adjusted because of the reduced glomerular filtration rate. Supplementation of vitamins (pyridoxine and folic acid) and minerals (iron and calcium) is usually necessary to offset dietary deficiencies. Ergocalciferol and calcitriol (vitamin D) are given to increase calcium absorption and treat renal osteodystrophy. Ascorbic acid is administered to enhance iron absorption. Erythropoietin is given to stimulate increased production of red blood cells, improve energy tolerance and school performance, and reduce the need for transfusions. Human growth hormone is given during the course of renal failure, until ESRD occurs, to increase muscle mass and total body weight gain.

Children who progress to ESRD require renal replacement therapy (see the following discussion). The timetable for dialysis or renal transplantation is different from that of adults; earlier initiation can prevent some complications of ESRD. Rather than use the absolute BUN or serum creatinine as the guide, nonspecific signs such as uremic syndrome, poorly controlled hypertension, renal osteodystrophy, failure of head circumference measurement to increase normally, developmental delay, and poor growth are used in determining when to initiate therapy. (Refer to the subsequent discussion of "Renal Replacement Therapy.")

CRF is irreversible. However, the course of the disease is variable. Some children progress quickly to renal failure, necessitating dialysis. Other children are managed with a combination of medication and diet therapy for some time before significant renal impairment occurs. Frequent modifications in the treatment plan are often necessary to address the child's changing status.

NURSING MANAGEMENT

Nursing Assessment and Diagnoses

Physiologic Assessment

The initial and ongoing assessment of the child focuses on identifying complications of renal failure. Observe for signs of edema, poor growth and development, osteodystrophy, and anemia. Assessment of vital signs helps to identify electrolyte alterations (see the clinical manifestations table on page 663).

Psychosocial Assessment

As renal disease progresses, the number of stressors on the child and family increases. Denial and disbelief are commonly the first reactions. A thorough family assessment can help to identify particular needs of the child and family (see Table 6-7). The development of

ESRD is particularly challenging during adolescence. Noncompliance with treatments can endanger the adolescent's life.

Nursing diagnoses for the child with CRF are similar to those previously listed for ARF. Additional diagnoses may include the following:

- *Altered growth,* related to decreased protein and caloric intake and loss of protein in dialysate
- *Impaired social isolation,* related to hemodialysis schedule during school hours
- *Activity intolerance,* related to renal disease, anemia, and fatigue
- *Ineffective management of therapeutic regimen,* related to complexity of care plan and economic difficulties
- *Body image disturbance,* related to short stature and visible external catheter for dialysis

Planning and Implementation

Children with CRF are usually hospitalized for initial diagnostic evaluation, to initiate dialysis treatment, to monitor problems that develop in the treatment plan, or to treat infection or another concurrent problem. Nursing care for the hospitalized child with CRF focuses on monitoring for side effects of medications, preventing infection, meeting nutritional needs, and providing emotional support and anticipatory teaching.

Monitor for Side Effects of Medications

Watch for signs of electrolyte imbalance such as weakness, muscle cramps, dizziness, headache, and nausea and vomiting in children who are taking diuretics. Supervise the child's activities closely to prevent falls resulting from dizziness, especially at the beginning of diuretic therapy. If antihypertensive medications such as hydralazine are being administered, monitor the child's weight to detect excessive gain resulting from water and sodium retention.

Prevent Infection

The child with CRF is extremely susceptible to infections. Be alert for signs of infection, such as elevated temperature; cloudy, strong-smelling urine; dysuria; changes in respiratory pattern; or productive cough. Emphasize to the child and family the importance of good handwashing practices. Make sure the child receives influenza, 23-valent pneumococcal, and meningococcal vaccines in addition to usual childhood immunizations.

Meet Nutritional Needs

Maintaining adequate nutritional intake in a child with CRF who has dietary restrictions is challenging. Provide small, frequent feedings and present meals attractively to encourage the child to eat.

Provide Emotional Support

Development of progressive CRF requires a total life-style change for the child and family. The parents and child need opportunities to express and work through their feelings related to the disease, prognosis, and treatment restrictions. Children can be assisted to express their feelings through drawings or therapeutic play.

The need for ongoing dialysis treatments and the wait for a suitable donor kidney are stressful for parents and child. Identification of effective coping methods and family support systems is needed to promote treatment compliance. The National Kidney Foundation and local support groups for kidney disease can provide the family with information or additional support.

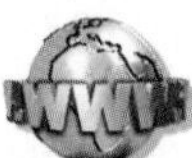

Chronic Renal Failure Resources

Discharge Planning and Home Care Teaching

Parents need to understand the necessity of long-term treatments and follow-up care. Help the family develop a schedule for medication administration that fits with their routine. Emphasize the importance of consistency in administration times. Teach parents how to recognize side effects and complications.

TABLE 18-7 Complications of Peritoneal Dialysis

COMPLICATION	CAUSE
Peritonitis	
Cloudy dialysate, abdominal pain, tenderness, leukocytosis, fever (neonatal hypothermia), constipation	*Staphylococcus aureus, Staphylococcus epidermidis,* fungal infections, gram-negative rods (risk is proportional to duration of dialysis and inversely proportional to age)
Pain	
During inflow	Too rapid a rate of infusion, too large a volume of dialysate, encasement of catheter in a false passage, extremes in temperature of dialysate
During outflow at end of emptying	Omentum entering catheter at end of outflow
Leakage	
Fluid around catheter, edema of penis or scrotum secondary to leakage into abdominal subcutaneous tissue, fluid leakage to pleural spaces through diaphragm	Overfilling of abdomen, catheter that has migrated from peritoneal cavity
Respiratory symptoms	
Shortness of breath, decreased breath sounds in lower lobes, inadequate chest expansion	Abdominal fullness that compromises diaphragm movement, hole in diaphragm allowing dialysate into chest cavity

Appropriate referrals should be made to the local visiting nurse association and to home care nursing agencies. Home care nurses will help the parents care for the child receiving dialysis as well as provide necessary support and reassurance. Parents of children receiving dialysis at home should be taught how to perform the treatment and how to identify complications (Table 18-7). Strict aseptic technique is necessary to prevent infection at the catheter site.

Care in the Community

Children with CRF require frequent outpatient visits to monitor the progression of signs and symptoms, and to evaluate the effectiveness of current treatments.

Assessment Compare the child's height, weight, and head circumference to age-specific norms to identify growth retardation and to plot progress. Assess developmental progress using the Denver II or another screening tool (see Chapter 6). Assess the adolescent for signs of delayed sexual maturation and, in girls, amenorrhea. Blood and urine tests will be performed to monitor renal function. Radiographs of the bones will be taken at 6-month intervals to assess changes caused by osteodystrophy.

Health Supervision Promote good dentition and oral hygiene. Regular dental visits are important to reduce infections. Make sure the family understands the need for antibiotic prophylaxis before certain invasive procedures, including dental care (see Table 14-4). If possible, all immunizations should be provided before renal transplantation, as long-term immunosuppressive therapy will then be prescribed. Live vaccines should not be given to the child taking immunosuppressive agents.

Nutrition Review any dietary restrictions with parents. Provide sample menus for meal planning to help parents incorporate dietary changes into daily meals. A renal dietitian usually assists the child to make food selections and to restrict fluids and sodium as necessary, taking into account the child's likes and dislikes and cultural background. High caloric supplements may be needed because of anorexia. School-age children may not understand the consequences of noncompliance with dietary restrictions and may perceive these restrictions as punishment. Adolescents often resent the dietary restrictions and ongoing dialysis treatments, which pose a threat to their independence and evolving sense of self. Noncooperation, depression, and hostility are common responses. Discuss possible behavioral responses to dietary restrictions and limitations imposed by the treatment plan.

Emotional Support School-age children and adolescents are often embarrassed about being perceived as different from peers. Ask them how they feel about the need to follow a special diet, take medications, and undergo dialysis treatments. To minimize the psychologic consequences of coping with a chronic disease, encourage parents to promote their child's participation in age-appropriate activities. Attendance at school and contacts with peers promote normal growth and development. Work to promote the child's self-worth and a healthy self-esteem. Prepare the child for peer conflict. Encourage adolescents to participate in a program that helps transition them to adult health services and job skill training.

Anticipatory Teaching Supply the parents with timely information about the disease process, dialysis treatments, and issues related to renal transplantation, as the child's renal impairment progresses.

Evaluation

Expected outcomes of nursing care include the following:

- The child is fully immunized with childhood and additional vaccines.
- The child's fluid status is maintained.
- The child eats foods that meet nutritional needs while adhering to dietary restrictions.

GROWTH & DEVELOPMENT

Adequate protein intake helps improve the child's growth and height velocity. Recommendations are as follows:

<3 years	2.5–3.0 gm/kg/day
3 years to puberty	2.0–2.5 gm/kg/day
puberty	2.0 gm/kg/day
postpuberty	1.5 gm/kg/day

(Warady, Alexander, & Watkins, et al., 1999)

Renal Replacement Therapy

Renal replacement therapy is the treatment for renal failure and includes both dialysis and renal transplantation. In 2000, approximately 5,300 children between birth and 19 years received some form of renal replacement therapy, and 1,602 children (200 children less than 2 years old) received regular dialysis. Approximately 41% of children managed at home with ESRD received peritoneal dialysis and 59% received hemodialysis (United States Renal Data System, 2000). Dialysis treatment can cost more than $50,000 per year.

PERITONEAL DIALYSIS Peritoneal dialysis is the preferred form of dialysis for small children because continuous removal of fluids and waste products is possible. A continuous steady state of dialysis clearance occurs, decreasing the toxic effects of waste products on the child's developing body. Dietary and fluid restrictions are less severe. The timing of the treatment can be set to minimize the interruption of school, play, or other social events.

Two types of peritoneal dialysis are commonly used: continuous ambulatory peritoneal dialysis and automated peritoneal dialysis. Buretrols or graduated cylinders are used to monitor the volume of fluid exchanged.

- Continuous ambulatory peritoneal dialysis uses gravity to instill prefilled bags of **dialysate** (dialysis solution) into the peritoneal cavity four or five times a day. The fluid remains in the cavity for 4 to 8 hours. An attached bag is folded under the child's clothes, permitting normal activity. After the allotted time, the dialysate is drained by hanging the bag lower than the pelvis. The repeated connections and disconnections with this method are time consuming for the child and family and increase the risk of infection.
- Automated peritoneal dialysis uses an automatic cycler to instill and drain the dialysate about five times over a 10-hour period, usually overnight. With this method, only one connection and disconnection is needed per day, which reduces demands on the family as well as the risk of infection. Of the peritoneal dialysis methods, this is preferred because it enables the delivery of more dialysate (Warady et al., 1999).

In children receiving peritoneal dialysis for ARF, a catheter can be placed percutaneously that can be used for a few weeks. In children with CRF, a catheter is placed surgically for long-term use.

The primary complications of peritoneal dialysis are peritonitis and abdominal hernia (see Table 18-7). Patients average one episode of peritonitis per year (Evans, Greenbaum, & Ettenger, 1995).

Teach the family to perform peritoneal dialysis and to use sterile technique when performing dialysis and doing catheter care. Peritoneal dialysis is time consuming, and commitment by family members is required to manage this procedure daily. Help the family to develop home routines that minimize disruptions to daily family life. For additional information, refer to the nursing care plan for the child receiving home peritoneal dialysis.

CLINICAL TIP

Signs and symptoms of peritonitis associated with peritoneal dialysis include fever, vomiting, diarrhea, abdominal pain, tenderness, and cloudy dialysate.

NURSING CARE PLAN The Child Receiving Home Peritoneal Dialysis

GOAL	INTERVENTION	RATIONALE	EXPECTED OUTCOME
1. Altered Nutrition: Less Than Body Requirements related to poor appetite, feeling of fullness after a small amount, and loss of protein in dialysate			
	NIC Priority Intervention: **Nutrition Management:** Assistance with or provision of a balanced dietary intake of foods and fluids.		NOC Suggested Outcome: **Nutrition Status:** Food and fluid intake: Amount of food and fluid taken into the body over a 24-hour period.
The child will obtain adequate nutrients each day.	■ With a nutritionist; develop a diet plan to identify the amounts of essential nutrients needed. ■ Provide small, frequent meals of needed nutrients. ■ Make mealtimes pleasant and avoid battles over the child's intake. ■ Provide supplements by tube feeding if adequate oral intake is not possible.	■ Parents need concrete guidelines for food preparation. ■ The child will feel full with smaller amounts of food because of the dialysate. ■ The child will be more inclined to eat if there is less stress. ■ Adequate nutrition is important for growth and development, and must be supported if oral intake is inadequate.	The child's intake is adequate for an expected growth pattern to be maintained.
2. Risk for Infection related to daily invasive procedure			
	NIC Priority Intervention: **Infection Control:** Minimizing the Acquisition and Transmission of infectious agents.		NOC Suggested Outcome: **Risk Control:** Actions to eliminate or reduce actual, personal, and modifiable health threats.
The child will not develop peritonitis.	■ Use aseptic technique for connection and disconnection of catheters. ■ Perform daily catheter site care.	■ Aseptic technique reduces chance of introducing bacteria into the abdomen. ■ Skin around the catheter site will have fewer organisms that could potentially cause infection.	The child does not develop peritonitis.
If peritonitis occurs, it will be treated appropriately.	■ Observe for signs of infection (fever, abdominal pain, cloudy dialysate). ■ Report signs of infection to physician immediately.	■ Early identification of infection will reduce complications. ■ Rapid intervention may reduce need for hospitalization.	Hospitalization will not be needed for peritonitis due to early identification and prompt treatment.
3. Caregiver Role Strain related to daily dialysis treatments			
	NIC Priority Intervention: **Caregiver Support:** Provision of necessary information, advocacy and support to facilitate primary patient care by someone other than a health care professional.		NOC Suggested Outcome: **Caregiver Performance:** Direct Care: Provision by family care provider of appropriate personal and health care for a family member or significant other.
The family copes with daily demands for the child's dialysis treatments.	■ Discuss the importance of daily, consistent dialysis treatments for the child's overall health status. ■ Collaborate with the family to identify strategies that could reduce the impact of dialysis on the family's life. ■ Refer the family to local support groups for emotional support, treatment strategies, and respite care.	■ If parents understand the need for consistent dialysis treatments, they are more likely to comply. ■ When the family participates in planning care, compliance is more likely. ■ Support groups may help the family develop effective coping strategies.	The family complies with daily dialysis treatment guidelines.

(continued)

NURSING CARE PLAN The Child Receiving Home Peritoneal Dialysis (continued)

GOAL	INTERVENTION	RATIONALE	EXPECTED OUTCOME
4. Body Image Disturbance related to small size and perception of being and looking different			
	NIC Priority Intervention: **Body Image Enhancement:** Improving a patient's conscious and unconscious perceptions and attitudes towards his/her body.		NOC Suggested Outcome: **Psychosocial Adjustment:** Life change: Psychosocial adaptation of an individual to a life change.
The child will develop a sense of self-worth and self-esteem.	■ Identify and emphasize strengths the child has (e.g., interaction style, skills, or cognitive abilities) despite being smaller than peers. ■ Assist the child and family to identify popular clothing styles that hide the dialysate bag and catheter. ■ Increase the child's participation in self-care as appropriate for developmental age. ■ Promote participation in safe activities with peers. ■ Encourage the child to participate in support groups with other children receiving dialysis when possible.	■ Perception of personal strengths should increase self-esteem. ■ Clothing that conforms to current styles, but still hides dialysate, will help the child feel less different from peers. ■ Ability to perform self-care increases the child's sense of control. ■ Social interaction with peers helps reinforce similarities with others. ■ Interactions with other affected children provide a chance to express feelings and frustrations, and to develop successful coping strategies.	The child effectively interacts with peers and participates in age-appropriate activities.
5. Altered Health Maintenance related to chronic condition			
	NIC Priority Intervention: **Health System Guidance:** Facilitating a patient's location and use of appropriate health services.		NOC Suggested Outcome: **Health-Seeking Behaviors:** Actions to promote optimal wellness, recovery, and rehabilitation.
The child's routine health maintenance visits will be integrated with the management of the chronic condition.	■ If a renal specialty team is not conveniently located and providing general health care, make sure the child has a primary care provider working in collaboration with the renal team. ■ Assess the child regularly for growth and developmental progress and signs that the chronic condition is being managed effectively. ■ Provide immunizations as recommended for the child with a chronic condition. ■ Provide anticipatory guidance related to safety, developmental progress, appropriate physical activities, and behavior management.	■ A source of health maintenance and acute minor illness care is important, especially if the family lives a distance from the tertiary care center. ■ Routine assessments will allow potential complications to be identified earlier. ■ Immunizations may reduce the risk of potentially life-threatening infections in a child at high risk. ■ Information will help the family support the child's health status and promote development.	The child is fully immunized at appropriate intervals and the family has a source of regular care in the community.

NURSING ALERT

Monitor the child receiving hemodialysis for complications that can occur suddenly.

- Hypotension—sudden nausea and vomiting, abdominal cramping, tachycardia, and dizziness
- Rapid fluid and electrolyte exchange—muscle cramping, nausea and vomiting, and dizziness
- Dysequilibrium syndrome—restlessness, headache, nausea and vomiting, blurred vision, muscle twitching, and altered level of consciousness

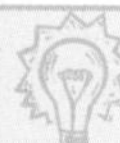

CLINICAL TIP

Carefully monitor fluid balance in the child undergoing hemodialysis. Check vital signs and blood pressure every half hour. Monitor oral intake and urinary output when on the dialysis equipment every half hour. Weigh the child before and after the dialysis to determine any fluid imbalances that must be adjusted in the next hemodialysis session.

HEMODIALYSIS Hemodialysis is used in the critical care setting, and for those children with CRF when peritoneal dialysis is not possible for technical reasons or when the family is unable to safely provide it. Hemodialysis for children is offered in a special center. In the opening scenario, Terrell's health care providers and his family decided to switch from peritoneal dialysis to hemodialysis after he developed several episodes of peritonitis in one year. Infants as small as 4 kg (8.8 lb) can be hemodialyzed with current technology. Treatment is usually performed three times a week, with each session lasting approximately 3 to 4 hours.

In emergency hemodialysis and for infants, a double-lumen cannula is inserted into a large vein (e.g., the femoral, jugular, or subclavian vein). Children over 20 kg (44 lb) often have an artificial blood vessel, an arteriovenous shunt or fistula, created. Blood is pumped out of the body and through a dialyzer, where waste products and extra fluids diffuse out across a semipermeable membrane. Dialysate is pumped in the direction opposite blood flow to promote waste extraction. Differences in osmolarity and concentration between the child's blood and the dialysate alter the intravascular electrolyte concentration and reduce the intravascular volume (Figure 18-8 ◆).

Hemodialysis is more efficient than peritoneal dialysis but requires close monitoring for symptoms related to hypotension or rapid changes in fluid and electrolyte balance. Uncommonly, a disequilibrium syndrome may occur during or soon after the dialysis procedure is first performed. Other complications include access thrombosis and infection. Heparin is used to achieve an active clotting time of 150%, which reduces the risk of thrombosis.

Nursing management focuses on teaching the child and family about the administration of heparin and the control of bleeding from minor trauma. Because dietary limitations are needed more often with hemodialysis than with peritoneal dialysis, make sure the family knows how to plan and provide for the child's daily nutritional needs. Methods to reduce the risk of infection should be reviewed, including the provision of daily care to the catheter site. Encourage showering rather than tub baths. Activities such as swimming may be discouraged.

RENAL TRANSPLANTATION Renal transplantation provides the only alternative to long-term dialysis for children with ESRD. It can normalize physiology and provide a potential for normal growth. Because of the adverse effects on growth and development resulting from delaying transplantation, children are given some priority over adults awaiting transplantation. To be successful, blood type compatibility between the kidney donor and

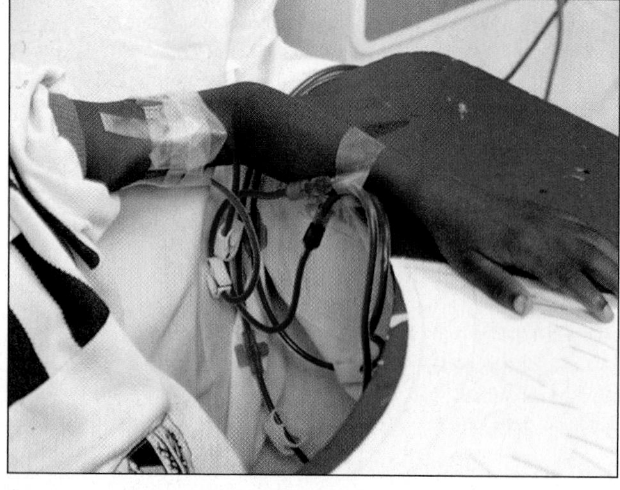

A

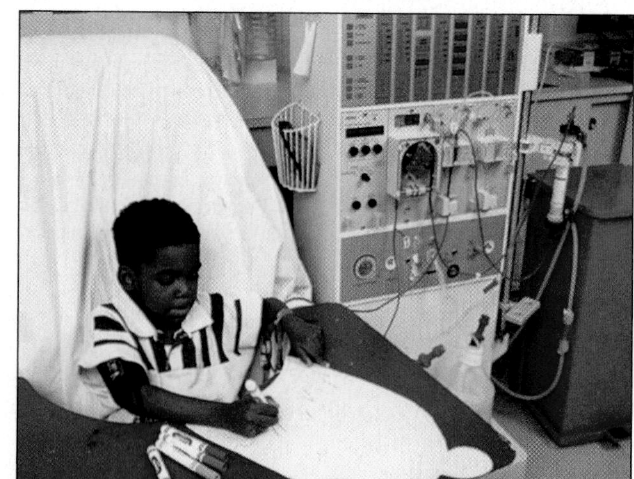

B

FIGURE 18-8 ◆

This child is undergoing hemodialysis. A, A surgically implanted vascular graft is being used here. One needle is placed in the arterialized end of the graft (red tubing), and one needle is placed in the venous end (blue tubing) for blood return. B, The child is able to draw or perform other quiet activities during dialysis treatment. Note that the child's blood pressure is monitored carefully throughout the treatment.

the recipient is necessary. A human leukocyte antigen (HLA) system match also improves survival of the graft. A living relative donor kidney has a higher survival rate than a cadaver kidney.

After transplantation, the child must take immunosuppressive medications such as corticosteroids, azathioprine, cyclosporine, and antilymphocyte antibodies to suppress rejection. Immunosuppression regimens use various combinations and sequences of these drugs to reduce the incidence of acute and chronic rejection. Signs of rejection include fever, increased BUN and serum creatinine levels, pain and tenderness over the abdomen, irritability, and weight gain.

Complications of immunosuppression therapy include opportunistic infection, lymphomas and skin cancer, and hypertension. Noncompliance with management is highest among families with instability, adolescents, females, and children and youth with low self-esteem (Bereket and Fine, 1995). Some primary kidney diseases, such as glomerulonephritis and hemolytic-uremic syndrome, can also recur in the transplanted kidney.

Nursing management includes teaching parents about the transplantation process before it occurs to help prepare them for the experience. Discuss all aspects of the child's care that will have an impact on the family's life, including follow-up appointments, medications, and general health promotion. Teach parents about the signs of acute rejection and infection, including when and how to notify the child's physician if immediate care is required.

CULTURE 

Racial differences exist with regard to access to the renal transplant waiting list. Black children are 12% less likely to be placed on the waiting list than whites at any point in time. It is unknown if these differences are due to physican bias in identifying transplant candidates, patient or family preference, or difference in the time to see a nephrologist (Furth, Garg, & Neu, et al., 2000).

POLYCYSTIC KIDNEY DISEASE

Polycystic kidney disease (PKD) is a genetic disorder that has autosomal recessive and dominant forms. Liver abnormalities are associated with both forms of the disease. They each have a spectrum of severity and may be detected in the fetus or become apparent during infancy or childhood. The incidence of the autosomal recessive form is 1 per 10,000 to 40,000, and is most often detected in fetuses and infants (Barratt, Avner, & Harmon, 1999). The autosomal dominant form is the most common inherited kidney disease, with a prevalence of 1 per 1,000 patients (Barratt et al., 1999). The most common PKD results from mutations on the PKD1 locus on chromosome 16 (Goodyer & Kashtan, 1998).

Cellular hyperplasia of the collecting ducts causes dilation of the ducts. Fluid secreted into these ducts enables cyst sacs to form. Initially, cysts are usually less than 2 mm in size and do not obstruct urinary flow. As the child grows, however, the cysts become larger and fibrosis occurs. Tubular atrophy may occur in some children, whereas others have minimal changes in renal function. Polycystic kidney disease is also associated with liver abnormalities that progress to fibrosis, portal hypertension, and biliary infection, which progress in severity with age.

Newborns with polycystic kidney disease may have enlarged kidneys, detected at birth. Those with the most severe form of the disease die shortly after birth as a result of pulmonary hypoplasia. Clinical manifestations in infants and children include hypertension, hematuria, frequent urination, poor growth, urinary tract infections, and proteinuria. Polyuria and polydipsia develop with progressive **renal insufficiency** (that is, as the kidneys' ability to conserve sodium and concentrate the urine decreases). As uremia develops, infants and children develop renal osteodystrophy and progressive developmental delay and growth failure.

Diagnosis is confirmed by sonogram or renal biopsy. The disease is often diagnosed on prenatal ultrasound. If identified, other family members should be screened for subclinical cases of the disease. Liver function tests are usually normal.

Treatment is supportive. Medications such as diuretics are prescribed for hypertension. Antibiotics are used to treat urinary tract infection. Erythropoietin is prescribed to prevent and treat anemia. Growth hormones may be used in some children to promote growth. Renal osteodystrophy is treated to suppress the parathyroid hormone. Chronic renal failure is managed as described earlier on pages 668–671. Surgery is performed for portal hypertension. Renal dialysis or a transplant will prolong survival; however, liver problems may continue to complicate the child's health, even when the renal condition is well controlled.

Nursing Management

Nursing care is the same as that for the child with renal insufficiency and chronic renal failure. Observe the child for signs of progressive renal impairment. Ensure that follow-up appointments are scheduled to assess growth, developmental progress, and the effectiveness of the treatment plan. Family teaching for home management focuses on medications, diet adequate in protein and calories to support growth, management of acute gastrointestinal illnesses, and care for the child with progressive renal insufficiency and a liver disorder.

HEMOLYTIC-UREMIC SYNDROME

Hemolytic-uremic syndrome (HUS) is a relatively rare, acute renal disease that occurs most often in children under 4 years. The syndrome is characterized by a classic triad of signs: hemolytic anemia, thrombocytopenia, and ARF. It is an important cause of CRF.

The development of HUS is often linked to enterohemorrhagic *Escherichia coli* strain 0157:H7, which produces a toxin that attaches to the kidneys and other organs. Hamburger is the vector in more than half of the epidemics. Damage to the lining of the glomerular arterioles results in swelling of the endothelial cells. In response, clotting mechanisms deposit fibrin in the renal arterioles and capillaries. This partial occlusion damages the red blood cells, resulting in hemolysis and subsequent anemia. Platelet agglutination occurs in areas of vascular endothelial damage, causing thrombocytopenia. ARF develops as a consequence of blood clotting in the arterioles as well as the toxic effect of hemolized red blood cells on renal tubular cells leading to acute tubular necrosis. Autosomal recessive and dominant forms of HUS also exist and account for <5% of cases (Varade, 2000).

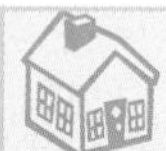

HOME CARE

HUS can be largely prevented by cooking of ground beef to 155°F throughout, meaning no more rare hamburgers. Wash hands carefully when handling raw ground meats, and make sure utensils touching raw meat do not come into contact with cooked meats.

An episode of mild gastroenteritis with diarrhea, upper respiratory infection, or urinary tract infection precedes the development of HUS by 1 to 2 weeks. Signs and symptoms of HUS are described in the clinical manifestations table. The child may also have hyperkalemia and metabolic acidosis as a result of renal failure.

A peripheral blood smear with fragments of red blood cells, fibrin split products, and a decreased platelet count (<140,000/μL[mm^3]) confirms the diagnosis. Treatment focuses on the complications of ARF and includes fluid restrictions, antihypertensive medications, and a high-calorie, high-carbohydrate diet that is low in protein, sodium, potassium, and phosphorus. Enteral nutritional support is sometimes needed (refer to the earlier discussion of ARF). Dialysis is needed for about 60% of children, and peritoneal dialysis is preferred unless the child has severe colitis and abdominal tenderness. It generally takes about 8 days to recover normal renal function (Varade, 2000). Chronic renal failure may develop in other children. Transfusions of fresh packed red blood cells may be ordered to treat severe anemia. Platelets are given if the child is bleeding or if surgery is needed. Transfusions should be administered carefully to prevent hypertension caused by hypervolemia. Mortality from HUS is now <5%.

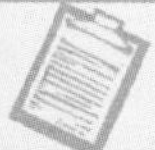

RESEARCH

A recent study revealed that antibiotic treatment of the child with exposure to E. coli 0157:H7 increases the risk of developing HUS due to the release of toxins and alteration of the intestinal flora (Wong, Jelacic, & Habeeb, et al., 2000).

CLINICAL MANIFESTATIONS OF HEMOLYTIC-UREMIC SYNDROME

STAGE	CLINICAL MANIFESTATIONS
Prodromal Stage (1–7 days)	Upper respiratory illness Abdominal pain with nausea, vomiting, and bloody diarrhea Pallor Fever and irritability Lymphadenopathy Skin rash Edema Severe gastroenteritis with bloody diarrhea in 90% of cases
Acute Stage	Hemolytic anemia Hypertension Purpura Neurologic involvement (irritability, seizures, lethargy, stupor, coma, cerebral edema) Hematuria and proteinuria Oliguria or anuria Edema and ascites

Nursing Management

Nursing care is the same as that for the child with ARF, as described earlier. Careful monitoring of neurologic signs, laboratory values, and fluid and electrolyte balance is essential. Observe the child carefully for signs of progressive renal impairment. Discharge planning focuses on teaching parents about medications and dietary and fluid restrictions. Follow-up visits are necessary to evaluate the effectiveness of the treatment plan.

CLINICAL TIP

Treatment of diarrhea with antimotility medications is contraindicated because they increase the risk of toxic megacolon or progression from hemorrhagic colitis to HUS (Varade, 2000).

ACUTE POSTINFECTIOUS GLOMERULONEPHRITIS

Glomerulonephritis is an inflammation of the glomeruli of the kidneys. In children, it is most often a response to a group A beta-hemolytic streptococcal infection of the skin or pharynx. It is also caused by other organisms including *Staphylococcus, Pneumococcus,* and Coxsackie virus. The incidence of acute postinfectious glomerulonephritis (APIGN) is highest in children who are 5 to 8 years of age, and the disorder is more common in boys than in girls. Early antibiotic therapy for streptococcal infection does not seem to prevent the development of APIGN.

CLINICAL TIP

Encourage prompt treatment of streptococcal infections with a full course of antibiotics to prevent APIGN when possible. Ensure that children with possible streptococcal infections, such as a severe or continuing sore throat, are seen by a health care provider.

Etiology and Pathophysiology

The child with APIGN usually becomes ill after a nephritogenic strain of group A beta-hemolytic streptococcal infection of the upper respiratory tract or the skin. Often the child becomes ill with strep throat, recovers, and then develops signs of APIGN after an interval of 8 to 14 days.

Glomerular damage occurs as a result of an immune complex reaction that localizes on the glomerular capillary wall. Antibody–antigen complexes become lodged in the glomeruli, leading to inflammation and obstruction. Damage to the glomerular membrane allows red blood cells and red cell casts to be excreted. Sodium and water are retained, expanding the intravascular and interstitial compartments. This process results in the characteristic finding of edema (Figure 18-9 ◆).

PATHOPHYSIOLOGY ILLUSTRATED

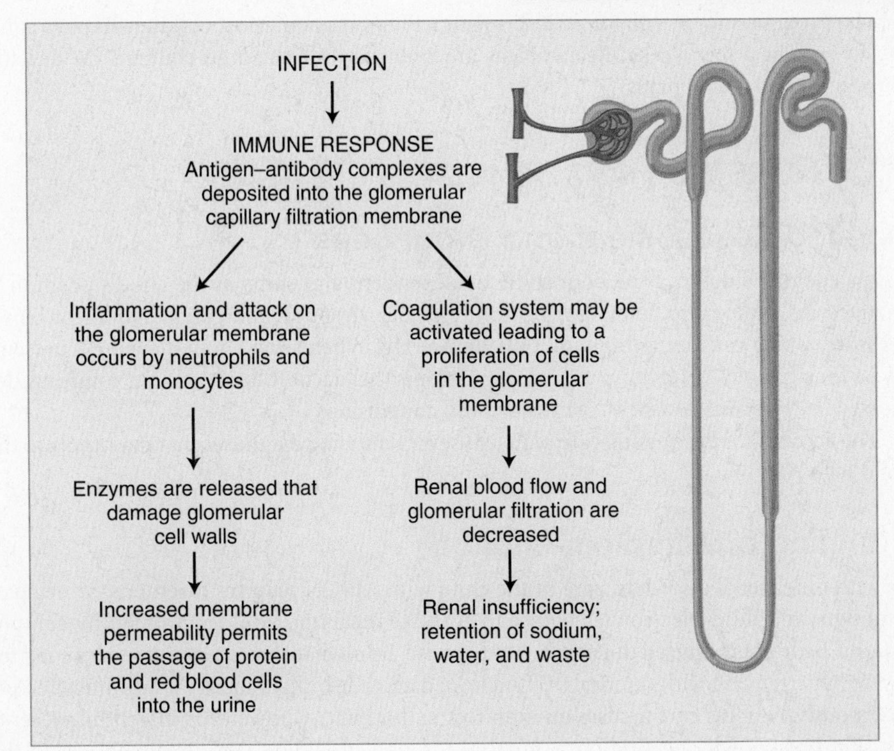

Acute Postinfectious Glomerulonephritis
FIGURE 18-9 ◆

Clinical Manifestations

Onset is usually abrupt. Microscopic hematuria is present in nearly all cases, while gross hematuria, resulting in tea-colored urine, is found in up to 50% of cases. Mild periorbital edema occurs early, but edema may become more severe if fluid intake is not restricted during the acute stage. Hypertension occurs in a majority of hospitalized children. As the disease progresses, the child becomes lethargic and feverish and may complain of abdominal pain, headache, and costovertebral tenderness (related to stretching of the renal capsule from edema).

Clinical Therapy

URINALYSIS RESULTS IN APIGN

- Acid pH
- Hematuria
- Proteinuria (trace to 2+)
- Discoloration (reddish brown to rusty color secondary to red blood cell and hemoglobin content)
- Leukocyturia

Blood tests may reveal elevated BUN and creatinine concentrations. The erythrocyte sedimentation rate is increased in the acute phase, and serum lipid levels are increased in about 40% of cases. An elevated antistreptolysin O (ASO) titer reflects the presence of antibodies from a recent streptococcal respiratory infection, but the ASO level associated with a recent skin infection is low. The anti-DNAse B titer is helpful for detecting antibodies associated with recent skin infections. Up to 90% of children have reduced serum C3. Anemia is common in the acute phase and is generally caused by dilution of the serum by the extracellular fluid. The hemoglobin level and hematocrit value may decrease during the late phase as a result of hematuria. The white blood cell count may be normal or slightly elevated.

Treatment focuses on relief of symptoms and supportive therapy. Bedrest is a key component of the treatment plan during the acute phase. Hypertension can be managed with a combination of an antihypertensive medication such as hydralazine (Apresoline) and a diuretic such as furosemide (Lasix). Mild to moderate hypertension should be treated with fluid and salt restriction. A course of antibiotics may be given to ensure eradication of the infectious agent.

Fluid requirements are determined by careful monitoring of urinary output, weight, blood pressure, and serum electrolytes. Initially, only insensible losses are replaced until the status of renal function is known. The degree of dietary restriction is determined by the severity of edema. Sodium and potassium intake are restricted. With severe azotemia, protein intake may have to be limited.

The prognosis for >95% of children with APIGN is good. Most children recover completely within a few weeks. Recurrences are unusual. Rarely, some children do develop chronic glomerulonephritis.

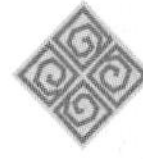

NURSING MANAGEMENT

Nursing Assessment and Diagnoses

Assess edema, which may be periorbital or dependent and shifts as the child's position is changed. Assess for circulatory congestion (crackles, dyspnea, and cough). Monitor blood pressure, which can rise as high as 200/120 mm Hg. When severe hypertension is present, assess for signs of central nervous system problems (headache, blurred vision, vomiting, decreased level of consciousness, confusion, and convulsions).

The accompanying nursing care plan lists several nursing diagnoses that may apply to the child with APIGN.

Planning and Implementation

As with other renal disorders, care of the child with APIGN requires careful monitoring of vital signs and fluid–electrolyte balance to evaluate renal functioning and identify complications. Bedrest is required during the acute phase. Immediate emergency care is needed for severe hypertension with cerebral dysfunction; diazoxide or hydralazine is administered intravenously. Nursing care focuses on monitoring fluid status, preventing infection, preventing skin breakdown, meeting nutritional needs, and providing emotional support to the child and family.

NURSING CARE PLAN The Child with Acute Postinfectious Glomerulonephritis

GOAL	INTERVENTION	RATIONALE	EXPECTED OUTCOME
1. Fluid Volume Excess related to decreased glomerular filtration and increased sodium retention			
	NIC Priority Intervention: **Fluid Management:** Promotion of fluid balance and prevention of complications resulting from abnormal or undesired fluid levels		NOC Suggested Outcome: **Fluid Balance:** Balance of water in the intracellular and extracellular compartments of the body.
The child will regain normal fluid balance.	■ Assess for edema (periorbital or dependent areas). ■ Calculate fluid intake and plan amounts to offer throughout the day. ■ Limit foods with moderate to high sodium content. ■ Document intake and output. ■ Perform daily weight measurement on the same scale at the same time of day. ■ Administer prescribed medications (diuretics and antihypertensives).	■ Sodium and water retention leads to edema. ■ An intake/output ratio of 1:1 reflects normal hydration and kidney function. ■ Further reduction in sodium intake will help balance fluid and sodium retention. ■ Prevents excessive fluid intake. ■ Weight gain is an early sign of fluid retention. Weight loss indicates improvement in condition. ■ Diuretics cause excretion of excess fluid by preventing reabsorption of water and sodium. Antihypertensives increase excretion of water and sodium and cause vasodilation.	The child maintains normal urine output of 0.5–1 mL/kg/hr. The child receives appropriate fluid each day.
2. Risk for Infection related to renal impairment and corticosteroid therapy			
	NIC Priority Intervention: **Infection Protection:** Prevention and early detection of infection in a patient at risk.		NOC Suggested Outcome: **Risk Control:** Actions to eliminate or reduce actual, personal, and modifiable health threats.
The child will be infection free.	■ Assess temperature every 4 hours. Observe for signs of infection. ■ Obtain throat and other cultures as ordered.	■ The child is at risk for secondary infection. ■ Culture can identify causative microorganism in secondary infection or presence of residual streptococcal infection.	The child's temperature remains within normal limits and child is free of secondary infection.
3. Risk for Impaired Skin Integrity related to tissue edema			
	NIC Priority Intervention: **Pressure Management:** Minimizing pressure to body parts.		NOC Suggested Outcome: **Risk Control:** Actions to eliminate or reduce actual, personal, and modifiable health threats.
The child will be free of skin breakdown.	■ Assess skin for breakdown secondary to edema and bedrest. ■ Encourage position changes every 1–2 hours. Provide skin care. Use a therapeutic mattress.	■ Ensures early identification and implementation of preventive measures. ■ Prolonged pressure leads to skin breakdown.	The child has unimpaired skin integrity.

(continued)

NURSING CARE PLAN The Child with Acute Postinfectious Glomerulonephritis (continued)

GOAL	INTERVENTION	RATIONALE	EXPECTED OUTCOME
4. Altered Nutrition: Less Than Body Requirements related to loss of appetite			
	NIC Priority Intervention: **Nutrition Management:** Assistance with or provision of balanced dietary intake of foods and fluids		NOC Suggested Outcome: **Food and Fluid Intake:** Amount of food and fluid taken into the body over a 24-hour period
The child will maintain adequate caloric intake.	■ Maintain meal schedule similar to that at home. Serve food in age-appropriate servings. Assess for food likes and dislikes. Provide favorite foods, as possible.	■ Normal routine and preferred food choices help to encourage the child to eat.	Child maintains weight and tolerates daily intake that meets nutritional requirements.
5. Activity Intolerance related to fluid and electrolyte imbalance, infectious process, and altered nutrition			
	NIC Priority Intervention: **Energy Management:** Regulations energy use to treat or prevent fatigue and optimize function		NOC Suggested Outcome: **Energy Conservation:** Extent of active management of energy to initiate and sustain activity
The child will progress in activity tolerance without excess fatigue as the disease process improves.	■ Maintain bedrest during acute stage. Encourage gradual activity increase as the condition improves. ■ Provide for quiet play according to the developmental stage of the child (e.g., coloring books, music, videotapes, television).	■ Rest decreases the production of waste materials, which place increased stress on the kidneys. ■ Quiet activities minimize energy expenditures and stress on the kidneys.	The child avoids fatigue and exhibits the ability to tolerate activity for longer period
6. Effective Management of Therapeutic Regimen (Parents) related to child's medication schedule and treatment regimen after discharge			
	NIC Priority Intervention: **Anticipatory Guidance:** Preparation of patient for an anticipated developmental and/or situational crisis		NOC Suggested Outcome: **Compliance Behavior:** Actions taken on the basis of professional advice to promote wellness, recovery, and rehabilitation.
The parents will state knowledge of the child's treatment regiment after discharge.	■ Assess parents' understanding of need for compliance with medication schedule. ■ Describe best schedule for giving medications to match child's and family's routines. ■ Inform parents about potential side effects of prescribed medications and signs and symptoms of complications.	■ Diuretics and antihypertensives are central to treatment plan. ■ Improves compliance. ■ Allows early intervention to prevent side effects.	The parents administer medications as prescribed.

MONITOR FLUID STATUS

Monitor vital signs, fluid and electrolyte status, and intake and output. Hypovolemia can occur as a result of fluid shifting from vascular to interstitial spaces despite the outward clinical signs of excess fluid retention. Monitor the degree of ascites by measuring abdominal girth. Document urine specific gravity.

PREVENT INFECTION

Impaired renal function places the child at risk for infection. Monitor for signs of infection, including fever, increased malaise, and an elevated white blood cell count. Instruct the family in good handwashing technique. Limit visitors, and screen for upper respiratory infections.

PREVENT SKIN BREAKDOWN

Dependent areas or areas prone to pressure are vulnerable to skin breakdown. Turn the child frequently. Pad bony prominences or susceptible areas with sheepskin, or protect skin with a transparent dressing. Make sure the child's bed is free of crumbs or sharp toys. Keep sheets tight and free of wrinkles.

MEET NUTRITIONAL NEEDS

A team approach (including the nurse, renal dietitian, parents, and child) is often needed to meet the child's nutritional needs. In most cases a "no added salt" and low-protein diet is implemented. Anorexia presents the greatest challenge to meeting daily nutritional requirements during the acute phase of the disease. Encouraging parents to bring the child's favorite foods from home, to serve foods in age-appropriate quantities, and to allow the child to eat with other children or with family members may increase the child's appetite.

PROVIDE EMOTIONAL SUPPORT

Guilt is a common reaction of parents of a child with APIGN. Parents may blame themselves for not responding more quickly to the child's initial symptoms or may believe they could have prevented the development of glomerular damage. Discuss the etiology of the disease and the child's treatment, and correct any misconceptions. Emphasize that APIGN develops in only a few children with streptococcal infection.

DISCHARGE PLANNING AND HOME CARE TEACHING

Children are hospitalized for a few days, but it may take 3 weeks for hypertension and gross hematuria to resolve and longer for complete resolution of the disorder. Discharge planning focuses on teaching parents about the child's medication regimen, potential side effects of medications, dietary restrictions, and signs and symptoms of complications. Teach parents how to take the child's blood pressure and how to test urine for albumin, if ordered. Have them demonstrate these procedures. Emphasize that it is important to avoid exposing the child to individuals with upper respiratory tract infections. Recommend family screening for streptococcal infection if this is found to be the cause of the child's APIGN. After discharge, parents should be advised to allow the child to return to his or her normal routine and activities, with periods allowed for rest.

Evaluation

Expected outcomes of nursing care are listed on the nursing care plan.

STRUCTURAL DEFECTS OF THE REPRODUCTIVE SYSTEM

PHIMOSIS

In phimosis, the foreskin over the glans penis cannot be pulled back, due to adhesions or infection. Circumcision, surgical removal of the foreskin, is often performed during the newborn period to prevent phimosis, for ease of proper male hygiene, and to prevent urinary tract infections, balanitis (inflammation of the glans penis), and penile cancer. Approximately 12% of males who are not circumcised as newborns will eventually need the surgery (Williamson, 1997). Bethamethasone cream 0.05% applied twice daily for a month to the glans is an effective alternative to surgery (Van Howe, 1998)

Nursing management involves preoperative preparation of the infant, including the advocacy for and assistance in giving the newborn local anesthesia. Teach parents to care for the surgical site, as newborns are discharged within 24 hours of surgery.

CRYPTORCHIDISM

Cryptorchidism (undescended testes) occurs when one or both testes fail to descend through the inguinal canal into the scrotum. Normally, the testes descend during the seventh to ninth month of gestation.

FAMILIES WANT TO KNOW

Care Following Circumcision

- Wash hands well before and after each diaper change.
- The penis is wrapped in a bandage with petroleum jelly for the first 24 hours. To remove the bandage, soak it by dribbling water from a wet washcloth. Wet the bandage until it can be removed without disturbing the crust or clot.
- To keep the penis from sticking to the diaper, apply petroleum jelly to the head of the penis with each diaper change until the redness goes away.
- A pale yellow crust around the incision site is normal for 3–4 days after surgery.
- Call the physician if any of the following occur: bleeding that will not stop, swelling that lasts for more than 2 days, or signs of infection (tenderness after healing has started, or foul-smelling drainage).

Note: From Ball, J. B. (1998). *Mosby's pediatric patient teaching guides.* St. Louis: Mosby; and L'Archevesque, C. I., & Goldstein-Lohman, H. (1996) Ritual circumcision: Educating parents. *Pediatric Nursing, 22*(3), 228–234.

COMPLICATIONS OF UNCORRECTED CRYPTORCHIDISM

- Infertility
- Malignancy in undescended testis
- Torsion of the undescended testis
- Atrophy
- Psychologic effects of "empty" scrotum

Cryptorchidism may be the result of a testosterone deficiency, an absent or defective testis, or a structural problem such as a narrow inguinal canal, short spermatic cord, or adhesions. The disorder occurs in 3% to 4% of term male infants and in approximately 30% of premature infants (Fonkalsrud, 1996). The higher temperature in the abdomen than in the scrotum results in morphologic change to the testis, beginning after the second birthday. Lower sperm counts are the ultimate result.

Cryptorchidism is usually detected during the newborn examination when palpation of the scrotum fails to reveal one or both testes (see Figure 4-43). It is not unusual for boys with cryptorchidism to have an inguinal hernia as well. In 75% of cases, the testes descend spontaneously by 3 months of age. If descent does not occur within the first year, human chorionic gonadotropin may be prescribed to detect the presence of nonpalpable testes. An orchiopexy is performed at 1 year of age before further damage to the testes occurs. An incision is made at the location of the testis, either in the abdomen or in the inguinal area. Blood vessels are disentangled to allow the testis to reach into the lower scrotum. A second incision is made in the scrotum at the point where the testis is stitched to the inside wall to keep it in place. If the testis is defective or undeveloped, it may be removed surgically to decrease the risk of later malignancies, and a prosthesis may be placed in the scrotum (Tanagho & McAninch, 1995). The goals of surgery are repair of any hernia, enhanced fertility, and psychologic benefit. The orchiopexy also makes it easier to examine the testis for the presence of a tumor. The risk of testicular cancer is 35 to 50 times greater in men with a history of cryptorchidism (Ferrer and McKenna, 2000).

Nursing Management

Preoperative nursing care includes preparing the parents and child for the procedure and addressing parents' concerns about the postsurgical outcome. Orchiopexy is often performed as an outpatient procedure. If the child is hospitalized, postoperative nursing care focuses on maintaining comfort and preventing infection. Encourage bedrest and monitor voiding. Apply ice to the surgical area and administer prescribed analgesics to relieve pain.

Discharge instructions should include demonstration of proper incision care. The diaper area should be cleaned well with each diaper change to decrease chances of infection. Teach parents to identify signs of infection such as redness, warmth, swelling, and discharge. All vigorous activity should be restricted for 2 weeks following surgery to promote healing and prevent injury.

INGUINAL HERNIA AND HYDROCELE

An inguinal hernia is a painless inguinal or scrotal swelling of variable size. A hydrocele is a fluid-filled mass in the scrotum. The condition is found in 1% to 5% of infants, more commonly in boys than girls by a 4:1 ratio. Inguinal hernias occur more commonly in premature infants.

During fetal development, a peritoneal sac precedes the testicle's descent to the scrotum. The lower sac enfolds the testis to become the tunica vaginalis, and the upper sac atrophies before birth. Fluid may become trapped in the tunica vaginalis and cause the hydrocele. When the tunica vaginalis does not atrophy, an abdominal structure may move into it.

Diagnosis is made by physical examination at birth or in early infancy. On palpation of the scrotum, a round, smooth, nontender mass is noted. Transillumination is used to help determine whether the mass is a hernia or hydrocele (see Chapter 4). Swelling associated with a hernia may become more apparent with straining. Some hernias reduce in size during sleep.

Outpatient surgery is performed at an early age (usually after 3 months of age to reduce anesthesia risks) to avoid incarceration, which is a medical emergency. A nerve block may be given in the operating room to reduce postoperative pain. The prognosis is generally excellent. Most hydroceles without inguinal hernia resolve spontaneously as the fluid reabsorbs by the time an infant is 1 to 2 years of age.

Nursing care for hydrocele and inguinal hernia includes explaining the disorder and its treatment and providing preoperative and postoperative teaching and care. Inform parents that the scrotum may be edematous and may appear bruised after surgery. Care of the incision involves careful cleaning of the diaper area. The incision is covered with a protective sealant rather than a dressing.

NURSING ALERT

Inguinal hernias can become incarcerated when a bit of bowel becomes trapped in the inguinal opening. The child has a sudden painful swelling in the groin, increased irritability, vomiting, and abdominal distention. A bowel obstruction is seen on x-ray. Efforts are made to reduce the hernia before surgery, by placing the child in the Trendelenburg position and applying firm manual pressure on the affected side. The child needs surgery within 24–48 hours.

TESTICULAR TORSION

Testicular torsion is an emergency condition in which the testis suddenly rotates on its spermatic cord, cutting off its blood supply. The arteries and veins in the spermatic cord become twisted and interrupt the blood supply, leading to vascular engorgement and ischemia. The incidence is highest at puberty; however, the condition may occur at any time between 3 and 20 years of age. Often the testicles are positioned horizontally in the scrotum, a congenital anomaly known as a bell clapper deformity, which predisposes the boy to this condition.

Manifestations include severe pain and erythema in the scrotum, nausea and vomiting, abdominal pain, and scrotal swelling that is not relieved by rest or scrotal support. The cremasteric reflex is absent. Symptoms generally start when the child is sleeping or inactive, but they can occur after trauma, sexual activity, or exercise. The testis is positioned higher in the scrotum than the unaffected testis because of the shortened vascular pedicle. A testicular scan or sonogram may be performed, if necessary, to confirm the diagnosis.

Torsion must be reduced within 6 hours to save the testis. Manual reduction with an analgesic is sometimes attempted. More often, emergency surgery is performed. During surgery, the testis is untwisted and stitched to the side of the scrotum in the correct position. The procedure is usually performed bilaterally to prevent future torsion in the other testis.

Nursing management involves psychologic support for the child and family related to the need for emergency surgery and concern about the child's future fertility. Reassure parents that as only one testis is usually affected, fertility should not be affected. The child often goes home within a few hours of surgery; thus, the child and family need to be taught about proper care of the incision and pain management. Explain to parents that the child should not lift heavy objects for 4 weeks or participate in strenuous activity for 2 weeks after surgery to promote healing. Teach the adolescent testicular self-examination.

SEXUALLY TRANSMITTED DISEASES

Over the past 10 years, sexually transmitted diseases (STDs) have become a major national public health concern. There are presently more than 25 organisms of bacterial, parasitic, and viral origin, including human immunodeficiency virus (HIV), that are identified as causative agents of sexually transmitted infections (Sharts-Hopko, 1997).

It is the combined responsibility of the federal, state, and local health departments to control and prevent STDs. On a national level, the Centers for Disease Control and Prevention (CDC) and the National Institutes of Health (NIH) coordinate control plans, provide surveillance, and fund basic science and clinical research. State and local health departments

TABLE 18-8 Sexually Transmitted Diseases

DISEASE	CLINICAL MANIFESTATIONS	CLINICAL THERAPY AND NURSING MANAGEMENT
Chlamydia Causative organism: *Chlamydia trachomatis* Incubation period: 5–10 days Reportable: National	*C. trachomatis* is the most frequent cause of nongonococcal urethritis with a prevalence of 6%–12% in adolescents. Common symptoms include: Adolescent females: yellow mucopurulent endocervical discharge, dysuria, pelvic pain, mild abdominal pain, vaginal spotting, cervicitis, salpingitis, pelvic inflammatory disease (PID); 70% are asymptomatic. Adolescent males: urethritis, mucoid gray or clear discharge, dysuria, proctitis, epididymitis; 10% are asymptomatic.	Recommended drug therapy includes doxycyline, or erythromycin for 7 days, or single-dose azithromycin. Sexual partners should be treated if adolescent has had sexual contact within 60 days of onset of symptoms. Avoid sexual contact for 7 days. Encourage use of condoms.
Genital Herpes Causative organism: *Herpes simplex virus* (HSV-2) Incubation period: 2–12 days. Reportable: No	Presentation can be variable and ranges from no symptoms to systematic involvement. Common symptoms include dull pain, itching, and small lesions or pimples on genitalia, buttocks, or thighs. Two types of lesions develop, either fluid-filled blisters on an erythematous base or more commonly, painful papules and ulcers. Ulcers can appear between vaginal folds, in posterior cervix, on glans penis, or shaft of penis, in rectum, or in anus. Ulcers heal within 2–4 weeks. Lymph nodes closest to lesions are frequently enlarged. Disease frequently recurs 4–5 times a year with episodes lasting 5–10 days. Triggers include stress, menses, or trauma. Of adolescents, 12% have HSV-2 antibodies indicating prior infection (McDermott-Webster, 1999).	There is no permanent cure. Recommended drug therapy is acyclovir given for 7–10 days. Discourage oral sex if ulcers are present in mouth, on lips, in vagina, or on penis. Discourage anal sex when lesions are active. Encourage use of condoms, although they may not prevent transmission. The patient remains contagious, even after lesions are healed.
Gonorrhea Causative organism: *Neisseria gonorrhoeae* Incubation period: 2–7 days Reportable: Mandatory	Symptoms and severity vary from mild to severe and are different for males and females. In females, areas that can be infected include urethra, cervix, fallopian tubes, and Bartholin and Skene glands. In males, areas include urethra, prostate, seminal vesicles, epididymis, and Littre and Cowper glands. Of females, 80% are asymptomatic, and 50% are co-infected with chlamydia (Stamm & McGregor, 2001). The classic sign is discharge from vagina and urethra; however, infections involving conjunctiva, pharynx, and anus area are also seen. Prepubescent girls: heavy, thick green or creamy vaginal discharge, vulvovagintis. Adolescent girls: purulent vaginal discharge, cervicitis, PID, Fallopian tube involvement can lead to sterility. Prepubescent and adolescent boys: yellow puslike urethral discharge, erythematous meatus, frequency, dysuria.	Recommended drug therapy includes ceftriaxone IM + azithromycin po given in 1 dose, or cefixime + azithromycin po in 1 dose. Sexual partners should be treated if adolescent has had sexual contact within 60 days of onset of symptoms. Encourage use of condoms or abstinence.

(continued)

are responsible for controlling the spread of STDs through health-promotion programs, staff training, reporting systems, diagnosis, treatment, patient counseling, and the notification of sex partners.

Children and adolescents can become infected with sexually transmitted organisms through sexual experimentation, sexual play, molestation, and sexual abuse. Adolescents are considered an at-risk population because of their inexperience and lack of knowledge about STDs. They may disregard the importance of using barrier protection, may have multiple sexual partners, may have sex frequently, and often do not seek medical treatment until symptoms are well advanced. The adolescent who acquires an STD has a 40% chance of acquiring another STD within a year, especially if gonorrhea is the first infection (Stamm & McGregor, 2001).

More than half of all school-age adolescents have had sexual intercourse during their lifetime, and 8.3% of students had initiated sexual intercourse before 13 years of age (Centers for Disease Control and Prevention, 2000a). Of the 15 million new STD cases each year, approximately 25% occur in adolescents (CDC, 2000b). The most frequently diagnosed STDs

LAW & ETHICS

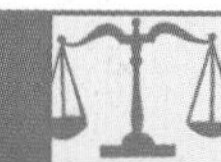

When a child is found to have an STD, the law requires that a report be made to social services and the local health department and that an investigation take place.

TABLE 18-8 Sexually Transmitted Diseases (continued)

DISEASE	CLINICAL MANIFESTATIONS	CLINICAL THERAPY AND NURSING MANAGEMENT
Genital Warts—Condyloma acuminatum Causal Organism: *Human papillomavirus* (HPV) Incubation period: 2–8 months, 3 months average Reportable: In some states	This is the most common STD in adolescents and has been found in 38% of sexually active females (American Academy of Pediatrics, 2000). Warts are small, flat, fleshy-colored with a cauliflower appearance. Adolescent females: warts clustered or alone on the vulva, perineal area, vagina, or cervix; itching, bleeding, burning, irritation. A subclinical infection may be detected through a Pap smear. Specific types of HPV cause 90% of cervical cancers. Adolescent males: warts on the penis, near base of penis on scrotal skin, or near anus.	No cure exists. Treatment includes cryotherapy, topical podophyllin, laser ablation, or chemical cautery with trichloracetic acid. Encourage abstinence or condom use, but condoms are not sufficient to prevent contact transmission. The disorder is transmissible even after treatment.
Trichomoniasis Causal organism: *Trichomonas vaginalis,* a unicellular flagellated protozoa Incubation period: 4–28 days, 1 week average Reportable: No	Adolescent females: pale yellow to gray-green discharge that may be frothy or have a fishy odor, dysuria, vulvar pruritis, occasional abdominal pain; symptoms worsen during menses. Adolescent males: most common site is the urethra; mucoid or purulent urethral discharge, pruritis, dysuria; however, males are usually asymptomatic.	Metronidazole orally as a single dose or for 7 days. Avoid alcohol during and for several days after treatment if a single dose is used. Sexual contact should be avoided until both partners are cured. No follow-up test is needed if symptoms resolve after treatment.
Syphillis Causal organism: *Treponema pallidum* Incubation period: 3 weeks Reportable: Mandatory	Appearance of classic signs and symptoms of syphilis depends on stage of disease. *Primary state* manifests an ulcer on labia, within vagina, on penis, in anus, or on lips or tongue that appears at invasion site approximately 2 weeks to 3 months after infection. Ulcer has an indurated border and smooth base (chancre), and it is painless. Lymphadenopathy is usually present. Ulcer spontaneously heals within 5 weeks. *Second stage* appears up to 10 weeks after initial infection with fever, malaise, lymphadenopathy, patchy alopecia, and diffuse rash. Rash can be macular, papular, papulosquamous, or bullous, and appearance on the palms and soles is classic. Flat mucous patches called condylomata lata appear on genitals. *Latent stage* is asymptomatic and follows the second stage by about 6 weeks. It can last for several years or be lifelong. *Tertiary stage* occurs more than 2 years after onset and manifests as neurosyphillis, cardiovascular disease, ophthalmic, or congenital syphilis.	Recommended drug therapy includes single IM injection of benzathine penicillin G. For children allergic to penicillin, erythromycin is given by mouth for 15 days. Saline compresses and a topical antibiotic are often used to treat lesions on skin. Treat all sexual contacts within 90 days to 1 year of diagnosis, depending upon stage when diagnosed. Encourage abstinence or the use of condoms plus spermicidal foams, cream, or jelly.

are chlamydia, genital herpes (herpes simplex type 2), gonorrhea, genital warts (Human papillomavirus), trichomoniasis, and syphilis (Table 18-8). Adolescents represent 0.5% of the population infected with HIV (CDC, 2000c). However, there are increased numbers of individuals in the 20- to 29-year-old population group who may have become infected initially during their teen years. Complications of STDs include pelvic inflammatory disease, infertility, high risk for ectopic pregnancy, and genital cancer. Lesions associated with STDs provide increased opportunity for HIV infection transmission (Sharts-Hopko, 1997).

The nurse usually encounters the child, adolescent, and family in the emergency department, outpatient clinic, or nursing unit. Because adolescents are often afraid of the consequences of reporting symptoms, it is important for the nurse to develop good assessment skills, particularly when asking questions about sexual activity, partners, and the possibility of abuse. When a child or adolescent is diagnosed with one STD, it is important to screen for others as these diseases may coexist. Adolescents who are symptomatic may postpone care because of the discomfort with examinations and cultures. Routine screening of sexually active adolescents is recommended as many have subclinical cases or are asymptomatic.

NURSING ALERT

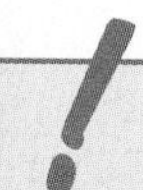

When a child younger than 10 years is found to have gonorrhea or other STD, consider the possibility of sexual abuse. When anorectal symptoms are found, suspect molestation (see Chapter 7).

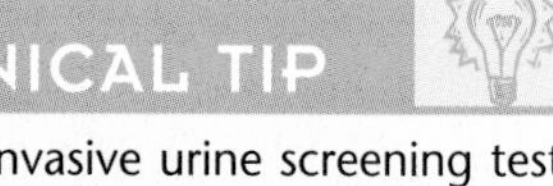

FAMILIES WANT TO KNOW

Preventing STDs and Their Consequences

- Abstinence is the best method to prevent STDs.
- Limit the number of sexual contacts; practice mutual monogamy.
- Always use condoms and spermicidal gels or foams for vaginal and anal intercourse.
- Refrain from oral sex if partner has active sores in mouth, vagina, or anus or on penis.
- Reduce high-risk sexual behaviors. Use of recreational drugs and alcohol can increase sexual risk taking.
- Seek care as soon as symptoms are noticed and make sure partner gets treatment.
- Seek annual screening for STDs.

CLINICAL TIP

A noninvasive urine screening test is now available for chlamydia and gonorrhea. Urine tests are also under development for other STDs (Blake & Woods, 2001).

Nursing care focuses on identifying the cause and the organism, providing appropriate treatment, preventing transmission and complications, and educating the child, adolescent, and family. Encourage sexually active adolescents to receive hepatitis B immunization. When counseling the adolescent, reinforce the importance of treating all sexual partners involved and modifying high-risk sexual behaviors. Be supportive and understanding—never judgmental.

Chapter Highlights

- Bladder capacity increases with growth, from 20 to 50 mL in newborns to 700 mL in adults.
- Structural defects of the urinary system—including bladder exstrophy, hypospadius and epispadius, and obstructive uropathy—generally require surgical treatment.
- Urinary tract infections are the second most common infection in children. Symptoms vary by the age of the child. Children who do not receive aggressive treatment may develop permanent kidney damage or sepsis.
- Nocturnal enuresis often occurs in children whose parents have a history of enuresis. A structural or neurological cause is identified in very few children.
- Minimal change nephrotic syndrome is characterized by edema that develops over several weeks, weight gain, hypertension, irritability, hematuria, malaise, anorexia, and foamy or frothy urine.
- Acute renal failure occurs when kidney function diminishes abruptly and is often reversible. It may occur as a complication of cardiac surgery or drug toxicity. It is also seen in critically ill neonates with asphyxia, sepsis, or shock.
- Chronic renal failure is progressive and irreversible reduced function of the kidneys, eventually resulting in end-stage renal disease. It often results from developmental abnormalities of the kidneys or urinary tract.
- Children with end-stage renal disease are treated with hemodialysis, peritoneal dialysis, or renal transplant.
- Polycystic kidney disease is a genetic disorder with both autosomal recessive and dominant forms that leads to chronic renal failure. It may be detected prenatally or in young children.
- Hemolytic-uremic syndrome is often associated with ingestion of E. coli strain 0157:H7 that produces a toxin that attacks the kidneys. The child develops hemolytic anemia, thrombocytopenia, and acute renal failure that can progress to chronic renal failure.
- Acute postinfectious glomerulonephritis results from a beta-hemolytic group A streptococcal infection of the respiratory tract or skin. Most children have a complete recovery of kidney function.
- Structural defects of the male reproductive system include phimosis, cryptorchidism, inguinal hernia and hydrocele, and testicular torsion.
- Nursing care of sexually transmitted diseases includes identifying the cause and organism, providing appropriate treatment, preventing transmission and complications, and educating the child, adolescent, and family.

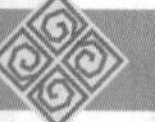

EXPLORE MediaLink

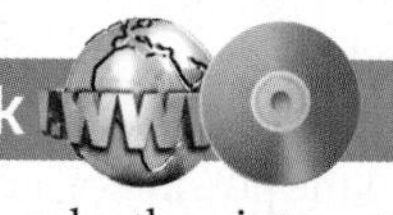

- NCLEX review, case studies, and other interactive resources for this chapter can be found on the Companion Website at **http://www.prenhall.com/ball.** Click on Chapter 18 to select the activities for this chapter.
- For animations, more NCLEX review questions, and an audio glossary, access the accompanying CD-ROM in this textbook.

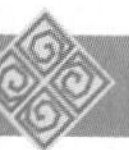

References

1. American Academy of Pediatrics. (2000). *The red book: Report of the committee on infectious diseases* (25th ed.). Elk Grove Village, IL: Author.
2. Anderson, J. E., & Anderson, K. A. (1999). What to tell parents about circumcision. *Contemporary Pediatrics, 16*(2), 87–102.
3. Balinsky, W. (2000). Pediatric end-stage renal disease: Incidence, management, and prevention. *Journal of Pediatric Health Care, 14*(6), 304–308.
4. Barratt, T. M., Avner, E. D., & Harmon, W. E. (1999). *Pediatric nephrology* (4th ed.). Philadelphia: Lippincott, Williams & Wilkins.
5. Becker, N., & Avner, E. D. (1995). Congenital neuropathies and uropathies. *Pediatric Clinics of North America, 42(6),* 1319–1341.
6. Ben-Chaim, J., Docimo, S. G., Jeffs, R. D., Gearhart, J. P. (1996). Bladder exstrophy from childhood to adult life. *Journal of the Royal Society of Medicine 89*(1), 39P-46P.
7. Bereket, G., & Fine, R. N. (1995). Pediatric renal transplantation. *Pediatric Clinics of North America, 42*(6), 1603–1628.
8. Blake, D. R., & Woods, E. R. (2001). The future is here: Noninvasive diagnosis of STDs. *Contemporary Pediatrics, 18*(2), 71–87.
9. Centers for Disease Control and Prevention. (2000a). Youth risk behavior surveillance—United States, 1999. *Morbidity and Mortality Weekly Report, 49*(SS05), 1–96.
10. Centers for Disease Control and Prevention. (2000b). *Tracking the hidden epidemic: Trends in STDs in the United States 2000.* Atlanta: Author.
11. Centers for Disease Control and Prevention. (2000c). *HIV/AIDS Surveillance Report, 12*(1), *www.cdc.gov/hiv/stats.*
12. Evans, E. D., Greenbaum, L. A., & Ettenger, R. B. (1995). Principles of renal replacement therapy in children. *Pediatric Clinics of North America, 42*(6), 1579–1602.
13. Ferrer, F. A., & McKenna, P. H. (2000). Current approaches to the undescended testicle. *Contemporary Pediatrics, 17*(1), 106–111.
14. Fonkalsrud, E. W. (1996). Current management of the undescended testis. *Seminars in Pediatric Surgery, 5*(1), 2–7.
15. Furth, S. L., Garg, P. P., Neu, A. M., Hwang, W., Fivush, B. A., & Powe, N. R. (2000). Racial differences in access to the kidney transplant waiting list for children and adolescents with end-stage renal disease. *Pediatrics, 106*(4), 756–761.
16. Gilman, C. M., & Mooney, K. H. (1998). Alterations in renal and urinary tract function in children. In K. L. McCance & S. E. Huether (Eds.), *Pathophysiology: The biologic basis for disease in adults and children* (3rd ed., pp. 1273–1287). St. Louis: Mosby.
17. Goodyer, P., & Kashtan, C. (1998). The genetic basis of pediatric renal disease. *Seminars in Nephrology, 18*(3), 244–255.
18. Hellerstein, S. (2000). Long term consequences of urinary tract infections. *Current Opinion in Pediatrics, 12,* 125–128.
19. Issenman, R. M., Filmer, R. B., & Gorski, P. A. (1999). A review of bowel and bladder control development in children: How gastrointestinal and urologic conditions relate to problems in toilet training. *Pediatrics, 103*(6), 1346–1352.
20. Kelleher, R. E. (1997). Day time and night time wetting in children: A review of management. *Journal of the Society of Pediatric Nurses, 2*(2), 73–82.
21. McDermott-Webster, M. (1999). The HPV epidemic. *American Journal of Nursing, 99*(3), 24L–24N.
22. Miller, K. L. (1996). Urinary tract infections: Children are not small adults. *Pediatric Nursing, 22*(6), 473–480, 544.
23. Paulozzi, L. J., Erickson, J. D., & Jackson, R. J. (1997). Hypospadias trends in two U.S. surveillance systems. *Pediatrics, 100*(5), 831–834
24. Saborio, P., Hahn, S., Hisano, S., Lotta, K., Scheinman, J. I., & Chan, J. C. M. (1998). Chronic renal failure: An overview from a pediatric perspective. *Nephron, 80,* 134–148.
25. Sharts-Hopko, N. C. (1997). STDs in women: What you need to know. *American Journal of Nursing, 97*(4), 46–53.
26. Shaw, K. N., & Gorelick, M. H. (1999). Urinary tract infection in the pediatric patient. *Pediatric Clinics of North America, 46*(6), 1111–1123.
27. Stamm, C. A., & McGregor, J. A. (2001). Diagnosing and treating STDs in young women. *Contemporary Pediatrics, 18*(2), 53–67.
28. Tanagho, E. A., & McAninch, J. W. (1995). *Smith's general urology* (14th ed.). Stamford, CT: Appleton & Lange.
29. Taylor, J. H. (1996). End-stage renal disease in children: Diagnosis, management, and interventions. *Pediatric Nursing, 22*(6), 481–490.
30. Tobias, N. E. (2000). Management of nocturnal enuresis. *Nursing Clinics of North America, 35*(1), 37–60.
31. Tune, B. M., & Mendoza, S. A. (1997). Treatment of idiopathic nephritic syndrome: Regimens and outcomes in children and adults. *Journal of American Society of Nephrology 8*(5), 824–832.
32. United States Renal Data System. (2000). *2000 Annual Data Report: Atlas of End-stage Renal Disease in the United States.* Minneapolis, MN: USRDS Coordinating Center.
33. Van Howe, R. S. (1998). Cost-effective treatment of phimosis. *Pediatrics, 102*(4), e43, *www.pediatrics.org.*
34. Varade, W. S. (2000). Hemolytic uremic syndrome: Reducing the risks. *Contemporary Pediatrics, 17*(9), 54–64.
35. Vogt, B. A. (1997). Identifying kidney disease: Simple steps can make a difference. *Contemporary Pediatrics, 14*(3), 115–127.
36. Warady, B. A., Alexander, S. R., Watkins, S., Kohout, E., & Harmon, W. E. (1999). Optimal care of the pediatric end-stage renal disease patient on dialysis. *American Journal of Kidney Diseases, 33*(3), 567–583.
37. Williamson, M. L. (1997). Circumcision anesthesia: A study of nursing implications for dorsal penile nerve blocks. *Pediatric Nursing, 23*(1), 59–63.
38. Wong, C. S., Jelacic, S., Habeeb, R. L., Watkins, S. L., & Tarr, P. I. (2000). The risk of HUS after antibiotic treatment of Escherichia coli 0157:H7 infection. *New England Journal of Medicine, 342*(26), 1930–1936.

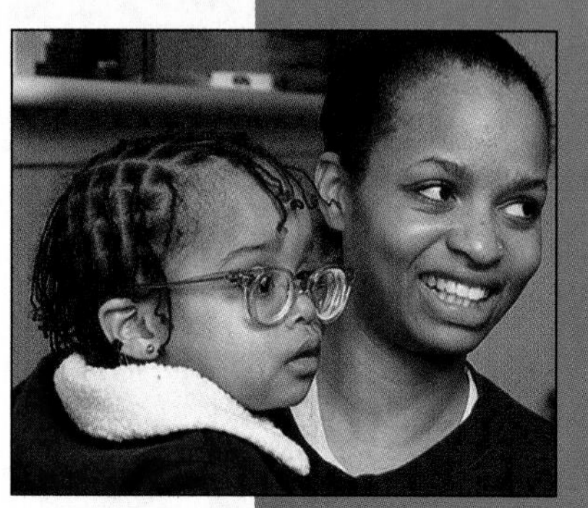

"THE EARLY-INTERVENTION PROGRAM THAT RAEANNE AND I ATTENDED HELPED HER DEVELOP THE SKILLS SHE'LL NEED FOR PRESCHOOL, BUT I KNOW THIS WILL STILL BE A BIG STEP FOR HER. THE NURSE HAS BEEN WORKING WITH US TO HELP PREPARE RAEANNE TO MEET THIS NEW CHALLENGE."

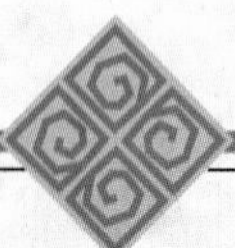

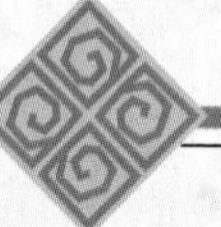

Raeanne, 3 years old, has a severe visual impairment. Born prematurely at 25 weeks gestation, she received oxygen therapy, which damaged her retinal blood vessels. As a result, Raeanne developed retinopathy of prematurity. While in the hospital, Raeanne was given frequent ophthalmoscopic examinations. She received cryotherapy to the retinal vessels—a treatment designed to prevent detached retinae and the resulting total vision loss. Although this treatment halted progression of the disorder, Raeanne was left severely myopic (nearsighted).

For the first 3 years of life, Raeanne and her mother attended an early-intervention program, which provided stimulation for Raeanne and helped teach her mother techniques for enhancing her developmental progress. Raeanne will soon begin attending preschool. Her speech is well developed for a 3-year-old; she is socially mature, converses readily, and shows no developmental delays. However, she has had little contact with other children.

As the nurse in the preschool Raeanne will be attending, how will you assist both her parents and the preschool staff in facilitating Raeanne's adaptation to the preschool experience? Your role includes helping her parents to prepare her for this new experience. You also provide information to the other preschool staff members to help them ensure a safe environment for Raeanne, assist her in adjustment to working and playing in a group of children, and foster her development.

CHAPTER

19

ALTERATIONS IN EYE, EAR, NOSE, AND THROAT FUNCTION

KEY TERMS

audiography A test used to assess hearing in which sounds of various pitches and intensity are presented to children through earphones.

binocularity Ability of the eyes to function together.

conductive hearing loss Hearing loss caused by inadequate conduction of sound from the outer to the middle ear.

decibels Units used to measure the loudness of sounds.

mixed hearing loss Hearing loss having a combination of conductive and sensorineural causes.

myringotomy A procedure whereby an incision is made in the tympanic membrane to drain fluid.

sensorineural hearing loss Hearing loss caused by damage to the inner ear structures or the auditory nerve.

tympanogram A graph showing the ability of the middle ear to transmit sound energy; measured by inserting an airtight probe into the external ear entrance and emitting a tone.

tympanotomy tubes Small Teflon tubes inserted surgically into the tympanic membrane to equalize pressure, promote fluid drainage, and ventilate the middle ear.

visual acuity Measurement of the ability to discriminate a letter or other object to test sight.

vision A complex process of acquiring meaning from what is seen, involving the eye, brain, and related neurologic and physiologic structures.

MediaLink 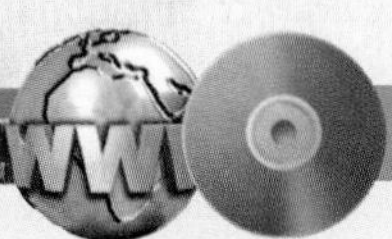

http://www.prenhall.com/ball

Resources for this chapter can be found on the CD-ROM accompanying this textbook, and on the Companion Website at http://www.prenhall.com/ball. Click on Chapter 19 to select the activities for this chapter.

CD-ROM

Animations
- Ear Abnormalities
- Eye Conditions

Audio Glossary

NCLEX Review

COMPANION WEBSITE

Web Links

NCLEX Review

MediaLink Applications
- Planning Interventions for Visual Disorders
- Early Identification and Intervention for Hearing Loss

How are conditions of the eye, ear, nose, and throat related? Which conditions have the potential to affect a child's growth, development, and behavior? In what settings do children with eye, ear, nose, and throat conditions receive care?

Because the eye, ear, nose, and throat are connected, a malformation, infection, or other condition in one of these structures may affect them all. Intact sensory structures are necessary for attainment of developmental milestones; thus alterations, especially to the eye and ear, may delay a child's development. In the preceding scenario, Raeanne's condition was diagnosed when she was very young, and she was enrolled in a program to help her develop normally. Although Raeanne received her initial diagnosis and treatment in the hospital, most children with eye, ear, nose, and throat disorders are treated at home or in the community rather than in the hospital.

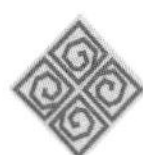

ANATOMY AND PHYSIOLOGY OF PEDIATRIC DIFFERENCES

EYE

How are the eyes of children different from those of adults? Chapter 4 provides a detailed discussion of the assessment of the eyes and **visual acuity,** the ability to discriminate letters or other objects. The eyes of neonates differ from the eyes of adults in several ways. Visual acuity in neonates ranges between 20/100 and 20/400. The lens is more spherical and cannot accommodate to both near and far objects, which means that the neonate sees best at a distance of about 20 cm (8 in.). Because the optic nerve is not yet completely myelinated, the ability to distinguish color and other details is decreased. If the infant is preterm, especially less than 32 weeks' gestation, retinal vascularization, particularly in the periphery of the retina, may be incomplete. The rectus muscles that control binocular vision may be somewhat uncoordinated at birth. The eyes should be aligned and movement coordinated by the age of 3 months.

The eyeball of the infant and young child occupies a larger portion of the orbit than in the adult. Because the eyeball is relatively unprotected laterally, it is more easily injured. The sclera of the neonate is thin and translucent with a bluish tinge, and the iris is blue or gray. Eye color changes during the first 6 months of life. Infants produce tears to nourish and oxygenate the outer layers of the cornea. Parents do not see tears when a young infant cries because the infant's lacrimal system drains them efficiently into the nasal cavity.

As infants grow, their eyes mature and their vision improves. By the age of 2 or 3 years, most children have a visual acuity of 20/50, and by the age of 6 or 7 years, it is 20/20. Visual acuity is measured using standardized letter or picture charts (see Chapter 4 and the Skills Manual). **Vision** refers to the complex process of acquiring meaning from what is seen, involving the eye, brain, and related neurologic and physiologic structures. Development interacts with a child's maturing physiologic system to bring increasing meaning to objects in sight (Table 19-1).

EAR

Why do infants and young children have more ear problems than adults? The eustachian tube, which connects the nasopharynx to the middle ear, is proportionately shorter, wider, and more horizontal in infants than in older children or adults (Figure 19-1 ◆). During sucking, yawning, and other movements, the tube opens for milliseconds, allowing free passage of air between the nasopharynx and the middle ear.

The external ear canal is small at birth, although the internal ear and middle ear are relatively large. As a result, the tympanic membrane is close to the surface and can be easily injured.

NOSE AND THROAT

Up to the age of 6 months, infants are primarily nasal breathers. Edema and nasal discharge may interfere with adequate air intake and feeding. Mucosal swelling and exudate may block the small nasal passages of young children.

The palatine tonsils, which are visible on oral examination, are located on each side of the oropharynx. The method for examining a child's throat is discussed in Chapter 4. Although tonsils vary in size considerably during childhood, they are normally large, espe-

TABLE 19-1 Visually Related Developmental Milestones

AGE	MILESTONE
Term neonate	Demonstrates alertness to visual stimulus presented 8–12 in. (20–30 cm) from eyes
1 month	Follows an object 60 degrees horizontally and 30 degrees vertically; blinks at an approaching object
2 months	Follows a person from 6 ft (2 m) away; smiles in response to a face; raises head 30 degrees from prone
3 months	Tracks an object through 180 degrees; regards own hand; begins visual-motor coordination
4–5 months	Social smile; reaches for a cube 12 in. (30 cm) away; notices a raisin 12 in. (30 cm) away
7–8 months	Picks up a raisin by raking
8–9 months	Pokes at holes in a peg board; neat pincer grasp; crawling
12–14 months	Stacks blocks; places a peg in a round hole; stands and walks

Note: From Scheiner, A. P. (1996). Vision problems: Impairment to blindness. In A. M. Rudolph, J. I. E. Hoffman, & C. D. Rudolph (Eds.), *Rudolph's pediatrics* (20th ed.). Stamford, CT: Appleton & Lange, Pg. 167.

AS THEY GROW 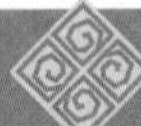 Eustachian Tube

FIGURE 19-1 ◆

Of the three anatomical differences in the eustachian tube between adults and small children (shorter, wider, more horizontal), which do you think could cause more problems for the child and why? Answer: More horizontal. Small children who are bottle-fed in a supine position have a greater probability of developing otitis media because the eustachian tube opens when the child sucks and the horizontal angle provides easy access to the middle ear. In older children the greater angle helps keep foreign substances and germs away from the middle ear.

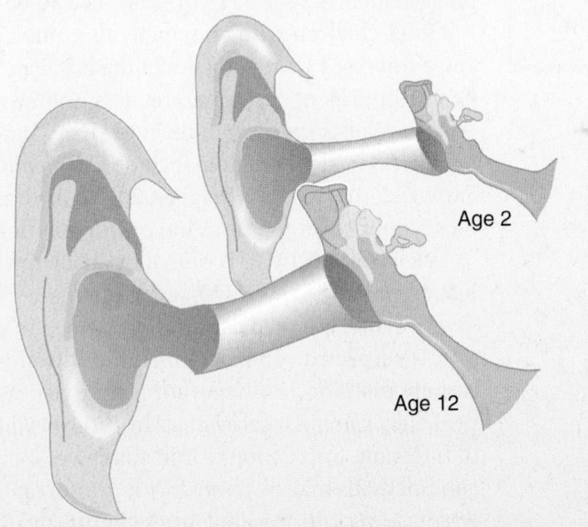

Position of eustachian tube is at less of an angle in the young child, resulting in decreased drainage. (more horizontal)

End of eustachian tube in nasal pharynx opens during sucking.

Eustachian tube equalizes air pressure between the middle ear and the outside environment and allows for drainage of secretions from middle ear mucosa.

cially in school-age children. The nasopharyngeal tonsils (adenoids) lie in the posterior wall of the nasopharynx, just above the oropharynx. In children, the adenoids may become enlarged, harboring bacteria and interfering with breathing.

 DISORDERS OF THE EYE

INFECTIOUS CONJUNCTIVITIS

Conjunctivitis is an inflammation of the conjunctiva, the clear membrane that lines the inside of the lid and sclera. Bacteria, viruses, allergies, trauma, or irritants cause the conjunctiva to become swollen and red with a yellow or white discharge (Figure 19-2 ◆).

Conjunctivitis in an infant under 30 days of age is called ophthalmia neonatorum. These infections are usually acquired from the mother during vaginal delivery as a result of contact

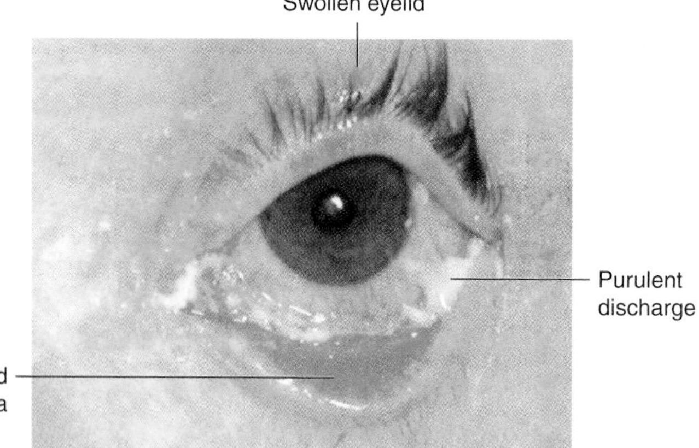

FIGURE 19-2 ◆
Acute conjunctivitis. The major difference between bacterial and viral conjunctivitis is that bacterial conjunctivitis has a purulent discharge that may result in crusting whereas the discharge from viral conjunctivitis is serous (watery). Allergic conjunctivitis produces watery to thick drainage and is characterized by itching.
Adapted from Newell, F. W. (1996). *Ophthalmology: Principles and concepts* (8th ed.). St. Louis: Mosby Year-Book.

LAW & ETHICS

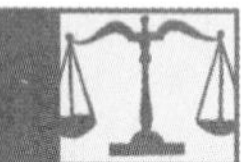

By federal law, all infants born in the United States are given prophylactic eye treatment soon after delivery to help prevent ophthalmia neonatorum. The nurse is responsible for administering this eye ointment. Penicillin, tetracycline, erthromycin, or povidone–iodine ointments are most commonly used.

CLINICAL TIP

Sometimes an infant can develop chemical conjunctivitis due to the prophylactic eye ointment. A chemical reaction should be considered as a possible cause when conjunctivitis develops within 24–48 hours after instillation of the medication.

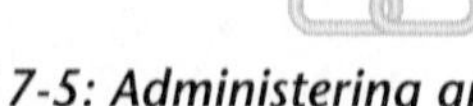

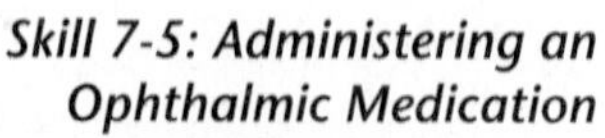

Skill 7-5: Administering an Ophthalmic Medication

CLINICAL TIP

Place a gloved index finger on the child's nose next to the inner corner of the eye and apply gentle pressure for several seconds. If mucopurulent drainage is discharged from the eye, conjunctivitis may be present.

with infected vaginal discharge containing organisms such as *Chlamydia trachomatis* and *Neisseria gonorrhoeae.* Antibiotics are instilled into the eyes of newborns in most states soon after birth as a prophylactic measure. For the infection caused by herpesvirus, prompt and vigorous treatment is needed to prevent eye injury or blindness, which can occur in children with recurrent herpesvirus infections as a result of antibody reaction to the viral antigen. Infants with herpesvirus infections of the eye are treated with intravenous acyclovir and topical drops. Chemical conjunctivitis occasionally occurs in newborns (Alcorn, 2001).

In infants who have frequent tearing and mattering (eyelid discharge that has formed a crust) on awakening, a plugged lacrimal duct may mimic conjunctivitis. Treatment involves massaging the tear duct every 4 hours when the infant is awake. Lacrimal ducts that remain plugged after the age of 1 year may have to be opened surgically.

Older children with conjunctivitis complain of itching or burning, mild photophobia, and a feeling of scratching under the lids. Parents may notice increased tearing or a mucoid or mucopurulent discharge, redness and swelling of the conjunctiva, a pink sclera, and crusty eyelids, especially in the morning. There is no change in vision. Common infectious organisms in older children include *Haemophilus influenzae, Streptococcus pneumoniae,* and *Staphylococcus aureus* (Wagner, 2000). A viral cause is also possible, with adenovirus the most common organism. Viral conjunctivitis is more often bilateral than unilateral.

When conjunctivitis is caused by an allergy, the child complains of intense itching. Examination reveals red eyes with watery discharge. The eyes may also appear puffy and swollen.

Antibiotic eye medication is prescribed in droplet or ointment form if a bacterial infection is suspected. Amoxicillin and erythromycin are common choices. When gonococcal conjunctivitis occurs in newborns, ceftriaxone is recommended, as the disease is resistant to penicillin. Careful total evaluation of the newborn is also performed to watch for other signs of infection. Instructions for instilling eye medications are given in the Skills Manual. Viral conjunctivitis may be treated with comfort measures such as cleaning drainage away with a warm clean cloth, avoiding bright lights, and avoiding reading, with ophthalmic antibiotics sometimes given to prevent bacterial invasion due to frequent rubbing of the eyes. If an allergen is believed to be the cause, antihistamines administered orally or ophthalmically may be prescribed. Topical steroids and vasoconstrictors may also be used (Alcorn, 2001).

Nursing Management

Nurses routinely instill antibiotics into the eyes of newborns after birth. A careful examination should occur so that any cases of ophthalmia neonatorum are referred promptly to an ophthalmologist. Women infected with gonococcus or chlamydia should be identified so their babies can receive attention and medication at birth to prevent infection (Brocklehurst & Rooney, 2000). Babies born at home should have ocular examinations soon after birth.

Because infectious conjunctivitis is extremely contagious, tell parents that children should not return to child care or school until they have been taking an antibiotic for 24 hours. Teach parents the importance of careful handwashing and the avoidance of shared towels. Tell parents that children should not rub their eyes; mittens may help prevent infants from doing so. Toddlers may be distracted by activities that keep their hands busy. Teach

FAMILIES WANT TO KNOW

Instilling Eye Medications

It can be challenging to safely instill eye medication into young children. Give parents the following suggestions:

- Wash hands well.
- Be sure the medicine is warmed at least to room temperature.
- Remove any drainage from the eye with a clean or sterile moist, warm cloth or gauze.
- Wash hands again.
- Have the child lying on the back with eyes closed.
- Gently pull the lower lid down to form a small pocket.
- Apply a thin string (for ointment) or drops of the medicine.
- Allow the eyelid to return to normal position.
- Have the child keep the eye closed for several seconds.
- Help prevent spread of the infection by keeping the child's hands clean.
- Enhance comfort by keeping the head elevated to decrease swelling and by avoiding exposure to bright light.

parents the proper techniques for instilling eye medications. For children with allergies, alert parents to signs of infection so if the child gets an eye infection, prompt treatment will be obtained.

PERIORBITAL CELLULITIS

Periorbital cellulitis is an infection of the eyelid and surrounding tissues that is usually caused by bacteria (Figure 19-3 ◆). Children present with swollen, tender, red or purple eyelids; restricted, painful movement of the area around the eye; and fever. Periorbital cellulitis should be treated promptly to prevent the spread of the infection to the posterior orbit. Management includes hospitalization for intravenous administration of antibiotics and the application of hot packs. Children usually respond favorably within 48 to 72 hours.

VISUAL DISORDERS

Vision, the complex process of acquiring meaning from what is seen, depends on many factors. The eyes must move quickly and in a coordinated manner (see Chapter 4 for discussion of eye movement assessment). They must function together for clear, single vision to occur. If this ability, called **binocularity,** is not present (perhaps due to strabismus or amblyopia), the child cannot make sense of the images the brain receives. Normally, the objects seen are integrated with other senses through eye–hand coordination, and with the brain through visual imagery and discrimination of objects seen. Although visual acuity is essential, the child's movements, mental processes, and other senses all interact to give meaning to objects that are viewed. Vision therefore influences learning and school performance.

Visual disturbances must be diagnosed and treated promptly to prevent impairment or loss of visual acuity (Altemeier, 2000). Most children undergo a simple test for visual acuity during health care visits as soon as they can cooperate with the examiner. Once in school, children's visual acuity is screened every 2 to 3 years during the elementary years. Nurses often organize vision screening programs for children. Table 19-2 provides a series of questions

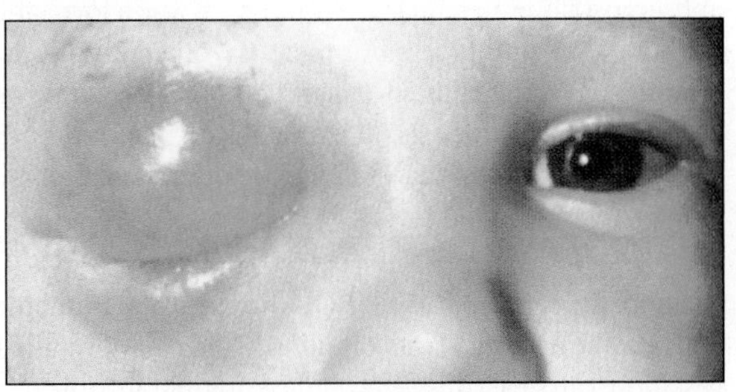

FIGURE 19-3 ◆
Periorbital cellulitis is an infection of the eyelid and surrounding tissues, not the eye itself. It is a serious bacterial infection that can spread to the optic nerve if not treated promptly with intravenous antibiotics.
From Malinow, I. & Powell, K.R. (1993). Periorbital cellulitis. *Pediatric Annals, 22*(4), 241–246.

TABLE 19-2 Assessment Questions for Identifying Visual Disturbances in Children

YOUNG CHILD	SCHOOL-AGE CHILD
Ask the parents:	Ask the parents:
Does your child follow you with his or her eyes as you come into a room?	Does your child like to look at pictures and read?
Are other objects followed with ease?	Does your child hold toys or books close, or sit very close to the television?
Do both eyes work together or does one seem to wander off?	Does your child squint or rub the eyes?
At what age did your baby sit, stand, walk?	Is he or she at grade level in all subjects?
Does your child have any difficulty picking up objects?	Has your child demonstrated any learning difficulties?
	Does he or she use a computer, watch television, or play computer games?
	Does your child play sports and games at the same level of ability as peers?

that can be asked to identify visual disturbances in children. A child who does not pass vision screening is referred to an ophthalmologist or optometrist for more detailed examination of near and far vision, eye structure and movement, and color discrimination.

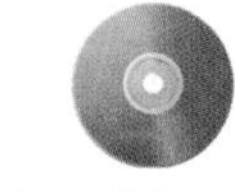

Eye Conditions

Common visual disorders in children are as follows (DeRespinis, 2001):

- *Hyperopia* (farsightedness): Light rays focus posterior to the retina, resulting in an inability to focus on nearby objects. All children have some degree of hyperopia until 9 to 10 years of age. However, their eyes can accommodate sufficiently to enable them to see near objects clearly. Blurring of vision occurs only in children with excessive hyperopia, or a difference in accommodation between the two eyes. Amblyopia, or a weakening of the poorer eye, can occur in these children if treatment is not obtained.
- *Myopia* (nearsightedness): Light rays focus anterior to the retina, resulting in an inability to see far-off objects. Although children of any age can manifest myopia, it most commonly develops at about 8 years of age. The child may complain of headaches and often squints to improve distance vision.
- *Astigmatism:* Light rays are refracted differently depending on their place of entry to the eye. The curvature of the cornea or lens is not uniformly spherical, causing blurred images. The child with astigmatism often holds pages very close to the face to obtain the best visual image.

For the clinical manifestations and management of four disorders that can significantly affect vision (strabismus, amblyopia, cataracts, and glaucoma), see pages 695–696.

Compensatory lenses are prescribed for most visual disorders. A significant difference in visual acuity between the eyes is often a result of amblyopia or strabismus, and further treatment may be needed. The visual acuity of a child with compensatory lenses should be reevaluated every 1 to 2 years. More frequent visits to an eye specialist are needed when a child is being treated for amblyopia or strabismus.

Color Blindness

Color blindness is an X-linked recessive disorder found in 8% of white and 4% of black males and almost never in females. The most common form affects the ability to distinguish between the colors red and green, but there are other variations. Preschool boys are tested for color blindness in some clinics to identify those with the disorder. Color blindness is not treatable and management focuses on issues of safety (e.g., problems in distinguishing red–green traffic signals) and techniques to improve discrimination of colors in the affected color groups.

RETINOPATHY OF PREMATURITY

Retinopathy of prematurity (ROP) occurs when immature blood vessels in the retina constrict and become necrotic. This condition, which may occur in infants of low birth weight or of short gestation, can heal completely or lead to mild myopia or retinal detachment and blindness.

CLINICAL MANIFESTATIONS OF VISUAL DISORDERS

ETIOLOGY	CLINICAL MANIFESTATIONS	CLINICAL THERAPY
Strabismus Can be congenital or acquired. Most common types: Esotropia: inward deviation of eyes ("crossed eyes") Exotropia: outward deviation of eyes ("wall-eyes") Strabismus Reprinted from *Paediatrics,* 2e, Thomas & Harvey, p. 130, 1997, by permission of the publisher Churchill Livingstone.	Eyes appear misaligned to observer. May occur only when child is tired. Symptoms include: squinting and frowning when reading; closing one eye to see; having trouble picking up objects; dizziness and headache. Corneal light reflex and cover-uncover tests confirm diagnosis.	Occlusion therapy (patching the fixating or good eye to force use of the weak eye) Compensatory lenses Surgery of the rectus muscles to correct muscle imbalance Eye drops to cause blurring of the good eye Prisms Vision therapy (eye exercises) If treatment is begun before 24 months of age, amblyopia (reduced vision in one or both eyes) may be prevented.
Amblyopia ("lazy eye") Reduced vision in one or both eyes Amblyopia can result from anything which causes visual deprivation to one eye. The most common causes are untreated strabismus, with the child "tuning out" the image in deviating eye, congenital cataract or visual differences between eyes.	Symptoms are the same as for strabismus. Vision testing can be used to diagnose condition.	Compensatory lenses Occlusion therapy Occasionally vision therapy (eye exercises) is used in an attempt to improve the weaker eye. Treatment is discontinued when visual acuity no longer improves; 20/20 acuity rarely attained. Treatment is most successful if done by 5-6 years of age.
Cataracts Occur when all or part of lens of eye becomes opaque, which prevents refraction of light rays onto retina Congenital cataract. From Vaughan, D., Asbury, T. & Riordan-Eva, P. (1992) *General ophthalmology.* (13th ed., p. 172). New York: McGraw-Hill Companies.	Can affect one or both eyes and may be congenital or acquired. Clouding of lens indicates presence of cataract; however, cataracts are not always visible to naked eye. Symptoms include: distorted red reflex; symptoms of vision loss (see strabismus).	Specific treatment depends on whether one or both eyes are affected, extent of clouding, and presence of other ocular abnormalities. Surgical removal of lens and corrective lenses; contact lenses frequently used; results of surgery are good; surgery before the age of 2 months is associated with the best results; visual acuity in 55% of children is 20/40 or better. Lens implant may be used. Eye protectors and restraints are used postoperatively to prevent injury; antibiotic or steroid drops may be used for several weeks; treatment for amblyopia may be necessary.

(continued)

CLINICAL MANIFESTATIONS OF VISUAL DISORDERS (continued)

ETIOLOGY	CLINICAL MANIFESTATIONS	CLINICAL THERAPY
Glaucoma Increased intraocular pressure damages eye and impairs visual function; ciliary body of eye produces aqueous fluid that flows between iris and lens into anterior chamber; if enough fluid accumulates, blindness results. May be congenital or acquired and affect one or both eyes Congenital glaucoma. From Vaughan, D., Asbury, T. & Riordan-Eva, P. (1992) *General ophthalmology.* (13th ed., p. 172). New York: McGraw-Hill Companies.	Symptoms of congenital glaucoma include: tearing, corneal clouding, eyelid spasms, and progressive enlargement of eye; photophobia (extreme sensitivity to light). Symptoms of acquired glaucoma include: constant bumping into objects in child's periphery (painless visual field loss); seeing halos around objects. Diagnosis is made using tonometer, which measures intraocular pressure.	Surgery to reduce intraocular pressure is treatment of choice, since medications used to combat glaucoma in adults are not effective in children. Compensatory lenses used following surgery Treatment is not always successful, especially if the child has congenital glaucoma, so parents' feelings regarding care of a visually handicapped child should be explored.

Note: Altemeier, W. A. (2000). Preschool vision screening: The importance of the two-line difference. *Pediatric Annals,* 29, 264–267; Bacal, D. A. & Wilson, M. C. (2000). Strabismus: Getting It Straight. *Contemporary Pediatrics,* 17, 49–60; and Starr, N. B. (2000). Vision Therapy for learning disabilities and dyslexia. *Journal of Pediatric Health Care,* 14, 32–33.

Etiology and Pathophysiology

Retinopathy of prematurity results from injury to the developing capillaries of the retina. Oxygen therapy is associated with the development of ROP (Figure 19-4 ◆), but other factors such as respiratory distress, artificial ventilation, apnea, bradycardia, heart disease, multiple blood transfusions, infection, hypoxia, hypercarbia, acidosis, shock, and sepsis have been linked with the disorder. It is most common in infants born before 28 weeks gestation and weighing under 1,600 g (3 lb, 8 oz) at birth.

The retina is normally vascularized by about 8 months gestation. For the premature infant, however, this process must continue after birth and the environmental and other conditions listed in the preceding paragraph appear to affect its course. Arteriole constriction, followed by vascular proliferation of abnormal vessels, occurs. In most cases, the abnormal vessels gradually regress and normal vascularization occurs. Sometimes, however, the abnormal vascularization continues into the vitreous cavity, causing abnormalities of the retina, optic disc, and macula. It is not known why the disease progresses in some cases, but progression is directly linked to lower birth weight, greater prematurity, and duration (not necessarily concentration) of oxygen therapy. Raeanne, the child described in the scenario at the beginning of this chapter, developed retinopathy of prematurity after receiving oxygen therapy to aid her underdeveloped lungs.

Although the developing capillaries are lost, in up to 90% of cases, some degree of revascularization occurs later. The degree of visual loss, varying from slight to total, is determined by the degree of revascularization that occurs.

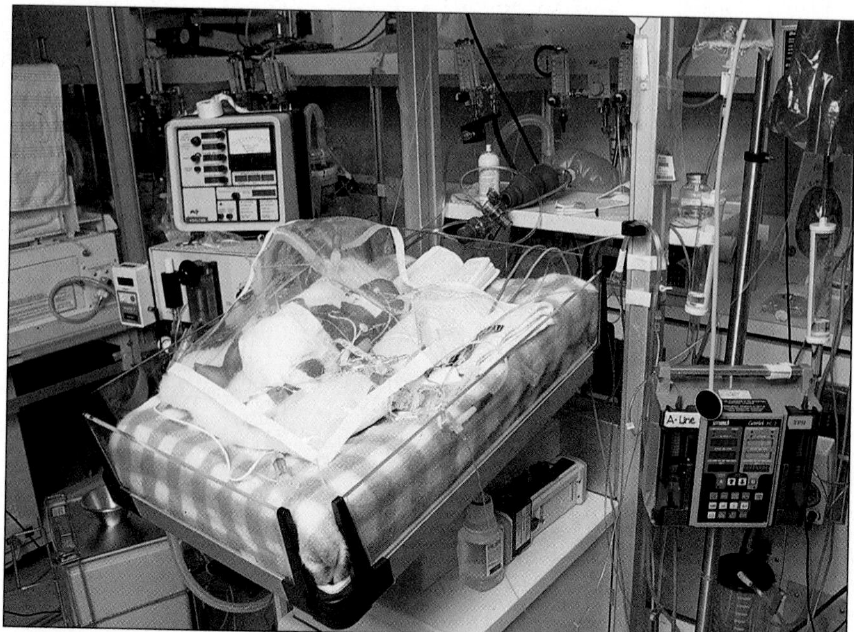

FIGURE 19-4 ◆
This premature infant in the neonatal intensive care unit is receiving artificial ventilation—a risk factor for retinopathy of prematurity. The infant will need careful management of oxygen exposure and periodic eye examinations.

Clinical Manifestations

Retinopathy of prematurity is characterized by progressive changes in the retinal blood vessels, and in severe disease, by retinal detachment. Premature and low-birth-weight infants at risk for the disease are given frequent ocular examinations to ensure early detection of these changes. For infants who do not receive ophthalmologic examinations, resulting visual impairment may be detected only later in infancy when the child progresses slowly in meeting developmental milestones, fails to reach for objects, and does not follow objects or faces with the eyes. When visual impairment is present, the child usually manifests myopia. Total loss of vision can occur in the child who suffers a retinal detachment.

Clinical Therapy

Diagnosis is made by ophthalmologic examination. A classification system is used to describe the location, extent, and severity of the disease (American Academy of Pediatrics, Section on Ophthalmology, 2001). All infants at risk, particularly those under 2,000 g (4 lb, 3 oz) at birth or born before 33 weeks gestation are assessed frequently by an ophthalmologist who is experienced with the condition. The disease does not manifest itself before 4 to 6 weeks after birth, so it is important that the infant receive regular eye examinations until the risk is discounted. If the infant shows signs of disease, eye examinations continue every 1 to 2 weeks. Involvement of blood vessels in the periphery of the retina rarely leads to visual impairment. With involvement in other areas of the retina, risk of visual problems is more common.

Treatment of infants with severe retinopathy of prematurity involves using cryotherapy or laser therapy to stop progression of the disease process. Other surgical procedures such as a scleral buckle procedure and vitrectomy have been used in retinal detachments. For children like Raeanne who have resulting visual impairment, it is important to treat problems such as strabismus, amblyopia, and myopia to promote maximal development.

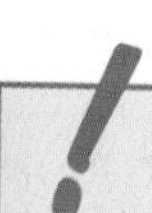

NURSING ALERT

Nurses should be aware of the dangers of oxygen therapy and ventilatory support. Constant monitoring of the oxygen delivery and testing equipment is essential. Newborns in special care units should be shielded from light as much as possible, as light exposure may increase their susceptibility to retinopathy of prematurity.

NURSING MANAGEMENT

Nursing Assessment and Diagnosis

Assessment of the infant at risk for retinopathy of prematurity begins at birth by identifying infants who may require oxygen therapy. Look for risk factors such as prematurity and low birth weight. Assess the infant's breathing efforts and report any changes. Be certain the

NURSING CARE PLAN The Child with a Visual Impairment Secondary to Retinopathy of Prematurity

GOAL	INTERVENTION	RATIONALE	EXPECTED OUTCOME
1. Sensory/Perceptual Alteration related to altered reception, transmission, and integration resulting from retinopathy of prematurity			
	NIC Priority Intervention: **Visual Deficit Enhancement:** Assistance in accepting and learning alternate methods for living with diminished vision.		NOC Suggested Outcome: **Developmental Progression:** Compensate for sensory deficits by maximizing use of impaired senses.
The child will receive adequate sensory input	■ Provide kinesthetic, tactile, and auditory stimulation during play and in daily care (e.g., talking and playing). Provide music while bathing an infant using bells and other noises on each side of infant. Verbally describe to a child all actions being carried out by adult.	■ Because visual sensory input is not present, the child needs input from all other senses to compensate and provide adequate sensory stimulation.	The child demonstrates minimal signs of sensory deprivation.
2. Risk for Injury related to impaired vision			
	NIC Priority Intervention: **Fall Prevention:** Instituting special precautions with patients at risk for injury.		NOC Suggested Outcome: **Risk Control:** Actions to eliminate or reduce modifiable health threats.
The child will be protected from safety hazards that can lead to injury.	■ Evaluate environment for potential safety hazards based on age of child and degree of impairment. Be particularly alert to objects that give visual cues to their dangers (e.g., stoves, fireplaces, candles). Eliminate safety hazards and protect the child from exposure. Take the child on a four of new rooms, explaining safety hazards (e.g., schools, hotel room, hospital room).	■ The child may be at risk for injury related both to developmental stage and inability to visualize hazards.	The child will experience no injuries.
3. Risk for Altered Growth and Development related to impaired vision			
	NIC Priority Intervention: **Developmental Enhancement:** Facilitating or teaching parents caregives to facilitate optional growth & development of children.		NOC Suggested Outcome: **Child Growth and Development:** Milestones of developmental progression.
The child has experiences necessary to foster normal growth and development.	■ Help parents plan early, regular social activities with other children. ■ Provide opportunities and encourage self-feeding activities. ■ Provide an environment rich in sensory input. ■ Assess growth and development during regular examinations to identify the child's strengths and needs.	■ The visually impaired child benefits developmentally from contact with other children. ■ To obtain adequate nutrients, the child needs to feel comfortable feeding self. ■ Sensory input is needed for normal development to occur. ■ Regular examinations aid in early identification of growth problems or developmental delays, so that appropriate interventions can be planned.	The child demonstrates normal growth and development milestones.

(continued)

NURSING CARE PLAN The Child with a Visual Impairment Secondary to Retinopathy of Prematurity (continued)

GOAL	INTERVENTION	RATIONALE	EXPECTED OUTCOME
4. Risk for Ineffective Family Coping related to child's prolonged disability from sensory impairment			
	NIC Priority Intervention: **Family Mobilization:** Utilization of family strengths to influence child's health positively.		NOC Suggested Outcome: **Positive Coping:** Extent to which family can mobilize resources to deal with the child's needs.
The family identifies methods for coping with their visually impaired child.	■ Provide explanation of visual impairment as appropriate.	■ The parents may feel guilt about the child's visual impairment, which can be allayed by knowledge of the cause.	The family successfully copes with the experience of having a visually impaired child.
	■ Refer parents to organizations, early intervention programs, and other parents of visually impaired children.	■ The parents will receive needed information and support from others.	
	■ Assist parents to plan for meeting developmental, educational, and safety needs of their visually impaired child. Offer resources for changing home environment to assist visually impaired child.	■ The child may require an enhanced environment in order to faster developmental progress.	

ventilation equipment is properly set to deliver the correct amount of oxygen. Note the cumulative risks in a particular case and suggest the need for a referral to an ophthalmologist, as necessary.

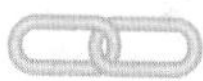

Skill 10-12: Assisted Ventilation

The accompanying nursing care plan outlines several nursing diagnoses for a child such as Raeanne with a visual impairment secondary to retinopathy of prematurity. Following are other nursing diagnoses that may be appropriate for an infant with the potential to develop ROP or a child with resulting visual impairment:

- *Sensory/perceptual alteration (visual),* related to altered transmission of impulses
- *Impaired gas exchange,* related to ventilation-perfusion imbalance
- *Alteration in growth and development,* related to effects of visual impairment
- *Altered family processes,* related to a child with a visual impairment

Planning and Implementation

The nurse plays an important role in preventing retinopathy of prematurity. Encourage early and regular prenatal care to prevent unnecessary premature births. Administer oxygen only to newborns who need it, and in the amount specified by the physician. Ensure that the proper ventilatory settings are used. Be alert for infants with multiple risk factors and refer them, when appropriate, for ophthalmologic examination. Parents of infants at risk for ROP require information about the disorder, as well as support, as the long-term effects on the child's vision are often identified only after subsequent examinations as the child grows.

The accompanying nursing care plan summarizes care for the child with a visual impairment resulting from retinopathy of prematurity. The nurse is instrumental in case management for such children. Reinforce to parents the importance of follow-up eye examinations. Teach methods of stimulating development for the visually impaired child (refer to the next section).

GROWTH & DEVELOPMENT

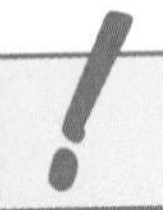

Infants with visual impairment use kinesthesia, touch, and language to socialize. They will appreciate and use touch more than other children and will respond to verbal explanations when others use non-verbal communication. Vision affects both fine and gross motor skills, so skills such as hand-to-mouth coordination and walking may be delayed in children who are visually impaired.

NURSING ALERT

Both the Food and Drug Administration (FDA) and the American Academy of Ophthalmology have issued warnings to keep laser pointers away from infants and children. These devices can cause retinal damage if stared at for more than 10 seconds. Young children are at greater risk than adults because they fail to blink and avert their gaze in less than 0.25 second (the typical adult response).

Evaluation

Expected outcomes of nursing care for the child with retinopathy of prematurity include:

- Early identification of visual impairment
- Normal developmental milestone achievement
- Positive management of child's visual condition by the family.

VISUAL IMPAIRMENT

Visual impairment accounts for 11% of chronic medical conditions in children. Legal blindness (defined as visual acuity of 20/200 or worse in the corrected eye or significantly reduced visual fields) occurs in 1 per 35,000 children. About 1 in 500 children have partial vision. About half of the children who are blind or have partial vision have other disabilities as well. One in 25 preschoolers and 1 in 4 school-age children have a vision problem that requires corrections (Burns, Brady, & Dunn, et al., 2000).

Many conditions discussed earlier in this chapter lead to temporary or permanent visual impairment. Infants who are premature; whose mothers were infected prenatally with rubella, toxoplasmosis, or other viruses; and who have certain congenital and hereditary conditions have a high risk of visual problems (Table 19-3). Fetal alcohol syndrome (FAS) is a major cause of visual disturbance; 90% of children with FAS have eye abnormalities.

The signs of visual impairment depend on the cause and degree of the problem and the age of the child (Table 19-4). The child's eyes may appear crossed or watery, and the lids may be crusty. Verbal children may complain of itching; dizziness; headache; or blurred, double, or poor vision.

Clinical therapy depends on the child's condition and may include surgery, medication, and supportive aids. In the case of a disorder that results in permanent visual impairment, an interdisciplinary team of specialists works with the child and family. Nurses have an important role in this team, as evidenced by the care provided to Raeanne.

TABLE 19-3 Common Causes of Visual Impairment in Children

Congenital or Hereditary	Acquired
Cataracts	Injury to eye or head
Glaucoma	Infections
Tay-Sachs disease	Rubella
Marfan syndrome	Measles
Down syndrome	Chickenpox
Fetal alcohol syndrome	Brain tumor
Prenatal infections (maternal infection)	Retinopathy of prematurity
Rubella	Cerebral palsy
Toxoplasmosis	
Herpes simplex	
Retinoblastoma	

TABLE 19-4 Signs of Visual Impairment

Infants	Toddlers and Older Children
May be unable to follow lights or objects	May rub, shut, or cover eyes
Do not make eye contact	Tilt or thrust head forward
Have a dull, vacant stare	Blink frequently
Do not imitate facial expressions	Hold objects close
	Bump into objects
	Squint

NURSING MANAGEMENT

Nursing Assessment and Diagnosis

Prevent visual deficits by teaching safety in activities that can injure the eye.

Vision screening facilitates early detection and treatment of conditions that can lead to vision loss. Visual testing can be done at any age, including immediately after birth. Developmental milestones that require vision, such as following bright lights, reaching for objects, or looking at pictures in a book, can be used to assess vision. For children over the age of 3 years, visual acuity is most frequently measured by means of an age-appropriate acuity test (see Chapter 4 and the Skills Manual). The photo screener is a device that can be used to take a photo of the child's eyes and is useful for infants, toddlers, and preschoolers. The photo can be used to diagnose refraction errors, eye opacities, and misalignment (Gomez & Davis, 2001). Visual fields and the ability to discriminate colors are tested at school age, when children can cooperate.

CLINICAL TIP

The American Academy of Pediatrics recommends that vision screening of all children should begin at 3 years of age during health care visits.

Skills 5-17 to 5-19: Visual Acuity Screening

Children who are visually impaired may lag in development of cognitive and other skills. Sighted children learn the word *cup* using four senses—sight, touch, hearing, and taste—to obtain the information necessary to connect words with the objects they represent. In contrast, children with visual impairments rely on only three senses—touch, hearing, and taste. They learn concepts through differences in sounds, textures, and shapes.

Many visual disorders are linked with conditions that influence development. Thus, a child with cerebral palsy or fetal alcohol syndrome should be assessed frequently to identify a visual disorder, as well as to evaluate normal developmental milestones.

Nursing diagnoses for the child with impaired vision may include the following:

- *Sensory/perceptual alteration (visual),* related to altered sensory perception
- *Risk for injury,* related to poor vision
- *Risk for altered growth and development,* related to visual impairment
- *Risk for ineffective family coping,* related to demands of a child with a sensory impairment

Planning and Implementation

Table 19-5 outlines several strategies that can be used by nurses who work with visually impaired children. Nursing care focuses on encouraging the child's use of all senses, promoting socialization, helping parents to meet the child's developmental and educational needs, and providing emotional support to parents. Refer the parents to an early intervention program upon diagnosis. Nearly all care will occur in community and home settings.

ENCOURAGE USE OF ALL SENSES

Children who are partially sighted or blind use other senses to a great extent. Encouraging the use of the eyes as much as possible is important even if a child has poor vision (Figure 19-5 ◆).

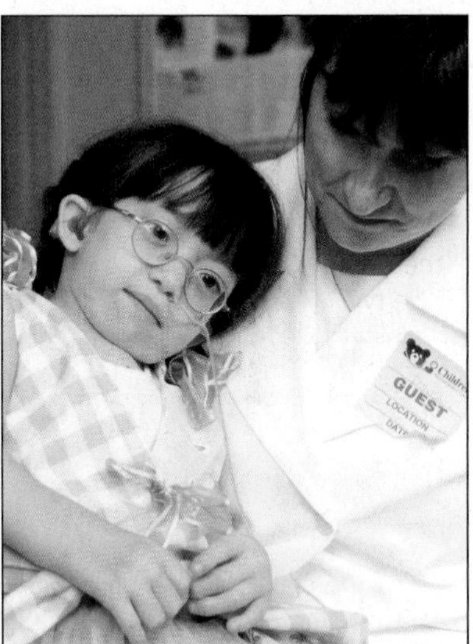

FIGURE 19-5 ◆ This child with a visual impairment needs ongoing developmental assessment and a comprehensive individual education plan. As is true with many children, she has several healthcare needs. Note that she is receiving tube feedings.

PROMOTE SOCIALIZATION

The child's interactions and socializations should be as normal as possible (similar to those of sighted children of the same age and development).

TABLE 19-5 Strategies for Nurses Working With Visually Impaired Children

- Call the child's name and speak before touching the child.
- Tell the child when you are leaving the room.
- Describe what each procedure will feel like (e.g., blood pressure cuff, otoscope).
- Let the child touch the equipment to establish familiarity.
- Describe what foods are present and their locations on the food tray.

FAMILIES WANT TO KNOW

Enhancing Development of the Visually Impaired Child

- Encourage a toddler or preschooler who is visually impaired to look at pictures in well-lit settings. Have a school-age child read large-print books. Computers designed for the visually impaired are also available. The Optacon (a device that raises print so it can be felt by the child) and View Scan (which magnifies print) are instruments that improve the ability to read.
- Expose the infant and child to everyday sounds.
- Encourage the infant to use the sense of touch to explore people and objects. Have the parents purchase toys with sound and texture in mind. Directional concepts can be taught using games. Responding to the infant's and child's vocalizations encourages the use of speech.
- Teach specific techniques for toileting, dressing, bathing, eating, and safety.
- When the child becomes mobile, furniture and other objects in the environment should be kept in the same positions so the child can safely move around independently. Extra care must be taken to prevent injuries when a child does not see.
- Emphasize the child's abilities. Adolescents can use seeing-eye dogs or a white cane to function independently.
- Encourage the child to function independently within normal developmental parameters.
- If in the hospital or another strange environment, orient the child to the placement of objects and do not rearrange them.
- Teach those around the child to:
  - Announce their presence to the child when approaching.
  - When walking with a blind child, walk slightly ahead of the child so he or she can sense your movements.
  - Let the child hold the seeing person's arm rather than the reverse.
  - Identify the contents of meals and encourage the child to feed self.

GROWTH & DEVELOPMENT

Children with visual impairment may take longer than expected to master self-help skills such as feeding and dressing.

CLINICAL TIP

Clean the child's glasses daily with warm water and a clean, soft dry cloth. Follow the prescriber's and family's directions for care of contact lenses. General guidelines include:

- Allow the child to wear the lenses for the recommended time only.
- Store each lens in the right or left containers as labeled.
- Wash hands carefully before contact with the child's eyes or lenses.
- Use a cleaning solution on the lens after its removal.
- Rinse the lens with the recommended rinsing solution.
- Keep the lenses in the case with the disinfecting solution.
- Note on the chart that the child wears lenses.

- Stroke, rock, and hug infants and children who are visually impaired. Sing and talk to them. These infants do not make eye contact and have rather blank expressions.
- Teach parents to read body language and vocalization as expressions of emotion. Facial expressions give a great deal of information, but infants and children with poor vision do not have the ability to learn by visual imitation. Show parents how to use tactile means to teach appropriate facial expressions. For example, a touch on the arm can be soft and stroking to indicate a smile, but firmer to indicate dismay or frown.
- Explain to parents that discipline and rewards for children with poor vision should be the same as those for other children in the family. The child should be given age-appropriate tasks.
- Encourage contact with peers as the child grows older. Teach the child to look directly at persons who are talking to him or her. Play, sports, and other activities can be modified to give the visually impaired child the same social experiences as a sighted child.

CARE IN THE COMMUNITY

Public laws require that each state provide educational and related services for children with disabilities (see Chapter 1). Parents and professionals should develop an individualized education plan (as discussed in Chapter 6) that maximizes the child's learning ability. If possible, the child with a vision problem should attend childcare and preschool with children who have normal visual acuity. What nursing actions are needed to help a child such as Raeanne, introduced at the beginning of this chapter, in adjusting to childcare or school?

- Provide parents with information about educational options before their child reaches school age. Education should take place in a setting that allows the child to have contact with other children and to participate in social activities.
- The child may be mainstreamed with a tutor, be partially mainstreamed in a resource room, attend special classes, or be tutored at home. If the child is to attend public

school, suggest to parents that they contact the school well before enrollment to ensure that school personnel understand the child's disability.

- Make sure that items such as large-print books, braille materials, audio equipment, or an Optacon (described earlier) is available. Ensure that frequent eye examinations are performed and assist with proper use and care of prescribed glasses or contact lenses, as necessary.
- Familiarize the child with the new environment.

PROVIDE EMOTIONAL SUPPORT

Family members often need help to understand the child's abilities and disabilities. Support them as they learn about the child's visual problems, tell friends and family, and then adjust to supporting the child.

- Encourage habilitation as soon as realistically possible. Make the adjustment easier by providing information about the child's specific type of visual impairment, available community services, and groups or associations for children with similar vision conditions. Suggest resources to families of children with visual disorders.
- Be supportive and listen to the family's concerns regarding the child's visual deficit.
- Ensure that parents meet their own physical and emotional needs so they are better able to care for and provide support to their child.

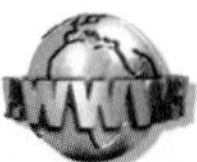

Resources for the Visually Impaired

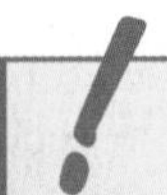

NURSING ALERT

Be sure to check the immunization status of the child with an eye injury. If the child has not had a tetanus booster within 5 years, this immunization should be given.

Evaluation

Expected outcomes of nursing care for the child with a visual impairment include:

- Prevention of injury
- Growth and development to maximum potential
- Establishment of successful individualized education plan.

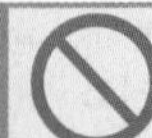

SAFETY PRECAUTIONS

Visual impairment caused by trauma is largely preventable. Dangerous chemicals and objects such as scissors and knives should be placed out of children's reach. When purchasing toys, parents should consider safety features. Protective eyewear should be encouraged during play or sports activities for children of all ages, especially in the child who already has a visual impairment. School nurses can ensure that students use protective eye gear in chemistry classes and that emergency treatment for injury is posted in classrooms.

INJURIES OF THE EYE

In the United States, eye injuries are common in boys 11 to 15 years of age and in all children aged 9 to 11 years (Coody, Banks, & Yetman, et al., 1997). Foreign bodies, blunt and sharp objects, chemical and thermal burns, physical irritants, and abuse may cause eye trauma. Recreational activities such as sports and projectile toys are common causes. Older children may be injured by chemicals in school science laboratories.

Some injuries can be treated at home, but many necessitate a trip to the emergency department or require hospitalization. Personnel take careful history of the injury, perform, assessment of the eye, and measure visual acuity. Table 19-6 summarizes emergency treatment of common eye injuries. Nurses should teach children and parents methods to prevent eye injuries, including use of protective eye wear, especially for children who participate in athletics and have poor vision or only one functional eye.

DISORDERS OF THE EAR

OTITIS MEDIA

Otitis media, or inflammation of the middle ear, is sometimes accompanied by infection. This condition is one of the most common childhood illnesses. Between 75% and 95% of all children have at least one episode by 6 years of age, with peak incidence at 2 years (Hoberman & Paradise, 2000). Otitis media occurs more frequently among boys and in children who attend child care centers. It is most common during the winter months.

Etiology and Pathophysiology

The specific cause of otitis media is unknown, but it appears to be related to eustachian tube dysfunction. Often an upper respiratory infection precedes the development of otitis media. This infection causes the mucous membranes of the eustachian tube to become edematous.

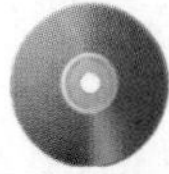

Ear Abnormalities

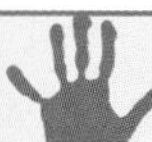

GROWTH & DEVELOPMENT

Fluid accumulation in the middle ear prevents the efficient transmission of sound and can result in hearing loss over time, potentially delaying speech and language development. These delays may manifest as cognitive deficits or behavior problems. Motor development has been found to be impaired in children with chronic ear infections.

CLINICAL TIP

The *Haemophilus influenzae* type B (Hib) vaccine, which is routinely given to children beginning at 2 months of age, has been influential in reducing the incidence of diseases such as otitis media that are caused by *H. influenzae* type B. Another, more recently recommended immunization for pneumococcal disease is expected to decrease cases of otitis media from that pathogen. Be sure to check the immunization status of each child to be sure it is up to date for Hib and pneumococcal vaccine. (See Chapter 12 for the recommended immunization schedule.)

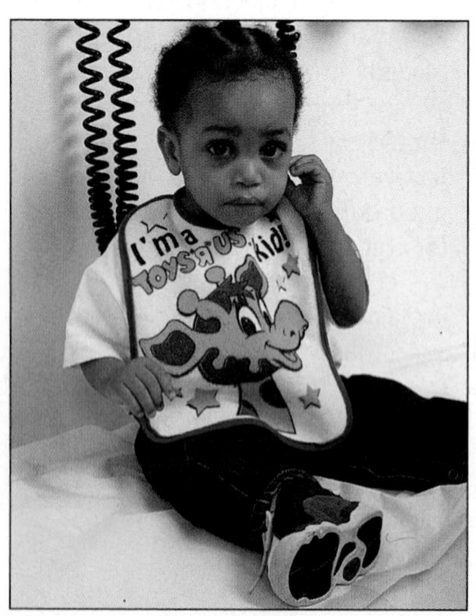

FIGURE 19-6 ◆
This young child is pulling at the ear and acting fussy, two important signs of otitis media. Ask the parents about the presence of fever and night awakenings, additional signs that are often observed in children with this condition.

TABLE 19-6 Emergency Treatment of Eye Injuries

INJURY	TREATMENT
Subconjunctival hemorrhage (caused by coughing, mild trauma, or increased physical activity)	Usually heals spontaneously; child should see ophthalmologist if most of sclera is covered or if condition does not clear up in 1–2 weeks
Periorbital ecchymosis ("black eye")	Apply ice to eye area (both eyes) for 5–15 minutes every hour for the first 1–2 days after injury (even if only one eye is affected, both eyes may discolor); then apply warm compresses
Foreign body on conjunctiva	Do not let child rub eye; remove material on surface of eye by closing upper lid over lower lid, irrigating or everting upper lid, visualizing material, and removing it with a slightly damp handkerchief; patch eye and transport child to emergency department if foreign body cannot be removed
Corneal abrasion	Superficial corneal abrasions are diagnosed by touching a sterile fluorescein strip to lower conjunctiva; dye remains where corneal epithelial cells are disrupted; most corneal abrasions heal spontaneously or antibiotic ointment may be prescribed and eyes patched in some children
Burns (alkaline burns readily penetrate cornea and are more serious than acid burns)	For child with chemical burn, irrigate eye for 15–30 minutes; transport child to emergency department, where irrigation should continue (see Skills Manual); pupils are dilated to reduce pain and prevent adhesions; after irrigation is complete, eyes are patched and antibiotics are prescribed
Penetrating and perforating injuries	Obtain medical assistance immediately; never try to remove an object that has penetrated the child's eye; such objects should be removed by an ophthalmologist; prevent the child from rubbing injured eye; cover both eyes with shield before transportation to emergency department
Eye injuries caused by severe blows to head and eye (blunt trauma can seriously injure all eye structures, including orbit, which can be fractured)	Transport immediately to ophthalmologist's office or emergency department for evaluation and treatment

As a result, air that normally flows to the middle ear is blocked, and the air in the middle ear is reabsorbed into the bloodstream. Fluid is pulled from the mucosal lining into the former air space, providing a medium for the rapid growth of pathogens. The tympanic membrane and fluid behind it become infected. The most common causative organisms are *Streptococcus pneumoniae, Haemophilus influenzae,* and *Moraxella catarrhalis* (Dowell, Butler, & Geibink, et al., 1999).

Conditions such as enlarged adenoids or edema from allergic rhinitis can also obstruct the eustachian tube and lead to otitis media. Because children with certain facial malformations (cleft palate) and genetic conditions (Down syndrome) usually have compromised eustachian tubes, these children are more vulnerable to the development of otitis media. Children who live in crowded conditions, those exposed to cigarette smoke, and those who attend child care with multiple children are at higher risk. Breastfeeding provides protection against otitis media (Dowell et al., 1999).

Clinical Manifestations

Otitis media is categorized according to symptoms and the length of time the condition has been present. Pulling at the ear is a sign of ear pain (Figure 19-6 ◆). Diarrhea, vomiting, and fever are typical of otitis media. Irritability and "acting out" may be signs of a related hear-

CLINICAL MANIFESTATIONS OF OTITIS MEDIA

TYPE	DURATION	CLINICAL MANIFESTATIONS
Acute otitis media (AOM)	Rapid onset; 1–3 weeks duration	Tympanic membrane (TM) red, retracted or media (AOM) bulging, and painful; ear pulling; fever; hearing loss caused by presence of fluid; possible spontaneous TM rupture resulting in fluid drainage and reduction of pain
Recurrent otitis media (ROM)	Similar onset and duration to AOM, but repeated episodes in succession (three in 6 months or four in 12 months)	Similar to those of AOM
Otitis media	May precede or follow any stage of OM	Ear popping; feeling of pressure in middle with effusion ear pain; hearing loss; TM retracted; fluid line (OME) or bubbles via otoscopy; symptoms of acute infection are absent
Chronic otitis media (COM)	Slow onset and persistence of 3 months of more	TM thick, immobile, retracted; if TM perforated, drainage from ear; tympanogram abnormal; hearing loss

ing impairment. Some children with otitis media are asymptomatic; therefore, an ear examination should be performed at every health care visit (see Chapter 4). A red, bulging, nonmobile tympanic membrane is a sign of otitis media (Figure 19-7 ◆). If fluid lines and air bubbles are visible, the child has otitis media with effusion (Figure 19-8 ◆).

Clinical Therapy

Diagnosis of otitis media is based on otoscopic examination. Redness, inflammation, or bulging of the tympanic membrane is usually present. The trained clinician can perform pneumatic otoscopy in which positive air pressure in the external canal is used to measure the movement of the tympanic membrane. Special gradient acoustic reflectometry (SGAR) measures the condition of the middle ear by introducing a sound and measuring the tympanic membrane response (Hoberman & Paradise, 2000).

A flat tympanogram is also suggestive of otitis media. (The tympanogram is described in the section on hearing impairment.)

Acute and recurrent otitis media have traditionally been treated with antibiotic therapy for 10 to 14 days. The choice of antibiotic depends on the probable organism, ease of administration, cost, previous effectiveness, and any history of allergies. First-line therapy is amoxicillin. Amoxicillin with clavulanate or cefuroxime axetil are second-line drugs, and ceftriaxome is used if other drugs are not successful (Dowell et al., 1999).

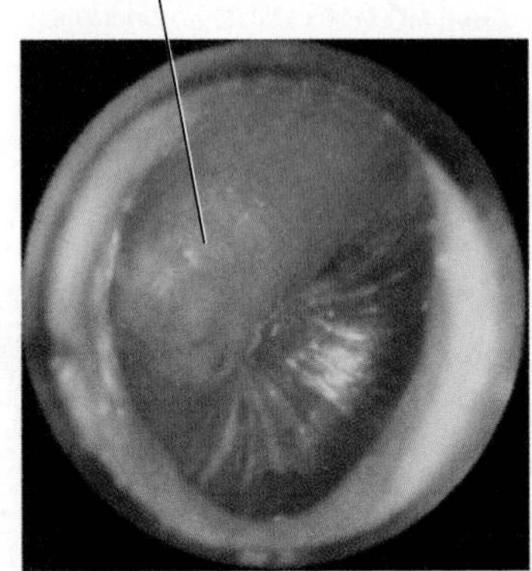

FIGURE 19-7 ◆
Acute otitis media is characterized by pain and a red, bulging nonmobile tympanic membrane.
From Malasanos, L., Barkauskas, V., & Stoltenberg-Allen, K. (1990). *Health assessment* (4th ed., Plate 2). St. Louis: Mosby-Year Book. Courtesy of Richard A. Buckingham, M. D., Clinical Professor, Otolaryngology, University of Illinois College of Medicine at Chicago, Chicago, IL.

Concern has developed about the increasing appearance of drug-resistant microbials as causative agents in otitis media. These organisms may explain the increase in otitis media observed in the last decade (Carlson & Fall, 1998). Because the specific pathogen is not usually known, wide spectrum antibiotics are used and microbial overgrowth is a known potential outcome. To learn if antibiotic treatment was essential, use of medication has been delayed in some cases, and children improved without drugs. Many clinicians now believe that a more cautious approach is warranted, with treatment delayed for 3 days to determine if the child improves, as long as the child does not appear extremely ill (Little, Gould, & Williamson, et al., 2001). Dosing with medication when needed for 5 or 7 days, rather than the traditional 10 days is also becoming more common. A one-dose injection is sometimes given rather than more extended therapy (Agency for Healthcare Research and Quality, 2001).

Chronic otitis media with effusion and recurrent otitis media may result in sensorineural or conductive hearing loss and cochlear damage, so treatment and follow-up with audiology are essential (Roddey & Hoover, 2000).

Neither decongestants nor antihistamines have been shown to be effective in the treatment of otitis media with or without effusion. If infection recurs despite antibiotic treatment, **myringotomy** (surgical incision of the tympanic membrane) may be performed and **tympanostomy** tubes (pressure-equalizing tubes) may be inserted to drain fluid from the middle ear. Tube insertion is generally recommended for children with bilateral middle ear

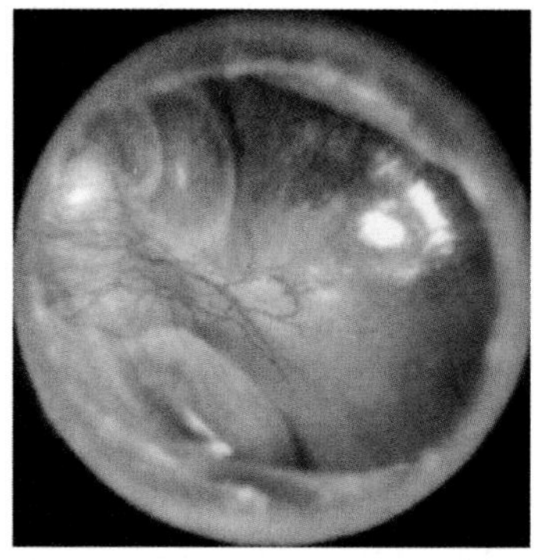

FIGURE 19-8 ◆
Otitis media with effusion is noted on otoscopy by fluid line or air bubbles. From Malasanos, L., Barkauskas, V., & Stoltenberg-Allen, K. (1990). *Health assessment* (4th ed., Plate 2). St. Louis: Mosby-Year Book. Courtesy of Richard A. Buckingham, M.D., Clinical Professor, Otolaryngology, University of Illinois College of Medicine at Chicago, Chicago, IL.

effusion and hearing deficiency of greater than 20 decibels (dB) for over 3 months. Enlarged and infected adenoids may be removed at the same time (Paradise, Feldman, & Campbell, et al., 2001). Alternatively, a tympanostomy may be done to extract middle ear fluid for culture and sensitivity so that antimicrobial therapy can be directed at the cause of infection.

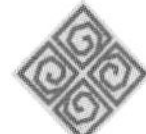

NURSING MANAGEMENT

Nursing Assessment and Diagnosis

The tympanic membrane is assessed for color, transparency, mobility, presence of landmarks, and light reflex. Ask the parents if the child has had a fever, been fussy, or been pulling at the ears. Observe for signs of impaired hearing.

Several nursing diagnoses that may apply to the child with otitis media are included in the accompanying nursing care plan. Additional nursing diagnoses may include the following:

- *Risk for altered body temperature: Hyperthermia,* related to infectious process
- *Fatigue (child and parent),* related to sleep deprivation
- *Sensory/perceptual alteration (auditory),* related to chronic ear infections and altered sensory reception

Planning and Implementation

Most children with otitis media are not hospitalized; therefore, nursing management centers on care of the child in the home. The child who is having tympanostomy tubes inserted is generally treated in a day surgery setting. Occasionally, children admitted to the hospital for other problems have a concurrent ear infection. The accompanying nursing care plan summarizes nursing care for the child with otitis media.

Preventive measures should be emphasized. Exposure to secondhand smoke in the home increases the incidence of otitis media in children; therefore, parents who smoke should be encouraged to avoid smoking near the child or in the home. If young children are in child care with fewer than 10 children, incidence decreases. Breastfeeding provides some protection from the disease. Placing babies to sleep with a pacifier may increase incidence and should be avoided in the infant with prior infections (Niemela, Pihakari, & Pokka, et al., 2000). Many cases of otitis media are related to microbials such as *Haemophilus influenzae* and *Pneumococcal pneumoniae,* so immunization against these pathogens (see Chapter 12) can be effective preventive measures.

Chronic otitis media can create many problems for the family. The child's waking at night with ear pain results in lack of sleep and parental fatigue. Parents often become frustrated

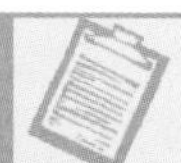

RESEARCH

Drug resistance to antibiotics has developed as some organisms evolve to produce beta lactamase, an enzyme that breaks through the beta-lactam ring of penicillin. Many cases of resistant otitis media relate to drug resistant *Haemophilus influenzae, Moraxilla catarrhalis,* and *Streptococcus pneumoniae.* The Centers for Disease Control and Prevention currently use surveillance techniques to track drug-resistant *S. pneumoniae* (DRSP) (Carlson & Fall, 1998)

FAMILIES WANT TO KNOW

Care of the Child With Tympanostomy Tubes

AFTER SURGERY

Encourage the child to drink generous amounts of fluids.
Reestablish a regular diet as tolerated.
Give pain medication (acetaminophen) as ordered for discomfort and at bedtime.
Place drops in child's ears if instructed.
Restrict the child to quiet activities.

FOLLOWING POSTOPERATIVE PERIOD

Follow the physician's instructions regarding swimming and water (some caution against swimming and other activities that might get water in ears; others do not).
Ear plugs can be used to prevent water from getting into ears.
Be alert for tubes becoming dislodged and falling out and alert physician (they usually fall out within 1 year).
Report purulent discharge from the ear, which may indicate a new ear infection. Contact the care provider.

NURSING CARE PLAN The Child with Otitis Media

GOAL	INTERVENTION	RATIONALE	EXPECTED OUTCOME
1. Pain related to inflammation and pressure on tympanic membrane			
	NIC Priority Intervention: **Pain Management:** Alleviation or reduction in pain to a level of comfort acceptable to patient and family.		NOC Suggested Outcome: **Pain Level:** Amount of reported or demonstrated pain.
The child or parent will indicate absence of pain.	■ Give analgesic such as acetaminophen. Use analgesic eardrops. ■ Have the child sit up, raise head on pillows, or lie on unaffected ear. ■ Apply heating pad or warm hot water bottle. ■ Have the child chew gum or blow on balloon to relieve pressure in ear.	■ Analgesics alter perception or response to pain. ■ Elevation decreases pressure from fluid. ■ Heat increases blood supply and reduces discomfort. ■ Attempts to open the eustachian tube may help aerate the middle ear.	Verbal child states that pain is relieved. Nonverbal child has improved disposition and comfort.
2. Infection related to presence of pathogens			
	NIC Priority Intervention: **Infection Control:** Minimizing the acquisition and transmission of infectious agents		NOC Suggested Outcome: **Risk Control:** Actions to eliminate or reduce health threats.
The child will be free of infection.	■ Encourage breastfeeding of infants. ■ Instruct the parents to administer antibiotics exactly as directed and to complete prescribed course of medication. ■ Telephone the parents 2–3 days after initial examination. ■ Examine ear 3–4 days after completion of antibiotic treatment, or if symptoms worsen in child on symptomatic treatment.	■ Breastfeeding affords natural immunity to infectious agents. ■ Taking antibiotics as prescribed minimizes chance for overgrowth of pathogens. ■ If symptoms have not improved in 36 hours, treatment should be evaluated. ■ Check-up determines if treatment is effective.	The child's temperature is normal, symptoms have disappeared, and tympanic membrane shows no signs of infection.
3. Risk for Caregiver Role Strain related to chronic disease			
	NIC Priority Intervention: **Caregiver Support:** Provision of necessary support, information, and advocacy to facilitate care by parents.		NOC Suggested Outcome: **Caregiver Performance:** Provision by family care provider of health care for child.
The parents will manage the child's condition with minimal stress.	■ Determine the parents' ability to manage condition. Provide frequent information and feedback. ■ Encourage parental input in managing care. ■ Listen carefully to parental expressions of frustration and fatigue and try to understand parents' feelings.	■ Many parents can treat children at home. Knowledge of condition allows parents to make informed decisions and to manage condition effectively. ■ Active participation increases confidence and ability to manage condition. ■ Reacting empathically encourages parents to communicate.	The parents express confidence about treating the child and state that stress is reduced.

(continued)

NURSING CARE PLAN The Child with Otitis Media (continued)

GOAL	INTERVENTION	RATIONALE	EXPECTED OUTCOME
4. Risk for Infection related to knowledge deficit about infection in children			
	NIC Priority Intervention: **Infection Control:** Minimizing the acquisition and transmission of infectious agents.		NOC Suggested Outcome: **Knowledge:** Extent of understanding conveyed about infectious disease prevention.
The parents will state understanding of preventive measures.	■ Teach family members to cover mouths and noses when sneezing or coughing and to wash hands frequently. Have parents isolate sick children.	■ Good hygiene prevents spread of pathogens.	Parents express understanding of measures to lead fewer to infections.
	■ Encourage optimal nutrition, rest, and exercise.	■ Physical well-being helps the body fight disease.	
	■ Position bottle-fed infants upright when feeding. Do not prop bottles.	■ Elevated position prevents injection of milk and pathogens into the eustachian tube.	
	■ Eliminate allergens and upper respiratory irritants such as tobacco, smoke, and dust.	■ Fewer irritants and allergens may decrease susceptibility to respiratory infections. Secondhand smoke contributes to higher incidence of otitis media.	
5. Risk for Altered Growth and Development related to hearing loss			
	NIC Priority Intervention: **Developmental Enhancement:** Facilitating optimal growth and development of the child.		NOC Suggested Outcome: **Growth and Development:** Milestones of developmental progression.
The child will have normal hearing.	■ Assess hearing ability frequently.	■ Monitoring detects hearing loss early.	The child's general health and hearing improve, and incidence of condition decreases.
The child will have normal motor and language development.	■ Assess motor and language development at each health care visit.	■ Early detection of developmental delays can lead to appropriate intervention.	The child has language and motor development within norms for age group.

and disillusioned because of the inability of the health care system to cure the child and may fear a permanent hearing impairment. Reassure parents that as the child grows older, the recurrent infections eventually cease. Teach them that asking for courses of antibiotics for every infection may not be the treatment of choice. Parents of children with tympanostomy tubes need to be taught how to care for the child and what symptoms to report.

Evaluation

Expected outcomes of nursing care for the child with otitis media include:

- Return to normal sleep and feeding patterns.
- Maintenance of normal hearing
- Effective pain and temperature management
- Understanding of treatment regimen by parents.

HEARING IMPAIRMENT

Approximately 1 million children in the United States have some form of hearing impairment. These hearing impairments are expressed in terms of **decibels (dB),** which are units of loudness, and rated according to severity (Table 19-7). Children who have only a mild hear-

TABLE 19-7 Severity of Hearing Loss

TYPE OF LOSS	HEARING ABILITY
Slight/mild	Some speech sounds are difficult to perceive, particularly unvoiced consonant sounds
Moderate	Most normal conversational speech sounds are missed
Severe	Speech sounds cannot be heard at a normal conversational level
Profound	No speech sounds can be heard; considered legally deaf
Deaf	No sound at all can be heard

ing loss (35 to 40 dB) may miss 50% of everyday conversation and are considered at high risk for school failure. Children with a hearing loss of more than 90 dB are considered legally deaf. From 2 to 6 children per 1,000 have a hearing loss (Bachman & Arvedson, 1998).

Etiology and Pathophysiology

About 50% of hearing loss is genetically caused, usually with a recessive inheritance pattern. Another 25% is due to environmental causes around the time of birth; the remainder is due to unknown causes. Infants and children at risk for hearing loss include those with a family history of hearing loss, recurrent otitis media, congenital perinatal infections such as rubella or herpes, anatomic malformations involving the head or neck, low birth weight (less than 1,500 g or 3 lb, 4 oz), hyperbilirubinemia, bacterial meningitis, severe asphyxia at birth, prolonged mechanical ventilation, and those who have received ototoxic medications (Bachman & Arvedson, 1998). Parents should be aware of excessive noise at home and at school. Teenagers who use earphones at high volumes or attend many rock concerts are at risk for hearing loss (Figure 19-9 ◆). Other noise hazards include firecrackers, guns, and power and farm equipment.

Clinical Manifestations

Hearing disorders can be classified according to the location of the deficit. **Conductive hearing loss** occurs when conditions in the external auditory canal or tympanic membrane prevent sound from reaching the middle ear. Common causes include impacted cerumen, the most frequent reason for conductive loss; outer ear infection ("swimmer's ear");

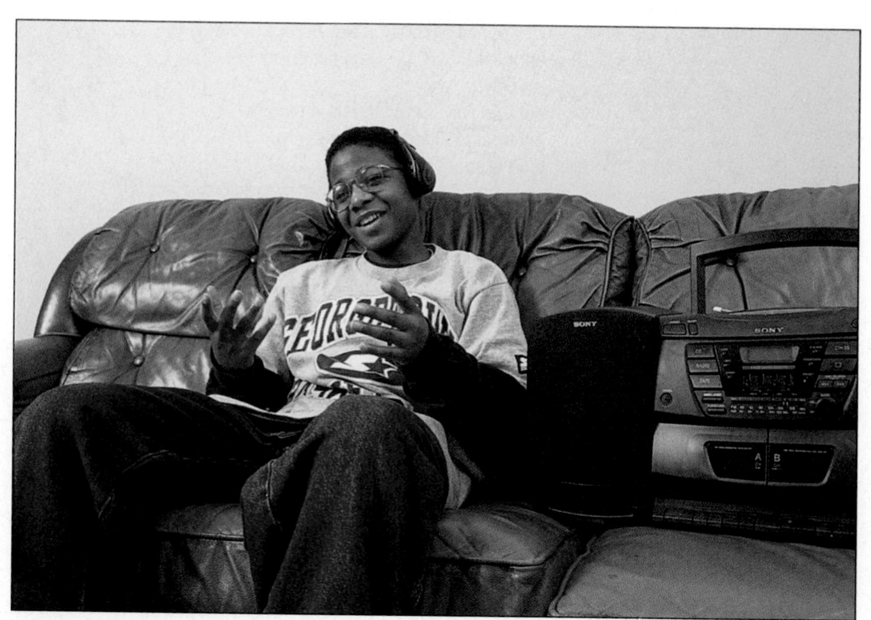

FIGURE 19-9 ◆ Listening to loud music with headphones or at rock concerts is a frequent cause of hearing loss among teenagers and young adults. This adolescent needs to be informed about the possible outcomes of this activity.

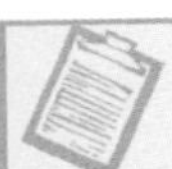

RESEARCH

Recent research has shown that 12% of school-age children may have hearing impairments due to noise exposure, often in ranges not screened during school auditory testing. Hearing loss is even more common among teens. Preventing these hearing losses is possible, so nurses should identify and find sources of noise in the child's environment. They may include stereos, airplanes, firearms, power tools, machinery, and toys. Encourage use of earplugs during hazardous activities (Niskar, Kieszak, & Holmes, et al., 2001).

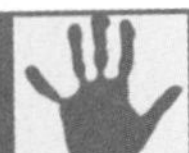

GROWTH & DEVELOPMENT

Infants and young children respond automatically with a blink or the startle reflex to unexpected or loud noises. As they mature, they localize the sound source, then understand speech, and then communicate verbally.

trauma; or a foreign body. Conductive loss also occurs if the tympanic membrane does not fully vibrate, as in otitis media. The loss of acuity may be gradual or rapid and results in diminished hearing in all ranges.

Sensorineural hearing loss occurs when the hair cells in the cochlea or along the auditory nerve (cranial nerve VIII) are damaged. This leads to permanent hearing loss. Conditions leading to this type of hearing loss may be congenital (maternal rubella), genetic (Tay-Sachs disease), or acquired (from ototoxic drugs or loud noise). In sensorineural hearing loss, high-frequency sounds are most affected.

A **mixed hearing loss** indicates a hearing loss having a combination of conductive and sensorineural causes.

Hearing is both an innate and a learned behavior. Infants and children who are hearing impaired exhibit a range of behaviors, depending on the child's age and the severity of the deficit. Infants who hear normally respond to sound in both obvious and subtle ways that do not occur in those who are hearing impaired (Table 19-8). As children with hearing impairments mature, language skills are affected. Hearing loss is often manifested as a cognitive deficit, a behavioral problem, or both.

Clinical Therapy

Early identification of hearing loss is a key element in successful treatment. Detection of hearing loss in infants is important to ensure optimal development. Universal screening of all infants and children is recommended with rescreening and monitoring of those at risk (American Academy of Pediatrics, Task Force on Newborn and Infant Hearing, 1999; Hayes, 1999). Observations of response to noise in all newborns should be accompanied by more sophisticated testing such as auditory brain stem response or transient evoked otoacoustic emissions in those at high risk of deficits (White & Maxon, 1999)

An otoscopic examination with a tympanogram can be performed on an older infant to determine conductive hearing loss. The **tympanogram** is a test that provides a graph of the ability of the middle ear to transmit sound. An airtight probe is inserted into the external ear canal and a tone is emitted. The pressure is measured by the probe and plotted on a graph. A flat tympanogram suggests conductive hearing loss (Figures 19-10A and B ◆). **Audiography** can be used with cooperative children over 3 years of age. Sounds of various frequencies and

TABLE 19-8 Behaviors Suggestive of Hearing Impairment

AGE	BEHAVIOR
Infant	Has a diminished or absent startle reflex to loud sound Does not awaken when environment is very noisy Awakens only to touch Does not turn head to sound at 3–4 months Does not localize sound at 6–10 months Babbles little or not at all
Toddler and preschooler	Speaks unintelligibly, in a monotone, or not at all Communicates needs through gestures Appears developmentally delayed Appears emotionally immature, yells inappropriately Does not respond to doorbell or telephone Appears more interested in objects than people and prefers to play alone Focuses on facial expressions rather than verbal communications
School-age child and adolescent	Asks to have statements repeated Answers questions inappropriately, except when able to view speaker's face Daydreams and is inattentive Performs poorly at school or is truant Has speech abnormalities or speaks in a monotone Sits close to or turns television or radio up loudly Prefers to play alone

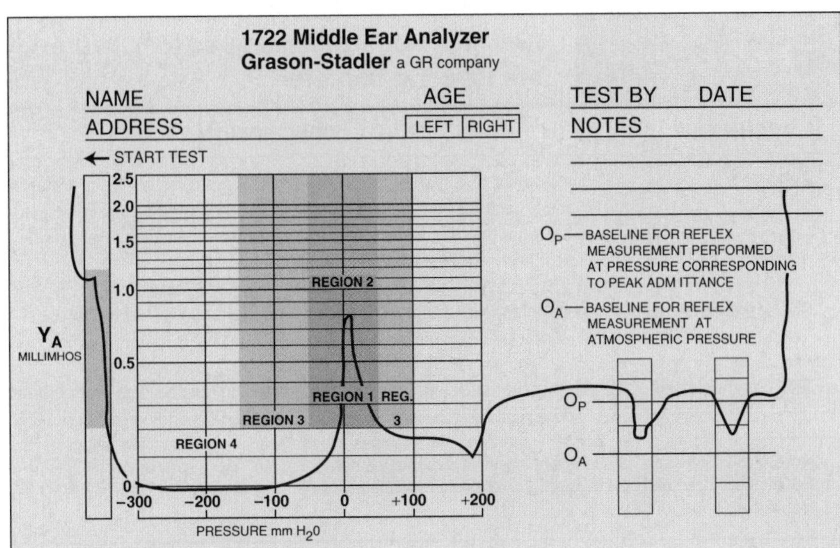

A

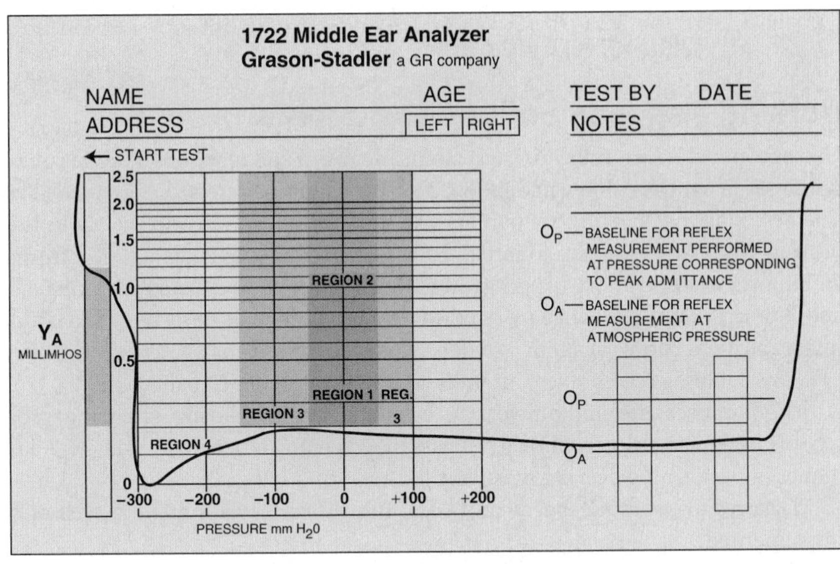

B

FIGURE 19-10 ◆
A, This tympanogram demonstrates normal hearing as evidenced by the curve showing the tympanic membrane's movement when a sound wave is emitted into the ear canal. Mobility is between 0.2 mL and 1.0 mL, the normal range. B, In contrast, note the flat pattern in the second tympanogram, which shows very restricted mobility of the tympanic membrane in response to sound.

intensities are presented to the child through earphones, and the child is instructed to raise a hand upon hearing the sound. Audiography cannot detect hearing loss caused by middle ear effusion but can indicate sensorineural loss. The hearing of preschool and school-age children is tested by asking them to repeat whispered words. Hearing of school-age children and adolescents also is assessed with the Weber and Rinne tests (see Chapter 4).

If a hearing loss is uncorrectable, a multidisciplinary team composed of pediatrician, audiologist, otolaryngologist, speech–language pathologist, nurse, teacher, and social worker should assist the child and family with adaptation to the disability (Brookhouse, Beauchaine, & Osberger, 1999). If the deficit is due to recurrent ear infections, tympanostomy tube insertion may improve hearing.

A hearing aid may be prescribed for a conductive loss. A sensorineural loss is more difficult to treat, but cochlear implants and bone conduction hearing aids have been used in some children. Cochlear implants are increasingly being used in children and have restored hearing in some who are profoundly deaf (Cheng, Rubin, & Powe, et al., 2000).

For children with uncorrectable hearing loss, several approaches are used to enhance communication (Table 19-9). Children with hearing impairment may receive speech therapy and instructions in lipreading, signing, cuing, and fingerspelling.

NURSING ALERT

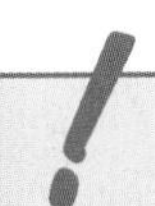

Although it is recommended that infants with significant hearing loss be identified by 3 months of age and receive treatment by 6 months, most children with hearing deficits are not identified until later in childhood. Early intervention is crucial for maximizing the ability of the child to use any hearing present and to learn communication methods. Development is profoundly impacted by difficulty in communication. Nurses must test all newborns and infants for signs of hearing disorders and refer as needed. Parents often are the first to notice a problem with hearing, so they should be asked their observations of the infant's hearing during each visit (Garganta & Seashore, 2000).

TABLE 19-9 Communication Techniques for Children Who Are Hearing Impaired

TECHNIQUE	DESCRIPTION
Cued speech	Supplement to lipreading; eight hand shapes represent groups of consonant sounds and four positions about the face represent groups of vowel sounds; based on the sounds the letters make, not the letters themselves; child can "see-hear" every spoken syllable a hearing person hears
Oral approach	Uses only spoken language for face-to-face communication; avoids use of formal signs; uses hearing aids and residual hearing
Total communication	Uses speech and sign, fingerspelling, lipreading, and residual hearing simultaneously; child selects communication technique depending on the situation

Note: From Schwartz, S. (1996). *Choices in deafness: A parent's guide* (2nd ed.). Rockville, MD: Woodbine House. Reprinted with permission. For publications related to hearing-impaired children, contact Woodbine House (see Appendix F).

NURSING MANAGEMENT

Nursing Assessment and Diagnosis

Nurses conduct newborn hearing tests soon after birth and make observations of the infant's responses to sound. As the child grows, hearing should be assessed at every well-child visit. The best judges of hearing are parents; ask them if they have concerns about their child's hearing. An infant's reaction to rattles, bells, or handclapping 30 cm (12 in.) from the ear is an important observation. Language milestones should be evaluated when the older infant and child are examined. Language development is a major area of focus in deaf children. Deaf infants begin to babble at about 5 to 6 months of age, the same age as hearing infants. However, this babbling ceases several months later in the hearing-impaired child.

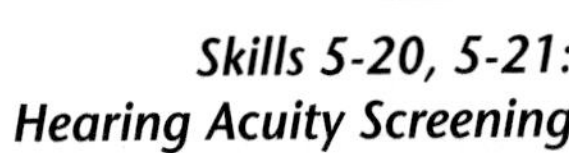

Skills 5-20, 5-21: Hearing Acuity Screening

School nurses use audiometers to evaluate hearing during screening programs in schools, and refer children who do not pass the screening test. See the Skills Manual for techniques in performing hearing screening.

Measures to promote speech and communication development as well as safety are implemented.

Following are common nursing diagnoses for the child with impaired hearing:

- *Sensory/perceptual alteration (auditory),* related to altered sensory perception
- *Risk for impaired verbal communication,* related to hearing loss
- *Risk for altered growth and development,* related to communication impairment
- *Risk for ineffective family coping,* related to caring for a child with a hearing impairment

Planning and Implementation

Nurses can encourage prevention of hearing loss from exposure to loud noises such as from music and power and farm equipment. Music should be turned down and ear protection worn for other activities. Early identification of hearing loss in infants and children is facilitated by newborn screening, developmental assessment, and childhood screening programs. Infants should be tested for hearing loss by 3 months of age and in cases of loss, intervention should begin before 6 months of age (Joint Committee on Infant Hearing, 2000).

Nursing care of the child with a hearing impairment focuses on facilitating the child's ability to receive spoken language and to send information, on helping parents to meet the child's schooling needs, and on providing emotional support to parents. Refer the parents to an early intervention program as soon as the diagnosis of hearing impairment is made, in order to foster the child's development. If a cochlear implant is planned, the child needs surgical care and follow-up to monitor results and integrate sound gradually into the child's life (Slattery & Fayad, 1999).

Facilitate Ability to Receive Spoken Language

Be aware of how the child compensates for hearing loss and use these strategies in communication:

- If hearing loss is mild or temporary or if the child reads lips, first obtain the child's visual attention by lightly touching the child or saying the child's name.
- Position your face 1 to 2 m (3 to 6 ft) from the child's face and make sure that the child's eyes are focused on your face and lips. Make sure the room is well lit, with no backlighting. Speak at a normal rate and tone, and use facial expressions that show caring or concern. If the child does not understand, rephrase the information in shorter, simpler sentences. Use specific, concrete explanations, and give the child time to comprehend. Watch for subtle signs of misinterpretations and give consistent and immediate feedback because only 30% of the English language is visible on the lips.
- Be familiar with the different types of hearing aids. Hearing aids, which are microphones that amplify all sounds, can be worn in or behind the ear, in the frame of glasses, or on the body with a wire attached to the ear. When talking to a child with a hearing aid, speak slowly and be positioned 15 to 45 cm (6 to 18 in.) from the microphone using a normal conversational tone. Talk to the child even if the child is not looking at you. Make sure the batteries are fresh for the best reception. All sound is amplified, so reduce background noise as much as possible.

Acoustic feedback, an audible whistling sound that cannot always be heard by the child, is a common problem with hearing aids. To eliminate this sound, readjust the hearing aid to ensure that it is inserted properly and that no hair or ear wax is caught between the ear mold and canal. Turning down the volume may also help.

A remote microphone system is another type of device designed to improve hearing. This is often used in the classroom situation because it eliminates background noise. The speaker wears a transmitter that picks up the voice and transmits it to a receiver worn by the child.

HOME CARE

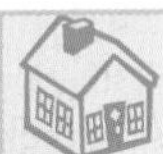

There are three types of hearing aids: those that fit totally in the ear canal, those that fit in the external ear canal, and those that fit behind the ear. The hearing aid should be cleaned each day with a damp cloth. Change the batteries as needed, usually about once a week. Disconnect the battery when not in use. Place the hearing aid in the ear with the volume off, then slowly turn up to half volume. Adjust as needed. Be sure the hearing aid fit is checked yearly, as the child's growth may necessitate a new fitting.

Facilitate Ability to Send Information

Maintain the child's hearing aid in proper condition. Many children with impaired hearing communicate using speech, which is enhanced through speech therapy. In addition, they are taught to sign, fingerspell, or use cued speech (Figure 19-11 ◆). Articulation may be difficult, and understanding what the child is trying to say may be frustrating for both the nurse and the child. Taking time to listen carefully is important.

Measures to promote speech and communication development as well as safety are implemented Ask the parents to explain the child's communication techniques and to help interpret words. Have younger children point to pictures. Use assisted technologies such as a computer or picture board, as well as drawings or gestures if necessary. This technique is especially helpful for communicating feelings of pain and hunger during hospitalization. If the child signs or fingerspells, be sure you understand the signs for important functions. Give older children paper and pencil to write requests. People other than parents should be able to understand what the child is trying to communicate. Have an interpreter available if the child uses American Sign Language. Learn some common signs yourself to communicate simple words or phrases. Orient the child carefully to new settings such as the hospital room or a new school.

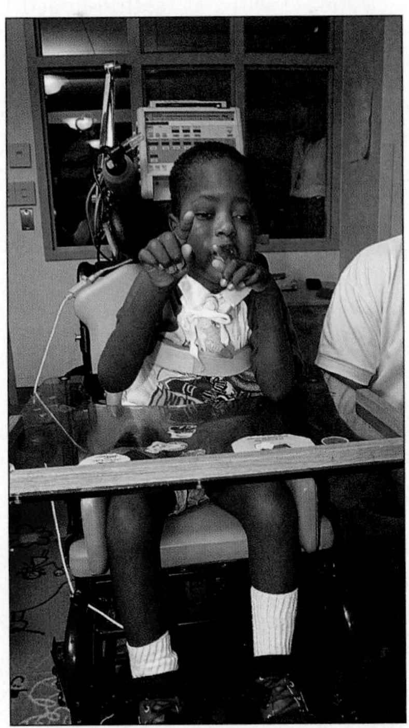

FIGURE 19-11 ◆
This child with a hearing impairment and tracheostomy is communicating by means of American Sign language.

Help Parents to Meet Child's Educational Needs

Public laws apply to the education of children who are hearing impaired (see Chapter 1). After diagnosis, the parents and professionals together agree on an individualized education plan (see discussion in Chapter 6). Childcare and preschool are recommended for children with hearing problems.

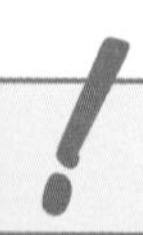

NURSING ALERT

If an alkaline button battery (like those found in many toys or watches) is inserted in a child's ear, it can rapidly destroy tissue, causing perforation of the tympanic membrane, destruction of the ossicles, and local tissue ulceration. Removal should be performed with the child under sedation or general anesthesia.

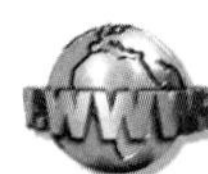

Resources for the Hearing Impaired

SAFETY PRECAUTIONS

Both parents and children should be instructed never to put any object in the child's ear. Some parents believe that the ear canal should be cleaned with a cotton-tipped swab. If the cleaning is too vigorous or the child moves unexpectedly, a ruptured tympanic membrane could result.

Skill 7-8: Performing an Ear Irrigation

- Provide parents with information about adjustments that may have to be made for the hearing-impaired child who attends public school. By sitting at the front of the classroom, the child can hear and see more clearly. The teacher should always face the child when speaking, and background noise should be reduced.
- Tell parents that children who are hearing impaired have the same intelligence quotient (IQ) distribution as children without hearing impairment. However, communication and learning can be difficult, and extra support is needed.
- Children with hearing impairment should reach their intellectual potential, although development in certain areas may take place more slowly than it does in children with no hearing impairment.

PROVIDE EMOTIONAL SUPPORT

By recognizing the effects of the diagnosis on the family, the nurse can help family members deal with their reactions to the child's hearing loss. Supporting healthy coping is an important intervention to help the parents carry on with their lives.

- Help the parents understand the child's disability and its effect on speech and language development. Provide accurate information about their concerns. Work jointly with other health care professionals and social service workers if necessary.
- Tell the family about the community services available for medical, nursing, psychologic, and financial assistance.

Evaluation

Expected outcomes of nursing care for a child with hearing impairment include:

- Successful establishment of communication method.
- Growth and development to maximum potential
- Establishment of successful individualized education plan
- Positive family coping

INJURIES OF THE EAR

Ear injuries of many types commonly occur in children. Lacerations, infections, and hematomas may occur in the external ear structures, especially the pinna. Children may place foreign objects in the ear, and insects may enter the ear canal. Rupture of the tympanic membrane may result from head injuries, blows to the ear, or insertion of objects into the ear canal.

See Table 19-10 for information on the emergency treatment of ear injuries. Any injury resulting in earache, decreased hearing, persistent bleeding, or other discharge should be seen by a physician.

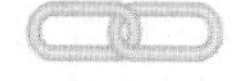

DISORDERS OF THE NOSE, THROAT, AND MOUTH

EPISTAXIS

Epistaxis, or nosebleed, is common in school-age children, especially boys. Kiesselbach's plexus, an area of plentiful veins located in the anterior nares, is a usual source of bleeding, commonly caused by irritation from nosepicking, foreign bodies, or low humidity. Other causes include forceful coughing, allergies, or infections resulting in congestion of the nasal mucosa. Bleeding from the posterior septum is more serious and may be life threatening. Hospitalization may be necessary. Posterior nosebleeds have a variety of causes, some of which may indicate systemic disease (i.e., bleeding disorder) or injury.

Children with nosebleeds are sometimes brought to the emergency department by a parent who has been unable to stop the flow of blood within a few minutes. Both parent and child may be frightened. Ask the parent briefly about any history of nosebleeds and other contributing factors, including medications. Take the child's pulse and blood pressure to as-

TABLE 19-10 Emergency Treatment of Ear Injuries

INJURY	TREATMENT
Pinna	
Minor cuts or abrasions	Wash thoroughly with soap and water and rinse well; leave exposed to air if possible or apply adhesive bandage, monitor for infection.
Hematomas	Needle aspiration should be performed and pressure dressing applied; undrained hematomas may become fibrotic; "cauliflower ear" deformity may develop.
Cellulitis or abscesses	Apply moist heat intermittently; make sure that prescribed antibiotic is taken; minor surgery may be performed for an abscess.
Deep lacerations	Apply pressure to stop bleeding transport to physician's office or emergency department for suturing.
Ear Canal	
Foreign bodies	Have child lie on back and turn head over edge of bed, with affected side down; wiggle earlobe and have child shake head; foreign object may fall out as result of gravity; if object remains in ear, call physician; do not try to remove foreign body with tweezers since this may push the object further into the ear.
Insects	Shine flashlights into ear to try to attract insect; instilling a few drops of mineral oil, olive oil, or alcohol kills insect, and irrigating ear canal gently may remove dead insect (see Skills Manual).
Tympanic Membrane	
Ruptures	Call physician if child has persistent ear pain after blow, blast injury, or insertion of foreign object; cover external ear loosely with piece of sterile cotton or gauze; if tympanic membrane has been ruptured, systemic antibiotics are prescribed.

sess for excessive blood loss. Carefully examine the nasal mucosa by asking the child to blow any clots out gently, if possible. Suctioning may be necessary.

Observing the flow may help determine if the blood is coming from an anterior or a posterior location. A nosebleed confined to one side of the nose is almost always anterior, but posterior bleeding can flow on one or both sides. If blood cannot be seen, the child may be swallowing it and may become nauseated. Suspect posterior bleeding in children who have sustained blunt trauma or in other children at high risk.

FAMILIES WANT TO KNOW

Prevention and Home Management of Epistaxis

PREVENTION

- Humidify the child's room, especially during the winter.
- Discourage the child from picking or rubbing the nose or inserting foreign objects in the nose.
- Instruct the child to blow the nose gently and release sneezes through the mouth.

HOME MANAGEMENT

- Keep the child calm.
- Sit the child upright with head tilted slightly forward so blood does not run down the nasopharynx.
- Press a roll of cotton under the upper lip to compress the labial artery.
- Apply steady pressure to both nostrils just below the nasal bone with the thumb and forefinger for 15–20 minutes. Time by the clock.
- Apply an ice pack or cold compress to the bridge of the nose or the back of the neck.
- Call health care provider if the bleeding does not stop.
- Avoid further bleeds by sleeping with the head elevated on pillows, avoiding hot showers and drinks, and avoiding aspirin or other noncoagulant drugs during the first few days after a nosebleed.

Note: Adapted from Newland, J. A., & Rich, E. (1998). Epistaxis. *American Journal of Nursing, 98,* 16HHH.

The child with anterior bleeding should sit upright quietly. The head should be tilted forward to prevent blood from trickling down the throat, which can lead to vomiting. The nares should be squeezed just below the nasal bone and held for 10 to 15 minutes while the child breathes through the mouth. If the bleeding does not stop, a cotton ball or swab soaked with Neo-Synephrine, epinephrine, thrombin, or lidocaine may be inserted into the affected nostril to promote topical vasoconstriction or anesthesia. Once the bleeding has stopped, the nostril may have to be cauterized with silver nitrate or electrocautery. If the bleeding cannot be stopped, absorbable packing may be used.

Posterior bleeding must also be stopped by packing, and the child must be monitored carefully. Arterial ligation is occasionally needed. Repeated or severe nosebleeds need further evaluation (Newland & Rich, 1998).

Nursing Management

Assess the child's hematocrit or hemoglobin if significant bleeding has occurred. Children with frequent epistaxis should have a complete history taken and physical examination performed to rule out systemic disease.

After the nosebleed has stopped, the child is more vulnerable to recurrent bleeding and should avoid bending over, stooping, strenuous exercise, hot drinks, and hot baths or showers for the next 3 to 4 days. Sleeping with the head elevated on two or three pillows and humidifying the air with a vaporizer may also prevent a recurrence. Provide parents with suggestions for prevention and home management of epistaxis.

NASOPHARYNGITIS

Nasopharyngitis, also known as the common cold, causes inflammation and infection of the nose and throat and is probably the most common illness of infancy and childhood. More than 200 viruses and numerous bacteria can cause this condition. The most common viruses include rhinovirus and coronavirus, and the most frequently occurring bacterium is group A *Streptococcus.* The organisms incubate in 1 to 3 days, and the infection is communicable several hours before symptoms develop and for 1 to 2 days after they begin. Symptoms may last 4 to 10 days or longer. The pathogens are believed to spread when the infected person touches the hand of an uninfected person, who then touches his or her mouth or nose, resulting in self-inoculation.

A red nasal mucosa with clear nasal discharge and an infected throat with enlarged tonsils may be apparent in children with nasopharyngitis. Vesicles may be present on the soft palate and in the pharynx. Accompanying symptoms may vary, depending on the child's age (Table 19-11).

Between episodes of nasopharyngitis, the child should be asymptomatic. If a child continues to have upper respiratory infections, the presence of an underlying condition such as allergy, asthma, or polyps should be ruled out.

TABLE 19-11 Symptoms of Nasopharyngitis

Infants Younger Than 3 Months of Age	Older Children
Lethargy	Dry, irritated nose and throat
Irritability	Chills, fever
Feeding poorly	Generalized muscle aches
Fever (may be absent)	Headache
Infants 3 Months of Age or Older	Malaise
Fever	Anorexia
Vomiting	Thin nasal discharge, which may later become thick and purulent
Diarrhea	Possible sneezing
Sneezing	
Anorexia	
Irritability	
Restlessness	

Nursing Management

For infants who cannot breathe through the mouth, normal saline nose drops can be administered every 3 to 4 hours, especially before feeding. (Refer to the Skills Manual for instructions on how to administer nose drops.) For infants over 9 months of age, nasal stuffiness can be treated with either normal saline nose drops or a decongestant such as phenylephrine (0.125% to 0.25%, depending on the child's age). Older children can use nasal sprays.

Skill 7-9: Administering a Nasal Medication

Although nose drops and sprays are more effective than systemic decongestants, they should not be used for more than 4 or 5 days or more often than recommended. Antihistamines may be helpful for children with allergic rhinitis or profuse nasal drainage. Long-acting nasal sprays and medications with several ingredients are not recommended.

Room humidification may help prevent drying of nasal secretions. Antipyretics such as acetaminophen reduce fever and make the child more comfortable. Aspirin is not recommended because of its association with Reye syndrome (refer to Chapter 20).

Children should avoid strenuous physical activity and engage in quiet play such as reading, listening to music or stories, or watching television or videotapes. Children should not be forced to eat, but the intake of favorite fluids to liquify secretions should be encouraged. Parents should be told that no medicine or vaccine can prevent the common cold, but eliminating contact with infected persons can reduce the spread of infection. Proper handwashing and disposal of tissues help to decrease the spread of the infection.

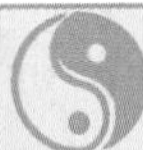

CULTURE

Many Hispanic and Asian cultural groups believe in the "hot and cold theory" of disease, in which health problems are viewed as the result of imbalance. For example, Mexican-Americans traditionally treat a "cold disease" such as an earache or common cold with "hot" substances. Ask families if they prefer to eat certain foods during an illness. Incorporating such preferences can help the child to get better and increase the confidence of the family in health care providers.

SINUSITIS

Sinusitis is an inflammation of one or more of the paranasal sinuses. These sinuses, which have respiratory epithelium and are continuous with the respiratory tract, include the maxillary, ethmoid, frontal, and sphenoid sinuses. The sinuses may become infected with bacteria following a viral upper respiratory infection. In most cases, the child's history reveals a cold for several days, followed by improvement in the cold symptoms, but an increase in purulent nasal drainage. There is accompanying facial pain, headache, and fever. Chronic sinusitis may occur in children with uncontrolled allergies and asthma.

Although most physicians treat suspected sinusitis with antibiotics, many cases will clear spontaneously without treatment. Amoxicillin is the first choice for therapy; amoxicillin/clavulanate and cephalosporins are also sometimes used (Sinus and Allergy Health Partnership, 2000; Kakish, Mahafza, & Batieha, et al., 2000).

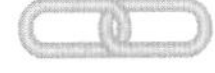

Skill 10-15: Performing Nasal Suctioning

Parents whose child has persistent and purulent nasal drainage should be told to see a health care provider, particularly if the drainage is accompanied by facial pain, headache, and fever. Teach parents to correctly administer antibiotics (e.g., to take medications for the full course) if prescribed, and to use saline nose drops if needed for comfort. Infants may need their nose cleared with nose drops and a bulb syringe prior to feedings. (Refer to the Skills Manual for correct use of a bulb syringe.) Antipyretics can be given for fever and to relieve pain.

PHARYNGITIS

Acute pharyngitis is an infection that primarily affects the pharynx, including the tonsils (Figure 19-12 ◆). It is seen most frequently in children 4 to 7 years and is rare in children less than 1 year. Approximately 80% of these infections are caused by viruses; the rest are caused by bacteria. Bacterial pharyngitis is commonly known as strep throat, because it is most often caused by group A beta-hemolytic *Streptococcus* (GABHS). Viral pharyngitis is caused by a large number of enteroviruses.

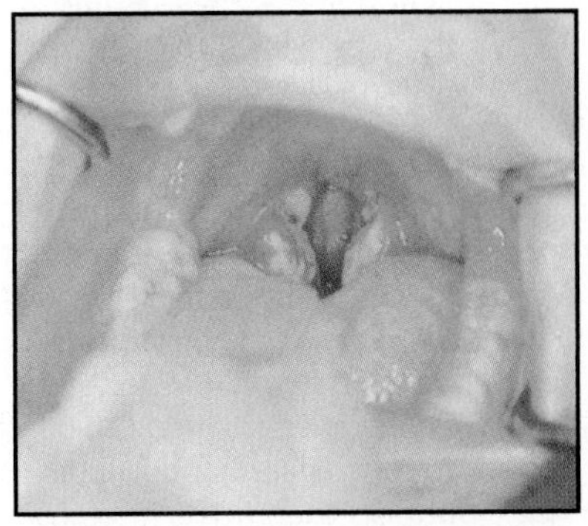

FIGURE 19-12 ◆

Acute pharyngitis primarily affects the pharynx but often involves the tonsils, as in this child.

From Malasanos, L., Barkauskas, V., & Stoltenberg-Allen, K. (1990). *Health assessment* (4th ed., Plate 2). St. Louis: Mosby-Year Book. Courtesy of Edward L. Applebaum, M.D., Chicago, IL.

The major complaint is a sore throat. See page 718 for clinical manifestations of viral pharyngitis and strep throat. Children with symptoms of strep throat who have minimal throat redness and pain, exudate, mild lymphadenopathy, and a low-grade fever, and who have been exposed to someone who has pharyngitis, should have a throat culture. The classic signs of purulent drainage and white patches are not present in all cases of strep throat. A child who finds swallowing difficult or extremely painful, who drools, or who exhibits

CLINICAL MANIFESTATIONS OF VIRAL PHARYNGITIS AND STREP THROAT (GROUP A BETA-HEMOLYTIC STREPTOCOCCUS [GABHS])[a]

VIRAL PHARYNGITIS	STREP THROAT
Nasal congestion	Tonsillar exudate[b]
Mild sore throat	Painful cervical lymphadenopathy[b]
Conjunctivitis	Abdominal pain
Cough	Vomiting
Hoarseness	Severe sore throat
Mild pharyngeal redness	Headache
Minimal tonsillar exudate	Fever >38.3°C (101°F)
Mildly tender anterior cervical lymphadenopathy	Petechial mottling of soft palate
Fever <38.3°C (101°F)	

[a]Children 6 months to 3 years of age may have streptococcus with symptoms that resemble those of viral pharyngitis. Children with scarlet fever have the symptoms of strep throat plus a sandpaper-textured erythemotous generalized rash and pallor around the lips.
[b]Classic signs of strep throat.

signs of dehydration or respiratory distress should be seen by a physician immediately. These signs could be indicators of serious conditions such as epiglottitis, peritonsillar or retropharyngeal abscess, or diphtheria.

The diagnosis of strep throat is made by throat culture, using the rapid or traditional strep tests. Results of the rapid strep test may be available within minutes; those for the traditional test are available in 24 to 48 hours. Early signs of strep throat should be treated with oral penicillin for 10 days or by long-acting penicillin given in one injection immediately, even before the result of the culture is available. If the child is allergic to penicillin, erythromycin is given. Acute symptoms should resolve within 24 hours of therapy, at which time the child is no longer contagious. For pharyngitis that is caused by a virus, symptomatic treatment alone is used.

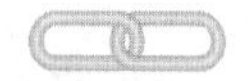

Skill 6-12: Obtaining a Sample for Throat Culture

CLINICAL TIP

Throat cultures must be properly performed for accurate diagnosis. A sterile cotton-tip applicator is swabbed across the tonsils, posterior edge of the soft palate, and uvula. Cooperative children can be asked to put their hands under their buttocks, open their mouth, and laugh or pant like a dog. The throat is quickly swabbed. Uncooperative and young children are placed on their back with their hands next to their head and held by a parent or an assistant. The tongue is gently depressed with a tongue blade and the throat is swabbed.

Nursing Management

Nursing care focuses on symptomatic relief. Acetaminophen reduces throat pain and generalized fever. Cool, nonacidic fluids and soft foods, ice chips, or frozen juice pops given frequently in small amounts facilitate swallowing and prevent dehydration. Humidification, chewing gum, and gargling with warm salt water (5 g to 250 mL water; 1 to 8 oz water) soothe an irritated throat. Commercial throat sprays or throat lozenges are not generally more effective than these home remedies. Encourage the child to rest, to conserve energy and promote recovery.

Teach parents the importance of completing the 10-day course of antibiotics if prescribed for bacterial pharyngitis. Reinforce to parents the importance of treating streptococcal infections, as untreated infections may lead to rheumatic fever, cervical adenitis, sinusitis, glomerulonephritis, or meningitis.

TONSILLITIS

Tonsillitis is an infection or inflammation (hypertrophy) of the palatine tonsils. Although most children with pharyngitis may have infected tonsils, they do not necessarily have tonsillitis.

Etiology and Pathophysiology

Like pharyngitis, tonsillitis may be caused by a virus or bacterium. The primary site of infection is the tonsils.

Clinical Manifestations

Symptoms suggestive of tonsillitis include frequent throat infections with breathing and swallowing difficulties; persistent redness of the anterior pillars; and enlargement of the cervical lymph nodes. If children breathe through their mouths continuously, the mucous membranes may become dry and irritated.

Clinical Therapy

Diagnosis is made on the basis of visual inspection and clinical manifestations. Symptomatic treatment for tonsillitis is the same as for pharyngitis. Surgical removal of tonsils (tonsillectomy) is often recommended when children have recurrent throat infections (about three per year for 3 years), chronic tonsillitis, obstructive sleep apnea, or malformations causing nasal speech or a facial growth abnormality. If the child is under 3 years of age, the surgery is postponed if possible because it may stimulate growth of other lymphoid tissue in the nasopharynx. If the pharyngeal tonsils (adenoids) are enlarged, as suggested by mouth breathing, cough, impaired taste and smell, a muffled quality to the voice, and chronic otitis media, then they may be removed at the same time.

CLINICAL TIP

Children may be more willing to gargle with salt water if the mixture is placed in a spray bottle and sprayed gently toward the throat. Do you know why? The salt water bypasses the salt sensation on the outer part of the tongue and is not as distasteful. The gentle spray does not stimulate a gag reflex; it delivers the salt solution directly to the throat area where it can be gargled and then spit out.

NURSING MANAGEMENT

Nursing Assessment and Diagnosis

Assess the throat carefully during each physical examination. Observe for tonsils that are simply large (a common finding in childhood) and those that are inflamed. Look for the degree of redness and presence of any exudate. Ask if the child has pain or difficulty swallowing. Ask about the history of past tonsillar infections and the length of time of the present discomfort.

If surgery is indicated, take a complete history of the child preoperatively. Monitor vital signs and observe for respiratory distress, hemorrhage, and dehydration postoperatively.

The following nursing diagnoses may apply to the child with tonsillitis:

- *Pain,* related to inflammation of the pharynx
- *Risk for fluid volume deficit,* related to inadequate intake
- *Risk for ineffective breathing pattern,* related to obstruction by enlarged tonsils
- *Impaired swallowing,* related to inflammation and pain
- *Knowledge deficit (Parents),* related to home care following discharge

FAMILIES WANT TO KNOW

Care After Tonsillectomy

After a child's tonsillectomy, the parent can institute measures to increase the child's comfort.

- Have the child drink adequate cool fluids or chew gum, as this reduces spasms in the muscles surrounding the throat.
- Give acetaminophen elixir, as ordered.
- Apply an ice collar around the child's neck.
- Have the child gargle with a solution of 2.5 g (0.5 t) each of baking soda and salt in 8 oz of water.
- Have the child rinse the mouth well with viscous lidocaine and then swallow the solution.

FAMILIES WANT TO KNOW

Complications of Tonsillectomy and Adenoidectomy

BLEEDING

- To prevent bleeding, aspirin or ibuprofen should not be given for pain for the first postoperative week. Use acetaminophen instead.
- Bleeding is most likely to occur within the first 24 hours or 7–10 days after the tonsillectomy, when the scar is forming. Report any trickle of bright red blood to the physician immediately.

INFECTION

- The back of the throat will look white and have an odor for the first 7–8 days after the surgery. The child may also have a low-grade fever. These are not signs of infection.
- For temperatures over 38.3°C (101°F), acetaminophen may be used.
- Call the physician if the child develops a fever above 38.8°C (102°F).

PAIN

- Administer acetaminophen as ordered.
- Offer frequent small amounts of cool liquids. Avoid citrus juice.
- Provide for rest and quiet activities for several days.

Planning and Implementation

The nurse provides general supportive care and, if medication is prescribed, encourages completion of the full course of treatment. The nursing management of children with tonsillitis is similar to that of children with pharyngitis (see earlier discussion).

If surgery is indicated, the parents are helped to prepare their child for a short-term surgical procedure with a possible overnight stay in the hospital (see Chapter 5). Children should be free of sore throat, fever, or upper respiratory infection for at least 1 week before surgery. They should not be given aspirin or ibuprofen for 2 weeks before surgery, as these medications can increase bleeding. Check if any herbal medications are taken and report them to the physician and anesthesiologist, because some may interfere with anesthetic drugs used in surgery.

Discharge Planning and Home Care Teaching

Discharge planning includes teaching parents about pain management, fluid and nutrition intake, activity restrictions, and possible complications in the postoperative period. Most children will have a sore throat for 7 to 10 days after tonsillectomy. Advise parents how to relieve the child's throat pain.

Children may experience ear pain, especially when swallowing, between 4 and 8 days after tonsillectomy. Advise parents that this pain is the result of referred pain from the tonsillar area and does not indicate an ear infection.

Emphasize to parents the importance of adequate fluid intake. Children should be given any liquid they prefer for the first week, except citrus juices, which may produce a burning sensation in the throat. Soft foods such as gelatin, applesauce, frozen juice pops, and mashed potatoes can be added as tolerated.

Children do not need to be confined to bed, but vigorous exercise should be avoided for the first week after surgery. Advise parents that the child may return to school approximately 10 days after tonsillectomy.

Any surgery carries with it the risk of postoperative complications. Teach parents the normal signs of healing in the postoperative period, as well as signs of complications.

Evaluation

Expected outcomes of nursing care for the child with tonsillitis include:

- Adequate intake of food and fluids
- Management of pain and fever
- Healing without impairment following tonsillectomy

FAMILIES WANT TO KNOW

Care of a Tooth Avulsion

When a tooth is removed during an injury, prompt treatment may influence the chance that it can be reimplanted. If the child's condition is stable, try to reimplant the tooth and then transfer the child to an emergency dental facility.

- Handle the tooth only by the crown (its top).
- Gently rinse the tooth in a bowl of tap water. Do not place it under running water.
- Insert into the socket.
- Have the child provide gentle pressure by biting a piece of gauze or a tea bag.

If child is unstable or has other injuries, enlist emergency medical transportation (call 9-1-1). In this case, the tooth is transported with the child.

- Place the tooth in milk, saline, saliva, or water. If a dental aid kit is available, it may contain a transport liquid called Hank's Balanced Salt Solution.

Note: Adapted from Rudy, C. A. (2001). Dental trauma. *School Nurse News, 18*(1), 33–35.

MOUTH AND DENTAL EMERGENCIES

Children may have trauma to the mouth and teeth during sporting activities and during other injuries. About 10% of children experience some dental trauma (Diangelis & Bakland, 1998). Nurses inform parents of proper treatment for injuries and may provide emergency treatment in schools and other community settings. Injury prevention is encouraged through use of protective gear during sports. See Chapter 16 for a discussion of oral care during treatment for cancer, and Chapter 7 for a discussion of protective sporting gear and of body piercing which may include the oral cavity.

Because the mouth has a profuse blood supply, bleeding may be extensive for even minor injuries. It is best to use clean cloths to absorb the blood and prevent choking on it, and get the child to an emergency facility to have the lesion carefully examined.

Dental injuries may involve fracture of a tooth, luxation (partial extrusion), or avulsion (complete removal). The child should be transported immediately to an emergency facility. If otherwise stable, an emergency dental visit is the best choice. When avulsion has occurred, fast care improves the chance that a permanent tooth can be reimplanted and kept alive. When reimplanted within 30 minutes, the chances of survival of tooth are best (Rudy, 2001). Nurses can perform care or teach parents what to do in case of dental emergency. Referral to dental resources may be needed.

HOME CARE

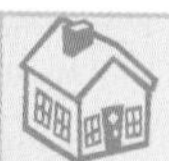

For families with financial constraints, dental care is often delayed or not available. Ask families about what they do for dental care, and how they would seek care if the child has a dental emergency. Many communities have an association of dentists and dental workers who provide care at clinics and other facilities for children without dental insurance. Nurses can help the families to find resources in their communities to provide regular dental visits and care for dental emergencies.

Chapter Highlights

- Health conditions affecting the eyes and ears are common in childhood, partially due to anatomical differences in structure.
- Disorders of the eye and ear can lead to developmental and communication delays.
- Conjunctivitis can occur throughout childhood, and can be caused by bacteria, viruses, and allergy.
- Conjunctivitis in the newborn, ophthalmia neonatorum, can be acquired during birth from the mother, and can provide a serious health threat.
- Children manifest a wide array of visual disorders such as hyperopia, myopia, and astigmatism.
- Conditions that can seriously affect vision are strabismus, amblyopia, cataracts, and glaucoma.
- An iatrogenically caused visual disorder is retinopathy of prematurity.
- Nurses commonly screen vision of children in schools and health facilities to identify those with visual impairment.
- Interventions for the child with visual impairment center on providing input through other senses to maximize child development.
- Otitis media is the most common childhood health condition, and has increased in incidence in the past decade.

- Overgrowth of resistant organisms has made treatment of otitis media difficult.
- Treatment may begin with up to 3 days of monitoring, followed by antibiotic therapy if the child's condition worsens.
- Newborns should be screened for response to sounds; those at high risk of hearing impairment should be carefully monitored in early childhood.
- Hearing loss may be conductive, sensorineural, or mixed.
- Nursing plan interventions maximize development and communication in the child with a hearing impairment.
- Common disorders of the nose and throat in children include epistaxis, nasopharyngitis, pharyngitis, and tonsillitis.

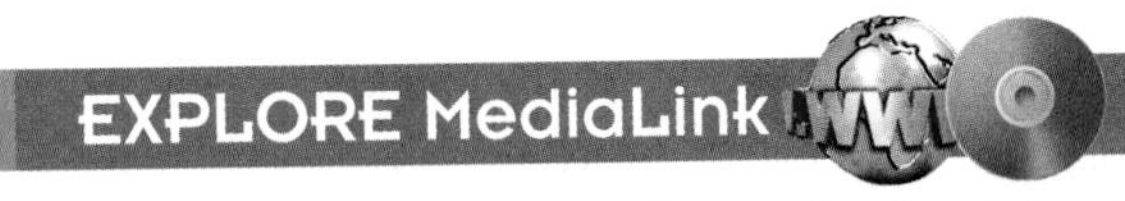

- NCLEX review, case studies, and other interactive resources for this chapter can be found on the Companion Website at **http://www.prenhall.com/ball.** Click on Chapter 19 to select the activities for this chapter.
- For animations, more NCLEX review questions, and an audio glossary, access the accompanying CD-ROM in this textbook.

References

1. Agency for Healthcare Research and Quality. (2001). *Management of acute otitis media* (AHRQ Publication No. 00-E010). Rockville, MD: Author.
2. Alcorn, D. M. (2001, March). Red eye: When to treat and when to refer. *Infectious Diseases in Children,* 3–8.
3. Altemeier, W. A. (2000). Preschool vision screening: The importance of the two-line difference. *Pediatric Annals, 29,* 264–267.
4. American Academy of Pediatrics, Section on Ophthalmology. (2001). Screening examination of premature infants for retinopathy of prematurity. *Pediatrics, 108,* 809–811.
5. American Academy of Pediatrics, Task Force on Newborn and Infant Hearing. (1999). Newborn and infant hearing loss: Detection and intervention. *Pediatrics, 103,* 527–530.
6. Bacal, D. A., & Wilson, M. C. (2000). Strabismus: Getting it straight. *Contemporary Pediatrics, 17,* 49–60.
7. Bachman, K. R., & Arvedson, J. C. (1998). Early identification and intervention for children who are hearing impaired. *Pediatrics in Review, 19,* 155–165.
8. Brocklehurst, P., & Rooney, G. (2000). Interventions for treating genital *Chlamydia trachomatis* infection in pregnancy. *Cochrane Database Systematic Review 2000, 2,* CD000054.
9. Brookhouse, P. E., Beauchaine, K. L., & Osberger, M. J. (1999). Management of the child with sensorineural hearing loss: Medical, surgical, hearing aids, cochlear implants. *Pediatric Clinics of North America, 46,* 121–142.
10. Burns, C. E., Brady, M. A., Dunn, A. M., & Starr, N. B. (2000). *Pediatric primary care,* (2nd ed.). Philadelphia: WB Saunders.
11. Carlson, L. H., & Fall, P. A. (1998). Otitis media: An update. *Journal of Pediatric Helath Care, 12,* 313–319.
12. Cheng, A. K., Rubin, H. R., Powe, N. R., Mellon, N. K., Francis, H. W., & Niparko, J. K. (2000). Cost-utility of the cochlear implant in children. *Journal of the American Medical Association, 284,* 850–856.
13. Coody, D., Banks, J. M., Yetman, R. J., & Musgrove, K. (1997). Eye trauma in children: Epidemiology, management, and prevention. *Journal of Pediatric Health Care, 11,* 182–188.
14. DeRespinis, P. A. (2001). Eyeglasses: Why and when do children need them? *Pediatric Annals, 30,* 455–461.
15. Diangelis, A. J., & Bakland, L. K. (1998). Traumatic dental injuries: Current treatment concepts. *Journal of the American Dental Association, 129,* 1401–1414.
16. Dowell, S. F., Butler, J. C., Geibink, G. S., and the Drug-resistant *Streptococcal pneumoniae* Therapeutic Working Group. (1999). *Pediatric Infectious Disease Journal, 18,* 1–9.
17. Garganta, C., & Seashore, M. R. (2000). Universal screening for congenital hearing loss. *Pediatric Annals, 29,* 302–308.
18. Gomez, S., & Davis, R. L. (2001). Photoscreening—A viable method for referral. *School Nurse News, 18*(1), 18–20.
19. Hayes, D. (1999). State programs for universal newborn hearing screening. *Pediatric Clinics of North America, 46,* 89–94.
20. Hoberman, A., & Paradise, J. L. (2000). Acute otitis media: Diagnosis and management in the year 2000. *Pediatric Annals, 29,* 609–620.
21. Joint Committee on Infant Hearing (2000). Joint committee on infant hearing 2000 position statement: Principles and guidelines for early hearing detection and intervention programs. *Pediatrics 106,* 798–817.
22. Kakish, K. S., Mahafza, T., Batieha, A., Ekteish, F., & Daoud, A. (2000). Clinical sinusitis in children attending primary care centers. *Pediatric Infectious Disease Journal, 19,* 1071–1074.
23. Little, P., Gould, C., Williamson, I., Moore, M., Warner, G., & Dunleavey, J. (2001). Pragmatic randomized controlled trial of two prescribing strategies for childhood acute otitis media. *British Medical Journal, 322,* 336–342.
24. Newland, J. A., & Rich, E. (1998). Epistaxis. *American Journal of Nursing, 98,* 16HHH.
25. Niemela, M., Pihakari, O., Pokka, T., Uhari, M. S., & Uhari, M. S. (2000). Pacifier as a risk factor for acute otitis media: A randomized, controlled trial of parental counseling. *Pediatrics, 106,* 483–488.
26. Niskar, A. S., Kieszak, S. M., Holmes, A. E., Esteban, E., Rubin, C., & Brody, D. J. (2001). Estimated prevalence of noise-induced hearing threshold shifts among children 6 to 19 years of age: The third national health and nutrition examination survey, 1988–1994, United States. *Pediatrics, 108,* 40–43.
27. Paradise, J. L., Feldman, H. M., Campbell, T. F., Dollaghan, C. A., Colburn, D. K., Bernard, B. S., Rockette, H. E., Janosky, J. E., Pitcairn, D. L., Sabo, D. L., Kurs-Lasky, M., & Smith, C. G. (2001). Effect of early or delayed insertion of tympanostomy tubes for persistent otitis media on developmental outcome at the age of 3 years. *New England Journal of Medicine, 344,* 1170–1187.
28. Roddey, O. F., & Hoover, H. A. (2000). Otitis media with effusion in children: A pediatric office perspective. *Pediatric Annals, 29,* 623–629.

29. Rudy, C. A. (2001). Dental trauma. *School Nurse News, 18*(1), 33–35.

30. Scheiner, A. P. (1996). Vision problems: Impairment to blindness. In A. M. Rudolph, J. I. E. Hoffman, & C. D. Rudolph (eds.), *Rudolph's pediatrics* (20th ed., p. 167). Stamford, CT: Appleton & Lange.

31. Sinus and Allergy Health Partnership. (2000). Antimicrobial treatment guidelines for acute bacterial rhinosinusitis. *Otolaryngology and Head and Neck Surgery, 123,* 5–31.

32. Slattery, W. H., & Fayad, J. N. (1999). Cochlear implants in children with sensorineural inner ear hearing loss. *Pediatric Annals, 28,* 359–363.

33. Starr, N. B. (2000). Vision therapy for learning disabilities and dyslexia. *Journal of Pediatric Health Care, 14,* 32–33.

34. Wagner, R. S. (2000). Management of conjunctivitis. *Contemporary Pediatrics Supplement 2000,* 3–14.

35. White, K. R., & Maxon, A. B. (1999). *Early identification of hearing loss: Implementing universal newborn hearing screening programs.* Rockville, MD: U.S. Department of Health & Human Services, Maternal & Child Health Bureau.

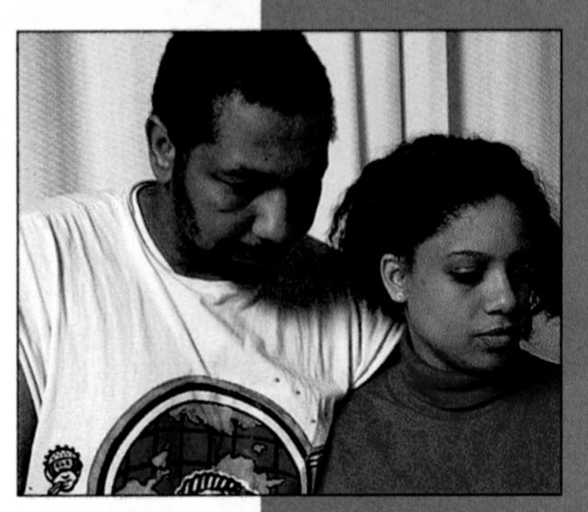

"It's so hard to watch your child experience an injury like this. All we can do is be here every day for Antwan and hope that he will fully recover."

Antwan, 7 years old, was injured when struck by a car and thrown several feet into the air. He was unconscious upon admission to the emergency department and showed some signs of increased intracranial pressure (dilated and fixed pupils). He was treated for shock, and his neurologic status and vital signs were frequently assessed. The initial evaluation revealed that Antwan had sustained several contusions of the brain, but no skull fracture. He was intubated and medicated to manage the increased intracranial pressure.

Antwan's intracranial pressure has now stabilized, but he still has not totally regained consciousness. He is restless and agitated, and unable to follow directions. His parents stay at his bedside and provide auditory and tactile stimulation, hoping he will eventually respond. Physical therapy has been initiated to prevent contractures and to maintain function. Long-term rehabilitation will be needed to help Antwan and his family achieve the best outcome possible after this injury.

What is the role of the nurse in acute care of the child who has a brain injury? What support does the family need to contribute to the child's care? How does the nurse work with other health care professionals to plan the long-term care of a child such as Antwan?

CHAPTER 20

ALTERATIONS IN NEUROLOGIC FUNCTION

KEY TERMS

areflexia No reflex response to verbal, sensory, or pain stimulation.

assistive technology A piece of equipment or system modified or customized to improve or maintain functional capabilities of individuals with disabilities.

aura Subjective sensation, often olfactory or visual in nature, that is an early sign of a migraine headache or a seizure.

cerebral edema Increase in intracellular and extracellular fluid in the brain that results from anoxia, vasodilation, or vascular stasis.

cerebral perfusion pressure Amount of pressure needed to ensure that adequate oxygen and nutrients will be delivered to the brain.

clonic Alternating muscular contraction and relaxation; often used to describe seizure activity.

coma State of unconsciousness in which the child cannot be aroused, even with powerful stimuli.

Cushing's triad Reflex response associated with increased intracranial pressure or compromised blood flow to the brainstem; characterized by hypertension, increased systolic pressure with wide pulse pressure, bradycardia, and irregular respirations.

encephalopathy Cerebral dysfunction resulting from an insult (toxin, injury, inflammation, or anoxic event) of limited duration; the tissue damage is often permanent, but the dysfunction may improve over time.

focal Specific area of the brain; often used to describe seizures or neurologic deficits.

intracranial pressure Force exerted by brain tissue, cerebrospinal fluid, and blood within the cranial vault.

intractable seizure Seizures that continue to occur even with optimal medical management.

level of consciousness (LOC) General description of cognitive, sensory, and motor response to stimuli.

postictal period Period after seizure activity during which the level of consciousness is decreased.

posturing Abnormal position assumed after injury or damage to the brain that may be seen as extreme flexion or extension of the limbs.

tonic Continuous muscular contraction; often used to describe seizure activity.

MediaLink

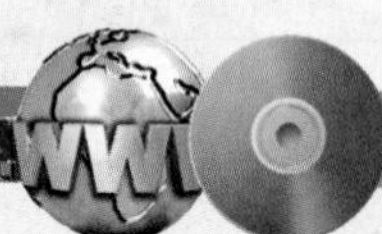

http://www.prenhall.com/ball

Resources for this chapter can be found on the CD-ROM accompanying this textbook, and on the Companion Website at http://www.prenhall.com/ball. Click on Chapter 20 to select the activities for this chapter.

CD-ROM

Audio Glossary

NCLEX Review

COMPANION WEBSITE

Web Links

NCLEX Review

MediaLink Applications

- Soothing Newborns with Neonatal Abstinence Syndrome
- Assessing a Child with a Concussion for Return to Competitive Play

Why do certain neurologic disorders occur more often in children than in adults? What effect do these disorders have on a child's growth and development? Why are some neurologic injuries more likely to be seen in children and why do children recover from these injuries more completely than adults? What role do nurses play in ensuring early diagnosis and treatment of neurologic disorders? This chapter will answer these questions by examining some of the more common disorders of neurologic function in children.

ANATOMY AND PHYSIOLOGY OF PEDIATRIC DIFFERENCES

Knowledge of the anatomy of the nervous system makes neurologic symptoms easier to understand. The brain, spinal cord, and nerves are the major structures of the nervous system (Figure 20-1 ◆). The spinal cord transmits impulses to and from the brain, conveying sensory information and relaying impulses that stimulate motor responses. Because the nervous system helps to control and coordinate many body functions, alterations in neurologic function can have widespread effects on the body's metabolism.

The brain and spinal cord are formed early in gestation from the neural tube. Any insult or critical event (teratogen, infection, substance abuse, or trauma) during this period can result in a central nervous system (CNS) malformation. Such defects account for approximately one-third of all apparent congenital malformations in live infants, and 90% of these are neural tube defects (Farley & Mooney, 1998). CNS defects are responsible for 40% of infant deaths in the first year of life (Farley & Dunleavy, 2000).

At birth, the nervous system is complete but immature. The infant is born with all of the nerve cells that will exist throughout life. However, the number of glial cells and dendrites, which enable receipt of nerve impulses, continues to increase until approximately 4 years of age. Myelination, which increases the speed and accuracy of nerve impulses, is also incomplete at birth. This process continues throughout childhood, proceeding in a cephalocaudal direction.

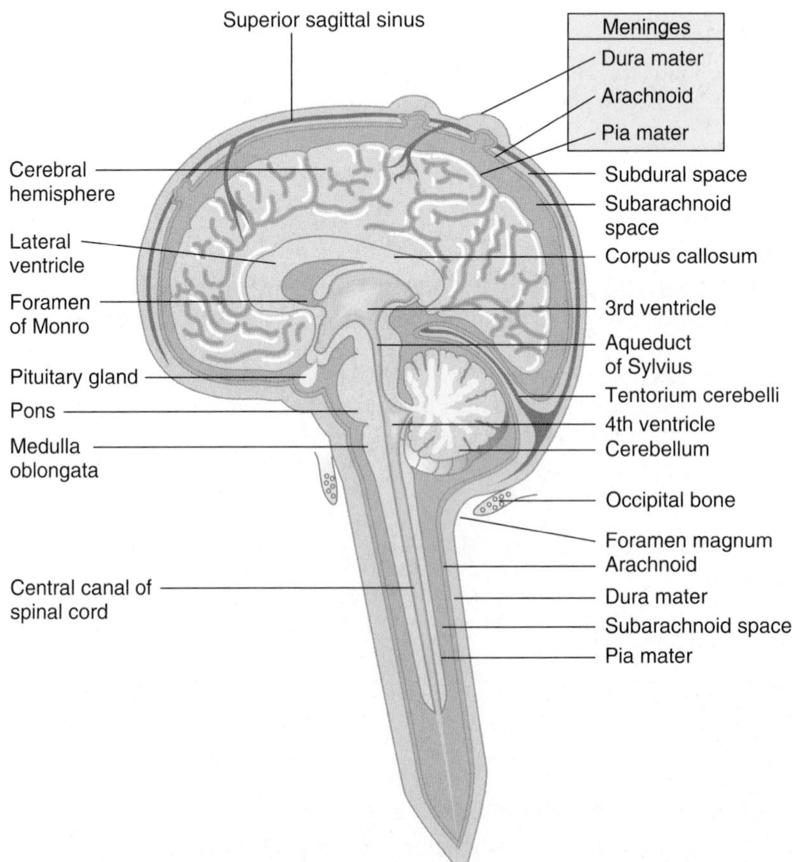

FIGURE 20-1 ◆
Transverse section of the brain and spinal cord. Knowledge of the anatomy of the brain is helpful in understanding the symptoms of neurologic dysfunction.

TABLE 20-1 Summary of Anatomic and Physiologic Differences Between Children and Adults

DIFFERENCE IN CHILDREN	SIGNIFICANCE
Top heavy; head is large in proportion to body; neck muscles not well developed	Prone to head injuries with falls; neck may not be able to support large head
Thin cranial bones that are not well developed; unfused sutures	Prone to fracture
Highly vascular brain; subarachnoid space small; dura firmly attached but can strip away from pericranium	Brain prone to hemorrhage; there is less cerebrospinal fluid to cushion the brain
Excessive spinal mobility; muscles, joint capsules, and ligaments of cervical spine immature	Greater risk for high cervical spine injury at C1–C2 level
Wedge-shaped, cartilaginous vertebral bodies; ossification of vertebral bodies incomplete	Greater risk for compression fractures of vertebrae with falls

The anatomic and physiologic differences between the nervous systems of children and adults help explain why children and adults have different neurologic problems (Table 20-1). For example, the brain and spinal cord are protected by the skeletal structures of the skull and vertebrae. In infants, however, the cranial bones and vertebrae are not completely ossified. The infant's brain and spinal cord are thus at greater risk for injury resulting from trauma.

GROWTH & DEVELOPMENT

The myelination process accounts for the progressive acquisition of fine and gross motor skills and coordination during early childhood.

ALTERED STATES OF CONSCIOUSNESS

Level of consciousness (**LOC**) is perhaps the most important indicator of neurologic dysfunction. Consciousness, the responsiveness of the mind to sensory stimuli, has two components: *alertness,* the ability to react to stimuli; and *cognitive power,* the ability to process the data and respond either verbally or physically. Unconsciousness, on the other hand, is depressed cerebral function, or the inability of the brain to respond to stimuli.

Levels of deterioration can be further categorized as follows:

- *Confusion*: disorientation to time, place, or person. The child may seem alert. Answers to simple questions may be correct, but responses to complex ones may be inaccurate.
- *Delirium*: state characterized by confusion, fear, agitation, hyperactivity, or anxiety.
- *Obtunded*: limited response to the environment. The child falls asleep unless given verbal or tactile stimulation.
- *Stupor*: response to vigorous stimulation only. The child returns to the unresponsive state when the stimulus is removed. For example, the child may react to a needle stick but not respond to a milder stimulus such as touching the skin.
- ***Coma***: state characterized by severely diminished response. The child cannot be aroused even by painful stimuli.

ETIOLOGY AND PATHOPHYSIOLOGY

Trauma, infection, poisoning, seizures, or any other process that affects the CNS may alter the level of consciousness (Table 20-2). Any of these pathologic processes can also cause increased **intracranial pressure** (force exerted by brain tissue, cerebrospinal fluid, and blood within the cranial vault). Discovering the cause of the decreased level of consciousness is essential so that immediate treatment can begin, to prevent possible secondary effects of the illness or injury.

CLINICAL MANIFESTATIONS

Decline in a child's level of consciousness often follows a sequential pattern of deterioration. A child may first appear awake and alert, and may respond appropriately. Initial changes may be

CAUSES OF ALTERED CONSCIOUSNESS

- Hypoxia
- Trauma
- Infection
- Poisoning
- Ventriculoperitoneal shunt
- Seizures
- Endocrine or metabolic disturbances (e.g., hypoglycemia)
- Electrolyte, acid–base, or biochemical imbalance
- CNS pathology (e.g., neoplasms or degenerative disorders)
- Congenital structural defect

TABLE 20-2 Signs of Increased Intracranial Pressure

Early Signs	Late Signs
Headache	Significant decrease in level of consciousness
Visual disturbances, diplopia	Cushing's triad
Nausea and vomiting	■ Increased systolic blood pressure and widened pulse pressure
Dizziness or vertigo	■ Brachycardia
Slight change in vital signs	■ Irregular respirations
Pupils not as reactive or equal	Fixed and dilated pupils
Sunsetting eyes	
Seizures	
Slight change in level of consciousness	
Infant has above signs plus:	
Bulging fontanel	
Wide sutures, increased head circumference	
Dilated scalp veins	
High-pitched, catlike cry	

subtle: a slight disorientation to time, place, and person. The child may become restless or fussy, and actions that normally calm or soothe the child only increase irritability. As responsiveness decreases, the child may become drowsy but still respond to loud verbal commands and withdraw from painful stimuli. Keeping the child awake is sometimes difficult. Then response to pain progresses from purposeful to nonpurposeful. Decorticate or decerebrate **posturing,** the abnormal positions assumed after injury or damage to the brain, may occur (Figure 20-2 ◆).

Clinical manifestations of increased intracranial pressure are provided in Table 20-2.

CLINICAL THERAPY

Clinical therapy focuses on early diagnosis, intervention, and prevention of complications. A thorough history is taken to identify a potential cause of altered consciousness. Assess whether the child had a recent head trauma, has an infection, has ingested toxins, or has a shunt, tumor, or other condition that could affect the level of consciousness.

Laboratory tests include a complete blood cell count, blood chemistry, clotting factors, and blood culture; toxicology assessments of both blood and urine; and urinalysis with culture. A lumbar puncture may be performed to assess the cerebrospinal fluid for protein, glucose, or blood cells. An electroencephalogram (EEG) identifies damaged or nonfunctioning areas of the brain.

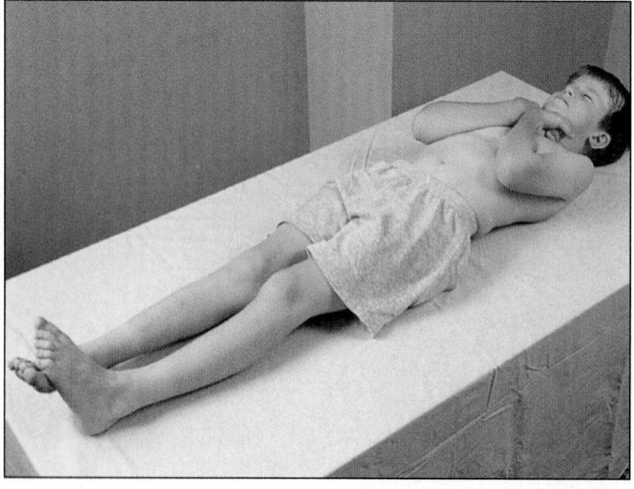

A

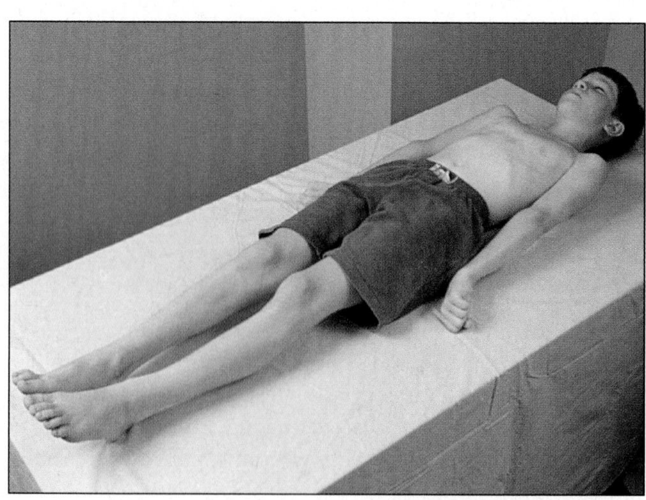

B

FIGURE 20-2 ◆

A, Decorticate posturing, characterized by rigid flexion, is associated with lesions above the brain stem in the corticospinal tracts. B, Decerebrate posturing, distinguished by rigid extension, is associated with lesions of the brain stem.

TABLE 20-3 Glasgow Coma Scale for Assessment of Coma in Infants and Children

CATEGORY	SCORE*	INFANT AND YOUNG CHILD CRITERIA	OLDER CHILD AND ADULT CRITERIA
Eye opening	4	Spontaneous opening	Spontaneous
	3	To loud noise	To verbal stimuli
	2	To pain	To pain
	1	No response	No response
Verbal response	5	Smiles, coos, cries to appropriate stimuli	Oriented to time, place, and person; uses appropriate words and phrases
	4	Irritable; cries	Confused
	3	Inappropriate crying	Inappropriate words or verbal response
	2	Grunts, moans	Incomprehensible words
	1	No response	No response
Motor response	6	Spontaneous movement	Obeys commands
	5	Withdraws to touch	Localizes pain
	4	Withdraws to pain	Withdraws to pain
	3	Abnormal flexion (decorticate)	Flexion to pain (decorticate)
	2	Abnormal extension (decerebrate)	Extention to pain (decerebrate)
	1	No response	No response

*Add the score from each category to get the total. The maximum score is 15, indicating the best level of neurologic functioning. The minimum is 3, indicating total neurologic unresponsiveness.
Note: From Teasdale, G., & Jennett, B. (1974). Assessment of coma and impaired consciousness. *Lancet, 2,* 81–84; and James, H. E. (1986). Neurologic evaluation and support in the child with acute brain insult. *Pediatric Annals,* 15(1), 17.

Computed tomography (CT) or magnetic resonance imaging (MRI) is used to detect any lesions, structural abnormalities, vascular malformations, or edema. Skull x-ray studies are used to detect fractures or bony malformations.

The Glasgow Coma Scale is used to quantify the level of consciousness, thus enabling future comparison of improvement or deterioration in the child's condition. Pediatric criteria, which take into account the child's developmental age for each category of the test, have been established to assess responses (Table 20-3).

The child is treated with oxygen, and assisted ventilation is provided when gas exchange is inadequate. Any metabolic, acid–base, or electrolyte imbalances are corrected. Antibiotics are initiated for suspected infection.

Efforts are made to maintain the **cerebral perfusion pressure** (the amount of pressure needed to ensure that adequate oxygen and nutrients will be delivered to the brain). In cases of hypovolemia, intravenous fluids are given. In cases of poor perfusion and fluid overload, dopamine or dobutamine is administered. If the intracranial pressure is markedly increased and results from the accumulation of cerebrospinal fluid because of obstruction, a ventricular tap can be performed to decrease the pressure, thus relieving a life-threatening condition that can lead to coma.

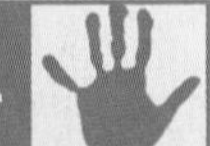

GROWTH & DEVELOPMENT

Glasgow Coma Scale Assessment

- Eye opening. Note if eye opening is spontaneous or occurs in response to stimuli.
- Verbal response. Crying in an infant is a positive response. The 2-year-old child who says no to each command is also responding in an age-appropriate way.
- Motor response. Motor score is probably the most critical aspect of this test, since the child cannot control reflexes. A fearful toddler may refuse to open the eyes or talk to strangers, but the child's reflexes should automatically respond to appropriate stimuli.

NURSING MANAGEMENT

Nursing Assessment and Diagnosis

Initially assess the child's physiologic status, focusing on the child's responsiveness to the environment or stimuli, ability to maintain the airway, vital signs, and breathing patterns. Use the Glasgow Coma Scale to assess the child at specified intervals.

Assess the child's cranial nerves (see Table 4-23). The child's responses may differ significantly when stress and anxiety are reduced. Encourage the parents to take part in the examination to reduce the child's anxiety. In the unconscious child, cranial nerve assessment and interpretation are more challenging (see Table 20-4).

Assess the child's respiratory effort and color. Monitor pulse oximetry or arterial blood gas measurements. Adequate air exchange to keep oxygen and carbon dioxide levels within normal ranges is critical to reduce the risk of increased intracranial pressure. If the child cannot maintain an adequate respiratory effort, mechanical ventilation will be necessary.

Skill 5-15: Glasgow Coma Scale

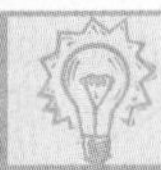

CLINICAL TIP

To make the toddler feel less threatened when assessing his or her motor skills, ask the child to reach for a finger puppet or doll rather than your hand. The toy serves as a reward.

TABLE 20-4 Assessment of Cranial Nerves in the Unconscious Child

CRANIAL NERVES	REFLEX	ASSESSMENT PROCEDURE AND NORMAL FINDINGS[a]
II, III	Pupillary	Shine a light source in eye. *Rapid, concentrically constricting pupils indicate intact cranial nerves II, III.*
II, IV, VI	Oculocephalic	Should be performed with eyes held open (doll's eyes) and head turned from side to side. *Eyes gazing straight up or lagging slightly behind head motion indicate intact cranial nerves. Precaution:* Cervical spine injury must be ruled out before this assessment is performed.
III, VIII	Oculovestibular	Place the head in a midline and slightly elevated position. Inject ice water into ear canal. *Eyes deviating toward the irrigated ear indicate intact cranial nerves III, VIII. Precautions:* Cervical spine injury must be ruled out before this assessment is performed. Tympanic membrane must be intact; otherwise brain may be filled with bacteria-laden fluid. *Note:* This assessment is usually performed by a physician.
V, VII	Corneal	Cornea is gently swabbed with sterile cotton swab. *A blink indicates intact cranial nerves V, VII.*
IX, X	Gag	Pharynx is irritated with tongue depressor or cotton swab. *Gagging response indicates intact* cranial nerves IX, X.

[a]Italic indicates normal findings.

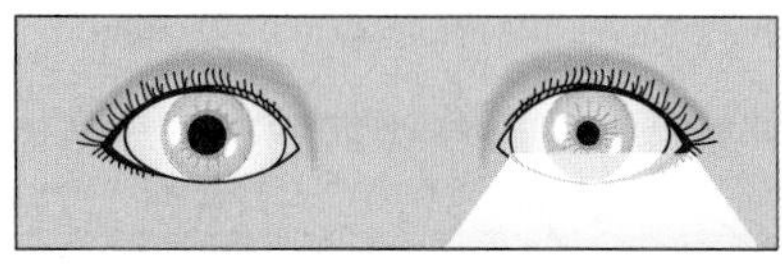

A

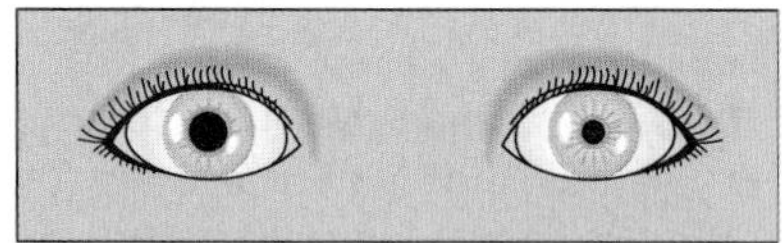

B

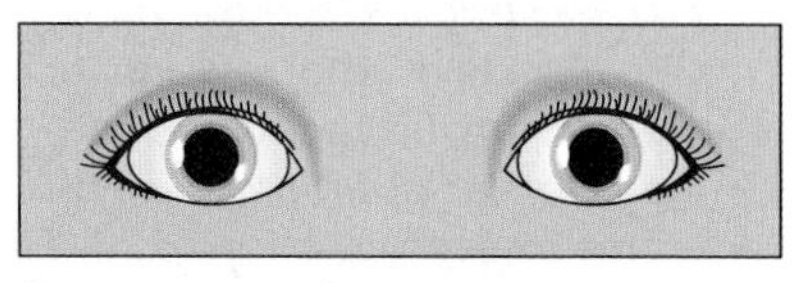

C

FIGURE 20-3 ◆
Pupil findings in various neurologic conditions with altered consciousness. A, A unilateral dilated and reactive pupil is associated with an intracranial mass. B, A fixed and dilated pupil may be a sign of impending brainstem herniation. C, Bilateral fixed and dilated pupils are associated with brainstem herniation from increased intracranial pressure.

Skill 10-17: Suctioning a Child with Decreased Level of Consciousness

Following are nursing diagnoses that may be appropriate for the child with an altered level of consciousness or increased intracranial pressure:

- *Ineffective breathing pattern,* related to neuromuscular dysfunction associated with increased intracranial pressure
- *Risk for aspiration,* related to decreased level of consciousness
- *Risk for impaired skin integrity,* related to decreased level of consciousness and impaired mobility
- *Impaired verbal communication,* related to physiologic condition of decreased level of consciousness
- *Altered family processes,* related to care of a child with an acquired disability

Planning and Implementation

Nursing care of the child with altered consciousness or increased intracranial pressure focuses on maintaining airway patency, monitoring neurologic status, performing routine care, providing sensory stimulation, and providing emotional support to parents.

Maintain Airway Patency

Make sure the child's airway is clear at all times. If the child is having difficulty swallowing secretions or does not have a gag reflex, intubation or a tracheostomy is performed. Frequent suctioning may be required. Keep suction apparatus with catheters, oxygen, resuscitation bag and mask, and extra tracheostomy tubes (if applicable) at bedside.

Pulse oximetry or arterial blood gas analysis is performed at regular intervals to ensure that gas exchange is adequate. Mechanical ventilation may be required.

Monitor Neurologic Status

Perform routine neurologic checks. Evaluate pupil size and reactivity, eye movements, and motor function (Figure 20-3 ◆). Monitor vital signs: Increased systolic blood pressure, a wide pulse pressure, and bradycardia indicate increased intracranial pressure. Observe for other signs of increased intracranial pressure listed in Table 20-2.

If seizures occur, the siderails should be padded to protect the child from injury.

Perform Routine Care

If the corneal reflex is absent, place artificial tears in the eyes and cover with gauze, taping over so they remain closed. Perform routine mouth care by brushing the teeth and using glycerine swabs.

TABLE 20-5 Care of the Immobile Child

- Help keep body in proper alignment with splints or rolls made of towels or blankets.
- Perform passive or gentle range-of-motion exercises 3–4 times per day according to physician's orders.
- Maintain skin integrity:
  - Change position every 2 hours.
  - Place child on foam or egg-crate mattress or sheepskin covering.
  - Massage child gently using lotion.

Provide adequate nutrition. Initially nutrients may be supplied intravenously. A nasogastric or gastrostomy tube may be inserted if the child remains unconscious or is not alert enough to take food by mouth.

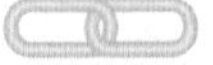

Skill 11-2: Inserting and Removing a Nasogastric Tube

Prevent complications associated with immobility (muscle atrophy, contractures, and skin breakdown) as described in Table 20-5. With Antwan, as discussed in the chapter opener, nurses support physical therapy efforts with extra passive range-of-motion exercises.

Provide Sensory Stimulation

Explain all procedures and actions. Because the child with a severely altered level of consciousness may still be able to hear, talking to him or her may be beneficial.

When the child becomes more alert, orient the child to time, place, and person, depending on age and level of understanding. Encourage parents to bring objects or toys from home to make the environment more familiar and promote a feeling of security.

CLINICAL TIP

Listening to music or tapes of family members talking or reading can soothe a child who has an altered level of consciousness.

Provide Emotional Support

Explain the child's condition in simple terms. Encourage parents to take part in the child's care and therapy as much as possible. If the child's normal functioning has been permanently impaired, refer the family to the appropriate psychologic and social services for emotional support. (See Chapter 8 for more information about helping families cope with a child's life-threatening illness.) Provide family members with opportunities to express their feelings.

Discharge Planning and Home Care Teaching

The child's transition from the hospital to home, a long-term care facility, or inpatient rehabilitation center must be planned well in advance of discharge. A case manager or social worker who can help plan the child's long-term care needs, including home health nursing, adaptation of the home, and the purchase of special equipment, should be identified.

Care in the Community

Home care nurses play a vital role in the care of such children as Antwan who have an acquired neurologic dysfunction and prolonged altered consciousness. Teach the family how to care for the child with severe neurologic dysfunction and to perform routine procedures such as maintaining the airway, skin care, feeding, positioning, exercises, and stimulation. Regular follow-up visits are needed to assess the child's progress and to modify the treatment plan.

The child also needs to be linked with community rehabilitation services through an early intervention program or school-based program. The home health nurse or case manager should assist the family to have an individualized education plan developed for the child (see Chapter 6).

Evaluation

Expected outcomes of nursing care include the following:

- The child's airway is maintained and the cerebral perfusion pressure is maintained to oxygenate the brain.
- The family provides appropriate care to the child with prolonged altered consciousness to promote minimal long-term disabilities.

CAUSES AND CLINICAL MANIFESTATIONS OF HEADACHES

TYPE OF HEADACHE AND CAUSE	CLINICAL MANIFESTATIONS	CLINICAL THERAPY
Migraine—vascular	■ Unilateral or bilateral pulsatile throbbing pain lasting for hours or days ■ Nausea and vomiting ■ Photophobia ■ Visual or motor aura several minutes before headache starts ■ Recurrent abdominal pain ■ Increased pain with activity ■ Relief with sleep	■ Food elimination trial ■ Medications to abort migraine (ergot, isometheptene, supatriptan) ■ Analgesic medication ■ Relaxation techniques and biofeedback
Tension—muscular contraction	■ Dull, achy pain in band around head, in neck and shoulders that may last for days ■ Intermittent or constant pain with fluctuations in degree of pain ■ Nausea, no vomiting ■ Sensitive to light or sound ■ Pain not aggravated by physical activity	■ Relaxation techniques ■ Analgesic and anti-inflammatory medications ■ Ice pack ■ Rest
Inflammatory—sinusitis or dental abscess	■ Frontal pain or tenderness over affected sinus ■ Fever	■ Analgesic, antipyretic, and anti-inflammatory medications ■ Antibiotic medications ■ Cold or heat application
Structural—space-occupying lesion, hemorrhage, increased intracranial pressure	■ Pain that awakens child in morning ■ Pain worse in morning, with coughing, sneezing, or straining ■ Morning vomiting, no nausea ■ Worsening pain with increasing frequency, abnormal neurologic signs within 2–6 months of headache onset (e.g., double vision, papilledema)	■ Surgery ■ Analgesic medications

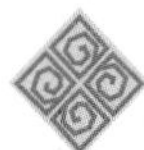

HEADACHES

Children commonly experience headaches. They may be the cause of school absence, decreased extracurricular activity, and poor academic achievement. Up to 82% of children experience a headache by late adolescence (O'Hara & Koch, 1998).

Headaches have both benign (migraine, inflammatory, and tension) and structural causes. Causes and clinical manifestations for various headaches can be found in the box above. Migraine headaches are the most common benign headaches in children, estimated to occur in 5% of patients. Most children are affected by 9 years of age. Migraines may be triggered by stress; foods containing nitrates, glutamate, caffeine, tyramine, and salt; menses; oral contraceptives; fatigue; and hunger. Another family member often has similar headaches, so genetic predisposition may also be a factor.

Clinical therapy involves obtaining a detailed history of the headache characteristics, onset, warning signs, duration, severity, and associated symptoms. The child is assessed for neurologic signs such as altered consciousness, abnormal cranial nerves, papilledema, and motor or sensory deficits. Radiologic studies (CT scan or MRI) are used only if a structural problem is suspected. Treatment includes relaxation techniques, analgesics, and anti-inflammatory medications. Food elimination diet trials are often initiated to identify foods that trigger headaches. Medications to abort migraines (ergot or isometheptene) are used in children old enough to identify an aura, or warning. Sumatriptan in oral or nasal spray form may be used to abort migraines in adolescents. Beta-blockers may be used prophylactically if headaches significantly interfere with usual activities.

Nursing management involves assessing the child for potential neurologic signs associated with headaches and assisting the child and family to identify strategies for relieving the

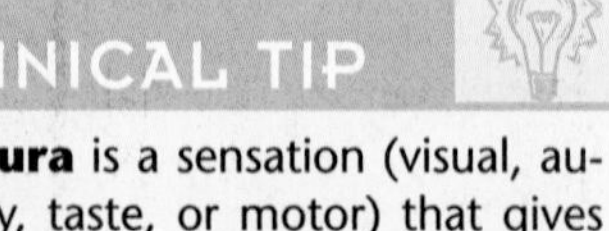

An **aura** is a sensation (visual, auditory, taste, or motor) that gives warning of an impending migraine headache or epileptic seizure. With migraine headaches, children may complain of seeing spots or a shimmery film that gets larger and affects their vision. In the case of the migraine, the child has time to take medications in an effort to abort the headache. In epilepsy, the child may have time to avoid injury by getting to the floor.

headaches. Assist the family and child to implement the food elimination trial and to gradually add foods to identify offending chemical triggers. Make sure the child learns to take the prescribed medications appropriately. Teach the child relaxation techniques (breathing control training, mental imagery, progressive relaxation, and biofeedback) to manage stress and the pain associated with the headaches.

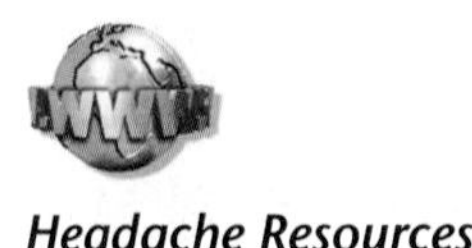

Headache Resources

SEIZURE DISORDERS

Seizures are periods of abnormal electrical discharges in the brain that cause involuntary movement, and behavior and sensory alterations. They are a common neurologic disorder in children. Approximately 2% to 4% of children have seizures during childhood, most often during infancy. Infants are susceptible to developing seizures in the first year of life with an incidence of 1 per 1,000. The incidence decreases with age. Approximately 20% of all epilepsy cases develop by 5 years of age (Farley & McEwan, 2000). Epilepsy is a chronic disorder characterized by recurrent, unprovoked seizures secondary to a CNS disorder. One in 100 people have epilepsy (Valente, 2000).

ETIOLOGY AND PATHOPHYSIOLOGY

Seizures are believed to be the result of abnormal electrical discharges of brain neurons. These cells can be triggered by either environmental or physiologic stimuli such as emotional stress, anxiety, fatigue, infection, or metabolic disturbances. The most common causes in children are CNS infection and head trauma.

Some seizures are idiopathic, or not provoked by known stimuli. Genetic factors may lower the seizure threshold by making brain cells more vulnerable to abnormal electrical discharges. Acquired seizures may be caused by underlying pathologic conditions such as trauma, infection, hypoglycemia, endocrine dysfunction, toxins, tumors, or lesions that may be manifested at any time. See page 742 for causes of various types of seizures.

Partial or **focal** seizures are caused by abnormal electrical activity in one hemisphere or a specific area of the cerebral cortex, most often the temporal, frontal, or parietal lobes. The symptoms that are displayed depend on the region of the cortex affected.

In contrast, generalized seizures are the result of diffuse electrical activity that begins in both hemispheres of the brain simultaneously and spreads throughout the cortex into the brainstem. As a result, movements and spasms displayed by the child are bilateral and symmetric.

The length of a seizure, especially that of a generalized seizure, is important, because the airway may be compromised during the tonic phase. The basal metabolic rate rises during the peak of seizure activity. This change, in turn, increases the demand for oxygen and glucose. During a seizure the child may become pale or cyanotic as a result of hypoxia or hypoglycemia.

Febrile seizures occur in connection with a sudden rise in temperature in association with an acute illness. No evidence of intracranial infection or other defined cause is found. They are usually seen between 3 months and 5 years with a peak incidence between 18 to 24 months of age. There is often a family history of febrile seizures. In addition, children who have one febrile seizure have a 30% to 50% greater chance of having future seizures (Sagraves, 1999). The lower convulsive threshold of infants may explain this type of seizure.

CLINICAL MANIFESTATIONS

The symptoms of a seizure depend on its type and duration. Seizures are classified into two types: partial (focal) seizures and generalized seizures of nonfocal origin. The specific characteristics of the various types of partial and generalized seizures are presented on page 742. The initial manifestations of the **tonic** phase of a generalized seizure are unconsciousness and continuous muscular contraction. The tonic phase is followed by the **clonic** phase, characterized by alternating muscular contraction and relaxation. The **postictal period** following seizure activity is a phase during which the level of consciousness is decreased. The length of the postictal period varies among children.

An olfactory or visual aura providing an early warning sign of a seizure occurs only in partial seizures (Vendanarayanan, 1999).

SAFETY PRECAUTIONS

During the postictal period, monitor the child's vital signs, perform neurologic checks, and keep the environment safe.

CLINICAL MANIFESTATIONS OF SEIZURES

TYPE OF SEIZURE AND CAUSE	CLINICAL MANIFESTATIONS
Partial Seizures ***Complex partial seizures (psychomotor seizures)*** Lesions, cysts, or tumors Perinatal trauma Focal sclerosis, i.e., scarring of the mediotemporal lobe from prolonged febrile seizures Vascular anomalies, i.e., arteriovenous malformations Head trauma	*Onset:* 3 years of age to adolescence Consciousness is impaired immediately or gradually after a simple partial onset. Lasts 5–10 seconds up to 1–2 minutes. Postseizure confusion Aura frequently present, unusual taste or odor Feelings of anxiety, fear, or déjà vu (sensation that event occurred before) Abdominal pain Staring into space, mental confusion Posturing **Automatisms**—lip smacking, lip chewing, sucking
Simple partial seizures (focal seizures) Focal damage (e.g., with cerebral palsy) Tumors or lesions Arteriovenous malformation Brain abscesses	*Onset:* any age No loss of consciousness. Lasts 5–10 seconds. No postseizure confusion No aura Motor responses may involve one extremity, part of extremity, or ipsilateral extremities with eyes and head turning in opposite direction Sensory responses involve paresthesias (decreased sensation or tingling); auditory, olfactory, or visual sensations; autonomic (sweating, papillary dilation) or psychic symptoms Motor and sensory involvement may be combined Jacksonian march (rare in children): tonic contractions of either fingers of one hand, toes of one foot, or one side of face become clonic or shows tonic–clonic movements; activity then "marches" up to adjacent muscles of either affected extremity or same side of body (such as face)
Generalized Seizures ***Tonic–clonic seizures (grand mal seizures)*** Cerebral damage from perinatal trauma, head trauma, tumors, structural lesions Metabolic and neuromuscular degenerative disorders Genetic link Many are idiopathic	*Onset:* any age, rare before 6 months of age, strong familial incidence Abrupt onset seizure, 1–2 minute loss of consciousness, postseizure confusion (few minutes to hours) May or may not have aura Falls to ground when all muscles contract Eyes roll upward or deviate to one side with pupils dilated Abdominal or chest wall rigidity with legs, head, and neck extended, and arms flexed or contracted Cry or grunt as air is forced out when diaphragm and chest muscles contract Urinary or bowel incontinence as muscles become flaccid during clonic phase Characterized by sleepiness, difficulty in arousal; hypertension; diaphoresis; headache, nausea, vomiting; poor coordination, decreased muscle tone; confusion, amnesia; slurred speech; visual disturbances; combativeness
Absence seizures (petit mal, or lapse seizures) Hyperventilation Genetic predisposition	*Onset:* age 4–5 years with remission in adolescence More prevalent in females May go on to develop other generalized seizures Brief loss of consciousness, usually lasts 5–10 seconds, rarely exceeds 30 seconds; no postseizure confusion, lethargy, or sleepiness Frequent attacks (50–100 per day), may cluster No aura Abrupt cessation of current activity Staring, episodes may be confused with daydreaming or inattentiveness Rolling of eyes, eye blinking, ptosis or fluttering of eyelids Slight increase or loss of muscle tone (head may droop, handheld objects may be dropped) Amnesia
Myoclonic seizures Progressive or degenerative encephalopathy	*Onset:* as early as 2 years, but more prevalent in school-age child or adolescent No loss of consciousness, child recovers in seconds, no postictal period Attacks occur most often upon falling asleep or awakening Quick involuntary muscle jerks, may appear to drop or throw object; head, extremity, or body contractions, may be limited to one body part or whole body

(continued)

CLINICAL MANIFESTATIONS OF SEIZURES (continued)

TYPE OF SEIZURE AND CAUSE	CLINICAL MANIFESTATIONS
Infantile spasms (myoclonic epilepsy of infancy, salaam seizures) Prenatal and perinatal encephalopathy Metabolic disorder Tuberous sclerosis Microcephaly	*Onset:* begin at age 3 months and resolve by 2 years Positive history of gestational difficulties, developmental delays, or other neurologic abnormalities Possible loss of consciousness Several seizures can occur throughout the day Episodes usually occur when infant is falling asleep or awakening Dropping of head, flexion of neck, extension of arms, and flexion of legs; sudden flexion or extension of trunk (or both) Eye rolling, either upward or downward Crying, pallor, or cyanosis Regression in development and irritability
Akinetic or atonic seizures (drop attacks) Gray matter degenerative diseases and subacute seizures Sclerosing panencephalitis Many are idiopathic	*Onset:* first seen at 2 years, disappear by 6 years. Momentary loss of consciousness Falls to ground with sudden loss of postural tone, inability to break fall

Febrile seizures—generalized seizures that usually occur in children as the result of rapid temperature rise above 39°C (102°F)—involve generalized tonic–clonic movements that last less than 15 minutes.

CLINICAL THERAPY

After the child's first seizure, it is essential that a thorough history be taken from the parent, primary caretaker, or witnesses to the event. Table 20-6 lists appropriate questions to ask. Details such as the description and length of the seizure, presence or absence of an aura, and if the child lost consciousness should be noted. This information is used to identify the type of seizure according to the International Classification of Epileptic Seizures.

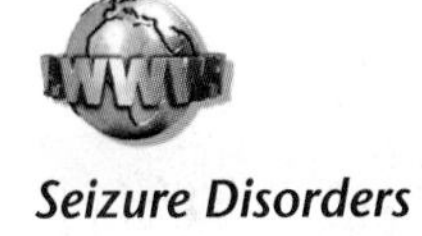
Seizure Disorders

A complete physical and neurologic examination is performed. Based on the physical findings and history, diagnostic tests are ordered. Laboratory tests include a complete blood cell count, blood chemistry, urine culture, and lumbar puncture. See Appendix C. If the child is taking any anticonvulsants, blood levels of the medication should be monitored. An EEG may be performed. A lead level, toxicology screening, and radiologic tests such as CT scanning or MRI and angiography may be performed to identify a cerebral lesion.

Many convulsions are self-limiting and require no emergency intervention. Children with febrile seizures may be treated with an anticonvulsant for the remainder of the presenting febrile illness. However, long-term anticonvulsants are not generally used. Instead,

TABLE 20-6 Questions to Ask about Seizures

- Did the child complain of not feeling well or feeling "funny" just before the seizure?
- Did the child complain of headache, nausea, muscle pain? Did the child vomit?
- Did the child suffer any trauma before the seizure?
- Did the child get into any medications or poisons before the seizure?
- Was the child sick or feverish before the seizure?
- What movements of the arms and legs were seen? Were the movements on one side of the body or in one extremity only?
- Was the child's vision normal?
- Were the pupils dilated or the eyes deviated to one side?
- Was the child aware of surroundings? Could the child respond to questions?
- Was the child incontinent of urine or stool?
- How long did the episode last? When did the child begin to wake up?
- Was the child lethargic, weak, or uncoordinated upon arousal?
- Was the child injured during the convulsion?
- Did the child's color change (pale, red, blue)?

CLINICAL TIP

Children under the age of 8 years with specific types of seizures may be put on a ketogenic diet, which consists of a ratio of 3–5 g of fat to 1 g of protein plus carbohydrates. This high-fat diet causes a mild state of starvation, resulting in ketosis as the body uses fat for metabolism. A mild state of dehydration is maintained so the level of ketones in the circulation is not diluted. Ketosis is believed to slow the electrical impulses that cause seizures. Medium-chain triglycerides may be given as a supplement to increase the acidosis.

TABLE 20-7 Management of Status Epilepticus

- Maintain a patent airway. Muscle rigidity may compromise the airway.
- Perform a jaw thrust maneuver if the airway is obstructed.
- Keep suction equipment at bedside in case secretions are excessive.
- Give oxygen by mask, as increased metabolic demands deplete oxygen stores.
- Monitor vital signs and circulation with pulse oximeter and cardiorespiratory monitor.
- Assess neurologic level.
- Establish an intravenous line to administer any necessary fluids or medications.
- Administer glucose if the child is hypoglycemic; the physical stress of the seizure may result in declining glucose levels.
- Insert a nasogastric tube.
- Protect the child from injury.
- Manage thermoregulation.
- Administer benzodiazepines such as diazepam, lorazepam, or midazolam. If there is no response, the dose may be repeated. Phenytoin or phenobarbital may be necessary if seizure activity continues. Cumulative doses of drugs may produce apnea, so be prepared to assist ventilations.

parents are taught to lower fevers by using antipyretics and keeping the child cool with light clothing, and to prepare for future seizures.

Any generalized seizure lasting longer than 10 minutes needs to be monitored for electrolytes, glucose, blood gases, increasing fever, and abnormal blood pressure. Anticonvulsants are given intravenously or rectally. Monitor for continued motor activity and the potential for status epilepticus (a continuous seizure that lasts for more than 30 minutes or a series of seizures during which consciousness is not regained). Motor activity may become less apparent after anticonvulsants are given, even though the child is still unconscious (Altmeier, 1999). The postictal period ranges from 30 minutes to 2 hours. Management of the child in status epilepticus is described in Table 20-7.

Most seizure disorders are treated with anticonvulsants. A single medication (monotherapy) is preferred for seizure control to minimize side effects. Monotherapy works for 80% of children with new onset epilepsy (Valente, 2000). See the medication table for first- and second-line medications. Serum drug levels are monitored to achieve therapeutic levels or when toxicity is possible. Therapeutic ranges of medications may be exceeded when tolerated by the child to achieve seizure control. Medication dosage adjustments are often needed as the child grows. Approximately 25% to 30% of children have refractory or **intractable seizures,** which continue to occur even with optimal medical management (Danielpour & Peacock, 2000). These children are often treated with multiple anticonvulsants. Surgery may occasionally be performed to remove a tumor, lesion, or portion of the brain that has been identified as causing the seizures.

A ketogenic diet is occasionally used for children with myoclonic and absence seizures. This diet involves a high intake of fat and low intake of carbohydrates and protein (Figure 20-4 ◆). Family motivation must be high to maintain the diet for 2 to 3 years and to frequently monitor the child's urine ketone values (Katyal, Koehler, & McGhee, et al., 2000).

A trial of medication withdrawal is attempted for some types of seizures (such as absence) during adolescence as some children have spontaneous remissions.

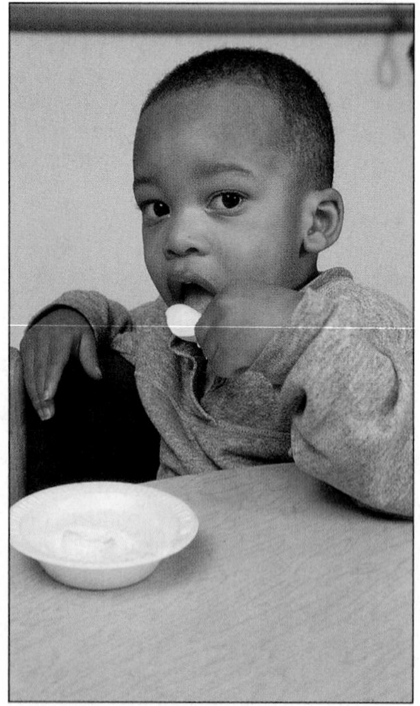

FIGURE 20-4 ◆
The family must make an effort to make the high-fat diet appealing to the child on a ketogenic diet, despite their personal feelings about eating large amounts of food such as mayonnaise, as this child is doing.

ANTICONVULSANTS USED TO TREAT SEIZURE DISORDERS

Emergency Medications	First-Line Medications	Second-Line Medications
Diazepam	Carbamazepine	Clonazepam
	Ethosuximide	Felbamate
	Phenobarbitol	Gabapentin
	Phenytoin	Lamotrigine
	Primidone	Tiagabine
	Valproic Acid	Topiramate

NURSING MANAGEMENT

Nursing Assessment and Diagnosis

Assess and monitor the child's physiologic status. Once the child is stable, a more definitive assessment can be made. Level of consciousness is a vital indicator of neurologic function. Remember that the child's lack of response may be the result of the postictal state.

Collect and analyze historical information about the seizure activity, clustering, aura, description of motor activity or changes in muscle tone, automatisms, and any changes in development or school performance to help determine the type of seizures the child experiences.

Common nursing diagnoses for the child with a seizure disorder include the following:

- *Ineffective breathing pattern,* related to neuromuscular dysfunction during the tonic phase of a seizure
- *Ineffective airway clearance,* related to inability to control secretions during seizure
- *Risk for trauma,* related to seizure activity
- *Chronic low self-esteem,* related to refractory seizures and loss of bowel and bladder control during seizure activity
- *Risk for anxiety,* related to unpredictable nature of seizure disorder
- *Ineffective management of therapeutic regimen (individual),* related to poor compliance with pharmacologic management of seizures
- *Altered family processes,* related to care of a child with a chronic disorder

Planning and Implementation

Nursing care focuses on maintaining airway patency, ensuring safety, administering medications, and providing emotional support. Both acute care and long-term management are involved.

MAINTAIN AIRWAY PATENCY

Be sure that nothing is placed in the child's mouth during a seizure. Monitor the child to ensure adequate oxygenation: The child's color should be pink, the heart rate at a normal or slightly elevated rate for age, and the pulse oximetry reading greater than 95%. Oxygen is usually given at levels below 95%.

ENSURE SAFETY

Protect the child from self-harm during violent seizures (Figure 20-5◆). If the child is in bed, the side rails should be padded to prevent injury.

ADMINISTER MEDICATIONS

Take special precautions when administering intravenous medications for the acute management of seizures. These medications should be given very slowly to minimize the risk of respiratory or circulatory collapse.

Medications for the management of chronic seizures are given orally. Crushing pills and mixing them in a teaspoonful of applesauce, pudding, or other soft food make them more palatable and easier for the child to swallow. For some medications flavored chewables are available.

When a child is NPO due to illness or on the day of surgery, seizure medications are usually given with a swallow of water. Check with the prescriber for clear orders in such cases.

PROVIDE EMOTIONAL SUPPORT

The loss of control of body movements and possible loss of consciousness make seizures frightening and difficult to accept for the child, parents, and other family members.

Parents often feel guilty about the child's seizure disorder and compensate by not disciplining or restricting the child appropriately. Stress the need to treat the child as normally as possible. Refer the child and family to support groups and counseling services if indicated.

CULTURE

Seizures may have a special meaning by different cultural groups. For example, the Hmong believe the child is experiencing *quag dab peg,* or "the spirit catches you and you fall down." Hmong view the condition as serious, but take pride in the child who has the condition. In 1997, Anne Fadiman wrote a compelling story about the cultural conflict between a Hmong family and health care providers over the treatment of their daughter's seizures, called *The Spirit Catches You and You Fall Down* (Fadiman, 1997, Spector, 2000).

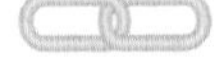

Skill 10-2: Pulse Oximetry

SAFETY PRECAUTIONS

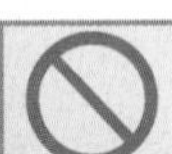

Do not put any object in the mouth or between the teeth of a child during a seizure. Loose teeth may be knocked out and aspirated.

SAFETY PRECAUTIONS

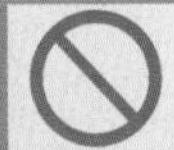

Children who have frequent, recurrent seizures should wear helmets to protect their heads in case they fall. All children with seizure disorders should wear some form of medical identification (e.g., a medical alert bracelet).

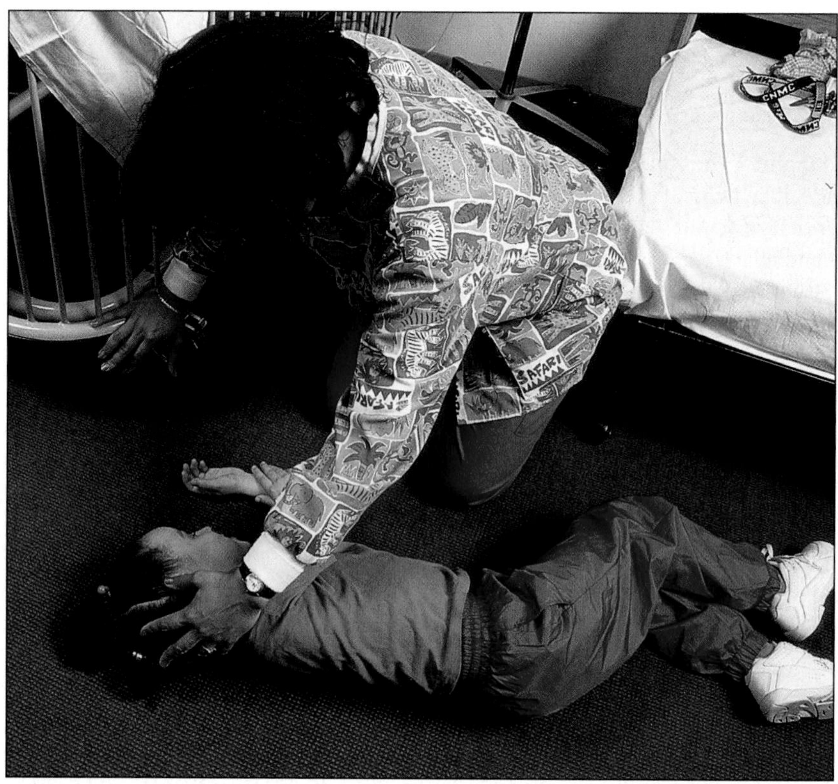

FIGURE 20-5 ◆
A child who has a seizure when standing should be gently assisted to the floor and placed in a side-lying position. Clear the area of any objects that might cause harm to the child.

Discharge Planning and Home Care Teaching

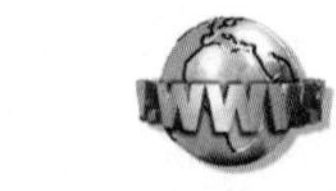

Epilepsy Support

Encourage parents to express their fears and anxieties. Answer their questions honestly, and refer them to organizations, such as the Epilepsy Foundation of America, where they can obtain more information about the child's disorder. Be sure parents know how to administer medications and provide for the child's safety. Discuss with them whom to call with questions and when to return for follow-up.

Care in the Community

Educate the child and parents about medication regimens. Explain the purpose of each drug, its schedule for administration, and the importance of giving all doses. Teaching the older child to take medications without parental intervention provides a sense of self-control. Provide information about the side effects of medications ordered, and alert parents to the signs of toxic reactions or undermedication. Regular dental care is important because of the effect of certain anticonvulsants on the gingiva. Explain the importance of follow-up visits to health care providers so the effectiveness of the child's medications can be monitored.

FAMILIES WANT TO KNOW

Safety for the Child with a Seizure Disorder

Children with epilepsy have more injuries of all sorts, including burns, falls, and drowning. Children are at increased risk for death due to drowning. Planning for safety includes the following:

- Do not leave the child alone in the bathtub.
- Children who bathe alone should use the shower.
- A buddy and lifeguard should always be present when the child swims.
- A life vest should always be worn when boating.
- The child should not play or stand around open flames or outdoor grills.
- The child should avoid areas where fall risks are increased.

Families of children with severe seizure disorders need to develop an emergency care plan so that emergency personnel are informed about their needs for care in advance (see Chapter 6).

Assist the family to develop an individual school health plan so the child can receive medications during school hours, if necessary. Teachers and school administrators should know what actions to take if the child has a seizure and what information to report about the seizure. Encourage participation in sports when good supervision is provided.

The child may be afraid of having a seizure in front of friends. Reassure the child and family that taking medications regularly should control seizures. Children should explain to peers what a seizure is and what to do if they are present when one occurs. Summer camps for children with seizures can be a safe and comfortable place for the child to enjoy outdoor activities. Tell parents to boost the child's self-image by emphasizing what the child can do, rather than focusing on contraindicated activities. Depending on state laws, most adolescents can drive after they have been seizure-free for at least 2 years.

Parents of children with recurrent febrile seizures should be taught how to give antipyretics in the proper dose. Antipyretic doses will need to be updated as the child grows. Parents must know that antipyretics and anticonvulsants may not prevent a future febrile seizure associated with an acute illness. The potential toxicity of an anticonvulsant in a child with febrile seizures often outweighs the risk of the seizures, and parents can be reassured that complications from febrile seizures are rare.

Evaluation

Expected outcomes of nursing management include the following:

- The child experiences no injuries when seizures occur because safety measures are used.
- The child's self-esteem is enhanced through participation in well-supervised sports and activities.

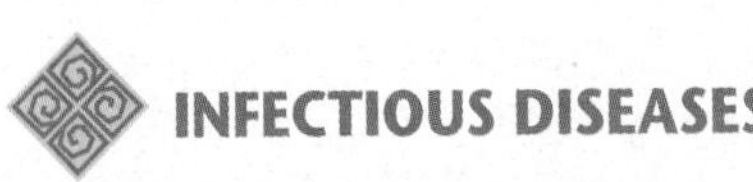

INFECTIOUS DISEASES

BACTERIAL MENINGITIS

Meningitis, an inflammation of the meninges, can be caused by either bacterial or viral agents. Bacterial meningitis is more virulent than viral meningitis and is sometimes fatal. The child who is less than 1 year of age is at greatest risk for acquiring bacterial meningitis. Of all cases, 70% appear before 5 years of age (Farley, et al., 1998).

Etiology and Pathophysiology

Meningitis may occur secondary to other infections such as otitis media, sinusitis, pharyngitis, cellulitis, pneumonia, or septic arthritis; head trauma; or a neurosurgical procedure. The majority of cases are caused by three organisms: *Haemophilus influenzae* type b, *Neisseria meningitidis,* and *Streptococcal pneumoniae* (Farley et al., 1998).

In many cases, bacteremia spreads the infectious agent to the CNS (Figure 20-6 ◆). An inflammatory response follows. White blood cells accumulate, covering the surface of the brain with a thick, white, purulent exudate. The brain then becomes hyperemic and edematous. If the infection spreads to the ventricles, they can become obstructed and impede the flow of cerebrospinal fluid, causing hydrocephalus.

CLINICAL TIP

The number of cases of bacterial meningitis caused by *Streptococcal pneumoniae* is expected to decline as more infants and children are immunized with the new heptovalent pneumococcal conjugate vaccine. Adolescents entering college should be encouraged to get the meningococcal vaccine to prevent meningococcal meningitis (see Chapter 12).

Clinical Manifestations

Symptoms are variable and depend on the child's age, the pathogen, and the length of the illness before diagnosis. Onset may be sudden or may develop over approximately a 1-week period. Symptoms in the young infant may include fever, change in feeding pattern, vomiting, or diarrhea. The anterior fontanel may be bulging or flat. The infant may be alert, restless, lethargic, or irritable. Rocking or cuddling, which normally calms a fussy infant, only irritates the infant with meningitis.

PATHOPHYSIOLOGY ILLUSTRATED

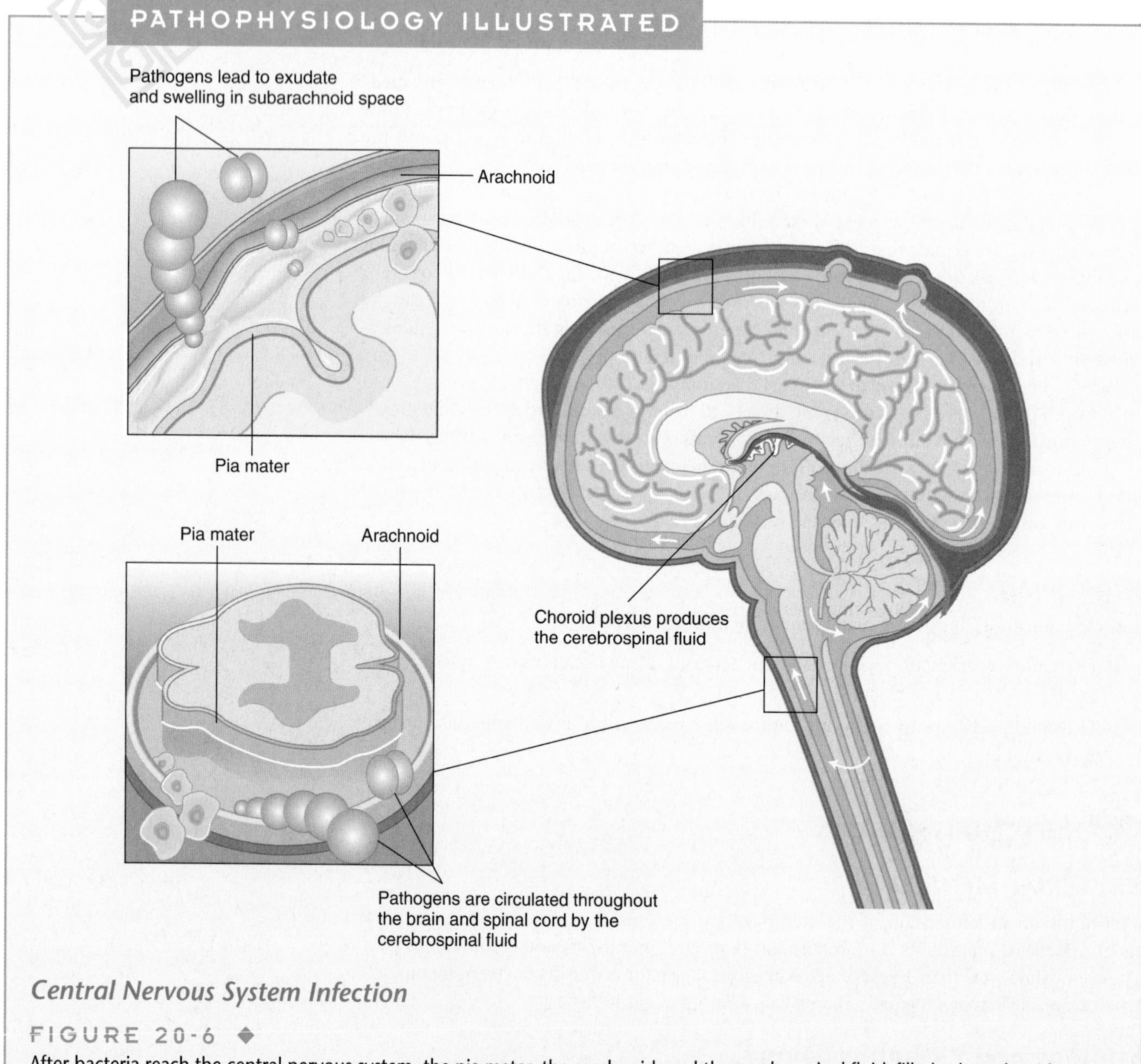

Central Nervous System Infection

FIGURE 20-6 ◆
After bacteria reach the central nervous system, the pia mater, the arachnoid, and the cerebrospinal fluid–filled subarachnoid space become infected. The cerebrospinal fluid then circulates the pathogens throughout the brain and spinal cord.

Older children are usually febrile; can be irritable, lethargic, or confused; have vomiting; and complain of muscle or joint pain. A hemorrhagic rash, first appearing as petechiae and changing to purpura or large necrotic patches, may be seen in meningococcal meningitis. The child displays other symptoms consistent with meningeal irritation: headache (most often frontal), photophobia, esotropia, and nuchal (resistance to neck flexion) rigidity. The child is comfortable only in an opisthotonic position (hyperextension of the head and neck to relieve discomfort; see Figure 20-7 ◆). The child may have a positive Kernig or Brudzinski sign, or both, on examination (Figures 20-8 ◆ and 20-9 ◆).

Symptoms can progress to include seizures, apnea, cerebral edema, subdural effusion, hydrocephalus, disseminated intravascular coagulation (DIC), shock, and increased intracranial pressure. The bacteria may also colonize within a joint, causing septic arthritis.

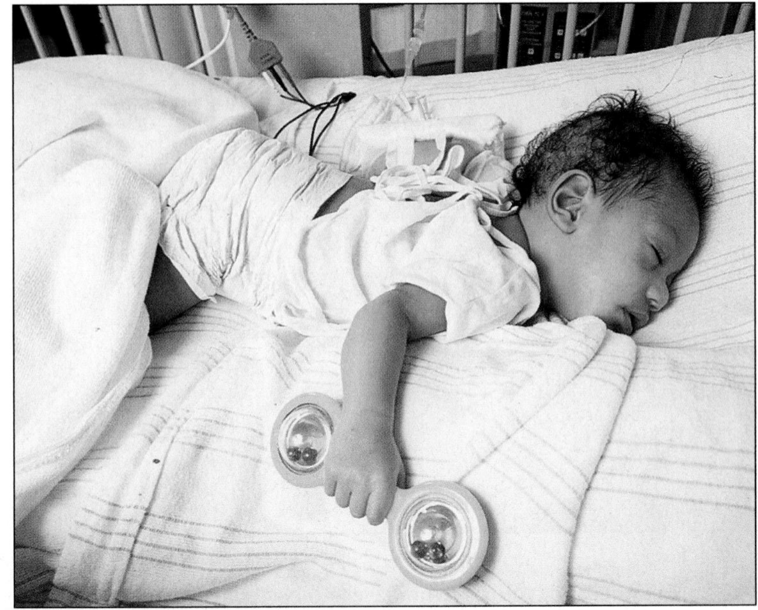

FIGURE 20-7 ◆
The child with bacterial meningitis assumes an opisthotonic position, with the neck and head hyperextended, to relieve discomfort.

Clinical Therapy

Diagnosis is based on the history, clinical presentation, and laboratory findings. A thorough history should be taken and a physical examination performed.

Laboratory tests include a complete blood count, blood cultures, serum electrolytes and osmolality, and clotting factors. A lumbar puncture is performed to evaluate the cerebrospinal fluid for number of white blood cells and protein and glucose levels. A Gram stain and culture are done on the cerebrospinal fluid.

Antibiotics are administered as soon as diagnostic tests are obtained. Those commonly used to treat bacterial meningitis include ampicillin, aminoglycosides, cefotaxime, ceftriaxone, and penicillin G. Antibiotics are often changed once culture and sensitivity results are known, especially as many organisms have resistance to certain antibiotics. These medications are administered intravenously for 7 to 21 days, depending on the organism and the child's clinical response. Depending on the causative organism, the disease may need to be reported to the local health department, and contacts may need to take prophylactic antibiotics, such as rifampin or ciprofloxacin. Corticosteroids (dexamethasone) are given as an adjunct to children over 6 weeks of age to reduce the risk of severe neurologic sequelae such as sensorineural hearing loss (Leake & Perkins, 2000). In some cases, anticonvulsants and antipyretics are given.

NURSING ALERT

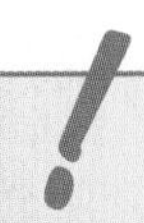

Remember that gastrointestinal bleeding is a potential complication of corticosteroid use. Monitor the child receiving these drugs for signs of intestinal discomfort and for blood in the stools.

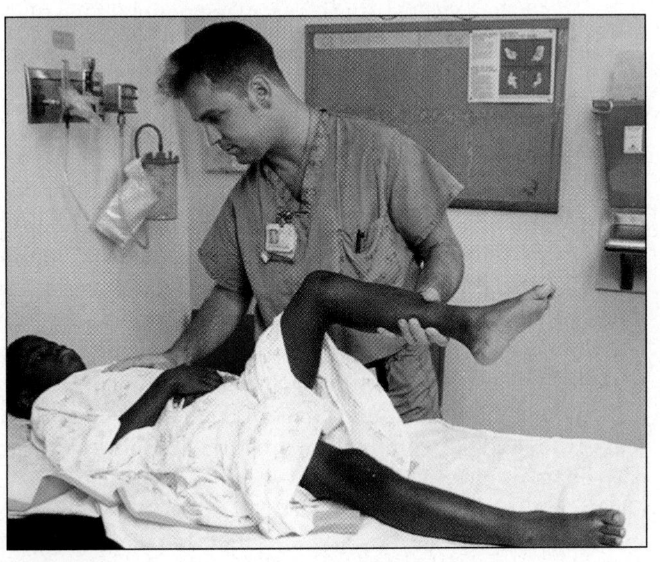

FIGURE 20-8 ◆
To test for Kernig sign, raise the child's leg with the knee flexed. Then extend the child's leg at the knee. If any resistance is noted or pain is felt, the result is a positive Kernig sign. This is a common finding in meningitis.

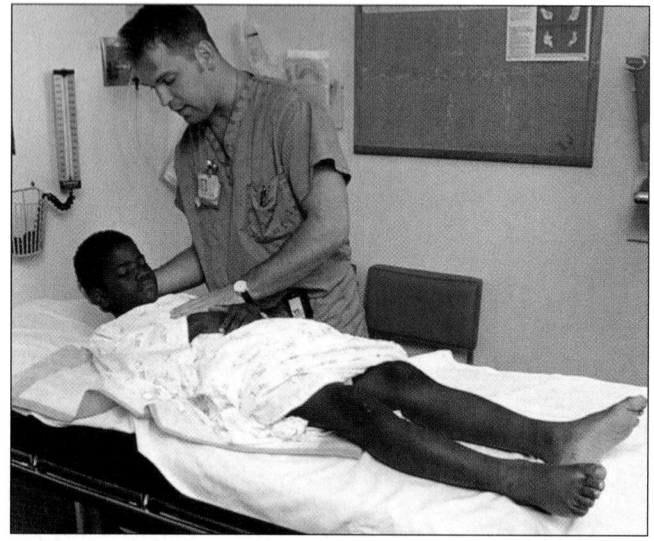

FIGURE 20-9 ◆
To test Brudzinski sign, flex the child's head while in a supine position. If this action makes the knees or hips flex involuntarily, a positive Brudzinski sign is present. This is a common sign in meningitis.

TABLE 20-8

Complications of Bacterial Meningitis

- Syndrome of inappropriate antidiuretic hormone secretion (SIADH)
- Disseminated intravascular coagulation (DIC)
- Subdural effusion
- Septicemia
- Septic arthritis
- Seizures
- Sensorineural hearing loss
- Hydrocephalus
- Behavior problems
- Learning problems

Some infants and children who have had bacterial meningitis suffer neurologic damage despite early, aggressive management. The most common sequelae involve cranial nerves, especially the eighth, resulting in hearing loss. In addition, seizures, developmental delay, and other complications may occur (Table 20-8). Another potential complication is meningococcal septicemia, which is characterized by high fever, hypotension, disseminated intravascular coagulation, and multisystem organ failure (Harrison, 2001). See the discussion about meningococcemia in Chapter 15.

NURSING MANAGEMENT

Nursing Assessment and Diagnosis

Assess the child's physiologic status, including vital signs and level of consciousness. Measure head circumference frequently in infants because of the potential for hydrocephalus to develop. Be alert for signs of a change in the child's condition and response to treatment. Monitor the child's ability to control secretions and to drink sufficient fluids. Monitor intake and output. Assess for any sensory deficits. Identify parents' concerns related to this potentially life-threatening condition.

Several nursing diagnoses that may apply to the child with bacterial meningitis are given in the accompanying nursing care plan. Additional nursing diagnoses might include the following:

- *Risk for aspiration,* related to altered level of consciousness and poor secretion control
- *Risk for fluid volume deficit,* related to poor oral fluid intake
- *Anticipatory grieving (parent),* related to the child's potentially life-threatening condition
- *Caregiver role strain,* related to a hospitalized child and other family responsibilities

NURSING ALERT

Maintenance and replacement fluids are usually given to children with bacterial meningitis. However, it is important to monitor the serum sodium concentration and urine specific gravity, because these children are at risk for developing the syndrome of insufficient antidiuretic hormone (SIADH; see Chapter 18). Fluids are restricted. Sodium chloride, potassium, and acetate or lactate is administered intravenously to balance sodium excretion.

Planning and Implementation

The nursing care plan summarizes care for the child with bacterial meningitis. Nursing care begins with emergency treatment and continues as the child's condition stabilizes. Monitor respiratory and neurologic status, maintain hydration, administer medications, and prevent complications. Promote the child's comfort with reduced stimulation (dim lights, quiet room) and by placing the child in a side-lying position. Monitor the child's response to antibiotic therapy. Isolate the child and use standard and droplet precautions until the causative organism is identified and effective treatment is underway.

Infection Control Methods

Respond to parents' concerns about their child's condition, explaining all measures to reduce the child's discomfort and provide adequate treatment. Identify ways parents can participate in meeting the child's comfort needs. Parents may also need assistance in identifying the best strategies for meeting the needs of other children at home while spending time with the hospitalized child.

NURSING CARE PLAN The Child with Bacterial Meningitis

GOAL	INTERVENTION	RATIONALE	EXPECTED OUTCOME
1. Inability to Sustain Spontaneous Ventilation related to level of consciousness			
	NIC Priority Intervention: **Respiratory Monitoring:** Collection and analysis of patient data to assure airway patency and adequate gas exchange.		NOC Suggested Outcome: **Vital Sign Status:** Pulse, respiration, and blood pressure are within expected range for age.
The child's respiratory failure does not progress to respiratory arrest.	■ Place the child on a cardiorespiratory monitor with a 20-second alarm. ■ Have resuscitation equipment, including oxygen, resuscitation bag with mask, and suction apparatus at bedside. ■ Stimulate child if apneic; if no response, begin manual ventilations and call for emergency resuscitation. ■ Monitor heart rate and perform compressions if necessary.	■ The alarm on the monitor alerts staff that the child is having bradycardia or an apneic spell. ■ Equipment should be at bedside in case of respiratory arrest. Bag-valve mask ventilation is recommended as the child's respiratory secretions contain bacteria. ■ Stimulation may encourage spontaneous respirations; if not, ventilation is necessary. Calling for emergency resuscitation ensures help in managing the child in a timely manner. ■ The apneic child may have bradycardia resulting from cardiac hypoxia.	The child's respiratory failure is easily managed with prompt assessment and treatment.
2. Risk for Injury related to infection of cerebrospinal fluid and potential sequelae			
	NIC Priority Intervention: **Complication Monitoring:** Evaluation of fever, shock, and consciousness responses to bacterial infection of the meninges.		NOC Suggested Outcome: **Risk Control:** Actions to eliminate or reduce actual personal and modifiable health threats.
The child will suffer minimal CNS injury secondary to infection.	■ Administer prescribed antibiotics and corticosteroids as scheduled. ■ Note return of fever, nuchal rigidity, or irritability. Monitor vital signs, assess for signs of increased intracranial pressure, measure head circumference once or twice daily, note changes in responsiveness. Notify the physician immediately if any signs are detected.	■ Administration of antibiotics helps eradicate the pathogen and prevent cerebral edema. Adminstration of corticosteroids diminishes inflammatory response and reduces the chance of neurologic sequelae. ■ Watching for common sequelae such as subdural effusions or septic arthritis ensures prompt treatment.	The child's condition improves significantly within 48–72 hours (fever decreases and no signs of neurologic sequelae are detected).
The child will not develop cerebral edema as a result of water retention.	■ Monitor for syndrome of inappropriate antidiuretic hormone secretion (SIADH) and watch for signs of increased intracranial pressure (ICP). ■ Perform strict intake and output measurements. Determine urine specific gravity. Check electrolytes and osmolality of both serum and urine. Weigh the child daily. Restrict fluids and give sodium chloride as ordered.	■ SIADH can be either avoided or quickly managed if early recognition is achieved. ■ Low urine output with a high specific gravity is a sign of fluid retention and SIADH. The child is maintained with lower fluids and provided sodium supplements to reduce the possibility for cerebral edema.	Cerebral edema does not develop. If SIADH or increased ICP occurs, the condition is treated promptly so effects on the child are minimal.

(continued)

NURSING CARE PLAN The Child with Bacterial Meningitis (continued)

GOAL	INTERVENTION	RATIONALE	EXPECTED OUTCOME
2. Risk for Injury related to infection of cerebrospinal fluid and potential sequelae (continued)			
The child will be free of injury resulting from disseminated intravascular coagulation (DIC).	■ Be aware of needle sticks that continue to bleed and lesions that continue to ooze. Monitor clotting times. ■ Administer blood products, vitamin K, or heparin as ordered.	■ Prompt recognition leads to management of the coagulopathy. ■ Prompt recognition allows for early initial treatment of DIC. The child may bleed to death if treatment is delayed.	The child does not sustain injury from DIC.
The child will be free of injury secondary to shock.	■ Monitor vital signs including pulse, respirations, and blood pressure. Note perfusion (capillary refill, central versus proximal pulses). Check level of consciousness. Note urine output. ■ Begin fluid resuscitation as ordered. ■ Administer inotropes if ordered.	■ Monitoring allows for prompt diagnosis of shock based on clinical signs. ■ Intravenous fluid bolus may improve perfusion. ■ Inotropes enhance perfusion when response to fluid challenge is minimal.	The child recovers from shock quickly with no complications. Prompt management of shock can enhance the child's recovery, since it prevents complications associated with poor perfusion (tissue acidosis and ischemia).
3. Impaired Social Interaction related to decreased level of consciousness, hospitalization, and isolation			
	NIC Priority Intervention: **Socialization Enhancement:** Facilitation of the child's ability to interact with others.		NOC Suggested Outcome: **Role Performance:** Congruence of the child's role behavior with role expectations.
The child's social interaction will be near normal despite isolation.	■ Educate parents and other visitors to use proper infection control techniques. ■ Encourage parents to help with daily activities such as feeding and bathing. ■ Have age-appropriate games and toys in the room. Play with the child. When the child is feeling better, encourage watching television/videotape or listening to the radio/audiotape.	■ Family members help fulfill the emotional and social needs of the ill and contagious child. ■ Parental involvement in the child's care provides the child with a sense of security and emotional well-being. Parents have a sense of control and a feeling that they are doing something to enhance the child's recovery. ■ Providing the child with toys and games as well as sensory stimulation helps the child achieve a sense of well-being.	The child's social and developmental needs are met by family members despite the child's illness and hospitalization.
The child with any degree of hearing loss will be identified.	■ Arrange for hearing assessment prior to discharge.	■ Hearing loss is a common complication. Early intervention is needed to promote growth and development.	The child with identified hearing loss is referred to appropriate specialist or program for intervention.
4. Pain related to meningeal irritation			
	NIC Priority Intervention: **Pain Management:** Alleviation of pain or reduction in pain to a level of comfort that is acceptable to patient.		NOC Suggested Outcome: **Comfort Level:** Feelings of physical and psychologic ease.
The child will be as comfortable as possible.	■ Minimize tactile stimulation.	■ Sensory stimulation increases discomfort.	The child is calm and expresses increased comfort.

(continued)

NURSING CARE PLAN The Child with Bacterial Meningitis (continued)

GOAL	INTERVENTION	RATIONALE	EXPECTED OUTCOME
4. Pain related to meningeal irritation (continued)			
	■ Allow the child to assume a position of comfort.	■ The child determines the most comfortable position. Opisthotonic position, with the head and neck hyperextended, may be the most comfortable.	
	■ Keep the lights dim.	■ Dim lights reduce the discomfort from photophobia.	
	■ Maintain a quiet environment. Keep doors closed.	■ Noise can disturb the child.	
5. Risk for Infection (Family and Close Contacts) related to pathogens in the cerebrospinal fluid			
	NIC Priority Intervention: **Infection Control:** Minimizing the acquisition and transmission of infectious agents.		NOC Suggested Outcome: **Risk Control:** Actions to eliminate an actual health threat.
Caretakers or family members will have no apparent evidence of infection.	■ Explain rationale and dose schedule for taking rifampin or ciprofloxacin.	■ Rifampin and ciprofloxacin provide prophlylaxis for many bacterial pathogens responsible for meningitis.	Family members and other close contacts verbalize schedule for rifampin or ciprofloxacin therapy.

Discharge Planning and Home Care Teaching

Home care needs should be identified and addressed well in advance of discharge. Follow-up visits are important to monitor for complications and sequelae. Help parents deal with any physical requirements resulting from the child's illness and any emotional, social, and financial repercussions of the child's condition. Teach parents what to do if the child has a seizure.

Infants and toddlers with neurologic sequelae should be referred to an early intervention program. If the child has had a hearing loss, referral to an otolaryngologist and speech and language specialist should be made. Early identification of other neurologic sequelae, such as learning problems, should be encouraged.

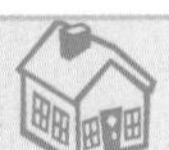

HOME CARE

Children with hearing, learning, or attention disorders need individualized education plans (see Chapter 6), and parents may need assistance in planning for the child's special educational needs. Refer parents to the appropriate social service agencies for support and assistance.

Evaluation

Expected outcomes of nursing care are provided on the nursing care plan.

VIRAL (ASEPTIC) MENINGITIS

Viral meningitis is an inflammatory response of the meninges characterized by an increased number of blood cells and protein in the cerebrospinal fluid. In the United States, an enterovirus is often the cause of aseptic meningitis (Cherry, 1999).

Generally, the child with aseptic meningitis does not appear to be as ill as the child with bacterial meningitis. The child may be irritable or lethargic and usually has a fever. Other symptoms include general malaise, headache, photophobia, gastrointestinal distress, upper respiratory symptoms, and a maculopapular rash. The child may also show signs of meningeal irritation such as stiff neck, back pain, and positive Kernig and Brudzinski signs (see Figures 20-8 and 20-9). The infant may have a tense anterior fontanel. Seizures are rare. Symptoms usually resolve spontaneously within 3 to 10 days.

The child with fever and meningeal signs is hospitalized. Blood, urine, and cerebrospinal fluid analyses are performed. Until the diagnosis of aseptic meningitis is confirmed, the child is treated aggressively, as if he or she has bacterial meningitis.

Nursing Management

Initial nursing care focuses on providing supportive care as described for the child with bacterial meningitis. Give acetaminophen as ordered to reduce fever, headache, and muscle or

TABLE 20-9

Causative Viruses of Encephalitis

Enteroviruses
- Poliovirus
- Echovirus
- Coxsackievirus

Adenoviruses and herpesviruses
Arboviruses
Measles
Mumps
Rubella
Rabies
Hepatitis B

joint pain. Keep the room dark and quiet (to decrease stimuli and meningeal irritation), give fluids either intravenously or orally, and promote comfort with proper positioning.

The child and family need information about the disease. Explain medical and nursing procedures in terms that the child and family can understand. Keep parents informed about the child's progress. Once the diagnosis of viral meningitis is made, discharge planning and teaching for home care must begin immediately. Explain that recovery may take several weeks but that complete recovery is expected.

ENCEPHALITIS

Encephalitis is an inflammation of the brain usually caused by a viral infection. Inflammation of the meninges is also common (Moe & Seay, 1997).

Viruses are believed to cause most cases of encephalitis (Table 20-9). Herpes simplex type I is the most common cause after the newborn period, and is associated with a high mortality rate.

Signs and symptoms depend on the causative organism and the location of the infection within the brain. An acute onset of a febrile illness with neurologic signs is the classic manifestation of encephalitis. Initially the child may have a severe headache, fever, signs of an upper respiratory infection, and nausea or vomiting. Meningeal irritation signs such as nuchal rigidity, photophobia, and positive Kernig and Brudzinski signs are uncommon. Other neurologic signs vary. The child may be disoriented or confused, with behavioral or personality changes. Speech disturbances; motor dysfunction such as hemiparesis, ataxia, or weakness; cranial nerve deficits; or alterations in reflex response may be present. Focal or generalized seizures may occur, alternating with periods of screaming, hallucinating, and moving in a bizarre fashion. The child's level of consciousness may deteriorate from stupor to coma.

Diagnosis is based on history and laboratory findings. Information about recent immunizations, insect bites, or travel to areas where vectors are present should be obtained. Cerebrospinal fluid analysis, blood serologic tests, and nasopharyngeal and stool specimens are evaluated to identify viral pathogens. A CT scan, MRI, and EEG may also be performed. The nucleic acid detection test is used to assay for herpes DNA in the spinal fluid. Brain biopsy may be performed to diagnose herpes simplex and parasitic infections.

The child with encephalitis is at risk for seizures, respiratory failure, and increased intracranial pressure and should be cared for in an intensive care unit. Treatment is both pharmacologic and supportive. The child with a suspected bacterial infection should be treated with antibiotics until bacterial pathogens have been ruled out.

Children with encephalitis have many permanent neurologic sequelae. Although some children recover completely, many more are left with intellectual, motor, visual, or auditory deficits. The cardiovascular system, lungs, or liver may also be affected. Generally, the younger the child, the more serious the illness and the more severe the residual effects.

Nursing Management

Nursing care focuses on monitoring cardiorespiratory function, preventing complications resulting from immobility, reorienting the child, and teaching the parents about the child's condition.

Monitor the child's cardiorespiratory function. Check the child's airway and ability to handle secretions. Monitor respiratory status by observing color, pulse oximetry readings, and arterial blood gas values. Observe cardiopulmonary status by monitoring heart rate, blood pressure, capillary refill time, and urine output. Provide seizure precautions, and have appropriate equipment for managing seizures at bedside.

Prevent complications resulting from immobility as described in Table 20-5. Maintain skin integrity. Proper positioning with frequent turning is important. When indicated by the physician, perform chest physiotherapy to prevent pneumonia.

Skill 10-20: Performing Chest Physiotherapy

The child whose level of consciousness begins to improve may at first be confused and disoriented and may have residual effects of the disease. Orient the child to the hospital environment. Have the family help to reorient the child by bringing favorite stuffed animals or music from home. Engage in therapeutic play (refer to Chapter 5 for techniques). Give the child age-appropriate toys to encourage a return to normal behavior.

Provide the parents with information about their child's condition and prognosis. If the child receives physical, occupational, or speech therapy, explain the treatment regimen to the parents.

DISCHARGE PLANNING AND HOME CARE TEACHING Encourage parents to take an active role in the child's physical and emotional care in the hospital, and give them written instructions concerning care for their child at home. Encourage the parents to learn specific physical, occupational, and speech therapies so they can work with their child at home between home care visits. Refer parents to home care, social services, family counseling, and support groups. Plan follow-up visits so the child can be evaluated for neurologic sequelae.

REYE SYNDROME

Reye syndrome is an acute **encephalopathy,** a cerebral dysfunction caused by a toxic, injury, inflammatory, or anoxic insult that may result in permanent tissue damage, although the dysfunction may improve over time. In Reye syndrome the encephalopathy is parainfectious, and it also affects the liver, causing hepatic dysfunction. It is characterized by cerebral edema and an enlarged, fatty, poorly functioning liver.

The etiology of Reye syndrome is unclear. The disorder usually develops after a mild viral illness, such as varicella or influenza. It has also been associated with aspirin use. Because most parents give children acetaminophen rather than aspirin for flulike symptoms and varicella, Reye syndrome has become rare, but the mortality rate for children who develop the condition is high.

Reye syndrome begins with nausea and vomiting, mental status changes, seizures, and progressive unresponsiveness (Ressler & Nelson, 2000). The condition has five stages, as described in Table 20-10. The condition is most severe in younger children.

The diagnosis of Reye syndrome is based on an abrupt change in the child's level of consciousness and diagnostic laboratory tests. The child has often progressed to coma or stage III by the time of diagnosis. Liver enzyme levels (aspartate aminotransferase [AST] or alanine aminotransferase [ALT]) are elevated to twice their normal levels, ammonia levels are elevated, blood glucose levels are below normal, and prothrombin time is prolonged. A liver biopsy is sometimes performed to confirm the diagnosis (by showing small droplet fat deposits).

The child with Reye syndrome should be placed in a pediatric intensive care unit because of the potential for rapid deterioration in his or her condition. The goal of medical management is to provide supportive treatment and to prevent the secondary effects of cerebral edema and metabolic injury. Assisted ventilation is often needed once the child is comatose. The child is monitored for signs of increased intracranial pressure, which can be secondary to cerebral edema. Hypoglycemia is treated with intravenous glucose; and electrolytes, blood chemistry, and blood pH are monitored.

CLINICAL TIP 

Make sure all parents know that aspirin must not be given when the child has a viral illness such as chicken pox or influenza, because aspirin is associated with the development of Reye syndrome. Instruct parents to check all over-the-counter medicines for the presence of aspirin compounds. Emphasize the importance of obtaining health care when a child's condition worsens at the end of a viral illness.

Nursing Management

Nursing care focuses on monitoring the child's physical status, providing emotional support, and teaching parents about disease prevention.

TABLE 20-10 Stages of Reye Syndrome

STAGE	CLINICAL MANIFESTATIONS
I	Vomiting; lethargy; appropriate responses to verbal commands; purposeful responses to pain; brisk pupillary reaction
II	Combativeness; stupor; inappropriate language; confusion; anxiety, fear; purposeful and nonpurposeful responses to pain; sluggish pupillary reaction; conjugate deviation with oculocephalic reflex; hyperactive reflexes; progresses to coma but interrupted by periods of screaming and ranting
III	Coma; decorticate rigidity; conjugate deviation with diminished oculocephalic reflex; sluggish pupillary reaction; decorticate posturing
IV	Coma with brainstem dysfunction; decerebrate rigidity; inconsistent or absent oculocephalic reflex; loss of corneal reflex; sluggish pupillary reaction; decerebrate posturing
V	Coma with seizures; flaccidity; loss of deep tendon reflexes; respiratory arrest

Check the child's respiratory and neurologic status frequently, and note any signs of improvement or deterioration. Orient the child who awakens from coma. Refer to the discussion of nursing management of altered states of consciousness at the beginning of this chapter for specific nursing interventions. Look for changes in laboratory values that indicate acidosis, an elevation of ammonia levels, or hypoglycemia. Monitor the child's intake and output. Correct imbalances by administering fluids, electrolytes, or medications as ordered. Prevent complications associated with immobility.

Provide emotional support to the parents, who may feel guilty because they did not seek medical attention sooner. Keep them informed about the child's condition, and prepare them for potential deterioration in the course of the disease. Explanations of treatments can help reduce anxiety. Encourage the parents to participate in the child's care when possible.

Once the child is discharged, monitoring is needed to observe for sequelae of the illness. Developmental and neurologic deficits may occur and are more severe in children under 2 years of age. Arrange for home nursing visits during the recovery period so that developmental and neurological status monitoring can be assessed. Be sure the parents are informed about resources in the community that can assist them in dealing with the child's recovery.

GUILLAIN-BARRÉ SYNDROME (POSTINFECTIOUS POLYNEURITIS)

Guillain-Barré syndrome is an acute inflammatory demyelinating polyneuropathy. This condition may lead to deteriorating motor function and paralysis that progresses in an ascending pattern. It is the most common cause of acute flaccid paralysis in infants and children (Jones, 2000). Guillain-Barré syndrome is caused by an immune response to an infectious organism, usually from a gastrointestinal or respiratory illness 2 to 3 weeks prior to onset. It has also been associated with immunizations and cytomegalovirus.

Infants have an onset of rapidly progressive severe hypotonia, possible respiratory distress, and feeding difficulties. Older children have rapidly progressive symmetric weakness and muscle pain with varying degrees of distal paresthesia and numbness in the legs. This weakness spreads to the upper extremities, trunk, chest, neck, face, and head. Deep tendon reflexes may be diminished or absent. The child may develop acute ataxia. Respiratory effort may be inadequate to ensure proper ventilation. Facial paresis and difficulty swallowing follow. Cranial nerves may be affected, thus causing, for example, Bell's palsy. A dysfunctional autonomic nervous system may cause such symptoms as hypertension, postural hypotension, sinus tachycardia or bradycardia, excessive diaphoresis, urinary and bowel incontinence, and facial flushing.

Diagnostic criteria of Guillain-Barré syndrome include progressive motor weakness (minimal weakness of the legs to total paralysis of all extremities), and areflexia of varying degrees. Two tests are used to diagnose. Lumbar puncture is performed to obtain cerebrospinal fluid; increased protein levels (80 to 200 mg/dL) with fewer than 50 lymphocytes per cubic millimeter are a positive indicator of the condition (Jones, 2000). Electroconduction tests such as electromyography are also used. An abnormal pattern of nerve conduction is indicative of Guillain-Barré syndrome.

Clinical therapy for Guillain-Barré syndrome is plasmapheresis or intravenous immune globulin if the child is unable to ambulate. Guidelines for administration of intravenous immune globulin can be found in Chapter 11. Responses to intravenous immune globulin are dramatic, often within days. If the child is able to ambulate, physical therapy and supportive care are provided. The condition is rarely fatal.

Nursing Management

Nursing care focuses on monitoring respiratory status, meeting nutritional needs, managing autonomic nervous system dysfunction, preventing complications associated with immobility, providing emotional support, and teaching the parents how to care for the child after discharge.

MONITOR RESPIRATORY STATUS Monitor the child's respiratory status closely, especially in the early phase of illness. Look for such signs as dyspnea, inability to handle secretions, inadequate respiratory effort, and color changes that may indicate the need for endotracheal intubation and mechanical ventilation.

MANAGE AUTONOMIC NERVOUS SYSTEM DYSFUNCTION Monitor the child's vital signs closely for episodes of tachycardia, bradycardia, and hypotension. Blood pressure fluctuations and autonomic instability are linked to fatal cardiac arrythmias (Jones, 2000). Observe frequently for decreased responsiveness. Intervene promptly if these or other signs of autonomic nervous system dysfunction are noted.

MEET NUTRITIONAL NEEDS Assess whether the child is having difficulty swallowing. If the child has no gag reflex, nutritional needs are maintained with intravenous supplements or nasogastric tube feedings.

PREVENT COMPLICATIONS Prevent complications associated with immobility (see Table 20-5). Ensure good postural alignment, and turn the child every 2 hours. Maintaining skin integrity is also important.

Evaluate the child's muscle tone, strength, and symmetry. When the child's condition begins to improve, recovery of lost strength is the priority. Active exercise is emphasized in physical therapy. Encourage family members to participate in the child's care, especially during the recovery phase. They can help with the activities of daily living and reinforce what the child has learned in physical therapy.

PROVIDE EMOTIONAL SUPPORT Explain the progression of Guillain-Barré syndrome to the parents during the initial stages. Witnessing a rapid deterioration in their child's physical status can be frightening; therefore, preparation is essential to reduce their anxieties. Be honest when discussing recovery and prognosis for the child.

Have parents bring in favorite toys, dolls, or books to make the child feel more secure. Playing with or reading to the child can be comforting.

DISCHARGE PLANNING AND HOME CARE TEACHING Home care needs should be identified and addressed well in advance of discharge. Support the parents as they prepare for the child's return home. Provide referral to home care nurses who can manage all aspects of treatment, rehabilitation, and follow-up. Refer the parents to social workers, who can help with financial arrangements and school considerations.

CARE IN THE COMMUNITY Help the child to adjust to any residual effects of Guillain-Barré syndrome. Help the child practice exercises learned in physical therapy sessions, and encourage the child to perform activities of daily living, such as brushing the teeth or combing the hair. Refer the child to outpatient rehabilitation programs to promote recovery.

To promote a positive self-image, praise any effort the child makes to be self-sufficient. The child may have feelings of frustration and anger. Allow the child to express these feelings in an appropriate way, either during play or in conversation.

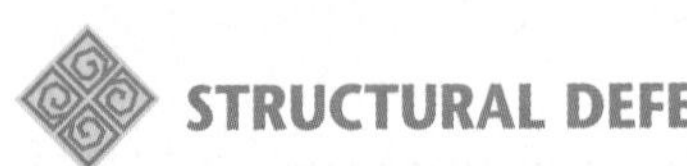

STRUCTURAL DEFECTS

HYDROCEPHALUS

Hydrocephalus is the body's response to an imbalance between the production and absorption of cerebrospinal fluid. The condition is often congenital, but may be related to prematurity. The incidence is 3 to 4 cases per 1,000 births. A recessive X-linked genetic hydrocephalus accounts for a small number of cases (Jackson & Harvey, 2000). Hydrocephalus can develop in older children as a complication of illness or trauma.

Etiology and Pathophysiology

Hydrocephalus may be either communicating or noncommunicating, and congenital or acquired. Communicating hydrocephalus is the blockage of flow or absorption of cerebrospinal fluid in the subarachnoid space and the arachnoid villi. It can be acquired from postinfectious meningitis or intraventricular hemorrhage, be congenital, or be of unknown etiology.

Noncommunicating hydrocephalus is responsible for the majority of cases in children. It results from a blockage in the ventricular system that prevents cerebrospinal fluid from entering the subarachnoid space (Figure 20-10 ◆). This obstruction can be caused by infection,

PATHOPHYSIOLOGY ILLUSTRATED

Hydrocephalus

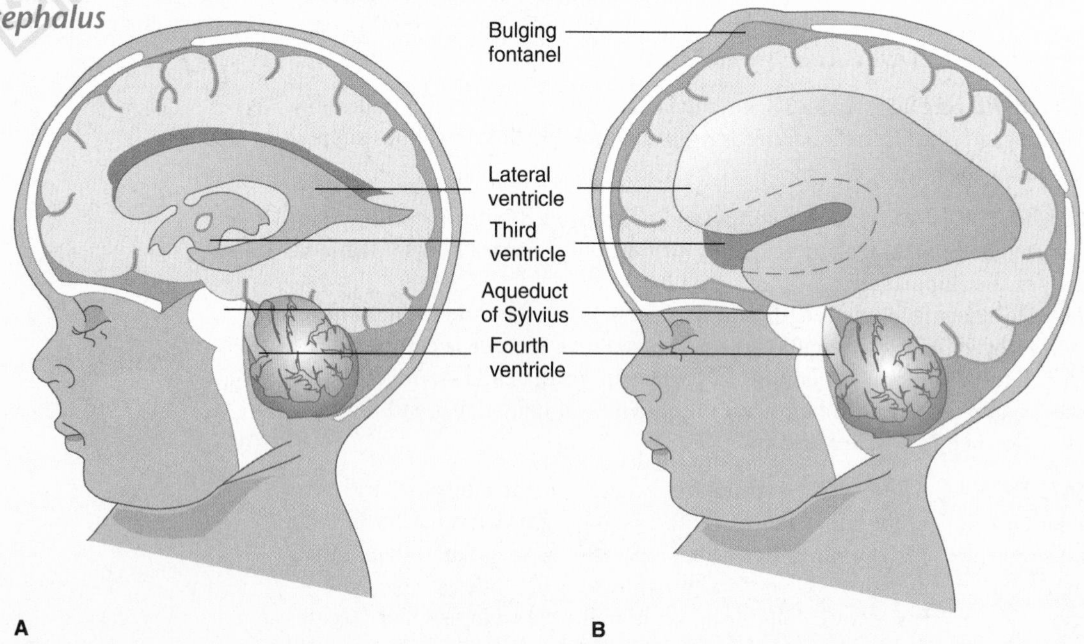

Bulging fontanel
Lateral ventricle
Third ventricle
Aqueduct of Sylvius
Fourth ventricle
A
B

FIGURE 20-10 ◆
A, Normal size of ventricle. B, Enlarged ventricles, characteristic of hydrocephalus.

hemorrhage, tumor, or structural deformity. Congenital structural defects such as the Arnold-Chiari II malformation (found in most children with myelomeningocele) and the Dandy-Walker syndrome have obstructions that block the flow of cerebrospinal fluid (Jackson & Harvey, 2000).

Clinical Manifestations

The signs and symptoms of hydrocephalus, which vary depending on the age of the child, are listed on page 751. The predominant manifestation of the condition in infants is rapid head growth (Figure 20-11 ◆). Older children show signs of increased intracranial pressure (see Table 20-2).

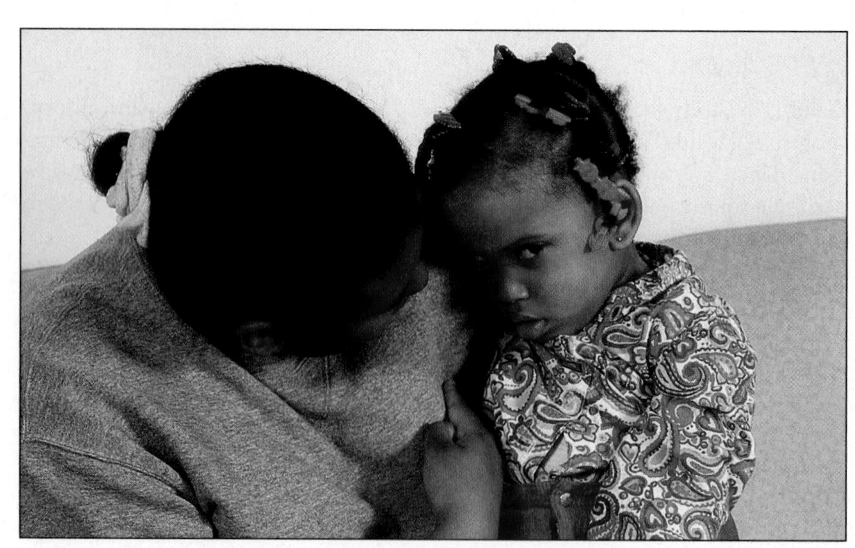

FIGURE 20-11 ◆
In communicating hydrocephalus, an excessive amount of cerebrospinal fluid accumulates in the subarachnoid space, producing the characteristic head enlargement seen here. Note the downward deviation of the eyes so that the lower half of the iris is hidden by the lower eyelid. This finding occurs in severe hydrocephalus.

CLINICAL MANIFESTATIONS OF HYDROCEPHALUS

CAUSES	CLINICAL MANIFESTATIONS
Congenital structural defect in infancy Dandy-Walker syndrome Arnold-Chiari II malformation	Early signs Rapid head growth Tense, bulging fontanel, split sutures Bossing (protrusion) of frontal area Prominent scalp veins Translucent skin Increased tone or hyperreflexia Irritability or lethargy, poor feeding Decline in level of consciousness Late signs Shrill, high-pitched cry Difficulty swallowing or feeding Macewen's or "cracked-pot" sign Sunsetting eyes (sclera visible above iris), cranial nerve VI palsy Vomiting Cardiopulmonary depression (severe cases)
Acquired hydrocephalus in older child Postinfectious Tumor Hemorrhage	No head enlargement Headache upon arising with vomiting Fussiness, sleepiness, confusion, or apathy Personality change, loss of interest in daily activities Poor judgment or verbal incoherence Ataxia, spasticity, or other alterations in motor development Visual defects secondary to pressure on cranial nerves II, III, and VI Signs of increased intracranial pressure

Clinical Therapy

The diagnosis of hydrocephalus in infants is based on clinical manifestations. In the hospital setting, daily measurements of the infant's head circumference are critical in any infant at risk of developing hydrocephalus. In older children, signs of increased intracranial pressure are noted.

CT scanning and MRI diagnose hydrocephalus, and in some cases reveal the anatomic cause. In the infant whose fontanel is still open, ultrasonography or echoencephalography may be used to confirm the diagnosis.

Clinical therapy for hydrocephalus involves removing the obstruction (e.g., surgical removal of a tumor) or creating a new cerebrospinal fluid pathway to divert excess fluid. A catheter or shunt is placed in the ventricle and passes the cerebrospinal fluid to the peritoneal cavity, atrium of the heart, or the pleural spaces. Ventriculoperitoneal shunts (Figure 20-12 ◆) are commonly used. Shunt systems consist of four parts: a ventricular catheter, a pumping chamber or reservoir, a one-way pressure valve, and a distal catheter. Initial shunt placement is usually performed early in infancy, with replacement two to four times as the child grows.

Mechanical complications may include blockage at either the proximal or the distal end of the catheter, kinking of the tubing, or valve breakdown. Infants or children with shunt failure show signs and symptoms of recurrent hydrocephalus and increased intracranial pressure. Shunt failure and ventricular size are confirmed by CT scanning or MRI. Shunt materials and systems continue to be refined in an attempt to reduce mechanical problems.

The most serious complication is shunt infection, which may occur at any time but is most prevalent in the first 2 months after placement. The infection rate is 4% to 12% per year, with infants under 6 months having the highest rates (Jackson, 2000). Antibiotics are usually prescribed, but if the infection is overwhelming, the shunt is removed and an external drainage device is placed. A new shunt is inserted when the infection resolves.

Some children, especially those with ventriculoatrial shunts, are placed on the same prophylactic antibiotic treatment regimen used for children with cardiac anomalies to reduce the risk of shunt infections (refer to Chapter 14).

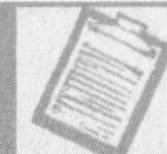

RESEARCH

Researchers in neuroendoscopy are developing techniques to create a new pathway for cerebrospinal fluid to flow between the ventricles and spinal cord in individuals with obstructive hydrocephalus. The new endoscopy procedure may be used in some patients in the future to avoid shunt placement (Jackson, 2000).

CLINICAL TIP

The most important signs of shunt infection are changes in responsiveness and irritability after fever is controlled. Other signs include low-grade fever, malaise, headache, and nausea (Jackson, 2000).

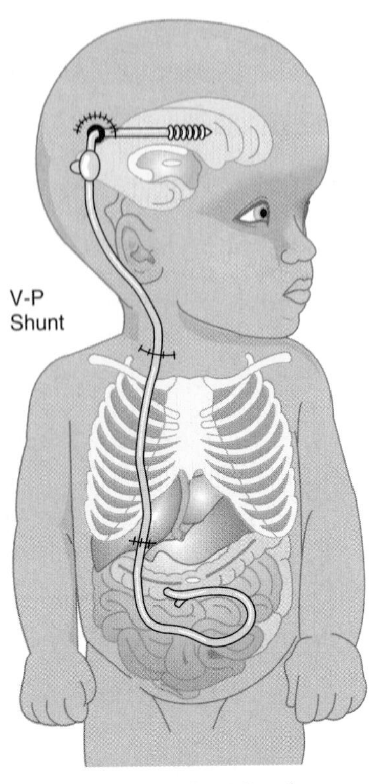

FIGURE 20-12 ◆
A ventriculoperitoneal shunt, commonly used to treat children with hydrocephalus, is usually placed at 3–4 months of age.

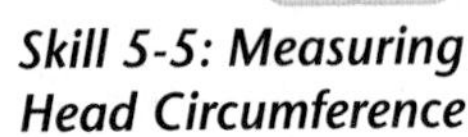

Skill 5-5: Measuring Head Circumference

NURSING MANAGEMENT

Nursing Assessment and Diagnosis

It is important for nurses to become familiar with the clinical manifestations of hydrocephalus to ensure prompt identification and treatment of children with this condition. Head circumference of all infants is measured at each well-child visit to detect the condition at an early stage.

Assess the child with a ventriculoperitoneal shunt for signs and symptoms of shunt failure and infection. Daily measurement of the infant's head circumference is performed when shunt failure is suspected. Report any abnormalities to the physician immediately.

Nursing diagnoses that may be appropriate for the child with hydrocephalus include the following:

- *Risk for infection,* related to presence of shunt
- *Impaired physical mobility (level 2),* related to decreased muscle mass to lift the increased weight of head
- *Risk for caregiver role strain,* related to care of a child with a chronic condition or life-threatening illness
- *Anxiety (parent),* related to repeated surgeries and life-threatening illness
- *Risk for injury,* related to potential shunt failure

Planning and Implementation

Nursing care in the hospital setting focuses on providing preoperative and postoperative care and providing emotional support.

Provide Preoperative Care

Measure the child's head circumference daily and watch for signs of increased intracranial pressure (see Table 20-2).

Measure fluid intake and output as ordered. Carefully assess respiratory status. Provide good skin care.

Position the child carefully; do not stretch or strain the neck muscles, as they must support the large head. Holding the child may be awkward because of the additional weight of the head. Reduce the chances for skin breakdown by placing sheepskin or a lamb's wool blanket under the head. Prevent any other complications associated with immobility (see Table 20-5).

Attend to the child's special nutritional needs. Because the infant is prone to vomiting, frequent small feedings with frequent burping are beneficial.

Provide Postoperative Care

The child is usually placed in a flat position to prevent rapid cerebrospinal fluid drainage. The head of the bed is elevated gradually.

Take vital signs every 2 to 4 hours. Monitor the child carefully for any signs of shunt malfunction, increased intracranial pressure, or infection.

Provide Emotional Support

Provide parents with explanations about the child's condition and all procedures to be performed. Encourage parents and family to help with the child's care in the hospital when appropriate. Be sympathetic and understanding, and allow parents to express their concerns. If hydrocephalus occurs during early infancy, the parents will be anxious about the impact of the chronic condition and subsequent surgical procedures. If hydrocephalus is secondary to neoplasm, however, the parents' anxieties are compounded by their child's life-threatening illness.

Assure parents that most children with shunts lead normal lives, attending school and interacting with others no differently than their peers.

Discharge Planning and Home Care Teaching

Home care needs should be identified and addressed well in advance of discharge. Parents must know how to care for a child with a shunt. Parents and other family members should be made aware of the signs and symptoms of both shunt failure (signs of increased intracranial pressure) and infection (changes in responsiveness, irritability, malaise, headache, nausea, and low-grade fever). Provide telephone numbers of the pediatrician and the neurosurgeon, and instruct parents to contact a physician immediately if they suspect a problem. Inform them that the shunt may need to be replaced one or more times in childhood as the child grows. Appropriate home care referrals should be arranged. Refer families to the appropriate psychologic and social services, such as the Hydrocephalus Association.

SAFETY PRECAUTIONS 

Infants with poor head control due to an enlarged head should not be placed in forward-facing car safety seats, regardless of their age. This position increases the risk of cervical spine injury and death to these children in the event of a car crash.

Care in the Community

Infants and children need frequent monitoring to ensure proper functioning of the shunt. Head circumference is measured at each visit to monitor growth. Assess the child for visual problems and cognitive, speech, and motor developmental delays. The child and family should be referred to an early intervention program to promote developmental progress. School-age children may need to have an individualized education plan developed (see Chapter 6). Intellectual functioning outcomes may be associated with the cause of the hydrocephalus. For example, children with uncomplicated congenital causes do better than those who have brain injury, infection, or intraventricular hemorrhage. About 70% of children function below the normal IQ range (Jackson, 2000).

Parents seeking child care for their infant should be encouraged to use a setting with fewer children to decrease exposure to infection. Review the signs of shunt failure and infection with parents at each visit and make sure they have a plan to manage the emergency of a shunt failure.

Encourage parents not to be overprotective and to allow the child to develop normally. Participation in sports with a high potential for head and abdominal impact should be discouraged.

Evaluation

Expected outcomes of nursing care include the following:

- The child develops adequate neck muscle control to interact with the environment.
- Shunt infections and malfunctions are identified by the parents and medical attention is sought quickly.
- Potential for growth and development is maximized by care and a stimulating environment.

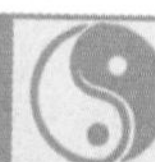
CULTURE

The rate of spina bifida varies with ethnicity and geographic location in the United States. Hispanic persons, especially those in Texas, have the highest rate. The rates of other ethnic groups in descending order are Caucasians, African-Americans, and Asian-Americans (Northrup & Volcik, 2000).

SPINA BIFIDA

Spina bifida, a congenital neural tube defect that affects the head and spinal column, is the most common developmental disorder of the central nervous system. It is a malformation of the neural tube that can occur anywhere along the spine. The condition occurs in about 1 per 2,000 births in the United States each year, but varies by region of the country (Northrup & Volcik, 2000).

The cause of spina bifida is unknown, although environmental factors such as chemicals, medications (e.g., valproic acid used for seizures), and maternal health conditions (insulin-dependent diabetes mellitus, gestational diabetes, folic acid deficiency, and maternal obesity) have been implicated. The increased incidence of the condition in families indicates a possible genetic influence.

There are several different types of spina bifida (Figure 20-13 ◆). A saclike protrusion on the infant's back indicates meningocele or myelomeningocele (Figure 20-14 ◆). The clinical manifestations seen depend on the location of the defect: the higher the defect, the greater the neurologic dysfunction. The lower extremities may be completely paralyzed with anesthesia of the skin, or there may be varying degrees of immobility with orthopedic problems of the hips, knees, and feet. Bowel and bladder sphincters may be affected. Renal

RESEARCH

By January 1998, mandatory fortification of all enriched grain products with folate had reduced the prevalence of neural tube defects by 19%. Educational efforts to increase folic acid supplementation to women of childbearing age has led to decreased cases of spina bifida (Honein, Paulozzi, & Matthews, et al., 2001).

PATHOPHYSIOLOGY ILLUSTRATED

Spina bifida occulta	Failure of posterior vertebral arches to fuse, most commonly at fifth lumbar or first sacral vertebrae; spinal cord and meninges entirely within vertebral canal; condition usually not visible externally; tuft of hair, a dermoid cyst, or hemangioma may be found over the site; mildest form
Spina bifida cystica	Defect in closure of posterior vertebral arch with protrusion through bony spine
Meningocele	Saclike protrusion through bony defect containing meninges and cerebrospinal fluid; sac covering defect may be translucent or membranous; spinal cord and spinal root in normal position
Myelomeningocele	Saclike herniation through bony defect holding meninges, cerebrospinal fluid, and a portion of spinal cord or nerve roots; fluid leakage may also occur; lesion poorly covered with imperfect tissue; handicap 99% of time; more common than meningocele

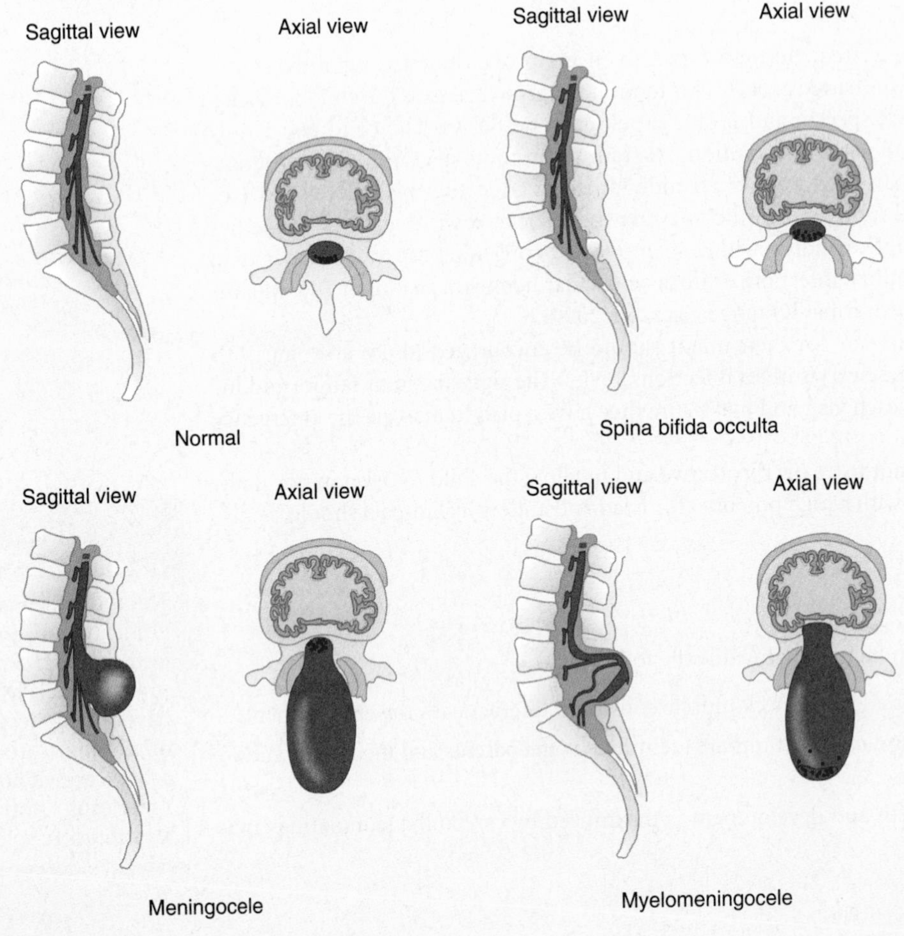

Types of Spina Bifida

FIGURE 20-13 ◆

involvement may occur secondary to neurologic impairment and urinary retention. Hydrocephalus is usually present in children with myelomeningocele because of the Arnold-Chiari II malformation. The range of potential problems for the child with spina bifida can be found on page 755.

Diagnosis is usually made prenatally, but after birth a multidisciplinary team examines the lesion and evaluates neurologic status. Radiologic imaging by CT scan, MRI, and flat films of the spinal column can pinpoint the bony defect. Surgery to close and repair the lesion usually occurs within 24 to 48 hours of the infant's birth to reduce infection. In some cases, uteromyelomeningocele repairs are performed. Early outcomes for carefully selected infants for this procedure show decreased shunting for hydrocephalus and resolution of the Arnold-Chiari II malformation (Sutton, Adzick, & Belaniuk, et al., 1999).

OTHER TYPES OF NEURAL TUBE DEFECTS

Anencephaly—exposed or absent brain

Encephalocele—protrusion of meningeal or skin-covered brain through the skull

Craniorachischisis—exposure of the entire CNS

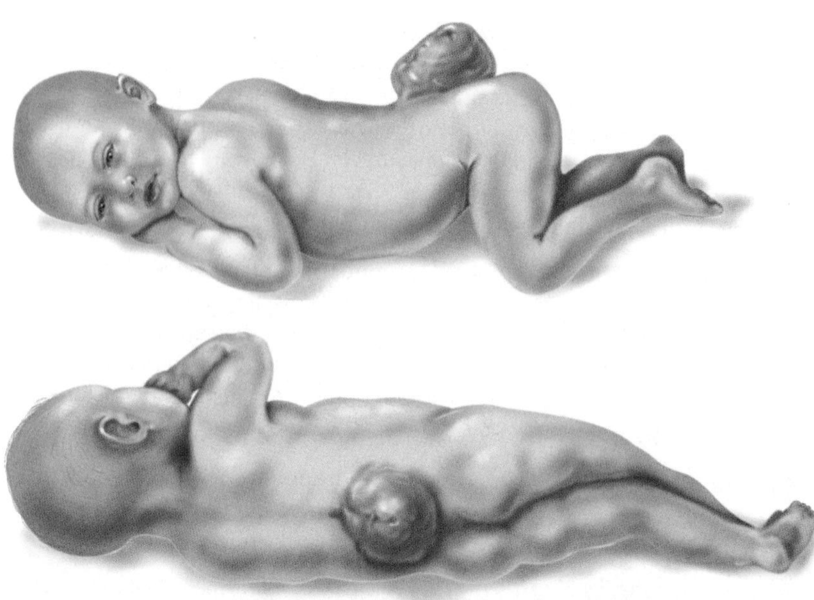

FIGURE 20-14 ◆ Lumbrosacral myelomeningocele is caused by a neural tube defect that results in incomplete closure of the vertebral column. As shown here, the meninges (and sometimes the spinal cord) protrude as a saclike structure.

Prognosis depends on the type of defect, the level of the lesion, and the presence of other complicating factors. Children need multiple surgeries and invasive procedures. A team of physicians, nurses, and therapists from the neurosurgery, orthopedic, urology, and physical medicine departments will work with the child and family to form a comprehensive care plan.

Nursing Management

Nursing care in the hospital focuses on providing preoperative and postoperative care, promoting mobility, and providing emotional support.

ARNOLD-CHIARI II MALFORMATION

The Arnold-Chiari malformation involves a downward displacement of the cerebellum, brainstem, and fourth ventricle. Because these structures control respiration and the protective reflexes, as well as house the cranial nerves, the displacement can have varying effects such as sudden death, respiratory difficulty, swallowing difficulties, and the need for assisted ventilation. Signs and symptoms may occur at any time. This malformation is the leading cause of death for children with spina bifida.

CLINICAL MANIFESTATIONS OF SPINA BIFIDA

CAUSE	CLINICAL MANIFESTATIONS
Interruption of the spinal cord at site of the spinal defect	Paralysis of legs Scoliosis or kyphosis Incontinence of urine and feces, constipation Anesthesia of skin
Muscle imbalance	Hip abnormalities, hip dysplasia Foot deformities (e.g., clubfoot)
Arnold-Chiari II malformation	Hydrocephalus *Infants:* Difficulty swallowing Apnea, respiratory difficulty, inspiratory stridor Weak or poor cry Sustained arching of head *Older children* Stiffness or spasticity of arms and hands Loss of feeling or sensation
Brain and spinal cord abnormalities	Learning problems, attention deficit disorder Problems with perceptual motor skills Memory and organization problems Problems with numerical reasoning

Note: Adapted from Northrup, H., & Volcik, K. A. (2000). Spinal bifida and other neural tube defects. *Current Problems in Pediatrics, 30*(10), 317–331.

GROWTH & DEVELOPMENT

Treat older children according to their intellectual level, not their motor development. Encourage them to take responsibility for self-care, and recognize their need to control their bodily functions. Promote interaction with peers in the hospital and participation in activities. If children are hospitalized for an extended time, schooling should be arranged.

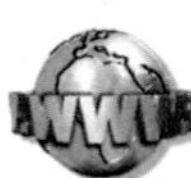

Hydrocephalus and Spina Bifida Resources

SAFETY PRECAUTIONS

Between 18% and 40% of children with spina bifida have a latex allergy (see Chapter 11). Cases in which latex exposure has caused anaphylaxis in a child have been reported. All children with latex allergy need to carry a kit with premeasured adrenaline for emergency treatment of anaphylaxis. Use nonlatex materials when providing care to the child in the hospital, in the outpatient setting, or at home. The Spina Bifida Association maintains an updated list of products containing latex and potential substitutes (Table 11-11).

PROVIDE PREOPERATIVE CARE Cover the sac with a sterile saline dressing to protect its integrity. Place the infant in a prone position with hips slightly flexed and legs abducted to minimize tension on the sac. Maintain this position using towel rolls placed between the knees. Assess the infant regularly for motor deficits as well as bladder and bowel involvement.

The infant is difficult to handle before surgery. Feed the infant with the head turned to one side until surgery has been performed. Comfort the infant before surgery with tactile stimulation such as touching, patting, and cuddling.

PROVIDE POSTOPERATIVE CARE Monitor the infant's vital signs carefully. Watch closely for symptoms of infection, especially meningitis. If a ventriculoperitoneal shunt was placed, watch for hydrocephalus, increased intracranial pressure, or infection. Inspect the surgical site for cerebrospinal fluid leakage. The infant should be placed in the prone or side-lying position, or in some cases may be held upright. Splints may be used to maintain extremity alignment.

PROMOTE MOBILITY Begin gentle range-of-motion exercises as soon as possible to prevent muscle contractures and atrophy. Extreme caution should be used because these children have brittle bones and are subject to idiopathic fractures.

PROVIDE EMOTIONAL SUPPORT Keep parents informed about their child's status. Allow them to express their frustrations and anger. As soon as parents are able to cope with the child's condition, encourage them to become involved in the child's care in the hospital.

DISCHARGE PLANNING AND HOME CARE TEACHING Home care needs should be identified and addressed well in advance of discharge. Make sure family members understand how to care for the child at home. Help them obtain special devices such as splints, wedges, and rolls, if indicated, to prevent complications. Instruct parents how to position, handle, feed, and perform range-of-motion exercises. Teach parents the signs and symptoms of increased intracranial pressure, hydrocephalus, shunt infection or malfunction, and urinary tract infection. Home care nursing should be arranged, if necessary. The home care nurse will reinforce the skills learned in the hospital setting and coordinate the numerous health care professionals who will be working with the child and family. Refer parents to resource groups such as the Spina Bifida Association of America.

CARE IN THE COMMUNITY To reduce complications and promote optimal development, children with spina bifida require comprehensive care that is planned and coordinated by a knowledgeable team of health care professionals. This care may be provided in partnership with the primary care physician.

Promote safety and independent mobility with proper use of braces, walkers, crutches, canes, and in some cases custom-designed wheelchairs and car safety seats (Figure 20-15 ◆). Encourage the use of latex-free products as the child is at risk for latex allergy (see Chapter 11). Other safety guidelines are provided below.

FAMILIES WANT TO KNOW

Safety for the Child with Spina Bifida

Due to the loss of sensation in the lower extremities, injuries to the skin may not be noticed by the child.

- Perform a daily check of all skin surfaces and pressure points associated with sitting, braces, shoes, etc. for abrasions, scrapes, reddened areas, and other lesions.
- Keep all skin surfaces clean and dry.
- Use a gel-filled cushion and teach the child to perform position shifts when in the wheelchair to avoid pressures sores.
- Avoid burns to the lower extremities by checking the temperature of bath water and car safety seats in a hot car.
- Take latex precautions as the child is at high risk for latex allergy. Inform all health care providers about the child's latex allergy.
- Use safe ambulation techniques with walkers, canes, and crutches

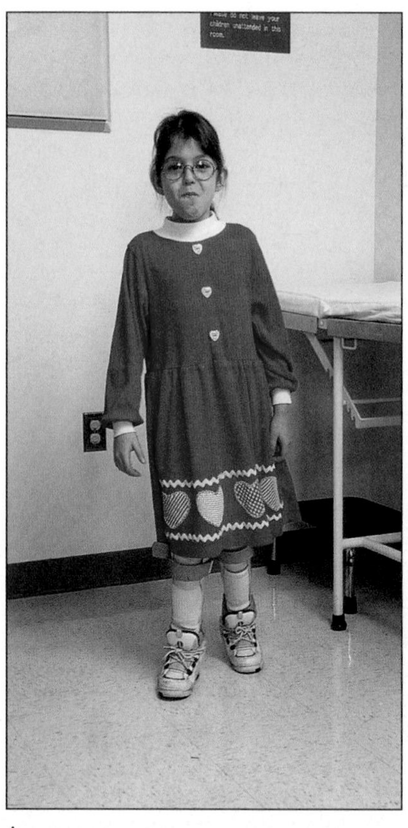

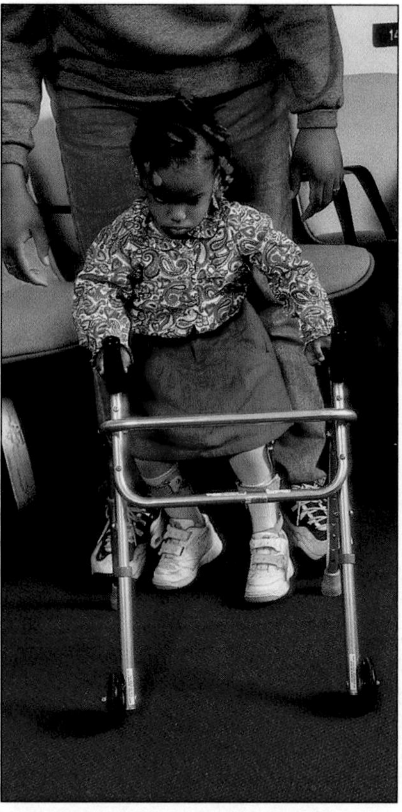

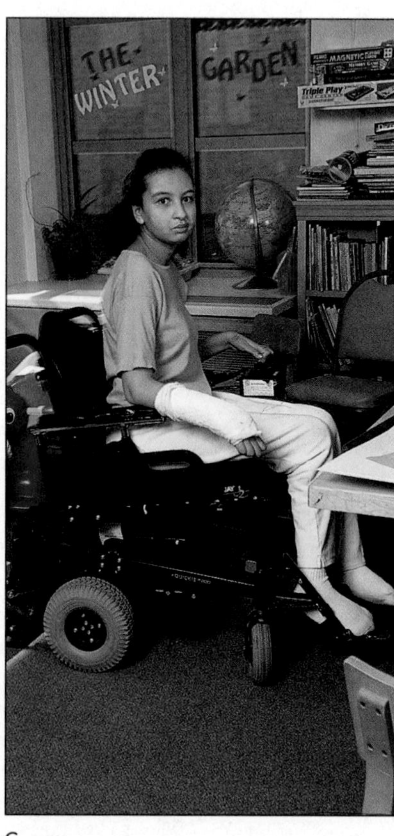

A B C

FIGURE 20-15 ◆

Help determine the best assistive device for the child to gain the most independence for mobilizing and to promote development. The child may change devices in different settings to promote optimal independence. A and B, Braces and walkers may be best for young children to promote an upright posture that encourages a normal interaction with the environment. C, A motorized wheelchair can assist the child with a significant neurologic impairment to achieve independence and mobility.

Parents may need to learn how to catheterize the child and then at an appropriate age teach the child intermittent self-catheterization to prevent urinary tract infections and other renal complications (see family information on page 655). Good nutrition planning is important to prevent obesity and to reduce constipation and complications such as fecal impaction. Surgery to create a channel between the skin and bowel (Malone antegrade continence enema) is sometimes performed. Children must learn to assume greater responsibility for self-care as they get older.

Parents are faced with the long-term financial issues of caring for the child who needs regular new adaptive equipment to match growth, as well as other medical supplies. At least 75% of children born with spina bifida generally survive to at least the early adult years (Bowman, McLone, & Grant, et al., 2001). Parents thus need to learn how to act as the child's case manager, or to work effectively with another individual in this role.

CRANIOSYNOSTOSIS

Craniosynostosis is the premature closing of the cranial sutures during the first 18 months of life. This condition occurs in up to 1 in 2,000 births (Renier, Lajeunie, & Arnaud, et al., 2000). Most children have no family history of the condition, although 15% have autosomal dominant inherited syndromes such as Alpert syndrome and Crouzon syndrome (Robinson, 1999).

The cause of craniosynostosis is unknown. Closure of the sutures usually takes place at predetermined times during the child's development. Problems arise if one or more sutures close early. Bone growth continues in a direction parallel to the suture line, which leads to compensatory overgrowth at normal suture lines and the classic skull deformities associated with craniosynostosis (Figure 20-16 ◆). Positional plagiocephaly, a totally flat occiput, is

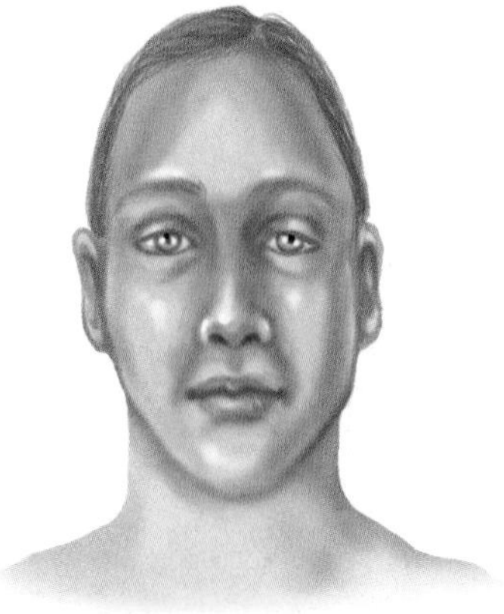

A

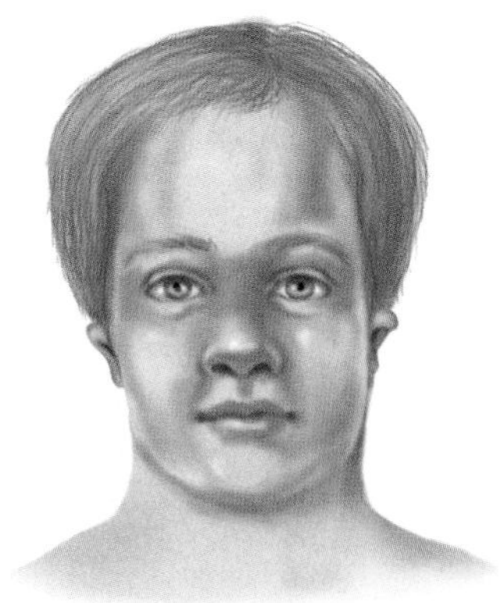

B

FIGURE 20-16 ◆
In craniosynostosis, the head shape is dependent upon which sutures are involved. Examples of different head shapes include those shown in A and B.

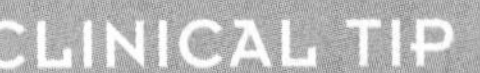

CLINICAL TIP

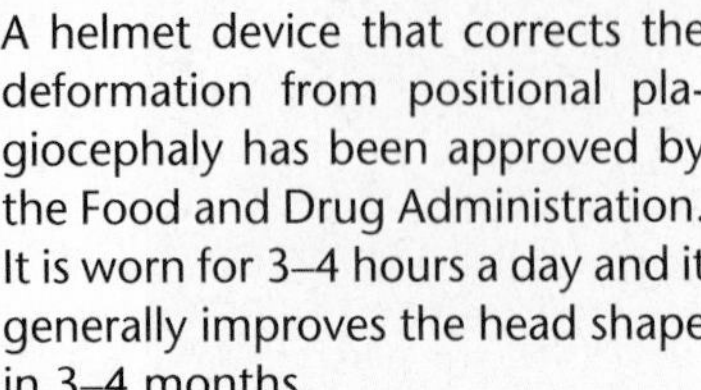

A helmet device that corrects the deformation from positional plagiocephaly has been approved by the Food and Drug Administration. It is worn for 3–4 hours a day and it generally improves the head shape in 3–4 months.

seen increasingly in healthy infants because they are put to sleep on their back to prevent sudden infant death syndrome. Since the infant's sleep position does not change, the weight of the head sometimes flattens the skull.

Diagnosis is made by clinical appearance. Palpation of the skull reveals a bony ridge along a suture. Skull x-ray films, CT scan, and MRI confirm the diagnosis. The hands and feet should be carefully examined to detect any skeletal defect that could be associated with a syndrome (Renier et al., 2000).

Reconstructive surgery, the most common form of treatment, is performed to protect mental development and vision. Many children need multiple procedures. Children having surgery before 1 year of age have a better outcome. After surgery, it is important for the incision to remain dry and intact. The nurse should also observe the child for symptoms of increased intracranial pressure (see Table 20-2).

Explain to parents that surgery will improve the child's appearance. Assure them that most children with craniosynostosis are healthy, and that their brains develop normally.

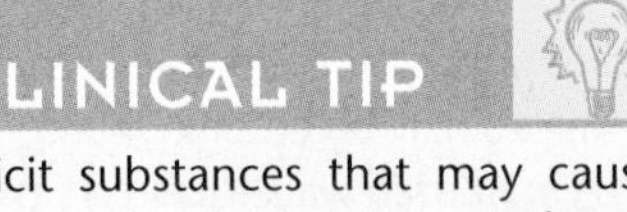

CLINICAL TIP

Illicit substances that may cause neonatal abstinence syndrome when used by the mother during pregnancy include opiates (heroine, meperidine, methadone), CNS stimulants (cocaine, propoxyphene, amphetamines), and CNS depressants (barbiturates, alcohol, and marijuana).

NEONATAL ABSTINENCE SYNDROME

More than 5% of all neonates (221,000) are exposed to illicit substances in utero, cocaine and marijuana being the most common (Robinson, 1999). Between 50% and 90% of infants born to drug-addicted mothers suffer withdrawal.

Repeated use of narcotics and other substances leads to tolerance and physical dependence. All narcotics, regardless of their mode of administration, readily cross the placenta, enter the fetal circulation, and have the same effects on the fetus that they do in the mother. When the mother stops taking drugs during pregnancy, both she and the fetus have withdrawal symptoms. If the infant is born to a mother who is still actively using drugs, then the neonate has signs of abrupt withdrawal from the illicit substance shortly after birth.

In the newborn, irritability and jitteriness are the most common symptoms of drug withdrawal. These infants may have excoriated skin, especially on the heels, toes, hands, elbows, nose, or chin, as a result of their continuous movements on the crib sheets (see clinical manifestations table below).

CLINICAL MANIFESTATIONS OF NEONATAL ABSTINENCE SYNDROME

SYSTEM INVOLVED	CLINICAL MANIFESTATIONS
Central nervous system	Irritability, restlessness, tremors, seizures, high-pitched cry, abnormal sleep patterns, drowsiness, yawning, and hypertonicity
Autonomic nervous system	Sneezing, stuffy nose, sweating, tachycardia, and tachypnea
Gastrointestinal system	Diarrhea, vomiting, and poor feeding

The onset of symptoms may be attributed to the type and amount of drug taken by the mother and how soon before birth it was taken. Withdrawal symptoms for opiates usually appear 24 to 48 hours after birth; however, it is not uncommon for barbiturate withdrawal symptoms to appear between 4 and 14 days after birth, or up to 7 days after birth if the mother was using cocaine or amphetamines. Opiates cause the most withdrawal symptoms, but consider the possibility of multiple drug use by the mother. Long-term exposure to these substances can result in intrauterine growth retardation, prematurity, small head circumference, shorter length, and low Apgar scores.

Diagnosis is based on the history of maternal substance abuse and physical signs in the infant. EEG abnormalities may be noted. Identification of the drug may be determined in some cases from maternal and infant urine. Meconium and hair of the infant may also be tested.

Treatment is generally supportive. Medications such as phenobarbitol, diazepam, methadone, clonidine, and paregoric may be prescribed to alleviate symptoms. The most serious and prevalent complication with drug abuse is human immunodeficiency virus (HIV) infection and hepatitis B.

CLINICAL TIP

Crying accompanied by poor feeding constitutes clinical signs that should increase the nurse's suspicion of neonatal abstinence syndrome.

NURSING MANAGEMENT

Nursing care focuses on monitoring withdrawal symptoms, administering prescribed medications, and meeting the infant's emotional needs.

The drug-addicted infant should be observed closely for poor sucking, seizures, vomiting and diarrhea, dehydration, and an increased metabolic rate. Many withdrawal symptoms are identical to those seen in other conditions such as infection, bowel obstruction, electrolyte disorder, hydrocephalus, and intracranial anomaly. The infant could potentially have both neonatal abstinence syndrome and another condition.

Administer prescribed medications, if ordered; however, many infants are managed without drugs. Provide frequent, small, high-calorie feedings, which are more readily tolerated by these infants. Special attention is given to dietary intake during hospitalization and at home for several months, as the infant may not eat well. Keep the infant in a quiet environment with subdued lighting and minimal stimulation.

Satisfy the emotional needs of the neonate by swaddling, rocking, holding, and cuddling along with decreased light and noise. Provide a pacifier for sucking needs. Volunteers or hospital-based foster grandparents, if available, may help fulfill these needs. Such positive interaction with adults promotes comfort and supplies necessary emotional support for the infant. Hold the infant with the spine flexed to decrease extensor tone.

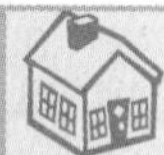

HOME CARE

Infants with neonatal abstinence syndrome are at a significantly higher risk (5–10:1) for sudden infant death syndrome when their mother used heroin or cocaine. The infant should sleep supine, and home apnea monitoring should be implemented (Blatt, Meguid, &Church, 2000).

Care in the Community

Long-term follow-up care of the child should be planned to ensure regular developmental testing and assessment for catch-up growth, neurobehavioral problems, and fetal alcohol syndrome. Interventions for any identified problem will need to be initiated. The mother will also need follow-up to determine if her drug problem has been overcome and if the infant is safe from neglect or other harmful situations. Mothers who continue to use cocaine should not breast-feed, because it is transferred in the breast milk. Care of the infant with neonatal abstinence syndrome and the substance-abusing mother often present complex family situations, and support from social services is often needed. The infant is at risk for neurobehavioral problems that a substance-abusing parent has difficulty meeting. Family resources and foster care may need to be considered if the infant does not have adequate growth. The long-term effects of this condition on cognitive function are not known at this time.

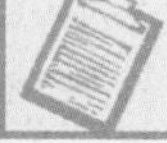

RESEARCH

A meta-analysis of 36 studies was performed to identify specific effects of uterine cocaine exposure. Less than optimal motor scores were found up to 7 months of age. No consistent negative associations were found between prenatal cocaine exposure and physical growth, developmental test scores, and receptive or expressive language. An association between cocaine exposure and decreased attentiveness and emotional expressivity was found possible. Actual long-term outcomes may be associated with the exposure dose (Frank, Augustyn, & Knight, et al., 2001).

CEREBRAL PALSY

Cerebral palsy is a nonprogressive motor and posture dysfunction that occurs secondary to CNS insults of congenital, hypoxic, ischemic, or traumatic origin, occurring in the prenatal, perinatal, or postnatal (up to 2 years) periods. Cerebral palsy is the most common chronic disorder of childhood, occurring in an estimated 1.4 to 3 per 1,000 births (Nehring, 2000). The four types of motor dysfunction seen with cerebral palsy—spastic, dyskinetic, ataxic, and mixed—are related to the location of brain insult.

CLINICAL MANIFESTATIONS OF CEREBRAL PALSY BY TYPE OF INSULT

CLASSIFICATION AND TYPE OF INSULT	CLINICAL MANIFESTATIONS
Spastic Cerebral cortex or pyramidal tract injury	Persistent hypertonia, rigidity Exaggerated deep tendon reflexes Persistent primitive reflexes Leads to contractures and abnormal curvature of the spine
Dyskinetic Extrapyramidal, basal ganglia injury	Impairment of voluntary muscle control Bizarre twisting movements Tremors, difficulty with fine and purposeful motor movements Exaggerated posturing Inconsistent muscle tone
Ataxic Cerebellar (extrapyramidal) injury	Lack of balance and position sense Hypotonia in infancy Muscle instability and gait disturbances
Mixed Injuries to multiple areas	Unique compensatory movements and posture to maintain control over specific neuromotor deficits Combination of characteristics from other types

LAW & ETHICS

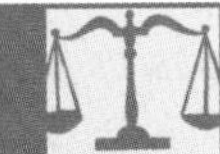

As the health care of women in labor and newborns has improved, new health issues have emerged. Fetal monitoring has led to the early diagnosis of fetal distress and improved the mortality rate of newborns. However, as more premature infants survive, more anoxic episodes also occur. Thus, the incidence of cerebral palsy has not decreased, and indeed the incidence of spastic diplegia has increased with technology improvements (Nelson & Grether, 1999). How should health care practitioners weigh the benefits and risks of certain procedures or interventions? Are parents always well informed about the benefits and risks of procedures involving their newborns? How can nurses deal with their feelings about these issues?

ETIOLOGY AND PATHOPHYSIOLOGY

The majority of cerebral palsy cases are believed to be caused by intrauterine insults or structural abnormalities of the CNS (Nelson & Grether, 1999). During gestation, insufficient nutrients and oxygen can cause damage to the developing brain of the fetus. Very premature infants are at high risk because of their immature CNS and the measures taken at birth to promote their survival. Injury at birth may be due to direct trauma to the brain or to asphyxia resulting from cord collapse, strangulation, or meconium aspiration. Asphyxia accounts for a small proportion of cerebral palsy cases. Neonatal sepsis and hyperbilirubinemia place the child at higher risk. In young children, CNS infection and head trauma are the major sources of acquired brain injury and subsequent motor dysfunction.

CLINICAL MANIFESTATIONS

Cerebral palsy is characterized by abnormal muscle tone and lack of coordination with spasticity found in the majority of cases (Table 20-11). Children have a variety of symptoms depending on their ages. See the table above for clinical manifestations by type of CNS injury. There is wide variability in symptoms depending on the area of the brain involved and the degree of anoxia. Children with cerebral palsy usually are delayed in meeting developmental milestones. For example, after 6 months of age, they may be unable to sit up, have persistent back arching, and little spontaneous movement. They frequently have other problems, including visual defects such as strabismus, nystagmus, or refractory errors; hearing loss; language delay; speech impediment; seizures; or mental retardation.

CLINICAL THERAPY

Diagnosis is usually based on clinical findings. Generally cerebral palsy is difficult to diagnose in the early months of life as it must be distinguished from other neurological conditions and signs may be subtle. Suspicious findings include an infant who is small for age; has a history of prematurity, low Apgar score (0–3 at 5 minutes), inflammatory, traumatic, or anoxic event; and also demonstrates abnormal positions and developmental delays (DeLuca, 1996). It is not uncommon for children who are delayed in meeting developmental milestones or have neuromuscular abnormalities at 1 year of age to show gradual improvement in function. In some cases, signs of dysfunction disappear entirely with physical maturation.

Clinical therapy focuses on helping the child develop to his or her maximum level of independence. Referrals are made for physical, occupational, and speech therapy, as well as

TABLE 20-11 Clinical Characteristics of Cerebral Palsy

CLINICAL CHARACTERISTICS	DEFINITIONS
Hypotonia	Floppiness, increased range of motion of joints, diminished reflex response
Hypertonia	
Rigidity	Tense, tight muscles
Spasticity	Uncoordinated, awkward, stiff movements; scissoring or crossing of the legs; exaggerated reflex reactions
Athetosis	Constant involuntary writhing motions that are more severe distally
Ataxia	Irregularity in muscle coordination or action
Hemiplegia	Involvement of one side of the body with the upper extremities being more dysfunctional than the lower extremities
Diplegia	Involvement of all extremities, but the lower extremities are more affected than the upper; usually spastic
Quadriplegia	Involvement of all extremities with the arms in flexion and legs in extension

special education to improve motor function and ability. Surgical interventions may be required to improve function by balancing muscle power and stabilizing uncontrollable joints. The Achilles tendon may be lengthened to increase range of motion in the ankle, which allows the heel to touch the floor and thus improves ambulation. The hamstrings may be released to correct knee flexion contractures. Other procedures may be performed to improve hip adduction or correct the natural position of the foot. Physical therapy and occupational therapy are provided to promote optimal independent functioning.

Medications are given to control seizures, to control spasms (skeletal muscle relaxants, baclofen, and benzodiazepines), and to minimize gastrointestinal side effects (cimetidine or ranitidine). Baclofen is administered by intrathecal pump to decrease muscle tone and vasospasms when oral administration is ineffective or causes side effects (Wiens, 1998).

The prognosis for infants and children with cerebral palsy depends on the level of physical involvement and on the presence of intellectual, visual, or hearing deficits. Many children with hemiplegia or ataxia show some improvement with maturation and are able to ambulate. Others will need assistance with mobility and activities of daily living. They are usually cared for in their homes, but in some cases receive care in long-term care facilities.

CLINICAL TIP

All infants who show symptoms of developmental delays, feeding difficulties caused by poor sucking, or abnormalities of muscle tone should be evaluated. Two simple screening assessments are as follows:

- Place a clean diaper on the infant's face. The normal infant will use two hands to remove it, but the infant with cerebral palsy will either use one hand or not remove the cloth at all.
- Turn the infant's head to one side. A persistent asymmetric tonic neck reflex (beyond 6 months of age) is an indicator of a pathologic condition. Cerebral palsy should be suspected in any infant who has persistent primitive reflexes.

NURSING MANAGEMENT

Nursing Assessment and Diagnosis

Be alert for children whose histories indicate an increased risk for cerebral palsy. Assess all children at each health care visit for developmental delays. Any orthopedic, visual, auditory, or intellectual deficits should be noted. Assess for the presence of newborn reflexes, which may persist beyond the normal age in a child with cerebral palsy. Record dietary intake and height and weight percentiles for children suspected to have or diagnosed with the condition.

Nursing diagnoses for the child with cerebral palsy vary, depending on the type, the particular child's symptoms and age, and the family situation. The accompanying nursing care plan includes several diagnoses that may be appropriate for the child with cerebral palsy. Additional nursing diagnoses may include the following:

- *Constipation,* related to low intake of fiber and fluids and insufficient physical activity
- *Impaired tissue integrity,* related to decreased physical mobility and limited self-care ability
- *Impaired verbal communication,* related to hearing and/or speech impairment

NURSING CARE PLAN The Child with Cerebral Palsy

GOAL	INTERVENTION	RATIONALE	EXPECTED OUTCOME
1. Impaired Physical Mobility related to decreased muscle strength and control			
	NIC Priority Intervention: **Exercise Therapy, Joint Mobility:** Use of active and passive body movement to maintain joint flexibility		NOC Suggested Outcome: **Joint Movement—Active:** Range of motion of joints with self-limited movement
The child will attain maximum physical abilities possible.	■ Perform development assessment and record age of achievement of milestones (e.g., reaching for objects, sitting) ■ Plan activities to use gross and fine motor skills (e.g., holding pen or eating utensils, toys positioned to encourage reaching and rolling over) ■ Allow time for the child to complete activities ■ Perform range-of-motion exercises every 4 hours for the child unable to move body parts. Position the child to promote tendon stretching (e.g., foot plantar flexion instead of dorsiflexion, legs extended instead of flexed at knees and hips) ■ Arrange for and encourage parents to keep appointments with a rehabilitation therapist. ■ Teach the family to maintain appropriate brace wear.	■ Delayed development milestones are common with cerebral palsy. Once one milestone is achieved, interventions are revised to assist in the next skill necessary. ■ Many activities of daily living and play activities promote physical development. ■ The child may perform tasks more slowly than most children. ■ Promotes mobility and increased circulation, and decreases the risk of contractures. ■ A regular and frequently reevaluated rehabilitation program assists in promoting development. ■ Adaptive devices are often necessary to maximize physical mobility.	The child reaches maximum physical mobility and all developmental milestones.
2. Sensory/Perceptual Alteration: Visual or Auditory related to cerebral damage			
	NIC Priority Intervention: **Communication Enhancement:** Visual Deficit or Auditory Deficit: Assistance with accepting or learning alternative methods for living with diminished vision or hearing.		NOC Suggested Outcome: **Body Image:** Positive perception of own appearance and body functioning
The child will receive and benefit from varied forms of sensory and perceptual input.	■ Facilitate eye and auditory examinations by specialist. Promote the use of adaptive devices (glasses, contact lenses, hearing aids), and encourage recommended return visits to specialists. ■ Maximize the use of intact senses (e.g., describe verbally the surroundings to a child with poor vision, allow touching of objects, provide visual materials to enhance learning in the child with impaired hearing, use computers to promote communication).	■ Adaptive devices often enhance sensory input. These devices need frequent changes as the child grows. ■ Other senses can compensate for those that are impaired.	The child receives adequate sensory/perceptual input to maximize developmental outcome.

(continued)

NURSING CARE PLAN The Child with Cerebral Palsy (continued)

GOAL	INTERVENTION	RATIONALE	EXPECTED OUTCOME
3. Altered Nutrition: Less than Body Requirements related to difficulty in chewing and swallowing and high metabolic needs			
	NIC Priority Intervention: **Weight Gain Assistance:** Facilitation of body weight gain.		NOC Suggested Outcome: **Nutritional Status:** Extent to which nutrients are available to meet metabolic needs.
The child will receive nutrients needed for normal growth.	■ Monitor height and weight and plot on a growth grid. Perform hydration status assessment. ■ Teach the family techniques to promote caloric and nutrient intake: ■ Position the child upright for feedings. ■ Place foods far back in the mouth to overcome tongue thrust. ■ Use soft and blended foods. ■ Allow extra time and quiet environment for meals. ■ Perform frequent respiratory assessment. Teach the family to avoid aspiration pneumonia. Teach care of gastrostomy and tube feeding technique as appropriate.	■ Insufficient intake can lead to impaired growth and dehydration. ■ Special techniques can facilitate food intake. ■ Aspiration pneumonia is a risk for the child with poor swallowing. Special feeding techniques may be needed.	The child shows normal growth patterns for height, weight, and other physical parameters.
4. Ineffective Management of Therapeutic Regimen: Family related to excessive demands made on family with child's complex care needs			
	NIC Priority Intervention: **Family Process Maintenance:** Minimization of family process disruption effects.		NOC Suggested Outcome: Not yet developed.
The family will adapt to growth and development needs of the child with cerebral palsy.	■ Allow opportunities for parents to verbalize the impact of cerebral palsy on the family. Provide referral to other parents and support groups. ■ Explore community services for rehabilitation, respite care, childcare, and other needs and refer family as appropriate. ■ During home and office visits review the child's achievements and praise the family for care provided. ■ Teach the families skills needed to manage the child's care (e.g., medication administration, physical rehabilitation, seizure management). ■ Teach case management techniques. ■ Involve siblings in the care for the child with cerebral palsy. Review for parents the needs of all children in the family.	■ The family needs an opportunity to explore the emotional and social impact of the child's care to integrate and grow from the experience. ■ Diverse services are available and will be needed due to the multiple impacts of cerebral palsy on the child. ■ The child's achievements are positive reinforcement of the family's efforts. ■ Complex skills must be learned before they can be performed with efficiency. ■ The child requires care by many specialists. Many parents become case managers to coordinate care. ■ Siblings of the child with cerebral palsy may feel left out because of the care provided. Special efforts contribute to meeting the developmental needs of all family members.	The family continues its development and provides support for all of its members.

(continued)

NURSING CARE PLAN The Child with Cerebral Palsy (continued)

GOAL	INTERVENTION	RATIONALE	EXPECTED OUTCOME
5. Diversional Activity Deficit (Child) related to poor social skills			
	NIC Priority Intervention: **Recreation Therapy:** Purposeful use of recreation to promote relaxation and enhancement of social skills.		NOC Suggested Outcome: **Play Participation:** Use of activities as needed for enjoyment, entertainment, and development by children.
The child will engage in adequate diversional activity to maximize growth and development.	■ Refer the family to early childhood stimulation programs. Encourage contact with other children. When hospitalized, place the child in a room with other children when possible.	■ The child needs a variety of activities and contact with other children and adults to maximize development.	The child engages in activities that maximize development.
	■ Work with the local school to develop an individualized education plan that allows the child contact with other children and a variety of activities.	■ Public schools must provide an individualized education plan. Parents may need assistance to interact effectively with the school system.	
	■ Investigate recreational programs for children with disabilities and share information with the parents.	■ Recreational programs for children with disabilities may promote social experiences and physical activity.	

- *Impaired home maintenance management,* related to child's developmental disability and inadequate support system
- *Altered growth and development,* related to lack of muscle strength or limited social interaction

Planning and Implementation

The accompanying nursing care plan summarizes care for the child with cerebral palsy. Because the condition can range from mild to severe and involve numerous manifestations, interventions need to be adapted to the particular child and family. Nursing care focuses on providing adequate nutrition, maintaining skin integrity, promoting physical mobility, promoting safety, promoting growth and development, teaching parents how to care for the child, and providing emotional support.

Provide Adequate Nutrition

Children with cerebral palsy require high-calorie diets or supplements to the diet because of feeding difficulties associated with spasticity. Many children have difficulty chewing and swallowing. Give the child small amounts of soft foods at a time. Feeding utensils with large, padded handles may be easier for the child to use.

Clinical Tip

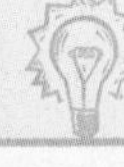

Provide audio and visual activities for the child who is quadriplegic. Encourage the use of a computer to interact with peers, participate in educational programs, and locate resources for adaptation to the disability. Television, videotapes, and music are good diversions. Encourage the child who is paraplegic to use his or her arms and hands in interactive games. Children can use special hand controls or pointers for computer or video game use and other adaptive devices to manipulate the television or radio.

Maintain Skin Integrity

Take special care to protect the bony prominences from skin breakdown. See Table 20-5 for specific nursing interventions.

Proper body alignment should be maintained at all times. Support the child with pillows, towels, and bolsters whether the child is in bed or in a chair. Support the head and body of a floppy infant. A spastic child with scissored, extended legs or an athetoid child who writhes constantly is difficult to carry and transport.

Promote Physical Mobility

Range-of-motion exercises are essential to maintain joint flexibility and to prevent contractures. Consult with the physical therapists who work with the child and assist with recommended exercises. Teach parents to position the child to foster flexion rather than extension so that interaction with the environment can be enhanced (e.g., the child can bring objects closer to the face). Encourage parents to bring the child's adaptive appliances (customized wheelchairs, braces) to the hospital to prevent deterioration during hospitalizations. Refer parents to the appropriate resources for help with the acquisition of adaptive devices (Figure 20-17 ◆).

Skill 3-3: Transporting the Child with a Disability

Promote Safety

Teach parents the importance of using safety belts with children in strollers and wheelchairs. A helmet should be worn by the child with chronic seizures to protect from further injury during seizures.

Promote Growth and Development

Remember that many children with cerebral palsy are physically but not intellectually disabled. Use terminology appropriate for the child's developmental level. Help the child develop a positive self-image to ensure emotional health and social growth. Children with a hearing impairment may need referral to learn American Sign Language or other communication methods.

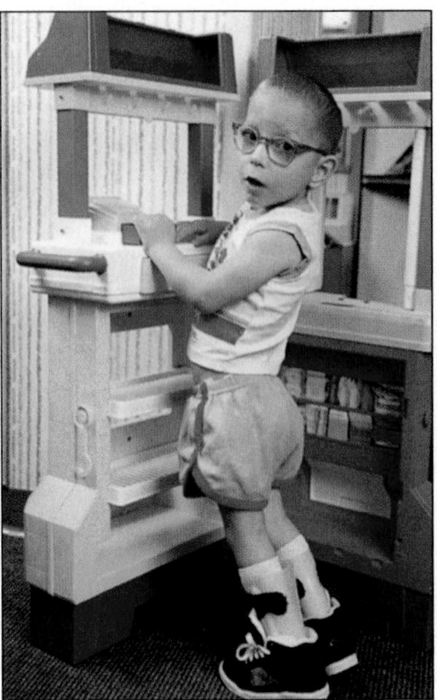

FIGURE 20-17 ◆
A child with cerebral palsy has abnormal muscle tone and lack of physical coordination.

Foster Parental Knowledge

Teach parents about the disorder and arrange sessions to teach them about all of the child's special needs. Teach administration, desired effects, and side effects of medications prescribed for seizures. Make sure parents are aware of the need for dental care when anticonvulsants are prescribed.

Provide Emotional Support

Refer parents to individual and family counseling if appropriate. Listen to the parents' concerns and encourage them to express their feelings and ask questions. Explain what they can expect regarding future treatment. Work with other health care professionals to help families adjust to this chronic disease.

Care in the Community

Children with cerebral palsy need continuous support in the community. A case manager such as the parent or nurse will likely be needed to coordinate care. As they grow, these children will need new adaptive devices, ongoing developmental assessment and care planning, and possibly surgery. Although the brain lesion does not change, it manifests itself in different ways as the child grows. For example, once the child begins to walk, the extensor tone may cause Achilles cord tightening. Braces may be used to decrease deformities, but surgery may eventually be needed. Later, surgery may be needed to loosen tight tendons in the knees or hips (Dzienkowski, Smith, & Dillow, et al., 1996). Speech therapy may be needed, as well as new glasses and eye examinations as the child grows. The child may need an individualized education plan to maximize learning potential (see Chapter 6). Other parents of children with cerebral palsy can provide needed support.

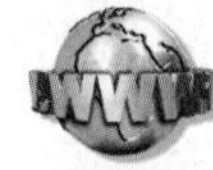

Cerebral Palsy Online

Early intervention programs can help parents learn how to meet their child's special needs, including physical, occupational, and speech therapy, as well as educational needs. Parents may need financial assistance to provide the care that the child needs and to obtain appliances such as braces, wheelchairs, or adaptive utensils. Technology offers many new strategies to promote communication and self-care by these children. The nurse can be instrumental in helping parents meet the needs of the child with cerebral palsy in preschools, schools, offices, clinics, and other settings. In addition, the nurse makes referrals as appropriate to early intervention programs, support groups, and organizations such as the United Cerebral Palsy Association and Shriners Hospitals. Recreational activities may be identified through the National Association of Sports for Cerebral Palsy.

CLINICAL TIP

Assistive technology is any item, piece of equipment, or product system modified or customized for use to improve or maintain functional capabilities of individuals with disabilities so that they are as independent as possible.

Transition programs assist the family and adolescent with cerebral palsy to develop plans for adult living. The young adult (18 to 21 years) may be able to move into a group home or live independently if desired. Vocational training options can be explored. Nurses in hospital programs may coordinate transition into smaller communities and settings and to assist the family in gaining access to available resources.

Evaluation

Expected outcomes of nursing care for the child with cerebral palsy are provided on the nursing care plan.

INJURIES OF THE NEUROLOGIC SYSTEM

TRAUMATIC BRAIN INJURY

A traumatic brain injury can be defined as any trauma involving the scalp, cranial bones, or structures within the skull resulting from force or penetration. Traumatic brain injuries are the most common injuries in childhood, with approximately 200,000 children hospitalized each year and 5,000 deaths. Approximately 30,000 children and adolescents under 19 years of age develop a permanent disability from a moderate or severe injury such as epilepsy, cognitive impairment, learning problems, and behavioral or emotional problems (Rosman, 1999).

Children are prone to skull fractures, often resulting in hematomas and brain injury. They may suffer from the secondary effects of trauma, such as diffuse cerebral edema, malignant brain edema, and increased intracranial pressure.

Young children with moderate and severe traumatic brain injury are at risk for long-term cognitive deficits. Most recovery occurs in the first 12 months following injury. With fewer well-established skills and knowledge and the slowed processing of information and attention impairment following the brain injury, the child has more challenges to develop cognitive and social competence (Anderson, Catroppa, & Morse, et al., 2000).

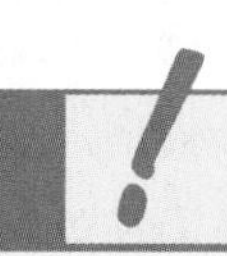

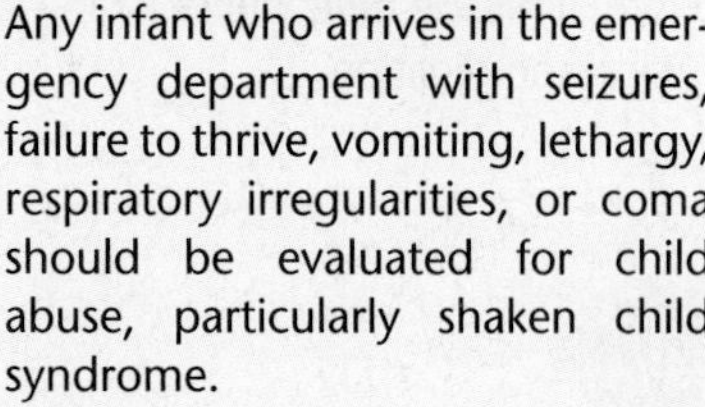

Any infant who arrives in the emergency department with seizures, failure to thrive, vomiting, lethargy, respiratory irregularities, or coma should be evaluated for child abuse, particularly shaken child syndrome.

Etiology and Pathophysiology

Falls are a major cause of unintentional head injuries in young children. Infants fall from dressing tables, beds, and sofas and also tumble down stairs, especially in walkers (American Academy of Pediatrics Committee on Injury and Poison Prevention, 2001). Child abuse accounts for a large number of traumatic brain injuries in children under 1 year of age. Toddlers and preschoolers lack good judgment, and so may run haphazardly into the street or lean out of windows and fall. School-age children may be injured in motor vehicle crashes, either as passengers or pedestrians, and they may also be injured in bicycle, roller-blading, scooter, or skateboard mishaps. Adolescents are frequently the drivers in motor vehicle crashes; often alcohol or drugs are involved. Teenagers are also injured in sports-related accidents (see Chapter 7).

Brain injuries can be categorized as either primary or secondary. Primary injuries occur at the time of the insult when the initial cellular damage occurs. These injuries result from either a direct blow to the head (coup injury) or acceleration-deceleration movement of the brain within the skull (contrecoup injury; Figure 20-18 ◆). At the time of impact, arterial and intracranial pressures increase, and apnea and loss of consciousness occur.

The secondary phase of head trauma is a biochemical and cellular response to the initial insult, and can be manifested immediately or over hours, days, or weeks. Damage usually results from destruction of brain tissue secondary to hypoxia, hypotension, edema, change in the blood-brain barrier, or hemorrhage (Rosman, 1999). The result is increased intracranial pressure.

Clinical Manifestations

The signs and symptoms of head injuries in children depend on the pathologic features and severity of the injury. The child with a mild head injury may remain conscious or have brief loss of consciousness. The child with a moderate head injury loses consciousness for 5 to 10 minutes. Following mild and moderate head injuries, children may have amnesia about the event, headache, nausea, and vomiting. A child with a severe head injury, such as Antwan in the opening scenario, is usually unconscious for more than 10 minutes and may rapidly show signs of increased intracranial pressure.

Unconsciousness may result from increased intracranial pressure, edema, hemorrhage, or parenchymal damage to both cerebral cortices or the brainstem. Posttraumatic seizures

PATHOPHYSIOLOGY ILLUSTRATED

Subdural vessels are torn
Contrecoup injury results from secondary impact as brain moves forward and then backward within skull
Coup injury results from initial impact
Bruising occurs as brain moves over skull floor

Brain Injury

FIGURE 20-18 ◆
Brain injury can result form a direct blow to the head (coup injury) or the acceleration-deceleration movement of the brain (contrecoup injury).

are common. Retinal hemorrhages are seen in 65% to 90% of children with inflicted traumatic brain injury (Schutzman & Greenes, 2001)

Vital signs are important indicators of head injury. Changes in respiratory effort or periods of apnea can occur secondary to shock, injury to the spinal cord above C4, or damage to or pressure on the medulla. Heart rate and blood pressure are indices of brainstem function. Tachycardia can be a sign of blood loss, shock, hypoxia, anxiety, or pain. **Cushing's triad,** associated with increased intracranial pressure or compromised blood flow to the brainstem, is characterized by hypertension, increased systolic pressure with wide pulse pressure, bradycardia, and irregular respirations. Refer to the earlier discussion of altered states of consciousness for more information about increased intracranial pressure.

Reflexes may be hyporesponsive, hyperresponsive, or nonexistent. The child may assume a decorticate, decerebrate, **areflexic** (no response to verbal, sensory, or pain stimulation), or flaccid posture (see Figure 20-2).

Clinical Therapy

Identifying the severity of a brain injury involves history, observation, examination, and diagnostic testing. Ask questions about how the injury occurred, the child's initial responses and current responses, any loss of consciousness, and the child's memory of the event.

Neurologic evaluation with the pediatric Glasgow Coma Scale is performed frequently to detect changes in the child's condition (see Table 20-3). Cranial nerves are assessed (see Table 20-4). See Chapter 4 and the earlier discussion of altered states of consciousness for further details.

Laboratory tests include a complete blood cell count, blood chemistry, toxicology screening, and urinalysis.

Radiologic examination is performed to identify the specific injury. Skull films are used to detect fractures. A CT scan is used to detect fractures, hematomas, lacerations, or contusions. An MRI scan may be performed to visualize subtle damage or injury. The presence of a fracture indicates a more serious injury.

NURSING ALERT

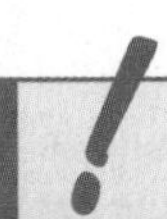

Most children with head injuries are the victims of multiple trauma, and even though cervical spine injuries are rare, all children should be suspected of having a cervical spine injury until this possibility has been ruled out by radiologic examination.

The initial management of a child with a brain injury is based on the child's physiologic status. The airway must be clear and stable, and hypoxia must be prevented. If indicated, the child is intubated, sedated, and chemically paralyzed.

Perfusion of the brain must be maintained to ensure that it gets adequate oxygen and nutrients. Shock is treated aggressively with fluid boluses. Keep the head of the bed flat until adequate cerebral perfusion pressure is ensured. Inotropes may be used to ensure perfusion if **cerebral edema** (the increase in intracellular and extracellular fluid in the brain that results from anoxia, vasodilation, or vascular stasis) is present.

Increased intracranial pressure must be controlled. Hypoxia and hypercapnia have disastrous effects on cerebral function, as they can cause vasodilation and increased intracranial pressure. Effective assisted ventilation with 100% oxygen at the child's normal respiratory rate is used in the first 24 hours after injury; however, hyperventilation may be used in subsequent days (Rosman, 1999). If there is no cervical spine injury, the head of the bed is elevated up to 30 degrees. The child's head is kept in the midline to promote venous (jugular) drainage. Hip flexion is avoided. Acetaminophen can be given for pain. The child's body temperature is kept within normal limits. The environment is kept as quiet as possible. Fluids may be restricted only after the child is hemodynamically stable. Diuretics such as mannitol or furosemide may be given to shrink brain volume. A urinary catheter is inserted to monitor output, and electrolytes should be checked frequently.

Invasive procedures may be necessary to reduce increased intracranial pressure. Burr holes may be made or more extensive surgery performed as a method of evacuating a lesion or hematoma. A ventricular catheter may be placed to drain cerebrospinal fluid and to monitor pressure.

Aggressive support continues until the child regains consciousness and rehabilitation can be initiated. Reliable predictions of outcome in the child who has suffered a severe brain injury cannot be made until 6 to 12 months postinjury.

NURSING MANAGEMENT

CLINICAL TIP

A child who has a decreased level of consciousness shortly after a head injury may have had a posttraumatic seizure and may still be in the postictal state.

Nursing Assessment and Diagnosis

Assess the child's neurologic status frequently. Evaluate the child's level of consciousness continually using the pediatric Glasgow Coma Scale (see Table 20-3). Monitor vital signs closely. Changes in these signs may indicate hypoxia, decreased perfusion, shock, or increased intracranial pressure. The child's neurologic status is compared with his or her previous state, with improvement, stability, or deterioration noted. The cause of any deterioration must be quickly determined and appropriate interventions taken.

The following nursing diagnoses may be appropriate for the child with a head injury:

- *Altered cerebral tissue perfusion,* related to hypoventilation, hypovolemia, and/or reduction of arterial blood flow to the brain due to increased intracranial pressure
- *Risk for aspiration,* related to decreased level of consciousness
- *Caregiver role strain,* related to 24-hour care responsibility of a child with neurologic complications
- *Altered family processes,* related to shift in health status of child
- *Altered growth and development,* related to serious brain injury

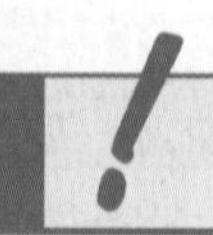

NURSING ALERT

In the child with moderate head injury, the oxygen saturation should remain over 95%. For the severely injured child who is intubated, monitor arterial blood gas results. The PaO_2 should be 70–100 mm Hg.

Planning and Implementation

Nursing care focuses on maintaining cardiopulmonary function, preventing complications, promoting recovery, and providing emotional support. Nursing management is based on prevention of secondary injury and return to an optimal level of function.

MAINTAIN CARDIOPULMONARY FUNCTION

In the moderately injured child, observe breathing patterns and check skin color and level of consciousness. Check the pulse oximeter. Report any sign of decreased oxygenation to the physician immediately.

Ensure that the siderails of the bed are padded to protect the child if a seizure occurs. Equipment for suction and ventilation should be at bedside.

Prevent Complications

Position the child properly, maintain a quiet environment, and control body temperature. Administer medications as ordered. Check intracranial monitors or surgical sites if invasive measures have been taken. Report any signs and symptoms of increased intracranial pressure (see Table 20-2) to the physician immediately.

Promote Recovery

Prevent physical deformities. Physical, occupational, and speech therapy should begin in the hospital. Work with these therapists to reinforce exercises and help teach parents the techniques so they can work with the child in the hospital and at home. The nurse can reinforce what has been done during these sessions, noting positive changes. Using toys, books, music, or games, provide stimulation based on the child's age and ability. Encourage parents to bring in favorite toys, stuffed animals, and tape recordings of the child's favorite music or of family members talking.

Provide Emotional Support

Nurses, social workers, physicians, psychologists, rehabilitation therapists, and members of the clergy can support and help parents adjust to having a child with a new disability.

Discharge Planning and Home Care Teaching

Home care needs should be identified and addressed well in advance of discharge. Children with significant injuries will benefit from inpatient or outpatient rehabilitation to promote optimal achievement of function. A case manager may be needed to coordinate services and resources during rehabilitation.

Give parents information about caring for children with head injuries at home and possible behaviors to expect from the child. For children with disabilities, determine what adaptations are needed in the home to care for the child, such as a wheelchair, walker, braces, or special bed. Social work and home health agencies can often help the parents make special arrangements.

Care in the Community

Arrange for home care nursing and follow-up care, if necessary. The home care nurse can assume the role of case manager for the disabled child and make sure the environment is safe. Many children with brain injuries are disabled enough to qualify for Social Security's Supplemental Security Income (SSI) benefits or the state program for children with special health care needs.

Parents of children with mild or moderate injuries need to be prepared for typical behavior after a head injury, until full recovery has occurred. If the child returns to school, help prepare the teachers, school administrators, and other children for how their classmate is "different." Such sensitivity training makes reintegrating the child into the classroom easier.

The child or adolescent who is facing long-term rehabilitation requires support to adjust to the disability and to find the strength to maximize his or her abilities. Identify recreational opportunities for the child with disabilities to promote exercise and self-esteem. The adolescent may need to gain vocational skills and learn to live independently. Refer parents to the Brain Injury Association for further information.

HOME CARE

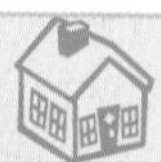

Even though the child looks normal within days of a mild or moderate head injury, brain healing takes up to 6 weeks. Parents and teachers should be made aware that typical behavior during this period may include any of the following behaviors: tiring easily, memory loss or forgetfulness, easy distractibility, difficulty concentrating, difficulty following directions, irritability or short temper, and needing help starting and finishing tasks. Educational assessment should be initiated if recovery takes longer than 6 weeks.

LAW & ETHICS

Public Law 104–166, the Traumatic Brain Injury Act, was enacted by Congress in 1996 to prevent brain injuries and to minimize the severity of dysfunction as a result of brain injury by providing funding to states to identify mechanisms to improve access to services (U.S. Congress, 1996).

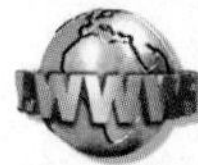

Traumatic Brain Injury Resources

Evaluation

Examples of expected outcomes of nursing care for the child with traumatic brain injury include the following:

- Cerebral perfusion pressure is maintained at an adequate rate to sustain oxygenation of the brain.

- Muscle function is maintained and physical deformities are prevented with range-of-motion exercises and splinting during the recovery stages of the brain injury.
- Parents are supported through the child's acute recovery phase and learn to provide appropriate care at home.

SPECIFIC HEAD INJURIES

SCALP INJURIES

Injuries to the scalp, which can be caused by falls, blunt trauma, or penetration of a foreign body, are usually benign. Although bleeding may be extensive, hypovolemia or shock is uncommon unless the patient is an infant.

Lacerations should be irrigated with copious amounts of sterile normal saline solution and inspected for bony fragments or depressions, cerebrospinal fluid leakage with a dural tear, or debris. If the injury is simple, the laceration can be sutured and the child discharged from the emergency department. If not, a neurosurgeon should be consulted.

CONCUSSION

A concussion can involve transient impairment of consciousness that usually results from blunt head trauma. It is secondary to stretching, compression, or shearing of nerve fibers. There is usually no gross structural damage or focal injury. The child will have an alteration in mental status (e.g., amnesia, dizziness, memory or orientation impairment, unsteady gait), but not necessary loss of consciousness. Concussions are categorized by three levels of severity, as discussed in Table 20-12.

CLINICAL TIP

Sports with a high risk for concussion include boxing, field hockey, football, ice hockey, lacrosse, martial arts, soccer, rodeo, wrestling, rugby, baseball, rollerblading, trampolining, and basketball. Up to 36% of high school football players experience a concussion each year. Athletes who sustain a concussion are nearly 3 times as likely to have a second concussion in the same season (Guskiewicz, Weaver, & Padua, et al., 2000).

Treatment is supportive. Children are observed in the emergency department for several hours before being sent home with instructions to the parents to watch them closely for decreased responsiveness. Any child who is unconscious for more than 5 minutes or has amnesia of the event may be admitted to the hospital or observed in a short-stay unit to rule out other injury.

Pediatric concussive syndrome, believed to be caused by an injury to the brainstem, is seen in children who are less than 3 years of age. Toddlers seem stunned at the time of injury, but do not lose consciousness. Later, however, these children become pale, clammy, and lethargic, and they may vomit. They are usually brought to the hospital for treatment when such symptoms appear. These children may be placed in a short-stay unit for observation and usually recover within 24 hours.

Postconcussive syndrome, common in both children and adults, may occur anytime after the initial head injury. Signs and symptoms can include headache, dizziness or vertigo, fatigue, irritability, photophobia, subtle changes in personality, poor concentration, poor memory, and ataxia. Treatment is supportive. Symptoms usually disappear within several weeks but may last

TABLE 20-12 Levels of Concussion Severity

GRADE 1
Transient confusion, no loss of consciousness, and a duration of mental status abnormalities of less than 15 minutes.
GRADE 2
Transient confusion, no loss of consciousness, and a duration of mental status abnormalities of 15 minutes or longer.
GRADE 3
Loss of consciousness, either brief (seconds) or prolonged (minutes or longer).
Note: Adapted from Quality Standards Subcommittee, American Academy of Neurology. (1997). Practice parameters: The management of concussion in sports. *Neurology, 48,* 581–585.

up to 6 months. Parents and teachers should be informed to expect altered behavior in the child. They should be encouraged to help the child maintain self-esteem.

Young athletes suffering a second concussion before complete recovery from the first develop *second impact syndrome.* This injury results in acute brain swelling, neurologic or cognitive deficits, and sometimes death from the cumulative effect of these concussions. Recommendations should be followed for the management of sports-related concussions to reduce the risk of disability and death. Removal from sports participation ranges from 1 week to the entire season, depending on the severity of concussion and neurologic symptoms (Guskiewicz et al., 2000).

SKULL FRACTURES

A fracture to any of the eight cranial bones is caused by a considerable force to the head. Any area of the skull with swelling or a hematoma should be evaluated for possible fracture. Diagnosis is made by visual inspection, palpation, radiologic study, or CT scan. Treatment should always include neurosurgical consultation.

Management of skull fractures depends on the type and extent of injury (Table 20-13 and Figure 20-19 ◆).

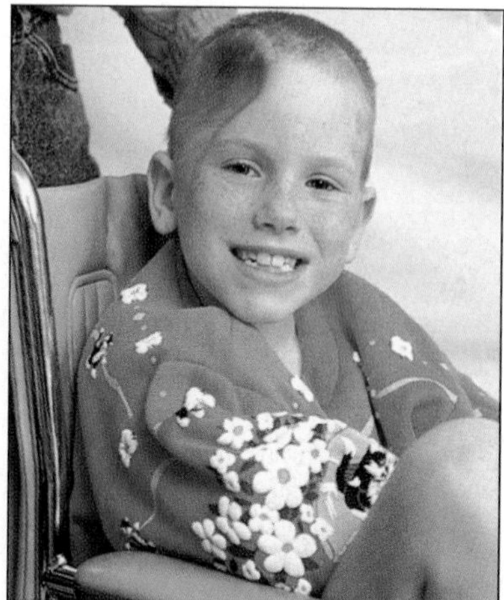

FIGURE 20-19 ◆
This child has had a significant depressed skull fracture that required removal of bony fragments over a section of the skull.

CEREBRAL CONTUSION

A cerebral contusion, or the bruising of brain tissue, is secondary to blunt trauma and can occur with either coup or contrecoup injuries (see Figure 20-18). Such injuries are rare in children less than 1 year of age. The temporal or frontal sections of the skull are the most

TABLE 20-13 Skull Fractures

INJURY	CLINICAL THERAPY
Linear fracture Results from impact to large area of the skull. Usually no symptoms. May have overlying hematoma or soft tissue swelling.	If fracture is on temporal bone or crosses sagittal suture line, a CT scan is performed to detect potential epidural hematoma. Consider the possibility of inflicted injury.
Depressed fracture Break in skull itself or an area shattered into many fragments. Pieces of bone may be depressed into brain tissue with hematoma forming on top.	Plain radiographic film or CT scan is performed. Surgery to elevate bone fragments when depression is greater than 5 mm. Tetanus prophylaxis is given as needed. Many are associated with intracranial injury and posttraumatic epilepsy.
Compound fracture Combination of a full-thickness scalp laceration and depressed skull fracture with the bone exposed. Injuries are considered penetrating fractures if the dura is torn.	Visual diagnosis is performed along with radiographic studies. Surgical debridement, a search for foreign bodies, and copious irrigation are performed. Parenteral antibiotics and tetanus prophylaxis are provided as needed.
Basilar fracture Fracture at the base of the skull that may involve the frontal, ethmoid, sphenoid, temporal, or occipital bones. A dural tear may be present.	Diagnosis is confirmed by signs of blood behind the tympanic membranes, cerebrospinal fluid leakage from the nose or ears, periorbital ecchymosis (raccoon eyes), or bruising of the mastoid (Battle sign). Radiographic imaging locates the fracture site. Antibiotics may be prescribed. Surgical repair of the site of the cerebrospinal fluid leak is performed if the leak persists after 7–10 days. Transient or permanent cranial nerve injuries occur (e.g., hearing loss).

Note: Adapted from Rosman, N. P. (1999). Acute head trauma. In J. A. McMillan, C. D. DeAngelis, R. D. Feigin, & J. B. Warshaw, *Oski's pediatrics: Principles and practice* (3rd ed., pp. 603–617). Philadelphia: Lippincott, Williams, & Wilkins.

common sites of this injury, which involves damage to the parenchyma with tears in vessels or tissue, pulping, and subsequent areas of necrosis or infarction.

The child may have focal symptoms depending on the area of injury. Altered levels of consciousness range from confusion and disorientation to being obtunded. A CT scan is used for diagnosis.

Treatment involves hospitalization for observation and to rule out other injuries. Surgical treatment is rarely necessary.

Sequelae are focal and specific to the area of the brain that was injured. For example, an injury to the left temporal area may affect speech.

INTRACRANIAL HEMATOMAS

Intracranial hematomas are space-occupying lesions that expand rapidly or slowly, depending on whether they are arterial or venous in origin. They must be located quickly.

TABLE 20-14 Intracranial Hematomas

TYPE OF HEMATOMA	DIAGNOSIS AND MANAGEMENT
Subdural Hematoma Result of severe head trauma such as falls, assaults, motor vehicle crashes, or shaken child syndrome Occurs most frequently in children less than 1 year of age Caused by laceration of the bridging veins; clot forms and presses directly on brain, leading to damage from two sources: original contusion and hematoma, usually venous Symptoms (may not appear until 48–72 hours after the injury) include: Change in level of consciousness (confusion, agitation, or lethargy) Nausea or vomiting Headache Retinal hemorrhages in both eyes Pupil on side of injury may be fixed and dilated Seizures Fever	Diagnosis confirmed by CT scan Treatment is usually surgical; subdural taps may be necessary after surgery to give the brain room to expand More than half of children with subdural hematomas die; those who survive have 75% chance of developing seizures 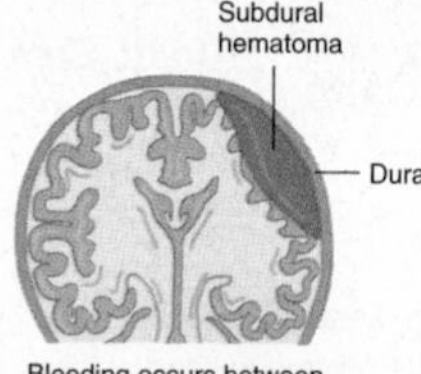 Bleeding occurs between dura and brain
Epidural Hematoma Rare in children and almost never occurs in children less than 4 years of age Results from blunt trauma (most often falls), motor vehicle crashes, assaults, or baseball to temporal area Temporal and parietal areas are most common sites May be associated with linear skull fracture May be fatal if bleeding is arterial Symptoms include: Brief loss of consciousness followed by lucid period and rapid deterioration Sleepiness or lethargy Headache Full fontanel Paresis of cranial nerves III and VI Papilledema Fixed and dilated pupil Signs of increased intracranial pressure	Diagnosis confirmed by CT scan Treatment involves immediate surgical intervention; craniotomy is performed followed by evacuation of the hematoma Prognosis is good, although 25% of children have seizures 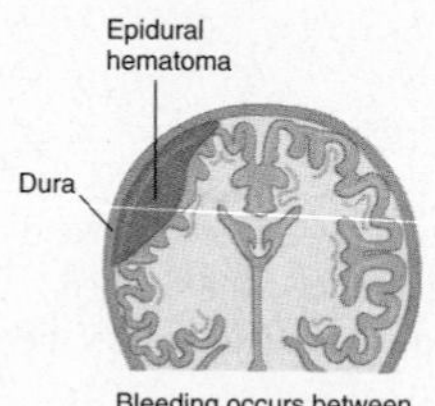 Bleeding occurs between dura and skull
Intracerebral Hematoma Result of deep confusion or intracerebral laceration (secondary to foreign body or bony penetration or impalement) Causes diffuse bleeding in parenchyma; there may be a hematoma with associated small areas of bleeding	Diagnosis confirmed by CT scan Surgical treatment not indicated Neurologic effects depend on size and location of lesion and whether bleeding can be controlled; hemiplegia or visual loss may result 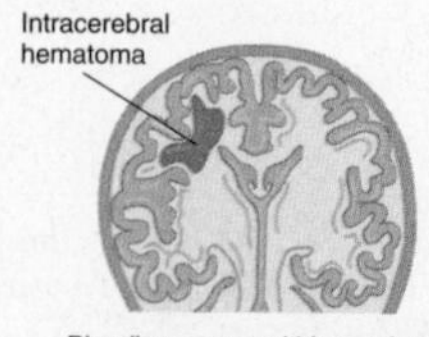 Bleeding occurs within cerebrum

Some lesions require evacuation as soon as possible to minimize the secondary effects of the injury. Table 20-14 describes types of intracranial hematomas and their treatment.

Subarachnoid hemorrhages, associated with severe head injuries such as intracranial hematomas or contusions, result from laceration of arteries or veins in the subarachnoid space. Symptoms include decreased level of consciousness, ipsilateral pupil dilation, diplopia, hemiparesis, nausea and vomiting, nuchal rigidity, and headache.

Diagnosis is confirmed by CT scan. There is no specific treatment, and the clinical course depends on associated injuries.

PENETRATING INJURIES

Gunshot wounds to the head can damage tissue, bone, and vessels. Low-velocity bullets enter but do not exit the skull; instead they ricochet within the cranial vault, destroying brain tissue and vessels. Although the child may be conscious just after the injury, the level of consciousness quickly deteriorates because of the edema surrounding the penetration tract. High-velocity bullets, on the other hand, cause immediate, severe damage on impact. See Chapter 7 for a discussion of violence in childhood. CT is used to evaluate gunshot trauma and to pinpoint the location of bullet and bone fragments as well as parenchymal damage. Treatment involves surgical debridement of the tract, evacuation of any hematomas, and removal of accessible bone or bullet particles. Approximately 50% of children with gunshot wounds to the head die. Those who survive may suffer multiple focal deficits and seizures.

Impalement injuries frequently occur in children in association with lawn darts or dog bites. All objects must be left in place and removed in the operating room by a neurosurgeon. The child with an impalement injury is at high risk for focal injury and infection. After surgery, children with this type of injury are managed as with other postoperative head injuries, with attention focused on level of consciousness, increased intracranial pressure, and infection control.

SPINAL CORD INJURY

Less than 5% of spinal cord injuries occur annually in children under 16 years of age (Massagli, 2000). Many children with these injuries die within the first hour of trauma or during the first 3 months after trauma.

Motor vehicle crashes are the leading cause of spinal cord injuries, either pedestrian–vehicular, bicycle–vehicular, passenger, or driver related. Other causes of spinal injuries, especially in toddlers and young children, include falls and child abuse. Recreation or sports-related trauma accounts for more injuries as children grow older. Penetrating injuries such as stabbings and gunshot wounds are becoming more prevalent.

The mechanism of injury determines the type of lesion that occurs (Figure 20-20 ◆). Hyperflexion injuries produce tears or avulsions and fractures of vertebral bodies, as well as subluxation and dislocation. Lateral flexion (rotation) may cause joint dislocations or unstable spinal fractures. Extension may result in the so-called hangman's fracture, ligament tears, avulsion fractures of vertebral bodies, and central or posterior spinal cord syndrome. Compression injuries cause anterior cord syndrome.

Spinal cord injuries are classified as complete or incomplete. Complete lesions are irreversible and involve a loss of sensory, motor, and autonomic function below the level of the injury. Incomplete lesions involve varying degrees of sensory, motor, and autonomic function below the level of injury.

Children are prone to specific kinds of spinal cord injuries because of the extreme mobility and flexibility of their spinal column. Table 20-15 describes the spinal cord injuries most common in children.

The higher the level of spinal cord injury, the more severe the neurologic damage. The child is often a victim of multiple trauma and may display signs of hypovolemic shock resulting from other injuries, increased intracranial pressure, or respiratory depression. Children can also experience neurogenic or spinal shock (see Chapter 14).

At the time of injury, the child is flaccid and areflexic below the lesion and responds only to stimuli above the level of injury. Priapism may be present. Muscle spasticity below the lesion occurs later. Respiratory compromise may be present due to paralysis of the diaphragm.

GROWTH & DEVELOPMENT

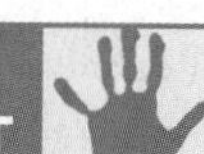

The vertebrae are incompletely ossified in children under 9 years. The facet joints are more shallow and horizontal. The young child's head is relatively large compared with the strength of the neck muscles. The fulcrum is at the C2–C3 level so injuries are more likely to occur at the C1–C3 level under 9 years and at the C4–C6 level for children 9–15 years (Massagli, 2000).

SCIWORA

Spinal cord injury without radiographic abnormality (SCIWORA) accounts for 15%–25% of all pediatric spinal cord trauma. SCIWORA occurs when initial films or CT scans show no bony deformity and the child is believed to be free of injury. Profound or progressive paralysis is found either immediately or within 48 hours. An MRI can detect the injury.

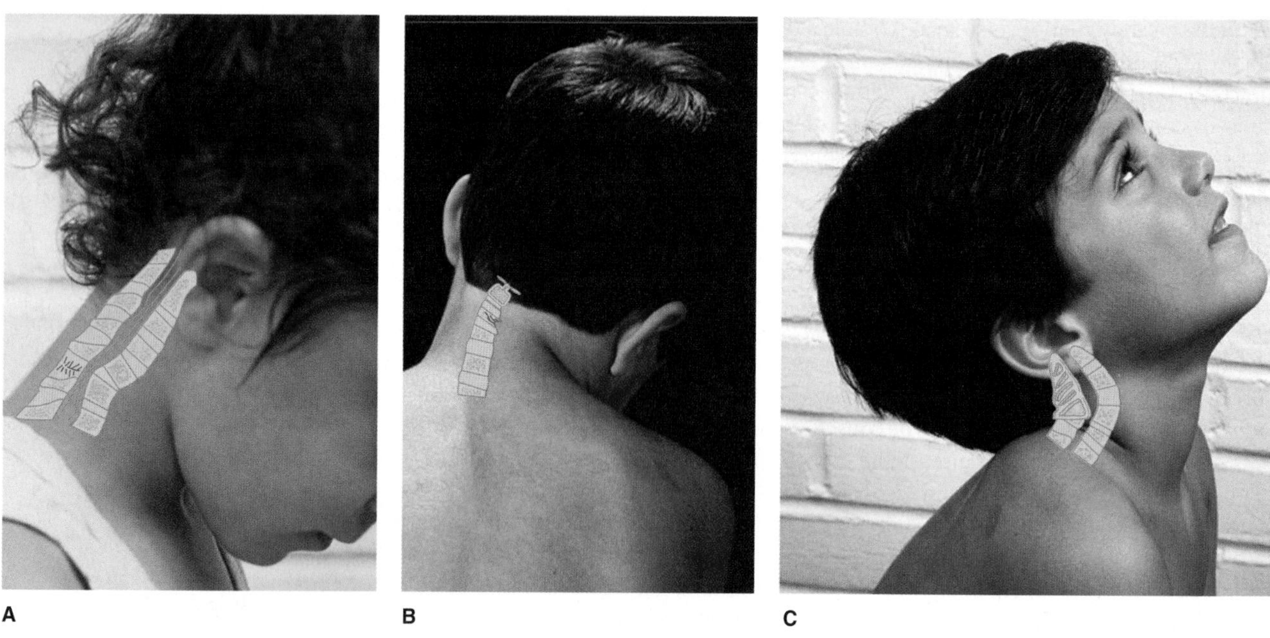

A B C

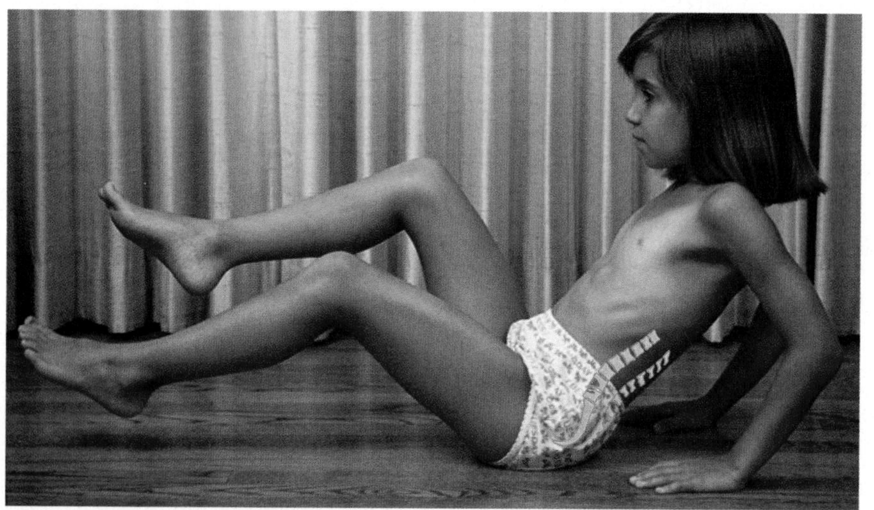

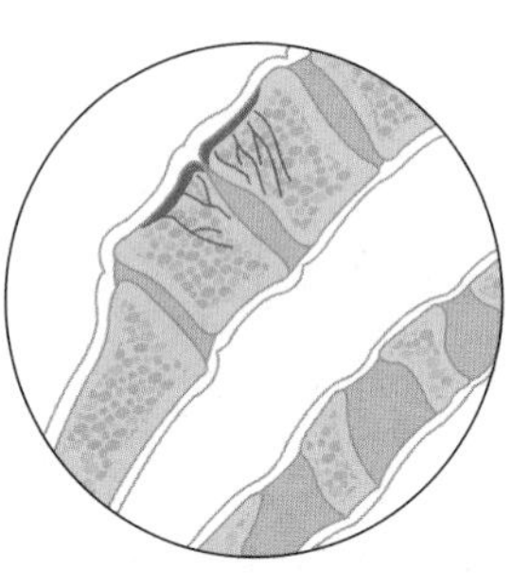

D

FIGURE 20-20 ◆

Mechanics of injury to the spinal cord. A, Hyperflexion. B, Lateral flexion. C, Extension. D, Compression.

Diagnosis is made by observation, neurologic examination, and x-ray studies. X-ray studies include lateral cervical spine and anteroposterior and lateral views of the thoracic and lumbosacral spine. In addition, CT scanning, MRI, fluoroscopy, or myelography may be performed. Many children have spinal cord injury without radiographic abnormality (SCIWORA) (Massagli, 2000).

Spinal injuries are managed aggressively. The child with a spinal cord injury may be placed in skeletal traction or a halo device. Further surgical management of the injury may be necessary. Debridement and decompression should be accomplished within the first 8 hours after penetrating injury. A fusion using bone from another part of the body may be performed to stabilize the spinal cord. If more drastic measures are necessary, an internal fixation device may be required.

To further decrease neurologic sequelae, methylprednisolone is administered in high doses to children with motor deficits. Administration must be started within 8 hours of the injury.

TABLE 20-15 Spinal Cord Injuries in Children
CERVICAL REGION
■ Site of 75% of spinal injuries in children through 8 years and 60% between 8 and 14 years ■ Highest incidence above C3 segment ■ Many of these injuries are fatal
THORACOLUMBAR REGION
■ Second most common area of injury; probably a result of improperly placed lap belts ■ Most injuries occur at the L2–L4 level
THORACIC REGION
■ Site of 20% of spinal injuries usually between 8 and 14 years

Complications of spinal cord injury include the following:

- Scoliosis if injury occurs before the skeleton is immature
- Impaired respiratory function due to a paralyzed diaphragm or diminished vital capacity
- Hip instability due to poor acetabular development
- Pathologic fractures of the long bones due to immobilization hypercalcemia
- Pressure sores
- Deep vein thrombosis
- Autonomic dysreflexia (hypertension, bradycardia, severe headaches, pallor below and flushing above the level of the cord lesion, and seizures)

An interdisciplinary approach is required to manage the rehabilitation and long-term care needs of the child and family.

Nursing Management

Nursing care focuses on monitoring vital signs, meeting nutritional needs, maintaining skin integrity, promoting independent functioning, encouraging therapeutic play, providing emotional support, and promoting rehabilitation.

MONITOR VITAL SIGNS Be alert for any changes in vital signs, especially those that may signify increased intracranial pressure (see Table 20-2) or autonomic dysreflexia. Monitor the child's respiratory status. Some children with cervical lesions have tracheostomies performed to help maintain airway patency; others with very high lesions are dependent on ventilators. Keep proper emergency equipment at bedside at all times.

MEET NUTRITIONAL NEEDS Ensure adequate nutrition. A child with complete paralysis may require a gastrostomy tube.

MAINTAIN SKIN INTEGRITY Prevent skin breakdown (see Table 20-5). Observe surgical sites for signs of infection or inflammation. Good skin care should be performed at the insertion of the external fixation device (see Table 21-5).

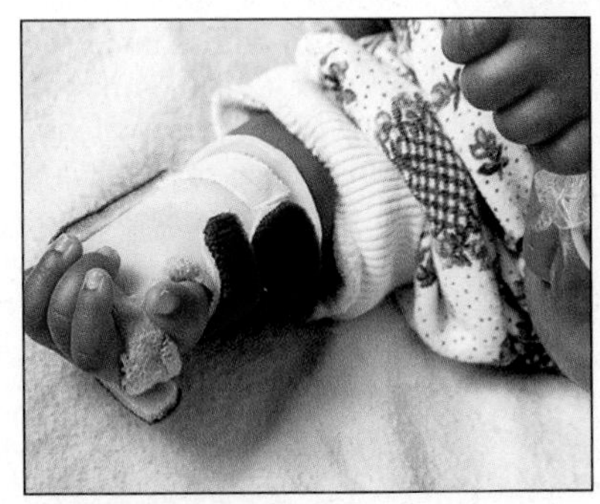

FIGURE 20-21 ◆ Splints are often used to prevent contractures, thus maintaining optimal functioning of the child's hands or feet.

PROMOTE INDEPENDENT FUNCTIONING Reinforce the exercises and skills learned in physical and occupational therapy. Use supports, boots, footboards, splints, and braces as recommended by therapists to prevent contractures (Figure 20-21 ◆). If hand mobility is limited, explore options for independence. Encourage the child to be as independent as possible in a wheelchair. An important mobility goal is to achieve wheelchair transfer and to perform self-care. Identify adaptive equipment that makes it possible to achieve those goals.

Bowel and bladder control may be hard to achieve. Intermittent catheterizations may be necessary (see page 655). Bowel training involves a diet high in fiber and the use of stool softeners.

Skill 12-1: Performing a Urinary Catheterization

ENCOURAGE THERAPEUTIC PLAY Therapeutic play appropriate for the child's developmental level is an important part of the healing process. Provide as many normal activities for the child as possible, but do not assign tasks that the child will have difficulty completing. Child-life teachers or tutors can help the child keep up with schoolwork.

Television, videotapes, and music can offer diversion for prolonged hospitalization. Paraplegic children can learn to use their arms and hands to play interactive games. Devices can also be adapted so that the child can play video games or manipulate the television or radio.

PROVIDE EMOTIONAL SUPPORT Support the child emotionally. Encourage the child to meet small, short-term goals, including those that involve self-care. Encourage the child to express fears and frustrations.

Be compassionate and understanding. Encourage siblings to visit, answer their questions honestly, and help them to discuss their feelings. Involve the parents and siblings in the care of the child as much as possible. When appropriate, encourage them to help with activities of daily living.

DISCHARGE PLANNING AND HOME CARE TEACHING Many children are discharged to inpatient rehabilitation facilities. Assist with arrangements for the child's transfer from the hospital to the rehabilitation facility. Work closely with the child, parents, and other members of the health care team concerning placement. Home care needs, reintegration into educational programs, and safety issues should be identified and addressed well in advance of discharge from the rehabilitation facility. Refer families to social services, family counseling, and support groups if indicated.

The young child's ultimate functioning will be related to cognitive development, the amount of upper body strength, and the family's expectations (Massagli, 2000).

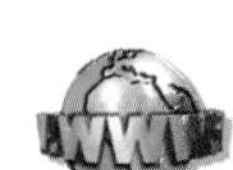

Spinal Cord Injury Support

HYPOXIC–ISCHEMIC BRAIN INJURY (DROWNING AND NEAR-DROWNING)

Drowning is defined as death within 24 hours of a submersion incident. Near-drowning is survival for at least 24 hours after submersion. Over 90% of drownings occur in fresh water such as ponds and residential swimming pools (Zuckerman & Conway, 2000). Drowning is the second leading cause of injury-related deaths in children. The majority of pediatric victims are either very young (under 4 years) or teenagers. Boys are 5 times more likely than girls to die from drowning.

There are two types of drowning. Wet drowning, which occurs more frequently, is the result of aspiration of fluid into the lungs. Dry drowning, as seen in 10% of cases, is due to hypoxemia resulting from laryngospasm, with small or insignificant amounts of liquid aspirated.

The events preceding drowning follow a sequential pattern. The child trapped in water panics, struggles, attempts to move using swimming motions, and holds his or her breath. Then the child swallows a small amount of fluid, vomits, and aspirates the vomitus. This leads to a brief period of laryngospasm, which lasts no more than 2 minutes. Because of the increasing panic and hypoxia, the child swallows more liquid. Then either the child goes into profound laryngospasm, becomes severely hypoxic, has a seizure, and dies (dry drowning), or the child becomes unconscious, the laryngospasm relaxes as reflexes are lost, and the child passively aspirates even greater amounts of water into the airway and stomach (wet drowning).

Anoxia is the major insult associated with drowning. Anoxia leads to cerebral edema and increased intracranial pressure. Little can be done to resuscitate the brain, but with aggressive cardiopulmonary resuscitation, more severely brain-injured children are surviving in a permanent vegetative state. Aspiration leads to impaired gas exchange and ultimately affects pulmonary, cardiac, cerebral, and renal functions. See Chapter 13 for a brief discussion of the effects of drowning on the respiratory system.

Prognosis and outcome are highly individual. Anoxic brain injury is the leading cause of mortality. Predictors of good outcome are submersion less than 5 minutes and cardiopulmonary resuscitation for less than 10 minutes (Zuckerman & Conway, 2000).

The child who has been immersed exhibits a wide variety of signs and symptoms depending on the length of time underwater, the temperature of the water, the response to the episode, and the initial treatment performed at the scene. Children who are submerged for

GROWTH & DEVELOPMENT

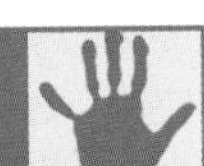

Between 40% and 50% of children who are injured in drowning incidents are under 4 years of age, with peak incidence between 1 and 2 years. The majority (55%) of infant drownings are in bathtubs. The most common drowning locations for children 1–4 years are artificial pools (56%) and other bodies of fresh water (26%). Among older children, 63% of drownings occur in natural bodies of fresh water (Brenner, Trumble, & Smith, et al., 2001).

NURSING ALERT

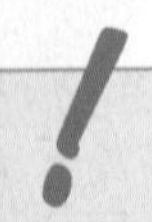

All near-drowning victims should be admitted to the hospital for at least 24 hours or observed in a short-stay observation unit for several hours, even when asymptomatic. Many life-threatening complications, including respiratory distress and cerebral edema, may not become evident for at least 12 hours after the incident.

short periods have few symptoms and recover without complication. The child with a longer submersion can experience the following symptoms: decreased level of consciousness ranging from stupor to total unresponsiveness, cerebral edema, increased intracranial pressure, seizures, respiratory acidosis, irregular respirations, apnea, and gastric distention.

Medical intervention begins at the scene of the drowning with immediate ventilation and compressions, when indicated. The sooner the treatment is started, the better the child's prognosis.

SAFETY PRECAUTIONS

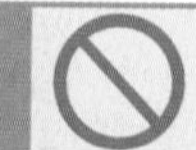

Drowning can be prevented by education, legislation, and changes in the environment. Pool owners should erect climb-proof 5-foot fences around all four sides of the pool. Local ordinances may require such fences. Adolescents should learn the dangers of mixing alcohol and swimming. Five- and 10-gallon buckets should be kept empty when not in use. The nurse should emphasize the importance of closely supervising children when near or in the water, whether at pools, at the beach, or in the bathtub.

Nursing Management

Nursing care of the child who survives a submersion incident focuses on monitoring the child's cardiopulmonary status and providing emotional support.

Monitor the child's respiratory status, cardiopulmonary function, and neurologic status. Administer prescribed medications and position the child properly. Other nursing interventions, especially for the comatose child, can be found in the earlier discussion of altered states of consciousness.

Provide emotional support to the family. Be nonjudgmental and provide a forum for parents to express their feelings. Reassure parents who exhibit guilt reactions that their child is receiving all possible medical treatment. Parents may be faced with an unknown prognosis. Encourage parents to seek assistance from social workers, members of the clergy, close friends, and relatives. Arrange for appropriate referrals.

Home care needs should be identified and addressed well in advance of discharge. Assist with arrangements for the child with minor deficits. Help the parents decide if the comatose child will go home or to a long-term care facility.

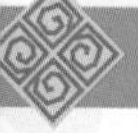

Chapter Highlights

- Altered level of consciousness is caused by trauma, infection, poisoning, seizures, or any other process that affects the CNS. Cerebral perfusion pressure (the amount of pressure needed to ensure that adequate oxygen and nutrients will be delivered to the brain) is decreased with hypovolemia and increased intracranial pressure.
- More than 80% of children experience a headache by late adolescence, and migraine is the most common type of benign head in children.
- Monitor any child with a generalized seizure lasting longer than 10 minutes for electrolytes, glucose, blood gases, increasing fever, and abnormal blood pressure to identify any conditions that can be treated and reduce the risk of significant CNS injury.
- Neurologic damage from bacterial meningitis often occurs in infants and young children despite early, aggressive management. The most common sequelae involve cranial nerves, especially the eighth, resulting in hearing loss, seizures, and developmental delay.
- Viral (aseptic) meningitis is not as virulent as bacterial meningitis; and the child with aseptic meningitis appears less ill than the child with bacterial meningitis.
- Encephalitis is usually caused by a virus, often herpes simplex I, and has a high mortality rate.
- Reye syndrome is an encephalopathy with a high mortality rate that is associated with aspirin use for a mild viral illness. Because most parents give children acetaminophen rather than aspirin for flulike symptoms and varicella, Reye syndrome has become rare.
- Guillain-Barré syndrome is the most common cause of flaccid paralysis in infants and children. It is caused by an immune response to an infectious organism, usually from a gastrointestinal or respiratory illness 2 to 3 weeks prior to onset.
- Hydrocephalus is caused by the blockage of flow or absorption of cerebrospinal fluid in the subarachnoid space and the arachnoid villi or blockage in the ventricular system. It can be associated with a congenital condition or acquired from meningitis or intraventricular hemorrhage, tumor, or structural deformity.
- Spina bifida, a congenital neural tube defect, is the most common developmental disorder of the CNS. Its prevalence is decreasing due to the fortification of all enriched grain products with folate.
- Positional plagiocephaly, a totally flat occiput, is seen increasingly because of the "Back to Sleep" campaign for sudden infant death syndrome.
- The most common symptoms of drug withdrawal in the newborn are irritability and jitteriness. The infant may also have excoriated skin, especially on the heels, toes, hands, elbows, nose, or chin, because of continuous rubbing against the crib sheets.
- Most cases of cerebral palsy are characterized by spasticity and a lack of coordination. The majority of cases are

believed to be caused by intrauterine insults, such as infection, or structural abnormalities of the CNS.

- Traumatic brain injuries are the most common injuries during childhood. They result from falls, motor vehicle crashes, sports injuries, and child abuse.
- Spinal cord injuries, although relatively rare in children, are often associated with the extreme mobility and flexibility of the spinal column. The cervical and lumbar regions are the locations most commonly affected.
- Children who have the best outcomes following a near-drowning include those submerged less than 5 minutes and those who need cardiopulmonary resuscitation for less than 10 minutes.

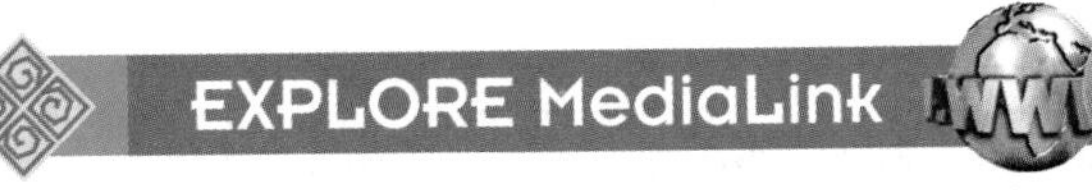

EXPLORE MediaLink

- NCLEX review, case studies, and other interactive resources for this chapter can be found on the Companion Website at **http://www.prenhall.com/ball.** Click on Chapter 20 to select the activities for this chapter.
- For animations, more NCLEX review questions, and an audio glossary, access the accompanying CD-ROM in this textbook.

References

1. Altmeier, W. A. (1999). Status epilepticus. *Pediatric Annals, 28*(4), 206–208.
2. American Academy of Pediatrics Committee on Injury and Poison Prevention. (2001). Injuries associated with infant walkers. *Pediatrics, 108*(3), 790–792.
3. Anderson, V., Catroppa, C., Morse, S., Haritou, F., & Rosenfeld, J. (2000). Recovery of intellectual ability following traumatic brain injury in childhood: Impact of injury severity and age at injury. *Pediatric Neurosurgery, 32*(6), 282–290.
4. Blatt, S. D., Meguid, V., & Church, C. C. (2000). Prenatal cocaine: What's known about outcomes? *Contemporary Pediatrics, 17*(5), 43–57.
5. Bowman, R. M., McLone, D. G., Grant, J. A., Tomita, T., &Ito, J. A. (2001). Spina bifida outcome: A 25-year perspective. *Pediatric Neurosurgery, 34*(3), 114–120.
6. Brenner, R. A., Trumble, A. C., Smith, G. S., Kessler, E. P., & Overpeck, M. D. (2001). Where children drown, United States, 1995. *Pediatrics, 108*(1), 85–89.
7. Cherry, J. D. (1999). Nonpolio enteroviruses. In J. A. McMillan, C. D. DeAngelis, R. D. Feigin, & J. B. Warshaw, *Oski's pediatrics: Principles and practice* (3rd ed., pp. 1102–1107). Philadelphia: Lippincott, Williams, & Wilkins.
8. Danielpour, M., & Peacock, W. J. (2000). Epilepsy surgery in children. *Clinical Neurosurgery, 47,* 400–421.
9. DeLuca, P. A. (1996). The musculoskeletal management of children with cerebral palsy. *Pediatric Clinics of North America, 43*(5), 1135–1150.
10. Dzienkowski, R. C., Smith, K. K., Dillow, K. A., & Yucha, C. B. (1996). Cerebral palsy: A comprehensive review. *Nurse Practitioner, 21*(2), 45–59.
11. Fadiman, A. (1997). The spirit catches you and you fall down. New York: Farrar, Strauss, Giroux
12. Farley, J. A., & Dunleavy, M. J., (2000). Myelodysplasia. In P. L. Jackson, & J. A. Vessey, (eds.). *Primary care of the child with a chronic condition,* (3rd ed., pp. 658–675), St. Louis: Mosby.
13. Farley, J. A., & McEwan, M. (2000). Epilepsy. In P. L. Jackson & J. A. Vessey, (eds). *Primary care of the child with a chronic condition,* (3rd. ed., pp. 475–494), St Louis. Mosby.
14. Farley, J. A., & Mooney, K. H. (1998). Alterations in neurologic function in children. In K. L. McCance & S. E. Huether (eds.), *Pathophysiology: The biologic basis for disease in adults and children* (3rd ed., pp. 591–624). St. Louis: Mosby.
15. Frank, D. A., Augustyn, M., Knight, W. G., Pell, T., & Zuckerman, B. (2001). Growth, development, and behavior in early childhood following prenatal cocaine exposure: A systematic review. *JAMA, 285*(12), 1613–1627.
16. Guskiewicz, K. M., Weaver, N. L., Padua, D. A., & Garrett, W. E. (2000). Epidemiology of concussion in collegiate and high school football players. *American Journal of Sports Medicine, 28*(5), 643–650.
17. Harrison, L. H. (2001, Spring). Meningococcal infection in adolescents and young adults. *Contemporary Pediatrics,* 4–15.
18. Honein, M. A., Paulozzi, L. J., Matthews, T. J., Erickson, J. D., & Wong, L. Y. (2001). Impact of folic acid fortification of the U.S. food supply on the occurrence of neural tube defects. *JAMA, 285*(23), 2981–2986.
19. Jackson, P. L., &Harvey, J. (2000). Hydrocephalus. In P. L. Jackson & J. A. Vessey (eds.), *Primary care of the child with a chronic condition* (3rd ed., pp. 560–582). St. Louis: Mosby.
20. Jones, H. R. (2000). Guillain-Barre syndrome: Perspectives with infants and children. *Seminars in Pediatric Neurology, 7*(2), 91–102.
21. Katyal, N. G., Koehler, A. N., McGhee, B., Foley, C. M., & Crumrine, P. K. (2000). The ketogenic diet in refractory epilepsy: The experience of Children's Hospital of Pittsburgh. *Clinical Pediatrics, 39*(3), 153–159.
22. Leake, J.A.D., & Perkins, B. (2000). Meningococcal disease: Challenges in prevention and management. *Infections in Medicine, 17*(5), 364–377.
23. Massagli, T. L. (2000). Medical and rehabilitation issues in the care of children with spinal cord injury. *Physical Medicine and Rehabilitation Clinics of North America, 11*(1), 169–182.
24. Moe, P. G., & Seay, A. R. (1997). Neurologic and muscular disorders. In W. W. Hay, J. R. Groothius, A. R. Hayward, &M. J. Levin (eds.), *Current pediatric diagnosis and treatment* (13th ed., pp. 686–689). Stamford, CT: Appleton & Lange.
25. Nehring, W. M. (2000). Cerebral palsy. In P. L. Jackson & J. A. Vessey (eds.), *Primary care of the child with a chronic condition* (3rd ed., pp. 305–330). St. Louis: Mosby.
26. Nelson, K. B., & Grether, J. K. (1999). Causes of cerebral palsy. *Current Opinion in Pediatrics, 11*(6), 487–491.
27. Northrup, H., & Volcik, K. A. (2000). Spina bifida and other neural tube defects. *Current Problems in Pediatrics, 30*(10), 317–331.
28. O'Hara, J., & Koch, T. K. (1998). Heading off headaches. *Contemporary Pediatrics, 15*(3), 97–116.

29. Renier, D., Lajeunie, E., Arnaud, E., &Marchac, D. (2000). Management of craniosynostosis. *Children's Nervous System, 16,* 645–658.

30. Ressler, J. A., & Nelson, M. (2000). Central nervous system infections in the pediatric population. *Neuroimaging Clinics of North America, 10*(2), 427–443.

31. Robinson, T.M.S. (1999). Perinatal substance abuse: Working with neonates and families. *Neonatal Network, 18*(2), 68–70.

32. Rosman, N. P. (1999). Acute head trauma. In J. A. McMillan, C. D. DeAngelis, R. D. Feigin, & J. B. Warshaw, *Oski's pediatrics: Principles and practice,* (3rd ed., pp. 603–617) Philadelphia: Lippincott, Williams, & Wilkins.

33. Sagraves, R. (1999). Febrile seizures—Treatment and prevention or not? *Journal of Pediatric Health Care, 13*(2), 79–83.

34. Schutzman, S. A., & Greenes, D. S. (2001). Pediatric minor head trauma. *Annals of Emergency Medicine, 27*(1), 65–74.

35. Spector, R. E. (2000). *Cultural diversity in health and illness* (5th ed., p. 71). Upper Saddle River, NJ: Prentice Hall Health.

36. Sutton, L., Adzick, N. S., Belaniuk, L. T., Johnson, M. P., Crombleholme, T. M., & Flake, A. W. (1999). Improvement of hindbrain herniation demonstrated by serial fetal magnetic resonance imaging following fetal surgery for myelomeningocele. *JAMA, 282*(19), 1826–1831.

37. United States Congress. (1996). Traumatic brain injury act of 1996. *Congressional Record, 142* (July 29, 1996), 110 STAT, 1445–1449.

38. Valente, L. R. (2000). Seizures and epilepsy: Optimizing patient management. *Clinician Reviews, 10*(3), 79–104.

39. Vendanarayanan, V. V. (1999). Diagnosis of epilepsy in children. *Pediatric Annals, 28*(4), 218–224.

40. Wiens, H. D. (1998). Spasticity in children with cerebral palsy: A retrospective review of effects of intrathecal baclofen. *Issues in Comprehensive Pediatric Nursing, 21,* 49–61.

41. Zuckerman, G. B., & Conway, E. E. (2000). Drowning and near-drowning: A pediatric epidemic. *Pediatric Annals, 29*(6), 360–366.

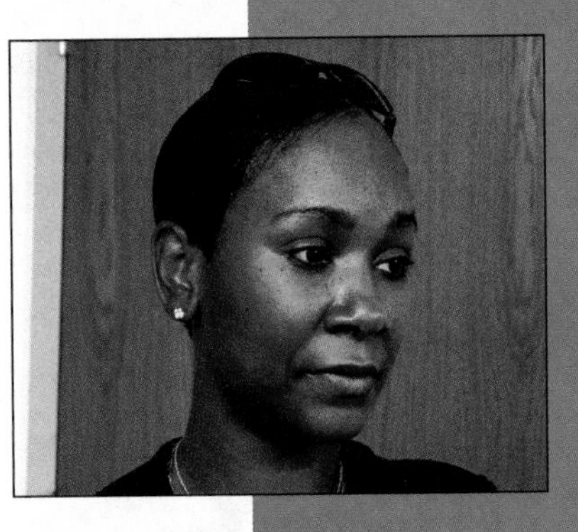

"When I got the call that Douglass was in the emergency room I was so scared. I guess we're lucky it was just a broken leg. I don't know what to do now though—should he go back to his friend's house? Should I tell him not to use the trampoline? And I never had a cast—what do you need to do with it?"

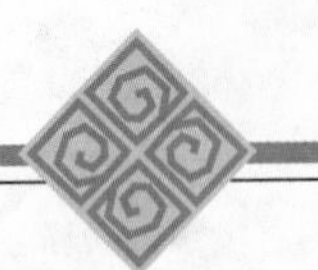

Douglass was admitted to the clinic today for application of a short leg cast. He broke his leg nearly a week ago when he was on a trampoline with three friends, trying to see who could jump the highest. Douglass slipped and his leg hit the frame on the side. His friends helped him off the trampoline and called his mother, who transported Douglass to the emergency room.

His mother states that he is now 12 years old and in middle school. He has been going to a friend's house nearly every day after school and spending time on activities such as the trampoline and roller blading, as well as watching television and playing video games. She felt this was safer than him being at home alone during her work hours, but is now starting to wonder about whether to allow Douglass to engage in activities with his friend.

In the emergency room after the accident, a splint was used to provide support for several days and allow the swelling to decrease before today's cast application. Douglass has been non-weight bearing on his leg and has been using crutches. He returned to school yesterday for part of the day and found it difficult to get to all of his classes.

CHAPTER 21

ALTERATIONS IN MUSCULOSKELETAL FUNCTION

KEY TERMS

chondrolysis The breaking down and absorption of cartilage.

compartment syndrome A condition of increased pressure in a limited space which compromises circulation and tissue function.

dislocation Displacement of a bone from its normal articulation with a joint.

dysplasia Abnormal development resulting in altered size, shape, and cell organization.

equinus A condition that limits dorsiflexion to less than normal; usually associated with clubfoot.

ossification Formation of bone from fibrous tissue or cartilage.

osteotomy Surgical cutting of bone.

pseudohypertrophy Enlargement of the muscles as a result of infiltration by fatty tissue.

sprain A tearing of ligaments usually caused when a joint is twisted or otherwise traumatized.

subluxation Partial or complete dislocation of a joint.

varus A condition in which the hindfoot turns inward; usually associated with clubfoot.

MediaLink 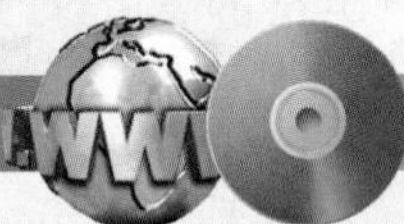 http://www.prenhall.com/ball

Resources for this chapter can be found on the CD-ROM accompanying this textbook, and on the Companion Website at http://www.prenhall.com/ball. Click on Chapter 21 to select the activities for this chapter.

CD-ROM

Audio Glossary
NCLEX Review

COMPANION WEBSITE

Web Links
NCLEX Review
MediaLink Applications
- Skeletal Assessment
- Home Care of Infant in a Spica Cast

What concerns will Douglass have once his cast is in place? What teaching does he need to keep the cast intact and to ensure his safety? Will any special adaptations be needed in his home and school? Is there any way his injury could have been avoided? The information in this chapter will provide answers to these questions and help to provide effective care for children like Douglass who have musculoskeletal disorders.

The musculoskeletal system helps the body to protect its vital organs, support weight, control motion, store minerals, and supply red blood cells. Bones provide a rigid framework for the body, muscles provide for active movement, and tendons and ligaments hold the bones and muscles together. Alterations in musculoskeletal functioning thus can have a significant impact on a child's growth and development.

Musculoskeletal disorders may be congenital, such as clubfoot, or acquired, such as osteomyelitis. They may require short- or long-term management, and may be treated on an outpatient basis or require hospitalization. Many musculoskeletal disorders require surgical correction, casting, or braces.

Table 21-1 reviews several terms used throughout this chapter in describing the positioning of a child's limbs.

ANATOMY AND PHYSIOLOGY OF PEDIATRIC DIFFERENCES

BONES

Several differences exist between the bones of children and those of adults. Although primary centers of **ossification** (bone formation) are nearly complete at birth, a fibrous membrane still exists between the cranial bones (fontanels) (see Figure 4-12). The posterior fontanel closes between 2 and 3 months of age. The anterior fontanel does not close until approximately 18 months of age, allowing for growth of the brain and skull. In addition, the ends of the long bones (epiphyses) remain cartilaginous (Figure 21-1 ◆). Long bone growth continues until approximately age 20, when skeletal maturation is complete.

Secondary ossification occurs as the long bones grow. Cartilage cells at the epiphyses are replaced by osteoblasts (immature bone cells), resulting in the deposition of calcium. Calcium intake during childhood and adolescence is essential to provide adequate bone density

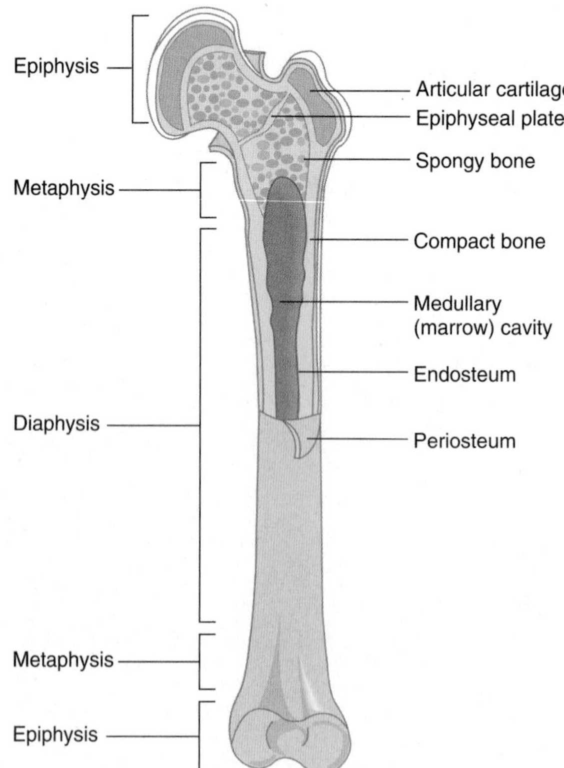

FIGURE 21-1 ◆ The parts of long bones.

TABLE 21-1 Musculoskeletal Positions

Varus
An abnormal position of a limb that involves bending inward toward the midline of the body

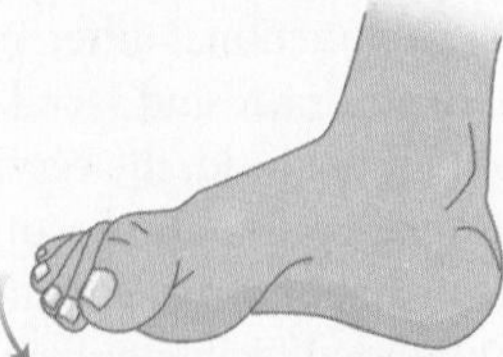

Valgus
An abnormal position of a limb that involves bending outward away from the midline of the body

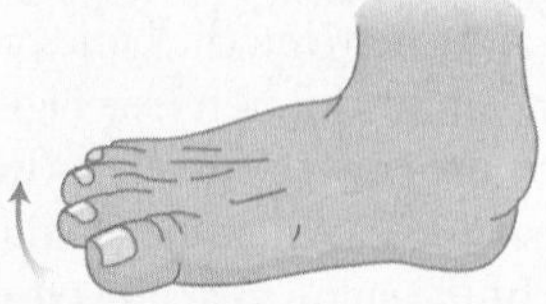

Adduction
Lateral movement of limbs toward the midline of the body

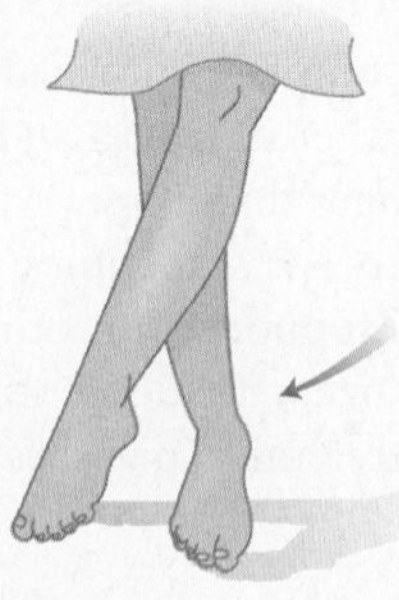

Abduction
Lateral movement of limbs away from the midline of the body

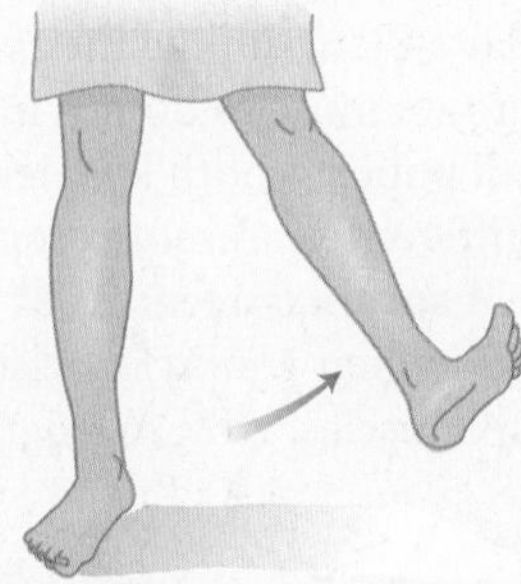

Inversion
Turning inward, usually more than normal

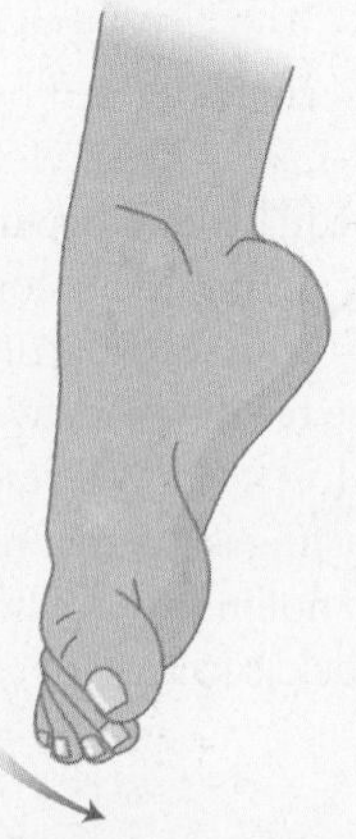

Eversion
Turning outward

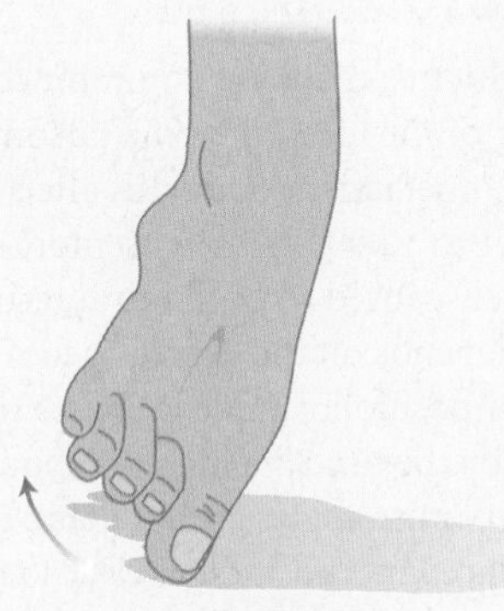

Supination
Lying on the back or placing the hand so the palm faces upward

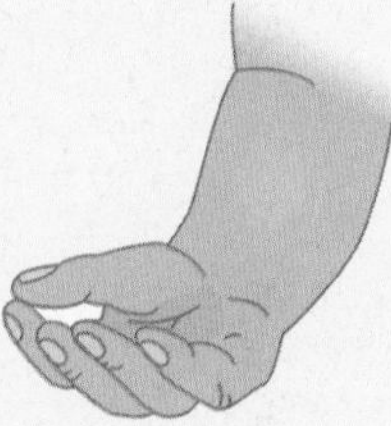

Pronation
Lying on the stomach or placing the hand so the palm faces downward

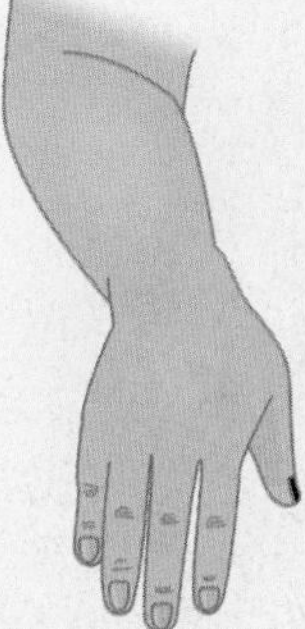

that will prevent osteoporosis and fractures in adulthood. See Chapter 3 for a discussion of inadequate calcium intake during school age and adolescence. Because growth takes place at the epiphyseal plates, injuries to this portion of a long bone are of particular concern in young children.

The long bones of children are porous and less dense than those of adults. For this reason, children's bones can bend, buckle, or break as a result of a simple fall. In addition to the structural differences between the bones of children and adults, are functional differences in the skeletal system of children (see Figure 4-1). Before birth, the thoracic and sacral regions of the spine are convex curves. As the infant learns to hold up the head, the cervical region becomes concave. When the child learns to stand, the lumbar region also becomes concave. Failure of the spine to assume these final curves results in an abnormal curvature of the spine (kyphosis or lordosis). The rapid bone growth of childhood facilitates healing after fractures, but may also lead to "growing pains," as muscles are pulled when bones grow quickly (Muscari, 1998).

MUSCLES, TENDONS, AND LIGAMENTS

The muscular system, unlike the skeletal system, is almost completely formed at birth. As a child grows, muscles do not increase in number, but rather in length and circumference. Until puberty, both ligaments and tendons are stronger than bone. When these structural differences are not recognized, a childhood fracture is sometimes mistaken for a sprain. A **sprain** is a tearing of ligaments, the structural support connecting bones, usually caused when a joint is twisted or otherwise traumatized. Tendons, which connect bones to muscles, grow in length and fibrous tissue as mechanical pressure is placed on them.

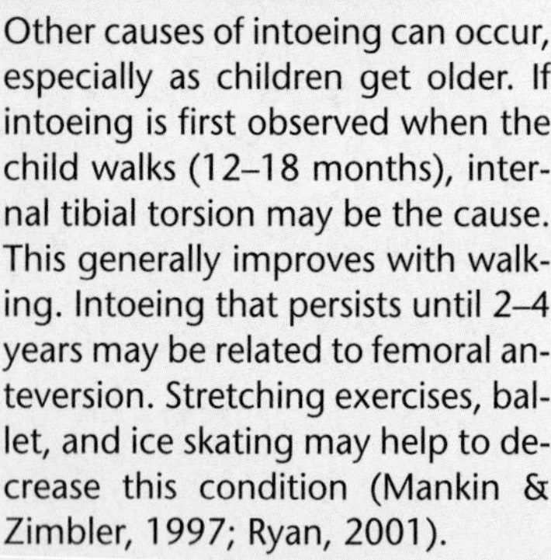

NURSING ALERT

Other causes of intoeing can occur, especially as children get older. If intoeing is first observed when the child walks (12–18 months), internal tibial torsion may be the cause. This generally improves with walking. Intoeing that persists until 2–4 years may be related to femoral anteversion. Stretching exercises, ballet, and ice skating may help to decrease this condition (Mankin & Zimbler, 1997; Ryan, 2001).

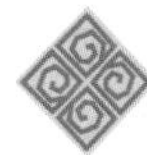

DISORDERS OF THE FEET AND LEGS

METATARSUS ADDUCTUS

Metatarsus adductus, the most common congenital foot deformity, is characterized by an inward turning of the forefoot at the tarsometatarsal joints (Figure 21-2 ◆). Often referred to as "intoeing," metatarsus adductus affects male and female infants equally and occurs in approximately 1 in 1,000 births, with more common incidence among siblings. This condition is most likely caused by both intrauterine positioning and genetic factors (Ryan, 2001).

Treatment depends on the degree of foot flexibility. If the foot can be readily maneuvered past the neutral position, simple exercises may correct the problem. Most cases will resolve spontaneously by the time the infant is about 3 months of age. Serial casting is the treatment of choice for curvature angles greater than 15 degrees, or in cases that do not improve. The infant's feet are placed in a position as close to neutral as possible and are held secure with casts.

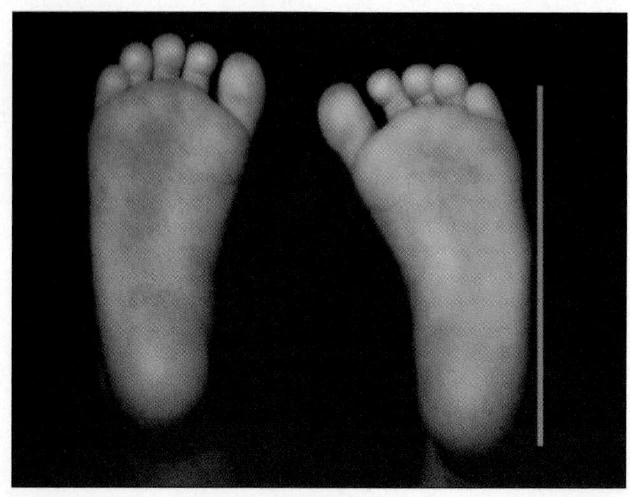

FIGURE 21-2 ◆
Metatarsus adductus is characterized by convexity (curvature) of the lateral border of the foot, as shown by the red line.
From Staheli, L.T., (1992). *Fundamentals of pediatric orthopedics* (p. 5.7). New York: Raven Press.

FAMILIES WANT TO KNOW

Stretching Exercises for Metatarsus Adductus

- Hold the infant's foot securely by the heel. Maintain the heel in this position.
- Move the forefoot outward away from the body with the other hand.
- Hold the foot in this position for 5 seconds.
- Repeat 5 times during each diaper change.

Casts are changed weekly until the desired correction is achieved. Braces and orthopedic shoes may also be used to maintain correction after casting (Mankin & Zimbler, 1997).

Nursing Management

Reassure parents that the child's condition can be corrected. If the child's deformity is mild, teach parents simple stretching exercises that can be performed at each diaper change. If casting is necessary, provide cast care as outlined in Table 21-2 and teach parents how to care for the child in a cast at home. If metatarsus adductus persists into childhood without correction, the challenge is to find shoes that accommodate the unusual shape of the foot.

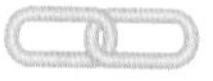

Skill 13-1: Providing Cast Care

CLUBFOOT

Clubfoot is a congenital abnormality in which the foot is twisted out of its normal position. It occurs in approximately 1 to 3 in 1,000 births and affects boys nearly twice as often as girls (Fernbach, 1998).

TABLE 21-2 Nursing Care of the Child in a Cast

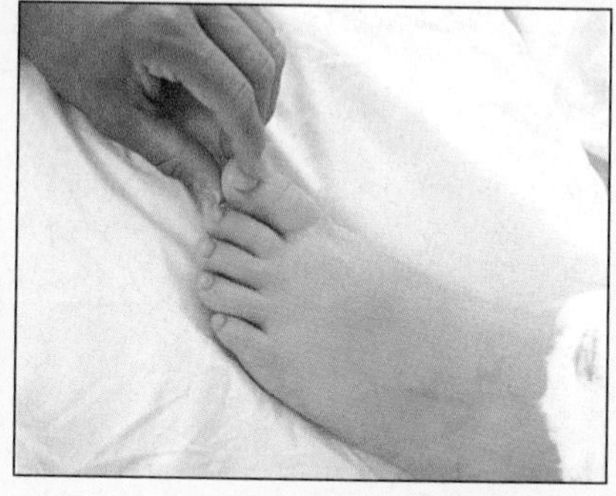

(1)

- A plaster cast takes anywhere from 24–48 hours to dry. When handling the cast, be gentle and use the palms of your hands, as fingertips can indent plaster and create pressure areas.
- After the cast is applied, elevate the extremity on a pillow above the level of the heart. Elevation helps to reduce swelling and increases venous return.
- If the cast is applied after surgery, there may be drainage or bleeding through the cast material. Circle the stain and note the date and time on the cast to provide a means of assessing the amount of fluid lost.
- Assess the distal pulses, and check the fingers and toes for color, warmth, capillary refill, and edema. Assess sensation as well as movement. Any deviation from normal may indicate nerve damage or decreased blood supply.
- During the first 24 hours, the casted extremily should be checked every 15–30 minutes for 2 hours, then every 1–2 hours thereafter. The skin should be warm. It should blanch when slight pressure is applied and then return to its normal color within 3 seconds **(1)**. For the next 2 days, the casted extremity should be assessed at least every 4 hours.
- Check the edges of the cast for roughness or crumbling. If necessary, pull the inner stockinette over the edge of the cast and tape.
- The rough edges of the cast may also be alleviated by "petaling." This is done by securing adhesive tape to the inside of the cast and pulling it over the edge, covering the jagged or broken pieces of plaster, and securing it to the outer surface of the cast **(2, 3, 4)**. Moleskin may be used on the cast as well.

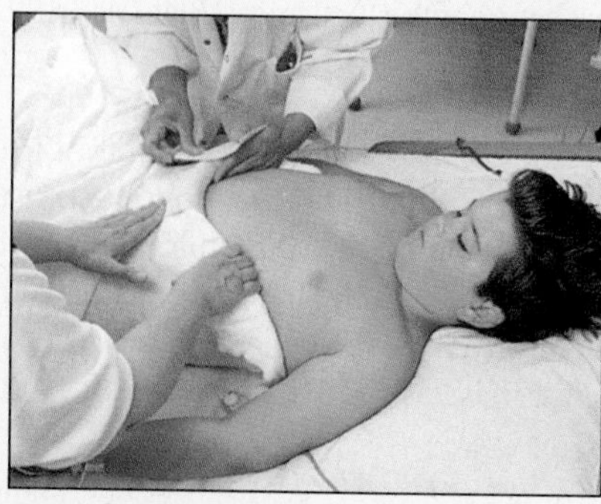

(2)

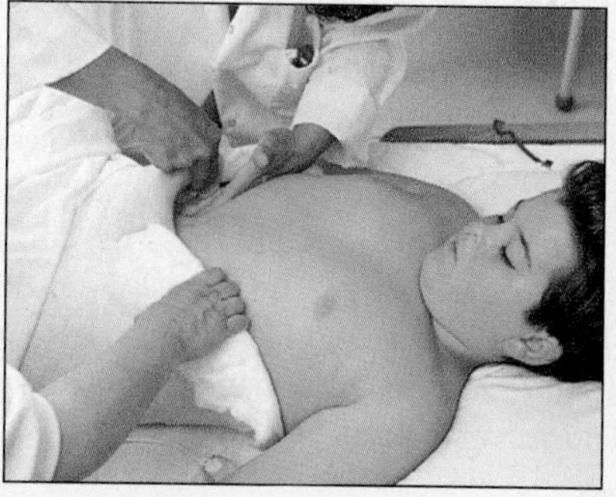

(3)

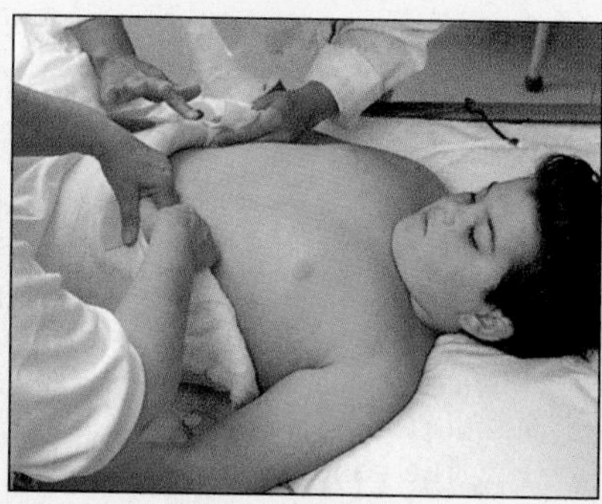

(4)

- Keep the cast as clean and dry as possible. Cover the cast with a plastic bag or plastic wrap when the child bathes or showers.
- The skin under the cast may itch; however, do not use powders or lotions near the edges or under the cast as they can cause skin irritation.
- Be sure that children do not put small objects between the casts and their extremities; these actions can cause skin irritation as well as neurovascular compromise.

FAMILIES WANT TO KNOW

Care of the Child with a Cast

SKIN CARE

- Check the skin around the cast edges for irritation, rubbing, or blistering. The skin should be clean and dry.
- Cleanse the skin just under the cast edges and between the toes or fingers with a cotton-tipped applicator and rubbing alcohol. Avoid using lotions, oils, and powders near the cast as they may cause caking.
- Avoid poking sharp objects down inside the cast as this may result in sores.

CAST CARE

- Keep the cast dry. Protect plaster with a cast shoe, thick sock, or sling.
- Allow a new, wet cast to air-dry for 24 hours.
- Begin walking on a leg cast only when the physician gives permission.

BE ALERT FOR POSSIBLE COMPLICATIONS

- Toes or fingers should be pink, not blue or white.
- Skin should be warm and the tips of the toes should blanch when pinched.
- Raise the casted arm or leg above heart level and rest it on pillows to prevent or reduce any swelling.

NOTIFY THE HEALTH CARE PROVIDER IF ANY OF THE FOLLOWING OCCUR

- Unusual odor beneath the cast
- Tingling
- Burning or numbness in the casted arm or leg
- Drainage through the cast
- Swelling or inability to move the fingers or toes
- Slippage of the cast
- Cast cracked, soft, or loose
- Sudden, unexplained fever
- Unusual fussiness or irritability in an infant or child
- Fingers or toes that are blue or white
- Pain that is not relieved by any comfort measures (e.g., repositioning or pain medication)

Note: Courtesy of Shriners Hospital for Children, Spokane, WA.

Etiology and Pathophysiology

The exact cause of clubfoot is unknown; however, several possible etiologies have been proposed. Some authorities believe abnormal intrauterine positioning causes the deformity. Neuromuscular or vascular problems are suspected as causes by others. Yet other experts believe there is a genetic component, either at the chromosomal level or by the arrest of normal fetal development. A positive family history increases the chance of the deformity (Blakeslee, 1997).

Clinical Manifestations

A true clubfoot (talipes equinovarus) involves three areas of deformity: the midfoot is directed downward (**equinus**), the hindfoot turns inward (**varus**), and the forefoot curls toward the heel (adduction) and turns upward in partial supination. Most children have this combination of findings. The foot is small with a shortened Achilles tendon. Muscles in the lower leg are atrophied, but leg lengths are generally normal. Clubfoot is bilateral in 50% of cases (Figure 21-3 ◆). Clubhand is a rare occurrence that has similar characteristics to the foot deformity (Figure 21-4 ◆).

CULTURE

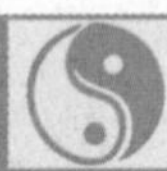

The incidence of talipes equinovarus (clubfoot) varies among ethnic groups. The condition is least common in Asian groups and whites, with a higher incidence in groups from the Middle East, South Africa, and Mexico. It is most common in Polynesian groups (Blakeslee, 1997).

Clinical Therapy

Diagnosis is made at birth on the basis of visual inspection. Radiographs are used to confirm the severity of the condition.

Early treatment is essential to achieve successful correction and reduce the chance of complications. Serial casting is the treatment of choice. Casting should begin as soon as possible after birth. Timing is critical, because the short bones of the foot, which are primarily carti-

PATHOPHYSIOLOGY ILLUSTRATED

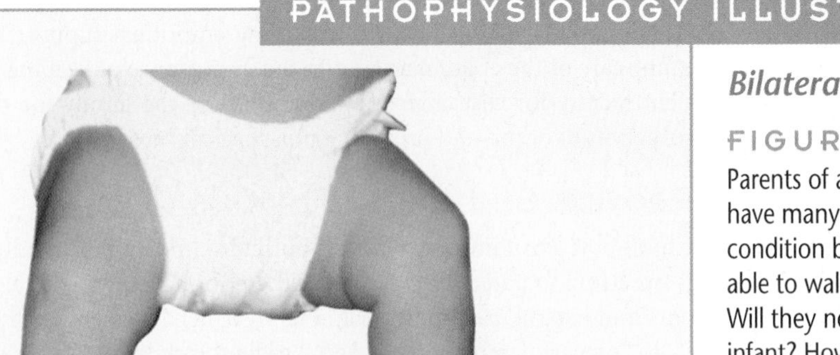

Bilateral Clubfoot Deformity

FIGURE 21-3 ◆

Parents of a child with clubfoot will have many questions. Can the condition be treated? Will the child be able to walk normally after surgery? Will they need help caring for the infant? How much will surgery and other care cost? Will any subsequent children have a clubfoot?

Modified from Staheli, L.T., (1992). *Fundamentals of pediatric orthopedics* (p. 5.10). New York: Raven Press.

laginous at birth, begin to ossify shortly thereafter. The foot is manipulated to achieve maximum correction first of the varus deformity and then of the equinus deformity. A long leg cast is applied to hold the foot in the desired position. The cast is changed every 1 to 2 weeks. This regimen of manipulation and casting continues for approximately 8 to 12 weeks until maximum correction is achieved. If the deformity has been corrected, the child may begin wearing a splint or reverse last corrective shoes to maintain the correction (Fernbach, 1998). If the deformity has not been corrected, surgical intervention is required. Casting is maintained to hold the foot in position until surgery is performed (Figure 21-5 ◆).

The age at which a child undergoes clubfoot surgery varies among surgeons. However, most children have surgery between 3 and 12 months of age. The one-stage posteromedial release procedure, which involves realignment of the bones of the foot and release of the constricting soft tissue, is most commonly performed. The foot is held in the proper position by one or more stainless steel pins. A cast is then applied with the knee flexed to prevent damage to the pin and to discourage weight bearing. Casting continues for 6 to 12 weeks. The child may then need to wear a brace or corrective shoes, depending on the severity of the deformity and the surgeon's preference.

More severe cases or those not corrected in infancy may require more than one surgery to correct the foot.

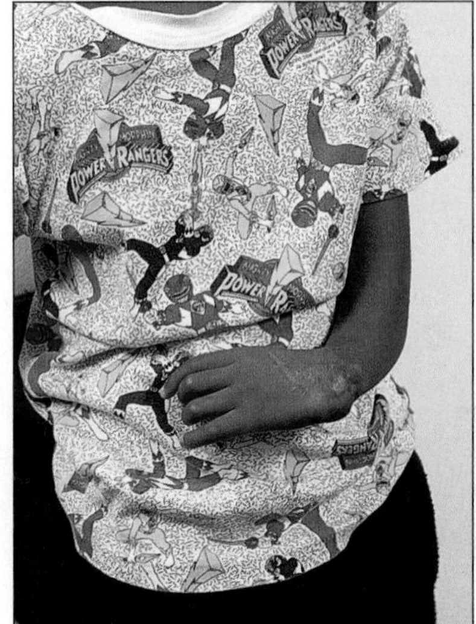

FIGURE 21-4 ◆

A clubhand deformity is a less common condition than clubfoot.

NURSING MANAGEMENT

Nursing Assessment and Diagnosis

Nursing assessment, which begins at birth and continues throughout the child's subsequent outpatient casting visits and hospitalization for surgery, includes taking a genetic and birth history, performing a physical examination (including position and appearance of the foot), and assessing the child's motor development and family's coping mechanisms. Because parents will need to bring the child for frequent cast changes, ask about transportation and other arrangements that are necessary to facilitate these visits.

Nursing diagnoses that may apply to the child with a clubfoot deformity are as follows:

- *Impaired physical mobility,* related to prescribed movement restriction of cast
- *Risk for impaired skin integrity,* related to cast
- *Altered parenting,* related to birth of a child with a physical defect
- *Health seeking behaviors,* related to lack of information about deformity, treatment, and home care

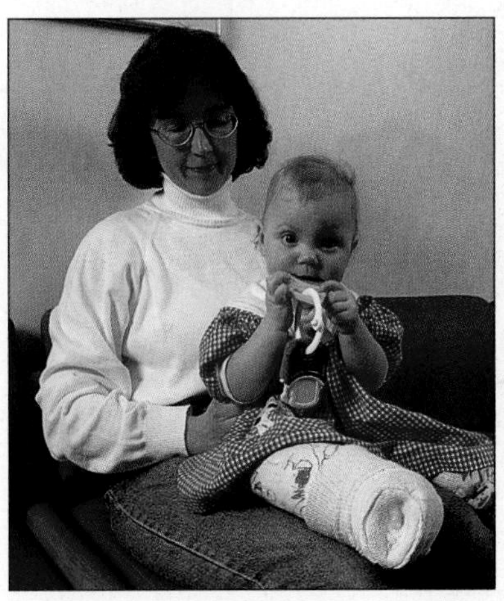

FIGURE 21-5 ◆

This girl has a long leg cast, which was applied after surgery to correct her clubfoot.

CLINICAL TIP

When an infant is receiving serial casting for clubfoot, recommend that the parent soak the cast off the night before a scheduled cast change. The baby can be placed in a warm bath, and the cast will start to disintegrate and can be unrolled. This avoids exposure of the baby to the loud sound of the cast cutter, and allows for the infant's leg to be washed and out of the cast overnight. Parents can also be encouraged to bring a bottle to the clinic. If the baby is hungry and feeding, the foot is more easily kept still for the cast application.

Planning and Implementation

Nursing management involves providing emotional support, educating the family about home care of the child in a cast and the importance of keeping appointments at the outpatient facility for cast changes, preparation of the family for the child's hospitalization if surgery is to occur, and providing postsurgical care.

Provide Emotional Support

Clubfoot is a condition that affects both the child and the family. The child's foot deformity is upsetting to parents, and they need emotional support to allay their fears. Helping parents understand the condition and its treatment is essential.

Encourage parents to hold and cuddle the child and to take an active role in the child's care to help promote bonding. Explain that, with treatment, the child will grow and develop normally.

Provide Cast and Brace Care

Routine cast care is outlined in Table 21-2. After serial casting is complete, or following surgery, the child may progress to wearing a brace or special shoe for 6 to 12 months. Braces should fit snugly but should not interfere with neurovascular function. Before the child begins to wear a brace, check the skin for any areas of redness or breakdown. Provide parents with guidelines for brace wear as outlined below. Emphasize that proper skin care is essential. If skin redness develops, arrange to have the fit of the brace evaluated and modified if necessary.

Provide Postsurgical Care

Routine postoperative care after surgical correction includes neurovascular status checks every 2 hours for the first 24 hours and observing for any swelling around the cast edges (see Table 21-2). Apply ice bags to the foot, and keep the ankle and foot elevated on a pillow for 24 hours to promote healing and help with venous return. Check for drainage or bleeding. Administer pain medication routinely for 24 to 48 hours. Popliteal or epidural blocks may be placed during surgery and used in the immediate postsurgical period for pain control (Figure 21-6 ◆). The nurse monitors these blocks for effectiveness and any undesired effects (see Chapter 9 for detailed instructions on pain management). See the Skills Manual for detail on monitoring nerve blocks.

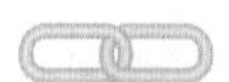

Skill 9-4: Local Pain Blocks

Discharge Planning and Home Care Teaching

Parents should be given written instructions for care of the child with a cast (see page 786). In addition, assist them in the following ways.

FAMILIES WANT TO KNOW

Guidelines for Brace Wear

- Braces should be as comfortable as possible and the child should have adequate mobility while wearing the brace.
- Begin wearing the brace for periods of 1–2 hours and then progress to 2–4 hours.
- Check the skin at 1–2-hour intervals initially, then lengthening to every 4 hours once skin has been clear for several days. If redness is apparent, leave the brace off and allow the skin to clear. If breakdown has occurred, the brace cannot be replaced until healing is complete. (See Chapter 23 for a discussion of pressure ulcers.)
- Always have the child wear a clean white sock, T-shirt, or other thin white liner beneath the brace. Be sure the liner is wrinkle-free under the brace. Avoid using powders or lotions that can cause skin to break down. Toughen any sensitive areas using alcohol wipes.
- Reapply the brace when the skin returns to its normal color.
- Return to the physician or orthotic specialist if discomfort or red areas persist or if the brace needs adjustment or repair or is outgrown.
- Check the brace daily for rough edges.

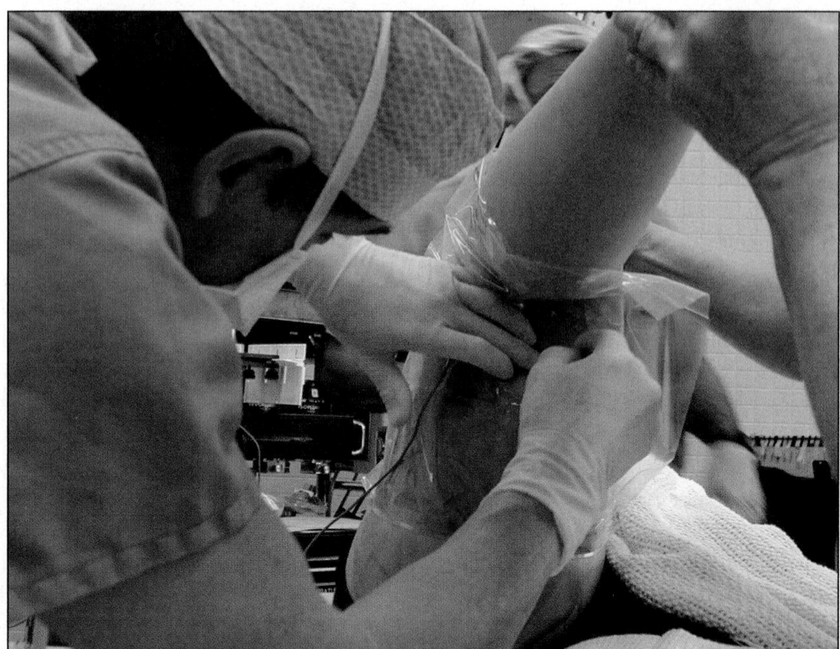

FIGURE 21-6 ◆
The insertion of a popliteal block during surgery. The site will be wrapped and the tubing connected to an infusion pump. The nurse will monitor the infusion and pain control after surgery.
Courtesy of Shriners Hospital, Spokane, WA.

- Demonstrate the use of a sponge bath to protect the cast from water breakdown.
- Discuss several options for clothing that accommodate a cast, for example, one-piece snap suits or sweatpants.
- Discuss potential safety hazards that may result from awkward positioning. Be sure the child is properly situated in a car safety seat for the trip home.
- Suggest that parents make an effort to place toys within the child's reach, because movements of a child in a cast may be slowed.

SAFETY PRECAUTIONS

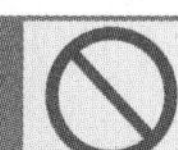

Advise parents that umbrella strollers may not be sturdy enough to support an infant's casted leg. Some infant swings do not provide a foot rest; its absence can contribute to cast slippage or breakdown.

Evaluation

Expected outcomes of nursing care include maintenance of skin integrity, recovery without complications after surgery, normal developmental progression of the child, and demonstrated knowledge by parents for care of braces or casts, as needed.

GENU VARUM AND GENU VALGUM

Genu varum (bowlegs) is a deformity in which the knees are widely separated and the lower legs are turned inward (varus). In genu valgum (knock-knees), the knees are close together and the lower legs are directed outward (valgus).

At certain stages of a child's development, the appearance of bowlegs or knock-knees is normal. Until 2 to 3 years, the knees are normally bowed, showing varus alignment, and by 4 to 5 years, some knock-knee or valgus alignment is common (Mankin & Zimbler, 1997). However, the persistence of knock-knees beyond the age of 4 or 5 years necessitates further evaluation. Chapter 4 discusses the assessment of bowlegs and knock-knees in children.

Braces are often used to correct mild deformities that could worsen as the child grows. Braces for bowlegs are worn at night; those for knock-knees are worn both day and night. Duration of brace wear is determined by the severity of the deformity, which is usually evaluated by radiographs. If the deformity continues to worsen, surgical intervention is necessary. An **osteotomy** (cutting of the bone) is performed and the tibiofemoral angle surgically corrected. The child is then placed in a cast for approximately 6 to 10 weeks, or until full healing has occurred.

Nursing Management

Reassure parents that bowlegs and knock-knees are usually a normal part of a child's growth and development. These conditions often resolve on their own and require no treatment other than monitoring.

NURSING ALERT

The most common pathologic causes of bowlegs are Blount disease (disruption of tibial growth plate) and rickets (see Chapter 3).

Nursing care focuses on educating the parents and child about the condition and its treatment. Provide the child and family with guidelines for brace wear and maintenance (see page 788).

CULTURE 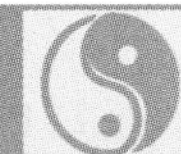

Infants who are positioned on cradle boards or traditionally swaddled, as in some Native American cultures, have a high incidence of developmental dysplasia of the hip (DDH). Among cultures in which mothers carry infants on their hips or backs with the infants' legs abducted—as in Korean, Chinese, and some African groups—the incidence of DDH is low (Novacheck, 1996).

DISORDERS OF THE HIP

DEVELOPMENTAL DYSPLASIA OF THE HIP

Developmental dysplasia of the hip (DDH) refers to a variety of conditions in which the femoral head and the acetabulum are improperly aligned. These conditions include hip instability, **dislocation** (displacement of the bone from its normal articulation with the joint), **subluxation** (in this instance, a partial dislocation), and acetabular **dysplasia** (abnormal cellular or structural development) (American Academy of Pediatrics, Committee on Quality Improvement and Subcommittee on Developmental Dysplasia of the Hip, 2000). In the past, DDH was referred to as congenital dislocated hip (CDH). The revised name of the disorder emphasizes that many cases of dislocation, subluxation, and dysplasia occur well after the neonatal period and involve more than a simple dislocation.

Hip instability is present in 1 in 100 newborns, while dislocation occurs in 1 to 2 in 1,000 births, and the condition affects girls 4 times as often as boys. It is unilateral in 80% of affected children, and the left hip is affected 3 times as often as the right (American Academy of Pediatrics, 2000).

Etiology and Pathophysiology

Although the exact cause of DDH is unknown, genetic factors appear to play a role. DDH is 20 to 50 times more common in first-degree relatives of an infant with the condition than in the general population. If one child of a set of identical twins has DDH, the other twin is affected 30% to 40% of the time.

Prenatal conditions may affect the development of DDH. The left hip is involved more often than the right hip as a result of intrauterine positioning of the left side of the fetus against the mother's sacrum. Maternal estrogen may cause laxity of the hip joint and capsule, leading to joint instability, especially in females who respond to these estrogen levels. DDH is more common in infants born in the breech position. Cultural factors may also be associated with DDH.

Clinical Manifestations

Common signs and symptoms of DDH include limited abduction of the affected hip, asymmetry of the gluteal and thigh fat folds, and telescoping or pistoning of the thigh (Figure 21-7 ◆). The older child with untreated DDH walks with a significant limp, which

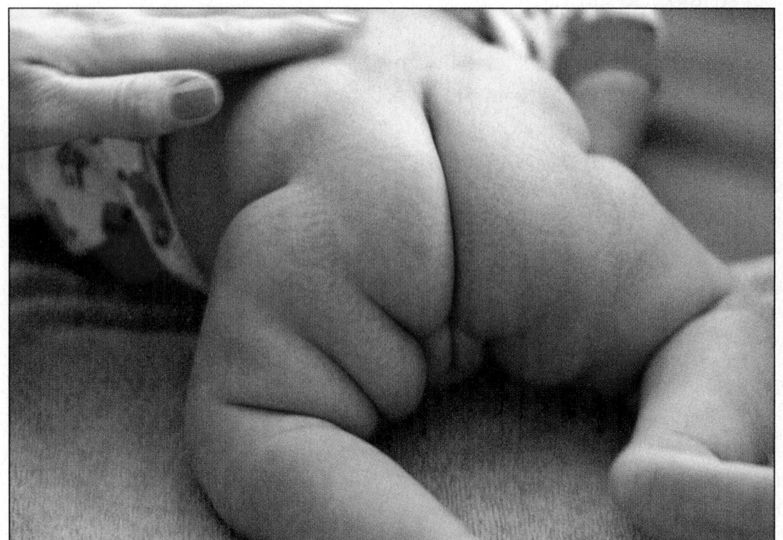

FIGURE 21-7 ◆
The asymmetry of the gluteal and thigh fat folds is easy to see in this child with developmental dysplasia of the hip.

results from telescoping of the femoral head into the pelvis. The longer the disorder goes untreated, the more pronounced the clinical manifestations become, and the worse the prognosis.

Clinical Therapy

Physical examination reveals Allis' sign (one knee lower than the other when the knees are flexed) and positive Ortolani–Barlow maneuver in babies under 8 to 12 weeks. Refer to Chapter 4 for a discussion of the assessment of hip dysplasia in newborns and infants. Radiographs are generally not reliable until approximately 4 months of age, because the pelvis in a newborn is still primarily cartilaginous. Before 4 months, ultrasonography may be useful for diagnosis. After that age, radiographs are used for diagnosis.

Treatment plans vary according to the child's age. For infants younger than 3 months, the Pavlik harness is the most commonly used method for hip reduction (Figure 21-8 ◆). The Pavlik harness is a dynamic splint, that is, a splint that allows movement. It ensures hip flexion and abduction and does not allow hip extension or adduction. For infants older than 3 months, skin traction is used (Figure 21-9 ◆). Correct positioning, which involves relocating the femoral head into the acetabulum while gently stretching the restrictive soft tissue, is essential. Surgery and the application of a spica cast may be necessary. In children over 18 months of age, surgery and casting are usually necessary and bracing may also be required.

Early screening, detection, and treatment enable the majority of affected children to attain normal hip function.

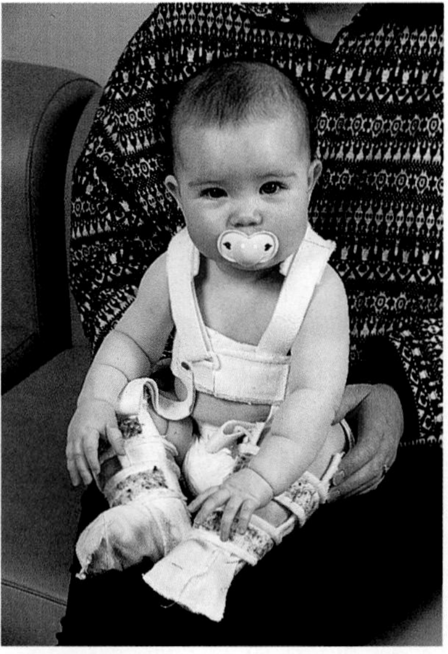

FIGURE 21-8 ◆
The most common treatment for DDH in a child under 3 months of age is a Pavlik harness. A shirt should be worn under the harness to prevent skin irritation (it was omitted for clarity in this photograph).

NURSING MANAGEMENT

Nursing Assessment and Diagnosis

Assessment for DDH begins at delivery and continues through all well-child checkups. The specific family history or birth data may indicate a high-risk infant. Instructions for performing the physical examination to assess the infant for DDH are given in Chapter 4. Further assessments are determined by the treatment provided. Skin assessments are performed on the child in traction or a cast. Respiratory and circulatory assessments are included when the child is immobilized. Ongoing assessment of the child's growth and development are needed. Weigh the casted child once the cast is dry so a baseline casted weight can be used for comparison during the weeks and months while the cast remains in place.

The following nursing diagnoses may apply to the child with DDH:

- *Impaired physical mobility,* related to prescribed movement restriction (Pavlik harness, traction, spica cast, brace)

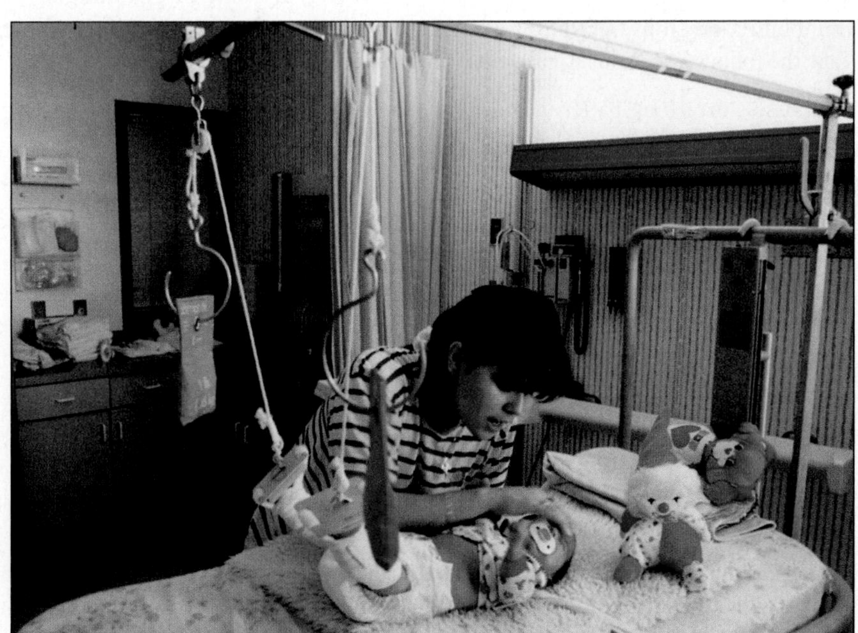

FIGURE 21-9 ◆
For infants older than 3 months of age, skin traction is commonly used for treatment of DDH.

- *Risk for impaired skin integrity,* related to irritation from harness straps or skin traction
- *Risk for altered urinary elimination or constipation,* related to immobility caused by treatment
- *Risk for altered nutrition,* related to decreased appetite
- *Risk for altered growth and development,* related to limited mobility and potential decreased exposure to stimulation
- *Health seeking behavior,* related to lack of information about disease process and treatment

Planning and Implementation

The infant with DDH is often cared for at home and in outpatient facilities. If surgery is performed, the child is hospitalized for surgery and the immediate postoperative period. Nursing care varies according to the medical treatment and the child's age. Management includes maintaining traction, if ordered; providing cast care; preventing complications resulting from immobility; promoting normal growth and development; and teaching parents how to care for a child in a cast, traction, or a Pavlik harness at home. Because treatment may interfere with the child's normal movement, the treatment plan should take into consideration the age and developmental stage of the child.

Maintain Traction

Bryant skin traction is the most common form of traction used in the treatment of DDH. (Types of traction are discussed later in the chapter and presented in Table 21-5) Check the traction apparatus frequently to ensure that proper alignment and healing occur. Traction may also be used as a treatment in the home. The family needs to be given careful instruction in how to care for the child in traction. In addition, arrangements should be made for a nurse to make several home visits to set up the traction apparatus and monitor the child's progress after discharge (see Table 21-5 later in the chapter).

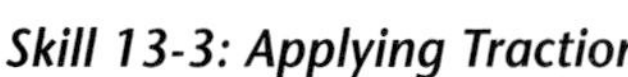

Skill 13-3: Applying Traction

Provide Cast Care

The principles of routine cast care presented in Table 21-2 apply to the care of spica casts. Special techniques should be used to help keep the cast clean and dry in children who are not toilet trained. Female and male urinals can be used for older children. Use a plastic lining to protect the cast edges during elimination for older children and use a small disposable diaper to cover the perineum in babies, tucking edges beneath the cast. Be sure to change the diaper frequently to prevent soiling of the cast.

Prevent Complications Resulting from Immobility

Immobilization from traction or a cast can cause alterations in physiologic functioning. Take the following actions to prevent complications:

- Assess breathing patterns and lung sounds frequently for congestion or respiratory compromise.
- Perform skin and neurovascular assessments approximately every 2 hours.
- Use adequate padding and skin wrapping to avoid placing pressure on the popliteal space. Such pressure could lead to nerve damage.
- For the child in a cast, change the child's position every 2 to 3 hours while awake to help avoid areas of pressure and promote increased circulation. The child can be placed either prone or supine or positioned on the floor and supported with pillows.
- Help prevent skin irritation and breakdown in the child with a cast. Use moleskin to provide protection from rough edges. Place tape around the perineal opening of the cast to prevent soiling.
- Increase fluids and fiber in the child's diet, as a change in bowel or bladder status is commonly associated with immobility.
- If permitted by physician's orders, release the child from traction for meals and daily care. The time out of traction should not exceed 1 hour per day. Encourage parents to hold and cuddle the child at this time to promote comfort and bonding.

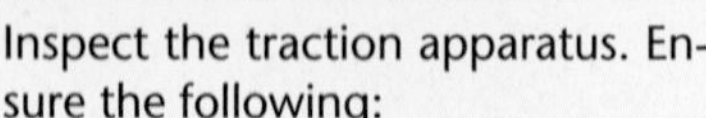

Inspect the traction apparatus. Ensure the following:

- Nuts and bolts are tight.
- Knots are well tied and secured with tape.
- Weight amounts are correct and weights are hanging free.
- Ropes are unfrayed.
- The line of pull is straight.

Promote Normal Growth and Development

Engage the child in activities that stimulate the upper extremities and all five senses. Provide stimulating toys such as stacking blocks, brightly colored mobiles, Koosh balls, or musical toys. Position toys within the child's reach and interact with the child as much as possible.

SAFETY PRECAUTIONS

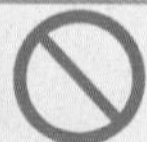

Use caution in selecting toys appropriate for the child's developmental age. If the child is in a cast, be sure that toys or parts cannot be swallowed or stuck inside the cast. Place a t-shirt over the cast so that the edges are securely covered and made difficult for the child to place something under them.

Discharge Planning and Home Care Teaching

Parents must learn how to care for a child in traction or a spica cast at home. The active participation of family members in the daily care of the child while hospitalized gradually increases their confidence in their ability to provide care at home. Home care needs should be identified and addressed well in advance of discharge. Before discharge, be sure the parents have the following information:

- Instructions about general cast care (see page 786), positioning, bathing, toileting, and age-appropriate diversional activities
- Appropriate referrals for periodic assessment by a visiting nurse or home health nurse
- Family resources to care for the child

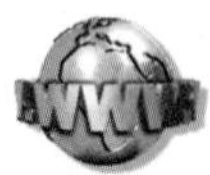

Adaptive Car Seats

Before discharge, have parents demonstrate how to dress and feed a child in a spica cast. Ensure that safe travel arrangements have been made for the day of discharge as described below. Help parents to obtain an appropriate car safety seat in advance of discharge. Encourage parents to let the child interact with other children at home, and to provide the child in a cast with similar opportunities for play and social activities.

Care in the Community

Have parents of an infant in a Pavlik harness demonstrate proper application of the harness and care of the infant while in the harness. Teach family members about daily care (bathing, dressing, and feeding) of the infant. Ideally, the harness is worn 23 hours per day and is removed only for skin checks and bathing. The hips and buttocks should be supported carefully when the infant is out of the harness. Demonstrate how to feed the infant in an upright position to maintain abduction and how to change a diaper without removing the harness. Double diapering may be recommended to provide support for the hips.

Instruct the parents of an infant with a harness or a child in a cast to look for any reddened or irritated areas near the harness or cast edges and to check toes frequently for proper circulation. Frequent repositioning reduces the risk of pressure sores or circulatory compromise. The infant should wear an undershirt and socks under the harness to prevent rubbing of the skin.

FAMILIES WANT TO KNOW

Transporting the Child with Orthopedic Devices

The American Academy of Pediatrics has established guidelines for transporting children with special health care needs.

- Placement in the rear seat is preferable.
- If the front seat must be used, the front passenger airbag should be disconnected.
- Use only approved car seat transport systems approved for use with special needs children.
- Install and use seats as instructed.
- A child should be moved from a wheelchair or other special device to be placed in the vehicle safety seat when reasonable.
- Pieces of medical equipment required during transportation (such as monitors or oxygen) or that are being transported with the child (such as wheelchair or walker) should be secured to the floor of the vehicle.
- If the child is transported by school bus, state and federal recommendations for school bus transportation of children with special needs should be followed.

Note: Adapted from American Academy of Pediatrics, Committee on Injury and Poison Prevention. (1999). Transporting children with special healthcare needs. *Pediatrics, 104*, 988–992.

FAMILIES WANT TO KNOW

Guidelines for Pavlik Harness Application

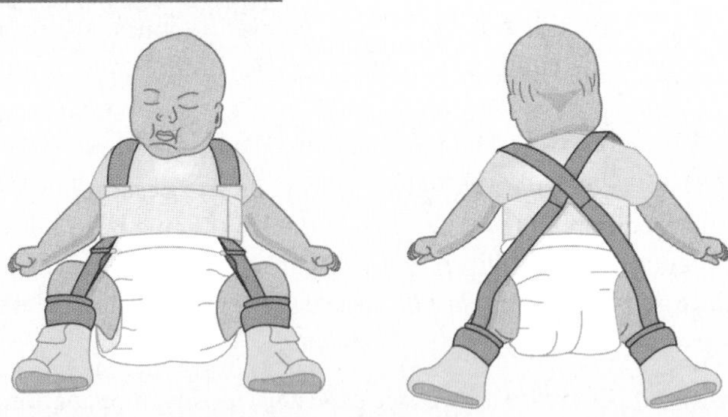

1. Position the chest halter at nipple line and fasten with Velcro.
2. Position the legs and feet in the stirrups, being sure the hips are flexed and abducted. Fasten with Velcro.
3. Connect the chest halter and leg straps in front.
4. Connect the chest halter and leg straps in back.

All the straps are marked at the first fitting with indelible ink so they can be reattached easily after the harness is rinsed and dried.

Safety precautions are important as the child will not have normal mobility. Parents will need to use a specially designed car seat that accommodates the child with abducted hips (see page 793). Strollers and cribs should provide sufficient room to protect the legs from injury and to prevent hip adduction.

Evaluation

Expected outcomes for nursing care of the child with developmental dysplasia of the hip include the following:

- Maintenance of skin integrity
- Absence of symptoms of immobility
- Knowledge of parents regarding the condition, treatment, and necessary home care
- Maintenance of a safe environment for the child

LEGG-CALVÉ-PERTHES DISEASE

Legg-Calvé-Perthes disease is a self-limiting condition in which there is avascular necrosis of the femoral head. The disease occurs in approximately 1 in 12,000 children and affects boys 4 times more often than girls. It usually occurs between the ages of 2 and 12 years, with a peak incidence between 4 and 8 years. The disease is bilateral in 10% of cases (Roy, 1999).

Etiology and Pathophysiology

The necrosis associated with Legg-Calvé-Perthes disease results from an interruption of the blood supply to the femoral epiphysis. How and why this occurs is not completely understood, but several predisposing factors have been identified. The incidence of this disease is up to 20% higher in families with a history of the disease than in the general population, which suggests that genetic factors may play a role. In 25% of the cases, onset of the disease is preceded by a mild traumatic injury. Trauma may cause a subchondral fracture and resultant synovitis, which in turn causes pressure that occludes the blood supply. Children with Legg-Calvé-Perthes disease often have delayed skeletal maturation, increased thyroid levels, and low somatomedin C (insulinlike growth factor). It is more common in those with low birth weight, increased parental age, and exposure to environmental tobacco smoke (Roy, 1999).

CULTURE

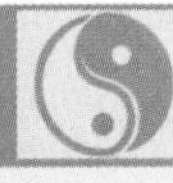

Legg-Calvé-Perthes disease is most common among white and Chinese children. It is less common among blacks and Native Americans.

CLINICAL MANIFESTATIONS OF LEGG-CALVÉ-PERTHES DISEASE

STAGE	CLINICAL MANIFESTATIONS
Prenecrosis	An insult causes loss of blood supply to the femoral head.
I—Necrosis	Avascular stage (3–6 months); the child is asymptomatic, bone radiographs are normal, and the head of the femur is structurally intact but avascular.
II—Revascularization	Period of 1–4 years characterized by pain and limitation of movement. Bone radiographs show new bone deposition and dead bone resorption. Fracture and deformity of the head of the femur can occur.
III—Bone healing	Reossification takes place; pain decreases.
IV—Remodeling	The disease process is over, pain is absent, and improvement in joint function occurs.

Clinical Manifestations

Legg-Calvé-Perthes disease progresses through four distinct stages after the original insult (usually unknown) occurs, over a period of 1 to 4 years. Early symptoms of the disease include a mild pain in the hip or anterior thigh and a limp, which are aggravated by increased activity and relieved by rest. The child favors the affected hip and limits hip movement to avoid discomfort (Davids, 1998).

As the disease progresses, range of motion becomes limited and weakness and muscle wasting develop. The affected thigh is 2 to 3 cm smaller than the unaffected thigh. Over time, prolonged hip irritability may produce muscle spasms.

Clinical Therapy

Because the child's initial symptoms are so mild, parents often do not seek medical attention until symptoms have been present for several months. Diagnosis is made using standard anteroposterior and frog-leg radiographs. As noted above, radiographs taken early in the course of the disease may be normal or show vague widening of the cartilage space. Bone scans and MRI may show the disease process earlier than radiographs. Laboratory studies of the blood, such as white blood cell count, help to rule out inflammatory synovitis of the hip.

Medical management and prognosis depend on the degree of femoral involvement. Early detection is important. The desired outcome is a pain-free hip that functions properly. To promote healing and prevent deformity, the femoral head must be contained within the hip socket until ossification is complete. Adequate containment will be achieved only if the hips remain in an abducted position. At the beginning of treatment, traction can be used to maintain the hips in an abducted and internally rotated position. Once abduction is accomplished, treatment consists of Petrie (leg abduction) casting, or surgical soft tissue releases such as adductor tenotomy, followed by bracing. Toronto (Figure 21-10 ◆) and Scottish-Rite braces are most commonly used. Prognosis is good if the femoral head can be contained long enough for proper healing to occur. Severe disease may be treated by surgery to release adductor muscles, treat the acetabulum or femur, and restore range of motion. Children with untreated disease or those diagnosed late in the disease process occasionally develop osteoarthritis and hip dysfunction later in life (Roy, 1999).

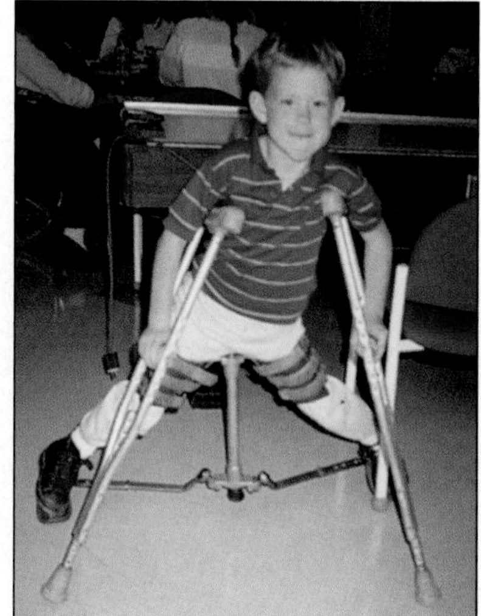

FIGURE 21-10 ◆
Although the Toronto brace may seem formidable for a child to wear, you can see by this photograph that, as usual, children adapt quite well to it.

NURSING MANAGEMENT

Nursing Assessment and Diagnosis

Legg-Calvé-Perthes disease should be suspected in any child, especially a boy age 2 to 12 years, who complains of hip discomfort accompanied by a limp. The school nurse may be the first person to observe the child with symptoms of the disease. The child may complain

GROWTH & DEVELOPMENT

Legg-Calvé-Perthes disease primarily affects boys with an average age of 6 years. These school-age children are industrious and independent. Offer suggestions for activities that redirect energy and promote normal development. These may include horseback riding, which promotes hip abduction; swimming to increase mobility; handcrafts to promote fine motor skills; and computer activities to stimulate cognitive development.

of pain and have to rest during physical education classes. Immediate referral should be made to the health care provider. Question the child who has an apparent limp about pain, and assess the child's range of motion. Ask if the child previously injured the hip.

Nursing diagnoses, which center on altered activities and compliance, may include the following:

- *Impaired physical mobility,* related to restriction of brace or cast
- *Risk for injury,* related to potential complications resulting from noncompliance with the treatment regimen
- *Risk for noncompliance,* related to duration of treatment
- *Diversional activity deficit,* related to forced inactivity
- *Potential body image disturbance,* related to brace

Planning and Implementation

Children with Legg-Calvé-Perthes disease often receive all of their treatment at home. Helping the child and family comply with the prescribed treatment plan may be challenging, because children develop the disease at an age when they are usually very active. The child, who may have little pain, often finds immobilization difficult.

Promote Normal Growth and Development

Parents should be given suggestions to help redirect the child's energy within the limitations in mobility imposed by treatment. A return to school promotes a feeling of normalcy. Coordinate the return to school by facilitating the child's use of elevator or ramp as needed in that setting. Activities that involve peers also help the child achieve developmental milestones. Help the child adjust to wearing a brace.

Care in the Community

Both the child and the family should be aware that treatment generally takes more than 2 years. Emphasize the importance of following the treatment plan to ensure adequate hip containment and proper healing. Teach the family how to care for a child in traction and how to check the child's skin for breakdown. Follow-up visits should be arranged at regular intervals, in addition to home care visits during the period of traction.

Evaluation

Expected outcomes of nursing care are elimination of hip pain and discomfort, normal development during the period of immobilization, and parent and child knowledge of treatment regimen.

SLIPPED CAPITAL FEMORAL EPIPHYSIS

Slipped capital femoral epiphysis (SCFE) occurs when the femoral head is displaced from the femoral neck. This condition is commonly seen during the adolescent growth spurt, between the ages of 8 and 16 years. Boys are more often affected than girls (Theophilopoulos & Barrett, 1998).

Etiology and Pathophysiology

The cause of SCFE is unknown. Predisposing factors include obesity, a recent growth spurt, and endocrine disorders such as hypothyroidism and hypogonadism. There may be a genetic predisposition to the development of the disorder.

Slippage of the femoral head occurs at the proximal epiphyseal plate, and the femur displaces from the epiphysis (Figure 21-11 ◆). Slippage is usually gradual (chronic), but may also result from acute trauma. The synovial membrane becomes inflamed, edematous, and painful. If untreated, callous formation occurs, resulting in a deformed hip with limited range of motion.

PATHOPHYSIOLOGY ILLUSTRATED

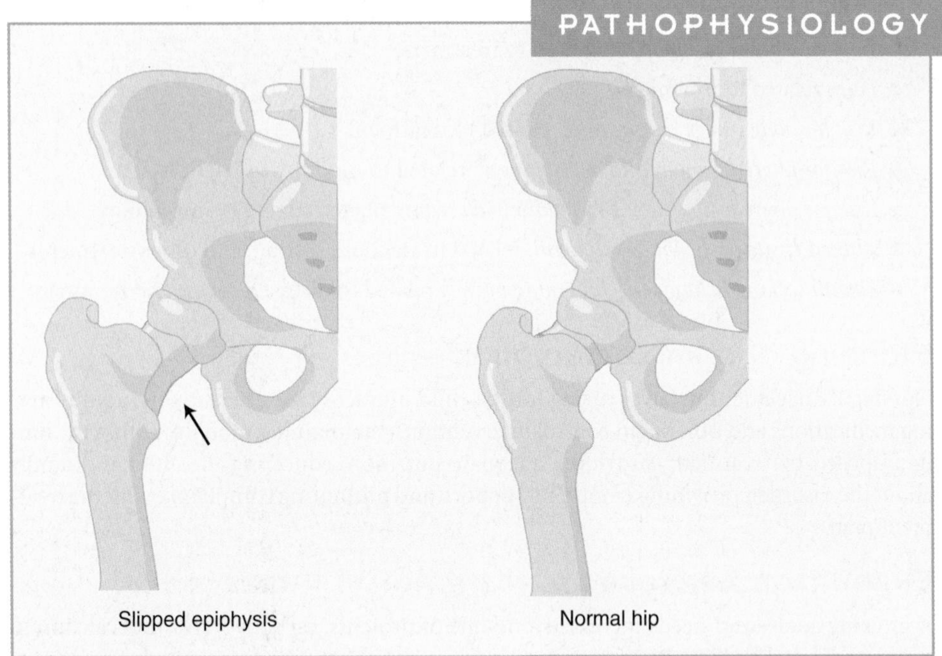

Slipped Epiphysis

FIGURE 21-11 ◆ In slipped capital femoral epiphysis, the femoral head is displaced from the femoral neck at the proximal epiphyseal plate.

Clinical Manifestations

Symptoms include limp, pain, and loss of hip motion. The condition is categorized as acute (sudden onset with less than 3 weeks' duration), chronic (longer than 3 weeks duration), or acute-on-chronic (an additional slippage in a child with a chronic condition), depending on the onset and severity of symptoms. The child with an acute slip has sudden, severe pain and cannot bear weight. An acute slip may be associated with traumatic injury.

A chronic slip presents with persistent hip pain, which is generally aching or mild and can be referred to the thigh, knee, or both. A limp and decreased range of motion may also occur.

When the child has had a chronic slip and then sustains a traumatic incident that causes further slippage of the femoral head, an acute-on-chronic slip is said to have occurred. The child experiences sudden, severe pain.

Clinical Therapy

A complete history provides information about risk factors and the development of the condition. Radiographs are used to confirm the diagnosis. A bone scan may also be performed.

The goal of medical management is to stabilize the femoral head while keeping displacement to a minimum and retaining as much hip function as possible. Surgical treatment is usually necessary; this involves fixation of the epiphysis with screws or pins. If treated early, a single screw into the hip in an outpatient procedure is sufficient for stabilization; in advanced cases, surgery becomes more complicated (Shaw, Gerardi, & Hennrikus, 1998). Medical treatment, which is occasionally used, includes a regimen of no weight bearing, bedrest, a spica cast, and Buck or Russell traction (see Table 21-4 later in the chapter).

Prognosis is related to the severity of the deformity and the occurrence of complications, such as avascular necrosis of the femoral head or **chondrolysis** (the breaking down and absorption of cartilage).

NURSING MANAGEMENT

Nursing Assessment and Diagnosis

The child usually presents with hip pain or referred pain to the groin, thigh, or knee, and limited mobility. A thorough history is needed to assess for injury as a cause. Assess the child's range of motion, pain, and limp, if apparent. Refer the child for treatment immediately if SCFE is suspected. This condition is considered to be an emergency, and it is essential that the child be treated immediately to keep weight off the affected joint.

Nursing diagnoses that may apply to the child with SCFE are as follows:

- *Impaired physical mobility,* related to treatment
- *Pain,* related to hip injury
- *Risk for body image disturbance,* related to treatment
- *Risk for altered growth and development,* related to mobility restrictions
- *Risk for altered nutrition: More than body requirements,* related to immobility
- *Altered tissue perfusion: Peripheral,* related to traction, casting, and other treatments
- *Health seeking behaviors (child and parent),* related to disease process and treatment

Planning and Implementation

Nursing management involves caring for the child in traction or after surgery, administering medications and other pain control interventions, maintaining mobility within the limits imposed by treatment, providing adequate nutrition, educating the child and family about the disorder, providing emotional support, and promoting compliance with the treatment plan.

Encourage Appropriate Nutritional Intake

A growing adolescent needs increased amounts of proteins, carbohydrates, and calcium to promote skeletal healing. Provide written instructions about nutritional requirements necessary to promote bone healing and maintain an ideal body weight. If a child is overweight, encourage weight loss by decreasing percent of fat in the diet. This decreases pressure on the femoral epiphysis and can also lead to a more positive self-image.

Provide Emotional Support

Because the onset of SCFE is usually unexpected, the child and family may find themselves facing surgery with little warning. Explain the treatment plan simply and thoroughly. Reassure the child and family that with proper compliance, treatment should be successful.

Discharge Planning and Home Care Teaching

Assist the family to plan for return to school. If attendance is not possible for a period of time due to traction or surgery, arrange for tutors and computer communication with school as needed. Follow-up visits are necessary until the child's epiphyseal plates close. It is not uncommon for SCFE to occur in the other hip. Make sure the child and family are aware of symptoms such as decreased range of motion or pain that could indicate onset of the disorder in the other hip. Tell parents to contact their health care provider immediately if these symptoms occur.

Evaluation

Expected outcomes of nursing care for the child with SCFE include maintenance of normal weight and recommended nutritional intake, absence of complications of immobility, successful adaptation to school following treatment, and family recognition of need for ongoing monitoring for complications.

DISORDERS OF THE SPINE

SCOLIOSIS

Scoliosis is a lateral S- or C-shaped curvature of the spine that is often associated with a rotational deformity of the spine and ribs. Many individuals exhibit some degree of spinal curvature, while curvatures of more than 10 degrees are considered abnormal. Curves are either structural or compensatory, as the spine curves to compensate for a structural deformity along its length. Idiopathic scoliosis occurs most often in girls, especially during the growth spurt between the ages of 10 and 13 years. Early onset of idiopathic scoliosis occurs before 10 years of age and comprises 15% of cases (Kautz & Skaggs, 1998).

Etiology and Pathophysiology

The cause of scoliosis is complex. Structural scoliosis may be congenital, idiopathic, or acquired (associated with neuromuscular disorders such as muscular dystrophy or myelodysplasia, or secondary to spinal cord injuries).

In idiopathic structural scoliosis (the most common type), the spine for unknown reasons begins to curve laterally, with vertebral rotation. The most common curve is a right thoracic and left lumbar deformity. As the curve progresses, structural changes occur. The ribs on the concave side (inside of the curve) are forced closer together, while the ribs on the convex side separate widely, causing narrowing of the thoracic cage and formation of the rib hump. The lateral curvature affects the vertebral structure. Disk spaces are narrowed on the concave side and spread wider on the convex side, resulting in an asymmetric vertebral canal (Figure 21-12 ◆).

Scoliosis can also occur in congenital diseases involving the spinal structure and in the musculoskeletal changes seen in conditions such as myelomeningocele, cerebral palsy (see Chapter 20), or muscular dystrophy. It can also be acquired after injury to the spinal cord. (The child in Figure 21-14, shown later in the chapter, acquired scoliosis after chemotherapy and radiation to the chest during treatment for cancer.)

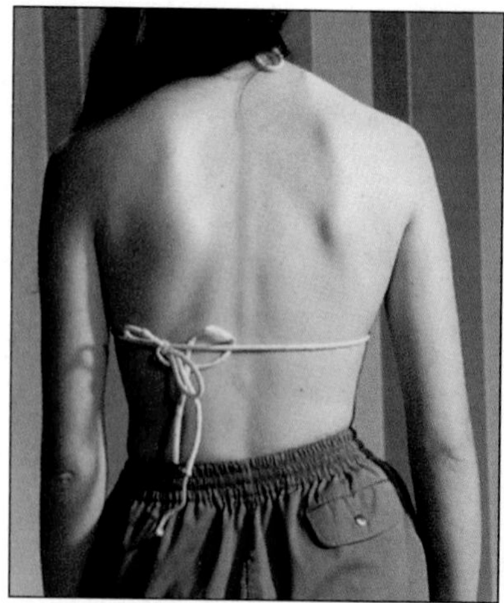

FIGURE 21-12 ◆
A child may have varying degrees of scoliosis. For mild forms, treatment will focus on strengthening and stretching. Moderate forms will require bracing. Severe forms may necessitate surgery and fusion. Clothes that fit at an angle, such as this teenage girl's shorts, and anatomic asymmetry of the back provide clues for early detection.

Clinical Manifestations

The classic signs of scoliosis include truncal asymmetry, uneven shoulders and hips, a one-sided rib hump, and a prominent scapula. The child does not complain of pain or discomfort.

Clinical Therapy

Generally, observation and radiographic examination are used to diagnose scoliosis. Additional diagnostic studies include MRI, CT scan, and bone scan, which are used occasionally to assess the degree of curvature. Moiré photography using a special screen and a point light source documents asymmetry of the spine and other bony landmarks (Figure 21-13 ◆).

The goal of medical management is to limit or stop progression of the curvature. Early detection is essential to successful treatment. Adequate treatment and follow-up maximize the child's chances for proper spinal alignment. The treatment regimen chosen depends on the degree and progression of the curvature and the reaction of the child and family to medical management.

Treatment of children with mild scoliosis (curvatures of 10 to 20 degrees) consists of exercises to improve posture and muscle tone and to maintain, or possibly increase, flexibility of the spine. Emphasis is placed on bending strength toward the outside of the curve while stretching the inside of the curve. These exercises are not a cure, however, and the child should be evaluated by a physician at 3-month intervals, with radiographic evaluation every 6 months.

Medical management of moderate scoliosis (curvatures of 20 to 40 degrees) includes bracing with either a Boston or Milwaukee brace. The goal of wearing a brace is to maintain the existing spinal curvature with no increase. Brace wear begins immediately after diagnosis. To achieve maximum effectiveness, the brace should be worn 23 hours per day. Brace treatment is lengthy and requires a high degree of compliance, which can be difficult for adolescents who view body image or sports involvement as important.

Electrical stimulation is used occasionally as an alternative treatment. An electric current stimulates the back muscles to contract, thus helping to correct the spinal curvature. This treatment, which is performed at night, eliminates the need for bracing. There is controversy about the usefulness of this therapy.

Children with severe scoliosis (curvatures of 40 degrees or more) require surgery, which involves spinal fusion. The majority of spinal fusions are performed using instrumentation with Luque wires or Coutrel-Dubosset (CD) instrumentation. These treatments stabilize the spine well during surgery, may be accompanied by bone grafting to the spine, and require no long-term therapy (Killian, Mayberry, & Wilkinson, 1999). Following surgery with wires or instrumentation, the child is on bedrest during a recovery period and then is generally fitted with anteroposterior plastic shells that are worn for several months to provide stability for the spine. Occasionally in severe cases, halo traction is used postoperatively to provide support for the unstable spine (Figure 21-14 ◆).

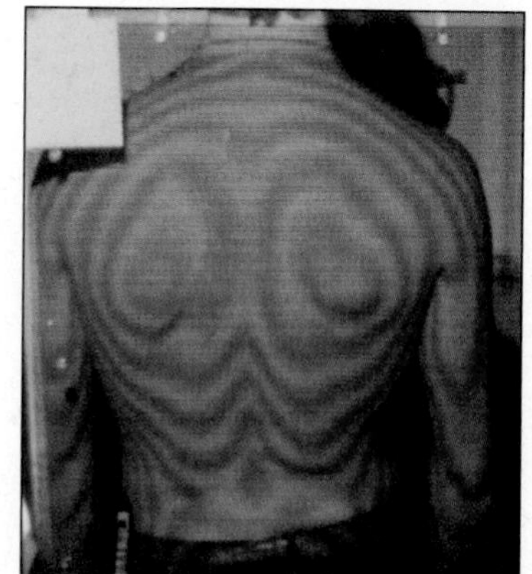

FIGURE 21-13 ◆
Moire photography is sometimes used to document the degree of spinal asymmetry.
From Staheli, L. T., (1992). *Fundamentals of pediatric orthopedics* (p. 8. 12). New York: Raven Press.

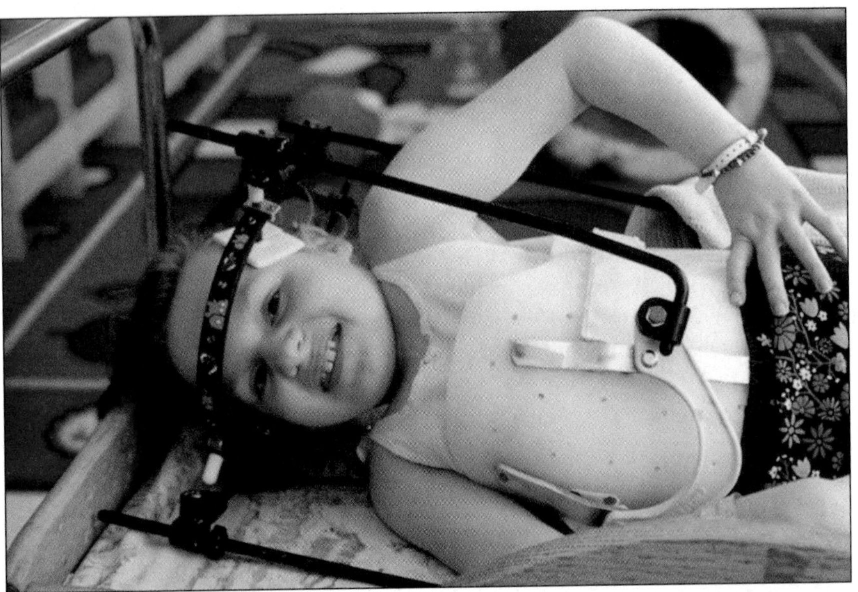

FIGURE 21-14 ◆
In severe scoliosis, the child may wear a halo brace, shown here, to hold the body in position after surgery.

NURSING MANAGEMENT

Nursing Assessment and Diagnosis

School nurses often screen children for scoliosis, generally in the fifth and seventh grades. This screening is mandated by law in several states. When abnormalities are noted, the child is referred to an orthopedic center for further evaluation. Children should be examined every 6 to 9 months thereafter. If scoliosis is detected, the child's brothers and sisters should be examined and observed closely. Chapter 4 discusses screening children for scoliosis.

Once scoliosis has been identified, the nurse's focus becomes education and follow-up. Any child with scoliosis should have a comprehensive neurologic, cardiac, and respiratory examination, since the rib cage deformity can influence the functioning of these systems.

The following nursing diagnoses may apply to the child with scoliosis who is not undergoing surgery:

- *Risk for noncompliance with exercise program,* related to duration and intensity of exercise
- *Impaired physical mobility,* related to brace
- *Risk for impaired skin integrity,* related to brace
- *Health seeking behaviors (child and parent),* related to unfamiliarity with disease process

Common nursing diagnoses for the child who is having surgery can be found in the accompanying nursing care plan.

Planning and Implementation

An important aspect of nursing care is patient education. Patient compliance is critical to the success of treatment. Children and their families need to understand the condition and the stages of treatment, particularly adolescents who are undergoing treatment for scoliosis. Children or adolescents facing surgery require education, reassurance, and support. The accompanying nursing care plan summarizes nursing care for the child undergoing surgery for scoliosis.

Promote Compliance with the Treatment Plan

Provide instructions about exercises that will help to decrease the severity of the spinal curvature. Demonstrate the exercises, and explain their purpose (e.g., to strengthen back muscles). Help the child adjust to wearing a brace. Adolescents, in particular, may be reluctant to wear an external device such as a brace. To promote a sense of control, allow the adolescent to choose when to exercise and when to be out of the brace, within the treatment guidelines.

NURSING CARE PLAN The Child Undergoing Surgery for Scoliosis

GOAL	INTERVENTION	RATIONALE	EXPECTED OUTCOME
1. Knowledge Deficit (Child and Parents) related to lack of information about surgery			
	NIC Priority Intervention: **Teaching, Disease Process and Preoperative:** Assisting the patient to understand information and mentally prepare for surgery and postoperative recovery.		NOC Suggested Outcome: **Knowledge:** Extent of understanding conveyed about scoliosis treatment.
The child and parents will verbalize understanding of the disease, its treatment, and the surgical procedure.	■ Teach the child and family about the course of the disease, its signs and symptoms, and treatment. Provide appropriate handouts. Encourage the child and parents to ask questions. ■ Begin preoperative teaching at the time of admission. Orient the child to hospital and postoperative procedures. Before surgery, have the child demonstrate log-rolling, range-of-motion exercises, and the use of an incentive spirometer. Discuss pain management.	■ Understanding and involvement increase motivation and compliance while reducing fear. ■ Preoperative teaching and familiarity with hospital procedures reduces the stress related to surgery and postoperative complications.	The child and family accurately verbalize knowledge about the disease and its treatment. The child and family ask appropriate questions about postoperative care.
2. Ineffective Breathing Pattern related to hypoventilation syndrome			
	NIC Priority Intervention: **Airway Management and Respiratory Monitoring:** Facilitation of patency of air passages and analysis of patient data.		NOC Suggested Outcome: **Respiratory Status: Ventilation:** Movement of air in and out of the lungs.
The child will show no signs of respiratory compromise.	■ Monitor respiratory status, especially after the administration of analgesics. Apply pulse oximeter. ■ Administer oxygen if ordered. ■ Have the child use an incentive spirometer. ■ Monitor intake and output. ■ Reposition the child at least every 2 hours.	■ Evaluation of the child's respiratory condition anticipates and avoids complications. Analgesics such as morphine may increase or potentiate respiratory compromise. ■ Oxygen increases peripheral oxygen saturation to 95%–100%. ■ Spirometry increases lung expansion and aeration of the alveoli. ■ Good hydration promotes loose secretions and helps prevent infection. ■ Repositioning ensures inflation of the lung fields.	The child has no respiratory complications.
3. Risk for Injury related to neurovascular deficit secondary to instrumentation			
	NIC Priority Intervention: **Injury Prevention:** Instituting special precautions with patient at risk.		NOC Suggested Outcome: **Risk Control:** Actions to eliminate or reduce modifiable health risks.

(continued)

NURSING CARE PLAN The Child Undergoing Surgery for Scoliosis (continued)

GOAL	INTERVENTION	RATIONALE	EXPECTED OUTCOME
3. Risk for Injury related to neurovascular deficit secondary to instrumentation (continued)			
The child's neurovascular system will remain intact as evidenced by circulation, sensation, and motor checks. The child will feel no numbness or tingling.	■ Monitor the child's color, circulation, capillary refill, warmth, sensation, and motion in all extremities. Perform neurovascular checks every 2 hours for the first 24 hours and then every 4 hours for the next 48 hours. Record presence of pedal and distal tibial pulses every hour for 48 hours. Report changes and abnormal findings immediately. ■ Have the child wear antiembolism stockings until ambulatory. The stockings may be removed for 1 hour 2-3 times daily. ■ Check for any pain, swelling, or a positive Homans' sign in the legs. Record any evidence of edema. ■ Monitor input and output. ■ Encourage and assist the child with range-of-motion exercises, both passive and active.	■ When the spinal column is manipulated during surgery, altered neurovascular status, thrombus formation, and paralysis are possible complications. Postoperative risks include loss of bowel or bladder control, weakness or paralysis, and impaired vision or sensation. ■ Antiembolism stockings prevent blood clots and promote venous return. Thrombus formation is a postoperative risk. ■ Swelling may indicate a tight dressing and tissue damage. A positive Homans' sign and pain may indicate thrombus formation. ■ Abnormalities may indicate a fluid shift problem. ■ Activity promotes mobility and reduces risk of thrombus formation.	The child exhibits only temporary alteration (pale skin, faint pulse, and edema occur but then resolve within the initial postoperative phase). The child returns to the preoperative baseline state by discharge.
4. Pain related to spinal fusion with instrumentation			
	NIC Priority Intervention: **Pain Management:** Alleviation of pain or a reduction of pain to a level of comfort acceptable to the patient.		NOC Suggested Outcome: **Pain Level:** Amount of reported or demonstrated pain.
The child will verbalize an adequate level of comfort or show absence of pain behavior within 1 hour of a specific nursing intervention.	■ Assess the level of pain and initiate pain management strategies as soon as possible. Use patient-controlled analgesia if ordered. ■ Administer pain medication around-the-clock to help ensure pain relief, especially during the first 48 hours. Monitor epidural blocks and patient-controlled analgesia or other methods used for pain control. ■ Use nonpharmacologic pain management techniques, such as imagery, relaxation, touch, music, application of heat and cold, and reduced environmental stimulation to supplement medications (see Chapter 9). ■ Document pain assessment, interventions, and the child's reactions. ■ Reassure the child that some discomfort is expected and that a variety of measures can be tried to reduce discomfort.	■ Adequate pain management allows for faster healing and a more cooperative patient. Patient controlled analgesics may be effective. ■ Medicating around-the-clock helps to maintain comfort. Monitoring ensures patient safety. ■ Alternative treatments also interrupt the pain stimulus and provide relief. Nonpharmacologic methods can be an effective adjunct to pain management. ■ Proper documentation guides the selection of the most effective means of pain control. ■ Realistic expectations decrease anxiety and give the child a sense of control.	The child experiences pain relief early in the postoperative period.

(continued)

NURSING CARE PLAN The Child Undergoing Surgery for Scoliosis (continued)

GOAL	INTERVENTION	RATIONALE	EXPECTED OUTCOME
5. Impaired Physical Mobility related to movement restrictions and pain			
	NIC Priority Intervention: **Positioning and Ambulation:** Moving the patient to provide comfort and promote healing, assist with walking.		NOC Suggested Outcome: **Ambulation:** Ability to walk from place to place.
The child will maintain proper body alignment and progress with activity as ordered by the physician. If no anteroposterior shell bracing is required the child will have active mobility by the third to fifth postoperative day.	■ Reposition the child every 2 hours using the log-roll technique. Support the back, feet, and knees with pillows. ■ Have the child do passive and active range-of-motion exercises every 2 hours for 48 hours and then every 4 hours while awake. Have the child dangle his or her legs at bedside by the second to fourth postoperative day. Begin ambulation by the third to fifth postoperative day. Note any complaints of dizziness, pallor, etc. Proceed slowly.	■ Proper positioning prevents twisting or turning the spine. ■ Exercises help maintain strength, circulation, and muscle tone. If the spine is stable and the physician has ordered no external support, the child may progress to full ambulation as tolerated. If the spine is not stable, great care must be taken until external supportive devices are used.	The child is as mobile as appropriate for condition with 3–5 days after surgery.
6. Risk for Body Image Disturbance related to treatment			
	NIC Priority Intervention: **Body Image Enhancement:** Improving conscious and unconscious perceptions toward the body.		NOC Suggested Outcome: **Body Image:** Positive perception of own appearance and body.
The child will verbalize feelings about body image and self-esteem in relation to the disease and its treatment. The child will be informed about available support services and use them as needed.	■ Encourage independence in daily activities within allowable limits. Use positive reinforcements. Encourage the child to participate in community activities, if possible. Involve the child in scoliosis support groups. ■ Provide contact with a peer resource person who has undergone treatment for scoliosis.	■ Involvement in activities demonstrates that a "normal" life is realistic. ■ Peers are an effective means of support.	The child has a positive self-image and is involved in community activities or support groups.
7. Risk for Knowledge Deficit (Child and Parent) related to lack of information about home care			
	NIC Priority Intervention: **Teaching: Prescribed Treatment:** Preparing family to understand and perform prescribed treatment.		NOC Suggested Outcome: **Knowledge:** Extent of understanding conveyed about postoperative treatment and follow-up care.
The child and family will verbalize reduced anxiety about home care. The child will demonstrate knowledge of self-care and permitted activities.	■ Teach cast or brace care as appropriate (see pp. 786 and 788). Provide oral and written instructions and a list of activity limitations (see Families Want to Know: Postoperative Activities after Spinal Surgery). Have the child and family demonstrate adequate knowledge. ■ Arrange for follow-up appointments as ordered by the physician. Encourage the child and family to notify the nurse or physician if they have any questions or concerns.	■ Providing education decreases anxiety and increases compliance with treatment plan. Demonstration reinforces the learning process. ■ Follow-up visits help the nurse and physician evaluate the effectiveness of the treatment plan and patient compliance.	The child and family demonstrate home care and implementation of discharge teaching.

FAMILIES WANT TO KNOW

Postoperative Activities after Spinal Surgery

RECOMMENDED
Lying
Sitting
Standing
Walking (including normal stair climbing)
Swimming, gentle (not with a cast); diving is not permitted

NOT RECOMMENDED
Bending or twisting at the waist
Lifting more than 10 pounds
Household chores such as vacuuming, unloading groceries, mowing the lawn, taking out the garbage
Sports such as bicycle riding, horseback riding, skiing, roller blading, skating
Physical education classes

COMMUNITY CARE

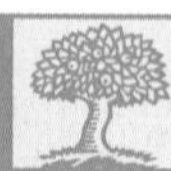

Some department stores will sponsor a fashion show for adolescents with scoliosis who must wear braces. Children with braces in place model and demonstrate how popular clothing can be worn to disguise the wearing of the brace. These events can have a positive impact on the self-esteem of adolescents who participate in and view the shows.

Provide reassurance and encouragement and promote interaction with peers. Suggesting that the adolescent work with a peer support person who is being treated for scoliosis or has had the condition in the past may be beneficial. Provide information about fashionable clothing that can be worn with the brace.

Discharge Planning and Home Care Teaching

Home care needs should be identified and addressed well in advance of discharge after spinal surgery. The child must learn to adapt to a new set of body mechanics. Show the child how to do simple tasks without bending or twisting the torso. Have the child demonstrate the ability to perform activities of daily living before discharge from the hospital.

Activities for the child who has had spinal surgery are commonly limited for a period of time. Restrictions usually should be followed for 6 to 8 months, depending on the type of surgery and the surgeon. Emphasize to both the child and the family the importance of compliance, and give them written discharge instructions. Follow-up visits are important. The child should be examined 4 to 6 weeks after discharge, then every 3 to 4 months for 1 year, and every 1 to 2 years thereafter.

Several organizations provide information and assistance to families of children with scoliosis. Referrals can be made as appropriate.

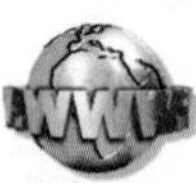

Scoliosis Resources and Support

COMMUNITY CARE

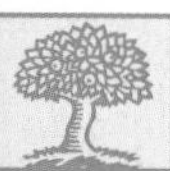

Children with metal hardware in their back after scoliosis surgery need to carry an explanation from the physician on airplane flights as they will set off metal detectors in airports.

Evaluation

Expected outcomes of nursing care for the child with scoliosis treated by brace are maintenance of intact skin and compliance with prescribed therapy. Expected outcomes after surgical correction are listed on the accompanying nursing care plan.

GROWTH & DEVELOPMENT

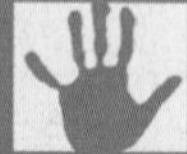

Postural lordosis is a characteristic finding in toddlers, but should disappear by the school-age years.

TORTICOLLIS, KYPHOSIS, AND LORDOSIS

Torticollis is tilt of the head caused by rotation of the cervical spine. Stretching exercises or surgical lengthening of the sternocleidomastoid muscle are usual treatments. Kyphosis (hunchback) and lordosis (swayback) are two other types of spinal curvature that may occur in children. Nurses can perform thorough musculoskeletal assessments of children (see Chapter 4) and refer any children with abnormalities for further evaluation. Clinical therapy depends on the cause and degree of the curvature, and the age of the child at onset. Refer to the table on page 805 for clinical manifestations and treatment of kyphosis and lordosis.

DISORDERS OF THE BONES AND JOINTS

OSTEOMYELITIS

Osteomyelitis is an infection of the bone, most often one of the long bones of the lower extremity. It may be acute or chronic and may spread into surrounding tissues. Although osteomyelitis may occur at any age, it is most common in children between the ages of 1 and

CLINICAL MANIFESTATIONS AND TREATMENT OF KYPHOSIS AND LORDOSIS

CONDITION	CLINICAL MANIFESTATIONS	CLINICAL THERAPY
Kyphosis Excessive convex curvature of the cervical thoracic spine.	*Clinical manifestations:* Visible hunchback or rounded shoulders; shortness of breath or fatigue; abdominal creases and light hamstrings in severe cases. *Diagnostic tests:* Spinal curvature is assessed by having the child bend 90 degrees at the waist and looking at the scapular area from side. Diagnosis is confirmed by radiograph.	*Medical therapy:* Exercises are prescribed for mild condition; bracing is commonly used; surgery is performed in severe cases. *Nursing management:* Provide support. Encourage exercises and diligent brace wear. Help the child to deal with the psychologic stress of altered body image.
Lordosis Excessive concave curvature of the lumbar spine with an angle of more than 60 degrees; most common in prepubescent girls and blacks.	*Clinical manifestations:* Presence of sway-back; prominent buttocks; hip flexion contractures; tight hamstrings. *Diagnostic tests:* Spinal curvature is assessed by looking at the standing child from the side. Lumbar lordosis is confirmed by visualizing the spine on standing, lateral radiograph.	*Medical therapy:* Treatment focuses on exercises and postural awareness. Bracing and surgery are rarely prescribed. *Nursing management:* Provide support. Reassure the child and family that the condition is often outgrown as the child matures. Encourage physical conditioning exercises and follow-up examinations on a yearly basis.

12 years. Boys are affected 2 to 3 times as often as girls, primarily because they have a greater incidence of trauma (Carek, Dickerson, & Sack, 2001).

Etiology and Pathophysiology

Osteomyelitis is caused by a microorganism, which is usually bacterial but can be viral or fungal. *Staphylococcus aureus* is the most common causative pathogen, followed by *Escherichia coli,* group *B* streptococci, *Streptococcus aureus, Streptococcus pyogenes,* and *Haemophilus influenzae.* A common source of infection is the upper respiratory system. Trauma to the bone or surgical interventions are other common causes of infection.

The infecting organism spreads through the bloodstream or via a penetrating injury to the bone, where it becomes established. Most infections in children begin in the metaphysis (see Figure 21-1), which has a sluggish blood supply. Eventually the infection may penetrate the bone cortex and periosteum. Inflammation and abscess formation can lead to interruption of the blood supply to the underlying bone, involvement of the surrounding soft tissue, and, if the infection is left untreated, to necrosis.

Clinical Manifestations

Symptoms include pain and tenderness with swelling, decreased mobility of the infected joint, and fever. Redness over the area may occur. Because the onset of acute osteomyelitis is generally rapid, it is sometimes misdiagnosed as a sports injury (Shaw, et al., 1998).

Clinical Therapy

A history suggestive of osteomyelitis includes an upper respiratory infection or blunt trauma followed by pain at the area of a growth plate. Laboratory evaluation shows leukocytosis and an elevated erythrocyte sedimentation rate (ESR) and C-reactive protein (Theophilopoulos & Barrett, 1998; Carek et al., 2001). The degree of ESR elevation is directly related to the severity of the infection. Radiographs and bone scans may identify the area of involvement. A needle aspiration of the site or a blood culture can confirm the diagnosis and provide a culture of the causative organism.

Medical management begins with the intravenous administration of a broad spectrum antibiotic, even before culture results are available. Once the culture results are obtained, the antibiotic may be altered. Oral antibiotics are given once an adequate response has occurred. However, extended intravenous home therapy may be used. Antibiotic therapy continues for about 6 weeks. When an adequate response is not obtained within 2 to 3 days, the area may be aspirated again, or surgical drainage may be carried out. Intravenous fluids may

CLINICAL TIP

When a child has a possible diagnosis of osteomyelitis, ensure that all cultures (blood, wound, etc.) are taken before antibiotic therapy begins.

GROWTH & DEVELOPMENT 

Osteomyelitis in a newborn is of great concern, as before 18 months of age the blood vessels cross the growth plates. This creates a higher risk of epiphyseal involvement with resultant limb length discrepancy.

be administered to ensure adequate hydration. In children with extensive orthopedic surgery, or in those with immunosuppression, a short course of prophylactic antibiotic may be administered after surgery (DeBaun, 1998).

Prompt diagnosis and treatment usually result in complete resolution of the infection. The prognosis is related to the initiation of therapy—the earlier treatment begins, the better the outcome. Long-term unfavorable outcomes include disruption of the growth plate, which can interrupt growth and damage the joints from septic arthritis.

NURSING MANAGEMENT

Nursing Assessment and Diagnosis

A thorough history, including information about the onset of symptoms and a history of recent infections or puncture wounds, is essential. Assess the affected area for signs of redness, swelling, pain, and decreased range of motion.

Nursing diagnoses that may apply to the child with osteomyelitis are as follows:

- *Pain,* related to biologic injury
- *Impaired physical mobility,* related to discomfort
- *Risk for sepsis,* related to spread of infection
- *Risk for altered nutrition: Less than body requirements,* related to loss of appetite
- *Risk for noncompliance,* related to duration of antibiotic therapy
- *Health seeking behaviors (child and parent),* related to lack of information about disease process

Planning and Implementation

Nursing management focuses on administering antibiotics, protecting the child from spread of the infection, and encouraging a well-balanced diet. Standard precautions should be used, with transmission-based precautions for any drainage from the site of infection.

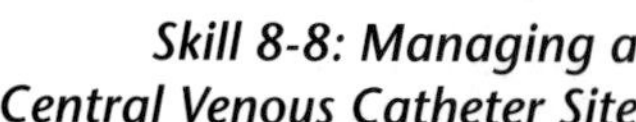

Skill 8-8: Managing a Central Venous Catheter Site

Administer Fluids and Medications

Administer intravenous fluids as ordered to maintain the hydration status of the child. Antibiotics are administered intravenously at first, then orally. Monitor the intravenous site and provide care for the central line, if used (refer to the Skills Manual). In the early stages of the infection, analgesics are prescribed to relieve the associated pain and joint tenderness.

HOME CARE 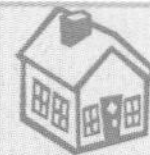

If the child is homebound for a period of time during treatment, assist the family in planning for completion of school tasks.

- Contact the school and ask that work be sent home.
- Arrange for a tutor if needed.
- Facilitate computer communication between child, teacher, and other students.
- Help family members to plan for help at home, to monitor the child when they are at work or performing other tasks.
- Refer to financial resources as appropriate for the services the child needs.
- Suggest activities that the child can do at home to foster developmental progression.

Protect from the Spread of Infection

Strict aseptic technique and transmission-based precautions should be used during all dressing changes. Children and family members should avoid direct contact with any dressings or drainage. Teach good hygiene practices, including handwashing, to maintain infection control. Take vital signs and evaluate the child frequently for symptoms indicating the spread of infection (e.g., increasing pain, difficulty breathing, increased pulse rate, fever).

Encourage a Well-Balanced Diet

Educate both the child and the parents about healthy dietary choices that promote the healing process. Providing a high-protein diet and extra vitamin C will contribute to this process. Encourage increased fluid intake to provide adequate hydration and circulation.

Discharge Planning and Home Care Teaching

Emphasize the importance of completing the full course of antibiotic therapy, especially for children who have undergone surgical drainage of an abscess or lesion. Explain that failure to follow the prescribed antibiotic therapy may result in chronic infection. Provide suggestions for the family if the child will be immobilized at home.

Evaluation

Expected outcomes of nursing care for the child with osteomyelitis include the following:

- Absence of signs of infection or sepsis

- Completion of prescribed course of antibiotics
- Prevention of infection in contacts
- Adequate intake of fluids and nutrients
- Absence of pain
- Return to normal activities of daily living

SKELETAL TUBERCULOSIS AND SEPTIC ARTHRITIS

Skeletal tuberculosis (Figure 21-15 ◆) and septic arthritis are two infections that, although infrequent, may affect children and adolescents. See page 808 for clinical manifestations, diagnostic tests, and medical and nursing management for these infections.

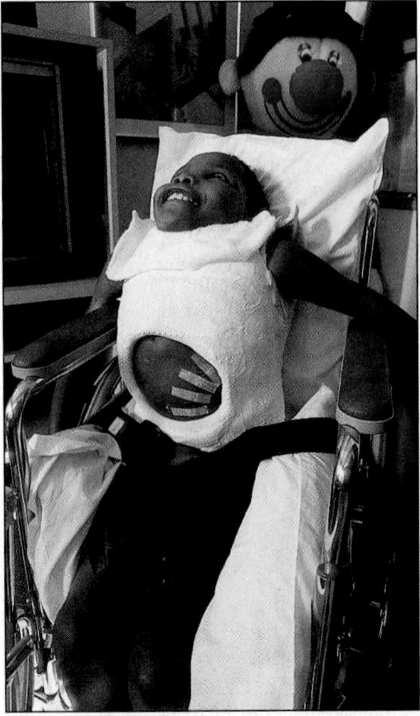

FIGURE 21-15 ◆
This boy from Kenya had surgery to correct severe kyphosis and scoliosis, caused by tuberculosis of the spine. A Risser cast has been applied to maintain stability of the spine and thoracic cage during healing. Notice the area cut out of the cast to allow for auscultation of the abdomen, as well as to facilitate the child's comfort and adequate intake of food.

OSTEOGENESIS IMPERFECTA

Osteogenesis imperfecta, also known as brittle bone disease, is a connective tissue disorder that primarily affects the bones. Children with this condition have fragile bones that are more likely to fracture. The major type of osteogenesis imperfecta occurs in 1 in 30,000 live births and affects boys and girls equally. Clinical manifestations include multiple and frequent fractures; blue sclerae; thin, soft skin; increased joint flexibility; enlargement of the anterior fontanel; weak muscles; soft, pliable, brittle bones; and short stature. Conductive hearing loss can occur by adolescence or young adulthood (Paterson, Monk, & McAllion, 2001).

The underlying disorder is a biochemical defect in the production of collagen. The disease is genetically transmitted, generally in an autosomal dominant inheritance pattern, although some types are transmitted in a recessive pattern.

The disease is classified into four types. In type I disease, the most common form, children have fragile bones, blue sclerae, weakened tooth dentin, and hearing loss that manifests in adolescence. In type II disease, the ribs and skeleton are extensively involved; most children with this form of the disease die in utero or shortly after birth. Type III disease is identified in the newborn period or in infancy when the child sustains numerous fractures and manifests blue sclera. Severe bone fragility and kyphoscoliosis are observed. Most children with type III disease die in childhood as a result of cardiorespiratory failure. Type IV disease is characterized by fractures without other symptoms of the disease. Bowing of the legs and other structural deformities can occur; however, the incidence of fractures decreases beginning in puberty.

Improved knowledge about the genetic transmission of this disease means that some cases of osteogenesis imperfecta can be identified before birth using ultrasound or collagen analysis of chorionic villus cells. In many cases, however, diagnosis of osteogenesis imperfecta is made only when the child has a delay in walking or sustains a fracture. Radiographic evaluation may detect both old and new fractures, and can lead to an erroneous diagnosis of child abuse.

There is no cure for osteogenesis imperfecta. Medical management consists primarily of fracture care and prevention of deformities. The goal is to maximize the child's independence and mobility while minimizing the risk of fractures. Treatment includes physical therapy; casting, bracing, or splinting; surgical stabilization; nutritional management with high vitamin D and calcium; and biphosphanate medication such as pamidronate. Bone marrow transplant has been used successfully in some children with severe osteogenesis imperfecta and is under further research (Horwitz, Prockop, & Gordon, et al., 2001).

RESEARCH 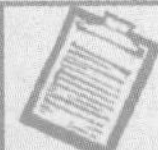

Pamidronate is a bone resorption inhibitor that is being used experimentally in children with osteogenesis imperfecta. Low-dose medication is given intravenously every 6 months, and appears to significantly reduce bone fractures and pain. Density of lumbar bones was improved in children receiving the medication (Gonzalez, Pavia, & Ros, et al., 2001).

Nursing Management

Nursing care is primarily supportive and focuses on educating the parents and child about the disease and its treatment. The family may have been suspected of child abuse before the disease was diagnosed, and they should be given an explanation about the similar presenting symptoms of these cases.

To prevent fractures, children with osteogenesis imperfecta must be handled gently. The trunk and extremities should be supported when the child is moved. Such tasks as bathing and diapering may cause fractures and should be performed carefully.

Emphasize the importance of maintaining normal patterns of growth and development. Toddlers should be helped to explore and interact safely in their environment. Socialization is

CLINICAL MANIFESTATIONS AND TREATMENT OF SKELETAL TUBERCULOSIS AND SEPTIC ARTHRITIS

CONDITION	CLINICAL MANIFESTATIONS	DIAGNOSTIC TESTS AND CLINICAL THERAPY	NURSING MANAGEMENT
Skeletal Tuberculosis Rare microbacterial infection that can be destructive. The spine is the most frequent site of infection (Pott's disease), with joints and other sites sometimes affected.	Depending on the site, pain, limp, severe muscle spasms, kyphosis, muscle atrophy, "doughy" swelling of joints, decreased joint motion, changes in reflexes, low-grade fever.	*Diagnostic tests:* Diagnostic studies include tuberculosis skin test, complete blood count, synovial fluid analysis, and radiographs of affected limb or joint. *Clinical Therapy:* Antibiotic therapy (using a combination of drugs) for 6–9 months is the treatment of choice. The affected site is immobilized. Disease may become resistant to these drugs, and additional drug therapy may be necessary.	Educate the child and family about the disorder and stress the importance of complying with long-term antibiotic therapy. Test all members of the family for tuberculosis. Report the disease to the local health department. Facilitate the immobilization and physical therapy of the child at home.
Septic Arthritis Joint infection of the synovial space most often caused by *Haemophilus influenzae, Staphylococcus,* and *Streptococcus*. The most common site of infection is the knee, followed by the hip, ankle, and elbow.	Fever, pain and local inflammation, joint tenderness, swelling, loss of spontaneous movement.	*Diagnostic tests:* Diagnosis is made based on joint aspiration findings. Radiographic changes may not be evident until later in the disease process. *Clinical Therapy:* This is a medical emergency requiring prompt treatment to avoid permanent disability. Treatment involves joint aspiration, open drainage, and irrigation, followed by intravenous antibiotic therapy for 3–4 weeks and then oral antibiotics. If the full course of antibiotic treatment is not completed, the child risks recurrent infection and further degeneration of the infected joint.	Educate the child and family about the disorder and emphasize the importance of proper antibiotic therapy. Carefully position the painful joint.

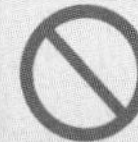

SAFETY PRECAUTIONS

Handle infants with osteogenesis imperfecta gently and use a blanket for additional support when lifting and moving them. Never pull the legs upward when changing a diaper as this can cause a fracture. Instead, gently slip a hand under the hips to raise them, sliding the diaper carefully in, and then bringing it up as the legs are slightly abducted.

essential during the school-age and adolescent years. Encourage exercise, such as swimming, to improve muscle tone and prevent obesity. Independent functioning is promoted by the use of adaptive equipment and motorized wheelchairs. Maintenance of function can depend on proper rehabilitation services. The nurse can arrange and manage such services for the family.

The Osteogenesis Imperfecta Foundation provides information about the disease and can put families in touch with others who have the disease. Parents should receive genetic counseling.

MUSCULAR DYSTROPHIES

The muscular dystrophies are a group of inherited diseases characterized by muscle fiber degeneration and muscle wasting. These disorders can begin early or late in life, and onset can be at birth or gradual.

Many kinds of muscular dystrophies affect children and adults (see page 809). The most common form of childhood muscular dystrophy is Duchenne's muscular dystrophy (pseudohypertrophic), which occurs in 1 in 3,500 live male births. **Pseudohypertrophy** refers to enlargement of the muscles as a result of their infiltration with fatty tissue. The gene for Duchenne's muscular dystrophy was identified in 1987; it is carried in the Xp21.2 region of the chromosome and is either absent or deleted in affected children.

Diagnosis and classification are most often based on clinical signs and the pattern of muscle involvement. Children with muscular dystrophy have generalized muscle weakness.

CLINICAL MANIFESTATIONS OF MUSCULAR DYSTROPHIES OF CHILDHOOD

TYPE OF DYSTROPHY	CLINICAL MANIFESTATIONS	CLINICAL THERAPY
Duchenne's Muscular Dystrophy X-linked recessive disorder seen in boys (on Xp21 gene); however, 30%–50% of affected children have no family history. Onset: within the first 3–4 years of life.	Delayed walking; frequent falls; easily tired when walking, running, or climbing stairs; toe walking, hypertrophied calves; waddling gait; lordosis; positive Gower's maneuver; mental retardation frequently seen.	Supportive care; physical therapy and braces to help maintain mobility and prevent contractures. Most children are wheelchair bound by 12 years of age; dealth usually occurs during adolescence from respiratory or cardiac failure.
Becker's Muscular Dystrophy X-linked recessive disorder. Onset: usually after 5 years.	Symptoms are similar to those of Duchenne's muscular dystrophy, but milder and delayed; child is mobile until late teens; normal intelligence; congestive heart failure; contractures.	Supportive care, same as for Duchenne's muscular dystrophy. Slow progression (same as for Duchenne's muscular dystrophy); death usually occurs by 30–50 years of age.
Fascioscapulohumeral Muscular Dystrophy Autosomal dominant disorder (on 4q35 chromosome). Onset: later childhood and adolescence.	Face, shoulder girdle, lower limbs affected; unable to raise arms over head; lordosis; cannot close eyes, whistle, smile, or drink from a straw because of inability to move face; characteristic appearance includes facial weakness, winging of the scapula, thin arms, well-developed forearms.	Physical therapy Slow progression; confined to wheelchair as older adult, but usually attains normal life span.
Emery-Dreyfuss Muscular Dystrophy X-linked recessive disorder (on Xq28 gene). Onset: childhood.	Early onset of contractures followed by weakness; Achilles tendon, elbow, and spine affected; muscle weakness in upper body follows, with lower body weakness occurring later; cardiac conduction defect may occur.	Physical therapy Surgery Pacemaker insertion
Congenital Muscular Dystrophies Autosomal recessive group of disorders.. Onset: present at birth.	Muscle weaknesses present at birth; motor development delay; contractures and joint deformities; hypotonia.	Correction of skeletal deformity (orthosis or surgery). Usually nonprogressive.

They compensate for weak lower extremities by using the upper extremity muscles to raise themselves to a standing position (Gower's maneuver) (Figure 21-16 ◆). Biochemical examinations such as serum enzyme assay, muscle biopsy, and electromyography confirm the diagnosis. Serum creatine kinase (CK) is elevated early in the disease. Dystrophin, the muscle protein that is deficient in muscular dystrophy, can be measured by muscle biopsy.

There is no effective treatment for childhood muscular dystrophy. At the present time, research is being directed at several techniques to repair mutations by gene therapy (Takeda & Miyagoe-Suzuki, 2001). Progressive weakness and muscle deformity result in chronic disability (Figure 21-17 ◆). The goal of medical management is to provide support and prevent complications such as infection or spinal deformities (Figure 21-18 ◆). The team approach to managing the child with muscular dystrophy ensures a comprehensive management plan. Team members should include physicians (pediatrician, orthopedic surgeon, neurologist), nurses, physical and occupational therapists, a nutritionist, and a social worker.

NURSING MANAGEMENT

Nursing care focuses on promoting independence and mobility and providing psychosocial support that helps the child and family deal with this progressive, incapacitating disease.

Monitor cardiac and respiratory functioning frequently. Administer oxygen or respiratory therapy as ordered. Perform periodic developmental assessments, and provide parents with suggestions for encouraging the child's development. Meet with teachers to evaluate the child's learning needs and functioning in the classroom.

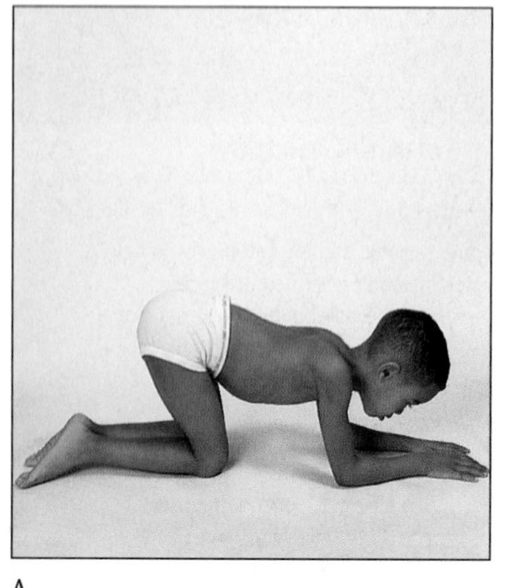

A

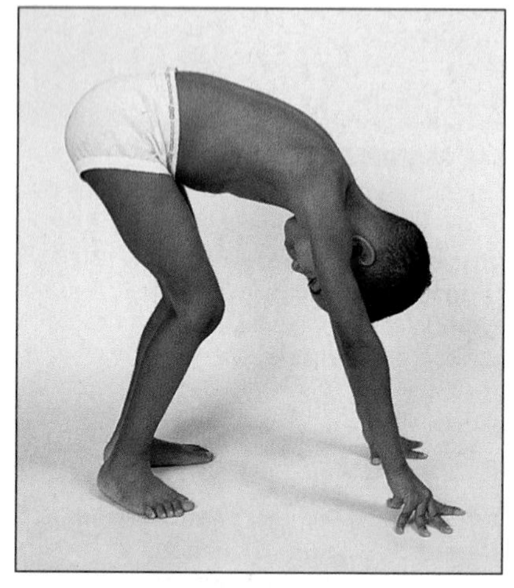

B

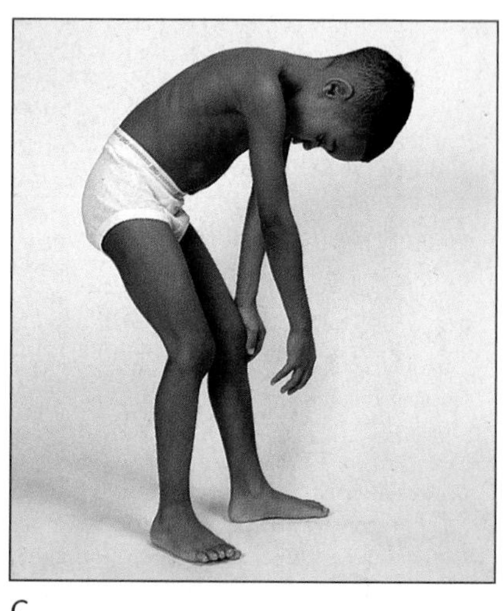

C

D

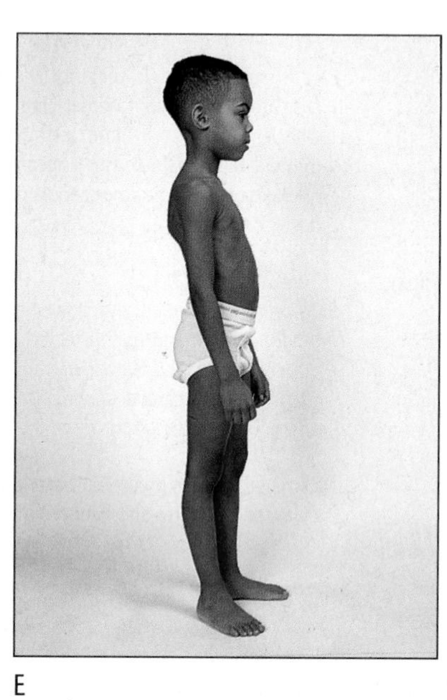

E

FIGURE 21-16 ◆

Since the leg muscles of children with muscular dystrophy are weak, these children must perform the Gower's maneuver to raise themselves to a standing position. A and B, The child first maneuvers to a position supported by arms and legs. C, The child next pushes off the floor and rests one hand on the knee. D and E, The child then pushes himself upright.

Encourage the child to be independent for as long as possible. Concentrate on what the child can accomplish and do not ask the child to complete tasks that may prove frustrating. Reading books to the child, listening to tapes, and watching television offer the child stimulation during hospitalization. Exercise as tolerated contributes to muscle strength. Physical therapy helps the child ambulate and prevents joint contractures. It is important to provide good back support and posture by keeping the child's body in alignment when confined to a wheelchair.

Parents may exhibit feelings of guilt and hopelessness. Encourage parents to express their feelings. Genetic counseling is recommended for the entire family, and it is especially important to identify women who are carriers of one of the X-linked disorders. Siblings may feel neglected because their brother or sister is receiving so much attention. They may be concerned that they will develop the disease. Encourage the parents to involve siblings in the child's care to reassure them of their importance.

Refer family members to resource and support groups such as the Muscular Dystrophy Association.

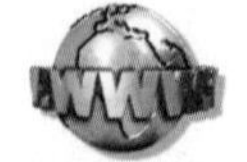

Muscular Dystrophy Online

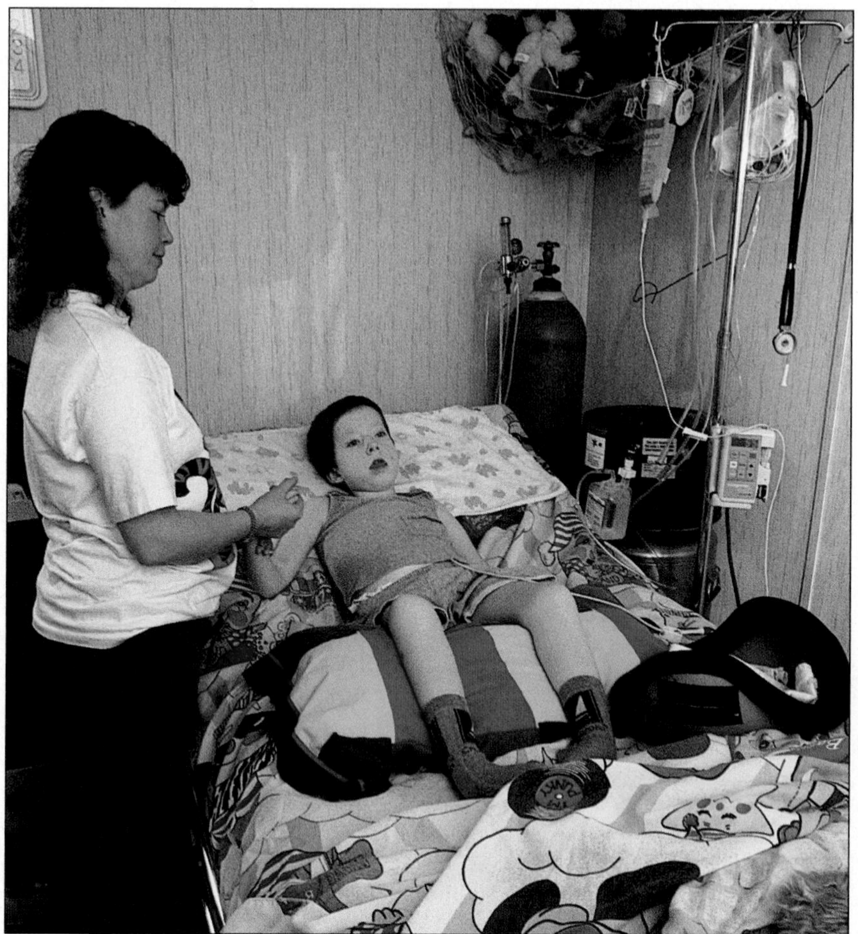

FIGURE 21-17 ◆
This young boy with muscular dystrophy needs to receive tube feedings and home nursing care. He attends school when possible and is able to use an adapted computer.

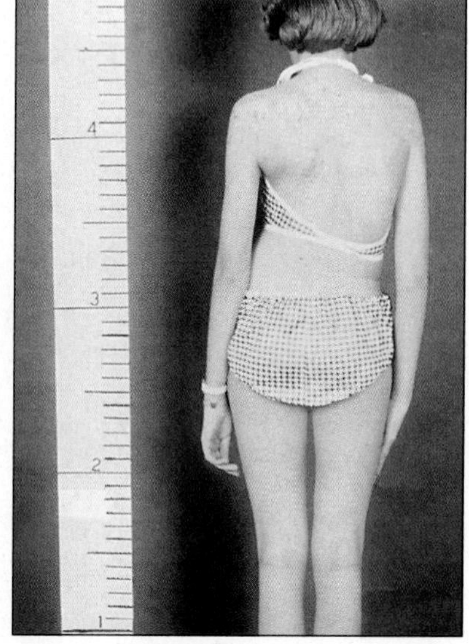

FIGURE 21-18 ◆
Spinal deviation with spinal muscular atrophy.
From Zitelli, B. J., and Davis H. W. (Eds.). (1997). *Atlas of Pediatric Physical Diagnosis* (3rd ed., p. 658) St. Louis, MO: Mosby, Inc.

INJURIES TO THE MUSCULOSKELETAL SYSTEM

Musculoskeletal injuries are classified according to the mechanism, the location, and the force of the injury. Strains, sprains, dislocations, and fractures are the most common musculoskeletal injuries in children. Distinguishing among these injuries is often difficult. See page 812 for management of strains, sprains, and dislocations. A detailed discussion of fractures follows.

FRACTURES

A fracture is a break in a bone that occurs when more stress is placed on the bone than the bone can withstand. Fractures, which may occur at any age, occur frequently in children because their bones are less dense and more porous than those of adults.

Etiology and Pathophysiology

Fractures in children may result from direct trauma to a bone (falls, sports injuries, abuse, motor vehicle crashes) or bone diseases (osteogenesis imperfecta) that result in weakening of the bone. Trauma may be caused by an acute injury, direct and forceful impact, or overuse such as in chronic and repetitive activities (O'Connor, 1998). In the opening scenario of this chapter, Douglass experienced an acute injury when his leg forcefully hit the trampoline frame.

Clinical Manifestations

Signs and symptoms of fractures vary depending on the location, type, and nature of the causative injury. Fractures are generally characterized by pain, abnormal positioning, edema, immobility or decreased range of motion, ecchymosis, guarding, and crepitus.

NURSING ALERT

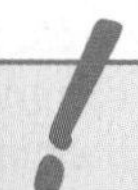

When in doubt about the nature of an injury, apply a splint. Splinting immobilizes the site, prevents further damage, and decreases pain. Be sure to immobilize both the joints above and below the injury.

CLINICAL MANIFESTATIONS OF STRAINS, SPRAINS, AND DISLOCATIONS

CONDITION	CLINICAL MANIFESTATIONS	CLINICAL THERAPY
Strain ■ Stretching or tearing of either a muscle or a tendon, usually from overuse (e.g., back strain resulting from improper or overly heavy lifting).	■ Vary according to the type and severity of the strain. Pain can be acute or chronic.	■ Rest and support of the injured part until the muscle or tendon heals and normal activity can occur.
Sprain ■ Stretching or tearing of a ligament, usually caused by a fall, sports injury, or motor vehicle crash.	■ Edema, joint immobility, and pain.	■ For the first 24–36 hours: **R**est **I**ce **C**ompression **E**levation ■ After the first 24–36 hours, mobility is gradually increased.
Dislocation ■ Complete displacement of an articular joint surface, usually associated with a fall, sports injury, or motor vehicle crash. Although almost any joint may be dislocated, most dislocations occur in the shoulder, knee, and hip.	■ Pain and tenderness, swelling and obvious deformity, and instability of the joint.	■ Varies according to the site and severity of the injury, and consists of: Shoulder: Open or closed reduction followed by the application of a sling. Knee: Closed reduction with gentle traction, then immobilization with a splint. Hip (posterior): Immediate closed reduction or possibly open reduction, traction, or hip spica cast. Hip (anterior): Immediate closed reduction, extension traction, and hip spica cast.

Childhood fractures most often involve the clavicle, tibia, ulna, and femur, with distal forearm fractures the most common type. Douglass had a fracture of his tibia. Fractures to the pelvis are often associated with motor vehicle crashes. Epiphyseal (growth plate) injuries are common in children. These injuries are described using the Salter-Harris classification system (Figure 21-19 ◆).

Clinical Therapy

Radiographs are useful for determining the exact location and type of fracture. Medical management consists of two basic steps: reduction to realign displaced or fragmented bones, and immobilization so that healing can take place.

A closed reduction aligns the bone by manual manipulation or traction. Conscious sedation or pain management may be used during closed reduction. An open reduction requires surgical alignment of the bone, often using pins, plates, wires, or screws. For open fractures, surgery must also be performed for debridement, to remove dead tissue and clean the wound. Casting is the most common external method of immobilization. Casts may be placed on extremities (short or long leg or arm cast) or the upper body to immobilize the spine, or may be applied from chest to legs to stabilize pelvis or hips (spica cast). Leg casts may be walking or nonwalking casts. Cast material is either plaster or a synthetic fabric. Other external methods of stabilization include traction and splinting (see Table 21-4 later in the chapter for types of traction). Pins may be inserted to stabilize the fracture, and can be used with or without casts or traction. A combination of treatments may be needed in the child with multiple fractures following a car crash or other trauma (Frye & Luterman, 1999). Healing of fractures is influenced by factors including age, size of the involved bone, and fracture site. Fractures heal in less time in children than in adults. Immobilization is essential for the bone healing process to take place. If a fracture is properly reduced, complications should be minimal (Table 21-3).

GROWTH & DEVELOPMENT

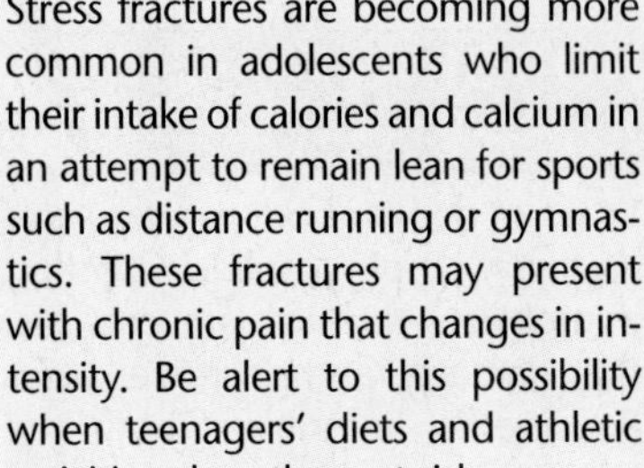
Stress fractures are becoming more common in adolescents who limit their intake of calories and calcium in an attempt to remain lean for sports such as distance running or gymnastics. These fractures may present with chronic pain that changes in intensity. Be alert to this possibility when teenagers' diets and athletic activities place them at risk.

PATHOPHYSIOLOGY ILLUSTRATED

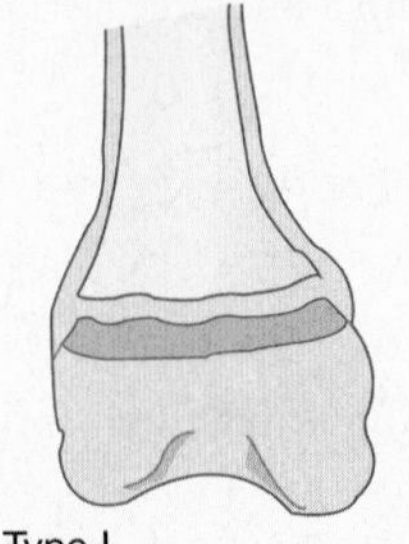

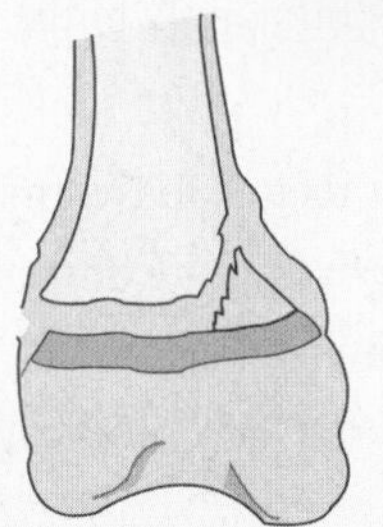

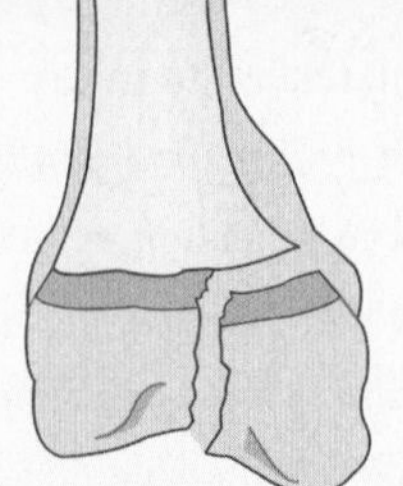

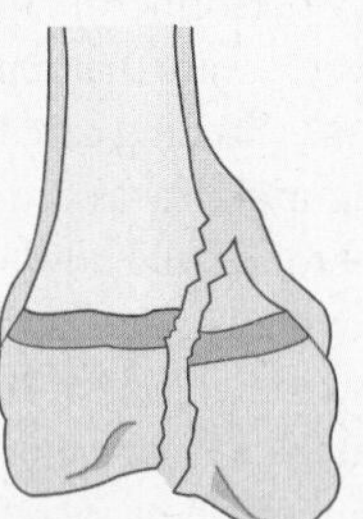

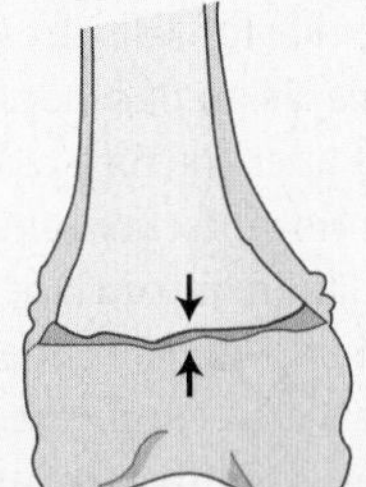

Salter-Harris Classification System

FIGURE 21-19 ◆ The Salter-Harris classification system is based on the angle of the fracture in relation to the epiphysis.

NURSING MANAGEMENT

Nursing Assessment and Diagnosis

When dealing with an injured child, be alert to the signs and symptoms of fractures before moving the child. Try to identify the cause of the injury by asking the child, parents, or other family members what happened. Evaluate pain, swelling, and any abnormal positioning of the injured area. When a child is admitted to the emergency department or hospital, nurs-

TABLE 21-3 Complications of Fracture Reduction

COMPLICATION	CLINICAL THERAPY
Infection Acute (may occur with open fractures) Chronic (osteomyelitis)	Debridement, drainage, culture, and treatment with antibiotics
Neurovascular injury resulting from physical nerve damage	Nerve repair
Vascular injury	Vascular repair, amputation, tendon lengthening
Malunion (undesired healed alignment of bone) or delayed union	Corrective osteotomy; prolonged immobilization
Nonunion	Surgical intervention; internal fixation
Leg length discrepancy	Shoe lift

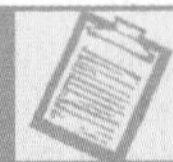

RESEARCH

The risk of bone fractures in adolescent females who consume carbonated beverages is 3 times higher than in those who do not consume such drinks. It is thought that the high phosphorus content of carbonated beverages fosters bone loss and that these beverages displace milk, a major calcium source, in the diet (Wyshak, 2000).

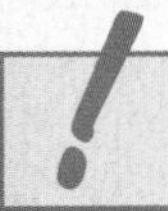

NURSING ALERT

Fractures involving the epiphyseal plate disrupt the growth process in children. If not treated properly, such injuries can cause limb length discrepancy, joint incongruity, and angular deformities.

ing assessment includes the extent of the injury, the degree of pain, and the child's vital signs (respiratory status, pulse, blood pressure).

The following nursing diagnoses may apply to the child with a fracture:

- *Pain,* related to injury
- *Risk for impaired skin integrity,* related to treatment
- *Risk for infection,* related to open fracture or trauma
- *Impaired physical mobility,* related to treatment
- *Health seeking behaviors,* related to lack of information about treatment and expected outcome

Planning and Implementation

Nurses may be in community settings when children experience a fracture, and need to provide emergency care and arrange for transport. Emergency personnel are informed of the assessment data to provide for safe care. In addition, nurses are aware that repeated fractures in the same child can be a sign of other health care conditions. Nursing care focuses on care of the child before and after fracture reduction, encouraging mobility as ordered, maintaining skin integrity, preventing infection, and teaching the parents and child how to care for the fracture. If conscious sedation or pain blocks are used, nursing care for these procedures is needed. When caring for a child who has undergone fracture reduction, it is important to be aware of the signs of complications. Notify the physician immediately if these signs occur. The major serious complication is **compartment syndrome,** or a condition of increased pressure in a limited space which compromises circulation and tissue function (Harvey, 2001).

Skill 9-3: Conscious Sedation Monitoring

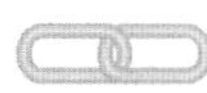

Skill 5-16: Neurovascular Assessment

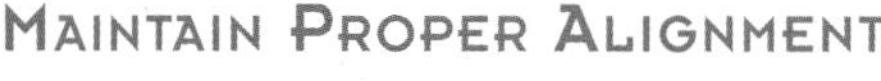

Maintain Proper Alignment

Immobilization is used to maintain proper alignment of the fracture. Casts and traction are methods used for immobilizing an injured child. Cast care guidelines are included in Table 21-2.

Different types of traction are used, depending on the location and type of fracture (Table 21-4). Nursing care for the child in traction is described in Table 21-5.

NURSING ALERT

It is uncommon for children to have repeated fractures. If they occur, make further assessments for their cause. The child may suffer from osteogenesis imperfecta. If attention deficit hyperactivity disorder (ADHD) is present or if the child has a mental health problem, excessive risky behavior may be the cause of fractures. When children are found on x-ray to have several old and healing fractures, or multiple fractures of the same or different bones, they may be victims of physical abuse, particularly if the caretaker explanation of fracture does not match the clinical picture. An example could be the parent who claims the child fell from a chair, but there is a severe arm fracture and skull fracture. See Chapter 7 for a description of child abuse and Chapter 24 for a discussion of ADHD.

Monitor Neurovascular Status

Neurovascular assessment is used for early detection of compartment syndrome, which may occur with a crush injury or when a fracture is reduced. Swelling associated with inflammation reduces blood flow to the affected area, and casting causes further constriction of blood flow. Douglass, in the opening scenario, had a splint applied for several days, with casting later, to allow swelling to decrease and to minimize risk for compartment syndrome. Monitor the child's sensation to touch, temperature, movement, strength of the pulse, and capillary refill time in the extremity distal to the injury. Monitor every 15 minutes after the cast is applied for at least 2 hours and then every 1 to 2 hours, depending on the care facility's policy and the child's condition. Keep the cast elevated above heart level to minimize edema.

Promote Mobility

The amount of mobility the child is allowed is ordered by the physician and restrictions depend on the extent and site of the fracture. Fractures of the hip or pelvis may involve body casts, and providing wheeled carts makes mobility possible. Children with leg fractures can sometimes bear weight on the cast; but if they cannot bear weight, they move around with crutches, walkers, or wheelchairs. See the Skills Manual for information on crutch walking.

Discharge Planning and Home Care Teaching

Most fractures can be easily managed at home. Activities are generally limited for approximately 8 weeks. Teach the parents and child cast care, activity restrictions, and how to identify problems that should be reported (see page 786). Help parents to identify any modifications that may be needed at home and school. The child who has to manage steps at home

Skill 13-2: Setting Crutch Height

TABLE 21-4 Types of Traction

TYPE

Skin Traction
Pull is applied to the skin surface, which puts traction directly on the bones and muscles. Traction is attached to the skin with adhesive materials or straps, or foam boots, belts, or halters.

Dunlop Traction (can be either skeletal or skin)
Used for fracture of the humerus. The arm, which is flexed, is suspended horizontally with straps placed on both the upper and lower portions for pull from both sides.

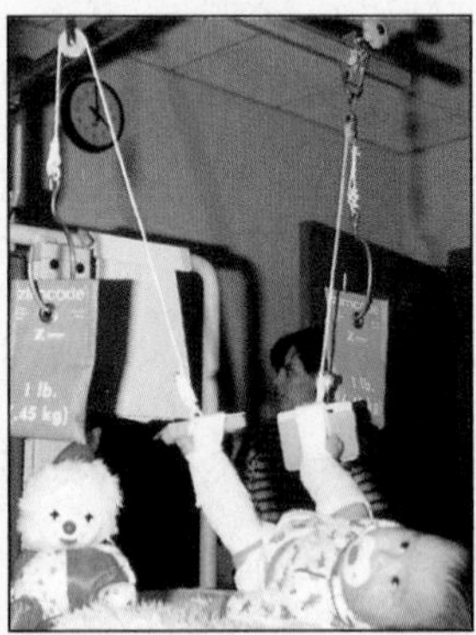

(1)

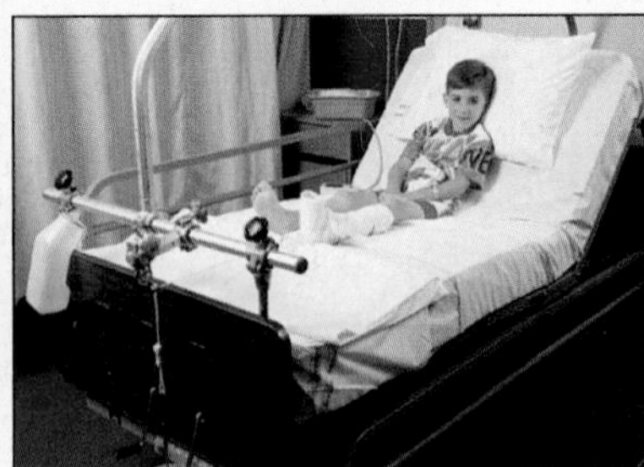

(2)

Bryant Traction (1)
Used specifically for the child under 3 years of age and weighing less than 17.5 kg (35 lb), who has developmental dysplasia of the hip or a fractured femur. This bilateral traction is applied to the child's legs and kept in place by wrapping the legs from foot to thigh with elastic bandages. The hips are flexed at a 90-degree angle, with knees extended. This position is maintained by attaching the traction appliance to weights and pulleys, which are suspended above the crib. The buttocks do not rest on the mattress, but are slightly elevated off the bed.

Buck Traction (2)
Used for knee immobilization; to correct contractures or deformities; or for short-term immobilization of a fracture. It keeps the leg in an extended position, withut hip flexion. Traction is applied to the extremity in one direction (straight line) with a single pulley system.

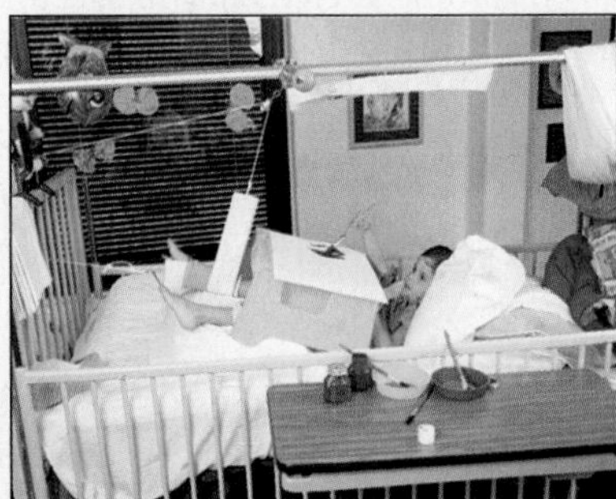

(3)

Russell Traction (3)
Used for fractures of the femur and lower leg. Traction is placed on the lower leg while the knee is suspended in a padded sling. The hips and knees, which are slightly flexed, are immobilized. One force is applied by a double pulley to the foot and another force is applied upward using a sling under the knee and an overhead pulley.

Skeletal Traction
Pull is directly applied to the bone by pins, wires, tongs, or other apparatus that have been surgically placed through the distal end of the bone.

Skeletal Cervical Traction
Used for cervical spine injuries to reduce fractures and dislocations, Crutchfield Gardner-Wells, or Vinke tongs are placed in the skull with burr holes. Weights are attached to the apparatus with a rope and pulley system to the hyperextended head.

Halo Traction
Used to immobilize the head and neck after cervical injury or dislocation. Also used for positioning and immobilization after cervical injury.

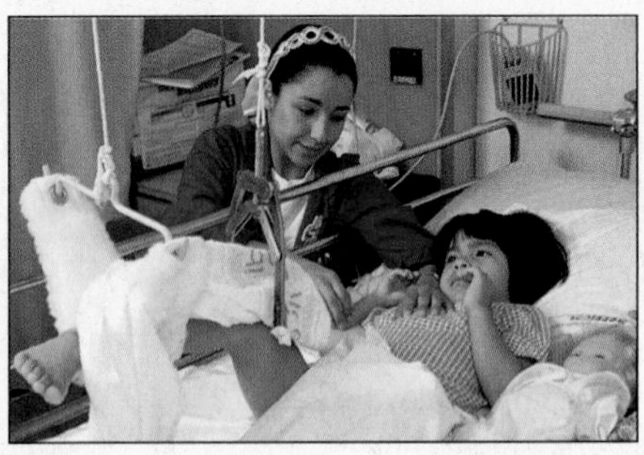

(4)

90-90 Traction (4)
Used for fractures of the femur or tibia. A skeletal pin or wire is surgically placed through the distal part of the femur, while the lower part of the extremity is in a boot cast. Traction ropes and pulleys are applied at the pin site and on the boot cast to maintain the flexion of both the hip and knee at 90 degrees. This traction can also be used for treatment of an upper extremity fracture.

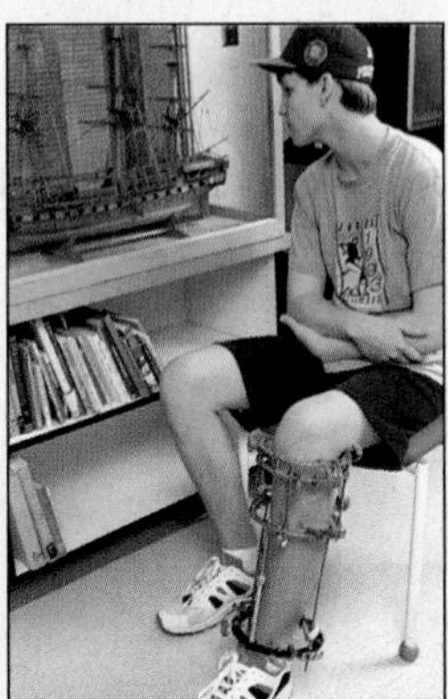

(5)

External Fixators (5)
These devices can be used in the treatment of simple fractures, both open and closed; complex fractures with extensive soft tissue involvement; correction of bony or soft tissue deformities; pseudoarthroses; and limb length discrepancy. They are attached to the extremity by percutaneous transfixing of pins or wires to the bone.

TABLE 21-5 Nursing Care of the Child with Traction or External Fixator

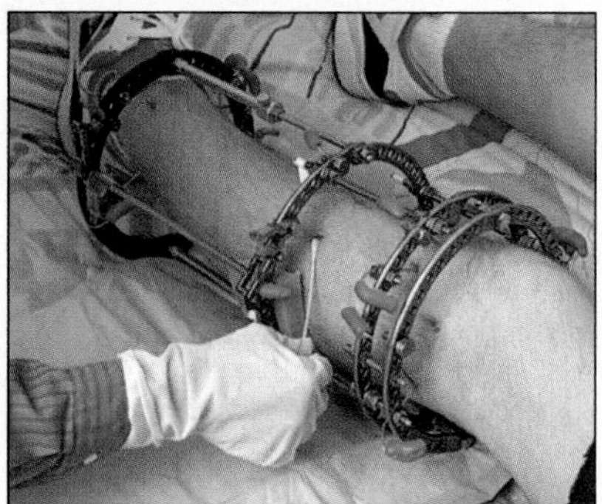
Providing pin care for external fixator

1. Assess the child in traction by first checking the equipment. Make sure that the equipment is in the proper position. Observe both the body appliance and the attached weights and pulleys. Make certain that the child's body is in proper alignment.
2. Assess the skin under the straps and pin insertion sites for any signs of redness, edema, or skin breakdown.
3. Assess the extremity by checking neurovascular status frequently (check warmth, color, distal pulses, capillary refill time, movement, sensation).
4. Provide pin care when ordered using sterile technique. Clean the area surrounding the pin with cotton-tipped applicators saturated with normal saline or half-strength hydrogen peroxide. Clean the area again with sterile water or more saline. Apply an antibacterial ointment, if ordered, using another cotton-tipped applicator.
5. When the traction equipment can be removed, skin care should be performed every 4 hours.
6. Place a sheepskin pad under the child's extremity if orders permit.

HOME CARE

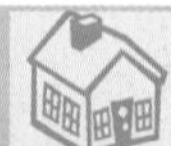

When a child has a fracture from sports or other activities, ask details about how the injury occurred. If protective gear is recommended and was not worn, reinforce the need for protection. Suggest financial resources as necessary.

or school may need special training with crutches or a temporary ramp. Refer parents to home health nurses or home teaching services if indicated. Provide pertinent teaching to prevent future injuries.

AMPUTATIONS

Amputation—the complete absence of a body extremity—can be either congenital or acquired. Approximately two-thirds of amputations in children are congenital and one-third are acquired. Congenital amputations can be caused by constrictive amniotic bands, drugs, or irradiation. Acquired amputations are generally associated with trauma or the result of a disease or disorder.

The child with an absent limb should be fitted with a prosthesis as soon as feasible, to foster a positive body image, independence, and self-confidence and to ensure that the child's motor skills develop as normally as possible. The prosthetic device should be reevaluated as the child progresses physically and developmentally. Frequent stump reconstructions are often necessary in children with traumatic amputations, because as children grow, so do their bones, and the skin tends to adhere to the bone. Bone may need to be cut and soft tissue added to keep the stump rounded. Joint fusions or stump lengthenings may also be needed to allow for the effective use of a prosthesis.

Nursing Management

Nursing care focuses on providing emotional support regarding altered body image, managing pain, maintaining skin integrity, and encouraging maximal independent functioning.

CLINICAL MANIFESTATIONS OF COMPARTMENT SYNDROME

Clinical manifestations begin about 30 minutes after tissue ischemia starts. Major manifestations are:

- Paresthesia (tingling, burning, loss of 2-point discrimination)
- Pain (unrelieved by medication, characterized by crying in the young child)
- Pressure (skin is tense, cast appears tight)
- Pallor* (pale, gray, or white skin tone)
- Paralysis* (weakness or inability to move extremity)
- Pulselessness* (weak or absent pulse)

Document results and report changes or abnormal results immediately.

Check extremities for:

- Color
- Temperature
- Capillary refill
- Peripheral pulses
- Edema
- Sensation
- Motor ability
- Pain

* = late sign

Note: Adapted from Kunkler, C. E. (1999). Neurovascular assessment. *Orthopaedic Nursing, 18(3),* 63–71; and Harvey, C. (2001). Compartment syndrome: When it is least expected. *Orthopaedic Nursing, 20(3),* 15–26.

Recovering from the loss of a limb is one of the most difficult challenges facing a child. Emphasize what the child can do rather than what he or she cannot do. Good listening skills are important.

The child who has had surgery or a traumatic injury experiences pain. Many of the techniques discussed in Chapter 9 are useful interventions. After surgery, an epidural may be the treatment of choice. Oral analgesics are used during the period of adaptation to a prosthesis if tenderness is present. Children can experience "phantom" limb pain in the lost extremity, although this phenomenon is less common in children than adults (Ray, 2000).

The child usually begins wearing the prosthetic device for 1 to 2 hours at a time. Check the skin for any redness or breakdown. If such conditions develop, leave the prosthesis off and allow the skin to clear before reapplying. Have the prosthesis adjusted if necessary, and increase wearing time as tolerated by the child.

Children with amputated limbs quickly learn how to accommodate to the prosthetic device. Make use of physical therapy programs that are specifically designed to help the child perform activities of daily living.

Answer any questions the family has about how to care for the prosthetic device and how to perform skin checks. Encourage parents to allow the child to participate in peer activities that are physically and emotionally challenging. Sporting activities that enable the child to participate using modified equipment are a good way to build self-confidence and motivation. For example, ski centers may offer programs that teach children with physical disabilities how to ski, or Special Olympics is a motivating option for some children. Assess the need for counseling and offer referrals as appropriate.

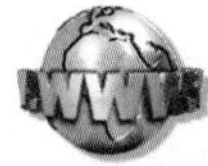

Sports Opportunities

Chapter Highlights

- Children may develop musculoskeletal conditions as a result of congenital conditions, developmental variations, or trauma.
- Talipes equinovarus (clubfoot) is a common unilateral or bilateral variation in newborns that is treated by casting, traction, and/or surgery.
- Genu varum and genu valgum are normal variations at certain times in development that may need treatment if they persist.
- The nurse may identify developmental dysplasia of the hip (DDH) during newborn assessments and must refer the child for care to a specialist.
- Mild DDH may be treated by a harness, but more severe cases may require surgery for the child to walk normally.
- Legg-Calvé-Perthes is a disease most commonly seen in school-age boys, and causes necrosis of the femoral head.
- Slipped capital femoral epiphysis is treated by casting, traction, or more commonly surgery with pinning, to stabilize the epiphysis.
- Scoliosis is a lateral curvature of the spine, and nurses commonly screen adolescents to identify the disorder.
- Osteomyelitis most commonly follows another infection and requires prompt treatment to prevent sepsis and serious injury to the bone.
- The child with osteogenesis imperfecta (brittle bone disease) requires careful handling by the nurse and parents to prevent fractures while fostering developmental progression.
- Muscular dystrophies are inherited diseases characterized by muscle wasting and degeneration.
- Children can experience a variety of fractures due to sports, car crashes, and other injuries.
- Cast and traction care are common interventions for fractures; nursing interventions minimize problem development from these treatments.

EXPLORE MediaLink

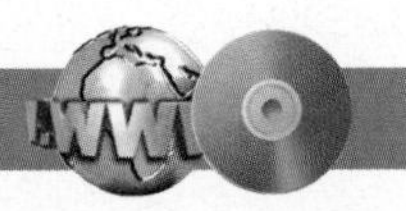

- NCLEX review, case studies, and other interactive resources for this chapter can be found on the Companion Website at **http://www.prenhall.com/ball.** Click on Chapter 21 to select the activities for this chapter.
- For animations, more NCLEX review questions, and an audio glossary, access the accompanying CD-ROM in this textbook.

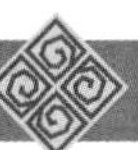

References

1. American Academy of Pediatrics, Committee on Quality Improvement and Subcommittee on Developmental Dysplasia of the Hip. (2000). *Pediatrics, 105,* 896–905.
2. Blakeslee, T. J. (1997). Congenital talipes equinovarus (clubfoot). *Clinics in Podiatric Medicine and Surgery, 14,* 9–55.
3. Carek, P. J., Dickerson, L. M., & Sack, J. L. (2001). Diagnosis and management of osteomyelitis. *American Family Physician, 63,* 2413–2420.
4. Davids, J. R. (1998). Limping. In L. T. Staheli (ed.), *Pediatric orthopedic secrets* (pp. 195–199). Philadelphia: Hanley & Belfus.
5. DeBaun, B. J. (1998). Prevention of infection in the orthopedic surgery patient. *Nursing Clinics of North America, 33,* 671–684.
6. Fernbach, S. A. (1998). Common orthopedic problems of the newborn. *Nursing Clinics of North America, 33,* 583–596.
7. Frye, K. E., & Luterman, A. (1999). Burns and fractures. *Orthopaedic Nursing, 18*(1), 30–35.
8. Gonzalez, E., Pavia, C., Ros, J., Villaronga, M., Valls, C., & Exxcola, J. (2001). Efficacy of low dose schedule pamidronate infusion in children with osteogenesis imperfecta. *Journal of Pediatric Endocrinology and Metabolism, 14,* 529–533.
9. Harvey, C. (2001). Compartment syndrome: When it is least expected. *Orthopaedic Nursing, 20*(3), 15–26.
10. Horwitz, E. M., Prockop, D. J., Gordon, P. L., Koo, W. W., Fitzpatrick, L. A., Neel, M. D., McCarville, M. E., Orchard, P. J., Pyeritz, R. E., & Brenner, M. K. (2001). Clinical responses to bone marrow transplantation in children with severe osteogenesis imperfecta. *Blood, 97,* 1227–1231.
11. Kautz, S. M. & Skaggs, D. L. (1998). Getting an angle on spinal deformities. *Contemporary Pediatrics, 15,* 111–128.
12. Killian, J. T., Mayberry, S., & Wilkinson, L. (1999). Current concepts in adolescent idiopathic scoliosis. *Pediatric Annals, 28,* 755–761.
13. Kunkler, C. E. (1999). Neurovascular assessment. *Orthopaedic Nursing, 18*(3), 63–71.
14. Mankin, K. P., & Zimbler, S. (1997). Gait and leg alignment: What's normal and what's not. *Contemporary Pediatrics, 14,* 41–70.
15. Muscari, M. E. (1998). Preventing sports injuries. *American Journal of Nursing, 98,* 58–60.
16. Novacheck, T. F. (1996). Developmental dysplasia of the hip. *Pediatric Clinics of North America, 43,* 829–848.
17. O'Connor, D. L. (1998). Preventing sports injuries in kids. *Patient Care Nurse Practitioner, 1*(4), 24–36.
18. Paterson, C. R., Monk, E. A., & McAllion, S. J. (2001). How common is hearing impairment in osteogenesis imperfecta? *Journal of Laryngology and Otolaryngology, 115,* 280–282.
19. Ray, R. L. (2000). Complications of lower extremity amputations. *Topics in Emergency Medicine, 22*(3), 35–43.
20. Roy, D. R. (1999). Current concept in Legg-Calvé-Perthes disease. *Pediatric Annals, 28,* 748–754.
21. Ryan, D. J. (2001). Intoeing: A developmental norm. *Orthpaedic Nursing, 20*(2), 13–18.
22. Shaw, B. A., Gerardi, J. A., & Hennrikus, W. L. (1998). Avoiding the pitfalls of orthopedic disorders. *Contemporary Pediatrics, 15,* 122–135.
23. Takeda, S., & Miyagoe-Suzuki, Y. (2001). Gene therapy for muscular dystrophies: Current status and future prospects. *Biodrugs, 15,* 635–644.
24. Theophilopoulos, E. P., & Barrett, D. J. (1998). Get a grip on the pediatric hip. *Contemporary Pediatrics, 15,* 43–65.
25. Wyshak, G. (2000). Teenaged girls, carbonated beverage consumption, and bone fractures. *Archives of Pediatrics and Adolescent Medicine, 154,* 610–613.

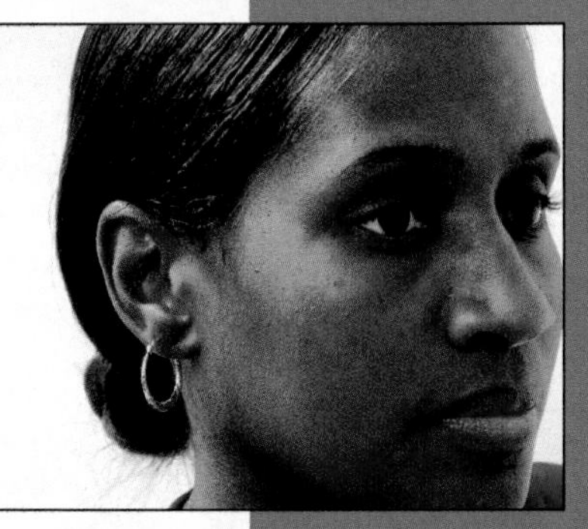

"I am really worried about how Anthony is going to learn to manage all these aspects of diabetes care. Learning to check his blood sugar is pretty easy compared to counting calories and figuring out how much insulin to take and when to take it. I hope we have some time to get into a routine before he gets sick, and we have to work hard to keep the diabetes under control."

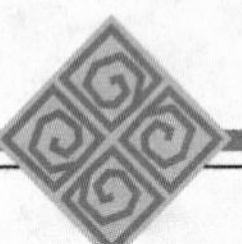

Anthony, 12 years old, has just been diagnosed with diabetes mellitus. His parents took him to their family physician after Anthony complained of being constantly thirsty and hungry for over a week. Despite this, he lost 5 pounds. They note that he had a viral illness about 1 month ago but seemed to recover from it. His mother says that Anthony has seemed lethargic for several days.

Anthony and his family must now learn to manage his diabetes using a combination of diet, exercise, and insulin therapy. Monitoring his blood glucose level is important in determining how much insulin he will need every day. Anthony and his mother will need to learn to schedule his meals and snacks, to have appropriate amounts of protein, fat, and carbohydrates at each meal, and to count carbohydrates. Anthony's meals and activities will need to be coordinated with his insulin doses. Anthony and his parents will need to watch closely for signs of hypoglycemia.

What causes diabetes? What potential problems need prompt treatment? What are the long-term implications of the diagnosis? During Anthony's short hospitalization and follow-up sessions, the nurse answers these questions and addresses other concerns raised by Anthony and his parents. As she begins to teach Anthony and his family about the condition, the nurse also reassures them that Anthony can live a normal life despite his disease.

ALTERATIONS IN ENDOCRINE FUNCTION

CHAPTER 22

KEY TERMS

acanthosis nigricans Hyperpigmentation and thickening of the skin associated with chronic hyperinsulinemia.

bone age A radiographic image of the bones of the wrist used to evaluate the stage of bone ossification.

euthyroid Normal thyroid state.

glucagon A hormone produced by the pancreas that helps release stored glucose from the liver.

glycosuria Abnormal amount of glucose in the urine.

goiter Enlargement of the thyroid gland.

hormone A chemical substance produced by a gland or organ and carried in the bloodstream to another part of the body where it has a regulatory effect on particular cells.

hyperinsulinemia Elevated insulin levels in the blood.

inborn errors of metabolism Inherited biochemical abnormalities of the urea cycle and amino acid and organic acid metabolism.

insulin resistance An alteration of the insulin receptor that signals the presence of insulin in the interior of cells.

karyotype A microscopic display of the 46 chromosomes in the human body lined up from the largest to the smallest. The human female is 46,XX and the human male is 46,XY.

polydipsia Excessive thirst.

polyphagia Excessive or voracious eating.

polyuria Passage of a large volume of urine in a given period.

pseudohermaphroditism Ambiguous development of the external genitalia.

puberty Period of life when the ability to reproduce sexually begins; characterized by maturation of the genital organs, development of the secondary sex characteristics, and (in females) the onset of menstruation.

thyrotoxicosis (thyroid storm) May occur when thyroid hormone is suddenly released into the bloodstream during surgery. The child experiences fever, diaphoresis, and tachycardia, progressing to shock and, if untreated, death.

MediaLink

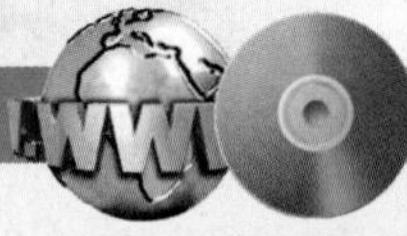

http://www.prenhall.com/ball

Resources for this chapter can be found on the CD-ROM accompanying this textbook, and on the Companion Website at http://www.prenhall.com/ball. Click on Chapter 22 to select the activities for this chapter.

CD-ROM

Animation

Hormone Regulation and Secretion

Audio Glossary

NCLEX Review

COMPANION WEBSITE

Web Links

NCLEX Review

MediaLink Applications

Identify Strategies to Help Girls Understand Early Pubertal Development

Develop a Plan: Child with Type 1 Diabetes Returning to Elementary School

Develop a Peer Strategy: Child with Inborn Errors of Metabolism and Diet

The endocrine system controls the cellular activity that regulates growth and body metabolism through the release of hormones. **Hormones** are chemical messengers secreted by various glands that exert controlling effects on the cells of the body. Overlapping with all body systems, the general functions of the endocrine system include the following:

- Differentiation of the reproductive and central nervous systems in the fetus
- Regulation of the pace of growth and development in concert with the central nervous system throughout childhood and adolescence
- Coordination of the male and female reproductive systems, enabling sexual reproduction
- Maintenance of an optimal level of hormones for body functioning
- Maintenance of homeostasis, a healthy internal environment, in the presence of a constantly changing external environment

Inborn errors of metabolism—inherited biochemical abnormalities of the urea cycle and amino acid and organic acid metabolism—often have a significant impact on the endocrine system's ability to support growth and development. Some chromosomal abnormalities also result in disturbances in growth and sexual development. Endocrine disturbances result in alterations in metabolism, growth and development, and behavior that may have significant implications for children. If not diagnosed and treated early, these conditions can result in delays in growth and development, mental retardation, and, occasionally, death. However, treatment, which usually consists of supplementation of missing hormones, adjustment of hormone levels, or dietary measures, allows most children to live a normal life.

ANATOMY AND PHYSIOLOGY OF PEDIATRIC DIFFERENCES

The hypothalamic-pituitary axis produces several releasing and inhibiting hormones that regulate the function of many endocrine glands including the thyroid, adrenal, and the male and female reproductive glands. In addition, growth is regulated by hormones originating from this axis. Other endocrine glands include the parathyroid glands and islets of Langerhans in the pancreas (Figure 22-1 ◆). These glands secrete hormones into the bloodstream that are carried to target organs or tissues. Most hormones exert their influence through interaction with receptors in the target cells of specific tissues (Table 22-1).

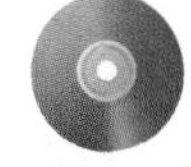

Hormone Regulation and Secretion

The regulation of hormone secretion occurs through a negative feedback mechanism that functions to maintain an optimal internal environment in the body. Negative feedback occurs when an endocrine gland or secretory tissue receives a message that an adequate amount of hormone has been received by the target cells. In response, further secretion is inhibited. Secretion is resumed only when the secretory tissue receives another message indicating that levels of the hormone are low.

The endocrine system is responsible for sexual differentiation during fetal development (Figure 22-2 ◆) and for stimulating growth and development during childhood and adolescence. This includes stimulating development of the reproductive system in both sexes.

Puberty (sexual maturation, lasting 2 to 3 years) occurs when the gonads secrete increased amounts of the sex hormones estrogen and testosterone. At the average age of 10 years in girls and 11 years in boys, the hypothalamus produces increased amounts of gonadotropin-releasing hormone. This hormone stimulates the anterior pituitary gland to increase the production of luteinizing hormone (LH) and follicle-stimulating hormone (FSH). These hormones in turn stimulate the gonads to secrete more sex hormones (Figure 22-3 ◆), resulting in the development of primary and secondary sex characteristics.

DISORDERS OF PITUITARY FUNCTION

GROWTH HORMONE DEFICIENCY (HYPOPITUITARISM)

Growth hormone deficiency (GHD) is a disorder caused by decreased activity of the pituitary gland. Because most children with this disorder secrete inadequate amounts of growth hormone, the term *growth hormone deficiency* is often preferred to *hypopituitarism.* As many as 10,000 school-age children have GHD (Shulman & Bercu, 1998).

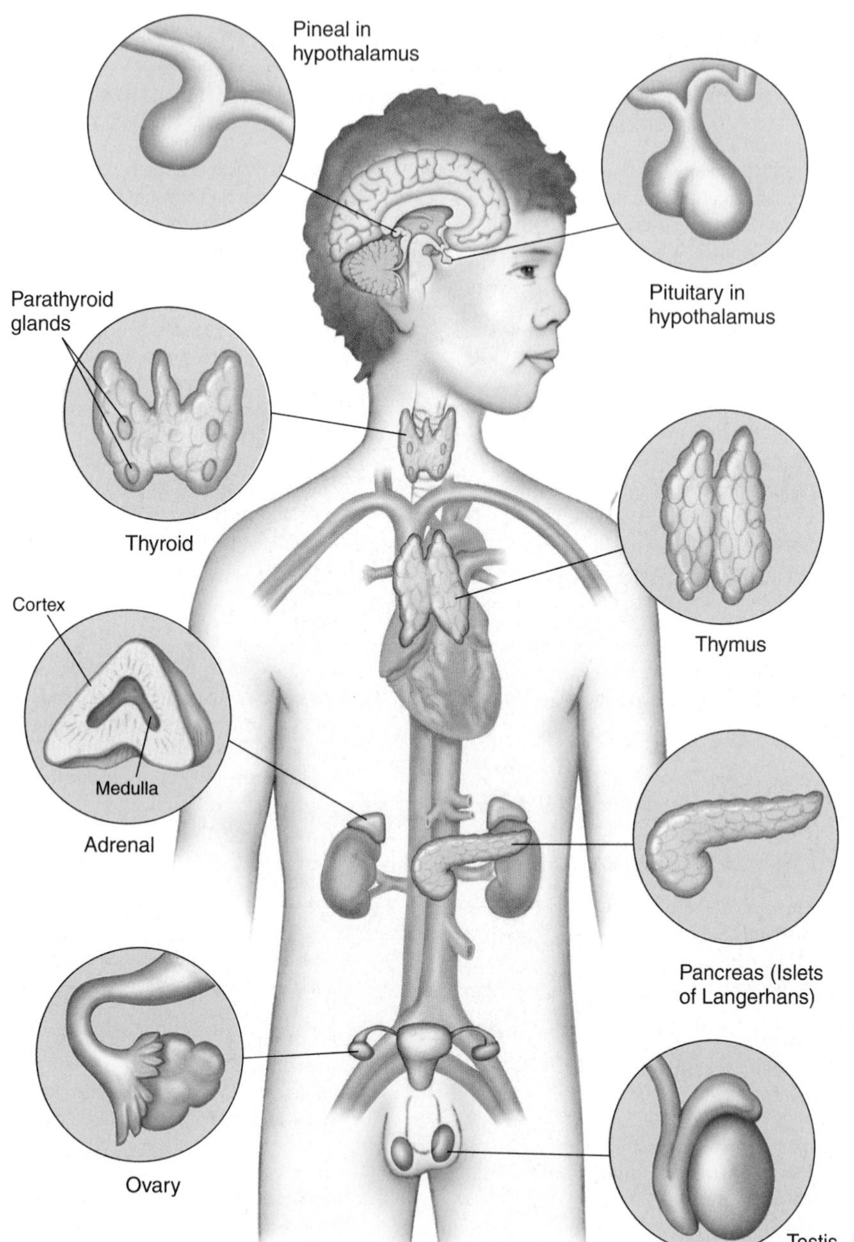

FIGURE 22-1 ◆
Major organs and glands of the endocrine system.

The release of growth hormone from the anterior pituitary gland is controlled by the hypothalamus, which secretes releasing and inhibitory factors. Growth hormone stimulates linear growth and bone mineral density, as well as the growth of all body tissues. It also stimulates the synthesis of proteins in the liver, among them the somatomedins or insulinlike growth factors (IGFs), which promote glucose utilization by the cells and cell proliferation.

Infection, infarction of the pituitary gland (related to sickle-cell disease), central nervous system disease, tumors of the pituitary gland or hypothalamus (primarily craniopharyngiomas and gliomas), other brain tumors, cranial irradiation, brain trauma, and psychosocial deprivation may cause growth hormone deficiency by interfering with the production or release of growth hormone. Deficiency of growth hormone or abnormalities of hormone receptors may be caused by dominant or recessive inheritance or by a genetic mutation (Finegold, 1997).

Children with GHD have normal birth weights and lengths. By the age of 1 year, however, they are below the 3rd percentile on the growth chart. They characteristically grow at a rate of less than 5 cm (2 in.) per year. Other characteristic findings in infants include hypoglycemic seizures, hyponatremia, neonatal jaundice, pale optic discs, micropenis, and

PSYCHOSOCIAL DWARFISM

Psychosocial dwarfism is a syndrome of emotional deprivation that causes suppression of production of pituitary hormones resulting in adrenocorticotropic hormone (ACTH) and growth hormone deficiencies. The child is often withdrawn, with bizarre eating habits and polydipsia, and may also gorge and vomit. Treatment involves removing the child from the stressful environment and providing for normal dietary intake. Pituitary secretion is usually restored, and dramatic catch-up growth in height is observed.

TABLE 22-1 Endocrine Glands and Their Functions

GLAND/HORMONE	FUNCTION
Anterior Pituitary	
Growth hormone	Stimulates growth of all body tissues
Thyroid-stimulating hormone (TSH)	Stimulates thyroid hormone secretion
Adrenocorticotropic hormone (ACTH)	Stimulates secretion of glucocorticoids and androgens
Follicle-stimulating hormone (FSH)	Stimulates secretion of estrogen; supports follicle development in ovaries
Luteinizing hormone (LH) and Interstitial cell-stimulating hormone (ICSH) (male analog)	Stimulates secretion of androgens in males and progesterone in females
Prolactin-releasing hormone	Stimulates secretion of prolactin that stimulates the secretion of milk during lactation
Melanocyte-stimulating hormone (MSH)	Stimulates skin pigmentation
Posterior Pituitary	
Antidiuretic hormone (ADH)	Stimulates permeability of distal renal tubules and collecting ducts
Oxytocin	Stimulates uterine contractions and breast milk let-down reflex
Beta endorphins	May regulate body temperature, food and water intake
Thyroid	
Thyroxine (T4) and triiodothyronine (T3)	Regulates metabolic rate of all cells, body heat production; protein, fat, and carbohydrate catabolism in all cells
Thyrocalcitonin	Stimulates bone ossification and development
Parathyroid	
Parathyroid hormone	Regulates serum calcium levels and excretion of phosphorus
Adrenal	
Aldosterone	Conserves sodium and excretion of potassium
Androgens	Stimulates bone development and secondary sexual characteristics
Cortisol	Stimulates anti-inflammatory reactions, protects from stress
Epinephrine	Activates sympathetic nervous system; stimulates increase in blood pressure and blood glucose levels
Pancreas (Islets of Langerhans)	
Insulin	Facilitates cellular glucose utilization
Glucagon	Increases blood glucose
Somatostatin	Stimulates inhibition of insulin and glucagon secretion; may prevent excess insulin secretion
Ovaries	
Estrogen	Stimulates development of breasts and ova
Progesterone	Stimulates breast glandular development; acts to maintain pregnancy
Testes	
Testosterone	Stimulates production of sperm, development of secondary sexual characteristics, and closure of epiphysis

undescended testicles. Children with GHD tend to be overweight and exhibit youthful facial features, higher pitched voices, delayed dentition, "ripply" abdominal fat, decreased muscle mass, delayed skeletal maturation, delayed sexual maturation, and hypoglycemia.

Any child whose height is 2 to 3 standard deviations below the mean height for age or whose measurement is falling off the normal growth chart should be evaluated for short stature (Table 22-2). A child whose screening tests reveal low levels of IGF-1 requires further

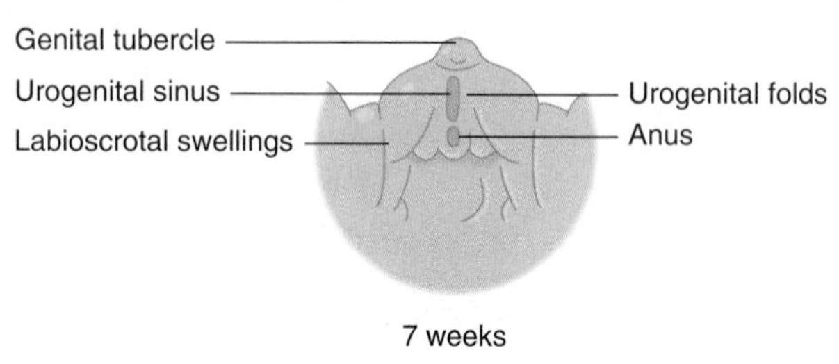

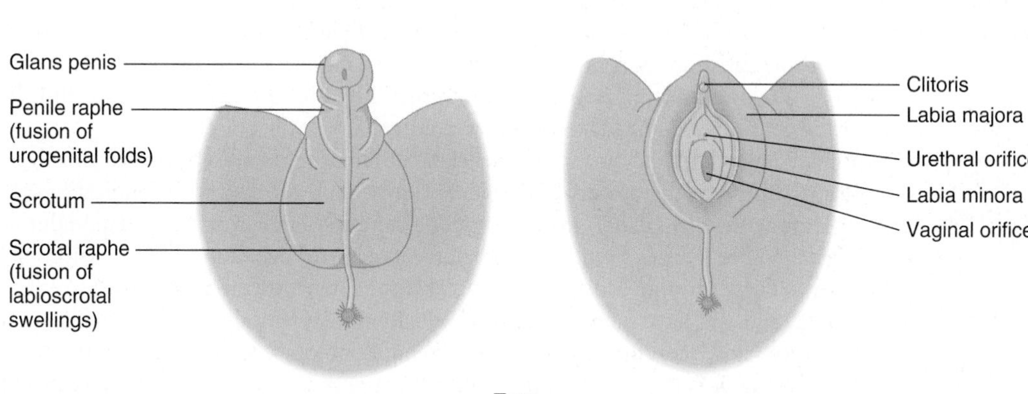

FIGURE 22-2 ◆
Sexual differentiation. A, At 7 weeks gestation, male and female genitalia are identical (undifferentiated). B and C, By 12 weeks gestation, noticeable differentiation begins to occur. D and E, Differentiation continues until birth, but is almost complete at term.

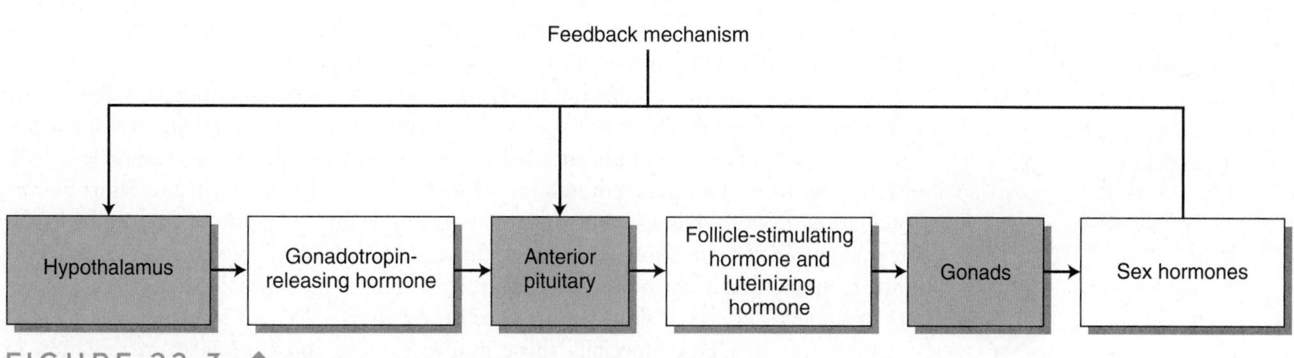

FIGURE 22-3 ◆
Feedback mechanism in hormonal stimulation of the gonads during puberty.

TABLE 22-2 Diagnostic Tests for Short Stature

TEST	PURPOSE RELATED TO SHORT STATURE
IGF-1 and IGFBP-3	Excludes growth hormone deficiency if normal
Radiographic views of the sella turcica (site of the pituitary gland)	Demonstrates size of the sella turcica or a tumor
Karotype (girls)	Detects Turner's syndrome (see page 855)
Thyroid function studies	Detects hypothyroidism (see page 829)
Urine creatinine, pH, specific gravity, urea nitrogen, electrolytes	Detects chronic renal failure (see Chapter 18)
Bone age	Identifies other potential causes of delayed growth
Complete blood count and erythrocyte sedimentation rate	Screens for inflammatory bowel disease with anemia
Antigliadin antibodies	Screens for celiac disease

Note: From D'Ercole, A.J., & Underwood, L. (1996). Anterior pituitary gland and hypothalamus. In A.M. Rudolph, J.I.E. Hoffman, & C.D. Rudolph (Eds.), *Rudolph's pediatrics* (20th ed., p. 1692). Stamford, CT: Appleton & Lange. Modified.

CLINICAL TIP

A radiographic image of the wrist bones is used to evaluate the stage of bone ossification, and thus the **bone age** (skeletal maturation) of the child. Using standardized norms for bone ossification, radiologists can determine if the child's chronologic and bone ages match. Bone age is used to evaluate the child with a growth problem. Significantly delayed (less than the child's age) or advanced (greater than the child's age) bone ages indicate that a problem such as a systemic chronic disease or hormone abnormality needs to be investigated.

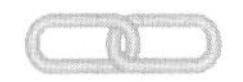

Skills 5-1 to 5-7: Growth Measurements

MAJOR CAUSES OF SHORT STATURE

Growth hormone deficiency
Familial short stature
Hypothyroidism
Turner syndrome
Constitutional growth delayed
Chronic renal failure
Cushing syndrome
Inborn error of metabolism
Severe cardiac disease
Pulmonary disease
Gastrointestinal disease

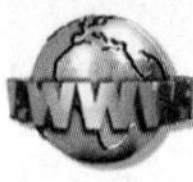

Growth Disorder Resources

evaluation by a pediatric endocrinologist. A careful history, physical examination, assessment of pubertal development and unusual facies, and radiologic studies are necessary to rule out familial short stature, constitutional growth delay, skeletal dysplasias, or psychosocial dwarfism. Provocative growth hormone testing, in which various medications (arginine, clonidine, glucagon, insulin, l-dopa) are administered to stimulate release of growth hormone, is the definitive diagnostic test in most children.

Treatment depends on the cause of the deficiency. Brain tumors must be treated effectively before growth hormone therapy can be considered (see Chapter 16). Approved indications for growth hormone therapy include growth hormone deficiency and growth retardation due to chronic renal failure, Turner's syndrome, small for gestational age, Russell Silver syndrome, and Prader Willi syndrome. Most children receive subcutaneous injections three to seven times a week, and will have increased growth velocity for 1 year, followed by more normal growth velocity. Close monitoring of growth and endocrinology visits every 3 to 4 months is needed. Replacement therapy is continued until either the child achieves an acceptable height or growth velocity drops to less than 2 cm (1 in.) per year (Willhaus, 1999). Early diagnosis and treatment are important to ensure attainment of maximum adult height potential. In some cases, the onset of puberty is delayed with gonadotropin-releasing hormone analogs to provide more time for growth hormone therapy to stimulate growth.

Nursing Management

Nursing care consists of monitoring growth, teaching the child and family about the disorder and its treatment, and providing emotional support. The child's height and weight are carefully measured and plotted on a growth chart (see Appendix A).

Teach the parents and child about the growth hormone replacement therapy and how to give injections. Provide the parents with ideas about how to minimize the trauma to the child who is receiving regular injections. Provide parents with educational resources such as information from the Magic Foundation, Human Growth Foundation, and Short Stature Foundation. Because replacement therapy is expensive and may not be covered by insurance, parents may need financial assistance that is sometimes available from the growth hormone manufacturers. The best results occur when treatment is initiated at an early age, before psychologic effects of short stature become apparent.

Children with GHD, especially those due to tumors and trauma from radiation or surgery, may have academic problems resulting from acquired learning disabilities. Before the child enters or returns to school, a comprehensive evaluation should be performed to identify potential problems.

If growth hormone therapy is not initiated early enough, attainment of near normal height may not be reached. People often treat short children on the basis of their size rather than their age, and such children experience social prejudice related to height. Teasing is a common problem. The teenage years may be particularly stressful because of the preoccupation with body image which is characteristic of adolescence.

Encourage parents and teachers to treat the child in an age-appropriate manner. The child should dress in clothing that reflects chronologic age. Emphasize the child's strengths, support independence, and encourage participation in age-appropriate activities to aid in the development of a positive self-image. Suggest that the child take part in sports in which ability does not depend on size (e.g., swimming, gymnastics, wrestling, ice skating, and martial arts). Identifying positive role models, short individuals who are successful in accomplishing their goals, is another approach that promotes a positive image. Refer the child for counseling if appropriate.

LAW & ETHICS

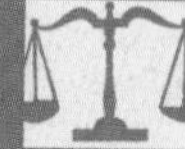

The increased availability of synthetic growth hormone has led to questions about its use for children who are below average for height but not growth hormone deficient. The medication is expensive (up to $15,000 per year) and its long-term effects, such as actually increasing adult height, are still being investigated. It is also an invasive therapy given by injection three to seven times a week for years.

HYPERPITUITARISM

Hyperpituitarism, a disorder in which excessive secretion of growth hormone increases the growth rate, is rare in children. Oversecretion of growth hormone is usually caused by a pituitary adenoma. If combined with precocious puberty, a tumor of the hypothalamus may be present. Affected children can grow to 7 or 8 feet in height when oversecretion occurs before closure of the epiphyseal plates. If the disorder occurs after closure of the epiphyseal plates, acromegaly occurs.

Because tall stature is valued in our society, assessment of children (particularly boys) with accelerated growth is often delayed. Any child whose predicted height exceeds that consistent with parental height should be evaluated for possible growth problems and underlying pathologic conditions.

A complete history is obtained, and physical examination and laboratory testing are performed. Increased levels of IGF-1 establish the diagnosis of hyperpituitarism. A bone scan is usually obtained to determine if the epiphyseal plates have begun to fuse. Radiologic studies are used to detect a tumor. Thorough evaluation is required to differentiate hyperpituitarism from familial tall stature.

Treatment depends on the cause of the excessive growth and may involve surgical removal of a tumor, radiation therapy, radioactive implants, or high doses of sex steroids given to close the epiphyseal plates. The child may need pituitary hormone replacement following surgery.

Nursing Management

Tall stature, like short stature, can be stressful for children. Tall children are often treated as if they are older than their chronologic age. Tall adolescents may have problems with self-image, and girls in particular may worry about their appearance.

Nursing care focuses on teaching the parents and child about the disorder and its treatment, providing emotional support, and, if surgery is required, providing preoperative and postoperative teaching and care (see Chapter 5).

DIABETES INSIPIDUS

Diabetes insipidus, a rare disorder of the posterior pituitary gland, may begin at any age. Two forms of diabetes insipidus occur in children: true (or central) antidiuretic hormone (ADH) deficiency and familial nephrogenic diabetes insipidus, in which the renal collecting tubules are unable to respond to the ADH that is present.

True ADH deficiency in children is usually familial or idiopathic. Secondary causes include CNS trauma, infection, tumor, hypoxic brain damage, vascular anomalies, or infiltrative diseases such as leukemia. Most cases of nephrogenic diabetes insipidus are familial, with either an X-linked or an autosomal recessive form. It may also result from drug toxicity or recurrent infection.

ADH facilitates concentration of the urine by stimulating reabsorption of water from the distal tubule of the kidney. When ADH is inadequate, the tubules do not resorb, leading to **polyuria** (passage of a large volume of urine in a given period).

CLINICAL MANIFESTATIONS OF DIABETES INSIPIDIS

CAUSE	CLINICAL MANIFESTATIONS	CLINICAL THERAPY
True Diabetes Insipidis ADH deficiency Familial or idiopathic	Polyuria, polydipsia Nocturia, enuresis Thirsty at night, irritable if fluids withheld Constipation, fever, dehydration	Desmopressin acetate
Nephrogenic Diabetes Insipidis Familial, decreased responsiveness of kidneys to ADH	Polyuria, polydipsia Hypernatremia in neonatal period Dehydration, fever, vomiting Mental status changes	Diuretics High fluid intake Salt and protein restricted diet

Polyuria and **polydipsia** (excessive thirst) are the cardinal signs of diabetes insipidus. See the table above for the clinical manifestations of diabetes insipidis by cause. Although the onset of symptoms is usually sudden, diagnosis is often delayed. Children who are able to quench their thirst may not complain to parents about symptoms. The child may have obesity due to an excessive intake of high caloric fluids.

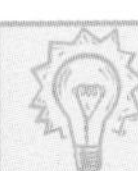

CLINICAL TIP

During the fluid deprivation test, advise parents that the child will be frustrated and irritable from thirst. No one should drink in front of the child during the testing period. Monitor the child's vital signs and intake and output carefully. The test is stopped if the child loses 3%–5% of body weight and develops a fever and hypotension (Dveirin & Tunnessen, 2000).

In all forms of diabetes insipidus, the urine cannot be concentrated, no matter how dehydrated the child becomes. Dehydration usually precipitates diagnosis. Serum sodium concentration and osmolality increase rapidly to pathologic levels. Often an unconscious child is admitted to the emergency department with dehydration accompanied by hypernatremia.

Serum electrolytes and both serum and urine osmolalities are tested. Diagnosis is confirmed by measuring the plasma arginine vasopressin (AVP) level before and during a fluid deprivation test, which is usually conducted in the hospital or in a carefully controlled outpatient setting for up to 7 hours. Urine osmolality, urine specific gravity, serum sodium, and serum osmolality are monitored hourly. The specific gravity will remain less than 1.010 even after dehydration. A dose of aqueous vasopressin is given after several hours. A decreased urine output and increased urine concentration confirms the diagnosis.

Treatment of true ADH deficiency consists of the subcutaneous, intranasal, or oral desmopressin acetate (DDAVP) with an effect lasting 8 to 12 hours. DDAVP reduces urinary output, enabling the child to live a more normal life with a decrease in thirst, urinary output, and nocturia. The dose of DDAVP must be titered so the child receives adequate caloric intake for growth and development. Because DDAVP is not effective in controlling nephrogenic diabetes insipidus, these children are treated with diuretics, a high fluid intake, and a salt- and protein-restricted diet. The child's sodium and potassium levels must be carefully monitored to prevent hypernatremia and hypokalemia (see Chapter 10).

Nursing Management

Nursing care centers on administering medications and teaching parents how to manage the condition and recognize signs of altered fluid status. Parent education is of primary importance. Infants usually need fluid intake even during the night. Many infants have coexisting brain damage and decreased thirst and require nasogastric or gastrostomy feeding to maintain adequate hydration and nutrition.

CLINICAL TIP

Administration of synthetic vasopressin (DDAVP) in small doses by intranasal insufflation (blowing the medication into the nasal cavity) in infants and young children often results in inconsistent absorption. If too large a dose is given, the child may swallow the medication, resulting in lack of absorption.

Help parents monitor fluid intake after DDAVP treatment is initiated. When the child has compensated for the condition with an excessive fluid intake, the diminished need for fluids must be learned. The child will not have the ability to excrete the excess water load with DDAVP treatment.

Teach parents to recognize signs of inadequate fluid intake (see Chapter 10) and to adjust the child's fluid intake to prevent dehydration. When the child with nephrogenic diabetes insipidis has an acute illness, the child's physician should be notified immediately, because the increased metabolic activity may cause dehydration and hypernatremia which may result in mental retardation, seizures, and cerebral calcification. Additional fluids are needed to prevent dehydration (Kirchlechner, Koller, & Seidl, et al., 1999).

Parents may need assistance to manage the child's care. Arrangements for a visiting nurse, a home health nurse, or respite care may be needed.

PRECOCIOUS PUBERTY

Puberty normally occurs between 8 and 13 years in girls and between 9.5 and 14 years in boys. Precocious puberty is defined as the appearance of any secondary sexual characteristics before 8 years in girls and 9 years in boys.

Early secretion of the normal hormones responsible for pubertal changes usually is not associated with abnormalities; however, a benign hypothalamic tumor may be present. Other causes include brain injury, brain tumor, postinfectious encephalitis or meningitis, congenital adrenal hyperplasia, tumors of the ovary, adrenal gland, or testicle, and exogenous sources or androgens (i.e., anabolic steroids). Children with precocious puberty have an advanced bone age (premature skeletal maturation) and may appear unusually tall for their age. Their growth ceases prematurely, however, as the hormones stimulate closure of the epiphyseal plates, resulting in short stature.

When the cause of the condition cannot be treated, the child's development may be monitored for 6 to 12 months to see how quickly pubertal changes are occurring. If development is stalled or slow, no treatment is initiated. If pubertal changes occur rapidly, a gonadotropin-releasing hormone analog is used to stop the development of secondary sexual characteristics, bone age progression, and rapid growth. The time for pubertal growth is extended. In some cases, growth hormone is given to increase the ultimate height of the child (Kohn, Julius, & Blethen, 1999).

CULTURE

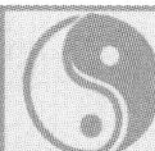

A national study of the age at which pubertal development begins in girls has revealed an earlier average age of puberty than described in texts. Black girls begin puberty between 8 and 9 years; white girls begin puberty by 10 years (Herman-Giddens, Slora, Wasserman, et al., 1997).

Nursing Management

Nursing care centers on teaching the child and parents about the condition and its treatment and providing emotional support. The child should be informed in age-appropriate terms that physiologic changes are normal but occurring at an earlier than usual age. Reassure the child that friends will go through the same stages of development eventually. Remember that the child's social, cognitive, and emotional development matches his or her age, even though the physical development is advanced.

Children with precocious puberty become self-conscious as body changes occur. Parents should be advised to dress the child in a manner appropriate to his or her chronologic age, even though the child may look older. Looser clothing may help hide some of the body changes that are occurring. Provide privacy during examinations. Encourage the child to express feelings about the changes. The child may need to practice role playing as a coping mechanism to manage teasing by other children.

Parents should be advised that they may need to discuss issues of sexuality with the child at an earlier age than normal. Refer the child for counseling if appropriate.

DISORDERS OF THYROID FUNCTION

HYPOTHYROIDISM

Hypothyroidism is a disorder in which levels of active thyroid hormones are decreased. It may be congenital or acquired. Congenital hypothyroidism occurs in approximately 1 in 4,000 live births and is twice as common in girls as in boys. It is less prevalent in black infants but more frequent in infants of Far Eastern and Hispanic origin (1 in 2,000 births). It also occurs more commonly in children with Down syndrome. Acquired hypothyroidism has an estimated prevalence of 1 in 500,000 school-age children, and is more common in girls than in boys (Donohoue, 1999).

Etiology and Pathophysiology

Thyroid hormones are important for growth and development and for the metabolism of nutrients and energy. When these hormones are not available for stimulation of other hormones or specific target cells, growth is delayed and mental retardation develops.

Congenital hypothyroidism is usually caused by a spontaneous gene mutation, an autosomal recessive genetic transmission of an enzyme deficiency, hypoplasia or aplasia of the thyroid gland, failure of the central nervous system–thyroid feedback mechanism to develop, or iodine deficiency. Mental retardation is irreversible if the disorder is not treated.

Acquired hypothyroidism can be idiopathic or result from autoimmune thyroiditis (Hashimoto's thyroiditis), late-onset thyroid dysfunction, isolated thyroid-stimulating hormone (TSH) deficiency due to pituitary or hypothalamic dysfunction, or exposure to drugs or substances such as lithium that interfere with thyroid hormone synthesis.

Clinical Manifestations

Infants with congenital hypothyroidism have few clinical signs of the disorder in the first weeks of life. In untreated infants, the characteristic cretinoid features (thickened protuberant tongue, thick lips, dull appearance) appear during the first few months of life. Other signs include prolonged neonatal jaundice, hypotonia, macroglossia, respiratory distress, bradycardia, decreased pulse pressure, cool extremities, mottling, umbilical hernia, a posterior fontanel larger than 1 cm in diameter, difficulty feeding, lethargy, constipation, and a hoarse cry.

Children with acquired hypothyroidism have many of the same signs as adults: decreased appetite, dry cool skin, thinning hair or hair loss, depressed deep tendon reflexes, bradycardia, constipation, sensitivity to cold temperatures, abnormal menses, and a **goiter** (a nontender enlarged thyroid gland). Manifestations unique to children include change in past normal growth patterns with a weight increase, decreased height velocity, delayed bone and dental age, muscle hypertrophy with muscle weakness, and delayed or precocious puberty.

Clinical Therapy

Congenital hypothyroidism is usually detected during newborn screening of thyroxine (T_4) and TSH levels, which is mandatory in every state. An elevated TSH level indicates that the disease originated in the thyroid, not the pituitary. Two tests are frequently performed so that the disorder is identified, before the newborn leaves the hospital and at the first health care visit at 1 to 2 weeks of age. Rapid responses from the laboratory that is testing the samples is important to reduce the time to diagnosis and the effects of hypothyroidism on the infant's development.

If the T_4 level is below normal and the TSH level is increased, the synthetic thyroid hormone levothyroxine (Synthroid) is prescribed. The dose is increased gradually as the child grows to ensure a **euthyroid** (normal thyroid) state. Treatment is monitored by a pediatric endocrinologist. Periodic evaluation of T_4 and TSH serum levels, bone age, and growth parameters is necessary to assess for signs of excess or inadequate thyroid hormone.

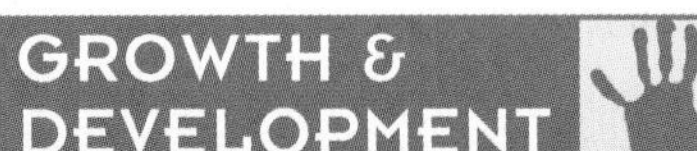

Treated children with the most severe form of congenital hypothyroidism lose 6 to 15 IQ points, whereas the less severely affected children have an IQ similar to their siblings (Van Vliet, 2001).

Antithyroid antibodies are measured in children with a goiter and suspected Hashimoto's thyroiditis, as increased titers of antithyroglobin and antimicrosomal antibodies are often found.

To ensure an adequate growth rate and prevent mental retardation, the hormone must be taken throughout life. Children with congenital hypothyroidism diagnosed before 3 months of age have the best prognosis for optimal mental development. Children with acquired hypothyroidism usually have normal growth following a period of catch-up growth. Many adolescents with Hashimoto's thyroiditis have a spontaneous remission.

NURSING MANAGEMENT

Nursing Assessment and Diagnosis

Routine neonatal screening is performed before discharge from the hospital and is often repeated at the infant's first health visit to evaluate levels of circulating thyroid hormones. Sometimes nurses make home visits a few days after discharge to assess the health of the mother and infant. Neonatal screening may be performed at that visit.

Skill 6-2: Newborn Screening

Serial measurement and recording of height and weight are performed at each follow-up visit. The child is assessed for signs of inadequate growth to determine if the dose of thyroid hormone needs to be adjusted and to monitor compliance with medication.

Following are nursing diagnoses that may be appropriate for the child with hypothyroidism:

- *Altered nutrition: Less than body requirements,* related to loss of appetite
- *Hypothermia,* related to decreased basal metabolic rate

- *Constipation,* related to decreased bowel motility
- *Fatigue,* related to altered body chemistry
- *Altered health maintenance,* related to lack of understanding about the treatment regimen

Planning and Implementation

Nursing care focuses on teaching the parents and child about the disorder and its treatment and monitoring the child's growth rate. When the cause is genetic, a referral for genetic counseling should be made. Explain how to administer thyroid hormone (e.g., tablets can be crushed and mixed in a small amount of formula or applesauce). Advise parents that the child may experience temporary sleep disturbances or behavioral changes in response to therapy. Teach the parents how to assess for an increased pulse rate, which could indicate the presence of too much thyroid hormone, and advise them to report problems such as fatigue, which could indicate an improper drug dose that needs to be readjusted.

Caution parents to dress the child appropriately for the season to prevent hypothermia. Modify the child's diet by increasing the amount of fruits and bulk if constipation is a problem.

Reassure the family that the child will develop normally with hormone replacement therapy. Reinforce the importance of follow-up visits to assess growth rate and response to therapy and to regulate drug dosages as the child grows. Periodic assessments of educational achievement is needed. Parents should be informed that therapy will be lifelong and is needed to promote the child's mental development.

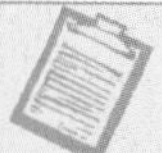

RESEARCH

Even with good control, adolescents have persistent visual-spatial deficits and memory and attention problems. Those with more severe disease or who take longer to get to euthyroid status have the poorest academic achievement and more behavior problems. Close monitoring and regular follow-up is important to promote learning (Rovet & Ehrlich, 2000).

Evaluation

Expected outcomes of nursing care of the child with hypothyroidism include the following:

- The child maintains adequate growth of height and weight, following a percentile curve throughout childhood.
- The child's diet contains adequate fruits and bulk to prevent constipation.
- The child's cognitive development is appropriate for age.

HYPERTHYROIDISM

Hyperthyroidism occurs when thyroid hormone levels are increased. It is rare in children and adolescents with a rate of 8 per 1 million children (Castiglia, 1997). It is most common in adolescent girls and is almost always due to Graves' disease.

Etiology and Pathophysiology

Graves' disease is an autoimmune disorder in which the body produces antibodies that attack the cells of the thyroid gland. It has a high familial incidence. Immunoglobulins produced by the B lymphocytes stimulate oversecretion of thyroid hormones, resulting in the clinical symptoms. Signs and symptoms are caused by hyperactivity of the sympathetic nervous system.

Other, more unusual forms of hyperthyroidism result from thyroiditis and thyroid hormone–producing tumors, including thyroid adenomas and carcinomas, and pituitary adenomas. Congenital hyperthyroidism can occur in infants of mothers with Graves' disease because of transplacental transfer of immunoglobulins.

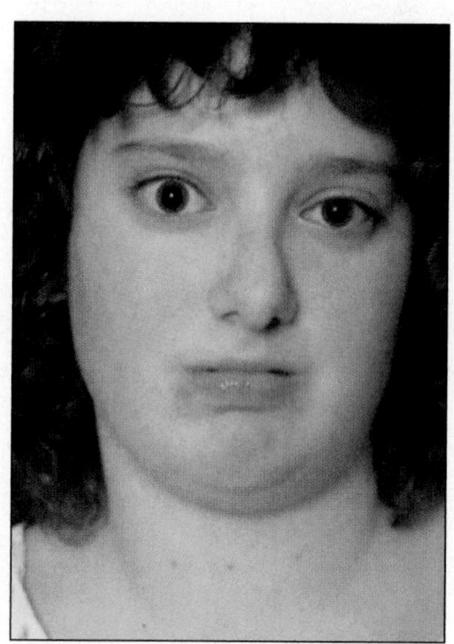

FIGURE 22-4 ◆

Exophthalmos and an enlarged thyroid in an adolescent with Graves' disease.
From Zitelli, B. J., & Davis, H. W. (eds.) (1997). *Atlas of pediatric physical diagnosis* (3rd ed., p. 271). St. Louis: Mosby-Wolfe.

Clinical Manifestations

Characteristic findings include an enlarged, nontender thyroid gland (goiter), prominent or bulging eyes (exophthalmos) (Figure 22-4 ◆), eyelid lag, tachycardia, nervousness, restlessness or irritability, increased appetite with weight loss, emotional lability, heat intolerance, increased sweating, insomnia, tremor, and muscle weakness. The thyroid gland may be slightly enlarged or grow to 3 to 4 times its normal size; feel warm, soft, and fleshy; and have an auditory bruit on auscultation. The disorder often presents in the preschool years, but with an increased incidence in adolescence. Onset is subtle, and the condition often goes unrecognized for 1 to 2 years.

Children with Graves' disease usually manifest behavioral problems and declining performance in school. They become easily frustrated in the classroom and overheated and fatigued during physical education class. It is difficult for them to relax or sleep. These symptoms usually prompt parents to seek medical treatment for them. Other symptoms include an increased appetite with weight loss, tremors, and tachycardia. Exophthalmos is less pronounced in children than in adults.

NURSING ALERT

Propylthiouracil therapy can cause temporary side effects, including skin rashes, urticaria, and lymphadenopathy. If fever or sore throat develops, the child should be evaluated by a health care professional to rule out granulocytopenia.

Clinical Therapy

Diagnostic studies include laboratory evaluation of serum TSH, T_3 (triiodothyronine) and T_4 levels, and a thyroid scan. Blood studies are also performed to detect autoantibodies specific for the various thyroid disorders.

The goal of clinical therapy is to inhibit excessive secretion of thyroid hormones. Treatment may include antithyroid drug therapy, radiation therapy, or surgery. Drug therapy is most often used as the initial treatment modality, but compliance is often a problem because of drug side effects. Methimazole (Tapazole) and propylthiouracil (PTU) are given to inhibit thyroid hormone secretion. Treatment continues for 18 months to 2 years or until the thyroid decreases in size. Symptoms usually improve within weeks of starting treatment. Approximately 25% of children have a remission of symptoms every 2 years (Castiglia, 1997).

If drug therapy is ineffective, radiation therapy using radioactive iodine (131I) is the next treatment choice. Current data do not indicate a relationship between radioactive iodine and cancer or leukemia. It also does not appear to increase the risk of birth defects in future offspring in those treated (Castiglia, 1997). Thyroidectomy is the third alternative; however, destruction or removal of the thyroid gland often results in permanent hypothyroidism, necessitating hormone replacement therapy.

NURSING MANAGEMENT

Nursing Assessment and Diagnosis

Assess the child's vital signs, as blood pressure and pulse may be elevated, and record food intake. Accurate measurement and recording of height and weight are important to establish baselines and identify patterns of growth. Observe the child's behavior, activity, and level of fatigue.

Common nursing diagnoses for the child with hyperthyroidism include the following:

- *Ineffective thermoregulation (elevated),* related to illness and excessive activity of the sympathetic nervous system
- *Altered nutrition: Less than body requirements,* related to high metabolic needs
- *Body image disturbance,* related to changes caused by illness (prominent eyes, excessive perspiration, and tremors)
- *Fatigue,* related to disease state and sleep deprivation
- *Self-esteem disturbance,* related to chronic illness and declining school performance

Planning and Implementation

Nursing care focuses on teaching the child and parents about the disorder and its treatment, promoting rest, providing emotional support, and, if the child requires surgery, providing preoperative and postoperative teaching and care. Promote increased caloric intake by providing five or six moderate meals per day. Encourage the child and family to express feelings and concerns about the disorder. Complimenting even slight improvements in the child's condition increases compliance with therapy.

Children with hyperthyroidism are easily fatigued. Rest periods should be scheduled at school and home and physical activities kept to a minimum until symptoms resolve. Encourage parents to provide a cool environment and allow the child to wear fewer clothes until symptoms subside.

Children who have partial or total removal of the thyroid gland receive antithyroid drugs, such as iodine, for approximately 2 weeks before surgery. Teach the child and parents about drug therapy and instruct parents to watch for side effects of antithyroid drugs, including fever, urticaria, and lymphadenopathy. Provide preoperative teaching (see Chapter 5). Young children in particular may be fearful about having their throat "cut." Postoperatively, observe for signs of severe **thyrotoxicosis** (thyroid "storm") and hypercalcemia, which can be life threatening. Treatment includes administration of antithyroid drugs and propranolol. Monitor the child's surgical site. Assess the child for bleeding, hoarseness, and difficulty breathing, which may be signs of inflammation.

Teach the family about the need for lifelong thyroid hormone replacement if radiation or surgery is performed. A medical alert bracelet should be worn. Make sure the child is monitored regularly to ensure that the T_4 level is adequate to sustain growth.

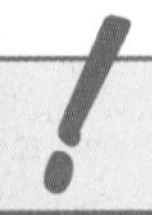

NURSING ALERT

Thyroid storm may occur when thyroid hormone is suddenly released into the bloodstream during surgery. The child experiences fever, diaphoresis, and tachycardia, progressing to shock and, if untreated, death.

Evaluation

Expected outcomes of nursing care for the child with hyperthyroidism include the following:

- The child regains lost weight and then follows the previously established growth curve because the T_4 level remains appropriate.
- Any difficulty breathing, bleeding, or hoarseness as a result of thyroid surgery is rapidly managed and controlled.

See Chapter 10 for parathyroid conditions.

DISORDERS OF ADRENAL FUNCTION

CUSHING'S SYNDROME

Cushing's syndrome, also called adrenocortical hyperfunction, is characterized by a group of symptoms resulting from excess levels of glucocorticoids (especially cortisol) in the bloodstream. It is uncommon in children and the true incidence is unknown. During infancy and childhood, most cases of Cushing's syndrome are due to malignant adrenal tumor. After 8 years of age, more than half of the cases are due to secretion of adrenocorticotropic hormone (ACTH) by a pituitary adenoma causing cortisol secretion. Another cause is hyperplasia of one or both adrenal glands. The increased secretion of cortisol alters metabolism.

CLINICAL TIP

The most common reasons for cushingoid features in children are receiving excessive doses of corticosteroids and prolonged use of corticosteroids as treatment for other diseases. Corticosteroids suppress adrenal function when given long term. These children do not have Cushing's syndrome.

The initial sign in most children is gradual excessive weight gain and growth retardation. It generally takes up to 5 years for the child to develop the characteristic "cushingoid" appearance, which includes a moon face (chubby cheeks and a double chin) and fat pads over the shoulders and back (buffalo hump). See box below for clinical manifestations caused by altered cortisol metabolism. Other signs include mental changes and delayed puberty.

Diagnosis is based on characteristic physical findings and laboratory values, including reduced serum levels of potassium and phosphorus; elevated serum calcium and sodium concentrations; increased 24-hour urinary levels of free cortisol and 17-hydroxycorticosteroid (17-OHC); and loss of diurnal rhythm in serum cortisol (usually elevated at night). The child has chronic hyperglycemia and an elevated glycolsylated hemoglobin concentration. See Appendix C for lab values.

The adrenal suppression test is used for the initial screening of children with suspected adrenocortical hyperfunction. If this test reveals that adrenal cortisol output is

CLINICAL MANIFESTATIONS OF CUSHING'S SYNDROME

CAUSE	CLINICAL MANIFESTATIONS
Catabolism of protein	Muscle weakness and wasting, capillary weakness and bruising, growth failure with delayed bone age, fatigue
Decreased absorption of calcium from the intestines	Demineralization of bones, osteoporosis
Increased appetite	Weight gain primarily on the trunk, striae on the abdomen, buttocks, thighs
Salt retention	Increased blood volume and hypertension

not suppressed overnight after a dose of dexamethasone, further diagnostic testing is necessary to determine the cause of hypercortisolism. CT and MRI are used to detect tumors in the adrenal and pituitary glands.

Surgical removal is the current treatment of choice for adrenal tumors or pituitary adenomas. Cortisol replacement is required when both adrenal glands are removed. The prognosis for children with malignant adrenal tumors is poor.

Nursing Management

The nurse usually encounters a child with Cushing's syndrome when the child is hospitalized for diagnostic evaluation or surgery. Nursing assessment includes monitoring the child's vital signs and fluid and nutritional status, and assessing muscle strength and endurance during hospital play activities.

Teach the child and family about the disorder and its treatment, and, for children undergoing surgery, provide preoperative and postoperative teaching and care. Answer any questions the child and family may have and explain all laboratory and diagnostic tests. Explain to parents that the child's cushingoid appearance is reversible with treatment. Provide nutritional guidance or refer the child and parents to a nutritionist to promote maintenance of an appropriate weight.

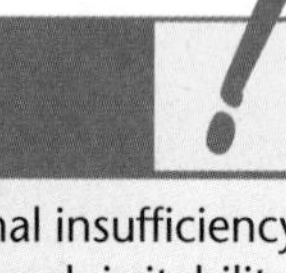

Signs of acute adrenal insufficiency may include increased irritability, headache, confusion, restlessness, nausea and vomiting, diarrhea, abdominal pain, dehydration, fever, loss of appetite, and lethargy. If untreated, the child will go into shock. In newborns, the symptoms include failure to thrive, weakness, vomiting, and dehydration. Hyponatremia and hyperkalemia are key signs.

Preoperative and postoperative teaching and care are similar to those for the child undergoing surgery (see Chapter 5). Refer to Chapter 16 for general nursing care of the child with cancer.

For children who require cortisol replacement therapy because both adrenal glands were surgically removed, administering the drug early in the morning or every other day causes fewer symptoms than daily administration and mimics the normal diurnal pattern of cortisol secretion. Cortisol replacement in the postoperative period must be explained carefully to parents. Hydrocortisone (Cortef, Solu-Cortef, cortisone acetate) comes in liquid, tablet, or injectable form. Teach parents how and when to administer the injectable form, usually when the child is vomiting or has diarrhea, or cannot take the oral medication. The oral preparations of cortisone have a bitter taste and can cause gastric irritation. Giving the dose at mealtimes and using antacids between meals helps reduce these side effects.

Teach parents to be alert to signs of acute adrenal insufficiency during the withdrawal of corticosteroid therapy, and to inform all health care providers of the child's condition and medication. A medical alert tag should be worn at all times.

CONGENITAL ADRENAL HYPERPLASIA

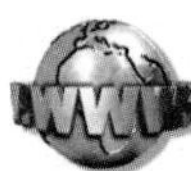

Congenital Adrenal Hyperplasia

Congenital adrenal hyperplasia, sometimes called adrenogenital syndrome, adrenocortical hyperplasia, or congenital adrenogenital hyperplasia, is an autosomal recessive disorder that causes a deficiency of one of the enzymes necessary for the synthesis of cortisol and aldosterone. The defective gene CYP21 is located on the short arm of chromosome 6. It occurs in 1 in 10,000 to 16,000 live births, and males and females are affected equally. The incidence is highest in Native Alaskans (American Academy of Pediatrics Section on Endocrinology and Committee on Genetica, 2000). Of the two classic forms of the disorder, 75% are salt losing, caused by the blockage of aldosterone production, and 25% are non salt losing, or simple virilization.

Etiology and Pathophysiology

More than 80% of children with congenital adrenal hyperplasia have partial or complete 21-hydroxylase enzyme deficiency in which deficient aldosterone synthesis leads to excessive renal excretion of salt (salt losing). This form has an autosomal recessive inheritance pattern. About 10% of children have 11-hydroxylase deficiency. The remainder have deficiencies involving five other enzymes. In its most severe form, the disorder can be life threatening. In all forms, increased secretion of ACTH occurs in response to diminished cortisol levels.

During fetal development, the lack of cortisol triggers the pituitary to continue secretion of ACTH. This in turn stimulates overproduction of the adrenal androgens. Female virilization of the external genitalia begins in week 10 of gestation. If untreated, the overproduction of androgens results in accelerated height, early closure of the epiphyseal plates, and premature sexual development with both pubic and axillary hair.

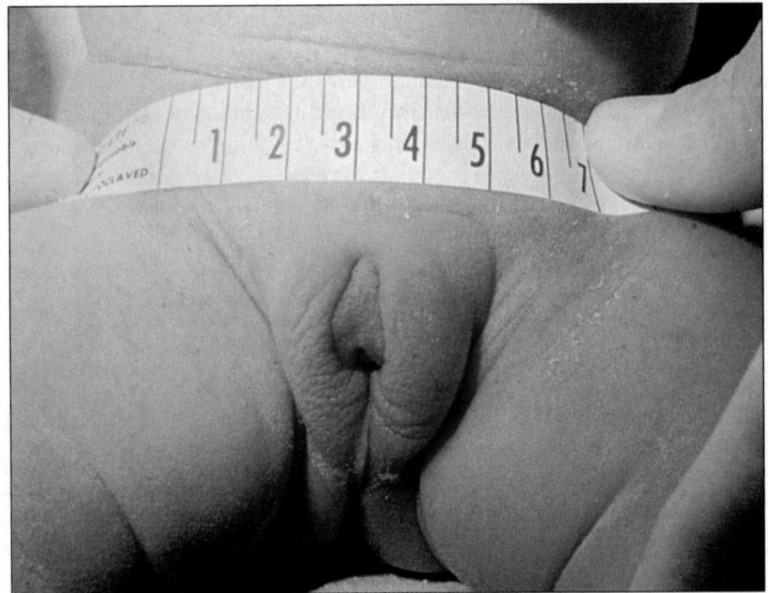

FIGURE 22-5 ◆
Newborn girl with ambiguous genitalia.
Courtesy of Patrick C. Walsh, M.D.

Approximately 65% to 75% of children have a disturbance in mineralocorticoid regulation that can lead to acute adrenal insufficiency with any serious illness or injury (Therrell, Berenbaum, & Manter-Kapanke, et al., 1998).

Clinical Manifestations

Congenital adrenal hyperplasia is the most common cause of **pseudohermaphroditism** (ambiguous genitalia) in newborn girls. Virilization begins in utero. The female infant is born with an enlarged clitoris and labial fusions (Figure 22-5 ◆). Severely virilized females may be mistaken for males with cryptorchidism, hypospadias, or micropenis. The male infant may look normal at birth or may have a slightly enlarged penis and hyperpigmented scrotum. The boy may have an adult-size penis by school age, but the testes are appropriately sized for age. Partial enzyme deficiency produces less obvious symptoms. Precocious puberty and tall stature for age may be noted later. Due to early epiphyseal fusion, adults have short stature.

Recurrent vomiting, dehydration, metabolic acidosis, hypotension, and hypoglycemia are characteristic signs of the salt-wasting form of the disorder. Hypertension with hypokalemic alkalosis is alternately found in children with 11-hydroxylase deficiency.

Clinical Therapy

Diagnosis in infants and children is usually confirmed by laboratory evaluation of serum 17-hydroxyprogesterone level. Routine newborn screening for congenital adrenal hyperplasia is performed in 19 states (American Academy of Pediatrics Committee on Bioethics, 2001). Prenatal screening is available. In instances of ambiguous genitalia, a **karyotype** (a microscopic chromosome study in which the 46 chromosomes of the child are lined up in pairs from largest to smallest to detect errors in chromosome number, shape, and size) is obtained to determine the gender of the infant. Ultrasonography may be used to visualize pelvic structures.

In the salt-wasting form of the disorder, the child may have hyponatremia, hyperkalemia, a high urine sodium level, and low serum and urinary aldosterone levels. Serum concentrations of testosterone in girls and androstenedione in boys and girls are elevated in affected infants. Elevated adrenocorticotropic hormone (ACTH) with measurement of serum cortisol and 17-OHP levels are necessary to confirm the diagnosis (American Academy of Pediatrics, 2000). Diagnosis may be delayed in the non salt losing form until 3 to 7 years.

The goal of treatment is to suppress adrenal secretion of androgens by replacing deficient hormones, which is accomplished by the lifelong oral administration of glucocorticoids (dexamethasone or hydrocortisone). The glucocorticoid replacement leads to a reduction in secretion of ACTH which had overstimulated the adrenal cortex. As a result, excessive

RESEARCH

A combination of flutamide and testolactone along with a reduced dose of glucocorticoids have shown promise in efforts to reduce excess androgen production that control the accelerated growth and slow bone maturation (Merke & Cutler, 1997).

Skill 5-22: Infant Intake and Output Measurement

adrenal androgen production is suppressed. The dose is individualized by monitoring growth parameters, bone age, and hormone levels. If the infant has the salt-wasting form of the disorder, salt is added to the infant's formula and a mineralocorticoid (Florinef) is given to replace the missing hormone. Hormone dosage must be doubled or tripled during acute illnesses or injury and for surgery. Injectable hydrocortisone is used for severe stress.

Reconstructive surgery of the enlarged clitoris is often performed on girls during the first year of life. Vaginal reconstruction is performed in a later procedure.

NURSING MANAGEMENT

Nursing Assessment and Diagnosis

Assess the infant and child for signs of dehydration, electrolyte imbalance, and shock in the salt-wasting form of the disease. Monitor vital signs and assess peripheral perfusion (capillary refill, distal pulses, color and temperature of the extremities) frequently to detect early changes in condition.

Assess the parents' emotional response to a child with ambiguous genitalia and a chronic condition. Explore their values and beliefs regarding gender roles and sexuality while awaiting results of the karyotype.

Nursing diagnoses for the child with congenital adrenal hyperplasia may include the following:

- *Risk for altered parenting,* related to a child with undetermined gender identity
- *Caregiver role strain,* related to care of a child with a chronic, potentially life-threatening condition
- *Risk for fluid volume deficit,* related to failure of regulatory mechanisms and excess excretion of salt by the kidneys
- *Risk for altered growth,* related to premature development of secondary sex characteristics and accelerated growth

Planning and Implementation

Nursing care of the newborn with congenital adrenal hyperplasia focuses on teaching parents about the disorder and its treatment, providing emotional support, and preoperative and postoperative teaching for parents of infants undergoing reconstructive surgery. Because of the risk for adrenal insufficiency, the child will most likely be hospitalized for surgery. The administration of glucocorticoids and mineralocorticoids must be carefully controlled.

It is often difficult for parents to accept that their infant, whose genitalia look male, is really female. With medication and surgery, the genitalia assume a female appearance and all organs necessary for future childbearing are usually functional. Several surgeries may be performed before 2 years of age and then during adolescence to dilate the vagina.

Nurses can assist parents in educating the child's siblings, grandparents, other family members, and daycare workers about the condition. In the newborn nursery, the infant should be referred to as "your beautiful infant," not "your son" or "your daughter," until gender identity is confirmed.

Inform parents that genetic counseling should be provided for the child during adolescence. Parents considering a future pregnancy should also be informed that prenatal testing may detect congenital adrenal hyperplasia in the fetus. Refer the family for counseling if indicated.

CARE IN THE COMMUNITY

Teach parents about the special problems that develop in the salt-wasting form of the disease during acute illness. Explain the medication regimen and help the family develop an emergency care plan. The child should wear a medical alert tag. Teach parents how to administer intramuscular injections of hydrocortisone for emergencies. Ensure that parents have an emergency kit of injectable hydrocortisone at home and at school to be used when the child is vomiting or has diarrhea. It should be carried wherever the child goes. If injectable hydrocortisone is not available, the child needs urgent treatment in an emergency department. The child may become dehydrated quickly and need intravenous fluid and electrolyte replacement in addition to higher doses of hydrocortisone.

Evaluation

Expected outcomes of nursing care for congenital adrenal hyperplasia are as follows:

- Parents learn to give glucocorticoids appropriately when the child is ill and prevent episodes of adrenal crisis.
- Families effectively cope with the virilized appearance of the child's genitalia and bond with the child.

ADRENAL INSUFFICIENCY (ADDISON'S DISEASE)

Adrenal insufficiency, also known as Addison's disease, is a rare disorder in childhood characterized by a deficiency of glucocorticoids (cortisone) and mineralocorticoids (aldosterone). It may be acquired after trauma; with tuberculosis, acquired immunodeficiency syndrome (AIDS), or fungal infections that cause destruction of the adrenal glands; or as the result of an autoimmune process.

Adrenal insufficiency usually develops slowly as the adrenal glands deteriorate. The early signs may not be noticed but include weakness with fatigue; anorexia and salt craving; poor weight gain or weight loss; hyperpigmentation at pressure points, lip borders and gingival margins, nipples, palms and soles, body creases, and scarred areas of the body; generalized bronzing of the skin or freckling without tan lines even in winter months; abdominal pain; nausea and vomiting; and diarrhea. Symptomatic hypoglycemia may also be present. If the child experiences a stressful period (illness, injury, or surgery), acute adrenal insufficiency may occur. Signs of an adrenal crisis include weakness, fever, abdominal pain, hypoglycemia with seizures, hypotension, dehydration, and shock.

Serum cortisol and urinary 17-hydroxycorticoid levels are measured in the early morning. Low levels are associated with adrenal insufficiency. The ACTH stimulation test is used to detect adrenal gland reserve. Electrolyte values generally reveal low serum sodium, elevated serum potassium, and low fasting blood glucose levels. CT may be used to visualize the adrenal glands.

Treatment involves replacement of the deficient hormones. Oral hydrocortisone is given in the lowest therapeutic dose to control symptoms and promote normal growth. Fludrocortisone acetate (Florinef) is administered to replace the missing mineralocorticoid in children with aldosterone deficiency. Adrenal crisis is treated by fluid and electrolyte resuscitation, treatment of the precipitating illness or injury, adequate doses of glucocorticoid, and maintenance doses of mineralocorticoid.

Nursing Management

Nursing management focuses on educating the child and parents about the disorder, providing emotional support, and caring for the child during acute episodes. See the earlier discussion of congenital adrenal hyperplasia for further detail.

PHEOCHROMOCYTOMA

Pheochromocytoma is a tumor of the adrenal gland, but it may be extra-adrenal with no anatomic connection. In most cases these tumors are benign and curable. They can occur in a familial pattern (autosomal dominant trait) with a 3:2 male to female ratio. The incidence is 1 to 500,000 children, and most tumors are diagnosed in children between the ages of 6 and 14 years (Reddy, O'Neill, & Holcomb, et al., 2000).

Clinical manifestations include labile hypertension with a systolic reading that may reach 250 mm Hg, tachycardia, arrhythmias, palpitations, profuse sweating with cool extremities, flushing, headache, abdominal pain, nausea and vomiting, weight loss, visual disturbances, weakness, polydipsia, and polyuria. The classic triad of signs includes new onset hypertension, new or worsening diabetes mellitus, and hypertensive crisis. Because release of catecholamines (norepinephrine and epinephrine) from the tumor is not continuous, these symptoms occur

NURSING ALERT

Pheochromocytoma crisis manifests with seizures, shock, altered level of consciousness, disseminated intravascular coagulation, rhabomyolysis (skeletal muscle destruction), and acute renal failure, which can result in death.

intermittently. Attacks may occur daily or monthly. In some cases the condition may be silent until a stressor such as surgery causes a hypertensive crisis.

Diagnosis is based on 24-hour urine studies to detect the presence of urinary catecholamines and VMA levels, and CT, MRI, and ultrasound studies to localize the tumor (see Appendix D). The treatment of choice is surgical removal of the tumor; however, the procedure is dangerous and may result in pheochromocytoma crisis. Alpha- and beta-adrenergic blocking agents to control hypertension and catecholamine release are given for 10 to 14 days before surgery. Plasma catecholamines are used to measure the effectiveness of the preoperative adrenergic blockade. Postoperatively, for several days, a 24-hour urine collection is measured for catecholamines to determine if all tumor sites were removed. With successful removal of all tumor sites, the prognosis is generally good. Follow-up is important to assess for recurrence.

Nursing Management

Nursing care is mainly supportive. Provide preoperative and postoperative teaching and care (see Chapter 5). Preoperatively, monitor vital signs and observe for signs of complications associated with pheochromocytoma crisis. Administer antihypertensives and watch for any signs of hyperglycemia (see page 851). Postoperatively, the child may be managed initially in an intensive care unit. Monitor blood pressure and observe for neurologic signs, respiratory distress, and signs of shock. Lifelong follow-up care with screening for hypertension and increased urinary catecholamine levels is required as symptoms have recurred in up to 20% of patients 2 to 7 years after surgery (Reddy et al., 2000).

DISORDERS OF PANCREATIC FUNCTION

DIABETES MELLITUS

Diabetes mellitus, the most common metabolic disease in children, is a disorder of carbohydrate, protein, and fat metabolism. There are two main types of diabetes. The majority of children have immune-mediated type 1 diabetes, formerly called insulin dependent diabetes mellitus or juvenile diabetes. However, a disturbingly large number of children are being diagnosed with type 2 diabetes, formerly called noninsulin dependent diabetes.

About 1.5 million children and adolescents in the United States have diabetes, 70% to 85% with type 1 and up to 30% with type 2 (Selekman, Scofield, & Swenson-Brousell, 1999). The national prevalence for diabetes of all types in 12- to 19-year-olds is 4.1 per 1,000 adolescents (American Diabetes Association, 2000).

Type 1 Diabetes

The majority of children with diabetes have immune-mediated type 1. The annual incidence of type 1 diabetes is 18 per 100,000 children under 20 years old. The peak age of onset is 10 to 12 years in girls and 12 to 14 years in boys (Boland & Grey, 2000).

GENETIC CONSIDERATIONS

The long arm of chromosome 14 at the 14q24 locus is the type 1 diabetes-11 marker. This is a polygenic multifactorial pattern of inheritance, as 18 different chromosomes show linkage to type 1 diabetes (Rennert & Francis, 1999). Inheritance of the DR3 and DR4 markers on the human leukocyte antigen (HLA) complex on chromosome 6 increase the likelihood of developing type 1 diabetes. If the child inherits one marker, the child's risk is 3–5 times higher than normal. If both markers are inherited, the child's risk is 10–20 times higher than normal (Selekman et al., 1999).

ETIOLOGY AND PATHOPHYSIOLOGY It is thought that type 1 diabetes is caused by a genetic component, environmental influences, and an autoimmune response. Type 1 diabetes has strong familial tendencies but does not show any specific pattern of inheritance. Approximately 5% of children with type 1 diabetes have a first- or second-degree relative with the type 1 diabetes (American Diabetes Association, 2000). The child inherits a susceptibility to the disease rather than the disease itself.

Insulin helps transport glucose into the cells so that this carbohydrate can be used as an energy source. It also prevents the outflow of glucose from the liver to the general circulation. Environmental factors such as enteroviruses or toxins are believed to lead to an autoimmune destruction of the beta cells in the Islets of Langerhans (Figure 22-6 ◆). Antigens are generated that lead to production of antibodies that indicate ongoing destruction of the islet cells. As the destruction continues, the child develops glucose intolerance. The preclinical stage may last up to 13 years as the autoimmune process begins early in life (Silverstein & Rosenbloom, 2000). Lack of insulin results in a rise in blood glucose level and a decrease in the glucose level inside the cells. When the renal threshold

PATHOPHYSIOLOGY ILLUSTRATED

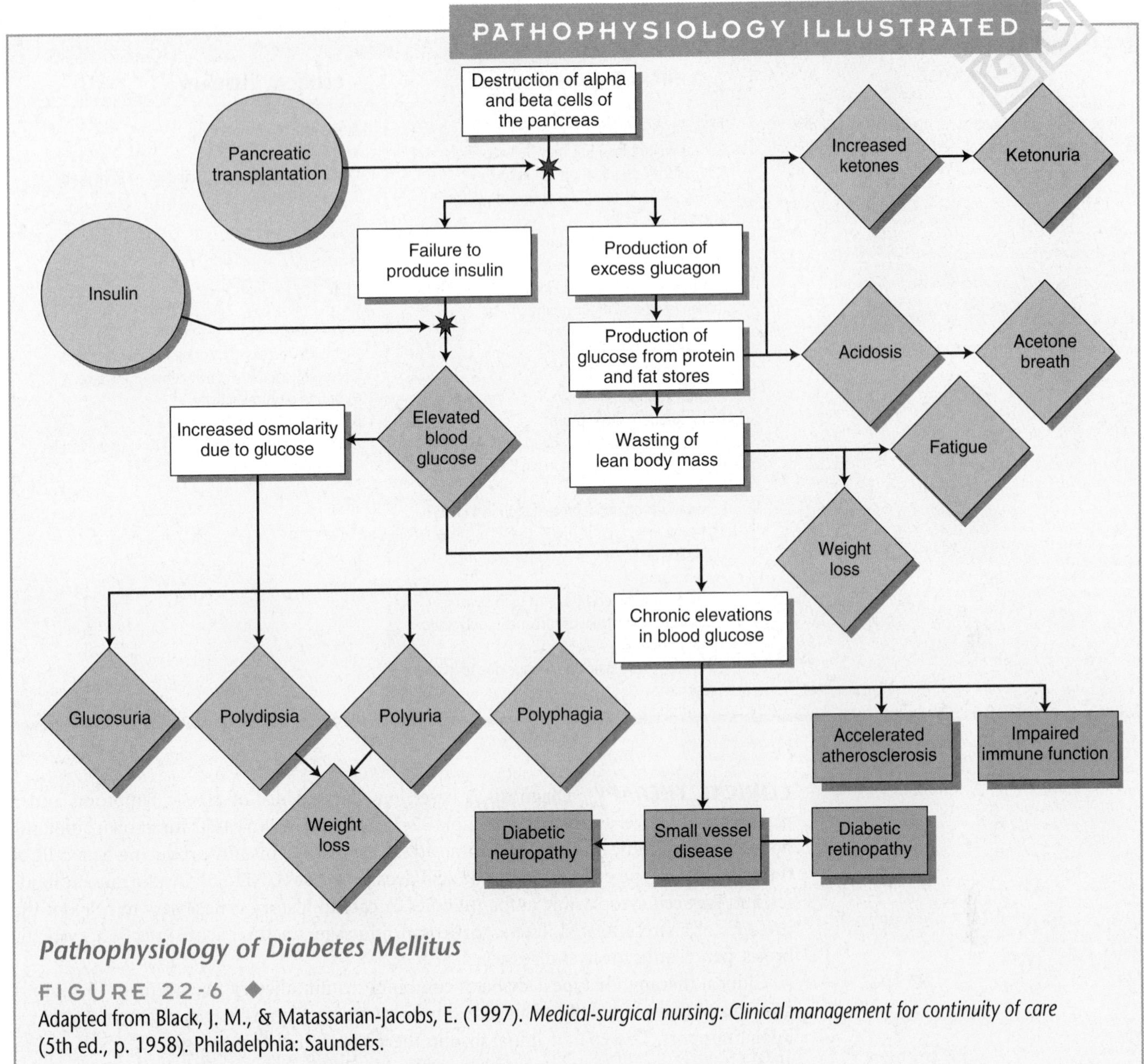

Pathophysiology of Diabetes Mellitus

FIGURE 22-6 ◆

Adapted from Black, J. M., & Matassarian-Jacobs, E. (1997). *Medical-surgical nursing: Clinical management for continuity of care* (5th ed., p. 1958). Philadelphia: Saunders.

for glucose (160 mg/dL) is exceeded, **glycosuria** (abnormal amount of glucose in the urine) occurs. Up to 1,000 calories per day can be lost in the urine.

When glucose is unavailable to the cells for metabolism, an alternate source of energy is provided by free fatty acids. They are metabolized at an increased rate by the liver, producing acetyl coenzyme A (CoA). The by-products of acetyl CoA metabolism (ketone bodies) accumulate in the body, resulting in a state of metabolic acidosis, or ketoacidosis. (Refer to Chapter 10 for discussion of metabolic acidosis.)

CLINICAL MANIFESTATIONS The classic signs of type 1 diabetes are polyuria, polydipsia, and **polyphagia** (excessive appetite) with significant weight loss, as occurred with Anthony in the opening scenario. See the clinical manifestations on page 848. Unexplained fatigue or lethargy, headaches, stomachaches, and occasional enuresis may also occur in a previously toilet-trained child. Adolescent girls may have vaginitis caused by candida, which thrives in the hyperglycemic tissues. Symptoms develop gradually and insidiously but have usually been present less than a month. In severe cases, diabetic ketoacidosis (DKA), a type of metabolic acidosis, may develop. This condition is discussed in more detail on page 849.

CLINICAL MANIFESTATIONS OF DIABETES BY TYPE

CAUSE	CLINICAL MANIFESTATIONS	CLINICAL THERAPY
Type 1—immune mediated, insulin deficiency due to pancreatic beta cell destruction	Polyuria, polydipsia Recent weight loss, but may be overweight Ketoacidosis on initial presentation in 30%–40% of cases, at continued risk for ketoacidosis Short duration of symptoms Ketosis Initial period of decreased insulin requirement, then need insulin for survival	Blood glucose monitoring Insulin Dietary management, balancing carbohydrate intake to insulin Exercise
Type 2—insulin resistance with relative insulin secretory defect	Obese, little or no weight loss, or may have significant weight loss Acanthosis nigranis Long duration of symptoms Polyuria, polydipsia, may be mild or absent Glycosuria without ketonuria in 33% of cases on initial presentation Ketoacidosis on initial presentation in 5%–25% of cases Lipid disorders Hypertension Androgen-mediated problems such as acne, hirsutism, menstrual disturbances, polycystic ovary disease Excessive weight gain and fatigue due to insulin resistance	Diet with decreased calories and low-fat foods Decrease sedentary activity time or increase routine physical activity Blood glucose monitoring Oral medication (metoformin) to improve insulin sensitivity

CLINICAL THERAPY Diagnosis is based on the presence of classic symptoms and a plasma glucose level as described in Table 22-3. Other laboratory tests for known autoantibodies that can indicate an autoimmune attack against the insulin-producing beta cells of the pancreas may be ordered: glutamic acid decarboxylase (GAD-65), insulin autoantibodies, and islet cell cytoplasmic autoantibodies. A careful history is necessary to rule out the presence of a stress-related illness, corticosteroid usage, fracture, acute infection, cystic fibrosis, pancreatitis, or liver disease.

Clinical therapy for type 1 diabetes combines insulin, dietary management to support growth and to maintain blood glucose at near normal levels, an exercise regimen, and physiologic support. The goal of initial insulin therapy is to lower blood glucose levels and to eliminate ketones. Blood glucose levels are then further lowered until stabilized. Long-term insulin therapy is calculated to maintain a blood glucose level as close to the normal range as possible and to minimize episodes of hyperglycemia and hypoglycemia (see page 851). Blood glucose levels are tested and recorded before meals and at bedtime. Insulin therapy is

TABLE 22-3 Criteria for the Diagnosis of All Types of Diabetes Mellitus

- Symptoms of diabetes (polyuria, polydipsia, unexplained weight loss for type 1, or acanthosis nigricans and obesity for type 2) *plus* plasma glucose concentration ≥200 mg/dL (11.1 mmol/L) taken at any time of day regardless of time of last meal.
- Fasting plasma glucose ≥126 mg/dL (7.0 mmol/L), no caloric intake for at least 8 hours.
- Two-hour plasma glucose ≥200 mg/dL (11.1 mmol/L) during an oral glucose tolerance test.

Repeat the testing on a second day if there is no unequivocal hyperglycemia with acute metabolic decompensation.

TABLE 22-4 Insulin Action, SQ

TYPE	ONSET	PEAK	DURATION
Rapid Acting Lispro/Humalog	5–15 min	1 hr	~4 hr
Short Acting Regular	1/2–1 hr	2–4 hr	6–8 hr
Intermediate Acting NPH Lente	1–2 hr 1–2 hr	6–12 hr 6–12 hr	18–26 hr 24–26 hr
Long Acting Ultralente Lantos/insulin glargine	4–8 hr	10–20 hr none/slight	16–24 hr 24 hr

CLINICAL TIP

Insulin is usually provided in prepackaged doses of 100 units/mL. Diluted insulin prepared by a pharmacist may be used for infants and toddlers who require a small insulin dosage.

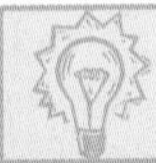

CLINICAL TIP

Advantages of rapid-acting insulin (Lispro) in therapy to achieve tight glucose control include:

- Decreased number of nocturnal hypoglycemic episodes
- Meal coverage for toddlers who have unpredictable food consumption
- Flexibility for adolescents concerned about weight gain who do not want to eat a mid-morning snack.

balanced by the child's dietary intake and exercise level. Stress, infection, and illness may either increase or decrease insulin needs. In addition, insulin doses must be adjusted for growth and at puberty.

Several forms of insulin are available (Table 22-4). Multiple approaches to insulin therapy for children and adolescents are available, and an approach that works for the child and family should be selected. In children, conventional insulin therapy is commonly used, requiring two or three injections a day. One example of conventional insulin therapy consists of daily administration of a combination of a short-acting (regular) insulin and an intermediate-acting (NPH or Lente) or long-acting insulin (Ultralente) before breakfast and before the evening meal (Figure 22-7 ◆). Older children and adolescents often use a regimen of tighter control that includes two injections a day of intermediate or long-acting insulin and an injection of rapid-acting insulin with each meal to match carbohydrate intake.

The American Diabetes Association recommends that all adolescents use the intensive therapy regimen with three or more insulin injections a day or a continuous subcutaneous insulin infusion (CSII) by an insulin pump. Research revealed that the risk for developing retinopathy, microalbuminuria, albuminuria, and clinical neuropathy was significantly lower with this treatment regimen over more conventional regimens. Advantages and disadvantages of an insulin pump are outlined in Table 22-5. A pen-shaped device that contains an insulin-filled cartridge that is easy to carry may also be used by adolescents taking frequent insulin injections during the day.

Intensive therapy for type 1 diabetes includes:

- Monitoring blood glucose four times a day and once a week at 3 A.M.
- Monitoring dietary intake
- Varying the insulin dose to fit the carbohydrates eaten at each meal or snack if doing carbohydrate counting
- Anticipating exercise in the routine

Laboratory evaluation of hemoglobin A_{1c} (HbA_{1c}) to measure glycosylated hemoglobin should be performed every 3 months. It provides an objective measurement of glycemic

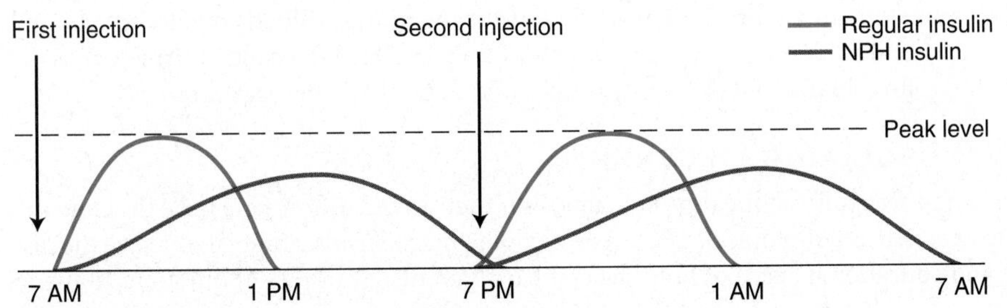

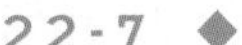

FIGURE 22-7 ◆ Conventional therapy. Insulin levels vary over a 24-hour period in relation to injections and mealtimes.

RESEARCH

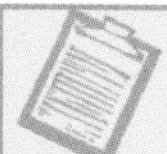

An implantable insulin infusion pump with a glucose sensing device that can work for years without being accessed is now being used experimentally. FDA approval has not yet been sought (Saudek, 1997).

Studies of the effectiveness of inhaled insulin for administration before meals also are being conducted. The goal is to find alternative methods of intensive insulin control without increasing injections (Silverstein & Rosenbloom, 2000).

Noninvasive or continuous glucose monitoring techniques are being investigated and have been approved by the FDA for adults (Silverstein & Rosenbloom, 2000).

TABLE 22-5 Advantages and Disadvantages of an External Insulin Infusion Pump

ADVANTAGES	DISADVANTAGES
■ Delivers a continuous infusion of insulin to match the basal rate needed plus an insulin bolus at mealtime ■ Helps maintain blood glucose control between meals ■ Improves growth in children ■ Reduces number of injections ■ Allows child to eat with less regard to a schedule ■ Reduces number of injection sites, so variation in absorption decreases ■ More closely simulates normal pancreatic function ■ Frequency of severe hypoglycemia has been decreased ■ More flexible lifestyle is permitted	■ Requires highly motivated child and supportive parents and health care professionals ■ Requires willingness to live connected to a device (can be disconnected for short periods by removing or clamping the catheter, however, DKA can occur within hours of interruption of insulin flow) ■ The site must be changed every 2–4 days, at least 1 inch from the last site. ■ Necessitates more time and energy to monitor blood glucose levels, dietary intake, and insulin bolus calculation ■ Involves changing syringe, catheter, and skin setup every 2–3 days ■ Infections can occur at the injection site ■ Weight gain is common when blood glucose control improves

Note: Based on information in Saudek, C. D. (1997). Novel forms of insulin delivery. *Endocrinology and Metabolism Clinics of North America, 26*(3), 599–610; and Maniatis, A. K., Klingensmith, G. J., Slover, R. H., Mowry, C. J., and Chase, H. P. (2001). Continuous subcutaneous insulin infusion therapy for children and adolescents: An option for routine diabetes care. *Pediatrics, 107*(2), 351–356.

control, because it represents the amount of glucose irreversibly attached to the hemoglobin molecule over an extended period (the life span of the red blood cell, approximately 120 days). The HbA_{1c} is below 6.2% for individuals without diabetes, and the goal for children with diabetes is 7.5% to 9.3% depending on age and physician preferences. It is also important to determine if the HbA_{1c} matches recorded blood sugars.

Physical activity is associated with increased insulin sensitivity. Regular exercise and fitness improve metabolic control with a lower insulin dose. Blood lipid levels are also positively affected. However, the child must have an adequate caloric intake to prevent hypoglycemia. Excessive exercise associated with sports requires careful planning and management.

Complications of type 1 diabetes (retinopathy, heart disease, renal failure, and peripheral vascular disease) result from long-term hyperglycemic effects on the blood vessels. Without careful management, diabetic children may develop renal failure and loss of vision in adulthood. Intensive therapy is expected to reduce the risk for or delay the development of these complications. Risk may be further reduced if the adolescent does not begin smoking and if the blood pressure is controlled.

NURSING MANAGEMENT

Nursing Assessment and Diagnosis

PHYSIOLOGIC ASSESSMENT

Children are generally admitted to the hospital at the time of diagnosis. Assess the child's physiologic status, focusing on vital signs and level of consciousness. Assess hydration by checking mucous membranes, skin turgor, and urine output. Blood initially is collected hourly to monitor blood gases, glucose, and electrolytes. Once the child is stable, assess dietary and caloric intake and the ability of the child or family to manage care.

PSYCHOSOCIAL ASSESSMENT

Parents may feel guilty at the time of diagnosis if they waited to seek care until the child began to experience symptoms of DKA. Assess coping mechanisms, ability to manage the disease, and educational needs of both the child and parents. Examples of questions to use in

TABLE 22-6 Questions to Ask When Planning Diabetic Education

- Do both parents work or does the single parent work? What hours?
- Who else is involved in the child's care?
- What is the child's usual daily schedule? Does the schedule vary on the weekend or any other days of the week?
- Does the child have health insurance? What coverage exists for diabetes education, treatment, and home management?
- Does the child have any cognitive, behavioral, motor, or visual problems coexisting with this condition?
- What other family stressors coexist with the diagnosis?

assessing the family's strengths and limitations in the child's disease management are provided in Table 22-6.

Developmental Assessment

Assess the child's developmental level, particularly fine motor skills and cognitive level. The child will need to learn how to obtain and read a blood glucose sample and how to draw up and administer insulin. Children are usually able to perform some of these tasks with supervision by 6 to 8 years of age. Self-management is the eventual goal, and the child's responsibilities are gradually increased.

Skill 6-3: Using a Blood Glucose Meter

Adolescents perceive type 1 diabetes as a disability and often deny having the disease so they can be like their peers when eating and exercising. Talk with the adolescent to evaluate motivation to manage diet, the exercise regimen, blood glucose testing, and insulin therapy. Although the adolescent is cognitively able to manage self-care, the desire to be like peers often interferes with compliance.

Several diagnoses that may apply to the child newly diagnosed with type 1 diabetes are provided in the accompanying nursing care plans. Additional diagnoses that may be appropriate are as follows:

- *Risk for fluid volume deficit,* related to active fluid loss associated with hyperglycemia
- *Ineffective breathing pattern,* related to neuromuscular dysfunction associated with metabolic acidosis
- *Ineffective denial,* related to inability to admit impact of disease on lifestyle

CLINICAL TIP

Testing strips for blood glucose meters cost between $0.50 and $1.00 each. Learn about the allowable expenses covered by health insurance. Try to work within those guidelines to reduce the family's out-of-pocket expenses.

Planning and Implementation

Nursing care focuses on teaching the child and parents about the disease and its management, managing dietary intake, providing emotional support, and planning strategies for daily management in the community. Refer to the accompanying nursing care plans, which summarize nursing care for the child who is hospitalized with newly diagnosed type 1 diabetes, and the child who is receiving care in the community. Some hospitals have developed clinical pathways to streamline and standardize diabetes care.

Provide Education

The nurse is an important member of the management team (physician, nurse, nutritionist, and social worker) and is usually responsible for educating the child and family. Teaching often is performed by a diabetic nurse educator in the clinic setting, since children may be hospitalized only briefly following diagnosis.

The timing and amount of information provided are especially important in the first days following diagnosis. Both the child and parents are very tired, and they are often in a state of shock and disbelief. Information presented during this period needs to be repeated. This time should be used to assess learning needs and to answer the family's questions. Initial teaching focuses on the survival skills necessary for home management (insulin administration, blood glucose testing, record keeping, dietary management, and the recognition and treatment of both hypoglycemia and hyperglycemia).

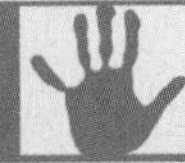

GROWTH & DEVELOPMENT

Education is ongoing, especially for children who develop diabetes at a young age. As they grow and assume more responsibility for their care, remember that they need to learn more about the pathophysiology of the disease and the rationale for its management.

NURSING CARE PLAN: The Child Hospitalized with Newly Diagnosed Type 1 Diabetes Mellitus

GOAL	INTERVENTION	RATIONALE	EXPECTED OUTCOME
1. Knowledge Deficit (Child and Parents) related to lack of exposure to diabetic management in the newly diagnosed child			
	NIC Priority Intervention: **Individual Teaching:** Planning, implementation, and evaluating a teaching program designed to address a patient's particular need.		NOC Suggested Outcome: **Knowledge:** Extent of understanding conveyed about treatment regimen.
The child and parents will acquire survival skills for home management.	■ Assess the child's developmental level and select an educational approach and self-care activities to match.	■ Learning goals for the child must match knowledge and skill expectations appropriate for developmental stage.	The child and parents demonstrate proper technique for blood glucose monitoring, urine testing for ketones, drawing up insulin doses and injection, and record keeping.
	■ Teach blood glucose monitoring, drawing up and injecting insulin, urine testing for ketones, record keeping, survival food guidelines, and when to call the doctor.	■ Diabetic management survival skills are needed for initial home management until more extensive education can be completed that permits more independent management.	
	■ Use demonstration/ return demonstration until the child and family are comfortable with procedures.	■ Evaluation permits positive reinforcement and guidance for modification of techniques.	
The child and parents will recognize signs and symptoms of hypoglycemia and hyperglycemia.	■ Teach signs and symptoms of hypoglycemic and hyperglycemic reactions.	■ Recognition of and treatment of poor glucose control will prevent progression of symptoms.	The child and family can describe symptoms of hypoglycemia and hyperglycemia.
	■ Teach child to test blood glucose when feeling different than usual, and record the reading and symptoms felt.	■ Permits child to learn his/her specific symptoms of hyper- and hypoglycemia.	
2. Risk for Injury related to periods of hypoglycemia and diabetic ketoacidosis			
	NIC Priority Intervention: **Hypoglycemia Monitoring:** Instituting special precautions with patient at risk for injury.		NOC Suggested Outcome: **Risk Control:** Actions to eliminate or reduce actual, personal, and modifiable health threats.
The child will experience few episodes of hypoglycemia during hospitalization.	■ Assess the child at least every 2 hours for signs of hypoglycemia. If signs are present, check blood glucose to verify and administer source of quick sugar.	■ Hypoglycemia commonly occurs during hospitalization because of change in diet, lack of food intake, or illness.	The child and staff manage episodes of hypoglycemia without a crisis developing.
	■ When the child is NPO for a special procedure, verify with physician when food, fluids, and insulin are to be given, or if an intravenous infusion with dextrose is to be given.	■ Giving insulin without food intake can lead to hypoglycemia. Intravenous dextrose and insulin can be used when the child must be NPO.	
	■ Have glucose paste or 50% dextrose solution readily available.	■ Dextrose is used for emergency intravenous treatment of severe hypoglycemia. Glucose paste is used for oral treatment.	

(continued)

NURSING CARE PLAN The Child Hospitalized with Newly Diagnosed Type 1 Diabetes Mellitus (continued)

GOAL	INTERVENTION	RATIONALE	EXPECTED OUTCOME
The child's condition is treated slowly, gradually reversing hyperglycemia and ketoacidosis to prevent cerebral edema.	■ Assess the child's mental status for improvement or deterioration.	■ Improvement in mental status may indicate successful treatment. Deterioration may indicate onset of cerebral edema.	The child's hyperglycemia and ketoacidosis resolves without additional complications.
	■ Check blood glucose and urine ketones frequently to confirm reduction in blood glucose level and ketosis, to identify the insulin dose for administration.	■ Frequent blood glucose and ketone level determination helps assess progress in treating ketoacidosis.	
	■ Monitor and control IV fluid intake. Measure output.	■ The child with ketoacidosis will be dehydrated. IV fluid intake needs to be carefully controlled to prevent cerebral edema.	
	■ Have insulin doses checked by a second nurse.	■ Doses are frequently small, and the possibility of error is great.	
The child and parents will demonstrate emergency management of hypoglycemia.	■ Identify sources of glucose to give in case of hypoglycemic reaction. Tell the child and parent to carry glucose tablets or paste with them at all times.	■ Access to sources of glucose and its rapid administration are important for emergency care.	The child and family can identify several glucose sources for emergencies. The child and family have a source of glucose with them at each visit. The child's hyperglycemic episodes do not progress to ketoacidosis.
The child and parents will demonstrate management of sick days.	■ Teach the child and family to test blood glucose and urine for ketones with acute symptoms and notify the physician.	■ When the child is ill, hyperglycemia needs special management to prevent progression to ketoacidosis.	
3. Risk for Altered Nutrition: Less than body requirements related to glycosuria			
	NIC Priority Intervention: **Nutrition Management:** Assistance with or provision of a balanced dietary intake of foods and fluids.		NOC Suggested Outcome: **Nutritional Status:** Extent to which nutrients are available to meet metabolic needs.
The child will eat a well-balanced diet and maintain normal height and weight proportions.	■ Encourage and serve meals and snacks with consistent carbohydrates at the same time each day.	■ Keeps blood glucose levels stable during initial disease management stages.	The child regains weight lost and demonstrates normal growth and stable blood glucose levels.
	■ Provide a calorie non-restricted diet.	■ Enables weight lost during onset of diabetes to be regained.	
The child and parents will state understanding of dietary management of diabetes mellitus.	■ Make an appointment with a nutritionist who can assess the child's favorite foods and promote their integration into the child's diet. Reinforce the dietary information taught.	■ The nutritionist can develop dietary recommendations that fit the specific needs of the child and include favorite foods, thereby increasing compliance with the diet.	The child and parents describe nutritional needs of the child and select the dietary management best suited to the family's and child's eating habits.
	■ Provide sample menus and food exchanges, or teach the use of carbohydrate counting.	■ Assists the family and adolescent with diet planning.	

NURSING CARE PLAN: The Child with Previously Diagnosed Type 1 Diabetes Being Cared For at Home

GOAL	INTERVENTION	RATIONALE	EXPECTED OUTCOME
1. Risk for Altered Nutrition: Less than body requirements related to chronic illness (diabetes mellitus)			
	NIC Priority Intervention: **Weight Management:** Assistance with or provision of a balanced dietary intake of foods and fluids.		NOC Suggested Outcome: **Nutritional Status:** Nutrient Value: Adequacy of nutrients taken into body.
The child will eat a well-balanced diet that maintains weight proportional to height.	■ Assess height and weight regularly and plot on growth chart. ■ Make an appointment with a nutritionist who can assess the child's favorite foods and integrate them into a diet plan that controls caloric intake. Encourage the child to keep a food diary.	■ Assesses change in body mass index to identify potential weight problem early. ■ Inclusion of child's favorite foods helps child adapt to changes in diet.	Diet records indicate meals and snacks have the appropriate distribution of carbohydrates, protein, and fats, and daily caloric intake goals are met.
2. Altered Family Processes related to management of a chronic disease			
	NIC Priority Intervention: **Family Process Maintenance:** Minimization of family process disruption effects		NOC Suggested Outcome: To be developed.
The child and family will manage the dietary modifications, exercise, blood glucose monitoring and medications regimen.	■ Assess the family's lifestyle and attempt to fit the child's care needs into the family's schedule. ■ Discuss the family's routines for special occasions and vacations. Identify ways to modify the child's management for these occasions.	■ Fitting the care to the family's lifestyle promotes compliance with regimen. ■ It is important for the child to participate in special events with the family and peers as a normal child to promote psychological development.	The child and family make minimal changes in usual lifestyle while managing the type 1 diabetes.
3. Ineffective Coping (Individual) related to inadequate level of confidence in ability to cope			
	NIC Priority Intervention: **Coping Enhancement:** Assisting a patient to adapt to perceived stressors, changes, or threats which interfere with meeting life demands and roles.		NOC Suggested Outcome: **Coping:** Actions to manage stressors that tax an individual's resources.
The child will demonstrate enhanced coping skills.	■ Ask how the child has solved problems in the past. Review possible problems the child may encounter. Together evaluate the effectiveness of solutions. Suggest other solutions to consider.	■ Children's success in mastering maturational conflicts and daily psychosocial problems will influence their pattern of coping.	The child demonstrates enhanced coping skills and expresses positive attitude toward self. The child displays warmth and affection toward family.
The child will develop positive self-esteem.	■ Role-play ways to talk about diabetes with friends and teachers. Encourage the child to express feelings about diabetes to those he or she trusts. ■ Encourage the child to attend diabetes camp. ■ Encourage the child to continue previous social activities and hobbies.	■ Sharing information about the condition helps others understand changes in lifestyle needed by the child. Expressing feelings decreases anxiety. ■ Learning and support networks developed at camp can promote self-esteem. ■ Increased social interaction, especially in group sessions, improves self-esteem.	

(continued)

NURSING CARE PLAN — The Child with Previously Diagnosed Type 1 Diabetes Being Cared For at Home (continued)

GOAL	INTERVENTION	RATIONALE	EXPECTED OUTCOME
4. Health-Seeking Behaviors (Child) related to learning self-management of chronic disorder			
	NIC Priority Intervention: **Self-Modification:** Assistance: Reinforcement of self-directed change initiated by the patient to achieve personally important goals.		NOC Suggested Outcome: **Health Promotion:** Actions to sustain or increase wellness.
The child will develop independent ability to manage diabetes care.	■ Allow the child to perform as many self-care procedures as possible at each developmental stage.	■ Normal growth and development are ensured if the child is encouraged to participate in care from the beginning.	The child is able to perform as many diabetic care techniques as possible for age.
	■ Encourage the child to make decisions regarding care. Review decisions and discuss possible alternative solutions. Role-play possible scenarios.	■ Feelings of trust are developed when children sense that their decisions are respected or at least considered by others.	
	■ Encourage parents to stay involved even when the adolescent takes primary responsibility for care.	■ The child's diabetic control is likely to be better when the parents continue to show interest and supervise care.	
	■ Provide 24-hour access to physician or diabetes nurse educator. Encourage the child to seek help early.	■ The child needs to overcome concerns about calling for guidance, and thus maintain better control.	

Explain the goals of insulin therapy. Teach the child and parents how to administer insulin and perform blood glucose tests (Figure 22-8 ◆). Rotating the injection sites is important to decrease the chances of hypertrophy (Figure 22-9 ◆). The absorption rate of insulin varies by the site used. Encourage the child to give the morning injections in one body area (e.g., an arm) and the evening injections in another (e.g., the thigh). An understanding of the different types of insulin and their actions is essential.

Once the child and parents demonstrate understanding of this information, guidelines for managing episodes of hyperglycemia during acute illness and using a sliding scale are taught. A sliding scale indicates specific insulin dosages appropriate for a particular blood glucose level. The family also needs to learn "sick day" care guidelines to prevent diabetic ketoacidosis.

Caution parents to check the blood glucose level of a toddler who is extremely sleepy or irritable, as these can be signs of either hypoglycemia or hyperglycemia.

Manage Dietary Intake

The preferred diet for children with type 1 diabetes is a low-saturated-fat, low-sodium diet. The total amount of carbohydrates consumed is more important than whether it is a simple or complex carbohydrate. A variety of carbohydrates should be eaten. The child needs adequate calories to reach or maintain a desirable body weight. Usually at the time of diagnosis the child needs to regain lost weight, so calorie limitation is not recommended.

For conventional treatment, dietary intake should include three meals per day, eaten at consistent intervals, plus a midafternoon carbohydrate snack and a bedtime snack high in protein. Some children need a morning snack depending on the time of morning the insulin dose is given, how much breakfast is eaten, and the scheduled lunchtime. A consistent intake of carbohydrates at each meal and snack is needed. The American Diabetes Association's exchange

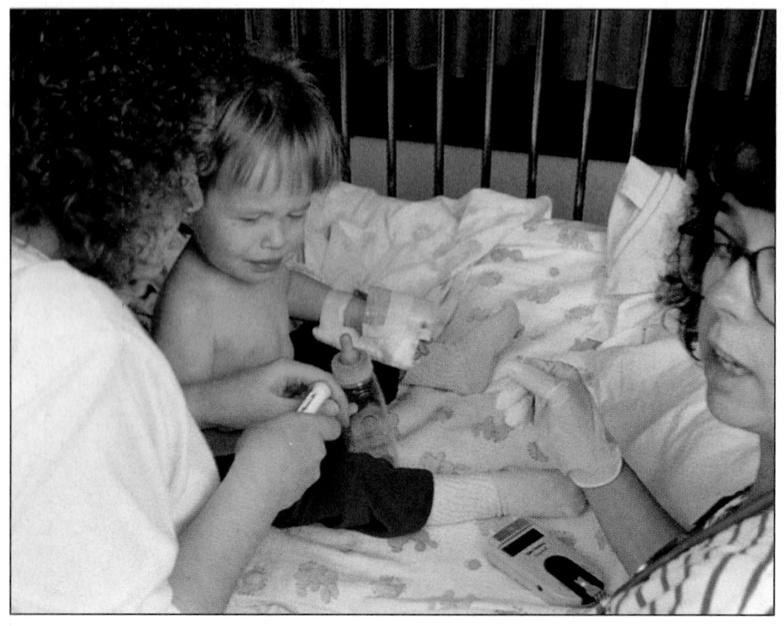

A

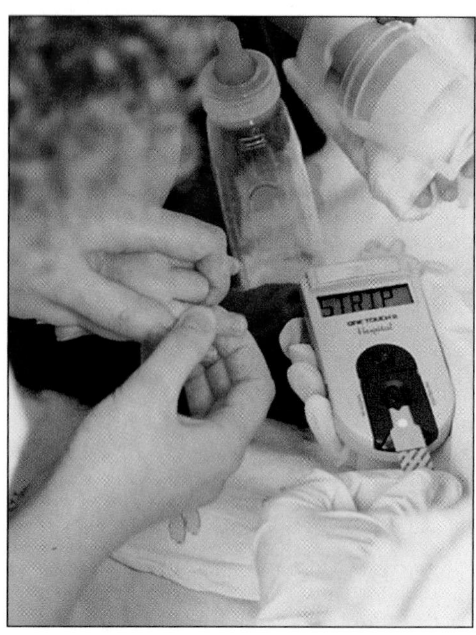

B

FIGURE 22-8 ◆
This mother is being taught how to test her child's blood glucose level.

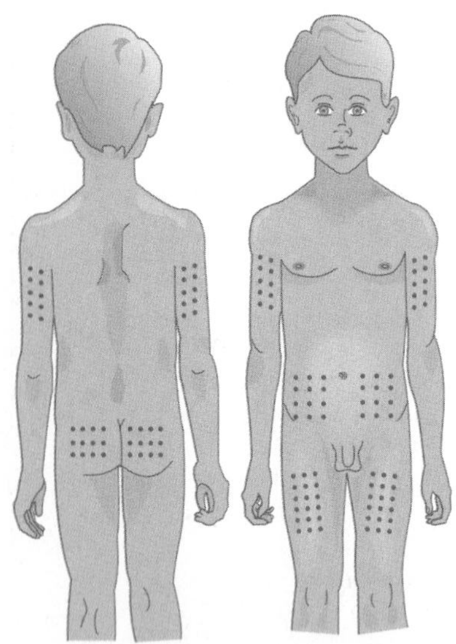

FIGURE 22-9 ◆
Insulin injection sites. Give all morning insulin in one site (e.g., arms) and all evening insulin in another (e.g., legs) because of different rates of absorption from these sites. Space injections about 1.25 cm (0.5 in.) apart.

lists facilitate dietary management by suggesting portions and types of foods and noting allowed substitutions.

Many adolescents find that carbohydrate counting for dietary management gives them more flexibility in disease management. One carbohydrate choice equals 15 g of carbohydrate. The number of units of insulin needed to cover the grams of carbohydrates eaten is then determined.

Provide Emotional Support

The diagnosis of type 1 diabetes often comes as a shock to the family. If there is a familial history, parents may feel guilty about having caused the disease. The diagnosis of a chronic disease that requires daily management can be difficult to accept. Give parents information about diabetes education programs, put them in touch with other parents of diabetic children, and help them to learn the role they can play in managing the disease.

Support for the child depends on age and developmental stage. Encourage the child to express feelings about the disease and its management. The adolescent may benefit from contact with other adolescents who have diabetes.

Discharge Planning and Home Care Teaching

Home care needs should be identified and addressed before discharge. Initial survival skills described above are taught with the plans for ongoing outpatient education.

Make every effort to incorporate the diabetic regimen (insulin administration, diet, blood glucose monitoring, and exercise) into the family's present lifestyle. The fewer changes the family has to make, the greater the chance of compliance.

Provide written materials and refer parents to books and other materials they can use in teaching the child about diabetes. The Juvenile Diabetic Research Foundation and the American Diabetes Association are good sources of information.

Care in the Community

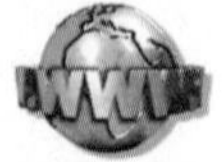

Diabetes Support and Resources

During follow-up visits, ask the child or parents about signs indicating problems of diabetic control (Table 22-7). Record growth measurements and vital signs in the child's chart. Assess the child's sexual development using Tanner staging guidelines (see Chapter 4). Puberty may be delayed if diabetic control is inadequate. Review the child's typical dietary intake and exercise regimens.

TABLE 22-7 Questions to Ask to Identify Problems in Diabetic Control

- Is the child hungry at meals? Between meals?
- How much fluid is the child drinking?
- Has the child been going to the bathroom frequently or had episodes of bedwetting?
- Does the child have dry skin?
- Are there sores on the feet? Do scratches or scrapes take a long time to heal?
- Has the child had any skin infections?
- Does the child have changes in mood (depression, unexplained sadness, irritability) or energy level from day to day or throughout the day?
- Have there been any changes in vision?

CLINICAL TIP

Although there are no foods that a child with diabetes must avoid, certain foods will need to be balanced by extra insulin. A nutritionist can help the family integrate preferred ethnic foods into the child's diet. The recommended distribution of total calories by food group for children with type 1 diabetes is as follows (Kaufman & Halvorson, 1999a):

Carbohydrates	50%–55%
Protein	20%–25%
Fat	25%–30%

Continually work with the child to help him or her assume responsibility for self-care, and with parents to promote the child's self-care (Figure 22-10 ◆). The child's developmental stage and cognitive level influence his or her readiness to take on responsibility for self-care. Summer camps and other programs for diabetic children are often helpful in providing education and support.

The preschool child's need for autonomy and control can be met by allowing the child to choose snacks or to pick which finger to stick for glucose testing and by helping parents to gather necessary supplies. School-age children can learn to test blood glucose, administer insulin, and keep records. They should be taught how to select foods appropriate for dietary management and how to plan an exercise program. School-age children need to learn to recognize the signs of hypoglycemia and hyperglycemia, and understand the importance of carrying a rapidly absorbed sugar product (see page 851).

Adolescents should take on total responsibility for self-care; however, they benefit from the ongoing supervision by the family. Although they understand explanations about the potential complications of diabetes, they are present-time oriented and may rebel against the daily regimentation of insulin injections and dietary management. Successful self-care depends in part on the adolescent's adjustment to the chronic nature of the disease and feelings of being different from peers.

Children with type 1 diabetes often learn manipulative behaviors, using their disease to obtain something they want. Teach parents to be alert to signs of manipulation, such as helpless, demanding, or whining behaviors, and any evidence of poor coping. Food may become a battleground for toddlers who are picky eaters, but must have adequate intake for the insulin dose. Referral for counseling may be appropriate for some families.

The child with type 1 diabetes may develop circulatory and neurologic changes over time. Emphasize the importance of good foot care from an early age, for example, wearing clean white cotton socks; changing socks and shoes when they are damp; washing, drying, and powdering feet; and keeping toenails short.

Explain to parents that the child should wear some type of medical alert identification. Assist them in having an individual school health plan developed (see Chapter 6) to ensure that school administrators and teachers can identify the signs of hypoglycemia or hyperglycemia and provide emergency management.

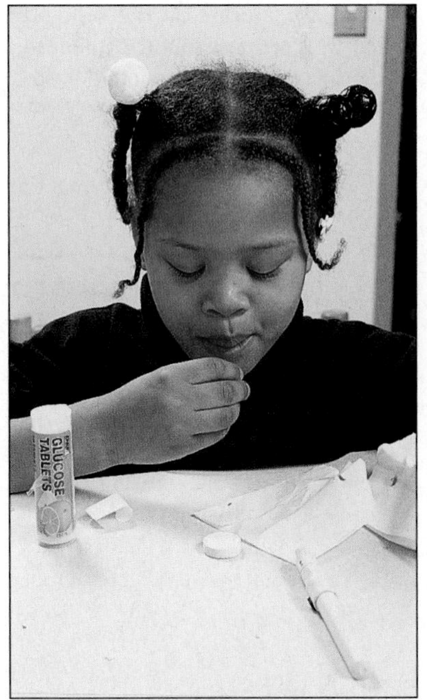

FIGURE 22-10 ◆
This girl is old enough to understand the need to take glucose tablets or another form of a rapidly absorbed sugar when her blood glucose level is low.

Evaluation

Expected outcomes of nursing care for children with Type 1 diabetes can be found on the nursing care plans.

Diabetic Ketoacidosis

Diabetic ketoacidosis (DKA) is the common and potentially life-threatening condition that occurs in children with type 1 diabetes when the body must burn fat for energy because no insulin is available to metabolize glucose.

Potential causes of DKA include incorrect or missed insulin doses or administration just under the skin, an illness, trauma, or surgery. Most have no clinical evidence of infection (Flood & Chiang, 2001). Insulin deficiency is accompanied by a compensatory increase in hormones (epinephrine, norepinephrine, cortisol, growth hormone, and glucagon) which leads to failure to deliver enough glucose to the cells. The muscle cells break down protein into amino acids that are then converted to glucose by the liver, leading to hyperglycemia. The adipose tissue releases fatty acids that are transformed by the liver into ketone bodies. Their accumulation leads to ketoacidosis. The hyperglycemia causes an osmotic diuresis resulting in dehydration, acidosis, and hyperosmolality. Altered consciousness occurs as symptoms progress (Hafeez & Vuguin, 2000).

Characteristic signs of DKA include dehydration, weight loss, tachycardia, flushed ears and cheeks, Kussmaul respirations, acetone breath, altered level of consciousness, and hypotension. The disorder may progress to electrolyte disturbances, arrhythmias, and shock. Children complain of abdominal or chest pain, begin to vomit, have labored breathing, and can slowly slip into a semiconscious state. Hyperglycemia, glycosuria, and ketonuria are also present.

DKA is present when the following findings are present: blood glucose level greater than 300 mg/dL, ketones in the serum, acidosis (pH less than or equal to 7.30 and bicarbonate less than 15 mEq/L), glycosuria, and ketonuria. Electrolyte disorders also occur (hyperkalemia, hyperchloremia, hyponatremia, hypophosphatemia, hypocalcemia, and hypomagnesemia). Diabetic coma occurs when the serum osmolality exceeds 350 mOsm/kg. Normal serum osmolality is 275 to 295 mOsm/kg. Cerebral edema is a life-threatening complication thought to be related to hyperosmolality.

NURSING ALERT

Bicarbonate is no longer used for treatment of DKA as it places the child at risk for increased CNS acidosis and hyperosmolality.

The child with ketoacidosis is usually hospitalized. Medical management includes intravenous fluids and electrolytes for dehydration and acidosis. Insulin is given by continuous infusion pump to decrease the serum glucose level at a rate not to exceed 100 mg/dL/hr. Faster reduction of hyperglycemia and serum osmolality may be related to the development of cerebral edema. Mannitol is kept on standby for treatment of neurologic deterioration.

Cerebral edema occurs in about 3% of children with DKA, but it accounts for 30% of DKA deaths and 20% of the overall childhood diabetes mortality (Felner & White, 2001). See Chapter 20 for information about cerebral edema.

CLINICAL TIP

Insulin binds to IV tubing. Let 50–100 mL run through the new IV tubing to saturate all the binding sites. This ensures that the full dose of insulin reaches the child from the outset.

NURSING MANAGEMENT The child's vital signs, respiratory status, perfusion, and mental status are continuously monitored. Frequently monitor the electrolytes and acid–base status, blood glucose levels, and urine ketone levels. Intake and output are monitored.

Intravenous fluids are given in boluses of 10 to 20 mL/kg per hour if the child is in shock. Adequate fluids are given to reverse the fluid deficit. Electrolytes are replaced as needed. The insulin infusion must be carefully maintained to control the gradual reduction in hyperglycemia. The child is weaned off of intravenous insulin when clinically stable.

FAMILIES WANT TO KNOW

Treating Hypoglycemic Episodes

- If the child shows signs of hypoglycemia (pallor, sweating, tremors, dizziness, numb lips or mouth, confusion, irritability, altered mental status), test the blood glucose level.
- Assist the child in performing the test, as skills needed to get an accurate reading deteriorate with altered mental status.
- If the blood glucose reading is ≤ 70 mg/dL, give glucose rapidly. Use one of the following:
  - 1/2 cup orange juice
  - 3/4 cup of sugar-sweetened beverage
  - 1 small box raisins
  - 3–4 glucose tablets
- Wait 15 minutes and recheck the blood glucose level. Repeat the glucose if it is still ≤ 70/mg/dL. Recheck the blood glucose level in another 15 minutes.
- Once blood glucose has returned to at least 80 mg/dL, give a more substantial snack such as cheese and crackers if the next meal will be more than 30 minutes later or an activity or exercise is planned.
- If the child is unconscious, administer IM or SQ glucagon.

CLINICAL MANIFESTATIONS OF HYPOGLYCEMIA AND HYPERGLYCEMIA

CAUSE	CLINICAL MANIFESTATIONS	CLINICAL THERAPY
Hypoglycemia ■ Insulin dose too high for food eaten ■ Insulin injection into muscle ■ Too much exercise for insulin dose ■ Too long between meals/snacks ■ Too few carbohydrates eaten ■ Illness, stress	Rapid onset Irritability, nervousness, tremors, shaky feeling, difficulty concentrating or speaking, behavior change, confusion, repetitive speech Unconsciousness, seizure, shallow breathing, tachycardia Pallor, sweating Moist mucous membranes, hunger Headache, dizziness, blurred vision, double vision, photophobia Numb lips or mouth	If conscious, give 15g of carbohydrate. Wait 15 minutes and recheck blood glucose level. Give another 15g of carbohydrate if ≤ 70 mg/dL. Recheck the blood glucose level in 15 minutes. If unconscious, give glucagon by injection.
Hyperglycemia ■ Insulin dose too low for food eaten ■ Illness or injury, stress ■ Too many carbohydrates eaten ■ Meals/snacks too close together ■ Insulin injected just under skin or injected into hypertrophied areas ■ Decreased activity	Gradual onset Lethargy, sleepiness, slowed responses, or confusion Deep, rapid breathing Flushed skin, dry skin Dry mucous membranes, thirst, hunger, dehydration Weakness, fatigue Headache, abdominal pain, nausea, vomiting Blurred vision Shock	Additional insulin given at usual injection time. Sliding scale insulin doses for specific blood glucose levels when ill or injured. Extra injections if hyperglycemia and moderate to large ketones. Increased fluids.

The prevention of future episodes of DKA is important. The parents and child need to learn strategies to keep hyperglycemic episodes from progressing to DKA. For example, the child's urine should be tested for ketones if three or four consecutive blood glucose readings are higher than 200 mg/dL, or if the child is sick. If the child has a high blood glucose and moderate or large amounts of ketones, treatment with extra insulin and fluids can be initiated. This monitoring is especially important when the child has significant stressors such as an illness. Insulin is needed even when the child is not eating to counter the hormones secreted in response to the stressor.

Hypoglycemia

Hypoglycemia can develop within minutes in children with diabetes mellitus. The symptoms outlined in the box above may occur when there is a sudden drop in blood glucose levels. Children are at risk of hypoglycemia due to their rapid growth rates and unpredictable eating habits and physical activity. Common causes include an error in insulin dosage, errors in injection technique, inadequate calories because of missed meals, or exercise without a corresponding increase in caloric intake.

Hypoglycemia can be diagnosed on the basis of the sudden onset of signs and symptoms. A blood glucose reading should be taken to confirm the diagnosis, because signs of hyperglycemia and hypoglycemia may be difficult to distinguish. Give glucose immediately in the form of a carbohydrate-containing snack or drink, sugar gel such as cakemate, glucose tablets, or glucose paste. In the hospital setting, administer an intravenous infusion of dextrose to prevent progression of symptoms. If the child becomes unconscious, sugar gel or glucose paste can be squeezed onto the gums.

NURSING MANAGEMENT Teach parents and children to recognize the signs of hypoglycemia and take appropriate action. Parents can be taught to give an intramuscular or subcutaneous dose of **glucagon** (a hormone produced by the pancreas that helps release stored glucose from the liver) for severe cases of hypoglycemia. Reinforce the importance of a daily balance of dietary intake, insulin, and exercise.

CLINICAL TIP

Do not use cake frosting or candy bars for treatment of hypoglycemia. The fat in the frosting and candy prevents the sugar from working quickly. Hard candy takes too long to dissolve to provide rapid treatment for hypoglycemia.

FAMILIES WANT TO KNOW

Preventing DKA

Call the health care provider if the child has the following signs (Kaufman & Halvorson, 1999b):

- Vomiting more than twice or for longer than 4 hours
- More than five diarrheal stools
- Sick and cannot eat
- Change in mental status
- Temperature over 38.4°C (101°F)
- Blood glucose >350 mg/dL on two separate readings, or >200 mg/dL and moderate to large ketones
- Large ketones present, acetone breath
- Evidence of bacterial infection
- Difficulty breathing

CULTURE

Children of African-American, American Indian, Hispanic, and Asian origins are at greater risk for developing type 2 diabetes (American Diabetes Association, 2000). The disease in children appears to be following the same racial and ethnic distribution as found in adults (Brosnan, Upchurch, & Schreiner, 2001). Particularly affected are members of some American Indian tribes that historically had a high level of exercise and hunter-gatherer types of diets. In some groups, such as the Pima Indians of the Southwest, the majority have diabetes and face complications from the disease.

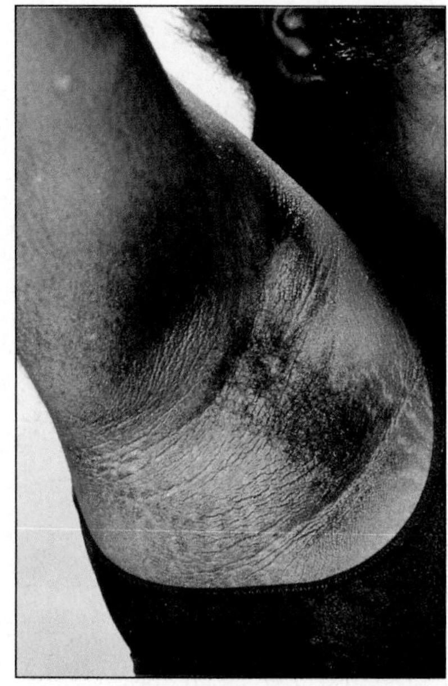

FIGURE 22-11 ◆
Acanthosis nigricans.
Courtesy of Audrey Austin, M.D., Children's National Medical Center, Washington, DC.

Type 2 Diabetes

Type 2 diabetes is a disease associated with **insulin resistance** (an alteration of the insulin receptor that signals the presence of insulin in the interior of cells), and it may be connected with an insulin secretory defect in the pancreas. Type 2 diabetes was formerly called noninsulin dependent diabetes. Risk factors include obesity, low physical exercise, and type 2 diabetes in a first-degree relative. Between 74% and 100% of children with type 2 diabetes have a first- or second-degree relative with the same type of diabetes (American Diabetes Association, 2000). The peak age of onset in children is at the time of puberty, and females are affected more than males with a 1.7:1 ratio (Pinhas-Hamiel & Zeitler, 2001). The increasing number of children being diagnosed with type 2 diabetes has caused significant concern in the health care community. Up to 45% of children with a new diagnosis of diabetes have type 2. The increasing rate of obesity among children is thought to be a contributing factor (American Diabetes Association, 2000). The true incidence in children is unknown as many children are undiagnosed.

ETIOLOGY AND PATHOPHYSIOLOGY Type 2 diabetes is a complex metabolic disorder in which the child has insulin resistance, and therefore, insulin fails to transfer glucose into the cells. With the increased weight, the visceral fat produces a cytokine homone (tumor necrosis factor) that desensitizes the insulin receptor to insulin. The pancreatic cells produce more insulin in an attempt to facilitate glucose transfer and overcome the insulin resistance. This results in **hyperinsulinemia** (elevated insulin levels in the blood). The child maintains a balance between hyperinsulinemia and insulin resistance and a normal glycemic state. As insulin resistance worsens, the islet of Langerhans beta cells fail in their ability to hypersecrete insulin. This leads to impaired glucose tolerance and overt diabetes develops. The growth hormone secretion may have a role during puberty in promoting insulin resistance.

CLINICAL MANIFESTATIONS Signs and symptoms of type 2 diabetes upon initial presentation are very different from type 1. **Acanthosis nigricans,** hyperpigmentation and thickening of the skin with velvety irregularities in the skin folds of the neck, axillae, elbows, knees, groin, and abdomen, is a common finding associated with chronic hyperinsulinemia (Figure 22-11 ◆). The child is usually obese, with truncal (or central) adiposity. The child may present in diabetic ketoacidosis. Other clinical manifestations can be found in the table on page 840.

CLINICAL THERAPY Obesity and the presence of acanthosis nigricans on physical exam are clues to the diagnosis. Blood glucose levels at 200 mg/dL without fasting or a fasting glucose at 126 mg/dL are diagnostic of diabetes. Urine is tested and ketones are found in about 50% of children. Islet cell autoantibodies, insulin levels, glutamic acid decarboxylase autoantibody test (GAD-65), and fasting C-peptid level are used to differentiate between type 1 and type 2 diabetes. The child with type 2 diabetes has higher insulin and fasting C-peptid levels than the child with type 1 diabetes. Islet cell and GAD-65 autoantibodies will not be present. A fasting lipid profile is obtained since dyslipidemia (primarily elevated LDL-C and triglycerides) is usually present. Elevated fasting insulin levels are present (see Appendix D).

The goal of clinical therapy is normal physical and emotional development, control of hypo- and hyperglycemia, and minimization of long-term complications. To accomplish this, the child requires gradual sustained weight loss, metabolic control of blood glucose levels, exercise, and emotional support. Oral medication is used when diet and exercise efforts are inadequate to control hyperglycemia. Metaformin enhances insulin sensitivity, slows the gastrointestinal absorption of glucose, and reduces the hepatic and renal glucose production. It can be used when there is normal liver and kidney function and no ketosis. If additional medication is needed, sulfonyluria may be used. The adolescent may ultimately need insulin for glycemic control.

If the child presents in ketoacidosis, insulin will be initially used to reverse the metabolic decompensation. Insulin may not be required after the metabolic deterioration is resolved.

CLINICAL TIP

Potential long-term health complications of diabetes mellitus include early-onset cardiovascular disease, atherosclerosis, neuropathy, retinopathy, and peripheral neuropathy.

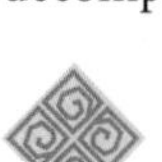

NURSING MANAGEMENT

Nursing Assessment and Diagnosis

Because the child does not often have an acute onset, assess any child with a BMI above the 85th percentile for age and gender for signs of insulin resistance (acanthosis nigricans, hypertension, and dyslipidemia). Family history of diabetes in an overweight child is a reason to begin screening for the condition. Once the child has been diagnosed, monitor blood glucose levels and blood pressure. Assess the child's diet and activity patterns to determine appropriate changes for disease management. Consider evaluating the siblings for diabetes.

Nursing diagnoses that may apply to the child with type 2 diabetes include the following:

- *Altered nutrition: More than body requirements,* related to obesity in one or both parents and ethnic and cultural norms
- *Activity intolerance,* related to sedentary lifestyle
- *Fatigue,* related to disease state (insulin resistance)
- *Ineffective management of therapeutic regimen (family and individual),* related to family conflict over changing eating patterns
- *Self-esteem disturbance,* related to situational crisis associated with diagnosis of new onset chronic illness

Planning and Implementation

The child with type 2 diabetes may be hospitalized at the time of diagnosis because ketoacidosis is present. However, the nurse in an inpatient setting is more likely to encounter this child when hospitalized for another condition or during visits for health care in clinics or schools. Nursing care focuses on managing the child's blood glucose levels and hypertension during the hospitalization, assessing growth and dietary intake, evaluating goals for weight loss and exercise programs, and reviewing the child's knowledge about diabetes and strategies for management at home.

Care in the Community

Since the child is initially diagnosed and managed on an outpatient basis, nursing care focuses on teaching the child and parents about the disease and its management, managing dietary intake, providing emotional support, and planning strategies for daily management in the community.

Educate the child and family about the disease and lifestyle changes required for effective management of the condition. Focus on the need to increase activity with routine exercise of at least 30 to 60 minutes daily and decrease sedentary activity time, such as computer and television viewing, to no more than 2 hours daily. Customize the activity strategy for each child with motivation to develop a regular routine.

Work with the family to decrease high-calorie and high-fat foods with a diet plan that is sensitive to the family's resources and ethnic preferences. Limit fast food to once weekly and snack on fruits and vegetables. Assess the child's height, weight, and BMI on each visit, and plot them on the appropriate growth curve for age and gender. A gradual sustained weight loss or decrease in BMI is the goal. If the child is going through a growth height spurt, maintenance of weight rather than weight loss is the goal. Make sure the child takes a multivitamin daily because of dietary restrictions. Encourage the entire family to make dietary changes, especially because other family members are also at risk for the condition.

Teach the child and family to perform home blood glucose testing to monitor glycemic control. This will provide feedback to the child and family that efforts to manage the disease are successful. HbA_{1c} levels should be taken at each visit to determine the average blood glucose level for the past 3 months. A HbA_{1c} level of 7% is the goal. When dietary control and exercise are not successful in reducing blood glucose levels, teach the child and family about the prescribed oral medication.

Provide the child and family with opportunities to talk about the impact of the disease on their lives. Identify resources for information about strategies that have worked for other families. Identify local support groups and peer groups for the family and child.

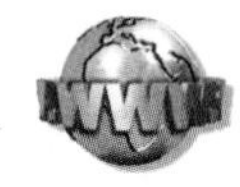

Diabetes Resources for Children

Make sure the child gets annual evaluations for potential complications of diabetes. The tests to be performed include blood for lipid levels, blood pressure, liver and renal function, urine for albumin, an eye exam for retinopathy, and a neurologic exam of the extremities for neuropathies.

Evaluation

Examples of expected outcomes of nursing care include the following:

- The child decreases sedentary activity time to under 2 hours a day.
- The child's daily intake of fruits and vegetables increases to five to eight daily and total fat intake decreases to less than 30% of total calories.
- The child's body mass index slowly and consistently decreases.

DISORDERS OF GONADAL FUNCTION

GYNECOMASTIA

Gynecomastia is the presence of unilateral or bilateral enlarged breast tissue in males. It is a common finding during adolescence and is sometimes confused with subcutaneous fat pads in obese boys. Gynecomastia occurs when the ratio of estrogen to testosterone is greater than the usual male ratio. It is also associated with drugs that increase the circulating concentration of prolactin such as marijuana and tricyclic antidepressants (Wilson, 1999). The amount of breast tissue varies among boys. The condition usually disappears in 1 to 2 years.

Nursing care focuses on reassuring the boy and his parents that gynecomastia is a common and transient condition. Because of the concerns about body image that are common during adolescence, embarrassment is a frequent problem. Alerting the teen's teachers may be necessary if teasing becomes a problem.

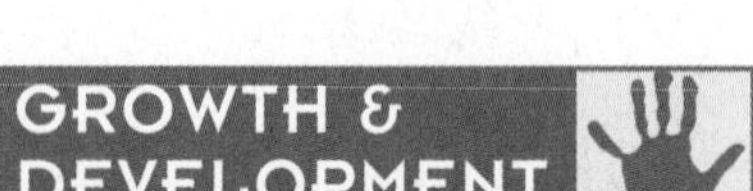

It is common for adolescents to have irregular menstrual cycles and duration of the menstrual period for 1–2 years after menarche. A large number of cycles are anovulatory for the first 2 years after menarche.

AMENORRHEA

Amenorrhea, or lack of menstruation, may be primary or secondary. Criteria for primary amenorrhea include the following:

- Absence of menarche by age 14 in association with no growth or development of secondary sexual characteristics
- Absence of menses by age 16 when secondary sexual characteristics and growth are present
- Absence of menarche 2 years after completing breast development and peak height velocity (Prose, Ford, & Lovely, 1998).

Secondary amenorrhea is the cessation of menstrual periods 6 months or three cycles after menstruation has begun; it is characterized by an absence of spontaneous bleeding for at least 120 days. Pregnancy is the most common cause of secondary amenorrhea in adolescents.

Primary amenorrhea is most often caused by structural defects of the reproductive system; chromosomal abnormalities (such as Turner's syndrome); or hypothalamic or pituitary tumors, thyroid dysfunction, or polycystic ovary disease. No underlying pathologic condition is found in some adolescents. Primary or secondary amenorrhea may be found in competitive athletes, particularly those who are pressured to be strong competitors, to maintain a perfect body type, and to have endurance.

A thorough history, physical examination, and laboratory evaluation are required to determine the cause of amenorrhea. The history focuses on asking questions about recent excessive weight loss or gain; excessive physical activity or sports training; chronic illness; use of illegal drugs, birth control pills, or phenothiazines; emotional problems; and age of the mother at menarche. The physical examination focuses on evaluating the adolescent's stage of sexual development and assessing for hirsutism (see Chapter 4). A vaginal exam is performed to determine vaginal patency and if the vaginal mucosa is estrogenized. A pregnancy test is performed. Bone age and hormone levels are evaluated (estrogen, LH, FSH, and prolactin).

Treatment of amenorrhea depends on the specific cause. The most common approach is to give birth control pills containing both estrogen and progesterone. Athletic teenagers are encouraged to eat a well-balanced, high-calorie diet. Calcium supplements may be ordered. Estrogen with progesterone in low doses may be prescribed for athletes to reduce the risk for osteoporosis. Nursing management centers on patient education and emotional support. The goal is to maintain normal growth and development.

GROWTH & DEVELOPMENT

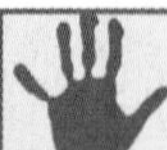

Girls competing in sports such as gymnastics, ballet, and long-distance running need to maintain a low weight and a perfect body type. The inadequate nutrition and strenuous activity may cause hypothalamic dysfunction and a low estrogen level. This results in amenorrhea (Prose et al., 1998). This, in turn, may increase the girl's risk of fractures and osteoporosis in young adulthood (see Chapter 3).

DYSMENORRHEA

Dysmenorrhea (menstrual pain or cramping) is a common complaint of adolescent girls. It is usually caused by an increased secretion of prostaglandins that are produced during the ovulatory cycle. Dysmenorrhea may also be caused by endometriosis and pelvic inflammatory disease. Dysmenorrhea usually occurs following the beginning of ovulation and ends on the second day of the menstrual cycle. The crampy pain in the lower abdomen and pelvic region can be mild or severe. Pain may radiate to the back or thighs. Other symptoms may include nausea, headache, vomiting, diarrhea, and urinary frequency.

Nonprescription analgesics, relaxation techniques, and application of a heating pad may relieve mild discomfort. Oral contraceptives may be prescribed to prevent ovulation and to decrease prostaglandin production. Nursing care centers on providing patient education and emotional support.

CLINICAL TIP

Nonsteroidal anti-inflammatory drugs (NSAIDs) such as ibuprofen and naproxen sodium inhibit prostaglandin synthesis and are effective if taken before cramping starts.

DISORDERS RELATED TO SEX CHROMOSOME ABNORMALITIES

TURNER'S SYNDROME

Turner's syndrome is the most common sex chromosome abnormality in females. Affected girls have a missing or abnormal X chromosome. It occurs in approximately 1 in 1,500 to 2,500 live female births (Prose et al., 1998). The cause of the chromosomal error is unknown.

Characteristic clinical findings include significant short stature (less than 5th percentile); undeveloped ovaries; a short, webbed neck with a low posterior hairline; cubitus valgus (increased angle at the elbow); broad chest with widely spaced nipples; lymphedema; hyperconvex fingernails; dark, pigmented nevi; delayed puberty; amenorrhea; and infertility (Figure 22-12 ◆). Few girls have all of these features. Pubertal development occurs spontaneously, but delayed, in up to 30% of affected girls (Ranke & Saenger, 2001).

Among the conditions that may be associated with Turner's syndrome are congenital heart disease; coarctation of aorta; structural abnormalities of the kidney; congenital lymphedema; hypothyroidism or Hashimoto's thyroiditis; chronic or recurrent otitis media;

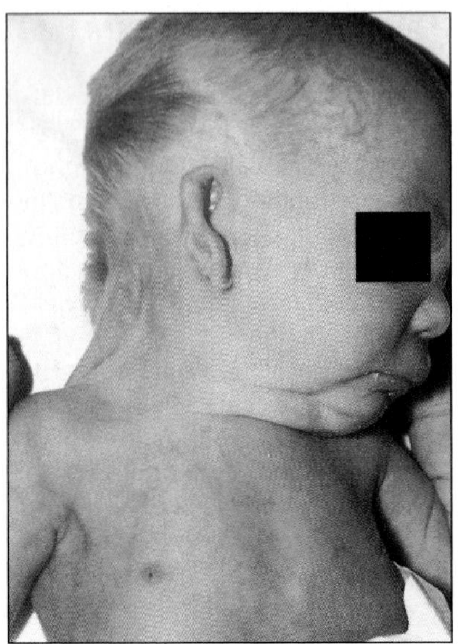

FIGURE 22-12 ◆
What characteristic physical manifestations of Turner's syndrome can you identify in this girl?
From Zittelli, B. J., and Davis, H. W. (Eds.). (1997). *Atlas of Pediatric Physical Diagnosis* (3rd ed., p. 14). St. Louis, MO: Mosby, Inc.

ptosis, myopia, or amblyopia (lazy eye); inflammatory bowel disease; idiopathic hypertension; and scoliosis (Sanger, 1996).

Growth usually proceeds at a normal rate for the first 2 to 3 years of life and then slows. Breast tissue, which begins to bud at about 10 to 12 years, fails to develop fully. Only in rare instances will a girl with Turner's syndrome menstruate spontaneously or be able to conceive. Without treatment, final height is approximately 1.4 m (56 in.).

The presence of characteristic physical findings may alert health care providers to suspect Turner's syndrome. Some infants, however, have few of these characteristics. In some instances, diagnosis is made only when short stature and delayed puberty become apparent in the teenage years. The condition is diagnosed definitively by a karyotype, which reveals the classic 45,XO chromosome pattern or 46,XX pattern with one misshapen X chromosome.

Treatment involves careful monitoring of the child's growth. A growth chart made especially for girls with Turner's syndrome is available. Growth hormone therapy may be prescribed to promote growth during childhood (Ranke & Saenger, 2001). Low-dose estrogen therapy is usually begun at about 15 years of age, with dosage increases over the next 2 to 3 years. Waiting until 15 years gives the girl the opportunity to achieve her maximum height before hormones cause the growth plates to close. This treatment produces pubertal changes such as breast development and pubic hair. Progesterone is added to the estrogen therapy to initiate menstrual periods.

Nursing Management

The lack of growth and sexual development associated with Turner's syndrome presents problems not only for physical growth but also for psychosocial development. Self-image, self-consciousness, and self-esteem are affected by the girl's perception of her body and how she differs from peers.

In the United States, cultural values place importance on attaining normal to tall stature. Short children tend to be treated according to their size rather than their age. Emphasis is also placed on sexual maturity. Television, advertisements, and movies encourage adolescents to dress and behave in a sexually mature manner. Girls with Turner's syndrome are often self-conscious, easily embarrassed, and suffer from low self-esteem. Even though their intelligence is generally normal, they have a higher incidence of learning problems because of visual–spatial deficits that affect performance on mathematical and manual dexterity tasks (Ranke & Saenger, 2001).

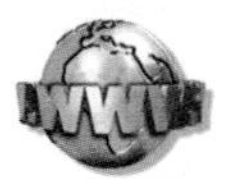

Turner's Syndrome Online

The nurse can be instrumental in helping the child adapt to the condition and gain self-esteem. Be an active listener and reinforce abilities and skills that the girl exhibits. Encourage parents to provide support. The Turner's Syndrome Society can provide additional information about the disorder for parents and adolescents.

KLINEFELTER'S SYNDROME

Klinefelter's syndrome is a genetic condition that occurs in boys who have an extra X chromosome (usually 47,XXY). It occurs in approximately 1 in 500 male births (Lewanda & Jabs, 1999). It is the single most common cause of hypogonadism (decreased secretory activity of the gonad) and infertility in males.

Most infants appear normal at birth. The condition is usually diagnosed during the school-age years when the boy's behavior becomes a problem in the classroom. Boys with Klinefelter's syndrome may have emotional problems because of delayed language development and auditory processing problems that are frustrating to the child. Intelligence quotient (IQ) scores are often 10 to 15 points below those of unaffected siblings, and IQs below 80 are not uncommon. Boys with Klinefelter's syndrome are tall and thin, with overly long arms and legs. The arm span to height ratio is normal. The onset of puberty may be delayed with an abnormal progression. Testicular size is decreased at all ages. Less facial and body hair may develop. Gynecomastia is a characteristic finding.

Diagnosis is confirmed by chromosomal analysis revealing one or more extra X chromosomes. The goal of treatment is to stimulate masculinization and the development of secondary sex characteristics when adolescence is delayed. Testosterone replacement is begun when the boy is 11 or 12 years of age. Depo-Testosterone is given by intramuscular injection every 3 to 4 weeks to maintain serum testosterone levels within the normal range. The dose is increased gradually until an adult dose is reached between 15 and 17 years of age; however, this medication does not improve fertility. Gynecomastia does not typically disappear with hormone treatment. Cosmetic surgery may be needed if breast size is distressing.

Nursing Management

Nursing care consists of educating the parents and child about the syndrome, evaluating the child's and family's coping mechanisms, assisting with school problems, and reinforcing the child's strengths. Encourage parents to channel their son's energy into areas that will provide opportunities for success and productive experiences. Emphasize the importance of rewarding the boy's successes in school, sports, or hobbies. Genetic counseling should be made available to adolescents, if indicated, because sexual functioning and fertility may be impaired.

INBORN ERRORS OF METABOLISM

Inborn errors of metabolism are inherited biochemical abnormalities of the urea cycle, amino acid, and organic acid metabolism. Individually they are rare disorders; however, as a group they are a significant health problem in infancy.

The biochemical defect usually causes an abnormal chemical by-product to accumulate in the blood, urine, or tissues or results in a decreased amount of normal enzymes. Most disorders are associated with a protein intolerance, with symptoms developing shortly after formula or breast milk feedings are begun.

Clinical manifestations usually occur within days or weeks of birth. Signs and symptoms may include lethargy and poor feeding, persistent vomiting, abnormal muscle tone and seizures, apnea and tachycardia, and an unusual urine or body odor (musty, sweet odor of maple syrup or burnt sugar, or cheesy or sweaty feet).

In many states, neonatal screening is used to detect several of these conditions before symptoms develop. Four million newborns are screened each year for metabolic disorders (e.g., phenylketonuria), hematologic disorders (e.g., sickle-cell anemia), and endocrinopathies (e.g., hypothyroidism) (Centers for Disease Control and Prevention, 2001). However, most inborn errors of metabolism are not detected until signs and symptoms are present. Initial laboratory tests include measurement of serum glucose, electrolytes, blood gases, and serum ammonia. Results of these tests make it possible to classify the disorder by the presence of hypoglycemia, metabolic acidosis, hyperammonemia, or liver dysfunction. Further diagnostic laboratory tests are then performed.

Treatment, when available, focuses on replacing or reducing the amount of the substance causing the biochemical abnormality.

Three of the more common inborn errors of metabolism, phenylketonuria, galactosemia, and maple syrup urine disease, are presented here. Congenital hypothyroidism and congenital adrenal hyperplasia, also considered inborn errors of metabolism, were discussed earlier in this chapter.

LAW & ETHICS

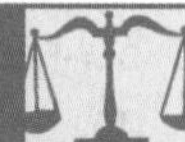

Neonatal screening for hypothyroidism and phenylketonuria is mandated by state law in every state. When a state law exists, signed informed consent of the parents is not required. All states but South Dakota permit parents to refuse screening for religious or personal reasons. If parents refuse the test, obtain a signature of "informed dissent" to include in the child's medical record (American Academy of Pediatrics, 2001).

PHENYLKETONURIA

Phenylketonuria (PKU) is an autosomal recessive inherited disorder of amino acid metabolism that affects the body's utilization of protein. It is caused by a mutation of the phenylalanine hydroxylase gene. The incidence is 1 in 10,000 live births per year, with great ethnic variability (Yule, 2000).

Children with PKU have a deficiency of the liver enzyme phenylalanine hydroxylase that normally breaks down the essential amino acid phenylalanine into tyrosine. As a result, phenylalanine accumulates in the blood, causing a musty or mousey body and urine odor, irritability, vomiting, hyperactivity, seizures, and an eczemalike rash. Persistence of elevated phenylalanine leads to disruption of cellular processes of myelination and protein synthesis and results in a seizure disorder and mental retardation without treatment.

Infants appear normal at birth. Screening for PKU is required by law in every state. For best results, the newborn should have begun formula or breast milk feeding before specimen collection. Early hospital discharge places newborns at risk for false negative screening

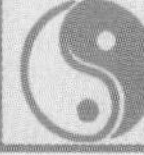

CULTURE

Phenylketonuria is rare in African, Jewish, and Japanese populations. It is more commonly found in isolated communities with numerous intermarriages between families over several generations.

tests if screened within 24 hours of birth. Screening must occur no sooner than 48 hours after birth, or the test should be repeated at 1 to 2 weeks of age. If the test shows elevated levels of plasma phenylalanine, a repeat test is performed. If the second test is positive, the family is referred to an outpatient treatment center.

PKU is treated using special formulas (e.g., lofenalac, minafen, and albumaid XP) and a diet low in phenylalanine to keep plasma phenylalanine levels between 2 and 6 mg/dL. The diet must also meet the child's needs for optimal growth. High-protein foods (meats and dairy products) and aspartame are avoided because they contain large amounts of phenylalanine. Elemental medical foods (modified protein hydrosylates in which the phenylalanine has been removed) are used instead. The low-phenylalanine diet should be maintained for life. If dietary control is lost before 6 years of age, there is a significant impact on IQ (Yule, 2000). If adults go off the diet, there is no change in their IQ, but they may perform less well on tasks requiring attention and processing speed (Phenylketonuria (PKU): Screening and Management. National Institutes of Health, 2000). The low phenylalanine diet is especially important for adolescent females and women prior to conception and during pregnancy to prevent congenital anomalies (low birth weight, mental retardation, microcephaly) in the fetus.

Nursing Management

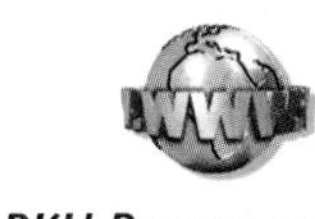

PKU Resources

Nursing care is mainly supportive and focuses on teaching parents about the disorder and its management. Serum levels of phenylalanine should be measured periodically throughout life.

The low-phenylalanine diet is a rigid, strict diet that excludes many foods. Parents and children need a great deal of support to promote compliance. The formula and elemental medical food costs are relatively high. Usually only the formula is reimbursed by insurance. Like children with diabetes mellitus, children with PKU may rebel against the dietary limitations in an effort to be like their peers. For this reason the low-phenylalanine diet may be discontinued during the late school-age years or adolescence. If the child has problems concentrating or sitting still, resumption of the low-phenylalanine diet may result in improvement of behavior and cognitive functioning.

Parents of an affected child who are considering a future pregnancy and adolescents with the disorder should be referred for genetic counseling.

GALACTOSEMIA

Galactosemia is a disorder of carbohydrate metabolism that has an autosomal recessive inheritance pattern. It occurs in 1 in 70,000 live births (Kirschner, Kolb, & Pandit, et al., 2000).

Galactosemia results from a deficiency of the liver enzyme galactose-1–phosphate uridyltransferase (GALT), one of three enzymes needed to convert galactose to glucose. The lack of enzyme leads to an accumulation of galactose metabolites in the eyes, liver, kidney, and brain, rapidly damaging the organs and causing life-threatening problems. Children become susceptible to gram-negative sepsis.

Early signs include feeding problems, failure to gain weight due to vomiting followed by diarrhea, hypoglycemia, and an enlarged liver. Later signs include mental retardation, jaundice, ascites, sepsis, lethargy, seizures, hypotonia, cataracts, and coma. Death may occur within 1 month of birth without treatment, usually due to sepsis.

Skill 6-2: Newborn Screening

Routine newborn screening for galactosemia is performed in 44 states and the District of Columbia (Kirschner et al., 2000). Infants in other states are identified once they become symptomatic. The diagnosis is based on history, physical examination, and laboratory tests (galactose, SGOT, and SGPT are abnormally high). Urines are checked for reducing substances (the clinitest is positive and the clinistix is negative). Infants with galactosemia are placed on a lactose- or galactose-free formula (e.g., nutramigen, a meat-based, or soybean formula), which remains the child's milk substitute for life. Improvement in the infant's condition is generally seen within 24 hours. A galactose-free diet (no milk or cheese products, including foods with dry milk products) is prescribed when the infant is ready for solids. In spite of compliance with the diet, complications (learning disabilities, speech defects, ovarian failure, and neurologic syndromes) develop in many children.

Nursing management focuses on educating the parents and child about the disorder and required diet, assessing coping abilities, and providing emotional support. Refer the family to a nutritionist for diet counseling. Families must learn to screen foods for added milk solids and to avoid medications, such as antibiotics, that have lactose fillers. Calcium supplementation may be needed. Advise parents that several galactose-free cheeses are sold commercially. Because the disorder is inherited, the family should be referred for genetic counseling.

MAPLE SYRUP URINE DISEASE

Maple syrup urine disease (MSUD) is a disorder of amino acid metabolism that has an autosomal recessive inheritance pattern. It is a rare disorder found in 1 in 225,000 live births, but has a high incidence in some Pennsylvania Mennonites (1 in 380 live births) (Robinson & Drumm, 2001).

In MSUD, three essential amino acids (leucine, isoleucine, and valine) cannot be broken down because of absent or defective enzyme branched chain alpha-keotacid dehydrogenase. This results in alpha ketoacidosis. All three amino acids are essential to form normal structures such as the hair, skin, and muscle. Leucine has the potential to accumulate in the brain and cause cerebral edema, progressive neurologic impairment, and death.

Within 3 to 7 days of life, the newborn develops symptoms of poor appetite, lethargy, vomiting, variable muscle tone, irritability, seizures, high pitched cry, and a sweet smell. Not all states require newborn screening for this condition. Diagnosis is made with laboratory tests of the urine for positive ketones and blood tests for elevated leucine, isoleucine, and valine. Specially designed medical formulas and foods rich in amino acids, calories, vitamins, minerals, and other nutrients are prescribed. These special medical foods have the three amino acids removed. The child needs special low-protein foods that are adequate for growth with enough calories to support twice the child's basal metabolic rate. Daily urine testing is required to determine if ketones are being excreted, an indication that the body is in a catabolic state.

Nursing care includes educating the families about the disorder and special dietary requirements. The parents need to learn how to mix the child's special formula with natural protein source, amino acid supplements, and water. The child needs formula even when ill, and a sick day plan should be provided to prevent ketoacidosis. The child should be permitted moderate exercise only to prevent increases in leucine levels. Help families identify sources of information or support groups who can share recipes and tips for managing the child's condition.

CLINICAL TIP

When the child starts child care or school, it is important for teachers and other care providers to know foods the child should avoid and have a list of snacks for special occasions. The child should have formula and other supplements available to ensure a steady intake of calories during the day. An individual school health plan should be developed with the school nurse so that teachers and other school personnel are informed.

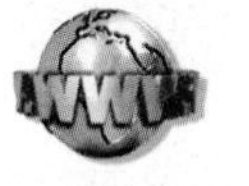

MSUD Resources

Chapter Highlights

- Puberty is the process of sexual maturation that occurs when the gonads secrete increased amounts of the sex hormones estrogen and testosterone, resulting in the development of primary and secondary sex characteristics.
- Children with hypopituitarism have short stature as a result of growth hormone deficiency. Treatment with growth hormone early in life enables these children to have near normal heights.
- An excessive secretion of growth hormone or hyperpituitarism may cause children to grow 7 or 8 feet in height when it occurs before the epiphyseal plates close.
- In diabetes insipidus, the urine cannot be concentrated, no matter how dehydrated the child becomes. Diagnosis rarely occurs until the child experiences hypernatremic dehydration.
- Precocious puberty is the appearance of any secondary sexual characteristics before 8 years of age in girls and 9 years of age in boys. If no treatment is provided, the hormones will stimulate closure of the epiphyseal plates and the child will have short stature as an adult.
- Untreated or ineffectively treated congenital hypothyroidism results in impaired growth and mental retardation.
- Signs of hyperthyroidism include an enlarged, nontender thyroid gland (goiter), prominent eyes, eyelid lag, tachycardia, nervousness, restlessness or irritability, increased appetite with weight loss, emotional lability, heat intolerance, increased sweating, insomnia, tremor, and muscle weakness.
- During infancy and childhood, most cases of Cushing's syndrome are due to a malignant adrenal tumor. It gen-

erally takes up to 5 years for the child to develop the characteristic cushingoid appearance.

- Congenital adrenal hyperplasia has two forms, salt losing or simple virilization. Approximately 65% to 75% of children have a disturbance in mineralocorticoid regulation that can lead to acute adrenal insufficiency with any serious illness or injury.
- Adrenal insufficiency, though rare in children, is characterized by weakness with fatigue, anorexia and salt craving, poor weight gain or weight loss, hyperpigmentation at pressure points, generalized bronzing of the skin, abdominal pain, nausea and vomiting, and diarrhea.
- Pheochromocytoma is a benign tumor of the adrenal gland, that causes labile hypertension and intermittent signs associated with epinephrine and norepinephrine secretion.
- The American Diabetes Association recommends that all adolescents with type 1 diabetes mellitus use an intensive therapy regimen with three or more insulin injections a day or a continuous subcutaneous insulin infusion (CSII) by an insulin pump.
- Treatment of the child with diabetic ketoacidosis includes intravenous fluids and electrolytes for dehydration and acidosis. Insulin is given by continuous infusion pump to decrease the serum glucose level at a slow but steady rate to prevent the development of cerebral edema.
- Common causes of hypoglycemia in children with type 1 diabetes include an error in insulin dosage, errors in injection technique, inadequate calories because of missed meals, or exercise without a corresponding increase in caloric intake.
- Type 2 diabetes mellitus is a new epidemic among children and adolescents that results from insulin resistance. Children most commonly affected are obese and the majority have family members with the same type of diabetes.
- Secondary amenorrhea is the cessation of spontaneous bleeding for at least 120 days and occurs 6 months or three cycles after menarche.
- Turner's syndrome is diagnosed definitively by a karyotype, which reveals the classic 45,XO chromosome pattern or 46,XX pattern with one misshapen X chromosome.
- Signs of Klinefelter's syndrome include a gynecomastia, delayed onset of puberty with an abnormal progression, decreased testicular size, and less facial and body hair than normal.
- Children with phenylketonuria (PKU) have a deficiency of the liver enzyme phenylalanine hydroxylase that normally breaks down the essential amino acid phenylalanine into tyrosine. It is treated with special formula and engineered foods.
- Galactosemia results from a deficiency of a liver enzyme needed to convert galactose to glucose. This leads to an accumulation of galactose metabolites in the eyes, liver, kidney, and brain, rapidly damaging the organs and causing life-threatening problems.
- Maple syrup urine disease is a rare inherited enzyme deficiency that results in ketoacidosis unless special formula, engineered foods, and extra calories are eaten.

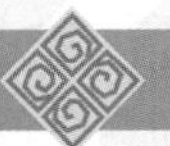

EXPLORE MediaLink

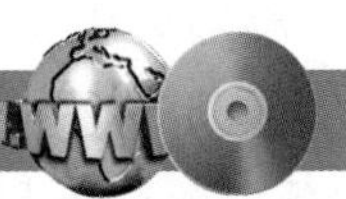

- NCLEX review, case studies, and other interactive resources for this chapter can be found on the Companion Website at **http://www.prenhall.com/ball.** Click on Chapter 22 to select the activities for this chapter.
- For animations, more NCLEX review questions, and an audio glossary, access the accompanying CD-ROM in this textbook.

References

1. American Academy of Pediatrics Committee on Bioethics. (2001). Ethical issues with genetic testing in pediatrics. *Pediatrics, 107*(6), 1451–1455.
2. American Academy of Pediatrics Section on Endocrinology and Committee on Genetics. (2000). Technical report: Congenital adrenal hyperplasia. *Pediatrics, 106*(6), 1511–1518.
3. American Diabetes Association. (2000). Type 2 diabetes in children and adolescents. *Diabetes Care, 23*(3), 381–389.
4. Boland, E. A., & Grey, M. (2000). Diabetes mellitus (type 1). In P. L. Jackson & J. A. Vessey (eds.), *Primary care of the child with a chronic condition* (3rd ed., pp. 426–444). St. Louis: Mosby.
5. Brosnan, C. A., Upchurch, S., & Schreiner, B. (2001). Type 2 diabetes in children and adolescents: An emerging disease. *Journal of Pediatric Health Care, 15*(4), 187–193.
6. Castiglia, P. T. (1997). Hyperthyroidism. *Journal of Pediatric Health Care, 11*(5), 227–229.

7. Centers for Disease Control and Prevention. (2001). Using tandem mass spectrometry for metabolic disease screening among newborns: A report of a work group. *Morbidity and Mortality Weekly Report, 50*(RR-31), 1–34.
8. Donohoue, P. A. (1999). The thyroid. In J. A. McMillan, C. D. DeAngelis, R. D. Feigin, & J. B. Warshaw, *Oski's pediatrics: Principles and practice* (3rd ed., pp. 1803–1812). Philadelphia: Lippincott, Williams & Wilkins.
9. Dveirin, K., & Tunnessen, W. W. (2000). A 14-month-old with polyuria and polydipsia: Searching for buried treasure. *Contemporary Pediatrics, 17*(10), 23–30.
10. Expert Committee on the Diagnosis and Classification of Diabetes Mellitus. (1999). Report of the expert committee on the diagnosis and classification of diabetes mellitus. *Diabetes Care, 22* (Suppl. 1), S5–S19.
11. Felner, E. I., & White, P. C. (2001). Improving management of diabetic ketoacidosis in children. *Pediatrics, 108*(3), 735–740.
12. Finegold, D. (1997). Endocrinology. In B. J. Zitelli & H. W. Davis (eds.), *Atlas of pediatric physical diagnosis* (3rd ed., p. 270). St. Louis: Mosby–Wolfe.
13. Flood, R. G., & Chiang, V. W. (2001). Rate and prediction of infection in children with diabetic ketoacidosis. *Journal of Emergency Medicine, 19*(4), 270–273.
14. Hafeez, W., & Vuguin, P. (2000). Managing diabetic ketoacidosis: A delicate balance. *Contemporary Pediatrics, 17*(6), 72–83.
15. Herman-Giddens, M. E., Slora, E. J., Wasserman, R. C., Bourdony, C. J., Bhapkar, M. V., Koch, G. G., & Hasemeier, C. M. (1997). Secondary sexual characteristics and menses in young girls seen in office practice: A study from the pediatric research in office settings network. *Pediatrics, 99*(4), 505–512.
16. Kaufman, F. R., & Halvorson, M. (1999a). New trends in managing type 1 diabetes. *Contemporary Pediatrics, 16*(10), 112–123.
17. Kaufman, F. R., & Halvorson, M. (1999b). The treatment and prevention of diabetic ketoacidosis in children and adolescents with type 1 diabetes. *Pediatric Annals, 28*(9), 576–582.
18. Kirchlechner, V., Koller, D. Y., Seidl, R., & Waldhauser, F. (1999). Treatment of nephrogenic diabetes insipidis with hydrochlorothiazide and amiloride. *Archives of Diseases in Children, 80,* 548–552.
19. Kirschner, C., Kolb, A., Pandit, S., & Tunnessen, W. W. (2000). A 4-week-old with poor weight gain and jaundice: A diagnosis in space. *Contemporary Pediatrics, 17*(11), 27–33.
20. Kohn, B., Julius, J. R., & Blethen, S. L. (1999). Combined use of growth hormone and gonadotropin-releasing hormone analogues: The National Cooperative Growth Study experience. *Pediatrics, 104*(4, Pt. 2), 1014–1017.
21. Lewanda, A. F., & Jabs, E. W. (1999). Dysmorphology: Genetic syndromes and associations. In J. A. McMillan, C. D. DeAngelis, R. D. Feigin, & J. B. Warshaw, *Oski's pediatrics: Principles and practice* (3rd ed., p. 2231). Philadelphia: Lippincott, Williams & Wilkins.
22. Merke, D. P., & Cutler, G. B. (1997). New approaches to the treatment of congenital adrenal hyperplasia. *Journal of the American Medical Association, 277*(13), 1073–1076.
23. NIH Consensus statement (2000, Oct. 16–18), *Phenylketonuria: Screening and management, 17*(3), 1–33.
24. Pinhas-Hamiel, O., & Zeitler, P. (2001). Type 2 diabetes: Not just for grownups anymore. *Contemporary Pediatrics, 18*(1), 102–125.
25. Prose, C. C., Ford, C. A., & Lovely, L. P. (1998). Evaluating amenorrhea: The pediatrician's role. *Contemporary Pediatrics, 15*(10), 83–110.
26. Ranke, W. B., & Saenger, P. (2001, July 28). Turner's syndrome. *The Lancet, 358,* 309–314.
27. Reddy, V. S., O'Neill, J. A., Holcomb, G. W., Neblett, W. W., Pietsch, J. B., & Morgan, W. M. (2000). Twenty-five year surgical experience with pheochromocytoma in children. *American Surgeon, 66*(12), 1085–1091.
28. Rennert, O. M., & Francis, G. L. (1999). Update on the genetics and pathophysiology of type 1 diabetes. *Pediatric Annals, 28*(9), 570–575.
29. Robinson, D., & Drumm, L. (2001). Maple syrup urine disease: A standard of nursing care. *Pediatric Nursing, 27*(3), 255–264, 270.
30. Rovet, J. F., & Ehrlich, R. (2000). Psychoeducational outcome in children with early-treated congenital hypothyroidism. *Pediatrics, 105*(3), 515–522.
31. Sanger, P. (1996). Turner's syndrome. *Current Concepts, 335*(2), 1749–1754.
32. Saudek, C. D. (1997). Novel forms of insulin delivery. *Endocrinology and Metabolism Clinics of North America, 26*(3), 599–610.
33. Selekman, J., Scofield, S., & Swenson-Brousell, C. (1999). Diabetes update in the pediatric population. *Pediatric Nursing, 25*(6), 666–669.
34. Shulman, D. I., & Bercu, B. B. (1998). Growth hormone therapy: An update. *Contemporary Pediatrics, 15*(8), 95–110.
35. Silverstein, J. H., & Rosenbloom, A. L. (2000). New developments in type 1 (insulin dependent) diabetes. *Clinical Pediatrics, 39*(5), 257–266.
36. Therrell, B. L., Berenbaum, S. A., Manter-Kapanke, V., Simmank, J., Korman, K., Prentice, L., Gonzalez, J., & Gunn, S. (1998). Results of screening 1.9 million Texas newborns for 21-hydroxylaxe-deficient congenital adrenal hyperplasia. *Pediatrics, 101*(4), 583–590.
37. Van Vliet, G. (2001, July 14). Treatment of congenital hypothyroidism. *The Lancet, 358,* 86–87.
38. Willhaus, J. (1999). Growth hormone therapy and children with idiopathic short stature: A viable option? *Pediatric Nursing, 25*(6), 662–665.
39. Wilson, M. D. (1999). Breast problems. In J. A. McMillan, C. D. DeAngelis, R. D. Feigin, & J. B. Warshaw, *Oski's pediatrics: Principles and practice* (3rd ed., pp. 536–539). Philadelphia: Lippincott, Williams & Wilkins.
40. Yule, K. S. (2000). Phenylketonuria. In P. L. Jackson & J. A. Vessey (eds.), *Primary care of the child with a chronic condition* (3rd ed., pp. 706–731). St. Louis: Mosby.

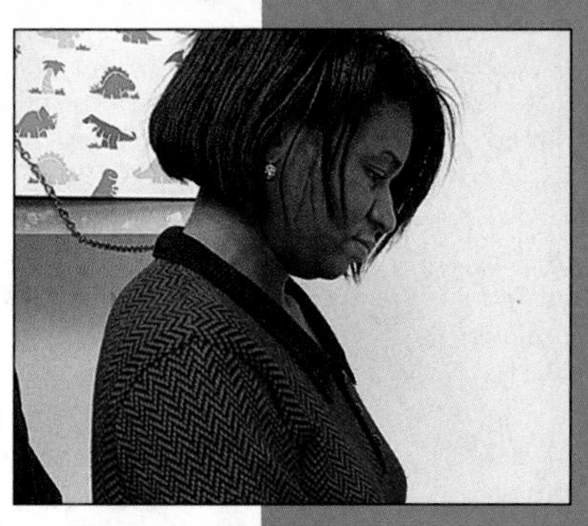

"I DIDN'T KNOW THAT SOUP COULD CAUSE SUCH A BAD INJURY. THE HARDEST THING FOR ME TO DEAL WITH IS ALL THE PAIN SHERRAY HAS WITH EACH DRESSING CHANGE."

Sherray, 6 years old, was admitted to the hospital with a deep partial-thickness burn after dropping a bowl of soup on her leg. By her second day of hospitalization, it is clear that Sherray's burn is not full thickness and that no skin grafting is needed. The amount of scarring she will have cannot be anticipated at this time.

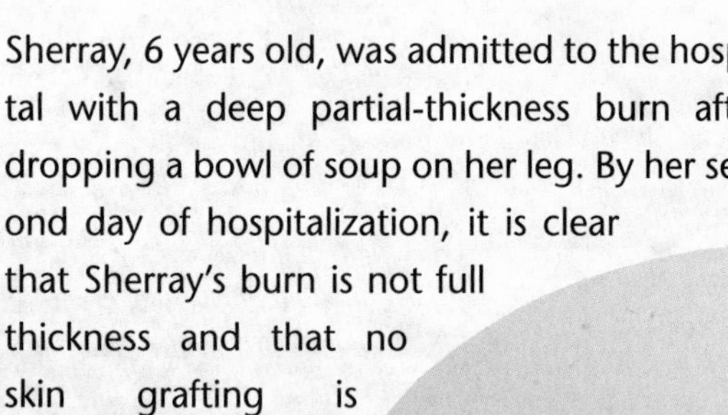

Sherray's treatment includes a bath with wound debridement and dressing changes twice a day. Although pain medication is provided, the debridement and dressing changes cause her much anxiety and pain. Sherray needs a high-protein, high-calorie diet to promote wound healing. She has a hard time extending her leg and walking, because movement stretches the burned skin, so she needs assistance to get out of bed and participate in child life activities.

Sherray's mother is rooming in, and remains at her side during the dressing changes. Her greatest concern now is to help Sherray deal with the burn injury and to reduce the chance of infection. Over the next couple of days, Sherray's mother will take more responsibility for the dressing changes in anticipation of continuing her daughter's care at home.

CHAPTER 23

ALTERATIONS IN SKIN INTEGRITY

KEY TERMS

atopy A hereditary allergic tendency.

autografting Use of healthy skin taken from a nonburned area of the child's body.

circumferential Injury completely surrounding the thorax or an extremity.

debridement Enzyme action to clean a lesion and dissolve fibrin clots or scabs; or removal of dead tissue to speed the healing process.

dermatophytoses Fungal infections that affect primarily the skin but may affect the hair and nails.

eschar Slough or layer of dead skin or tissue.

escharotomy Incision into constricting dead tissue of a burn injury to restore peripheral circulation.

intertriginous areas Skin folds of the neck, axillae, and antecubital fossa.

lichenification Thickening of the skin.

melanin Skin pigment.

phototoxic A rapid nonimmunologic reaction of the skin when exposed to sunlight.

xerosis Generally dry skin that is more likely to crack and fissure.

MediaLink 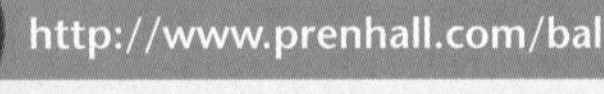 http://www.prenhall.com/ball

Resources for this chapter can be found on the CD-ROM accompanying this textbook, and on the Companion Website at http://www.prenhall.com/ball. Click on Chapter 23 to select the activities for this chapter.

CD-ROM

Audio Glossary
NCLEX Review

COMPANION WEBSITE

Web Links
NCLEX Review
MediaLink Applications
- Adolescents and Acne Management
- Develop an Educational Program to Reduce Potential for Burns in Young Children

What is the role of the nurse in providing care to the child with a burn injury? What nursing support may help the child deal with painful dressing changes and a disfiguring injury? What other health care team members are important in ensuring an optimal recovery for Sherray? What teaching must be provided to her mother to enable her to provide care at home? The information in this chapter will prepare you to answer these questions and to provide care to children such as Sherray with burn injuries or other alterations in skin integrity.

Skin disorders are seen frequently by nurses who work in outpatient clinics, schools, emergency departments, and pediatric units of hospitals. Many of these disorders are not unique to children, but children are at greater risk for some skin conditions for reasons that are discussed in this chapter.

The skin is the largest organ in the body. It performs several essential functions, among them perception, protection, temperature regulation, vitamin D synthesis, and excretion. The skin protects underlying tissues from invasion by microorganisms and from trauma. The nerves in the skin enable us to perceive pain, heat, and cold.

Temperature regulation of the body is achieved by dilation or constriction of blood vessels and sweat glands that act under the control of the CNS. The skin also supplements the body's intake of vitamin D by synthesizing this vitamin from ultraviolet light. Excretion is performed by the sweat glands, which secrete a solution of water, electrolytes, and urea, thus helping to rid the body of toxins.

ANATOMY AND PHYSIOLOGY OF PEDIATRIC DIFFERENCES

The skin is made up of three distinct layers: the epidermis, the dermis, and the subcutaneous fatty layer that separates the skin from the underlying tissue (Figure 23-1 ◆). Within the

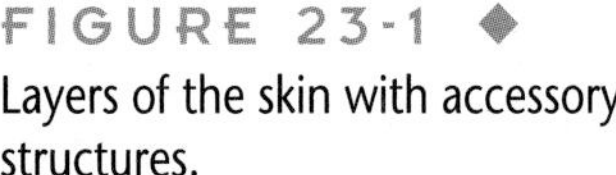

FIGURE 23-1 ◆ Layers of the skin with accessory structures.

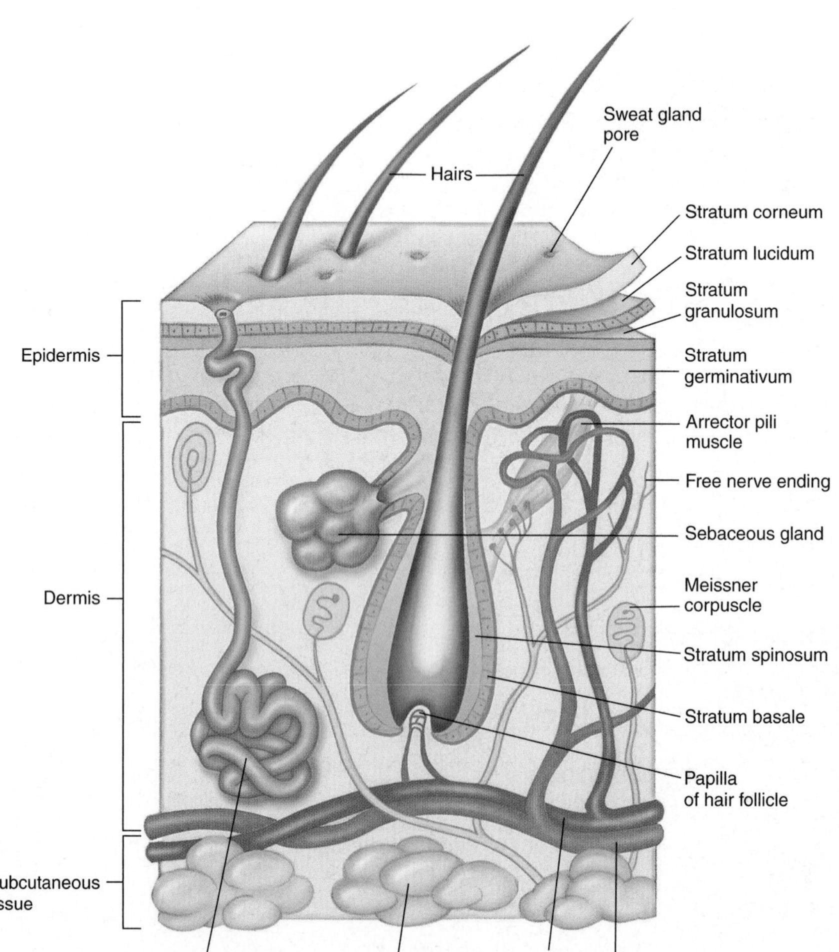

dermis are nerves, muscles, connective tissue, hair follicles, sebaceous and sweat glands, lymph channels, and blood vessels.

At birth the skin is thin, with little underlying subcutaneous fat. Because of this the infant loses heat more rapidly, has greater difficulty regulating body temperature, and becomes more easily chilled than an older child or an adult. The thinner skin also leads to increased absorption of harmful chemical substances. The newborn's skin contains more water than an adult's skin and has loosely attached cells. As the infant grows, the skin toughens and becomes less hydrated, making it less susceptible to bacteria.

The accessory structures of the skin (hair, sebaceous glands, eccrine glands, and apocrine glands) are present at birth. Like other body structures, however, they are still immature.

At birth, the infant may have soft, downy hair, called lanugo, on the shoulders and back. Lanugo is usually shed by 2 to 3 weeks of age. The amount of hair on the head varies. Scalp hair usually is shed within a few months and replaced, sometimes with hair of a different color.

Sebaceous glands function at birth, although somewhat immaturely. They vary in size and appear all over the body except on the hands and soles of the feet. Sebum, a lipid substance produced and secreted into the hair follicle or directly onto the skin, provides lubrication to the skin and hair.

Eccrine glands, located in the dermis, open onto the skin surface. They secrete an odorless, watery fluid, primarily in response to emotional stress. They also respond to changes in body temperature. As body temperature increases, the glands increase production of sweat. The result is decreased heat as the sweat evaporates. Because the eccrine sweat glands usually are not fully functional until middle childhood, infants and young children are unable to regulate temperature as effectively as older children and adults.

Apocrine glands, located mainly in the axillary and genital areas, do not function until puberty. Decomposition of the fluid secreted by these glands leads to body odor. Their biologic function, however, is unknown.

SKIN LESIONS

Skin lesions vary in size, shape, color, and texture characteristics. The two major types of skin lesions are primary lesions and secondary lesions. Primary lesions arise from previously healthy skin and include macules, patches, papules, nodules, tumors, vesicles, pustules, bullae, and wheals (see Figure 4-9). Secondary lesions result from changes in primary lesions. They include crusts, scales, **lichenification** (thickening of the skin), scars, keloids, excoriation, fissures, erosion, and ulcers (Table 23-1). It is important for the nurse to be able to identify and describe the primary and secondary skin lesions and understand their underlying cause and treatment. Some families may use complementary therapies to treat skin lesions (Table 23-2).

WOUND HEALING

Wound healing is a process that occurs in three overlapping phases: inflammation, reconstruction, and maturation (Figure 23-2 ◆) (Rote, 1998; Valencia, Falabella, & Schachner, 2001).

Inflammation, the initial response at the injury site, lasts approximately 3 to 5 days. This phase prepares the injury site for the repair process. Coagulation occurs as platelets, red blood cells, and fibrin gather to form a clot. This seals the wound, preventing bacterial invasion and joining the wound edges. Vasodilation, which occurs shortly after injury, allows leukocytes to travel to the injury site, where they ingest bacteria and debris.

Reconstruction or re-epithelialization, the second phase, may last from 5 days to 4 weeks, depending on the extent of the injury. Capillary budding to reestablish the blood flow and natural **debridement** (enzyme action to clean the lesion and dissolve the clot or scab) occur. The wound contracts. Fibroblasts multiply, producing collagen and granulation tissue to fill the wound to skin level. A fine layer of epithelial cells forms over the site.

Maturation or remodeling, the third phase, involves continued collagen production for scar production. Although the scar gradually strengthens and devascularizes, it will never be as strong as normal skin. Maturation can take months to years, depending on the extent of the injury.

TABLE 23-1 Common Secondary Skin Lesions and Associated Conditions

LESION NAME	DESCRIPTION	EXAMPLE
Crust	Dried residue of serum, pus, or blood	Impetigo
Scale	Thin flake of exfoliated epidermis	Dandruff, psoriasis
Lichenification	Thickening of skin with increased visibility of normal skin furrows	Eczema (atopic dermatitis)
Scar	Replacement of destroyed tissue with fibrous tissue	Healed surgical incision
Keloid	Overdevelopment or hypertrophy of scar that extends beyond wound edges and above skin line due to excess collagen	Healed skin area following traumatic injury
Excoriation	Abrasion or scratch mark	Scratched insect bite
Fissure	Linear crack in skin	Tinea pedis (athlete's foot)
Erosion	Loss of superficial epidermis; moist but does not bleed	Ruptured chickenpox vesicle
Ulcer	Deeper loss of skin surface; bleeding or scarring may ensue	Chancre

TABLE 23-2 Complementary Therapies for Skin Lesions

CONDITION	COMPLEMENTARY THERAPY	USE
Poison ivy	Aloe, calendula, oatmeal (topical)	Relief from itching
Atopic dermatitis	Evening primrose oil (oral)	Decreases excoriations and lichenification Decreases need for antihistamines for itching
Accelerated wound healing, burns, abrasions	Aloe vera gel (topical)	Antimicrobial effects, bacteriostatic, bacteriocidal
Skin inflammation	Chamomile (topical)	Wound drying, antimicrobial properties
Acne	5% Tea tree oil (topical)	Antibiotic, decreases open and closed comedomes

Note: Adapted from Gardner, P., Coles, D., & Kemper, K. J. (2001). The skinny on herbal remedies for dermatologic disorders. *Contemporary Pediatrics, 18*(7), 103–114.

DERMATITIS

Many skin inflammations occur in early childhood. Most are easily treated and have no long-term consequences. Dermatitis is a condition in which changes occur in the skin in response to external stimuli. The four most common types of dermatitis that occur in infants, children, and adolescents are contact dermatitis, diaper dermatitis, seborrheic dermatitis, and eczema (atopic dermatitis). It is important for the nurse to understand that these skin disorders bring with them emotional problems for the family and child. Be sympathetic; remember that the family and child can see the skin condition and need to be reassured that the child is not infectious.

PATHOPHYSIOLOGY ILLUSTRATED

Inflammation (3–5 days)
Clot formation and wound sealing
Increased blood flow to area
Increased capillary permeability, causing swelling
Phagocytosis

Reconstruction (5 days to 4 weeks)
Debridement
Collagen production
Epithelialization with granulation tissue
Capillary budding
Wound contraction

Maturation (Months to Years)
Remodeling
Scar formation and strengthening
Capillary disappearance

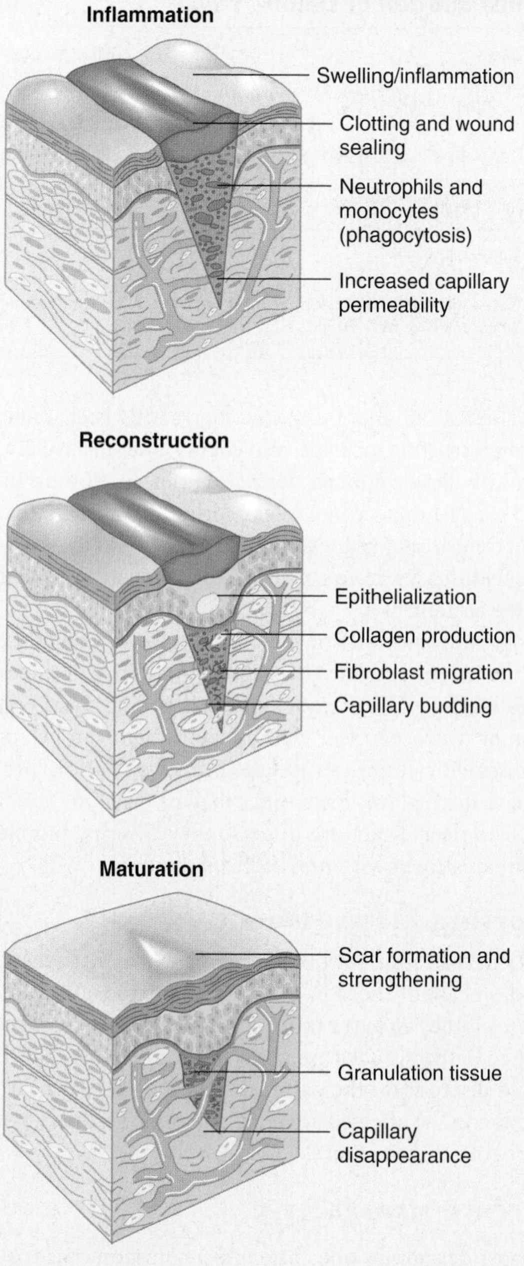

Phases of Wound Healing

FIGURE 23-2 ◆

Based on information in O'Hanlon-Nichols, T. (1995). Commonly asked questions about wound healing. *American Journal of Nursing,* 95 (4), 22–24; and Rote, N. S. (1998). Inflammation. In K. L. McCance & S. E. Huether (Eds.), *Pathophysiology: The basis for disease in adults and children* (3rd ed., pp. 205–236). St. Louis: Mosby.

CONTACT DERMATITIS

Contact dermatitis is an inflammation of the skin that occurs in response to direct contact with an allergen or irritant. Up to 35% of the infant population is affected, most commonly between 9 and 12 months of age (Kazaks & Lane, 2000).

At least 20% of children are at risk for allergic contact dermatitis (Weston & Bruckner, 2000). Generally, repeated or a long-term exposure is required to cause the immune response and the dermatitis. An irritant does not require an immune response. Common allergens include poison ivy, poison oak, lanolin, neomycin, rubber, chemicals in shoe leather, and nickel. Common irritants include soaps, detergents, fabric softeners, bleaches, lotions, urine, and stool. Both irritant and allergic reactions to latex, which can be found in many types of hospital equipment and supplies, as well as in products in the home and community, have been reported (see Chapter 11).

TABLE 23-3 Distribution of Lesions by Type of Allergen

DISTRIBUTION OF LESION	ALLERGEN
Linear	Plant exposure
Ear lobes, neck	Nickel
Dorsal aspects of toes and feet	Rubber or leather chemical in shoes
Face, eyelids	Cosmetics
Subumbilical	Snaps on pants

Note: Adapted from Weston, W. L., & Bruckner, A. (2000). Allergic contact dermatitis. *Pediatric Clinics of North America, 47*(4), 897–907.

CLINICAL TIP

Photodermatitis can result when the child has contact with citrus rinds and juice or fig leaves followed by sun exposure. The child develops erythema and blistering at the site of the exposure that then becomes hyperpigmented. The hyperpigmentation fades over time (Friedlander, 1998)

The rash of allergic contact dermatitis is characterized by erythematous papules with oozing, crusting, pruritis, and edema, and it is usually limited to the area of contact. Symptoms of allergic contact dermatitis can develop up to within 12 to 72 hours after contact, and can last up to 3 to 4 weeks without treatment. In contrast, irritant contact dermatitis is a discrete area of redness that corresponds to the exposure location. The rash usually develops within a few hours of contact, peaks within 24 hours, and quickly resolves with removal of the irritant.

Sweating and friction enhance the absorption of the allergen or irritant. The distribution of the lesions provide clues about the source and identity of the allergen (see Table 23-3). Treatment involves removing the offending agent (e.g., clothes, plant, soap). Calamine lotion or hydrocortisone cream or ointment can be applied to the affected skin. Cool compresses with aluminum acetate (Burrows solution) promote drying. Colloidal oatmeal soaks relieve itching. Antihistamines may be given for a sedative effect when the child is too irritable to sleep. Reactions to poison ivy covering more than 10% of the body surface area require treatment with oral corticosteroids.

Nursing Management

Patient education for home care management focuses on ways to avoid the offending agent and on care of the skin. Advise parents to wash all clothes before the first wearing and to rinse clothes an extra time to remove all soap. Mild soap should be used to clean the skin. When oatmeal soaks are used, caution parents that the tub will be slippery, and to pat the child dry to leave the oatmeal film in place. Familiarize parents with the symptoms of infection in the affected area (e.g., increased redness, oozing, fever) and tell them when to return for follow-up care.

DIAPER DERMATITIS

Diaper dermatitis, one of the most common causes of irritant contact dermatitis, occurs in approximately one-third of young children, usually in a mild form. It is most common in infants from 4 to 12 months of age.

FAMILIES WANT TO KNOW

Exposure to Poison Ivy or Poison Oak

- React quickly after contact. Wash off sap with soap and water and scrub under the nails.
- Do not rub fingers against broken skin or in eyes.
- Avoid hugging a pet exposed to poison ivy until after it has been bathed.
- Launder clothing worn during exposure, and wash hands after handling exposed clothing.
- Wear vinyl gloves to handle plants (cloth and rubber gloves allow sap to penetrate).
- Search the yard and remove all plants. Do not burn the plants. An individual with a sensitivity may inhale the smoke and develop airway inflammation.

Diaper dermatitis is a primary reaction to urine, feces, moisture, or friction. Urine and feces interact to cause dermatitis. The urine increases the wetness and pH of the skin, increasing abrasion and its permeability to irritants and microbes. Fecal organisms provide more irritants. Candida albicans, a secondary infection, is a common complication of diaper dermatitis or antibiotic therapy for another condition. It is frequently the underlying cause of severe diaper rash. Diaper candidiasis often occurs simultaneously with oral candidiasis (see later discussion).

The rash is characterized by erythema, edema, vesicles, papules, and scaling that appear in areas in direct contact with the diaper. Usually the perineum, genitals, and buttocks are affected, and the skin folds are spared. In severe cases, the infant develops a rash that is fiery red, raised, and confluent. Pustules with tenderness can also be present (Figure 23-3 ◆).

Mild diaper dermatitis is treated with a barrier or protective sealant such as zinc oxide, Desitin, or Balmex. Treatment for moderate or severe diaper dermatitis involves application of low potency (0.25% or 0.5%) hydrocortisone cream with each diaper change for 5 to 7 days and good basic hygiene. The cream must be applied before any protective sealant is used. Diaper candidiasis is treated with alternating applications of 1% hydrocortisone cream and antifungal creams (nystatin) applied to the affected areas at diaper change. An oral antifungal agent may be given to clear the candidiasis from the intestines. Fluorinated topical corticosteroids should not be used because of the higher rate of absorption through damaged skin.

CLINICAL TIP

Breast-fed babies have stools with a lower pH, which helps reduce the incidence of diaper rash (Kazaks & Lane, 2000).

Nursing Management

Severe diaper dermatitis can be a major source of stress for parents who must deal with a child in constant discomfort. Instruct parents to change the diaper as soon as the infant is wet, or at least every 2 hours during the day and once during the night.

Encourage parents to use superabsorbent disposable diapers, which tend to reduce the frequency and severity of diaper dermatitis. When wet, these diapers form a gel that keeps the skin drier than cloth diapers. However, this should not be an excuse for waiting until the diaper is saturated to change it. Tell parents to avoid using tight diapers and waterproof pants. A&D ointment, zinc oxide, Desitin, and Balmex can be used to protect the skin from urine and stool.

Advise parents to wash the perianal area with warm water and a mild soap (such as Dove or Tone) or a cleanser not needing water (Acquanil HC lotion or Cetaphil) only after a bowel movement. If baby wipes are preferred, advise parents to use those without alcohol. Cornstarch or zeaSORB powder helps to decrease friction and moisture, but it is important to keep these powders away from the infant's face. Exposing the diaper area to air helps aid healing; for example, allowing the child to go without a diaper, while lying on an absorbable pad or cloth. Observe for signs of infection since the skin is damaged and can allow infectious organisms to grow. If this occurs, additional treatment will be needed.

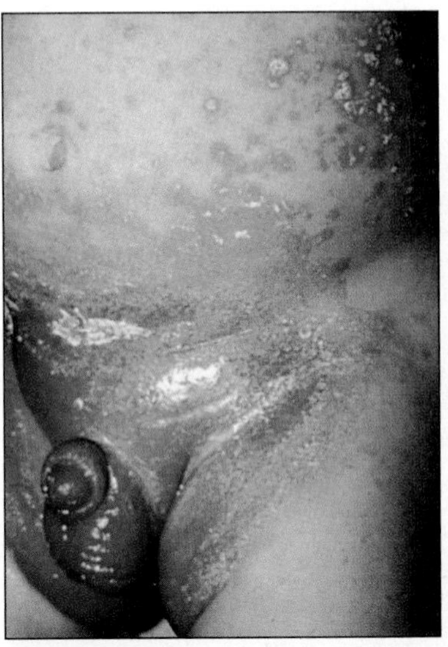

FIGURE 23-3 ◆
Diaper dermatitis.
Courtesy of the Centers for Disease Control, Atlanta, GA.

SEBORRHEIC DERMATITIS

Seborrheic dermatitis is a recurrent inflammatory skin condition thought to be caused by an overgrowth of *Pityrosporum* yeast, commonly found in areas of sebaceous gland activity (Armsmeier & Paller, 1997). The condition is also thought to be influenced by hormones and associated with an oily complexion. The rash is found over the areas of the body where the sebaceous glands are most plentiful: scalp (cradle cap), forehead, and postauricular and periorbital areas. It may also occur on the skin of the eyelids, inguinal area, or nasolabial folds. The condition is frequently seen in infants up to 3 months of age and adolescents.

Common symptoms are pruritus and a mildly erythematous, adherent waxy scaling of the scalp (or "dandruff"). Yellow-red patches with greasy scaling may be present, typically on the scalp and nasolabial folds on the face, behind the ears, on the upper chest, and sometimes the **intertriginous** (skin folds of the neck, axillae, antecubital fossa) areas (Figure 23-4 ◆).

Treatment for seborrheic dermatitis consists of daily shampooing with a medicated shampoo (e.g., Selsun or Head and Shoulders). An emollient is left on the scalp for about 20 minutes to soften the crusts. The scales are removed by brushing with the fingertips or with a baby hairbrush. The hair is then rinsed thoroughly. Lesions on the body can be treated with shampoos containing selenium sulfide or salicylic acid. Use baby shampoo to

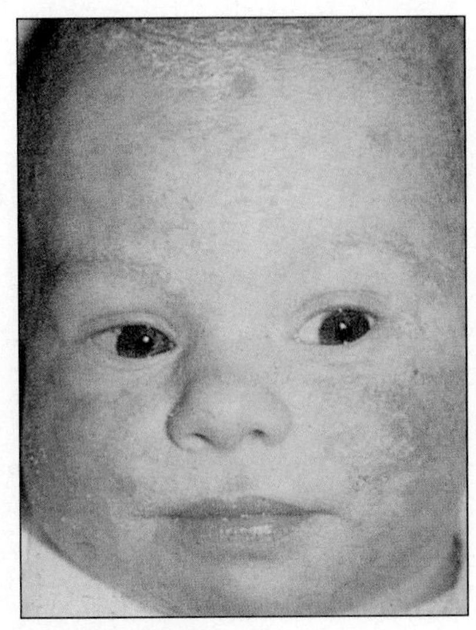

FIGURE 23-4 ◆
Seborrheic dermatitis.

wash lesions on the eyelids and eyelashes. Treatments are continued for several days after the lesions disappear. Topical corticosteriods are used to treat seborrhea that is not on the scalp.

Nursing Management

Seborrheic dermatitis in newborns can often be prevented with proper scalp hygiene. Teach new parents that the infant's hair should be washed regularly with each bath. Reassure parents that gentle cleansing will not harm the infant's "soft spot." Provide a bath demonstration to show them the proper technique, if necessary. Follow-up is seldom necessary, as the condition resolves with treatment. Advise adolescents that emotional distress may trigger future flare-ups and to initiate treatment promptly when symptoms begin.

DRUG REACTIONS

Adverse reactions to over-the-counter or prescription medications are relatively common. Children with drug allergies usually have reactions after ingestion (e.g., aspirin, antibiotics, sedatives), injection (e.g., penicillin), or direct skin contact with medications. Drug sensitivities may result from variations in an individual's ability to tolerate a particular drug or concentration of a drug or from allergic responses. (See Chapter 11 for a description of allergic reactions.)

NURSING ALERT

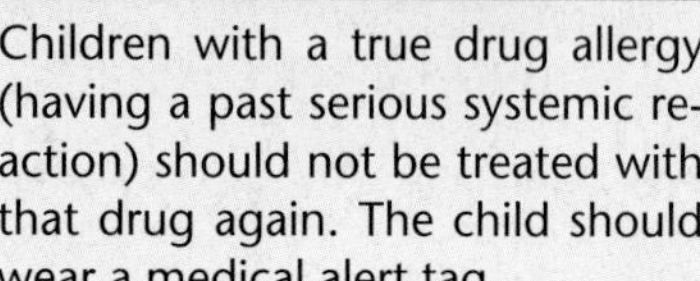

Children with a true drug allergy (having a past serious systemic reaction) should not be treated with that drug again. The child should wear a medical alert tag.

Sensitivity reactions to a drug not previously administered may take up to 7 days to develop. If the child has been sensitized to a drug, the reaction is almost immediate. The most common reactions in children are the development of erythematous macules and papules or urticaria, which may be pruritic. Drugs most likely to cause maculopapular eruptions, urticaria, and pruritis include the following: amoxicillin, ampicillin, cephalosporins, erythromycin, penicillin G, semisynthetic penicillins, sulfamethoxazole, and trimethoprim (Vanderhooft, 1998). Some drug reactions can be life threatening. Be alert to the possibility of serious drug reactions that may become a medical emergency.

The treatment of choice for most drug sensitivity reactions is discontinuation of the causative drug. In some cases, a drug may be continued when the child has a sensitivity reaction because it is the best treatment choice. Supportive measures should be taken to decrease the intensity of the reaction. An antihistamine may be used to block the release of histamine, which causes the rash. Topical corticosteroids, cool compresses, and baths may also be prescribed for pruritis.

Nursing Management

Nurses can play an important role by teaching parents to be alert for the signs of drug sensitivity reactions. Obtain a careful history of the child's past reactions to medications before starting new therapies. If a reaction occurs, discontinue the medication until the physician is notified. Prominently mark the child's records so that all allergies are easily identified.

ECZEMA (ATOPIC DERMATITIS)

Eczema, also called atopic dermatitis, is a chronic, superficial inflammatory skin disorder characterized by intense pruritus. The condition affects infants, children, and adolescents. It is a common skin condition, believed to affect 10% of children. Up to 75% of children who develop the condition do so during the first 6 months of life, and 80% to 90% develop it by 5 years of age (Nicol, 2000). An increasing prevalence has been noted in developed countries that also exhibit an increased rate of asthma, demonstrating the allergic tendency for this condition (Raimer, 2000).

Etiology and Pathophysiology

The etiology of eczema is unknown, but the disorder tends to occur in children with hereditary allergic tendencies (**atopy**). If one parent has allergies (e.g., hay fever, asthma, or contact dermatitis), then the child has a 60% greater chance of having allergies. This chance increases to 80% if both parents have allergies (Nicol, 2000). A family history of asthma or hay fever frequently predisposes a child to eczema. Infantile eczema is more likely to be food induced when the condition is severe (Hebert, Rakes, & Loach, et al., 1997). Several factors exacerbate the condition: triggers (house mites, animal dander, pollens), food allergies, irri-

CLINICAL MANIFESTATION OF DRUG REACTIONS

TYPE OF REACTION	CLINICAL MANIFESTATIONS	CLINICAL THERAPY
Allergic drug reaction	Erythematous macules and papules Pruritis Urticaria, move from one part of body to another	Remove offending drug Topical antipruritics Oral antihistamines Lubricate skin when scaly Systemic corticosteroids if no response to other treatment
Stevens-Johnson syndrome (erythema multiform major) Hypersensitivity reaction to the drug or reaction to an infectious agent	Target lesions coalesce to form large areas of erythema and bullae Fever, malaise Headache, muscle aches, joint pain Itching Cough, coryza, sore throat Vomiting and diarrhea	Remove offending drug Balance intake and output Gentle debridement of crusts Oral antihistamines Topical antipruritics Nutritional support Ophthalmic consultation Corticosteroid use is controversial—may delay wound healing and increase risk of secondary infection or sepsis
Toxic epidermal necrolysis Potential life-threatening hypersensitivity reaction to NSAIDS, sulfa, antibiotics, and anticonvulsants	Rash similar to Stevens-Johnson syndrome Appearance of tender skin, then bullae or erosions occur over more than 20% of body surface area Full-thickness epidermis peels off in sheets	May be cared for in a burn center, see page 889 Debridement of blisters may be performed Gentle cleaning with saline or Burrows solution (aluminum acetate) compresses Topical antibiotic ointment Sterile nonadherent dressings Wounds may be covered with biosynthetic dressing Intensive nutritional support Ophthalmic consultation No corticosteroids No creams with sulfa as this may be the cause of original toxicity
Erythema multiform Hypersensitivity reaction to anticonvulsants, penicillins, salicylates, and sulfa antibiotics	Fixed annular erythematous papules and placques Target lesions with dusky centers, may become bullae Edema	Remove offending drug Oral antihistamines Topical antipruritis Use of corticosteroids are controversial

Note: Adapted from Vanderhooft, S. L. (1998). Is the rash really an adverse drug reaction? *Contemporary Pediatrics, 15*(5), 118–137; and Valencia, I. C., Falabela, A. F., & Schachner, L. A. (2001). New developments in wound care for infants and children. *Pediatric Annals, 30*(4), 211–218.

tants (soaps, detergents, chemicals, solvents, abrasive clothing), hormonal changes, and emotional stress. Increased IgE levels are found in 80% to 85% of patients (Nicol, 2000). See Chapter 11 for a discussion of IgE.

Children with eczema have **xerosis,** generally dry skin that is more likely to crack and fissure. The barrier function of the skin is impaired, leading to increased water loss from the epidermis and decreased elasticity. When the skin is chronically dry, irritants have a greater chance to penetrate, and the child is more susceptible to infection.

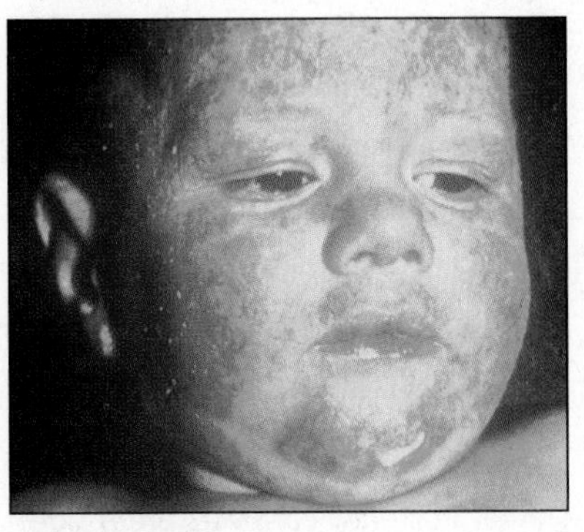
FIGURE 23-5 ◆ Chronic eczema.

Clinical Manifestations

Acute eczema is characterized by pruritus and erythematous patches with vesicles, exudate, and crusts (Figure 23-5 ◆). Subacute eczema is characterized by scaling with erythema and excoriation. There are often postinflammatory pigment changes. Symptoms of chronic eczema are pruritus, dryness, scaling, and lichenification (thickening of the skin with increased visibility of normal skin furrows). Inflammation usually occurs on the face, upper arms, back, upper thighs, and back of the hands and feet.

Eczema occurs in three forms: infantile (ages 2 months to 2 years), childhood (ages 2 years to puberty), and adolescent (puberty and onward).

CLINICAL MANIFESTATIONS OF ECZEMA

TYPE	CLINICAL MANIFESTATIONS	OUTCOME
Infantile (2 months to 2 years)	Exudative, crusty, papulovesicular, and erythematous lesions on cheeks, scalp, forehead, neck, trunk, and extensor surfaces of extremities Intensely pruritic Lichenification after the child can scratch at about 2 months of age	50% of cases resolve by age 2–3 years
Childhood (2 years to puberty)	Erythematous, dry scaly, well-circumscribed, papular, more thickened and lichenified lesions on flexor surfaces of extremities, neck, and retroauricular folds	Subacute and chronic 75% of cases have no recurrence after adolescence
Adolescent (puberty and onward)	Much the same as childhood eczema Large plaques thickened and lichenified on face, neck, back, hands, feet, and upper arms	May recur often as it is primarily a chronic inflammation

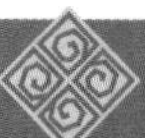

MEDICATIONS USED TO TREAT ECZEMA

■ ***Moisturizing Ointments and Creams for Eczema***

Eucerin cream
Aquaphor ointment
Vanicream
Cetaphil cream
SBR-Lipocream
White petrolatum

CLINICAL TIP

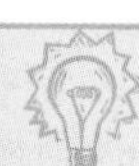

Newer corticosteroid ointments such as fluticasone propionate bind better with the glucocorticoid receptor. This maximizes the penetration and its anti-inflammatory properties. They also have fewer adverse effects (Nicol, 2000).

NURSING ALERT

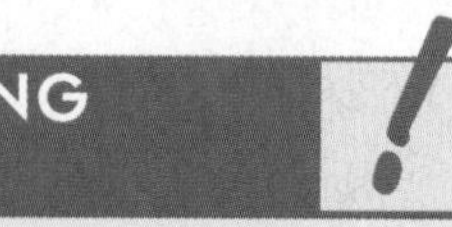

Teach parents to avoid use of topical corticosteroids in the periorbital area. Posterior cataracts are a side effect of this exposure.

Clinical Therapy

Eczema is distinguished from other forms of dermatitis by its history and clinical manifestations. See Table 23-4. No laboratory tests are diagnostic. Eczema is more likely to have a generalized distribution with no known exposure to an allergen.

As there is no cure, the goals of treatment are to hydrate and lubricate the skin, reduce pruritus, minimize inflammatory changes, and try to determine what triggers flare-ups. The cardinal principle of topical therapy for oozing or weeping is "wet on wet." If lesions are weeping, wet compresses (cotton cloths) soaked in aluminum acetate solution sometimes are used. Lubrication is achieved by applying occlusive topical ointment after bathing to trap moisture and prevent drying of the skin. Moisturizing ointments and creams should be applied 3 to 4 times a day or whenever the skin feels dry.

Topical corticosteroids are used to reduce inflammation. Ointments are preferred over creams because of their occlusive effect, which ensures a stronger barrier and absorption into the skin. Hydrocortisone 1% to 2.5% or triamcinolone 0.1% is usually the drug of choice. Corticosteroids are used twice daily for 2 weeks and must be applied before the skin moisturizer is used. Lower potency ointments are used for thinner skin areas, such as the face and skin folds. A higher potency ointment is used for flare-ups, with tapering to lower potency as the dermatitis improves. When the dermatitis resolves, only moisturizers are used. Steroids are not used on healthy skin. Oral corticosteroids may be used for an acute exacerbation; however, there is often a rebound effect (i.e., after the medication is discontinued, the rash returns). Systemic antibiotics are given only if the child has a superimposed infection.

Antihistamine agents such as hydroxyzine (Vistaril and Atarax) can be given to relieve itching at night. Nonsedating antihistamine agents have a limited effect on itching. Methods to reduce pruritus include environmental controls, such as humidification in the winter and air conditioning in the summer. Use of a humidifier counteracts dryness of the

TABLE 23-4 Diagnostic Criteria for Eczema (Atopic Dermatitis)

Itching skin condition with three additional factors from the following list:

- History of flexural dermatitis (knees, ankles, neck, or cheeks) if less than 4 years old
- History of asthma or hay fever in a child, or in a first-degree relative, if less than 4 years old
- History of dry skin in past year
- Skin rash occurring before 2 years of age
- Visible flexural dermatitis; dermatitis on cheeks, forehead, and outer limbs if less than 4 years old

Note: Adapted from Raimer, S.S. (2000). Managing pediatric atopic dermatitis. *Clinical Pediatrics, 39*(1), 1–14.

surrounding air, minimizing loss of skin moisture. Air conditioning limits unnecessary sweating that can exacerbate inflamed areas.

Because of the high rate of food allergies in infants under 2 years of age, a food elimination test may be suggested for infants and young children with moderate to severe eczema needing daily treatment. Milk, wheat, eggs, soy products, citrus, and peanuts are the foods most often withheld for 2 or more weeks to determine if any change in skin condition occurs. Foods withheld are then introduced one at a time to determine which ones are the allergens. A radioallergosorbent test (RAST) is sometimes used to exclude allergens (see Chapter 11).

NURSING MANAGEMENT

Nursing Assessment and Diagnosis

A thorough history, including any family history of allergy, environmental or dietary factors, and past exacerbations, is necessary. Note distribution and type of lesions.

Common nursing diagnoses that may be appropriate for the child with eczema include the following:

- *Impaired tissue integrity,* related to chemical irritants and mechanical factors (abrasive clothing)
- *Sleep deprivation,* related to prolonged physical discomfort (itching)
- *Risk for infection,* related to breaks in skin barrier
- *Self-esteem disturbance,* related to chronic illness and peer reaction to visible skin lesions
- *Ineffective management of therapeutic regimen (families),* related to excessive demands made on the family to keep the condition under control.

Planning and Implementation

Nursing management focuses on education and emotional support. Although no cure has been found for eczema, the condition can be controlled. Advise parents that the lesions are not contagious and will not result in scarring. Help parents and adolescents deal with the frustration of the acute flare-ups of the condition by reinforcing that remissions do occur with good home care.

Instruct parents or adolescents to avoid using harsh or perfumed soaps. Use a mild soap such as Dove or Tone, but only where the skin is dirty. Washing clean skin with soap only dries it out. Use wet wraps for severely affected skin to replace moisture. Hot water can exacerbate the condition and increase itching. Recommend tepid baths and patting dry or air-drying afterward. Moisturizers should be applied within 3 minutes of exiting the bath to help retain moisture. This should be performed once or twice daily. Wool clothing should be avoided because it can increase skin irritation and pruritus. Encourage the wearing of loose cotton clothing.

Teach parents and adolescents appropriate application of topical ointments or creams. Instruct parents to place clean cotton gloves or socks over the infant or young child's hands and to keep the child's fingernails cut short to decrease scratching and reduce the chance of secondary infection.

Eczema produces visible changes that can affect a child's self-confidence and self-esteem. Children need to be educated about the disorder and its treatment. Emphasize the importance of following the treatment plan to promote healing of existing lesions and to reduce the risk of secondary infections. Eczema that is difficult to manage is more stressful and has a more profound effect on the child's and family's quality of life than diabetes mellitus (Su, Kemp, & Varigos, et al., 1997).

Once the condition is under control, counsel the parents about the method for introducing a food that was previously eliminated when an allergen cause of eczema was suspected (see Chapter 11). Emphasize that increased itching within hours of eating a food may be associated with the eczema flare-up. Teach parents how to control the skin inflammation that results, as previously described. Once a specific food allergy has been identified, refer

CLINICAL TIP

Wet occlusive dressings increase penetration of corticosteroid ointments and help decrease itching. Apply the topical ointment and then wrap the child in a wet towel for 10 minutes, then reapply the topical ointment followed by an emollient (Raimer, 2000).

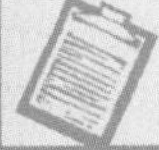

RESEARCH

A study of the effectiveness of massage in treating eczema showed positive benefit for the child and parent. Daily massage of the child for 20 minutes over 1 month resulted in improvements in redness, scaling, lichenification, excoriation, and pruritis. The child's activity level and disposition also improved. Parents doing the massage reported decreased anxiety (Schachner, Field, & Hernandez-Ruif, et al., 1998).

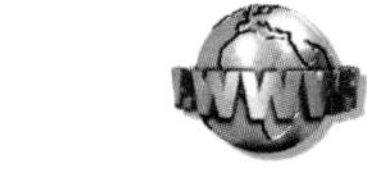

Eczema Resources

the parents to a nutritionist for counseling related to alternative food options that will fulfill daily nutritional requirements. Caution parents that food allergies can change, so foods connected with eczema can sometimes be safely eaten at a later time. Different food sensitivities may also develop. Refer the family to the Food Allergy Network.

Evaluation

Expected outcomes of nursing care include the following:

- Control of the child's eczema is maintained and no infection occurs.
- Parents identify triggers of the child's eczema and avoid or eliminate them.
- The child's sleep is minimally disturbed by itching.

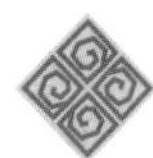

ACNE

Acne is an inflammatory disorder of the sebaceous hair follicles located on the face and trunk. It is the most common skin disorder in the pediatric population. It is believed to be triggered by the increased androgen production of puberty and the overproduction of sebum. The prevalence in adolescents aged 12–15 is estimated to approach 85% (Sidbury & Paller, 2000). The condition is often more severe in the winter. Acne may also occur in neonates in response to maternal androgen hormones. This form of acne usually develops between 2 and 4 weeks of age and resolves by 4 to 6 months.

ETIOLOGY AND PATHOPHYSIOLOGY

Acne is caused by the interaction of several factors: an overgrowth of residential bacteria on the skin, increased sebum production, and abnormal follicular skin cell shedding that is more adherent than normal. The extra sebum caused by androgen secretion mixes with the shed skin cells and causes them to clump together. The keratin and sebum that usually flow to the skin surface are obstructed in the follicular canal, causing comedones (whiteheads and blackheads). The sebum behind the comedone is an ideal environment for the anerobic *Propionibacterium* acnes, and this bacterium metabolizes the sebum causing an inflammatory reaction. When the inflammatory reaction is close to the surface, a papule or pustule develops. If the inflammatory reaction is deeper, a larger papule or nodule develops. Although familial trends are recognized, hard data to define a pattern of inheritance are not conclusive.

CLINICAL TIP

Medications associated with the appearance of acne lesions include corticosteroids, barbiturates, phenytoin, lithium, isoniazid, and cyclosporin.

CLINICAL MANIFESTATIONS

The three main types of acne are comedomal (characterized by open and closed comedones), papulopustular (characterized by papules and pustules) (Figure 23-6 ◆), and cystic (characterized by nodules and cysts). Lesions occur most often on the face, upper chest, shoulders, and back.

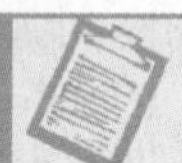

CLINICAL TIP

Increasing numbers of cases of bacterial resistance to antibiotics have been noted. A recurrence or flare-up of acne after control has been achieved may be an indication that the bacteria has developed resistance to the antibiotic.

CLINICAL THERAPY

Diagnosis is based on examination of the skin. The severity of skin lesions is graded, and treatment is customized to the severity level (see Table 23-5).

Treatment depends on the type of lesion. Most adolescent acne is treated with topical and oral medications, alone or in combination. The goal of treatment is to suppress lesions until the condition is outgrown, thus preventing infection, scarring, and minimizing psychologic distress. Gels and liquids prescribed to dry the skin, and dryness and scaling, are typical after several days of treatment. The initial response may look like the condition is worsening for the first 1 to 3 weeks of treatment (Sidbury & Paller, 2000).

Isotretinoin (Accutane) is reserved for the most serious cases of acne because of its teratogenicity. Patients started on isotretinoin need two negative pregnancy tests and a monthly pregnancy test. A 1-month supply is provided to promote compliance. In addition, two forms of contraception must be used when taking isotretinoin (Buck, 2001). Oral contraceptives with norgestimate and ethinyl estradiol are FDA approved for the treatment of acne (Sidbury & Paller, 2000).

RESEARCH

A recent study examining the association between isotretinoin (accutane) and mental health problems found no increased risk for depression, suicide, or other psychological problems (Jick, Kremers, & Vasilakis-Scaramozza, 2000).

TABLE 23-5 Treatment Protocols for Acne

APPEARANCE	TREATMENT
Grade I Comedomal acne	Tretinoin (Retin-A) 0.025% cream daily, in the (comedones only) evening, salicylic acid, adapalene, tazarotene)
Grade II Papulopustular acne (red papules, pustules)	2.5% benzoyl peroxide gel, Tretinoin (Retin-A) in evening, topical clindamycin and erythromycin, topical tetracycline, acaleic acid cream twice a day.
Grade III Cystic acne (red papules, many pustules, cysts)	Tretinoin (Retin-A) and benzoyl peroxide twice a day, with oral antibiotics (tetracycline, minocycline, or doxycline)
Grade IV Pustulocystic nodular (severe, resistant to other treatment)	Isotretinoin (Accutane)

Note: Adapted from Sidbury, R., & Paller, A.S. (2000). The diagnosis and management of acne. *Pediatric Annals, 29*(1), 17–24.

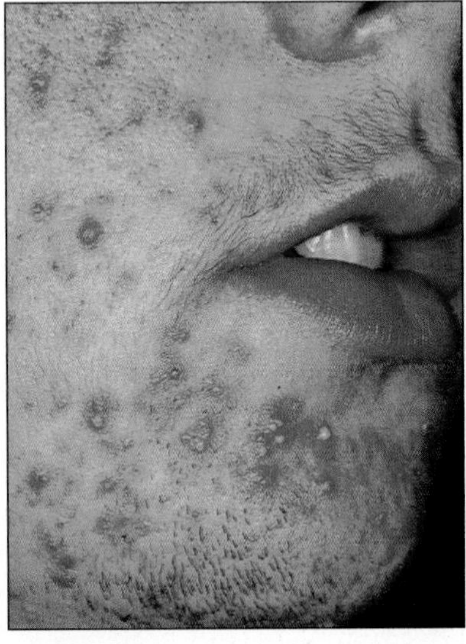

FIGURE 23-6 ◆ Pustular acne can have a significant effect on an adolescent's self-esteem. From Habif, T. P. (1990). *Clinical dermatology: A color guide to diagnosis and therapy* (2nd ed., p. 113). St. Louis: Mosby-Year Book.

NURSING MANAGEMENT

Nursing Assessment and Diagnosis

Physical assessment should include documentation regarding distribution, type, and severity of acne lesions. Assess the adolescent's and parents' knowledge about the cause and treatment of acne. Also explore the amount of emotional distress the acne is causing the adolescent.

Common nursing diagnoses are presented in the accompanying nursing care plan.

Planning and Implementation

Nursing care for the adolescent with acne is summarized in the accompanying nursing care plan. Nursing management focuses on educating the child and parents about acne and its treatment. Advise adolescents not to touch the affected areas and to avoid picking or squeezing the lesions. Remind them that the inflammation occurs with the rupture of lesions below the skin surface, which picking and squeezing may cause. In addition, advise them to avoid using any cleansing products that have a greasy base, to shampoo hair regularly (to treat seborrhea that can accompany acne), to expect flare-ups despite treatment, and to eat a well-balanced diet.

Instruct adolescents to wash the face no more than 2 to 3 times a day with a mild soap, then wait about 20 to 30 minutes before applying tretinoin (Retin-A), if prescribed. Topical

FAMILIES WANT TO KNOW

Caring for Acne

- Avoid picking and squeezing pimples.
- Avoid hats or gear that can cause friction and occlusion of the skin.
- Greasy foods may leave a residual oil on the face and hands that can be occlusive.
- Avoid touching the face.
- Limit the use of pomades or petrolatum-based hair products.
- Use noncomedonic sunscreen and emollients for the skin.
- Use oil-free or water-based makeup.
- Use sunscreen even on cloudy days.

NURSING CARE PLAN The Adolescent with Acne

GOAL	INTERVENTION	RATIONALE	EXPECTED OUTCOME
1. Management of Therapeutic Regimen: Individual, Effective			
	NIC Priority Intervention: **Anticipatory Guidance:** Preparation of patient for an anticipated developmental and/or situational crisis.		NOC Suggested Outcome: **Symptom Control Behavior:** Personal actions to minimize perceived adverse changes in physical and emotional functioning.
The adolescent will verbalize proper hygiene, nutrition, and treatment of acne.	■ Teach good skin care: ■ Wash skin with mild soap and water twice a day. ■ Do not use astringents. ■ Avoid vigorous scrubbing.	■ Good hygiene and appropriate skin care reduce surface oils and bacteria, which intensify inflammatory reactions.	The adolescent exhibits habits of good hygiene.
	■ Praise good habits.	■ Positive reinforcement encourages continued effort.	
	■ Advise the adolescent to wash hair with antiseborrheic shampoo, avoid oil-based cosmetics or lotions.	■ Treats seborrhea, which frequently accompanies acne. Oil-based preparations can obstruct sebaceous glands, exacerbating acne.	
	■ Encourage a balanced diet, adequate fluids, exercise, and adequate rest.	■ Adequate nutrients, water, and exercise promote healthy skin.	
	■ Encourage the adolescent to keep a diary of health and diet habits.	■ A record may help identify associations with flare-ups that can be avoided in the future.	
The adolescent will verbalize understanding of treatment regimen.	■ Educate the adolescent about medications (action, side effects, dosage, method of application).	■ Proper application of medication enhances healing of lesions.	The adolescent implements the treatment regimen as outlined, resulting in a noticeable reduction in lesions.
	■ Encourage application of tretinoin at night. Encourage use of nonoil sunscreens of at least SPF 15.	■ Helps reduce sensitivity to sun and avoid sunburn.	
	■ Educate the adolescent about time needed for response and importance of daily compliance.	■ May take up to 3 months for significant improvement to occur. The adolescent needs a reason to continue with the care plan.	
2. Body Image Disturbance related to biophysical factors (visible facial lesions)			
	NIC Priority Intervention: **Body Image Enhancement:** Improving a patient's conscious and unconscious perceptions and attitudes toward his/her body.		NOC Suggested Outcome: **Self-Esteem:** Personal judgment of self-worth.
The adolescent will demonstrate increased self-confidence and self-esteem.	■ Establish a rapport with the adolescent.	■ A trusting relationship promotes verbalization of concerns and fears.	The adolescent freely discusses concerns and fears.
	■ Provide education about the condition and therapy modalities.	■ Providing information better enables the adolescent to take control of the condition.	The adolescent demonstrates active involvement in own care.
	■ Encourage the adolescent to be responsible for treatment and follow-up, and give positive reinforcement.	■ Responsibility reinforces sense of self-esteem.	
	■ Encourage the adolescent to become involved with school activities and peers.	■ Involvement in activities helps enhance self-esteem and allows the adolescent to explore new experiences and friendships.	The adolescent shows increased confidence, as demonstrated by involvement in extracurricular activities.

medications should be spread in a thin film over the skin, according to directions. Emphasize that treatment is often long term. Significant improvement may not be seen until at least 6 to 12 weeks after the start of treatment.

Correct misconceptions about dietary causes. Although no food has been found to cause acne or an increase in severity of lesions, good nutrition is important. Teach parents and children that increased sweating, as well as heat and humidity, may exacerbate acne. Emotional stress may increase adrenal androgen production, resulting in increased sebum production and acne flare-ups.

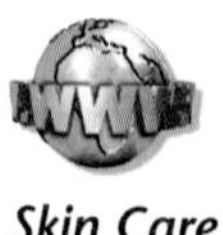

Skin Care

Caution patients who are using tretinoin that this medication is **phototoxic** (causes a rapid nonimmunologic reaction of the skin when exposed to sunlight), resulting in sunburn with even minimal exposure. Teach correct procedures for taking other prescribed drugs, such as tetracycline and isotretinoin (Accutane), and discuss possible side effects. Emphasize the importance of return visits to the adolescent's health care provider to monitor side effects of medications.

Psychologic support is an important aspect of care. Because adolescents are preoccupied with their body image and peer relationships, they often find having acne embarrassing. Encourage them to express their feelings and refer for counseling, if necessary.

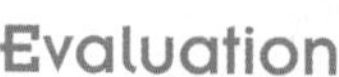

Evaluation

Expected outcomes of nursing care can be found on the accompanying nursing care plan.

INFECTIOUS DISORDERS

IMPETIGO

Impetigo is a highly contagious, superficial (epidermal) infection caused by streptococci, staphylococci, or both. The most common sites are the face, around the mouth, the hands, the neck, and the extremities. It is the most common bacterial skin condition in children and accounts for nearly 10% of all skin problems (Darmstadt, 1997).

Minor skin abrasions, lacerations, insect bites, burns, and dermatitis provide the portal for the infectious agent commonly present in the environment. Group A beta-hemolytic *Streptococcus* and *Staphylococcus aureus* are usually responsible. This infection occurs more commonly in children who are in close physical contact with others, such as in child care settings, or who have poor hygiene.

Clinical manifestations include a lesion, pruritus, and regional lymphadenopathy. There is little erythema. The lesion begins as a vesicle or pustule that is surrounded by edema and redness, usually at a site that has been injured. This progresses to an exudative and crusting stage. The initially serous vesicular fluid becomes cloudy, and the vesicle ruptures, leaving a honey-colored crust covering an ulcerated base (Figure 23-7 ◆). Common sites include the **intertriginous** areas. The rash may spread to the face and extremities by self-innoculation. Less commonly, bullous impetigo develops in which the vesicles enlarge into bullae with straw-colored fluid and then rupture. A moist, erythematous erosion with a collar of skin around the erosion is seen in this localized scalded skin syndrome.

CLINICAL TIP

If the child has a history of recurrent impetigo, determine if an individual who is in contact with the child is a nasal carrier of *Staphylococcus aureus.* The carrier can be effectively treated with topical mupiricin ointment applied to the nares 4 times daily (Mancini, 2000).

Impetigo is diagnosed by a Gram stain and bacterial culture. Local treatment involves removal of the crusts and application of a topical antibiotic. Crusts are soaked in warm water and gently scrubbed off with an antiseptic soap. A topical bactericidal ointment (such as bacitracin or mupirocin) is applied for 5 to 7 days. If there is no response to topical antibiotics, a systemic antibiotic (e.g., dicloxacillin or erythromycin) may be needed. The infection is communicable for 48 hours after antibiotic ointment treatment is begun.

Nursing Management

Advise parents that oral or topical medications must be continued for the full number of days prescribed. Tell the parents to observe all close contacts and family members for lesions. Caution parents that an infected child should not share towels or toiletries with others and that all linens and clothing used by the child should be washed separately with detergent in hot water. Fingernails should be kept short and clean to prevent the spread of infection from scratching.

CLINICAL TIP

Inform the child care center about the child's infection, so toys and surfaces can be sanitized.

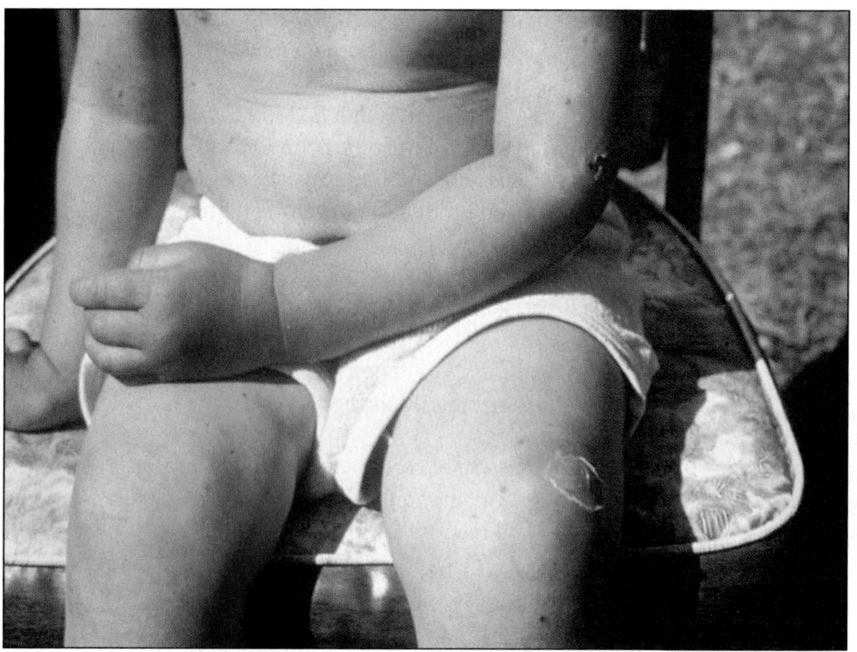

FIGURE 23-7 ◆
Characteristic lesions of impetigo.
Courtesy of the Centers for Disease Control, Atlanta, GA.

FOLLICULITIS

Folliculitis is a superficial inflammation of the pilosebaceous follicle caused by infection, trauma, or irritation. The causative organism is usually *Staphylococcus aureus.* The condition is common in children and teenagers because of increased sweat production. Folliculitis may be associated with *Pseudomonas* exposure in a poorly chlorinated pool or hot tub.

Symptoms include tenderness, localized swelling, and the formation of tiny dome-shaped, yellowish pustules and red papules at follicular openings with surrounding erythema. Individual lesions may become deeper and form an abscess (furuncle). Lesions are usually seen in clusters on the face, scalp, trunk, and extremities. Ruptured lesions heal with hyperpigmentation and no scarring.

Treatment of inflamed follicles consists of washing the affected area with a topical antibiotic cleanser and water, followed by application of hot compresses for 20 minutes, 4 times a day. Complications are rare. If lesions do not resolve within 1 week, the child may need systemic antibiotics (e.g., cephalexin or dicloxacillin) and, if the infection is deep, incision and drainage.

Nursing Management

Nursing management focuses on educating the parents and child about prevention. Advise children to shower daily and shortly after exercise, to cleanse with an antibacterial soap, and to wear loose cotton clothing.

CELLULITIS

Cellulitis is an acute inflammation of the dermis and underlying connective tissue characterized by red or lilac, tender, warm, edematous skin that may have an ill-defined, nonelevated border. The condition usually occurs on the face and extremities as a result of trauma or compromise of the skin barrier.

Etiology and Pathophysiology

Children with cellulitis often have a history of trauma, impetigo, folliculitis, or recent otitis media. Common causative organisms are *Staphylococcus aureus, Streptococcus pneumoniae, Hemophilus influenza,* and beta-hemolytic and group A *Streptococcus.* The condition may also result from a nearby abscess or sinusitis. Onset is usually rapid.

Clinical Manifestations

Children with cellulitis have a rapid onset and they appear ill. Classic signs and symptoms include erythema, edema of the face or infected limb, warmth, and tenderness around the infected site (Figure 23-8 ◆). Other symptoms include fever, chills, malaise, and enlargement and tenderness of regional lymph nodes. In some cases, a rapidly progressive lesion may result in septicemia.

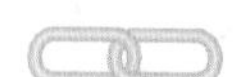

Skill 6-5: Obtaining a Blood Culture

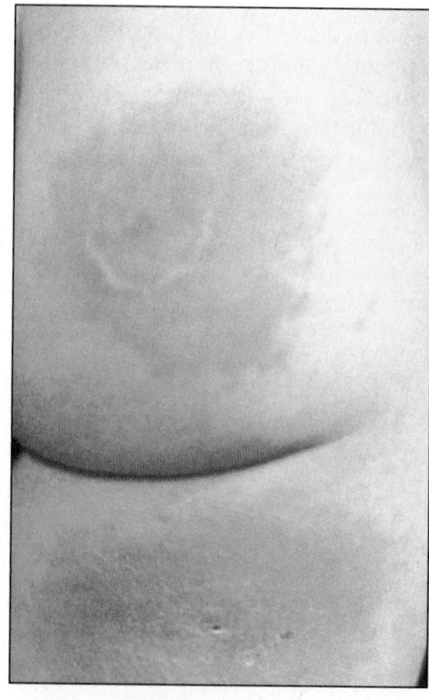

FIGURE 23-8 ◆
Characteristic appearance of cellulitis.
From Ben-Amitai, D., & Ashkenazi, S. (1993). Common bacterial skin infections in children. *Pediatric Annals, 22*(4), 226. Photograph courtesy of Dr. Aryeh Metzker.

Clinical Therapy

Blood studies may show an increase in white blood cells. Cultures are taken by needle aspiration, if possible, to identify the causative organisms. Blood cultures are taken if the child has a toxic (very ill) appearance. If the face is involved, antibiotic therapy is administered to avoid serious complications. (Periorbital cellulitis is discussed in Chapter 19.)

Children with cellulitis on the trunk, limbs, or perianal area may be treated on an outpatient basis with oral antibiotics. Recovery begins within 48 hours, but therapy should continue for at least 10 days.

Children with severe cases or a large affected surface area are hospitalized to prevent sepsis. Systemic antibiotics and analgesics are administered. Untreated cellulitis or cellulitis that does not respond to treatment can lead to osteomyelitis, arthritis, or serious systemic infection.

NURSING MANAGEMENT

Nursing Assessment and Diagnosis

Assessment centers on recognition of infection, documentation of location and related symptoms, and monitoring of vital signs.

The following nursing diagnoses may be appropriate for the child with cellulitis:

- *Impaired skin integrity,* related to mechanical factors (injury, the inflammatory process, and presence of infection)
- *Pain,* related to injury agents (swelling and inflammation of the skin)
- *Parental role conflict,* related to home care needs of child with special needs

Planning and Implementation

Because of the risk of sepsis, cellulitis should be managed carefully. Administer prescribed antibiotics. Supportive care includes warm compresses to the affected area 4 times daily, elevation of the affected limb, and bed rest. Outpatient follow-up is crucial.

Advise parents about possible complications, such as abcess formation. Instruct parents of children who are treated at home to contact their health care provider if the child displays any of the following:

- Spread of the infected area in the 24- to 48-hour period after the start of treatment
- Temperature over 38.3°C (101°F)
- Increased lethargy

Reinforce to parents the importance of compliance with the treatment regimen and the seriousness associated with complications.

Evaluation

Expected outcomes of nursing care include pain control, compliance with administration of antibiotics, and resolution of the infection without progression to systemic infection.

PEDICULOSIS CAPITIS (LICE)

Pediculosis capitis is an infestation of the hair and scalp with lice. Head lice live and reproduce only on humans and are transmitted by direct hair-to-hair contact or indirect contact such as sharing of hair accessories, brushes, hats, towels, and bedding. Lice do not fly or

CLINICAL TIP

Instruct parents that children infested with lice should not return to childcare or school until after the first pediculicide treatment is completed. Parents of other children exposed to the infected child should be notified so they can watch for signs of infestation.

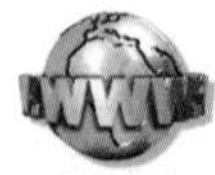

Head Lice Education

NURSING ALERT

Use of an insecticide in the home to kill the lice on carpets, furniture, and other items with which young children and pets come into contact is not recommended.

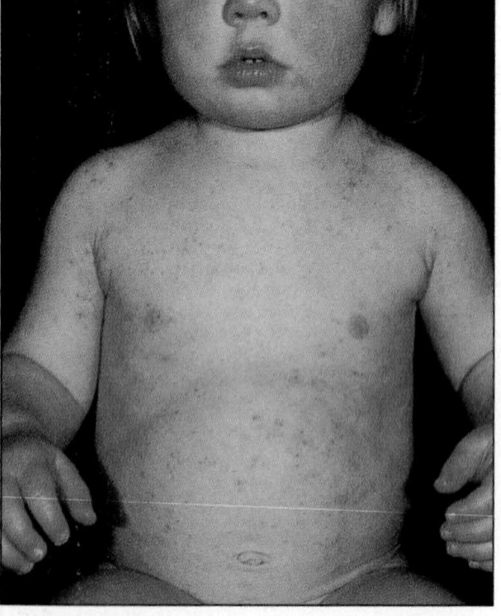

FIGURE 23-9 ◆
Diffuse scabies in an infant. The lesions are most numerous around the axillae, chest, and abdomen.
From Habif, T. P. (1990). *Clinical dermatology: A color guide to diagnosis and therapy* (2nd ed., p. 298). St. Louis: Mosby-Year Book.

jump, but they can crawl quickly. The female louse lays her eggs (nits) on the hair shaft, close to the scalp (see Figure 4–10). The incubation period is 8 to 10 days. Children between 3 and 10 years are most often affected.

Infestation occurs among children of all socioeconomic levels. The presence of lice may be noted by parents or teachers, or by health care providers during routine examination of the child (see Chapter 4). Outbreaks occur periodically among preschool and school-age children, particularly those in childcare and elementary school.

Clinical manifestations include intense pruritus and complaints of "dandruff" that sticks to the hair (actually the nits) and "bugs" in the hair. Nits look like silvery white 1-mm teardrops adhering to one side of the hair shaft. Secondary effects of scratching include inflammation, pustules, and bacterial infection. Nits are found most commonly behind the ears and at the base of the head. Lice move quickly away from light and are not commonly seen. Posterior cervical nodes are frequently palpable.

Treatment involves the use of a pediculicide shampoo, such as pyrethrum with an enzymatic lice egg remover, or an ovicidal rinse, such as permethrin (Nix). Permethrin resistance has been reported, but a 5% concentration is effective. An alternate therapy is malathion (ovide); however, problem's involve flammability, odor, and higher cost. Lindane shampoo is not recommended because of lice resistance and toxicity (Angel, Nigro, & Levy, 2000).

Permethrin cream rinse is applied to washed and towel-dried hair. The preparation is applied, left in place for 10 minutes, and then rinsed. The hair is towel dried, and the nits are removed with a fine-toothed comb. Distilled white vinegar or an over-the-counter formic acid solution helps loosen the nit's bond to the hair shaft. A second treatment is needed in 7 days.

Nursing Management

Carefully assess children who have been exposed to head lice (see Chapter 4). To avoid potential reinfestation of other children, change gloves frequently when assessing several children in a classroom setting.

Infestation with lice can be upsetting for both the child and family. Emphasize to the family that anyone can get lice. Thorough interventions and education are essential for effective treatment. All contacts of the child should be examined for infestation and should be treated as necessary. Teach the child not to share clothing, headwear, or combs.

Explain to parents that the shampoo and rinses prescribed are pesticides and must be used as directed. Keep these products out of the eyes and mouth of the child during their use. When combing the hair to remove nits, a creme rinse or oil may make the combing easier. Comb 1-in. sections from the scalp outward and pin these out of the way when done. All nits should be removed. Put the child under a bright light and use techniques such as a video to keep the child entertained during the procedure.

Although lice can survive for only about 3 days away from a human host, nits that are shed are capable of hatching 8 to 10 days later. For this reason, bedding and clothing used by the child should be changed daily, laundered in hot water with detergent, and dried in a hot dryer for 20 minutes. Nonessential bedding and clothing can be stored in a tightly sealed bag for 2 to 3 weeks and then washed. Hair accessories, brushes, and combs should be discarded or soaked in hot soapy water (54.4°C [130°F]). Furniture and carpets should be vacuumed and treated with a hot iron when possible. Seal toys and other personal items that cannot be washed or dry cleaned in a plastic bag for 2 weeks.

SCABIES

Scabies is a highly contagious infestation caused by the mite *Sarcoptes scabiei.* It is spread by skin-to-skin contact. Children of all ages and both sexes can be affected. The highest prevalence is in children under 2 years of age (Angel et al., 2000).

The female mite burrows into the outer layer of the epidermis (stratum corneum) to lay her eggs, leaving a trail of debris and feces. The larvae hatch in approximately 2 to 4 days and proceed toward the surface of the skin. The cycle is repeated 14 to 17 days later. The irritation and intense pruritus is caused by hypersensitivity to the ova and mite feces, which occurs approximately 1 month after infestation. Nodules, which can persist for weeks after effective treatment, develop as a granulomatous response to the dead mite antigens and feces. Because the mite usually takes at least 45 minutes to burrow into the skin, transient contact is unlikely to cause infestation.

Symptoms include a rash with various types of lesions, severe pruritus that worsens at night, and restlessness. Lesions are usually located in the webs of the fingers, in the intergluteal folds, around the axillae, or on the palms, wrists, head, neck, legs, buttocks, chest, abdomen, and waist (Figure 23-9 ◆). In infants the palms, insteps of the feet, and scalp and face can be affected. Lesions appear as linear, threadlike, grayish burrows 1 cm to 10 cm in length, which may end in a pinpoint vesicle. The lesion may have been obliterated by the child's scratching and secondary infection.

Diagnosis is confirmed by examination under the microscope of scrapings from a burrow, which reveals actively moving mites, fecal pellets, and eggs or nits. Treatment involves application of a scabicide, such as 5% permethrin lotion, over the entire body from the chin down. Apply scabicide only to the scalp and forehead of infants. The lotion can be applied to the face of older children if lesions are present.

Application of 5% permethrin lotion or malathion (ovide) is preceded by a warm soap and water bath. Skin must be cool and dry before the lotion is applied. The lotion is left in place for 8 to 12 hours (overnight) before washing it off. A second treatment is used 1 week later. All members of the household and child care contacts should be treated at the same time, even if not symptomatic. Itching may persist for 1 to 2 weeks after treatment. An oral antihistamine (e.g., Benadryl, Atarax) may be prescribed to help relieve itching.

NURSING ALERT

Lindane is no longer recommended for full-body application in infants and young children because of toxicity (Angel et al., 2000)

Nursing Management

Advise parents that scabies is transmitted by close contact and is highly contagious. All clothing, bedding, and pillowcases used by the child should be changed daily, washed with hot water, and ironed before reuse. Nonwashable toys and other items should be sealed in plastic bags for 5 to 7 days.

Family members who are not infected should avoid touching the affected child until after treatment is completed. If contact is made, hands should be washed well. Inform the parents about signs of secondary infections and that itching and nodules may persist for weeks after effective treatment.

Scabies, like pediculosis, can be embarrassing or upsetting for the child and family. Educate them about the condition, its spread, and treatment measures to prevent recurrence.

GROWTH & DEVELOPMENT

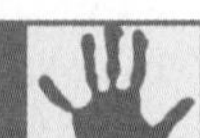

Precipitated sulfur in petrolatum for 3 successive nights is used to treat scabies in infants under 2 months of age who should not be exposed to the more toxic scabicide lotions (Metry & Hebert, 2000). It is malodorous, messy, and stains the bedding and clothing, so parents do not like using it.

FUNGAL INFECTIONS

Oral Candidiasis (Thrush)

Oral candidiasis (moniliasis or thrush) is a fungal infection that occurs as an acute condition in newborns (usually acquired during birth from the vaginal canal of an infected mother) and a chronic condition in young children who have an immune disorder, regularly use a corticosteroid inhaler, or are receiving antibiotics, which have disturbed the normal flora, allowing the growth of the fungus.

Thrush is characterized by white patches that resemble coagulated milk on the oral mucosa and may bleed when removed (Figure 23-10 ◆). The infant may refuse to nurse or feed because of discomfort and pain. The infant may also have diaper dermatitis superinfection with candidiasis. Fever is usually not present.

Treatment involves oral nystatin suspension, which is applied to the mouth and tongue after feedings. For infants, parents should use a swab to apply the suspension to the buccal mucosa and tongue surfaces, allowing the infant to swallow the remaining suspension. Older children are instructed to swish the solution around in the mouth before swallowing.

CLINICAL TIP

The white patches of candidiasis are easily differentiated from coagulated milk. Milk residue can be removed from the oral mucosa with gentle swabbing. With candidiasis, however, attempts at gentle removal are unsuccessful. (Avoid scraping the patches, as this will result in bleeding.)

If infection is severe, occurs in the esophagus, or invades other body systems, oral fluconazole or intravenous amphotericin B may be prescribed.

NURSING MANAGEMENT To prevent a reinfection, educate parents about the appropriate sterilization technique for bottle nipples and pacifiers the infant puts in the mouth. A commercial antiseptic spray may be used on toys that cannot be autoclaved, but follow directions carefully so the child does not ingest any harmful residue. Teach parents and older children with asthma to rinse the mouth well with water after using a corticosteroid inhaler to prevent candidiasis. If the child uses a spacer, that should also be rinsed with water after use.

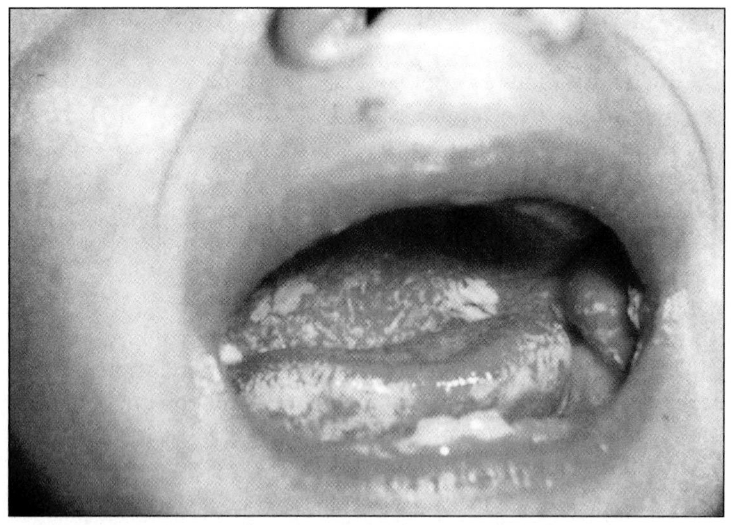

FIGURE 23-10 ◆
Thrush, an acute pseudomembranous form of oral candidiasis, is a common fungal infection in infants and children. From Zitelli, B. J., and Davis H. W. (Eds.). (1997). *Atlas of Pediatric Physical Diagnosis* (3rd ed., p. 104). St. Louis, MO: Mosby, Inc.

Dermatophytoses (Ringworm)

Dermatophytoses are fungal infections that affect the skin, hair, or nails. Children of all ages may be affected. Dermatophytoses may be spread from person to person or from animal to person. The most common infections are tinea capitis, tinea corporis, tinea cruris, and tinea pedis. The clinical manifestations table compares and contrasts these infections.

Diagnosis is confirmed through microscopic examination of the hair and scale scrapings using a potassium hydroxide (KOH) wet mount to reveal rows and chains of spores within the hair shaft. A fungal culture can also be taken. A Wood's lamp is also useful in identifying some forms of tinea that fluoresce under ultraviolet light. However, *Trichophyton tonsurans,* the most common cause of tinea capitus, does not fluoresce with a Wood's lamp (McDonald & Smith, 1998). An oral antifungal agent (e.g., griseofulvin) is usually prescribed for tinea capitus, but resistance is developing. Other drugs not yet approved for use in children include itraconazole, fluconazole, and terbinafine (American Academy of Pediatrics Committee on Infectious Disease, 2000).

CLINICAL TIP 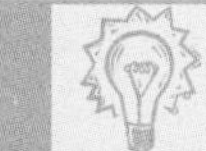

To take a fungal culture from a scalp lesion, rub a cotton-tipped applicator across the scalp and place in a throat culture tube.

NURSING MANAGEMENT All members of the family and household pets should be assessed for fungal lesions. Advise parents to give oral griseofulvin with fatty foods such as whole milk or peanut butter to enhance absorption. The medications must be used for the entire prescribed period, even if the lesions are gone, to prevent recurrence of the infection. Teach parents and older children or teenagers that fungi are found in soil and animals and are transmitted through direct contact.

Because person-to-person transmission is common, personal contact with hair and the sharing of hair accessories, brushes, and hats should be avoided. In some cases, there may be an asymptomatic carrier among the family, in which case all members of the family should be treated. For children with tinea cruris, encourage the use of loose-fitting undergarments to promote dryness. With tinea pedis, feet should be kept clean and dry and nails clipped short. Discourage the wearing of occlusive footwear or nylon socks, which trap moisture.

Parents of children with tinea capitis should be told that hair regrowth is slow and may take 6 to 12 months. In some cases hair loss is permanent, which can be particularly stressful for older children or adolescents. Provide emotional support.

INJURIES TO THE SKIN

PRESSURE ULCERS

An increasing number of children with disabilities are cared for in hospital, community, and home care settings. Many of these children are at risk for skin breakdown and pressure ulcer formation. Children at greatest risk are those with limited mobility, sensory deficits, or the inability to change positions (Table 23-6).

Etiology and Pathophysiology

Soft tissues can be compressed for a prolonged period of time between a bony prominence and another surface. Tissue ischemia occurs when high pressure is maintained over a short period of time or low pressure is maintained over a prolonged time. The cells are deprived of oxygen and nutrients, and metabolic waste products accumulate, resulting in soft tissue injury. Without appropriate intervention, the injury becomes rapidly progressive and a pressure ulcer forms.

CLINICAL MANIFESTATIONS OF TINEA INFECTIONS

SITE AND INCIDENCE	CLINICAL MANIFESTATIONS	CLINICAL THERAPY
Tinea capitus (scalp) Usually prepubertal children between 1 and 10 years	Circumscribed hair loss Broken hairs; black, dotted stubbed appearance where weakened hair has broken off. Diffuse fine scaling Many scaly pustular bald areas with indistinct margins Mild itching Boggy nodules with superficial pustules as an allergic response to fungus Suboccipital or posterior cervical nodes	Griseofulvin orally for 8–12 weeks Selenium sulfide shampoo 2–3 times weekly, leave on for 10 minutes before rinsing
Tinea corporis (trunk) Children and adolescents	One or several circular erythematous patches, may be scaly or erythematous throughout Slightly raised borders with a clearing center	Topical cream (e.g., clotrimazole, miconazole, tolnaftate, naftifine, terbinafine) twice a day for 4 weeks Wash with selenium sulfide shampoo
Tinea cruris (jock itch) (inner thighs, inguinal creases) Rare before adolescence	Scaly, erythematous eruption symmetric bilaterally Possibly elevated lesions, possible papules or vesicles	Same as for tinea corporis
Tinea pedis (athlete's foot) (feet and toes)	Itching Vesicles or erosions on instep or between toes (fissures, red scaly) Peeling maceration and fissures in lateral toe web spaces Dry scaly patches or plaques with mild erythema on plantar and lateral surfaces of foot	Same as for tinea corporis and cruris Keep feet dry with absorbent talc Allow to air dry Use 100% cotton socks, change twice daily

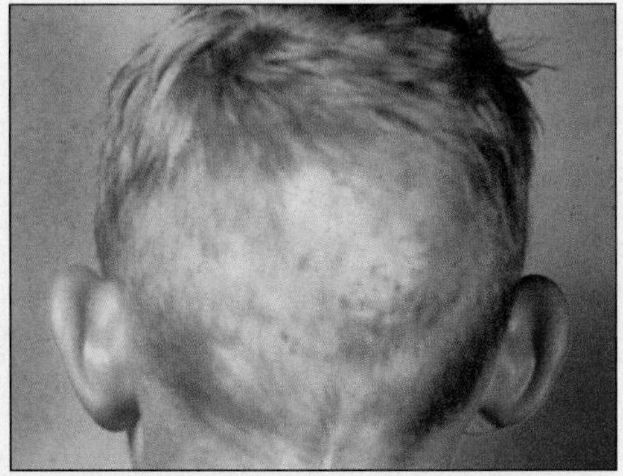

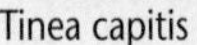

Tinea capitis

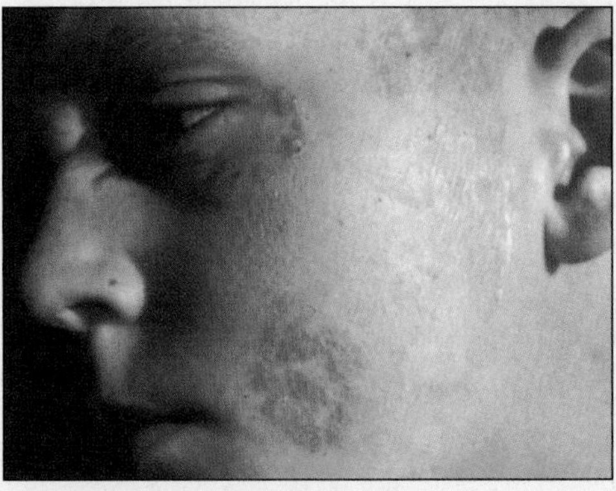

Tinea corporis

Photographs of tinea capitis and tinea corporis courtesy of the Centers for Disease Control and Prevention, Atlanta, GA.

CLINICAL TIP

Various factors place the child at greater risk for skin breakdown, including the following (Loman, 2000):

- Prolonged pressure
- Decreased mobility and activity
- Decreased sensory perception of pressure-related discomfort or injury
- Increased exposure to moisture
- Incontinence of urine and feces
- Friction and shearing forces
- Poor nutritional status
- Extended pediatric intensive care stay
- Impaired tissue perfusion and oxygenation requiring ventilator support

TABLE 23-6 Sites and Potential Causes of Pressure Ulcers

SITES	POTENTIAL CAUSES
Occipital region of scalp	Inability to lift head
Sacrum and buttocks	Confinement to bed or wheelchair
Legs and feet	Leg braces
Spine and neck	Scoliosis brace
Knees and elbows	Rubbing against bed sheet

Clinical Manifestations

The earliest sign of skin damage is an area of redness that does not dissipate within 30 minutes of removing the pressure or skin irritant. In the next stage, the skin looks rubbed or raw (superficial or partial-thickness injury), similar to an abrasion or blister. If intervention does not occur, the skin damage extends through the epidermis and dermis (full-thickness injury) and an ulcer forms. Injury deepens to underlying tissue (muscles, bone, or connective tissue) without intervention (Quigley & Curley, 1996; Ball, 1998) (see Figure 23-11 ◆).

Clinical Therapy

Initial treatment for early stages of skin damage involves removing pressure from the affected site until the skin has healed. Children who use leg braces for alignment and mobility are often put in wheelchairs. Children who use wheelchairs are often put on bed rest on a pressure-reducing surface. Frequent repositioning is needed. A transparent film may be applied to affected red skin to minimize friction. Pressure ulcers are treated with various dressings, such as hydrocolloids, gels or hydrogels, and calcium alginates (Quigley & Curley, 1996).

NURSING MANAGEMENT

Nursing Assessment and Diagnosis

Carefully inspect the dependent skin surfaces of all infants and children confined to bed at least 3 times in each 24-hour period. Evaluate the risk for skin damage based on factors that can contribute to skin breakdown.

Identify the size (diameter and depth) and character of the skin lesion. Note any signs of infection, the appearance of wound edges, and the type of tissue at the wound base. Describe drainage amount, color, and type.

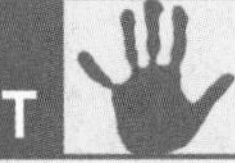

GROWTH & DEVELOPMENT

The site of greatest pressure in infants and young children is the occiput. Older children have increased pressure on the sacral and occipital areas.

The following nursing diagnoses may be appropriate for the child at risk for pressure sores:

- *Risk for impaired skin integrity,* related to infant's inability to shift position
- *Risk for injury,* related to sensory/perceptual alterations
- *Impaired physical mobility,* related to decreased muscle strength and control

Planning and Implementation

Develop protocols for pressure ulcer prevention so that children at high risk are identified and appropriate interventions are initiated. Such interventions may include increased ambulation, frequent position changes, use of pressure-reducing surfaces, and use of moisture barriers. If the child is incontinent, change the diaper frequently to keep the skin clean and dry.

Provide wound care and dressing changes according to agency guidelines. These guidelines may include irrigating the site with saline, debridement, and the application of a dressing appropriate for the wound condition. Avoid the use of tape to hold dressings in place unless a protective skin barrier is used.

Skill 6-10: Obtaining a Wound Culture

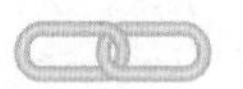

Skill 6-11: Wound Irrigation

Care in the Community

Teach parents of children with impaired mobility and diminished pain sensation to inspect the braces and skin under the braces daily for signs of irritation (redness or blisters). Take the braces off and help the child to use a mirror with a long handle to inspect skin on the bottom and sides of the feet, behind the knees, and lower legs. Check all edges of the braces

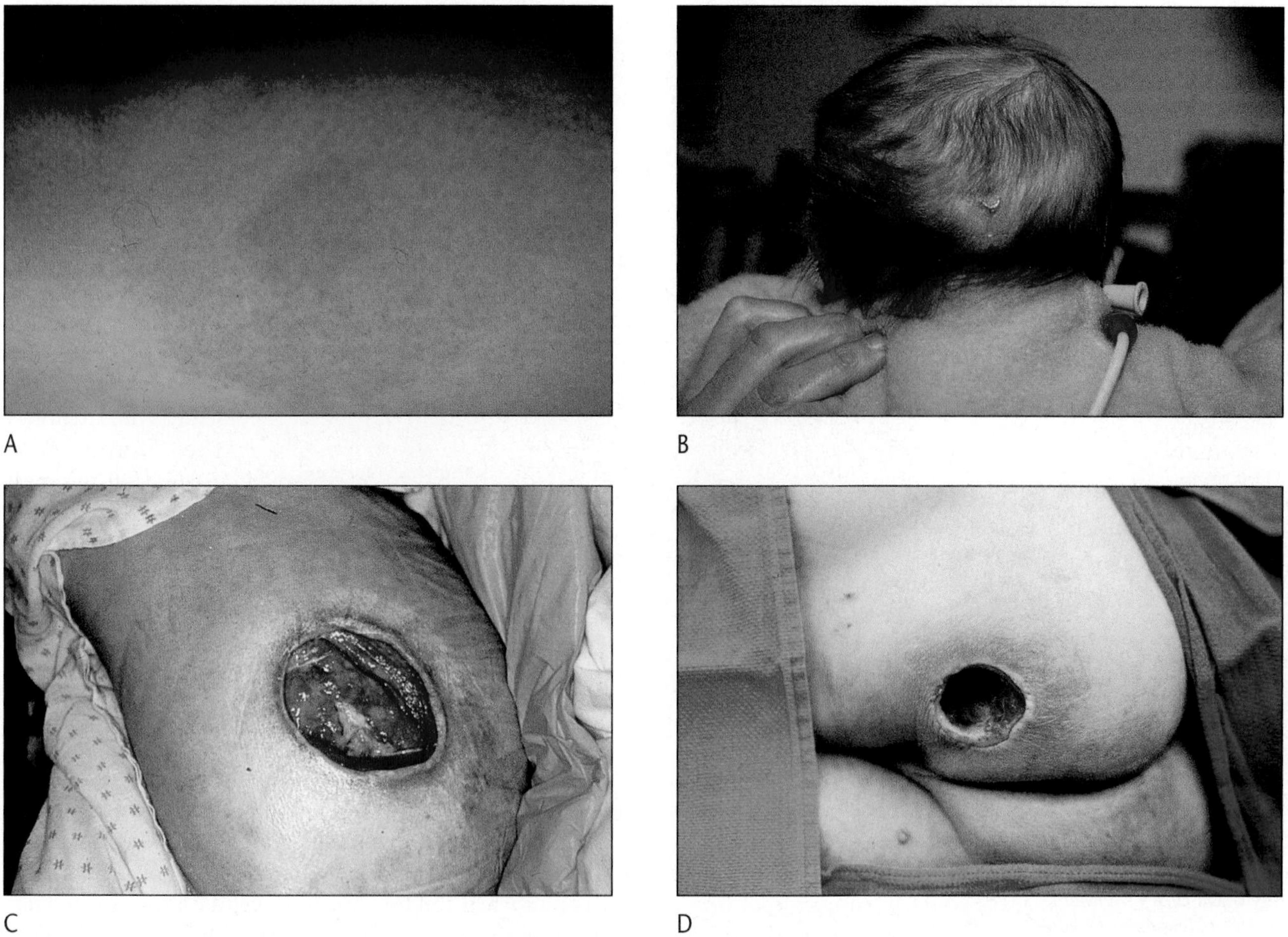

A

B

C

D

FIGURE 23-11 ◆
The four stages of ulcer formation. A, Stage 1, abrasion or blister appearance; nonblanchable erythema of intact skin. B, Stage 2, damage through the epidermis, dermis, or both. C, Stage 3, damage and necrosis of subcutaneous tissue; deep crater with or without undermining of adjacent tissue. D, Stage 4, extensive destruction to muscle, bone, or supporting tissues.
Courtesy of Sandra Quigley, Children's Hospital, Boston, MA.

for roughness or breakage that can pinch or scrape the skin. If any sign of skin irritation is seen and redness does not diminish within 30 minutes, do not wear the brace until the skin heals. Inform the child's physician so that an appropriate treatment regimen can be started immediately. To prevent braces from rubbing on bare skin, have the child wear cotton socks under the braces. To avoid irritation of the foot, shoes should be purchased that are large enough to accommodate the brace and the foot in the shoe. Advise parents to return to a prosthetist regularly for refitting as the child grows.

Children who are confined to a wheelchair are at risk for skin breakdown on the buttocks and lower back because of the pressure from sitting for hours. A wheelchair cushion can distribute and shift the child's weight when sitting in the chair. Frequent position changes need to be made to relieve the pressure on the skin. Teach the child to do wheelchair push-ups or to shift the weight by leaning to the side or forward for several minutes every 10 to 15 minutes. Make sure the child wears a safety belt when sitting in the wheelchair. Teach school personnel about the child's recommended protocol so they can provide opportunities in school to change positions and reinforce the routine.

BURNS

Burns are the second leading cause of injury deaths (after motor vehicle crashes) in children between 5 and 14 years of age (Murphy, 2000). Boys between the ages of 1 and 4 years are twice as likely as girls to be burned; however, the national average age of pediatric burn

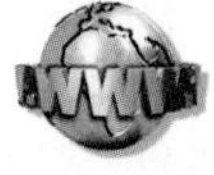

Burn Prevention and Resources

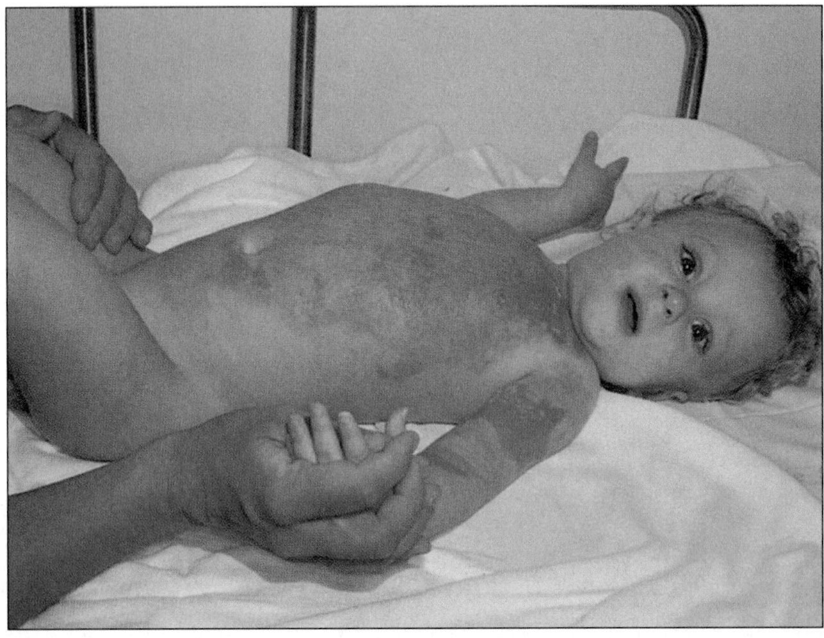

FIGURE 23-12 ◆
Thermal (scald) burns are the most common burn injury in infancy.

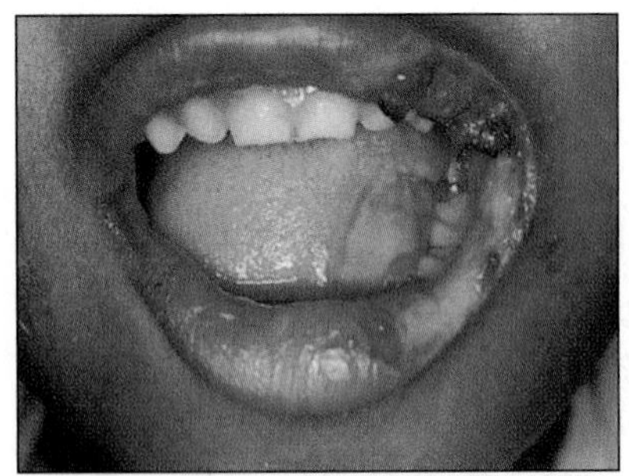

FIGURE 23-13 ◆
Electrical burn caused by biting an electric cord.
Courtesy of Dr. Lezley McIlveen, Department of Dentistry, Children's National Medical Center, Washington, DC.

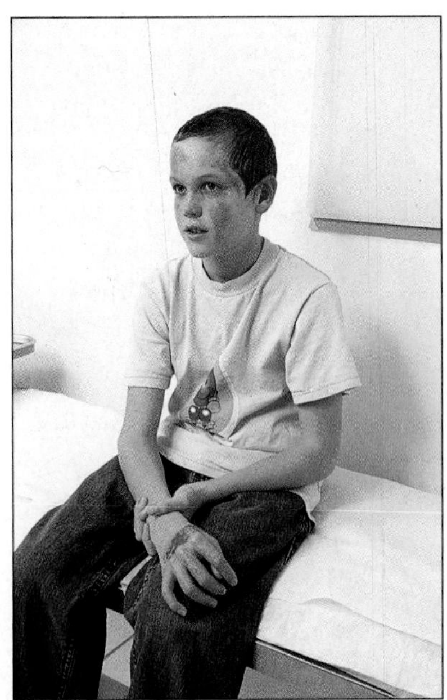

FIGURE 23-14 ◆
The burns on the face and hands of this school-age boy were the result of a flash burn caused by igniting gasoline.

patients is 32 months. In 1997, 83,000 children were hospitalized for burns (Hernandez-Reif, Field, & Largie, et al., 2001). About 440,000 children are treated for burns each year (Stewart, 2000).

The four main types of burns are thermal, chemical, electrical, and radioactive. Thermal burns, the most common burns in children, may occur through exposure to flames or scalds (such as coffee or grease), or contact with a hot object (such as a wood stove or curling iron). Sherray, described in the opening vignette, sustained a scald burn when a bowl of hot soup fell onto her leg. Chemical burns occur when children touch or ingest caustic agents. Electrical burns occur from exposure to direct or alternating current in electrical wires, appliances, or high-voltage wires. Radiation burns result from exposure to radioactive substances or sunlight. About 10% of all burns in children are due to child abuse (Rodgers, 2000). See Chapter 7 for a description of child abuse.

Etiology and Pathophysiology

Children at different developmental stages are at risk for different types of burns.

- Infants are most often injured by thermal burns (scalding liquids, house fires) (Figure 23-12 ◆).
- Toddlers are at risk for thermal burns (pulling hot liquids or grease onto themselves), electrical burns (biting electrical cords) (Figure 23-13 ◆), contact burns, and chemical burns (ingesting cleaning agents and other substances) associated with exploring the environment.
- Preschool-age children are most often injured by scalding or contact with hot appliances (curling irons, ovens).
- School-age children are at risk for thermal burns (playing with matches, fireworks), electrical burns (climbing high-voltage towers, climbing trees, and contact with electrical wires), and chemical burns (combustion experiments) associated with their curiosity and interest in experimentation (Figure 23-14 ◆).
- Adolescents also experience thermal, chemical, and electrical burns.

Immediately after the burn, intense vasoconstriction occurs in response to substances released by the injured cells; then vasodilation and capillary permeability allow plasma to seep into the wound. Ischemia due to vasoconstriction may increase the depth of the burn injury. The child experiences increased water and heat loss through the injured epidermis. The child's metabolic rate and need for calories increases as the child tries to maintain body temperature.

Clinical Manifestations

Burns are classified by depth. Burn depth may be defined as partial thickness or full thickness. Partial-thickness burns, in which the injured tissue can regenerate and heal, encompass first- and second-degree burns. Full-thickness burns, in which the injured tissue cannot regenerate, are known as third-degree burns. The depth of the burn depends on the temperature and duration of the heat application, and on the ability of tissues to dissipate the transferred energy. See Figure 23-15 ◆ for clinical manifestations by burn depth.

Signs of infection include purulent drainage, focal areas of necrosis, edema, erythema, discoloration of wound margins, and conversion from partial-thickness to full-thickness injury depth (Rodgers, 2000).

Clinical Therapy

ASSESSMENT OF BURN SEVERITY Burn severity is determined by the depth of the burn injury, percentage of body surface area (BSA) affected, and involvement of specific body parts (Table 23-7). A Lund and Browder chart with BSA distributions for various body

CLINICAL TIP

A full-thickness burn can occur in adults after only a 2-sec immersion in water with a temperature of 65°C (149°F). The amount of time for a burn to occur increases to 10 min when water temperature is 50°C (122°F). Because infants and children have more sensitive skin, less time is needed for them to receive a serious burn (Stewart, 2000).

PATHOPHYSIOLOGY ILLUSTRATED

Superficial Partial Thickness (first degree)
Damages only outer layer of skin; burn is painful and red; heals in a few days (e.g., sunburn)

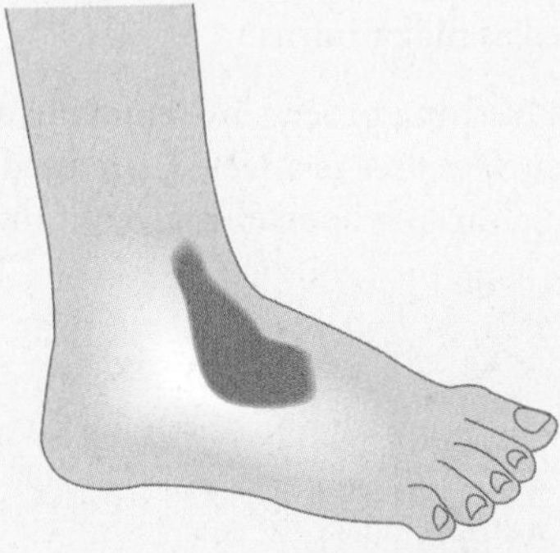

Erythema, blanches on pressure, no bullae, peeling after a few days due to premature cell death

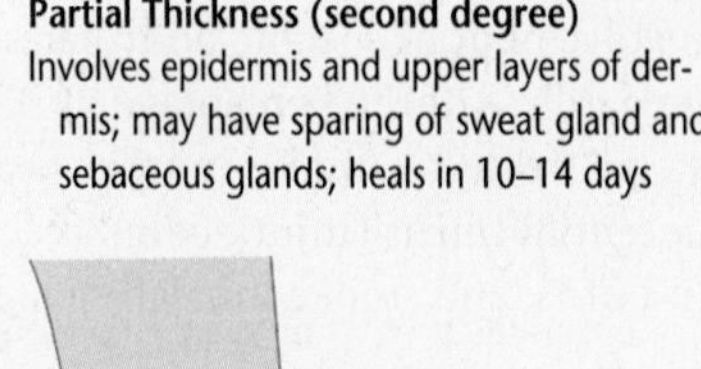

Partial Thickness (second degree)
Involves epidermis and upper layers of dermis; may have sparing of sweat gland and sebaceous glands; heals in 10–14 days

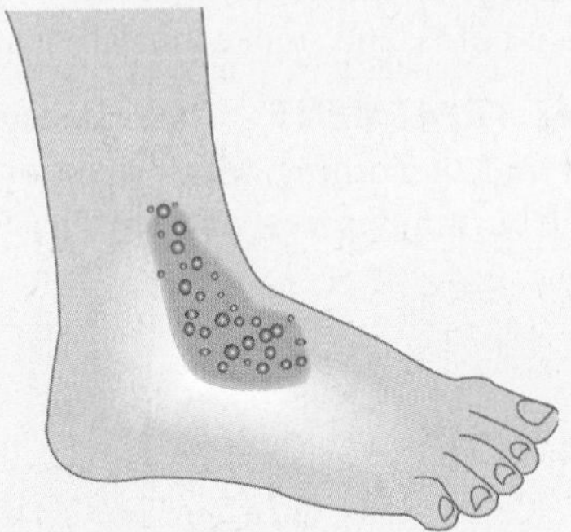

Blisters or bullae, erythema, blanches on pressure, pain and sensitivity to cold air, minimal scar formation

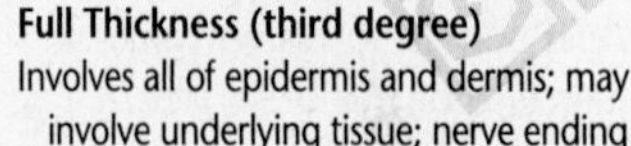

Full Thickness (third degree)
Involves all of epidermis and dermis; may also involve underlying tissue; nerve ending usually destroyed; requires skin grafting

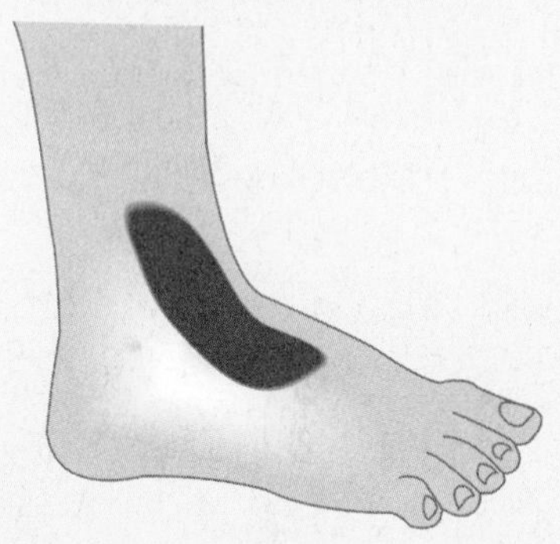

Skin may appear brown, black, deep cherry red, white to gray, waxy or translucent, usually no pain, injured area may appear sunken

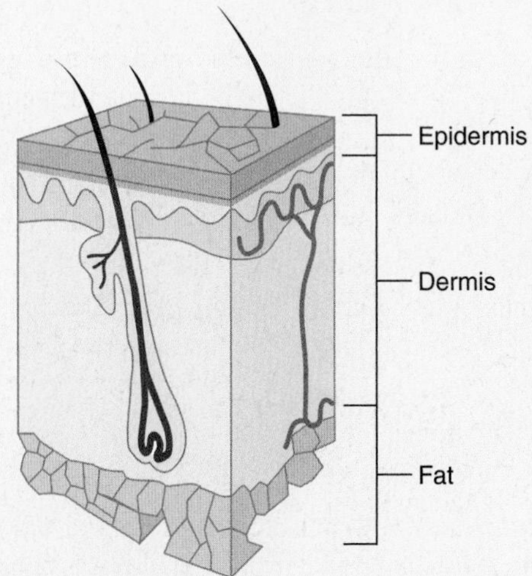

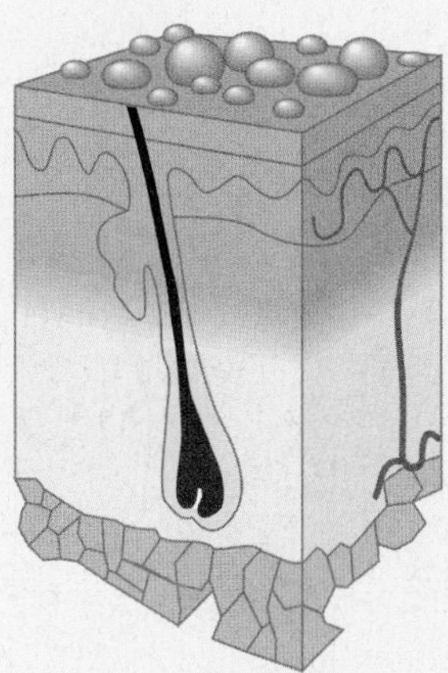

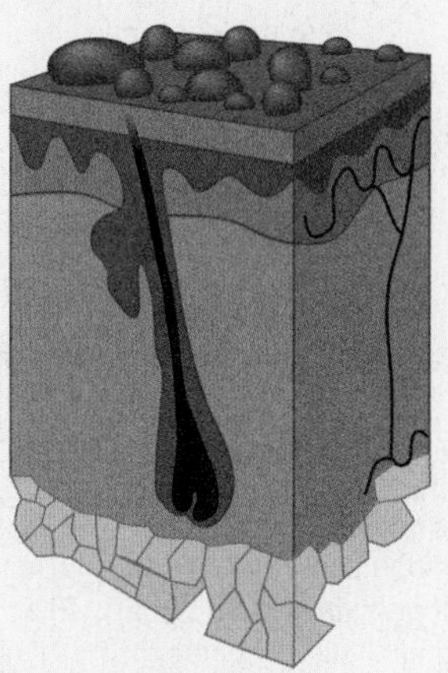

Classification of Burns

FIGURE 23-15 ◆

TABLE 23-7	Classification of Burn Severity
Minor	Partial thickness <10% BSA Full thickness <2% BSA
Moderate	Partial thickness 10%–20% BSA Full thickness 3%–10% BSA
Major	Partial thickness >20% BSA Full thickness >10% BSA Burns involving face, eyes, ears, hands, feet, and perineum Electrical burns, inhalation injury, other injuries, and preexisting chronic conditions

Note: Adapted from Stewart, C. (2000). Emergency care of pediatric burns. *Pediatric Emergency Medicine Reports, 5*(10), 101–112.

CLINICAL TIP

The palm of a child's hand is 1% of the BSA. It can be used to make a quick estimate of the burn size.

parts at different ages is used to calculate the area affected by the burn injury (Figure 23-16 ◆). Once the affected BSA is calculated, the burn can be classified as minor, moderate, or major. Children with moderate and major burns require hospitalization, and those with major burns will usually be transferred to a burn center.

The involvement of specific body parts or specific burn distributions increases the burn severity, regardless of the percentage of BSA affected. Burns to the face, hands, feet, or perineal area are treated as major injuries because of the potential for functional impairment. **Circumferential** burns (injury completely surrounding the thorax or an extremity), anterior chest burns, and smoke inhalation are also classified as major burns.

INITIAL TREATMENT The first step is to stop the burning process by removing any jewelry and all clothing. Moist soaks or ice (if small surface area is affected) are used to stop the burning process and to relieve pain. A tetanus vaccine booster is given if more

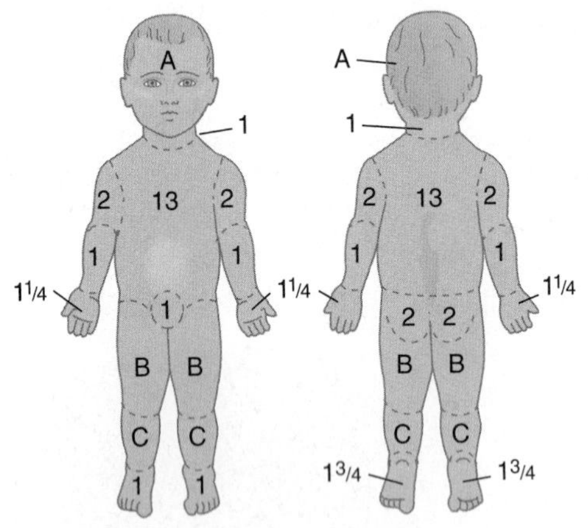

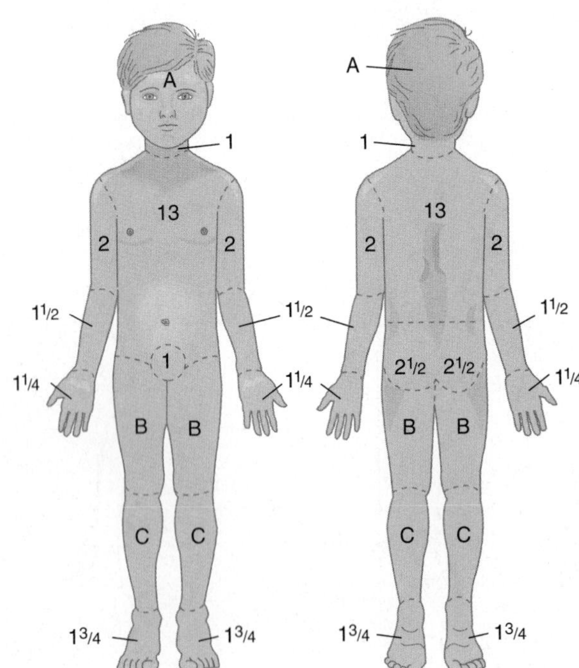

Relative Percentages of Areas Affected by Growth

	Age in years					
Area	0	1	5	10	11	Adult
A = 1/2 of head	9 1/2	8 1/2	6 1/2	5 1/2	4 1/2	3 1/2
B = 1/2 of one thigh	2 3/4	3 1/4	4	4 1/2	4 1/2	4 3/4
C = 1/2 of one lower leg	2 1/2	2 1/2	2 3/4	3	3 1/4	3 1/2

FIGURE 23-16 ◆

Lund and Browder chart for determining percentage of body surface areas in pediatric burn injuries.
Adapted from Artz, C. P., & Moncrief, J. A. (1969). *The treatment of burns* (2nd ed.). Philadelphia: Saunders.

than 5 years have passed since the last vaccine, or when the child has not completed the full vaccine series.

TREATMENT OF MAJOR BURNS The goals of treatment include decrease burn fluid losses, prevent infection, control pain, and salvage all viable burn tissue.

Fluid replacement is necessary to prevent hypovolemic shock in cases of major burn injury. Fluid shifts from the vasculature to the interstitial spaces (third spacing) occur soon after the burn. Fluid replacement for the first 24 hours after the injury is based on a fluid volume formula calculated from the child's body weight, affected BSA, and normal maintenance needs. Several formulas exist for this calculation. Lactated Ringer's or normal saline solution is the preferred fluid. Half of the total volume calculated for the 24-hour period is infused over the first 8 hours, and the remainder is distributed evenly over the next 16 hours. Resuscitation efforts are also focused on maintaining the child's temperature, because heat is lost rapidly through burned skin. Vascular integrity is usually restored after the first 24 hours.

Fever is a normal, expected outcome of any significant thermal injury, but it is not always a sign of infection. Treatment may include analgesics, ice packs, cooling blankets, or cool hydrotherapy sessions. Infection of the burned area is, however, a frequent complication, and can cause a partial-thickness burn to convert to full thickness (Rodgers, 2000).

Enteral feedings are often initiated within 6 hours of the burn injury to support the child's increased nutritional requirements, which result from the increased metabolic rate needed to support healing and the body's stress response to injury (Herndon & Spies, 2001). These children often need nearly twice the basal metabolic caloric requirements and nearly 2 g/kg body weight of protein (Smith, 2000).

Aggressive pain management with intravenous opioids is needed as all procedures cause pain. In addition, the burns cause a significant emotional overlay that increases the pain perceived. See Chapter 9 for a discussion of pain management. Cimetidine or other H_2 blockers may be ordered to prevent a burn stress ulcer.

Special consideration is needed when burns involve certain areas of the body:

- Deep partial-thickness and full-thickness burns develop **eschar** (the tough leathery scab that forms over severely burned areas) with no elasticity. When the burn is circumferential, blood flow can become restricted due to edema and cause tissue hypoxia. An **escharotomy** (incision into the constricting tissue) may be necessary to restore peripheral circulation.
- Facial burns usually cause significant edema. Care must be taken to ensure airway patency. For burns to the eye, an ophthalmologist should be consulted to assess damage and prescribe treatment. If the lips are burned, an infant may be unable to suck.
- Burns of the hands require careful management to maintain function. Special splinting and physical therapy are usually necessary.
- Perineal burns are at higher risk for infection because of frequent contamination with urine and stool. Frequent dressing changes are required. A urinary catheter is usually inserted but is removed once hydration status is stable to minimize the risk of urinary tract infection.

WOUND MANAGEMENT Burn wound care has several goals: (1) to speed wound debridement, (2) to protect granulation tissue and new grafts, (3) to conserve body heat and fluids, and (4) to control scarring and prevent scar contracture. Several treatment regimens are used to achieve these goals.

The entire body is bathed to initiate debridement (removal of dead tissue to speed the healing process). Conscious sedation and anesthesiology support may be ordered for pain management during debridement. Intact blisters provide a natural, pain-free, sterile dressing. If blisters break open, the tissue should be carefully cut away. After initial cleansing, antibacterial agents, such as Silvadene, are applied to prevent bacterial infection and dressings are added to cover the burned area (Table 23-8).

CLINICAL TIP

The most dramatic fluid shifts happen in the first 8–12 hours after the burn. Calculate fluid replacement formula for the first 8 hours starting at the time of the burn, not the time of arrival in the emergency department (Stewart, 2000).

NURSING ALERT

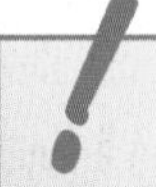

Hypotonic intravenous solutions such as D5W increase the risk of hyponatremia and subsequent cerebral edema and seizures (Stewart, 2000).

NURSING ALERT

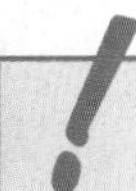

Assess for increases in cyanosis, deep tissue pain, and capillary refill time, and a decreased pulse distal to a circumferential burn. Detection of these signs requires immediate notification of the physician.

Skill 7-12: Burn Wound Care

TABLE 23-8 Burn Wound Care

PREPARATION

1. Check the physician's orders. Since burn care is often a painful procedure, check for pain medication orders and administer medication at least 30–60 minutes before starting burn care. Conscious sedation may be used for some debridement procedures.
2. Wash your hands. Gather supplies, including gloves (clean and sterile), a basin, sterile normal saline solution, a large supply of 4 × 4 gauze pads, forceps, scissors, a sterile tongue blade, the prescribed topical medication, tape, and an absorbent pad.
3. You may need an assistant to hold the child and the burned extremity during care.

PROCEDURE

1. Place the absorbent pad under the area to be cleaned. Put on clean gloves. Soak the wound for about 10 minutes in normal saline solution, or apply a wet dressing to the area. This will soften the wound. Remove the gloves.
2. After approximately 10 minutes, put on sterile gloves and wash the burn with the gauze pads using a *firm,* circular motion, moving from the inside to the outer edges. As you do this, be sure to remove any medication or crusting. Bleeding may occur, but this is a sign of healing, healthy tissue. Rinse with more normal saline solution. Pat dry with sterile gauze.
3. Remove (per physician's orders) any loose or dead skin around the edges of the burn by gently lifting it with the forceps and snipping it. This is not painful to the child. You may rinse and dry again.
4. Place a thin layer of prescribed medication (about 1/8-inch thick) on the burn or gauze with fingers or a tongue blade. Place the medicated gauze on the burn and cover with a dry, sterile dressing.

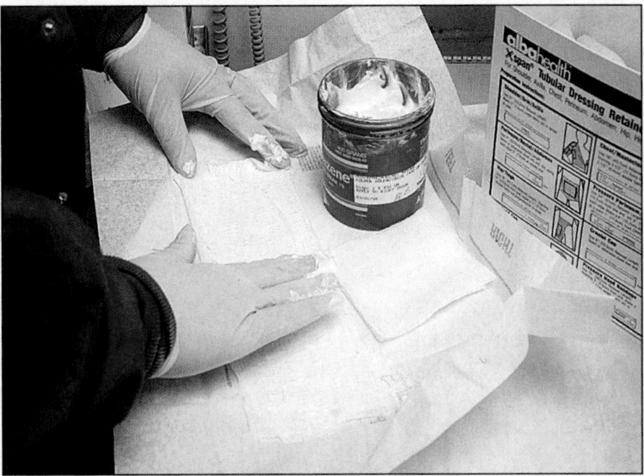

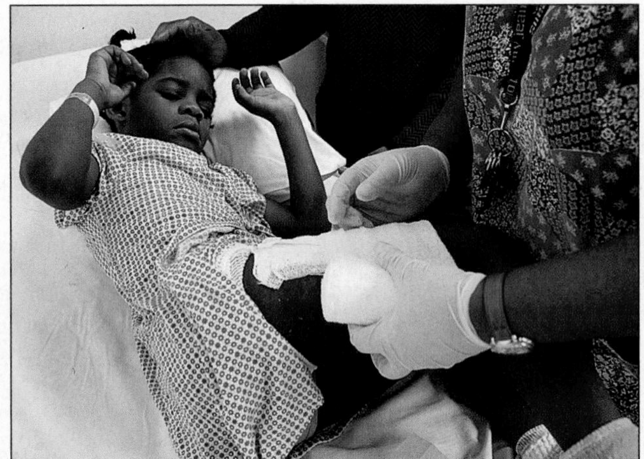

Burn wound care written by Marcia Wellington, R.N., M.S.

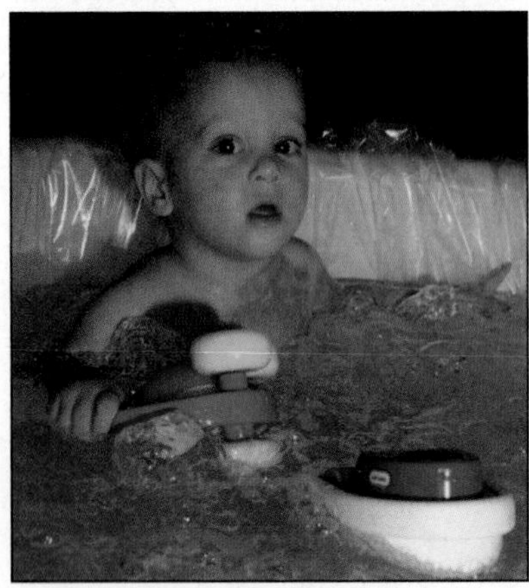

FIGURE 23-17 ◆
A whirlpool bath is being used to increase this child's circulation and speed the healing of his burns.

Dressing changes are performed once or twice daily. These changes are often very painful. When an old dressing is removed, a layer of eschar is also debrided.

Hydrotherapy (whirlpool) baths are given before debridement to loosen eschar. Hydrotherapy is performed twice daily to increase vasodilation and circulation and to speed healing (Figure 23-17 ◆). As a rule, tap water is used for debridement. Gentle washing is necessary to protect new epithelial cells. Granulation tissue forms as a result of daily debridement. Superficial second-degree burns re-epithelialize within 3 weeks.

Skin grafting is necessary with any deep second- or third-degree burn. Often a temporary skin substitute is used to cover a second-degree burn until healing occurs or a deep second- and third-degree burn until **autografting** (use of healthy skin taken from a nonburned area of the child's body). The graft is placed after the wound is debrided in the operating room to reveal healthy, bleeding tissue. This forms a protective barrier over the wound surface to decrease infection risk and to protect against fluid loss (Figure 23-18◆). It is applied with a surgical adhesive or staples and covered with a bulky dressing or pressure dressing.

An autograft is permanent. The donor site (where the autograft was harvested) is a new wound, causing pain and requiring close monitoring for signs of infection. A temporary skin substitute may be used to cover that wound until healing occurs.

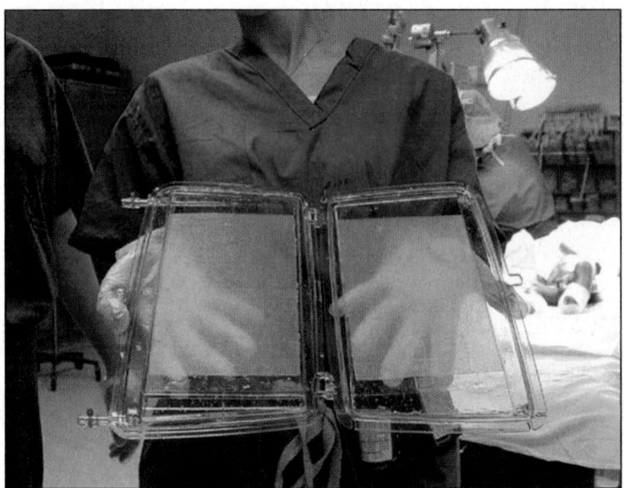

A

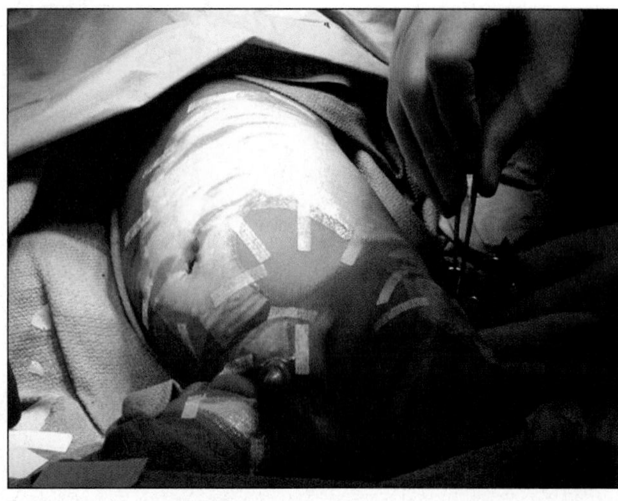

B

FIGURE 23-18 ◆

A, Trans-Cyte, a temporary skin substitute, prior to application. B, Application of Trans-Cyte after debridement of a scald burn.
Photos A and B Courtesy Martin R. Eichelberger, M.D., Children's National Medical Center, Washington, DC.

NURSING MANAGEMENT

Nursing Assessment and Diagnosis

Emergency assessment is based on the ABCs of basic life support (airway, breathing, and circulation). Assessment of the airway patency is necessary, especially when signs of smoke inhalation or burns to the face and neck are present. The child is assessed for other potential injuries when the mechanism of injury also includes a fall or explosion. Identify signs of respiratory distress and any potential bleeding source. A weak, thready pulse, tachycardia, and pallor are important signs of early shock that may provide clues to an internal injury.

Obtain information about the type of burn (e.g., thermal, electrical, chemical) and a complete history. Thorough documentation is essential to rule out child abuse. Be alert to signs of abuse (e.g., glove and stocking burns, burns that spare flexor surfaces, contact burns from cigarettes or irons, zebra burn lines from contact with a hot grate (Figure 23-19 ◆). Child neglect can be a factor in the burn of a child who was not adequately supervised. If a burn injury was preventable, parents may be emotionally stressed by feelings of guilt. Caution is needed to avoid sounding accusatory when questioning parents about the injury.

Physical assessment should be thorough, including frequent monitoring of vital signs, pain control, and daily weight measurement. A head-to-toe assessment is performed at the beginning of every shift followed by system-specific assessments, depending on clinical findings and changes in the child's status. Be alert to signs of infection such as purulent drainage and edematous, red or discolored wound margins.

Assess the child's concerns over appearance and the stress of hospitalization. Determine if the child has memories or nightmares about the burn so psychologic support can be provided as needed.

Common nursing diagnoses for the child with a major burn injury are included in the accompanying nursing care plan. Additional nursing diagnoses for the child with a major burn may include the following:

- *Impaired physical mobility,* related to prescribed movement prescriptions (limb immobilization) and pain
- *Body image disturbance,* related to burn injury
- *Anxiety,* related to situational crisis and threat of death or disfigurement

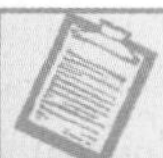

RESEARCH

Trans-Cyte is a temporary skin substitute approved by the Food and Drug Administration that is bioengineered from newborn foreskin tissue. Research conducted in children indicates that it promotes healing more rapidly than silvidene, decreases infection risk, avoids painful burn dressings, and reduces length of hospital stay (Wiebelhaus & Hansen, 2001; Lukish, Eichelberger, & Newman, et al., 2001).

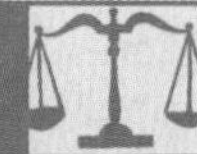

LAW & ETHICS

When taking a burn history, carefully document the following:

- Type of injury
- Time of injury
- People present at the time of injury
- First aid administered
- History of other unusual injuries or emergency department visits

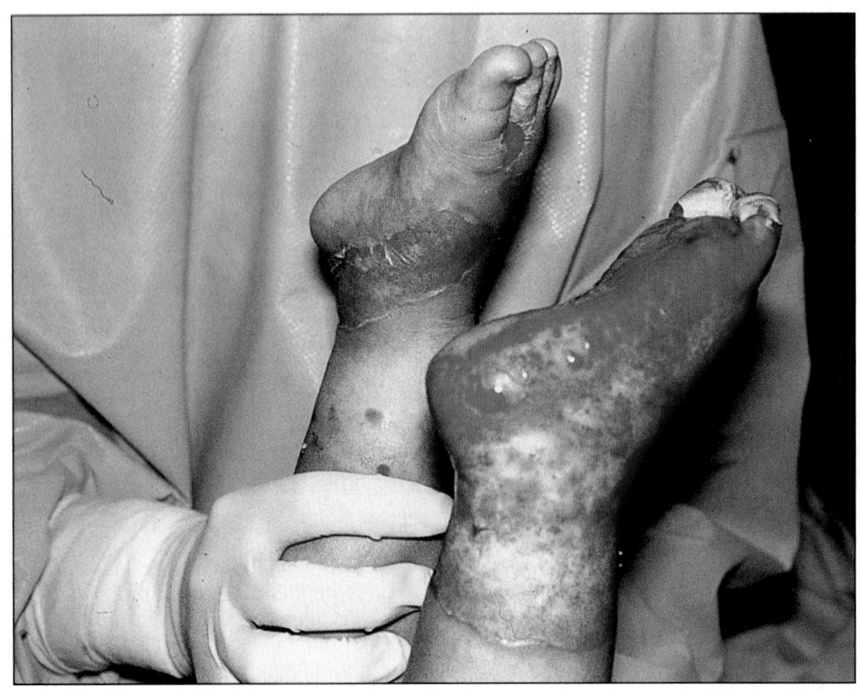

A

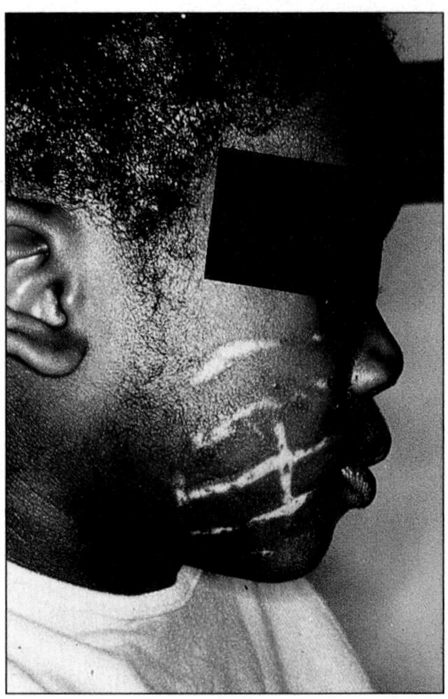

B

FIGURE 23-19 ◆

Burn injuries associated with child abuse. A, Burns of the hands or feet that are distributed like gloves or stockings. B, Zebra burns from a grate.
Courtesy American Academy of Pediatrics, Elk Grove, Il, and the Kempe Children's Center.

CLINICAL TIP

Be sure to follow all agency guidelines for patient assessment and monitoring of conscious sedation during the debridement process (see Chapter 9).

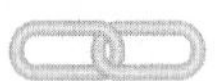

Skill 12-1: Performing a Urinary Catheterization

CLINICAL TIP

For superficial burns covering a small area, use moist soaks or ice to stop the burning process and to relieve pain. Pain management is initiated as soon as possible. Soak charred clothing off with sterile saline and clip any hair within 2 in. of the burn to keep it out of the burn site. Cleanse the burn with mild soap and water and remove any foreign matter. If a chemical is the burning agent, remove the clothing and wash with lots of water. Elevate burned extremities.

Planning and Implementation

Nursing care focuses on performing burn care, preventing complications, and providing emotional support. Care of the burned child involves various treatments designed to promote healing and prevent complications. These include dressing changes, hydrotherapy, antibiotic therapy, analgesic support, physical therapy, play therapy, and possibly skin grafting. The accompanying nursing care plan summarizes nursing care of the child with a major burn.

Severe morbidity is likely with major burns. Significant scarring may occur regardless of autografting. Contractures and loss of function are also possible. If fluid replacement is inadequate, irreversible renal damage or cardiac damage may ensue, necessitating close follow-up unrelated to the actual burn injury. Intake and output must be monitored closely. A urinary catheter may be inserted to enable close monitoring of urine output.

Children with major burns require comprehensive follow-up, sometimes involving repeated hospitalizations for surgery to release burn contractures, perform new grafting, or provide scar revision.

Prevent Complications

Severe complications of burns include infections, pneumonia, and renal failure, as well as possible irreversible loss of function of the burned area. The goal of the health care team is to prevent complications. Parents need to be involved in their child's care and to learn how to change dressings, assess for infection and dehydration (see Chapter 10), and perform range-of-motion exercises to aid in the child's recovery.

Wound Care

When a synthetic skin cover such as Trans-Cyte is used, the area must be protected from moisture and ointments, as these interfere with adherence. Trans-Cyte is transparent, so the site can be monitored for signs of infection and wound healing. The skin covering is assessed for air bubbles or fluid, which are aspirated or drained as ordered. If the covering is used over a joint, a splint will prevent movement. When healing occurs, the skin covering loosens, permitting it to be trimmed.

NURSING CARE PLAN The Child with a Major Burn Injury

GOAL	INTERVENTION	RATIONALE	EXPECTED OUTCOME
1. Pain related to physical injury agents			
	NIC Priority Intervention: **Pain Management:** Alleviation of pain or a reduction in pain to a level of comfort that is acceptable to the patient.		NOC Suggested Outcome: **Comfort Level:** Feelings of physical and psychological ease.
The child will verbalize adequate relief from pain and will be able to perform activities of daily living (ADLs).	■ Assess the level of pain frequently using pain scales (see Chapter 9). ■ Cover burns as much as possible. ■ Change the child's position frequently. Perform range-of-motion exercises. ■ Encourage verbalization about pain. ■ Provide diversional activities. ■ Promote uninterrupted sleep with use of medications. ■ Use analgesics before all dressing changes and burn care.	■ Pain scale provides objective measurement. Pain is always present, but changes location; intensity may indicate complications. ■ Temperature changes or movement of air causes pain. ■ Reduces joint stiffness and prevents contractures. ■ Provides outlet for emotions and helps the child cope. ■ Helps lessen focus on pain. ■ Sleep deprivation can increase pain perception. ■ Helps to reduce pain and decreases anxiety for subsequent dressing changes.	The child verbalizes adequate relief from pain and is able to perform ADLs.
2. Risk for Infection related to trauma and destruction of skin barrier			
	NIC Priority Intervention: **Infection Protection:** Prevention and early detection of infection in a patient at risk.		NOC Suggested Outcome: **Risk Control:** Actions to eliminate or reduce actual, personal, and modifiable health threats.
The child will be free of infection during healing process.	■ Take vital signs frequently. ■ Use standard precautions (gown, gloves, mask) when wounds of a major burn are exposed. Limit visitors (no one with an upper respiratory infection or other contagious disease). ■ Clip hair around burns. ■ Keep biosynthetic burn dressing dry. ■ Do not place the IV in any burned area. ■ Administer oral or IV antibiotics for diagnosed infections as prescribed.	■ Increased temperature is an early sign of infection. ■ Reduces risk of wound contamination. ■ Hair harbors bacteria. ■ Helps reduce the number of bacteria introduced to the burn site. ■ Reduces risk of wound contamination. ■ Antibiotics administered as prescribed help to clear the infection quickly.	The child either stays free of secondary infection, or has infection diagnosed and treated early.
3. Risk for Fluid Volume Imbalance related to loss of fluids through wounds and to subsequent excess fluid intake			
	NIC Priority Intervention: To be developed.		NOC Suggested Outcome: To be developed.
The child will maintain adequate urine output.	■ Monitor vital signs, central venous pressure, capillary refill time, pulses.	■ The child is initially at risk for hypovolemic shock and needs fluid resuscitation (see Chapter 10).	The child maintains normal urine output and burn site edema is not excessive.

(continued)

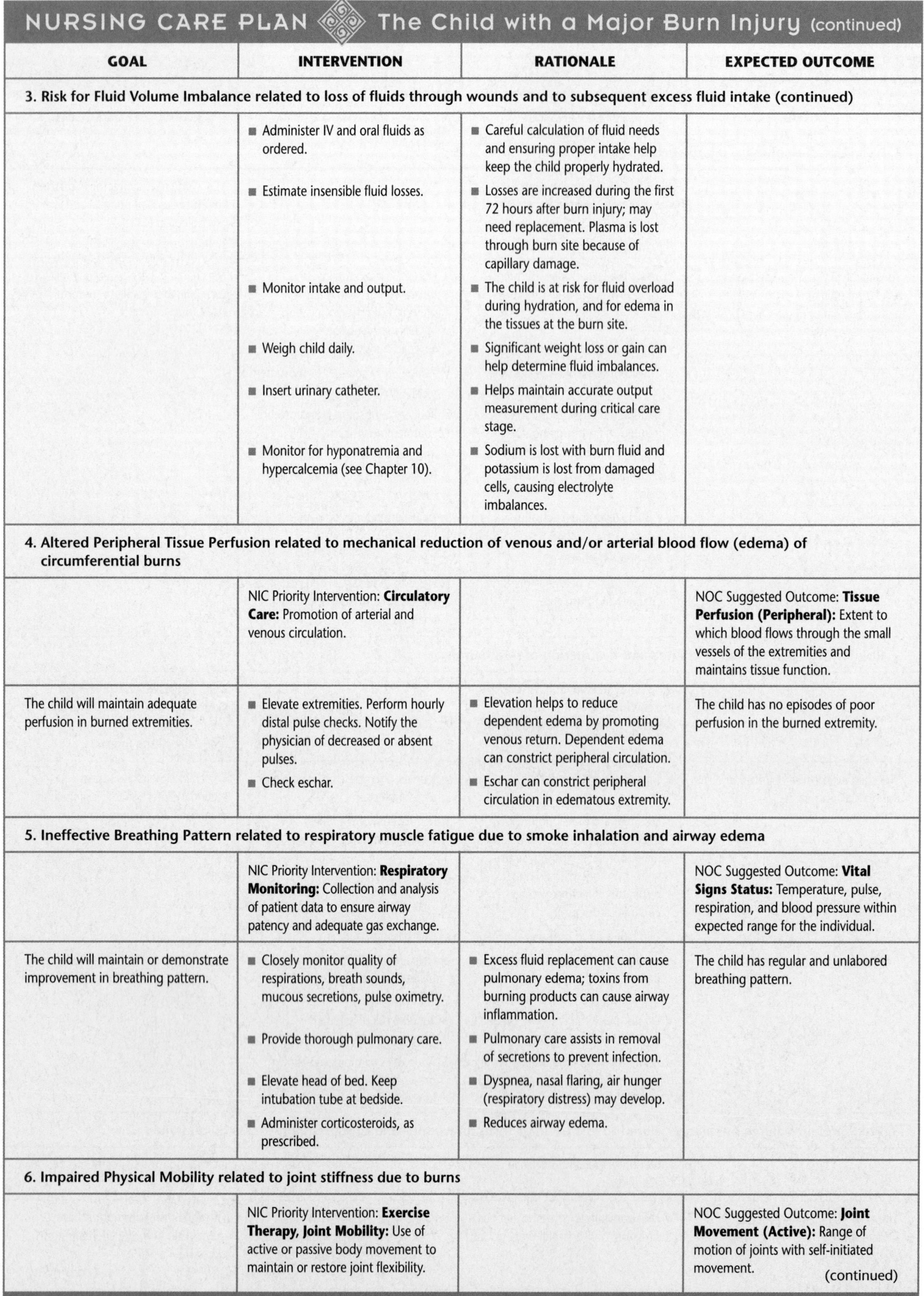

NURSING CARE PLAN The Child with a Major Burn Injury (continued)

GOAL	INTERVENTION	RATIONALE	EXPECTED OUTCOME
3. Risk for Fluid Volume Imbalance related to loss of fluids through wounds and to subsequent excess fluid intake (continued)			
	■ Administer IV and oral fluids as ordered.	■ Careful calculation of fluid needs and ensuring proper intake help keep the child properly hydrated.	
	■ Estimate insensible fluid losses.	■ Losses are increased during the first 72 hours after burn injury; may need replacement. Plasma is lost through burn site because of capillary damage.	
	■ Monitor intake and output.	■ The child is at risk for fluid overload during hydration, and for edema in the tissues at the burn site.	
	■ Weigh child daily.	■ Significant weight loss or gain can help determine fluid imbalances.	
	■ Insert urinary catheter.	■ Helps maintain accurate output measurement during critical care stage.	
	■ Monitor for hyponatremia and hypercalcemia (see Chapter 10).	■ Sodium is lost with burn fluid and potassium is lost from damaged cells, causing electrolyte imbalances.	
4. Altered Peripheral Tissue Perfusion related to mechanical reduction of venous and/or arterial blood flow (edema) of circumferential burns			
	NIC Priority Intervention: **Circulatory Care:** Promotion of arterial and venous circulation.		NOC Suggested Outcome: **Tissue Perfusion (Peripheral):** Extent to which blood flows through the small vessels of the extremities and maintains tissue function.
The child will maintain adequate perfusion in burned extremities.	■ Elevate extremities. Perform hourly distal pulse checks. Notify the physician of decreased or absent pulses. ■ Check eschar.	■ Elevation helps to reduce dependent edema by promoting venous return. Dependent edema can constrict peripheral circulation. ■ Eschar can constrict peripheral circulation in edematous extremity.	The child has no episodes of poor perfusion in the burned extremity.
5. Ineffective Breathing Pattern related to respiratory muscle fatigue due to smoke inhalation and airway edema			
	NIC Priority Intervention: **Respiratory Monitoring:** Collection and analysis of patient data to ensure airway patency and adequate gas exchange.		NOC Suggested Outcome: **Vital Signs Status:** Temperature, pulse, respiration, and blood pressure within expected range for the individual.
The child will maintain or demonstrate improvement in breathing pattern.	■ Closely monitor quality of respirations, breath sounds, mucous secretions, pulse oximetry. ■ Provide thorough pulmonary care. ■ Elevate head of bed. Keep intubation tube at bedside. ■ Administer corticosteroids, as prescribed.	■ Excess fluid replacement can cause pulmonary edema; toxins from burning products can cause airway inflammation. ■ Pulmonary care assists in removal of secretions to prevent infection. ■ Dyspnea, nasal flaring, air hunger (respiratory distress) may develop. ■ Reduces airway edema.	The child has regular and unlabored breathing pattern.
6. Impaired Physical Mobility related to joint stiffness due to burns			
	NIC Priority Intervention: **Exercise Therapy, Joint Mobility:** Use of active or passive body movement to maintain or restore joint flexibility.		NOC Suggested Outcome: **Joint Movement (Active):** Range of motion of joints with self-initiated movement.

(continued)

GOAL	INTERVENTION	RATIONALE	EXPECTED OUTCOME
The child will maintain maximum range of motion.	■ Arrange physical and occupational therapy twice daily for stretching and range-of-motion exercises. Splint as ordered. Encourage independent ADLs.	■ Good positioning, range-of-motion exercises, and alignment prevent contractures.	The child maintains maximum range of motion without contractures.
7. Altered Nutrition: Less than Body Requirements related to high metabolic needs			
	NIC Priority Intervention: **Nutrition Management:** Assistance with or provision of balance dietary intake of foods and fluids.		NOC Suggested Outcome: **Nutritional Status:** Extent to which nutrients are available to meet metabolic needs.
The child will maintain weight and demonstrate adequate serum albumin and hydration.	■ Provide an opportunity to choose meals. Offer a variety of foods. Provide snacks. ■ Encourage the child to have meals with other children. ■ Provide a multivitamin supplement. ■ Substitute milk and juices for water. ■ Provide nasogastric feedings as needed. ■ Weigh the child daily.	■ Encourages intake. General malaise and anorexia lead to poor healing. ■ Socialization improves intake. ■ Vitamin C aids zinc absorption; zinc aids in healing. ■ A child with a burn greater than 10% of BSA cannot usually meet nutrition requirements without assistance. ■ Provides objective evaluation.	The child maintains weight, adequate hydration, normal serum albumin.
8. Anxiety (Child) related to threat to or change in health status			
	NIC Priority Intervention: **Anxiety Reduction:** Minimizing apprehension, dread, foreboding, or uneasiness related to an unidentified source of anticipated danger.		NOC Suggested Outcome: **Coping:** Actions to manage stressors that tax an individual's resources.
The child will verbalize reduced anxiety.	■ Provide continuity of care providers. ■ Encourage parents to stay with the child; calls from home; pictures from classmates. ■ Group tasks and activities.	■ Helps to build a trusting relationship. ■ Familiar surroundings, people, and items encourage relaxation. ■ Reduces overstimulation and encourages rest.	The child expresses and shows signs of reduced anxiety.
9. Anxiety (Parent) related to situational crisis			
	NIC Priority Intervention: **Anxiety Reduction:** Minimizing apprehension, dread, foreboding, or uneasiness related to an unidentified source of anticipated danger.		NOC Suggested Outcome: **Anxiety Control:** Ability to eliminate or reduce feelings of apprehension and tension from an unidentified source.
Parents will verbalize decreased anxiety.	■ Provide educational materials about healing, grafting, dressing changes, and course of action. ■ Be flexible when teaching parents about wound care. ■ Provide referral to social services or parent support group	■ Knowledge reduces anxiety. ■ Adults learn in many different ways. ■ Allows for venting of fears and guilt feelings, and provides exchange of ideas on dealing with hospitalization and long-term care.	Parents state decreased anxiety.

Provide Emotional Support

Burned children have received a profound insult to their body and their self-image. Fear and anxiety related to disfigurement and scarring are common responses, especially among adolescents. Increased stress occurs as a result of the shock and pain of the injury, as well as the unfamiliar surroundings and presence of health care providers.

An attitude of genuine interest and concern on the part of the nurse is essential. The child should be oriented to his or her surroundings frequently and given ample preparation for procedures, when possible. Continuity of care providers is important in developing a trusting relationship with the child. Encourage the child to voice concerns, and show understanding and support.

Play therapy is encouraged for children, even if they can only observe initially. Play therapy serves several purposes for the child with a major burn:

- It provides an outlet for frustration, independence, and creativity.
- It promotes activities that challenge range of motion.
- It normalizes the child's daily routine.
- It encourages the child, who sees the progress that other children make day by day.

Families are at risk for emotional stress. They should be forewarned about the expected edema and the resulting gross changes in the child's body. Parents often feel guilty and responsible for the child's injury. It is important to help parents focus on recovery rather than on past actions. Fear usually results from lack of knowledge about the severity of the burn and the child's status, especially in the early stages of burn care and admission to the hospital ICU. Include the family in the child's care when possible. The family must be given information and frequent updates. This promotes the development of trust between the family and the health care team.

Autografting procedures enable the child to recover from major burns, but the operation leaves visible scarring. Psychologic support is therefore essential to the child's recovery. Social workers, chaplains, art therapists, child life specialists, and play therapists are trained to help the child and family deal with the stressors of recovery. Appropriate referrals should be made to ensure that the child and family receive necessary services.

Discharge Planning and Home Care Teaching

Home care needs should be identified and addressed well in advance of discharge. Thorough assessment is necessary to identify the family's needs related to the child's discharge home or to a rehabilitation facility. Discharge planning may include instructing parents in nutrition and diet needs, safety in the home, burn wound care, and range-of-motion exercises to prevent contractures.

Provide support and encouragement to parents when they are learning how to care for the burned child. Many parents find it difficult to perform dressing change procedures they know will inflict pain on their child. Provide pain medication for dressing changes, and outline specific guidelines so that parents and health care team members will have the same focus. Parents should first observe care being performed and then provide repeat demonstrations until competent.

Care in the Community

Care of the child with a burn requires long-term therapy and rehabilitation. Nurses in clinic and home care settings continue the care provided during hospitalization. Long-term care commonly occurs in the home, with frequent visits to health care professionals. In some cases, children return to the hospital clinic for dressing changes on a regular basis. Children with extensive burns or with burns in locations that have the potential to cause functional limitations related to scarring must often wear an elasticized (Jobst) garment, and sometimes a face mask if the face was burned. The Jobst garment may present a threat to the child's body image, but it is an important means of decreasing scarring. Scar management may also be handled through drug injections or surgery (e.g., revision, grafting, or Z-plasty). Help families understand the need for the special garments and masks and how to clean and care for them.

Continued physical therapy and occupational therapy are often needed to increase strength and dexterity in performing ADLs and to prevent contractures. Emphasis is placed on returning to normal ADLs as soon as possible, such as returning to school as soon as health permits. Some children have home tutors for a time to decrease their risk of exposure to infection.

School reentry is often a traumatic experience, especially for older children and adolescents, because of the fear of rejection, decreased self-esteem, and impaired body image. The child's primary nurse, social worker, and child life specialist may visit the school of a child with a burn injury before the child returns to school—bringing photographs of the child, pressure garments, or other items—to desensitize the class and allow them to explore their emotions relating to the child's burn injury. Several communities offer support groups for families and children with burn injuries. Referral to these groups may be beneficial.

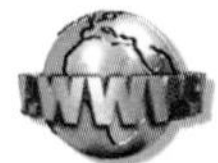

Burn Rehabilitation and Support

Management of Minor Burns

Many children with minor burns are cared for at home after an initial visit to the emergency department or urgent care clinic. Any open blisters are debrided, and a thin layer of silver sulfadiazine is applied over the burn. Do not place this medication close to the eyes or mouth. The burn is then covered with one or two layers of gauze. Burn dressings should be changed twice daily. This involves cleaning the burn and reapplying antibiotic cream.

Instruct parents to increase the child's fluid intake to compensate for loss of fluid through damaged skin. A high-calorie, high-protein diet is necessary to meet the increased nutritional requirements of healing. Acetaminophen (Tylenol) with codeine is often given, especially before dressing changes. Infection is a common complication. The child should be seen within 48 hours of treatment to monitor progress. Reinforce to parents the importance of follow-up appointments.

Moisturizing creams can be used after healing to relieve residual drying. The healed skin is highly sensitive to sunburn, so cover the area or use a sunscreen. Use of a sunscreen will also help prevent hyperpigmentation after burn healing.

SUNBURN

Sunburn is a burn injury to the outer layer of skin caused by excess sun exposure, or sun exposure after taking phototoxic drugs (acne medication, chlorpheniramine, diphenylhydramine, sulfonamides, tetracycline) (Laughlin-Richard, 2000). It occurs more often in fair-skinned children, who have less **melanin** (skin pigment) to protect their skin against these harmful rays. Repeated sunburns during childhood correlate strongly with the development of malignant melanoma in adulthood. Melanoma is the most common cancer in women between 25 and 29 years (Schachner, 2000). Avoiding sunburn during childhood is believed to be more important than actions taken to protect skin during adulthood.

Erythema and skin tenderness usually develop between 30 minutes and 4 hours after exposure to sunlight. Increased vasodilation and vascular permeability result in the extravasation of fluid to the tissues and white blood cell migration to the damaged skin. The erythema peaks at 24 hours. Prolonged exposure can result in edema, vesiculation, bullae, or ulceration. Systemic complaints include malaise, insomnia (because of skin tenderness), fatigue, headaches, and chilling (because of rapid heat loss).

CLINICAL TIP

It is estimated that 80% of a person's lifetime exposure to sunburns occurs before 21 years of age. This occurs at a time when the epidermis is relatively thin. Melanin is also present in low levels during infancy and childhood (Laughlin-Richard, 2000). For these reasons, it is recommended that children use a sunscreen with an SPF of 15 or higher during outdoor activities.

FAMILIES WANT TO KNOW

Caring for Minor Burns

- Place burn under cool, running water to stop the burning process and to help pain.
- Do not use ice as it can cause more damage to the injured skin.
- Remove all clothing and jewelry from the burned area.
- Apply a topical antibiotic such as Neosporin.

Treatment is generally supportive. Pain can be relieved by cool compresses followed by the application of a topical corticosteroid to relieve discomfort. Children with severe sunburn may require nonsteroidal anti-inflammatory drugs for pain relief and reduced inflammation (see Chapter 9).

Nursing Management

Educate parents and children about ways to prevent sunburn. Advise that repeated sunburns may lead to permanent skin damage and skin cancer. Recommend to parents that children use sunscreens of at least sun protection factor (SPF) 15, reapplied several times daily, wear protective clothing, and limit the amount of time they spend in the sun. Children should also wear sunglasses with 99% ultraviolet blockage.

HYPOTHERMIA

Hypothermia is a condition in which the core body temperature falls below 35°C (95°F). This occurs when the heat produced by the body is less than the heat lost. Hypothermia is a life-threatening emergency.

Hypothermia is associated with near-drowning episodes, because body heat is lost quickly in water, as compared with air. Children are at greater risk for hypothermia because of their thinner skin, limited subcutaneous fat, and high surface area to body mass ratio. As the core temperature falls, the body tries to conserve this temperature at the expense of the extremities. Increased muscle tone and an increased metabolic rate occur. Shivering occurs to try to rewarm the blood before it returns to the core of the body. Other causes of hypothermia include exposure to a cold environment, ingestion of alcohol or barbiturates, trauma or a brain disorder that interferes with temperature regulation, and overwhelming sepsis (Eichelberger, Ball, & Pratsch, et al., 1998).

Symptoms of mild hypothermia include slurred speech, incoordination, poor judgment, and shivering. Symptoms of moderate hypothermia include depressed respirations, slow pulse, low blood pressure, pale or cyanotic color, shivering, dilated pupils, and confusion. Profound hypothermia (body temperature below 29°C [84°F]) may result in absence of respirations and pulse, ventricular arrhythmia, dilated pupils, and loss of consciousness.

FAMILIES WANT TO KNOW

Preventing Sunburn

- Keep children out of direct sunlight as much as possible, especially the midday sun. Avoid scheduling outdoor activities during the hours of maximum exposure (10 A.M. to 2 P.M.).
- When outdoors, minimize exposed areas by wearing hats and long-sleeve, closely woven cotton clothing and pants; wear T-shirts while swimming. Special sun protection clothing is now available from some manufacturers.
- Be aware that water, concrete, and sand reflect sunlight and increase exposure up to 90% by reflecting up to 85% of the ultraviolet rays.
- Use sunscreen (of at least 15 SPF). For optimal protection, apply as thickly as directed to all exposed areas 30–45 minutes before sun exposure. Reapply every 2 hours as needed, or sooner if swimming, toweling off, or perspiring heavily.
- Use a waterproof sunscreen when swimming; this provides protection in water for approximately 60–80 minutes. Then reapply. Avoid placing waterproof sunscreen in the eyes as it causes severe pain and a chemical burn. Call the poison control center immediately for guidance.
- Avoid using sunscreens in infants less than 6 months of age because of the possibility of absorption of the chemicals through their skin.
- Remember that a child can be burned even on a cloudy day. Up to 80% of ultraviolet rays can penetrate the cloud cover.
- If the child is taking any medications, check with your health care practitioner before exposure (some medications cause hypersensitivity to sunlight).

Clinical therapy focuses on resuscitation, if necessary, and gradual rewarming of the body. The child who has been immersed in cold water for a long time (30 to 45 minutes) should receive CPR until the body temperature returns to normal because the diving reflex may preserve vital organs. Body temperature is assessed with a rectal thermometer. For mild hypothermia (temperature above 35°C [95°F]), external heat lamps, immersion in warm water, and an electric blanket may be all that are necessary. More aggressive techniques are required for profound hypothermia, including use of humidified, warm oxygen; warmed intravenous fluids; hemodialysis; or application of warmth to core circulation areas (axilla, groin, and posterior neck).

If a child becomes hypothermic during an outing such as a camping trip, a warm person should get into a sleeping bag (or under the blankets) next to the child. This action will warm the child and prevent further heat loss.

CLINICAL TIP

The diving reflex is a series of changes in the cardiovascular system that occurs when the face and nose are immersed in cold water. Heart rate decreases and blood flow is decreased to all body areas except the brain, thus conserving oxygen.

Nursing Management

Monitor vital signs and urine output during rewarming. Prevention is geared toward educating parents to layer children's clothing in cold climates, recognize signs of hypothermia, decrease time of exposure to cold, and be aware of actions to take for mild hypothermia. Teach school-age children and adolescents who go on camping and hunting trips how to recognize and manage hypothermia in themselves and others. Teach preventive techniques such as not riding snowmobiles or walking on ice that may be thin.

CLINICAL TIP

First aid for hypothermia: If mild hypothermia occurs at home, move the child to a dry area and remove any wet clothing. Replace with warm, dry clothing, and encourage the child to drink a warm, high-calorie liquid, if able.

FROSTBITE

Frostbite is an extreme form of hypothermia that results from overexposure to extremely low temperatures. Areas of the body at high risk for frostbite include the hands, feet, cheeks, nose, and ears. Skin cells have a high concentration of water. Ice crystallizes in the tissues, resulting in cellular dehydration and ischemic damage.

Clinical manifestations depend on the severity of the cellular damage. The skin at first appears pale and is numb. Rapid rewarming causes a flush and the sensation of tingling, burning, or prickling in the affected area. The erythema and mild swelling develop into bullae. The extent of injury usually is not initially apparent.

If frostbite is suspected, loosen all constricting clothing and remove any wet clothes. Obtain health care as soon as possible. Rewarming is done slowly to decrease the chance of cellular damage. Immerse the affected part for 10 to 15 minutes in water warmed to between 38° and 40°C (100.4° and 104°F). Analgesics may be given to manage pain. Elevate the affected part, if possible, to improve venous return. Encourage the child to drink warm fluids to aid in the warming process. Because the frostbitten area is numb, extreme caution is needed to protect it from any trauma.

Lengthy treatment and amputation are sometimes necessary when tissues are permanently damaged.

Nursing Management

As with hypothermia, the goal of management is prevention. Teach parents to layer children's clothing for warmth and to pack extra blankets and clothing if cold temperatures are expected during outdoor activities. Teach adolescents how to avoid frostbite during hunting and other cold weather expeditions. Wet clothing should be changed quickly. Early care is instrumental in minimizing permanent injury. Severe frostbite will require hospitalization, with fluid management, dressing changes, antibiotic therapy, and careful attention to diet.

BITES

Animal Bites

Each year, 5 million people are bitten by animals in the United States, of which 80% are dog bites. Other animals that may bite include cats, birds, turtles, and wild animals such as bats, squirrels, and raccoons. Children, especially less than 8 years old, are at higher risk for animal bites, and boys are bitten more than twice as often as girls (Bernardo, Gardner, & O'Connor, et al., 2000). The majority of dogs are known by the child.

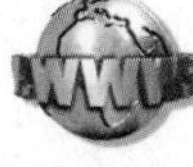

Dog Bite Statistics

LAW & ETHICS

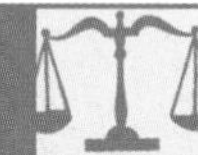

If a child sustains an animal bite, a complete and accurate history is essential, and should include the following:

- Extent of injury
- Circumstances surrounding attack
- Present location of animal
- Attempts to assess animal's health

CLINICAL TIP

Human Rabies immune globulin (HRIG) or human diploid cell rabies (HDCV) vaccine should be given to all children bitten by wild animals in which rabies cannot be excluded, as well as to children bitten by domestic animals (cats and dogs) suspected or proven to be rabid. See Chapter 12 for a description of rabies treatment.

Assessment includes noting location and number of puncture wounds, abrasions, lacerations, and crushing injuries, redness or swelling at entry sites, redness extending from site (possible cellulitis), and any drainage related to the bite. Check for nerve, muscle, tendon, or vascular damage. Findings should be carefully documented. Head and neck bites require radiographic examination to rule out any associated injury, such as trauma to the airway or breathing structures or a depressed skull fracture.

To decrease infection, initial treatment involves high-pressure wound irrigation with large quantities of sterile saline or lactated Ringer's solution rather than scrubbing. A 19-gauge needle on a 60-cc syringe may be used. Any devitalized tissue is debrided. Conscious sedation may be needed for some children. A clean pressure dressing is applied, and the affected part is elevated to reduce bleeding. Small wounds may be closed with adhesive strips rather than suturing because of the potential for infection. Severe bites sometimes require surgical closure or reconstruction. Wounds over joints should be immobilized and elevated. Puncture wounds should not be irrigated or sutured.

Dog bites tend to be crushing, rather than clean, sharp lacerations. The major complication of bites is infection. Antibiotics and early treatment of the wound can greatly decrease this sequela. Dog bites should be reported to the police, and the dog should be observed for 10 days for signs of rabies. Cat bites are also dangerous because they tend to be puncture wounds and are therefore associated with a higher rate of infection, cellulitis, and abscesses. Bites by wild animals in areas with endemic rabies will require rabies prophylaxis. Check the child's immunization record to determine if a tetanus booster is necessary. (Refer to Chapter 12 for information about rabies and the immunization schedule.) Instruct parents about how to care for the wound.

Human Bites

Human bites are more common than most people realize. They usually occur in toddlers and young children. Because the mouth harbors many bacteria, infection is fairly common. Assess the risk for hepatitis B and HIV infection. Antibiotics may be prescribed to prevent systemic complications. Initial treatment includes irrigating with sterile saline and debridement. Instruct parents about how to care for the wound. Follow-up is important to watch for infection.

NURSING MANAGEMENT Educate parents about ways to prevent animal and human bites and the importance of teaching children appropriate behavior around other children and animals. When these bites occur in a childcare or school setting, inform parents about the human bite so they can discuss potential risks and follow up with a health care provider.

FAMILIES WANT TO KNOW

Preventing Animal Bites

- Teach children the following rules:
  Avoid all unfamiliar animals and report them to a parent.
  Avoid contact with all wild animals.
  Do not touch an animal when it is eating, sleeping, or nursing.
  Never overexcite an animal, even in play. Do not rough house or play games that stimulate aggressive behavior.
  Never tease or throw objects at an animal.
  Never put your face close to an animal. Seek permission before hugging or petting an animal.
  If approached by a dog, stay calm, stand still, talk softly, and back away slowly until the dog loses interest; do not run.
  If attacked, pretend to be a tree or a log and protect the face.
- If an animal is sick or acting strangely, notify the health department.
- Never leave a young child alone with an animal.
- Do not buy a pet unless you are confident of your child's ability to respect it.
- Spay or neuter the pet to reduce aggression.

As these children are often cared for at home, teach the parents about the normal healing process, proper wound care, and the signs and symptoms of infection.

Children who receive traumatic animal bites often experience significant psychologic trauma. They may develop a fear of strange animals and a decreased capacity to enjoy the presence of household pets. Counseling and follow-up may be necessary to evaluate such concerns.

Insect Bites and Stings

Insect bites and stings occur frequently in children and usually are not a cause for concern. Exceptions include bites or stings by insects that carry parasites or communicable diseases (ticks, mosquitos), those of venomous nature (spiders), and those that produce an allergic reaction. About 4% of the population is sensitized to bee stings (Herman & Skokan, 1999). (For a discussion of Lyme disease and Rocky Mountain spotted fever, see Chapter 12.)

CLINICAL TIP

A dash of meat tenderizer (papain powder) and a drop of water massaged into the skin for 5 minutes quickly relieves the pain of most insect bites and stings. Ice is also effective.

Reactions to mosquito and flea bites can be localized or systemic. Local reactions include discrete, red papules and edema at the bite site, as well as itching, burning, pain, and hives. Local inflammation results from injected foreign protein or chemicals. Most bites produce minimal discomfort. Systemic reactions can include wheezing, urticaria, laryngeal edema, and shock.

Treatment is usually supportive and focuses on relieving itching and reducing inflammation. Pruritus is treated with cold compresses or ice applied to the site and an antihistamine. In children who are sensitized to insect bites, pruritic wheals and bullae tend to develop with repeat exposure. In rare cases, exposure can lead to an anaphylactic reaction. If large wheals, swelling of extremities, or respiratory difficulty occurs, emergency medical treatment is needed.

CLINICAL TIP

Remove a bee stinger as soon as possible, but do not use tweezers or squeeze the venom sack. This pushes more venom into the skin. Use a straight edge, such as a piece of cardboard, to pull the stinger out in a scraping motion.

Bees and fire ants (Hymenoptera) inject a hemolytic, neurotoxic venom that causes a histaminelike response. Fire ants bite repeatedly in a small area. A black center is seen at the point of the bite along with pustules and local swelling. Reactions to either bee stings or fire ant bites may be local inflammation or a systemic allergic response (wheezing, urticaria, diarrhea, vomiting, and dizziness). In some cases an anaphylactic response occurs. Treatment of local reactions includes antihistamines. For systemic reactions, treat with glucocorticoids and antihistamines or intravenous or subcutaneous 1:1000 epinephrine solution. Desensitization for the Hymenoptera group should also be considered when the child has a systemic reaction.

Black widow spider bites are characterized by a stinging sensation at the time of the bite followed by swelling, redness, and pain at the site. Red fang marks can be seen in a target lesion. Systemic symptoms can occur 15 minutes to 2 hours after the bite and include dizziness, fever, regional lymph node tenderness, severe abdominal pain (abdominal muscle rigidity), and weakness. Profuse sweating, vomiting, hypertension, and tachycardia may also be seen. Muscle cramps begin near the bite and can involve all skeletal muscles. If large doses of venom are absorbed, the bite may lead to paralysis and death. A neurotoxin produced by the spider is responsible for the symptoms. The black widow spider can be recognized by the red and orange hourglass-shape markings on its underside. It usually bites in self-defense and avoids light areas. Treatment involves cleansing the wound, elevating the extremity, and immediately applying ice packs. Sedatives, analgesics, or muscle relaxants may be prescribed. Intravenous calcium gluconate may be given for muscle spasms. Antivenom (produced in horse serum) is used only in severe or high-risk cases because of the risk for anaphylaxis (Metry & Hebert, 2000). Hydrocortisone may decrease the inflammatory response. Symptoms generally peak in 3 to 12 hours and diminish within 72 hours.

The brown recluse spider bite is characterized by a sharp pain resembling a sting. Most bites are mild and cause only minimal edema and mild erythema. Severe bites can become necrotic over 48 to 72 hours in 10% of cases. (Metry & Hebert, 2000). The child experiences mild to severe pain and tenderness. Within 3 to 4 days, a purple star-shaped area forms at the site with a white ischemic halo and outer ring of erythema progressing to black eschar that is sloughed off. The wound usually heals with scar formation in 6 to 8 weeks. Severe progressive reactions may include associated fever, chills, restlessness, malaise, joint pain, and nausea and vomiting. Intravascular hemolysis may also occur with a severe reaction that results in anemia. The brown recluse spider is recognized by the fiddle-shape marking on its head. It is usually unaggressive and bites only when provoked. Treatment involves prophylactic antibiotics, analgesics, application of cool compresses to the site, and corticosteroids for inflammation. In some cases a skin graft is needed.

CLINICAL TIP

Use insect repellent containing DEET (diethyltoluamide) in concentrations less than 10% for children. If combined with sunscreen, the effectiveness of the sunscreen is reduced by a third or half, so use sunscreen with an SPF of 30 (Metry & Hebert, 2000). However, caution parents to avoid overuse of products containing DEET, especially with infants and small children. Cases of toxic encephalopathy have been reported following repeated use on children's bedding and clothing (Metry & Hebert, 2000).

NURSING MANAGEMENT The goal of nursing care is prevention. Become familiar with the harmful insects in your geographic area, so you can identify them and recognize their effects. Children should be taught to avoid spiders and other biting or stinging insects. Many commercial repellents (OFF, Cutter's, Deep Woods OFF) are available. Most products contain DEET (diethyltoluamide) and are effective against many insects including mosquitos, fleas, ticks, and chiggers. DEET does not repel stinging insects. Warn parents against using heavily perfumed shampoos, powders, soaps, or lotions, or dressing children in bright clothing when outdoors, as these may attract insects. Household pets may be a source of fleas or ticks. Encourage frequent inspection of pets and preventive treatments against fleas and ticks before pets are allowed prolonged contact with children. When a known allergy to Hymenoptera has occurred, the child should wear a medical alert identification and carry an emergency kit with epinephrine. Desensitization injections may be given. Teach parents and school personnel how to administer epinephrine.

Snake Bites

Venomous snakes are found in most areas of the country. During warm months of the year, snakes are active and likely to bite if disturbed. Fortunately many bites are dry, delivering no venom. Fatalities are rare. Rattlesnake, copperhead, and cottonmouth venom affects the blood coagulation system (Bond & Burkhart, 1997). Coral snake venom causes neuromuscular paralysis.

Puncture marks, white wheal, and severe pain are noted at the site. Erythema and edema rapidly develop and extend from the site. Numbness may occur. Systemic signs include dizziness, nausea and vomiting, sweating and chills, weakness, hematemesis and bleeding from the nose, intestines, or bladder. Numbness of the tongue and perioral areas may develop. Death may occur from intracranial hemorrhage. Clinical therapy involves immobilization of the extremity and a cold compress to slow the spread of the venom. Excision of the bite is no longer recommended. Laboratory studies include complete blood count, platelet count, coagulation studies, electrolytes, and renal function. Specific antivenom is quickly administered, but because antivenom contains a horse serum base, a skin test may be performed first to detect hypersensitivity. A tetanus booster is given if vaccination status is unknown or the tetanus series is incomplete.

NURSING MANAGEMENT Nursing care involves assessment of the child for initial and progressive signs of envenomation. First aid involves immobilizing the extremity, keeping it in dependent position to slow the spread of venom, and cold compresses. Remove any jewelry from the injured extremity. Keep the child quiet and calm to slow the circulation. Help the child identify the snake from pictures of snakes common to the geographic area; however, keep in mind that other venomous snakes may be kept as exotic pets.

Administer the antivenom intravenously after tests for sensitivity to horse serum are completed. Assist in locating additional antivenom if the hospital does not have an adequate supply. Monitor the child for progressive signs of envenomation and for hypersensitivity responses to antivenom. Provide emotional support to the child and family, and teach them how to avoid future snakebites.

CONTUSIONS

Contusions are soft tissue injuries that result from a variety of causes. Often it is difficult to assess whether an injury has caused underlying tissue damage. An injury does not have to break the skin to result in internal damage. Radiographic examination may be necessary to rule out broken bones or further tissue damage. Signs and symptoms that indicate a need for treatment include swelling that does not subside within 72 hours, intense pain, inability to move the injured part, and infection. Elevate the injured extremity and apply ice as soon as possible after injury to reduce inflammation and swelling in the area.

FOREIGN BODIES

Many skin injuries result from penetration of foreign particles. Common substances include gravel from abrasions, bee stingers, and splinters. Treatment of superficial foreign bodies involves irrigating the wound to try to forcibly dislodge the debris. A deeply embedded foreign body is best removed under medical supervision to avoid permanent injury or scarring.

Chapter Highlights

- The skin has several essential functions: perception of pain, heat, and cold; protection from invasion by microorganisms and trauma; temperature regulation; vitamin D synthesis; and excretion.
- Wound healing has three phases: inflammation, reconstruction, and maturation.
- Contact dermatitis is an inflammation of the skin that occurs in response to direct contact with an allergen, causing an immune response or an irritant without an immune response.
- Superabsorbent disposable diapers reduce the frequency and severity of diaper dermatitis because, when wet, a gel forms and keeps the skin drier than cloth diapers.
- Seborrheic dermatitis is an inflammatory skin condition due to an overgrowth of *Pityrosporum* yeast in areas of sebaceous gland activity. It is commonly found on the scalp, forehead, and postauricular and periorbital areas.
- Treatment of atopic dermatitis involves hydration and lubrication of the skin with moisturizing ointments. Inflammation is treated with wet compresses and corticosteroid ointments.
- Acne medications, tretinoin or isotretinoin, are phototoxic. Avoidance of sun exposure or the use of sunscreen is important to prevent a significant sunburn.
- The classic impetigo lesion begins as a vesicle surrounded by edema and redness. The vesicle fluid turns cloudy and ruptures, leaving a honey-colored crust on an ulcerated base.
- Folliculitis, a superficial inflammation of the pilosebaceous follicle, may be associated with *Pseudomonas* exposure in a poorly chlorinated pool or hot tub.
- Children with cellulitis appear ill with fever, chills, malaise, and enlarged lymph nodes. The infected site is erythematous, warm, and tender.
- Treatment for lice includes a pediculicide shampoo, distilled white vinegar to loosen the nits' bonds to the hair shafts, and combing the hair with a fine-toothed comb to remove all the nits. A second treatment is needed in 7 days.
- Scabies lesions appear as linear, threadlike, grayish burrows 1 cm to 10 cm in length that may end in a pinpoint vesicle. Often the child's scratching and secondary infection will change the appearance of the lesions.
- Children using oral inhalers with corticosteroids are at risk for thrush (oral candidiasis). Rinsing the mouth well with water after using the inhaler helps to prevent thrush.
- Treatment for tinea capitus involves 8 to 12 weeks of oral griseofulvin. Giving this medication with fatty foods such as whole milk or peanut butter enhances its absorption.
- Children at greatest risk for pressure ulcers are those with limited mobility, sensory deficits, or the inability to change positions.
- Of the four main types of burns (thermal, chemical, electrical, and radioactive), thermal burns are most common in children. They occur through exposure to flames or scalds and contact with a hot object.
- Repeated sunburns during childhood increase the risk for development of malignant melanoma in early adulthood.
- Children are at greater risk for hypothermia because of their thinner skin, limited subcutaneous fat, and high surface area to body mass ratio.
- Frostbite occurs when ice crystallizes in the tissues, causing cellular dehydration and ischemic damage.
- Dog bites account for 80% of animal bites treated in the United States. Children at greater risk for animal bites are boys less than 8 years old. Most children know the dog that bites them.
- Insects and spiders with venomous bites include bees, fire ants, black widow spiders, and brown recluse spiders.
- Venomous snakes living in the wild in the United States include rattlesnakes, copperheads, cottonmouths, and coral snakes.

EXPLORE MediaLink

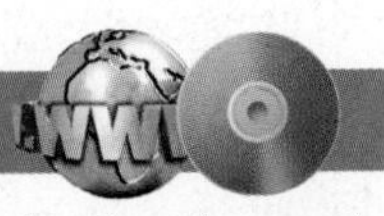

- NCLEX review, case studies, and other interactive resources for this chapter can be found on the Companion Website at **http://www.prenhall.com/ball.** Click on Chapter 23 to select the activities for this chapter.
- For animations, more NCLEX review questions, and an audio glossary, access the accompanying CD-ROM in this textbook.

References

1. American Academy of Pediatrics Committee on Infectious Disease. (2000). *Red book, report of the committee on infectious disease* (25th ed). Elk Grove Village, IL: author.
2. Angel, T. A., Nigro, J., & Levy, M. L. (2000). Infestations in the pediatric patient. *Pediatric Clinics of North America, 47*(4), 921–935.
3. Armsmeier, S. L., & Paller, A. S. (1997). Getting to the bottom of diaper dermatitis. *Contemporary Pediatrics, 14*(11), 115–129.
4. Ball, J. W. (1998). *Mosby's pediatric patient teaching guides.* St. Louis: Mosby.
5. Bernardo, L. M., Gardner, M. J., O'Connor, J., & Amon, N. (2000). Dog bites in children treated in a pediatric emergency department. *Journal of Society of Pediatric Nurses, 5*(2), 87–95.
6. Bond, R. G., & Burkhart, K. K. (1997). Thrombocytopenia following timber rattlesnake envenomation. *Annals of Emergency Medicine, 30*(1), 40–44
7. Buck, M. L. (2001). Isotretinoin: Improving patient education and reducing risk. *Pediatric Pharmacology, 7*(7), 1–6.
8. Darmstadt, G. L. (1997). A guide to superficial strep and staph skin infections. *Contemporary Pediatrics, 14*(5), 95–116.
9. Eichelberger, M. R., Ball, J. W., Pratsch, G. L., & Clark, J. R. (1998). *Pediatric emergencies* (2nd ed., p. 182). Upper Saddle River, NJ: Prentice Hall.
10. Friedlander, S. F. (1998). Contact dermatitis. *Pediatrics in Review, 19*(5), 166–170.
11. Gardner, P., Coles, D., & Kemper, K. J. (2001). The skinny on herbal remedies for dermatologic disorders. *Contemporary Pediatrics, 18*(7), 103–114.
12. Hebert, P. W., Rakes, G. P., Loach, T. C., & Murphy, D. D. (1997). Recognizing the young atopic child. *Contemporary Pediatrics, 14*(4), 131–139.
13. Herman, B. E., & Skokan, E. G. (1999). Bites that poison: A tale of spiders, snakes, and scorpions. *Contemporary Pediatrics, 16*(8), 41–65.
14. Hernandez-Reif, M., Field, T., Largie, S., Hart, S., Redezepi, M., Nierenberg, B., & Peck, M. (2001). Children's distress during burn treatment reduced by massage therapy. *Journal of Burn Care Rehabilitation, 22*(2), 191–195.
15. Herndon, D. N., & Spies, M. (2001). Modern burn care. *Seminars in Pediatric Surgery, 10*(1), 28–31.
16. Jick, S. S., Kremers, H. M., & Vasilakis-Scarmozza, C. (2000). Isotretinoin use and risk of depression, psychotic symptoms, suicide, and attempted suicide. *Archives of Dermatology, 136*(10), 1231–1236.
17. Kazaks, E. L., & Lane, A. T. (2000). Diaper dermatitis. *Pediatric Clinics of North America, 47*(4), 909–919.
18. Laughlin-Richard, N. (2000). Sun exposure and skin cancer prevention in children and adolescents. *Journal of School Nursing, 16*(2), 20–26.
19. Loman, D. G. (2000). Assessment of skin breakdown risk in children. *Journal of Child and Family Nursing, 3*(3), 234–238.
20. Lukish, J. R., Eichelberger, M. R., Newman, K. D., Pao, M., Nobuhara, K., Keating, M., et al. (2001). The use of a bioactive skin substitute decreases length of stay for pediatric burn patients. *Journal of Pediatric Surgery, 36*(8), 1118–1121.
21. Mancini, A. J. (2000). Acne vulgaris: A treatment update. *Contemporary Pediatrics, 17*(12), 122–133.
22. McDonald, L. L., & Smith, M. L. (1998). Diagnostic dilemmas in pediatric/adolescent dermatology: Scaly scalp. *Journal of Pediatric Health Care, 12*(2), 80–84.
23. Metry, D. W., & Hebert, A. A. (2000). Insect and arachnid stings, bites, infestations, and repellents. *Pediatric Annals, 29*(1), 39–48.
24. Murphy, S. A. (2000). Deaths: Final data for 1998. *National Vital Statistics Reports, 48*(11). Hyattsville, MD: National Center for Health Statistics.
25. Nicol, N. H. (2000). Managing atopic dermatitis in children and adults. *The Nurse Practitioner, 25*(4), 54–76.
26. Quigley, S. M., & Curley, M. A. Q. (1996). Skin integrity in the pediatric population: Preventing and managing pressure ulcers. *Journal of the Society of Pediatric Nurses, 1*(1), 7–18.
27. Raimer, S. S. (2000). Managing pediatric atopic dermatitis. *Clinical Pediatrics, 39*(1), 1–14.
28. Rodgers, G. L. (2000). Reducing the toll of childhood burns. *Contemporary Pediatrics, 17*(4), 152–173.
29. Rote, N. S. (1998). Inflammation. In K. L. McCance & S. E. Huether (eds.), *Pathophysiology: The biologic basis for disease in adults and children* (3rd ed., pp. 205–236). St. Louis: Mosby.
30. Schachner, L. A. (2000, May). Sun protection in three ways. *Contemporary Pediatrics,* (Suppl.), 8–11.
31. Schachner, L., Field, T., & Hernandez-Ruif, M., Duarte, A. M., & Krasnegor, J. (1998). Atopic dermatitis symptoms decreased in children following massage therapy. *Pediatric Dermatology, 15*(5), 390–395.
32. Sidbury, R., & Paller, A. S. (2000). The diagnosis and management of acne. *Pediatric Annals, 29*(1), 17–24.
33. Smith, M. L. (2000). Pediatric burns: Management of thermal, electrical, and chemical burns and burnlike dermatologic conditions. *Pediatric Annals, 29*(6), 367–378.
34. Stewart, C. (2000). Emergency care of pediatric burns. *Pediatric Emergency Medicine Reports, 5*(10), 101–112.
35. Su, J. C., Kemp, A. S., Varigos, G. A., & Nolan, T. M. (1997). Atopic eczema: Its impact on the family and financial cost. *Archives of Diseases in Children, 76*(2), 159–162.
36. Valencia, I. C., Falabella, A. F., & Schachner, L. A. (2001). New developments in wound care for infants and children. *Pediatric Annals, 30*(4), 211–218.
37. Vanderhooft, S. L. (1998). Is the rash really a drug reaction? *Contemporary Pediatrics, 15*(5), 118–137.
38. Weston, W. L., & Bruckner, A. (2000). Allergic contact dermatitis. *Pediatric Clinics of North America, 47*(4), 897–907.
39. Wiebelhaus, P., & Hansen, S. L. (2001). Another choice for burn victims. *RN, 64*(9), 34–37.

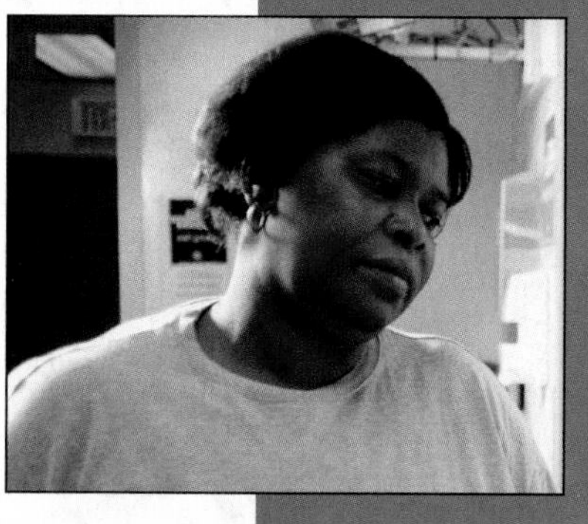

"WE'VE BEEN SO WORRIED ABOUT CASSANDRA. AFTER THE CAR CRASH, SHE BECAME SO FRIGHTENED OF EVERYTHING. SHE WAKES UP AT NIGHT SCREAMING AND HAS LOST INTEREST IN SCHOOL AND FRIENDS. WE HOPE THAT HER WORK WITH THE THERAPIST WILL HELP TO DECREASE HER FEARS AND GET HER INVOLVED IN ALL OF HER ACTIVITIES AGAIN."

Cassandra is a 9-year-old girl who has recently become fearful about attending school and awakens crying each night. She is in the third grade at a school she has attended for 2 years. A few weeks ago she was in a car crash as her mother drove her to school. She received only minor injuries and returned to school the next day. Her mother believes that Cassandra's behavior has been worsening since the car crash. She spoke with the school nurse, who is aware of no trauma at school, but did learn from the teacher that Cassandra has not been paying attention in class. Cassandra cannot explain why she does not want to go to school, only that her stomach aches or some other part of her body hurts.

Cassandra visited her pediatrician who ruled out any physical cause for her complaints, and referred her to a child psychologist. The psychologist has scheduled several sessions with Cassandra to help her learn to verbalize her fears and learn strategies to deal with them. She uses dolls in an attempt to help Cassandra act out her fears and gain some understanding. The psychologist communicates Cassandra's progress to the school nurse who helps to support her and makes sure she attends each day.

CHAPTER 24

ALTERATIONS IN MENTAL HEALTH FUNCTION

KEY TERMS

adaptive functioning The ability of an individual to meet the standards expected for his or her age by his or her cultural group.

affect Outward manifestation of feeling or emotion; the tone of a person's reaction or response to people or events.

agoraphobia Anxiety of being in places or situations from which escape may be difficult or embarrassing, or in which help may not be available.

behavior modification A technique used to reinforce desirable behaviors, helping the child to replace maladaptive behaviors with more appropriate ones.

cognitive therapy A therapeutic approach that attempts to help the person recognize automatic thought patterns that lead to unpleasant feelings.

echolalia A compulsive parroting of what is heard.

evidence-based practice Use of a body of scientific knowledge to plan health care services.

pervasive developmental disorders Conditions that begin in early childhood and are characterized by impaired social interactions and communication, with restricted interests, activities, and behaviors.

play therapy A therapeutic intervention often used with preschool and school-aged children. The child reveals conflicts, wishes, and fears on an unconscious level while playing with dolls, toys, clay, and other objects.

stereotypy Repetitive, obsessive, machine-like movements, commonly seen in autistic or schizophrenic children.

MediaLink

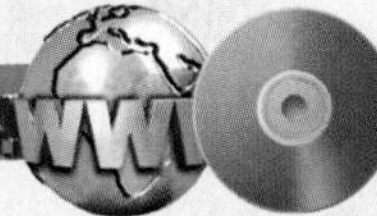

http://www.prenhall.com/ball

Resources for this chapter can be found on the CD-ROM accompanying this textbook, and on the Companion Website at http://www.prenhall.com/ball. Click on Chapter 24 to select the activities for this chapter.

CD-ROM

Audio Glossary
NCLEX Review

COMPANION WEBSITE

Web Links
NCLEX Review
MediaLink Applications
- Nursing Practice: Putting National Goals into Local Community Action
- Helping Families to Evaluate Mental Health Information on the Internet

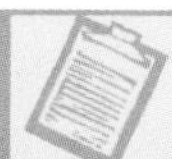

RESEARCH

Evidence-based practice refers to a body of scientific knowledge and its relationship to health care services (see Chapter 1). While the research basis for care in all areas of pediatric health is generally scant, there is even less scientific basis to support interventions in mental health services. Nurses must seek to apply evidence-based practice to enhance mental health care when possible, and to participate in research and outcomes measurement so that additional strong evidence can be gathered on the best approaches to care (Hoagwood, Burns, & Kiser, et al., 2001).

The purpose of this chapter is to provide the knowledge and tools that can help you to provide appropriate care for children with alterations in mental health. Because much of this care will be provided by psychiatric–mental health specialists, the nurse's role often centers on identification, support of the therapy, teaching, and referral.

Some mental health conditions in children originate from a genetic or physiologic cause. Examples include mental retardation and childhood schizophrenia. Often the environments in which children live influence their characteristics and contributes to dysfunctions such as anxiety, depression, and posttraumatic stress disorder.

Most mental health conditions are treated in community settings, and nurses in these settings play an active role in the treatment and support of the child and family. Nurses may function as case managers, assisting a family to deal with all areas of the child's care. Occasionally a child is hospitalized for treatment of a significant mental health disruption, or is hospitalized for treatment of another health problem and requires continued mental health services.

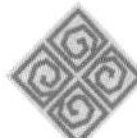

PSYCHOTHERAPEUTIC MANAGEMENT OF CHILDREN AND ADOLESCENTS

Mental health is foundational to a sense of personal well-being. However, 10% of children in the United States suffer from mental illness that is severe enough to impair functioning, and only 50% of those children receive any mental health services. Further, some of the services received are not comprehensive or multidisciplinary, leading to unmet mental health needs (Navon, Nelson, & Pagano, et al., 2001). In other cases, the interventions used are not based on evidence supported by theory and research investigation.

The surgeon general is leading an initiative to examine mental health in the United States and has identified a series of goals and steps toward improving mental health care for children (Department of Health and Human Services, 2000). From the ages of 10 to 21 years, mental health issues are among the top two leading causes of hospitalization in all age groups (see Chapter 1). This high rate of hospitalization infers that children are not receiving mental health services early, when outpatient care is appropriate and prognosis is best. To confront this childhood mental health crisis, the surgeon general's agenda has established a commitment to promote mental health as an essential part of child health, to integrate mental health services into all health services provided to children, to engage families and youth in planning for mental health care, and to develop and enhance the infrastructure to support child and youth mental health services (Department of Health and Human Services, 2000). See Table 24-1 for a list of the goals established in the surgeon general's report.

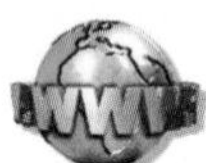

National Mental Health Goals and Organizations

The primary treatment goal in the management of children and adolescents with psychosocial disorders is to assist the child and family to achieve and maintain an optimal level of functioning through interventions designed to reduce the impact of stressors. Therapeutic interventions and communication are based on the principle that feelings motivate behaviors.

TABLE 24-1 Goals of the Surgeon General's National Action Agenda for Children's Mental Health

1. Promote public awareness of children's mental health issues and reduce stigma associated with mental illness.
2. Continue to develop, disseminate, and implement scientifically proven prevention and treatment services in the field of children's mental health.
3. Improve the assessment and recognition of mental health needs in children.
4. Eliminate racial/ethnic and socioeconomic disparities in access to mental health care.
5. Improve the infrastructure for children's mental health services, including support for scientifically proven interventions across professions.
6. Increase access to and coordination of quality mental health care services.
7. Train frontline providers to recognize and manage mental health issues and educate mental health providers in scientifically proven prevention and treatment services.
8. Monitor the access to and coordination of quality mental health care services.

Note: From Department of Health and Human Services. (2000). *Report on the surgeon general's conference on children's mental health: A national action agenda.* Washington, DC: U.S. Department of Health and Human Services.

Parents and others who are close to the child often fall into the habit of reacting to the child's behaviors rather than trying to find out what feelings may be precipitating the undesirable actions. Although behaviors may be considered in treatment, feelings and life experiences are often explored to provide insight and to lead to behavior change. Medication may be used to enhance and support other therapy, or may be the major therapeutic measure.

TREATMENT MODES

Three basic treatment modes are used: individual, family, and group therapy. The choice of treatment mode must take into account the child's age and developmental stage. Most therapists incorporate several intervention strategies simultaneously within these modes. Different strategies are more or less effective and appropriate for children and adolescents in various stages of development. A thorough understanding of developmental needs, expectations, and abilities is therefore essential for mental health professionals.

Individual Therapy

Individual therapy involves only the child and the therapist. Treatment of specific emotional problems or disorders may involve various techniques such as play therapy, psychodrama, art therapy, and **cognitive therapy** (a technique used to help a person recognize automatic negative thinking). Individual therapy may be short term (four to six sessions) or long term (lasting for several years).

Family Therapy

Family therapy involves the exploration of a particular emotional problem and its manifestations among the family members. Family therapy is based on the idea that the emotional symptoms or problems of an individual are an expression of emotional symptoms or problems in the family. The focus is on the relationships among the family members, not the psychologic conflict within each individual member.

Group Therapy

Group therapy involves an ongoing or limited number of sessions in which several individuals participate. The emphasis is on the interpersonal styles of relating to one another in the group. Group therapy is particularly effective with adolescents because of the importance of the peer group at this age. An advantage of group therapy is that stimuli and feedback come from multiple sources (the group members) instead of just one person (the therapist).

THERAPEUTIC STRATEGIES

Play Therapy

Play is often called the language or work of the child. From a developmental perspective, children progressively learn to express feelings and needs through action, fantasy, and finally language. The special quality of play buffers children against the pressures and demands of daily life. Play facilitates mastery of developmental stages by strengthening physical and neurologic processes. Play also assists in cognitive learning, setting the stage for problem solving and creativity.

Play therapy is a technique that reveals problems on a fantasy level through the use of toys, dolls, clay, art, and other creative objects. It is often used with preschool and school-age children who are experiencing anxiety, stress, and other specific nonpsychotic mental disorders. Play therapy encourages the child to act out feelings such as anger, hostility, sadness, and fear. It also provides the opportunity for the therapist to help the child understand, on a conscious or unconscious level, personal responses and behavior in a safe, supportive environment. This type of therapy was helpful for Cassandra, in the opening scenario, who was able to gain some control over a frightening environment by acting out fears and trying solutions during play with a therapist.

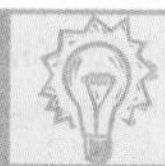

CLINICAL TIP

Play therapy, a technique used with children who have psychosocial disorders, is different from therapeutic play, which may be used with many hospitalized children (see Chapter 5). Although some techniques overlap, only a specialist is qualified to provide play therapy.

Art Therapy

Children who may be apprehensive about playing can sometimes be encouraged to participate in art therapy, using brief drawing exercises. This technique is appropriate for children of all ages, including adolescents. The drawings can help the therapist gain information about the child, the family, and the interactions between the child and family. However, children's drawings should never be used solely to form a definitive diagnosis.

When used in conjunction with a thorough history and appropriate psychologic testing information, art therapy can guide the child's treatment. These drawing exercises provide an opportunity to help in the healing process. The therapist can assist the child to release feelings of anger, pain, or fear onto paper, where they can be examined objectively. (Figures 24-1 ◆ to 24-4 present examples of this technique.)

Behavior and Cognitive Therapy

Behavior modification is a therapeutic technique that uses stimulus and response conditioning to alter inappropriate behaviors. It is used to reinforce desirable behaviors, helping the child to replace maladaptive behaviors with more appropriate ones. This technique is based on the assumption that any learned behavior can be unlearned. Thus, if parents,

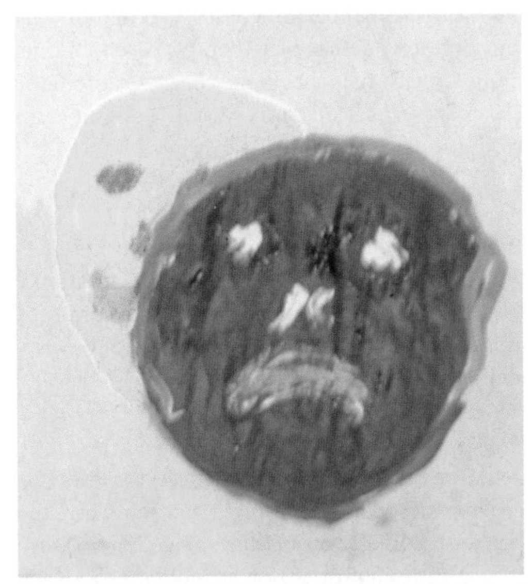

FIGURE 24-1 ◆
"Me." Drawn by a 14-year-old girl with major depression, anxiety, and school phobia who had experienced multiple losses over several years. Her mother had severe chronic lung problems and diabetes, and the girl had stopped attending school for fear that something would happen to her mother. This drawing represents the girl's obvious feelings of sadness and depression but also indicates a glimmer of hope (represented by the yellow mask coming from behind the dark mask of depression).

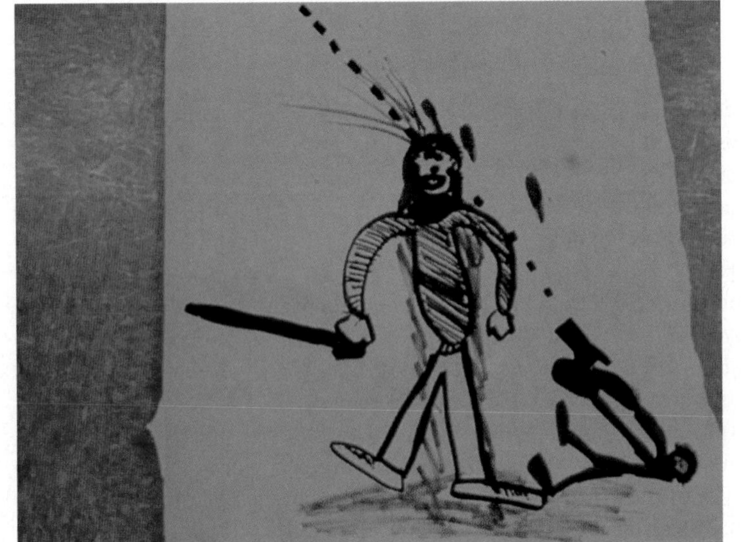

FIGURE 24-2 ◆
"Self-Portrait." Drawn by a 15-year-old boy who was admitted through the emergency department after a failed suicide attempt by hanging. He had a psychiatric diagnosis of depression and polysubstance abuse (including inhalants and alcohol) and insisted that he was a member of a satanic cult in his hometown. Most of his drawings depicted a preoccupation with violence and suicide. The boy said he always felt a "darkness" like a shadow that followed him around and wanted him dead. His family history was significant for depression and suicide on both his mother's and his father's side. His father also had a lengthy history of polysubstance abuse and alcoholism. The boy was discharged to a long-term residential treatment facility for adolescents.

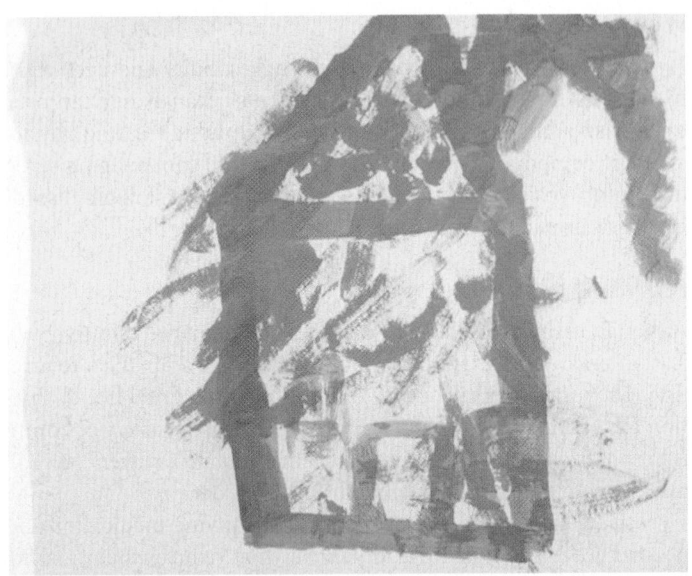

FIGURE 24-3 ◆
"An Activity." Drawn by an 8-year-old boy who was initially admitted to the medical-surgical floor of a pediatric hospital for dehydration resulting from vomiting and diarrhea. Psychiatric evaluation was ordered for extreme anxiety. These drawings, completed during the initial interview, led to further investigation, which revealed that the child had started a house fire in which his grandmother was killed. The family's home and all their belongings were lost. No one had known that the child had set the fire. Further sessions indicated that he had been setting neighborhood garage fires and watching them burn from a distance.

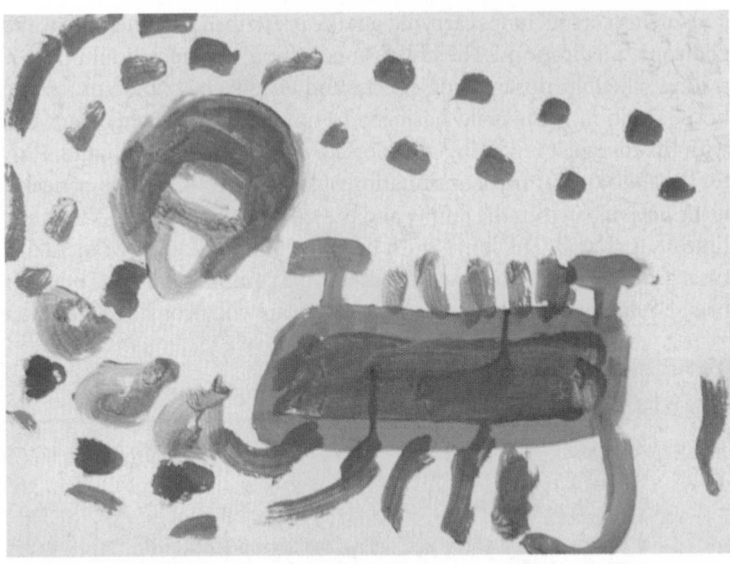

FIGURE 24-4 ◆
"A Family Activity." By the same boy who drew Figure 24-3. This drawing depicts a recurring incident of physical and emotional abuse by his mother's live-in boyfriend. It shows the family bathtub with feces and blood smeared on the floor and walls. The boy reported that when either he or his 3-year-old brother had a toileting accident the boyfriend would make them go into the bathroom and stand in the bathtub while he smeared the feces on the walls. He would then hit the children and make them clean up the mess. The boy had previously been removed from the mother's custody for neglect. He was transferred from the medical-surgical area to the inpatient children's psychiatric unit, where he received a diagnosis of depression, overanxious disorder, and child abuse (physical and emotional). Charges were filed against the mother's boyfriend and custody of both children was temporarily revoked.

nurses, teachers, and other adults consistently reinforce desirable behaviors, the child will eventually alter or discontinue undesirable behaviors.

Behavior modification may include (1) removing the child from the home to a more structured environment, such as a hospital, for a brief time, and (2) instructing the parents, teachers, and other appropriate adults to be agents of behavioral change. Several ongoing sessions may be required with the adults involved, using role play and other techniques. Consistency is the most important principle in the successful use of behavior modification.

Cognitive therapy teaches thinking patterns to change reactions to situations that cause anxiety or other undesirable conditions. The child is taught how their brain and body are working; this understanding assists them in having control over the experience. Often a combination of cognitive and behavioral approaches are useful in treating children.

Visualization and Guided Imagery

The techniques of visualization and guided imagery begin with specific directions for progressive relaxation according to the child's ability. This form of therapy uses the child's own imagination and positive thinking to reduce stress and anxiety, decrease the experience of pain or discomfort, and promote healing. The techniques are especially useful in the management of anxiety disorders and chronic pain. It is not easy for every child to use his or her imagination in this way, so the technique may not work or be appropriate for everyone.

COMPLEMENTARY AND ALTERNATIVE THERAPIES

In many cultures care of the "spirit" is believed necessary to promote mental health. An identity with one's community and spiritual wholeness is promoted by story telling, singing, and rites of passage. Use of certain objects such as bags of herbs may be considered important.

CULTURE

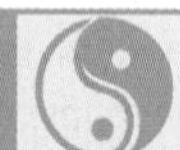

Mental health is defined in different ways by various cultural groups. For most it is a sense of well-being, peace, and productive use of the mind. An array of therapies are used to support and restore mental health. They may include healers, family and community support, relaxation or meditation, teas and other herbal products, and exorcism. Find out how individuals and groups define mental health and how they believe health is maintained. Be alert to learn if mental disorders are viewed as a negative stigma or are openly accepted and discussed.

Hypnosis

Hypnosis involves varying degrees of suggestibility and deep relaxation effects. This technique is useful for children and adolescents because they can usually be hypnotized more easily than adults. Hypnosis is especially helpful in treating physical symptoms with a psychologic component, anxiety, and phobias and in managing severe physical symptoms or discomfort (pain or nausea) associated with a physiologic disorder or its treatment (e.g., cancer or juvenile rheumatoid arthritis).

NURSE'S ROLE

Although many mental health disorders are managed effectively with therapy and/or medication on an outpatient basis, some necessitate admission to an inpatient psychiatric setting. The nurse may encounter the child with a mental health disorder during hospitalization for a concurrent physiologic problem, or in a variety of community settings. If a child is hospitalized for a concurrent problem, the child's current level of functioning needs to be assessed in relation to the mental health disorder.

Nursing assessment also focuses on identifying medications being taken, common abnormal behaviors (what triggers them, what reduces them), family interactions, and routines to maintain appropriate behaviors (Table 24-2). The nurse then considers how to support the child within the hospital environment.

Nursing care includes carrying out the prescribed treatment plan and administering psychotropic medications. The child's medication regimen should be evaluated for administration schedule, dosage, side effects, and effectiveness. Inform the therapist of the child's hospitalization if the child has been hospitalized for a concurrent condition, and consult with the therapist regarding appropriate approaches for the child. Provide supportive care for the child and family. Continuation of family involvement is critical. The nurse frequently is the liaison between the family and the therapist in making follow-up arrangements at the time of discharge. The nurse must be aware of the meaning of mental illness in various cultural groups and the treatments that may be commonly used. These complementary therapies should be integrated within the care plan when considered safe and families must feel

TABLE 24-2 Mental Health Assessment

The nurse gathers information about the child's mental health by asking questions and making observations. The following components may be helpful:

- Appearance
  - Clothing appropriate for age, setting, and developmental level
  - Facial expression and response to nurse
  - Body size and posture
  - Interactions with parents or others
  - Interest in surroundings
- Behavior
  - Level of consciousness and interaction with surroundings
  - Recent reported changes in behavior (e.g., sleep, eating patterns, communication with others, school performance, friendships, risky activities)
  - Problem behaviors identified by child or parent
  - Events associated with problem behaviors
- Development
  - Results of developmental testing
  - Progression of skills reported by family
  - Unusual capabilities or deficits
  - Progression in school and extracurricular activities
- Life events
  - Recent stress or trauma
  - Changes in family structure
  - Chronic health conditions in family members
- History
  - Prenatal events or birth trauma
  - Diagnosed mental health disorder in child or other family members
  - Neurological injuries or diseases

that their responses and approaches to the child with a mental disorder are not judged by health professionals.

The nurse in the community assesses how a child with a mental health disorder is functioning in each microsystem (see Chapter 2), such as home, childcare, school, and with friends. Risk and protective factors of the child and family are assessed (see Chapter 7). Involvement in therapy sessions and ability to manage prescribed pharmacologic interventions are evaluated.

DEVELOPMENTAL AND BEHAVIORAL DISORDERS

AUTISTIC SPECTRUM DISORDER

Pervasive developmental disorders (PDDs)begin in early childhood and are characterized by impaired social interactions and communication, with restricted interests, activities, and behaviors (Baird, Charman, & Cox, et al., 2001). Autism or autistic spectrum disorder (ASD) is the most common of the pervasive developmental disorders. (Rett syndrome and Asperger's syndrome are two examples of nonautistic PDDs.) Autistic disorder is a complex childhood disorder that involves abnormalities in behavior, social interactions, and communication. The essential features typically become apparent by the time a child is 3 years of age. For every 1,000 births, one to two children are found to have autistic disorder, and an increasing incidence has been noted in the last few years (American Academy of Pediatrics, 2001a). The disorder occurs 4 times more often in boys than in girls.

Etiology and Pathophysiology

The cause of autistic disorder is unknown. Genetic transmission, immune responses, and neuroanatomy are being investigated as causes (Williams, Dalrymple, & Neal, 2000). Neurotransmitters such as dopamine, serotonin, and opioids are abnormal in some children and a focus of present research (Cade & Tidwell, 2001). Congenital rubella syndrome and tuberous sclerosis can lead to autism (American Academy of Pediatrics, 2001a). Autistic children are frequently cognitively impaired but can demonstrate a wide range of intellectual ability and functioning.

Clinical Manifestations

Autistic children may manifest disturbances in the rate or sequence of development. A primary finding is impairment in social interactions. Autistic children are unable to relate to people or to respond to social and emotional cues. In addition, they engage in **stereotypy,** or rigid and obsessive behavior. Characteristically these repetitive behaviors in affected children include head banging, twirling in circles, biting themselves, and flapping their hands or arms. Frequently a child's behavior is self-stimulating or self-destructive. Responses to sensory stimuli are frequently abnormal and include an extreme aversion to touch, loud noises, and bright lights. Emotional lability is common.

Difficulties or delays in speech and language are common and are often the first symptoms that lead to diagnosis. Abnormal communication patterns include both verbal and nonverbal communication. Autistic children may eventually learn to talk, in some cases well, but their speech is likely to show certain abnormalities: use of "you" in place of "I"; **echolalia** (a compulsive parroting of what is heard); repeating questions rather than answering them; and fascination with rhythmic, repetitive songs and verses.

About 75% of children with ASD are mentally retarded (Koenig, 1998). While 25% have microcephaly, most children have normal appearance. Cognitive impairment may become manifested early in life by slow developmental progression, particularly in social skills.

Clinical Therapy

Diagnosis is based on the presence of specific criteria, as described in the American Psychiatric Association's *Diagnostic and Statistical Manual of Mental Disorders,* 4th edition (DSM-IV-TR), outlined in Table 24-3. Additional testing is done to rule out other causes of the child's behavior. Tests may include neuroimaging (CT scan or MRI), lead screening, DNA analysis, and electroencephalogram. See Chapters 4 and 20 for further descriptions related to the neurological system.

RETT SYNDROME

Rett syndrome is a pervasive developmental disorder similar in some ways to autistic disorder. Rett syndrome, however, occurs only in girls. The child usually appears normal until 6 to 18 months of age. Symptoms of increasing ataxia, handwringing, intermittent hyperventilation, dementia, and growth retardation then progress until the child requires total care.

ASPERGER'S SYNDROME

Asperger's syndrome is manifested by impaired social interaction and repetitive behavior. Pitch, tone, and other characteristics of speech may be abnormal; however, cognition and language skills are usually normal for age.

RESEARCH

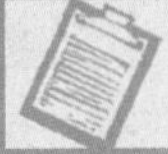

Some scientists proposed that since there has been an increase in cases of autism in the last few decades and an increase in numbers of children immunized for measles, mumps, and rubella (MMR), perhaps autism could be caused by the MMR vaccine. Recent comprehensive studies have demonstrated that there is no link between the MMR vaccine and autism (Dales, Hammer, & Smith, 2001). Nurses should share this information with parents who are concerned about a possible link, and encourage immunization for all children.

TABLE 24-3 DSM-IV Diagnostic Criteria for Autistic Disorder

A. A total of six or more items from 1, 2, and 3, with at least two from 1, and one each from 2 and 3:
  1. Qualitative impairment in social interaction, as manifested by at least two of the following:
     a. Marked impairment in the use of multiple nonverbal behaviors such as eye-to-eye gaze, facial expression, body posture and gestures to regulate social interaction
     b. Failure to develop peer relationships appropriate to developmental level
     c. A lack of spontaneous seeking to share enjoyment, interests, or achievements with other people
     d. Lack of social or emotional reciprocity
  2. Qualitative impairments in communication as manifested by at least one of the following:
     a. Delay in, or total lack of, the development of spoken language (not accompanied by an attempt to compensate through alternative modes of communication such as gesture or mime)
     b. In individuals with adequate speech, marked impairment in the ability to initiate or sustain a conversation with others
     c. Stereotyped and repetitive use of language or idiosyncratic language
     d. Lack of varied, spontaneous make-believe play or social imitative play appropriate to developmental level
  3. Restricted repetitive and stereotyped patterns of behavior, interests, and activities, as manifested by at least one of the following:
     a. Encompossing preoccupation with one or more stereotyped and restricted patterns of interest that is abnormal either in intensity or in focus
     b. Apparently inflexible adherence to specific, nonfunctional routines or rituals
     c. Stereotyped and repetitive motor mannerisms (e.g., hand or finger flapping or twisting, or complex whole-body movements)
     d. Persistent preoccupation with parts of objects

B. Delays or abnormal functioning in at least one of the following areas, with onset prior to age 3 years: (1) social interaction, (2) language as used in social communication, or (3) symbolic or imaginative play.

C. The disturbance is not better accounted for by Rett syndrome or childhood disintegrative disorder.

Early intervention assists in maximizing the child's potential and establishing helpful support for parents. Treatment focuses on behavior management to reward appropriate behaviors, foster positive or adaptive coping skills, and facilitate effective communication. The goals of treatment are to reduce rigidity or stereotypy (repetitive, obsessive, machinelike movements) and other maladaptive behaviors. Often the child must be physically restrained from aggressive or self-destructive behaviors. Some parents choose to use complementary therapies such as vitamin supplements and dimethylglycine. Foods such as sugar, aspartame, milk products, and wheat are sometimes eliminated from the diet (Hyman & Levy, 2000).

The overall prognosis for autistic children to become functioning members of society is guarded. The extent to which adequate adjustment is achieved varies greatly. Successful adjustment is more likely for children with higher IQs, adequate speech, and access to specialized programs.

COMPLEMENTARY AND ALTERNATIVE MEDICINE (CAM)

Some parents who have a child with autism will choose to use CAM in an attempt to help the child. Some CAM approaches include vitamin therapy, elimination of some additives from the diet, or providing medicines such as secretin (a pancreatic hormone), Pepcid, or other antacids. Nurses can help parents to evaluate studies on CAM and encourage them to initiate only one treatment at a time to measure any effectiveness seen (Hyman & Levy, 2000).

NURSING MANAGEMENT

Nursing Assessment and Diagnosis

The nurse may encounter the autistic child when parents seek care for a suspected hearing impairment, speech difficulty, or developmental delay. Early and frequent developmental screening of all children can help in referral for thorough assessment and identification of cases. Parents may report abnormal interaction such as lack of eye contact, disinterest in cuddling, minimal facial responsiveness, and failure to talk. Initial assessment focuses on language development, response to others, and hearing acuity (see Chapters 4 and 19). Specialized screening tests for autism are available online and are being evaluated for their usefulness.

When a child with a diagnosis of autistic disorder is hospitalized for a concurrent problem, obtain a history from the parents regarding the child's routines, rituals, and likes and dislikes, as well as ways to promote interaction and cooperation. Autistic children may carry a special toy or object that they play with during times of stress. Ask parents about these objects and their use.

Ask about the child's behaviors as well as observing them on admission. Obtain a history of acute and chronic illnesses and injuries. Ask about eating patterns and food restrictions. Inquire about CAM in a nonjudgmental and supportive manner.

Nursing diagnoses must be tailored to fit the individual needs of the child. Examples of diagnoses that may be appropriate for autistic children include the following:

- *Impaired verbal communication,* related to psychological condition
- *Impaired social interaction,* related to developmental disability
- *Altered thought processes,* related to mental disorder
- *Risk for injury,* related to cognitive impairment
- *Risk for caregiver role strain,* related to chronicity and demands of child's condition
- *Ineffective family coping: Compromised or disabling,* related to having a child with prolonged disability

Planning and Implementation

Nursing care focuses on stabilizing environmental stimuli, providing supportive care, enhancing communication, maintaining a safe environment, giving the parents anticipatory guidance, and providing emotional support.

Stabilize Environmental Stimuli

Autistic children interpret and respond to the environment differently from other individuals. Sounds that are not distressing to the average person may be interpreted by autistic children as louder, more frightening, and overwhelming. The child needs to be oriented to new settings such as a classroom or the hospital room and may adjust best to a small classroom or a hospital room with only one other child. Encourage parents to bring the child's favorite objects from home, and try to keep these objects in the same places, because the child does not cope well with changes in the environment.

Provide Supportive Care

Developing a trusting relationship with the autistic child is often difficult. Adjust communication techniques and teaching to the child's developmental level. Ask parents about the child's usual home routines, and maintain these routines as much as possible. Because self-care abilities are often limited, the child may need assistance to meet basic needs. School programs and individualized education plans (see Chapter 6) can help the child to learn self-care skills. When possible, schedule daily care and routine procedures at consistent times to maintain predictability. Encourage parents to remain with the hospitalized child and to participate in daily care planning. Parents are integral parts of the treatment team when the child's learning goals are established in early intervention or school programs. Identify rituals for naptime and bedtime, and maintain them to promote rest and sleep. Integrate patterns that facilitate intake of nutritious foods at mealtimes.

Enhance Communication

Because children with autism have impaired communication, nursing care focuses on utilizing and improving communication with the child (Cade & Tidwell, 2001). Speech is used when possible. If the child responds well to visual cues, then pictures, computers, and other visual aids may form an important part of interaction. Sign language is used with some children.

Maintain a Safe Environment

Monitor autistic children at all times, including bath time and bedtime. Close supervision is needed to ensure that the child does not obtain any harmful objects or engage in dangerous behaviors.

SAFETY PRECAUTIONS

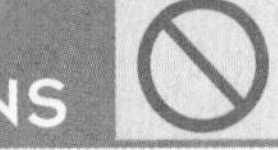

If the autistic child or adolescent is particularly aggressive or self-abusive, bike helmets and mitts can be the least restrictive method used for the safety of the child, other patients, and staff. This may enable the child to participate in activities and engage in the social environment to the degree capable.

PROVIDE ANTICIPATORY GUIDANCE

Approximately half of all children with autistic disorder require lifelong supervision and support, especially if the disorder is accompanied by mental retardation. Some children may grow up to lead independent lives, although they will have social limitations with impaired interpersonal relationships. Encourage parents to promote the child's development through behavior modification and specialized educational programs. The overall goal is to provide the child with the guidance, education, and support necessary for optimal functioning.

CARE IN THE COMMUNITY

Families of autistic children need a great deal of support to cope with the challenges of caring for the autistic child. Help them to identify resources for child care, such as special toddler programs and preschools. The child will need an individualized education plan. The parent or primary caretaker often has difficulty obtaining respite care and may need assistance to find suitable resources. Siblings of the autistic child may need help to explain the disorder to their friends or teachers. Family support programs are available in some states to provide assistance to parents.

Genetic counseling should be offered to the family. Information on immunizations is necessary, because parents may have heard about a potential connection between immunization and the disorder. They should be encouraged to have the child immunized on the recommended schedule. Parents may have questions about where to find information on complementary and alternative therapies.

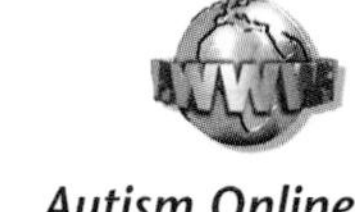

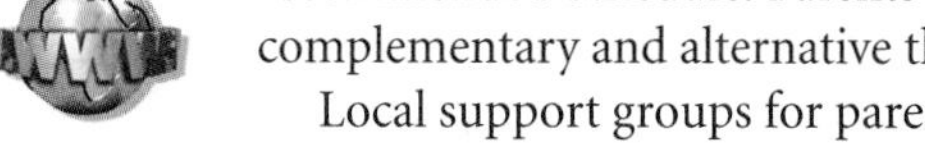

Autism Online

Local support groups for parents of autistic children are available in most areas. Parents can also be referred to the Autism Society of America for information.

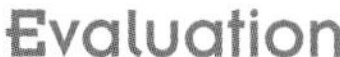

Evaluation

Expected outcomes of nursing care for the child with autism are as follows:

- Management of behavioral symptoms
- Maximization of self-care
- Maintenance of safe environment
- Consistent developmental progression
- Successful communication strategies

ATTENTION DEFICIT DISORDER AND ATTENTION DEFICIT HYPERACTIVITY DISORDER

Attention deficit disorder (ADD) is a variation in central nervous system processing characterized by developmentally inappropriate behaviors involving inattention. When hyperactivity and impulsivity accompany inattention, the disorder is called attention deficit hyperactivity disorder (ADHD). The latter is the more common condition and affects approximately 5% of all children, boys more commonly than girls (Hunt, Paguin, & Payton, 2001).

Etiology and Pathophysiology

Although a variety of physical and neurologic disorders are associated with ADHD, children with identifiable causes represent a small proportion of this population. Examples of known associations include exposure to high levels of lead in childhood and prenatal exposure to alcohol. There may be a deficit in the catecholamines dopamine and norepinephrine in some children, lowering the threshold for stimuli input. Probably there are many types of attention deficit, resulting from several different mechanisms. Genetic factors may be important, as well as family dynamics and environmental characteristics. Although ADHD occurs more commonly within families, a single gene has not been located and a specific mechanism of genetic transmission is not known. It is believed that a genetic predisposition interacts with the child's environment, so that both factors contribute to the appearance of the condition. Some children exhibit additional problems such as aggressive behaviors, learning disabilities, and motor disorders (Fletcher, Shaywitz, & Shaywitz, 1999; Blondis, 1999).

Clinical Manifestations

Children with ADD and ADHD have problems related to decreased attention span, impulsiveness, and/or increased motor activity. Symptoms can range from mild to severe. The disorders often coexist with various developmental learning disabilities. The child has difficulty completing tasks, fidgets constantly, is frequently loud, and interrupts others. Sleep disturbances are common. Because of these behaviors, the child often has difficulty developing and maintaining social relationships and may be shunned or teased by other children. This only increases the anxiety of the already compromised child, whose behavior is set on a downward-spiraling course (American Academy of Pediatrics, 2000).

Typically, girls with ADHD show less aggression and impulsiveness than boys, but far more anxiety, mood swings, social withdrawal, rejection, and cognitive and language problems. Girls tend to be older at the time of diagnosis. Children are frequently diagnosed with the disorder soon after beginning school, when demands increase for attentive behavior.

Clinical Therapy

Children are usually brought for evaluation when behaviors escalate to the point of interfering with the daily functioning of teachers or parents. When children have learning disabilities or anxiety disorders, the problem is commonly misdiagnosed as ADHD without further evaluation of the child's symptoms. Obtaining an accurate diagnosis by a pediatric mental health specialist is vital (American Academy of Pediatrics, 2000).

Specific diagnostic criteria (Table 24-4) must be applied to all children with the potential diagnosis. Behaviors both at home and school or child care must be evaluated, because abnormal patterns in two settings are needed for diagnosis. Based on the findings, desired outcomes are established for the child's performance and management of the disorder.

Treatment is established to meet the desired behavioral outcomes, and includes a combination of approaches, such as environmental changes, behavior therapy, and pharmacotherapy (American Academy of Pediatrics, 2001b). It is expected that treatment will be long term.

Children often benefit from environmental changes. Decreasing stimulation, for example, by turning off television, keeping the environment quiet, and maintaining an orderly and clutter-free desk or study area without distraction, may help the child to stay focused on the task at hand. Another relatively simple change is appropriate classroom placement, preferably in a small class with a teacher who can provide close supervision and a structured daily routine. Consistent limits and expectations should be set for the child. Children living in chaotic homes and communities may function better if the environment can be simplified. When aggressive behaviors occur, therapeutic approaches such as play and group therapy may be useful.

Behavior therapy involves rewarding the child for desired behaviors and applying consequences for undesirable behaviors. Children may be rewarded by praise or earn points toward a movie or other desired outing for staying seated during meals or quietly listening in a classroom.

Children with moderate to severe ADHD are treated with pharmacotherapy. Methylphenidate (Ritalin, Concerta) is most often prescribed. Usually a favorable response (a decrease in impulsive behaviors and an increase in the ability to sit still and attend to an activity for at least 15 minutes) is seen in the first 10 days of treatment and frequently with the first few doses. Other medications that may be used include dextroamphetamine (Dexedrine or Adderall), the tricyclic antidepressants desipramine and imipramine, and the antidepressant bupropion (Wellbutrin) (American Academy of Pediatrics, 2001b).

A variety of other treatments have been attempted for ADHD, and are commonly used by families. Chiropractic manipulation, biofeedback, and dietary interventions (both elimination diets and supplement use) are examples of common complementary or alternative therapies.

Although ADHD was once thought to be a disorder of childhood that gradually improved with age, it is now believed that symptoms continue into adulthood and that careful management in childhood assists in lessening problems of social functioning later in life.

TABLE 24-4 DSM-IV-TR Diagnostic Criteria for Attention Deficit Hyperactivity Disorder

A. Either 1 or 2:
1. **Inattention:** Six (or more) of the following symptoms of inattention have persisted for at least 6 months to a degree that is maladaptive and inconsistent with developmental level:
   a. Often fails to give close attention to details or makes careless mistakes in schoolwork, work, and other activities
   b. Often has difficulty sustaining attention in tasks or play activities
   c. Often does not seem to listen when spoken to directly
   d. Often does not follow through on instructions and fails to finish schoolwork, chores, or duties in the workplace (not due to oppositional behavior or failure to understand instructions)
   e. Often has difficulty organizing tasks and activities
   f. Often avoids, dislikes, or is reluctant to engage in tasks that require sustained mental effort (such as schoolwork or homework)
   g. Often loses things necessary for tasks or activities (e.g., toys, school assignments, pencils, books, or tools)
   h. Is often easily distracted by extraneous stimuli
   i. Is often forgetful in daily activities
2. **Hyperactivity-impulsivity:** Six (or more) of the following symptoms of hyperactivity-impulsivity have persisted for at least 6 months to a degree that is maladaptive and inconsistent with developmental level:
   Hyperactivity
   a. Often fidgets with hands or feet or squirms in seat
   b. Often leaves seat in classroom or in other situations in which remaining seated is expected
   c. Often runs about or climbs excessively in situations in which it is inappropriate (in adolescents or adults, may be limited to subjective feelings of restlessness)
   d. Often has difficulty playing or engaging in leisure activities quietly
   e. Is often "on the go" or often acts as if "driven by a motor"
   f. Often talks excessively
   Impulsivity
   g. Often blurts out answers before questions have been completed
   h. Often has difficulty awaiting turn
   i. Often interrupts or intrudes on others (e.g., butts into conversations or games)

B. Some hyperactive-impulsive or inattentive symptoms that caused impairment were present before age 7 years.
C. Some impairment from the symptoms is present in two or more settings (e.g., at school [or work] and at home).
D. There must be clear evidence of clinically significant impairment in social, academic, or occupational functioning.
E. The symptoms do not occur exclusively during the course of a pervasive developmental disorder, schizophrenia, or other psychotic disorder and are not better accounted for by another mental disorder (e.g., mood disorder, anxiety disorder, dissociative disorder, or a personality disorder).

NURSING MANAGEMENT

Nursing Assessment and Diagnosis

The nurse may encounter the child with ADHD in the hospital when parents bring the child for treatment of an injury (e.g., fracture) or other problem. Explore the parent's report of the child's attention span in detail. Usually within a few minutes in an unstructured setting or waiting area, the child with ADHD becomes restless and searches for distraction. Gather information about the child's activity level and impulsiveness. Be alert for information that reveals a serious problem, such as hurting animals or other children. Obtain information about distractibility, attention deficit in activities of daily living, characteristic ways of reacting, and the extent of impulsiveness when the child is receiving medication. Find out how the family manages at home. Ask about a family history of the disorder, as that is a common finding among children with ADHD.

Examples of nursing diagnoses that may be appropriate for a child with ADHD include the following:

- *Impaired verbal communication,* related to altered perceptions
- *Impaired social interaction,* related to chronic episodes of impulsive behavior
- *Chronic low self-esteem,* related to behaviors associated with ADHD
- *Risk for injury,* related to high level of impulsiveness and excitability
- *Risk for caregiver role strain,* related to management of child with unpredictable moods and high energy

Planning and Implementation

Nursing care of the hospitalized child with ADHD focuses on administering medications, managing the child's environment, implementing behavioral management plans, providing emotional support to the child and family, promoting self-esteem, and ensuring ongoing care.

Administer Medications

Methylphenidate and other medications increase the child's attention span and decrease distractibility. Be alert for the common side effects of these medications, including anorexia, insomnia, and tachycardia. Administering medication early in the day helps to alleviate insomnia. Anorexia can be managed by giving medication at mealtimes. Careful monitoring of weight, height, and blood pressure is necessary.

Minimize Environmental Distractions

The child may need to be placed in an environment with minimal distractions. When hospitalized, this may mean a room with only one other child. Potentially harmful equipment should be kept out of reach. Television and video game time needs to be monitored and limited. Use shades to darken the room during naps or at bedtime and minimize noise. Teach parents to minimize distractions at home during periods when the child needs to concentrate, for example, when doing schoolwork. Visits to areas such as shopping malls and playgrounds may need to be limited. Plenty of daily exercise and minimal use of television/video games may assist the child in being able to concentrate when needed for schoolwork.

Implement Behavioral Management Plans

Behavior modification programs can help to reduce specific impulsive behaviors. An example is setting up a reward program for the child who has taken medication as ordered or completed a homework assignment. The rewards may be daily as well as weekly or monthly, depending on the child's age. (For example, one completed homework assignment might be rewarded with 30 minutes of basketball or a bike ride; assignments completed for a week might be rewarded with participation in an activity of the child's choice on the weekend.)

If punishment is necessary, the behavior should be corrected while simultaneously supporting the child as a person. Punishment is generally withdrawal of a privilege, and should follow the offense quickly as the child may not otherwise connect the punishment with the behavior.

Provide Emotional Support

Children with ADHD offer a special challenge to parents, teachers, and health care providers. Parents must cope simultaneously with managing the difficult needs and demands of a hard-to-handle child, obtaining appropriate evaluation and treatment, and understanding and accepting the diagnosis, even when the child exhibits different behaviors with different people. Family support is essential. Educate both the parents and the child about the importance of appropriate expectations and consequences of behaviors. Teach skills that will help as the child grows older: making lists of tasks to accomplish; having routines for eating, sleeping, recreation, and schoolwork; minimizing stimuli in the environment when completing work; and asking teachers and friends to identify when behavior is inappropriate.

Promote Self-Esteem

Help the child to understand the disorder at an appropriate developmental level, and facilitate a trusting relationship with health care providers. Assist the child with social skills through the use of role play, small-group play, and modeling. Promote the child's self-esteem by emphasizing the positive aspects of behavior and treating instances of negative behavior as learning opportunities. Help the child to develop ego strengths (the conscious ability to screen outside stimuli and to control internal demands), which will result in better impulse control and thus increase self-esteem over time.

Care in the Community

Most children with ADHD are only hospitalized when needing care for another condition. Parents need support to understand the diagnosis and to learn how to manage the child. Emphasize the importance of a stable environment, at home as well as at school. At home the child may have difficulty staying on task. Parents need to consider age and developmental appropriateness of tasks, give clear and simple instructions, and provide frequent reminders to ensure completion. Routines in the evening can promote good sleep patterns.

The nurse can serve as a liaison to teachers and school personnel, or as the case manager for the child. An individualized education plan may be needed (see Chapter 6), with clear expected outcomes stated for the child's behaviors. Special classrooms or periods of instruction free from the distractions of the entire class may enable the child to improve school performance. Parents may have difficulty understanding the need for these approaches because the child often tests with above-average intelligence. Reinforce the importance of providing a structured environment free from unnecessary external stimuli. Be sure that parents understand behavioral approaches that will help the child, how to administer prescribed medications, and the importance of returning for health care visits to monitor for side effects. Medication should be locked safely away at home to keep it away from other children and prevent illegal use of this controlled substance. An individualized school health plan may be needed for medication management.

Parents may have heard about ADHD in the media and can have many questions about its cause and management. Providing information about complementary and alternative treatments is a nursing role.

As the child grows older, provide explanations about the disorder and information about techniques that will assist in dealing with problems. Emphasize the importance of doing homework or other tasks requiring concentration in a quiet environment without background noise from a television or radio. Encourage children with ADHD to keep assignment notebooks and use checklists to help them accomplish specific tasks.

CLINICAL TIP

Many families who have a child with ADHD or another mental health disorder are embarrassed and feel shame because of the diagnosis, especially in certain cultures such as some Asian groups, and in very structured and highly achieving families. When taking histories from family members, it is best to be sensitive to the stigma some may feel. Ask questions in a private setting and ask about the family's feelings regarding a mental health disorder. Provide information in a nonjudgmental manner and provide support if appropriate from other families with similar experiences.

COMPLEMENTARY AND ALTERNATIVE MEDICINE (CAM)

ADD and ADHD are common diagnoses and there are many claims in the media about what causes these conditions. Parents may wish to try a variety of approaches in addition to or instead of traditional behavioral therapy and medication. Some common alternative therapies include elimination of dietary components such as highly processed foods, sugar, aspartame, or yeast. Other therapies include use of supplements such as iron, magnesium zinc, and vitamin B_6. Herbs such as pycnogenol, melatonin, and gingko biloba are sometimes used. Visual and auditory training are used with some children. Ask parents about alternative therapies used and investigate what is known about them in order to share this information with parents. (Baumgaertel, 1999).

Evaluation

Expected outcomes of nursing care for the child with ADD or ADHD include the following:

- Understanding of disorder by parents and child
- Management of medication administration
- Increase in attentiveness and decrease in hyperactivity, impulsivity, and sleep disturbance
- Formation of positive self-image in the child

MENTAL RETARDATION

Mental retardation is defined as significantly subaverage general intellectual functioning (IQ below 70 to 75), as well as impairments in **adaptive functioning** (the ability of an individual to meet the standards expected for his or her cultural group). The mentally retarded child has adaptive deficits in at least two areas such as communication, self-care, home living, social/interpersonal skills, use of community resources, self-direction, functional academic skills, work, leisure, health, or safety. A low IQ score by itself does not necessarily correlate with impairment in the ability to carry out adaptive skills. The IQ score and the level of adaptive skills together determine the degree of severity of mental retardation.

Etiology and Pathophysiology

Mild retardation occurs in 3 to 6 per 1,000 people, and mental retardation affects about 3% of the population (Baralle, 2001). The causes of mental retardation can be grouped into three general categories: prenatal errors in the development of the CNS, prenatal or postnatal changes in the biologic environment of the person, and external forces leading to CNS damage. In each instance, the precipitating factor causes a change in the form, function, and adaptation of the CNS. Table 24-5 provides examples of common causes of mental retardation for each category.

Three common causes of retardation from the prenatal category are Down syndrome, fragile X Syndrome, and fetal alcohol syndrome. In the United States, about 1 in 1,000 infants, or 4,000 infants each year, are born with Down syndrome (Zickler, Morrow, & Bull, 1998). The condition is caused by an extra chromosome; the child has 47 rather than 46 chromosomes (see discussion of genetic transmission in Chapter 2). The most common chromosome affected is 21, so that the child often has trisomy 21, or the child has 3 instead of 2 chromosome 21s. In addition to mental retardation and physical signs, the child with Down syndrome is at higher risk of developing other conditions such as cardiac defects, hearing loss, thyroid disease, and leukemia (Van Riper & Cohen, 2001).

Fragile X syndrome is caused by a single recessive gene abnormality on the X chromosome. A permutation to the X chromosome may occur in males or females. When a father or mother give the faulty X chromosome to a daughter, it may remain as a permutation or may change into a true mutation. The daughter has two X chromosomes and therefore does not manifest this recessive disorder; however, she can give the mutated X chromosome to her son who becomes affected with fragile X. The mutation of fragile X is on gene FMRP-1, which instructs cells to make a protein necessary for normal brain development (Bailey, Roberts, & Mirrett, et al., 2001).

Fetal alcohol syndrome (FAS) is caused by the effect of ethyl alcohol on the developing fetus. Alcohol ingestion by the pregnant woman can influence development of many body organs and effects can range from mild to severe.

Chapter 22 discusses phenylketonuria and hypothyroidism, two common biochemical causes of mental retardation. Other causes involve traumatic brain injury and infections of the CNS (see Chapter 20).

Clinical Manifestations

Mild mental retardation was originally described as an intelligence quotient (IQ) between 50 and 70, moderate retardation with IQ of 35 to 50, severe retardation with IQ of 20 to 35, and profound retardation with IQ below 20. Although an IQ below 70 is generally considered indicative of retardation, the functional assessment of the child is now considered to be a more accurate identification of children's performance and needs. Children who are mentally retarded manifest delays in all areas of development, including motor movement, language, and adaptive behavior. They usually achieve developmental milestones more slowly than the average child. These developmental delays may be the first indication to parents and care providers of the child's condition.

Mental retardation is sometimes accompanied by sensory impairment, speech problems, motor and orthopedic disabilities, and seizure disorders. Of children with mental retardation, 10% to 30% manifest one such disorder. Table 24-6 lists several physical characteristics associated with Down syndrome, fragile X syndrome, and fetal alcohol syndrome.

Clinical Therapy

Mental retardation is diagnosed and initial treatment is planned in a multistep process, and by involving a multidisciplinary team (Frederic & Williams, 1998). See Table 24-7 for a description of the DSM-IV-TR for mental retardation. First, a comprehensive history and evaluation of the child's physical characteristics, developmental level, and intellectual and adaptive functioning is carried out. Laboratory tests such as chromosome analysis, blood enzyme levels, lead levels, or cranial imaging provide valuable information in some circumstances.

Developmental screening using a test such as the Denver II (see Chapter 6) can help to identify children who may be at risk. Tests of intellectual and adaptive functioning are performed when mental retardation is suspected. A neurologic examination may indicate asymmetry of movement or strength, irritability or lethargy, or abnormal pitch to an infant's cry. Because mental retardation may be accompanied by physical abnormalities, it is important to observe the child for facial symmetry, distance between the eyes, level of the ears, hair growth, and palmar creases. These abnormalities may be cues to other health problems.

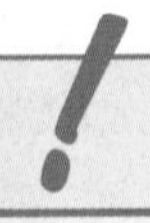

NURSING ALERT

Prematurity places the child at risk of displaying below-normal cognitive development. The premature infant needs frequent, thorough neurologic and developmental examinations, particularly in the first 2 years of life.

TABLE 24-5 Common Causes of Mental Retardation

PRENATAL CONDITIONS
Down syndrome Fragile X syndrome Fetal alcohol syndrome Maternal infection (e.g., rubella, cytomegalovirus)
BIOLOGIC ENVIRONMENT
Inborn errors of metabolism (e.g., phenylketonuria, hypothyroidism)
EXTERNAL FORCES
Traumatic brain injury (e.g., accident) Poison ingestion (acute or chronic) Hypoxia/anoxic insult Infection (e.g., meningitis) Environmental deprivation

CULTURE

Fetal alcohol syndrome is more common in groups with higher intake of alcohol. Because some Native American tribes have a high rate of alcoholism, the federal government and some tribes have joined to lower that risk among this ethnic group. On some reservations, such as the Yakama Nation in Washington State, alcoholic beverages are not sold and educational programs are in place.

TABLE 24-6 Characteristics Associated with Three Common Types of Mental Retardation

DOWN SYNDROME (SEE FIGURES 4-15, 4-46)
Small head (microcephaly)
Flattened forehead
Wide, short neck
Epicanthal eye folds
White spots on eye iris (Brushfield spots)
Congenital cataracts
Flat nose
Small, low-set ears
Protruding tongue
Short broad hands
Simian line on palm
Wide space between first and second toes
Hearing loss
Increased incidence of diabetes, congenital heart defect, and leukemia
Hypotonia
FRAGILE X SYNDROME
Long face
Prominent jaw
Large ears
Frequent otitis media
Large testicles
Epicanthal eye folds
Strabismus
High-arched palate
Scoliosis
Pliable joints
FETAL ALCOHOL SYNDROME (SEE FIGURE 2-5)
Flat midface
Low nasal bridge
Long philtrum with narrow upper lip
Short upturned nose
Poor coordination
Failure to thrive
Skeletal and joint abnormalities
Hearing loss

CLINICAL TIP

The diagnosis of mental retardation and the planning for early intervention should include a multidisciplinary team. Members of the team are generally a developmental specialist, physician, geneticist, nurse, teacher, language therapist, occupational therapist, and physical rehabilitation specialist.

TABLE 24-7 DSM-IV-TR Diagnostic Criteria for Mental Retardation

A. Significantly subaverage intellectual functioning: an IQ of approximately 70 or below on an individually administered IQ test (for infants, a clinical judgment of significantly subaverage intellectual functioning)
B. Concurrent deficits or impairments in present adaptive functioning (i.e., the person's effectiveness in meeting the standards expected for his or her age by his or her cultural group) in at least two of the following areas: communication, self-care, home living, social/interpersonal skills, use of community resources, self-direction, functional academic skills, work, leisure, health, and safety
C. The onset is before age 18 years

Based on the results of the evaluation, a multidisciplinary team plans the support needed to maximize the child's potential for development. Management focuses on early intervention to improve the degree of adaptive functioning. Simultaneous treatment of associated physical, emotional, and behavioral problems is provided. Depending on the child's condition, special education programs and physical or occupational therapy may be necessary (Figure 24-5 ◆). The child may require supportive care and assistance with ADLs. The plans for intervention change as the child grows and family situations evolve.

NURSING MANAGEMENT

Nursing Assessment and Diagnosis

Nurses can help to identify children with mental retardation through history taking, observation, and developmental screening during early childhood. The history should provide information about the mental and adaptive functioning of birth parents and other family members, as mental retardation may cluster in some families and conditions such as fragile X syndrome are genetic in origin. The pregnancy and birth history can provide important information relating to alcohol and drug use by the mother during pregnancy. Be alert for a history of difficult pregnancy and problems during delivery. When genetic conditions in the family predispose family members to mental retardation, careful assessment of the child is needed. Children from deprived environments or those at risk because of environmental factors such as lead poisoning (see Chapter 17) are more likely to manifest mental retardation.

Many children with mental retardation are not diagnosed with the condition until they reach school age, particularly if the condition is mild or moderate. Early intervention, however, can help to enhance the child's functioning later. During home visits, clinic appointments, in child care centers, and during hospitalization, be alert for signs of developmental delays, multiple (more than three) physical anomalies associated with a specific condition (see Table 24-6), or neurologic alterations. Developmental assessment should be part of each health care visit.

Once the diagnosis of mental retardation has been made, assess the adaptive functioning of the child and family. A functional assessment of the child should be performed, including toileting, dressing, and feeding skills. Assess the child's language, sensory, and psychomotor functioning. Assess the home and community for safety hazards. Observe how the family is managing with the child. Assess the availability of services such as support groups for parents and special education opportunities for children. Evaluate the coping skills of family members.

Several nursing diagnoses may be appropriate for the child with mental retardation, depending on the degree, cause, and outcome of the condition. Diagnoses that relate to impairments in adaptive functioning and family impact include the following:

- *Altered growth and development,* related to neonatal disease or condition
- *Altered nutrition: Less than body requirements,* related to inability to ingest sufficient food
- *Self-care deficit: Dressing, toileting, bathing,* related to developmental disability

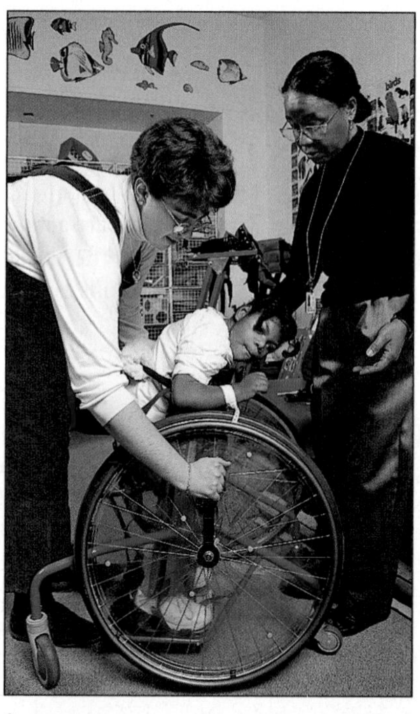
A

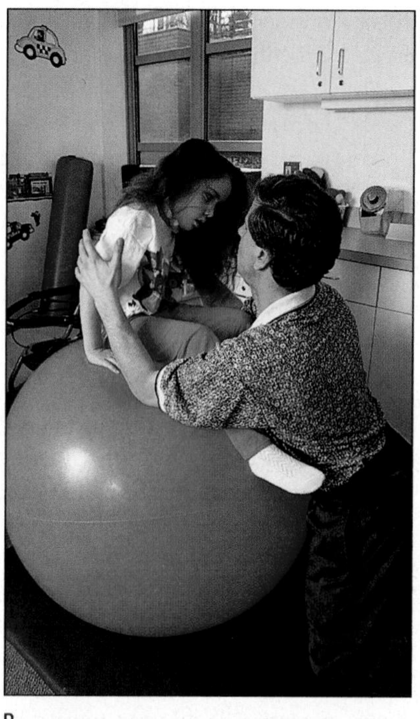
B

FIGURE 24-5 ◆
Physical therapy is an important component of medical management for many children who are mentally retarded. A, This girl with severe retardation, is wheelchair bound, and is being positioned in a mobile prone stander, which enables her to interact in a different manner with her therapists and the environment. B, Physical therapists also provide outpatient care in the community to children with varying degrees of disability.

- *Impaired verbal communication,* related to developmental disability
- *Risk for injury,* related to lack of understanding of environmental hazards
- *Ineffective family coping: Compromised,* related to the child's developmental variations

Planning and Implementation

Nearly all children who are mentally retarded are cared for in the community; however, they may have conditions that require periodic hospitalization or frequent health care visits. When needed, nursing care focuses on providing emotional support and information to family members, assisting the child with adaptive functioning, and fostering parental management of the child's activities. When possible, the nurse uses preventive teaching to lower the risk of mental retardation.

Provide Emotional Support and Information

Family members need empathy and support both at the time of diagnosis and in the ensuing years. Parents may be in an acute or chronic state of grief over the loss of the perfect child. Encourage them to verbalize their feelings. Introducing them to parents of other mentally retarded children may provide assistance and support as they learn how to manage the child's needs. Discuss the availability of respite care to provide parents with a break from caretaking. Other family members such as grandparents and siblings may also be experiencing grief or guilt and should be given an opportunity to talk about their feelings.

Parents need honest information and answers to their questions about the child's condition. Reinforce information provided by genetic counselors and other health care professionals. Parents need to be informed about community resources designed to assist children with mental retardation. Such resources include the Zero to Three Project, special education preschools and schools, county health services, and respite care. Refer parents to internet sources, and help them to interpret information received and analyze its strengths and limitations.

Maintain a Safe Environment

Children with mental retardation require close supervision because they may lack an understanding of common hazards. Ensure safety in the hospital environment. Assist parents to provide safety at home and school and to teach their child necessary skills such as pedestrian

CLINICAL TIP

To determine the impact of the child with mental retardation on the family, ask parents to describe (1) family activities that include the child, (2) strategies that parents and siblings use to deal with community attitudes about the child, and (3) in the case of a child with other disabilities, methods of managing the child's care and planning for future care needs.

COMMUNITY CARE

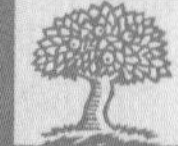

Fetal alcohol syndrome (FAS) is a totally preventable cause of mental retardation. Teach all pregnant women that total abstention from alcohol for the entire length of pregnancy is the only completely effective method of preventing FAS. Include this in teaching to all adolescent girls, so they are aware of how alcohol can harm their infant if they become pregnant. Emphasize that the most dangerous time may be early in pregnancy before women commonly know they are pregnant.

safety. Consider both physical and emotional safety. This type of child may be trusting of others and sometimes is at risk for physical or sexual abuse.

Provide Assistance with Adaptive Functioning

Encourage parents' efforts to maximize the child's areas of strength and identify needs related to adaptive behaviors. Refer them to resources to assist in the areas of adaptive functioning in which the child has impairment, such as communication, self-care activities, or social skills. During hospitalization, support parents' efforts to maintain the child's skills in toileting, dressing, and self-care by planning interventions to use the skills being taught at home.

LAW & ETHICS

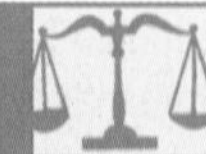

The Education for All Handicapped Children Act, P.L. 94-142, provides free appropriate education to all handicapped children between 2 and 21 years of age. Amendments to this act in 1986 (P.L. 99-457) encouraged states to provide early intervention services for handicapped infants and toddlers by providing federal funding.

Care in the Community

The child with mental retardation needs ongoing care throughout childhood, and adaptation of interventions as development occurs and the family's needs evolve. Parents often act as case managers for the child's care. Assist parents as necessary to acquire the skills required to coordinate the child's plan of care. Evaluate the child's needs regularly and assist parents with the treatment plan as necessary. Assist with plans for education and for services such as physical or speech therapy. Most children with mental retardation have an individualized education plan designed to meet their specific learning needs. Parents, nurses, and others such as teachers and language therapists are part of the team that establishes this plan. Promote optimal development and socialization. As the child reaches adolescence, education is directed toward a vocation, issues of sexuality, and the goal of independent living, when appropriate.

Specific guidelines for care are available for the child with Down syndrome. These guidelines suggest times for evaluation of hearing, growth, cardiac function, and other areas designed for early identification and treatment of associated disorders (Van Riper & Cohen, 2001). There are specific growth grids for children with Down syndrome, and specific topics to suggest for anticipatory guidance during health care visits (American Academy of Pediatrics, 2001c).

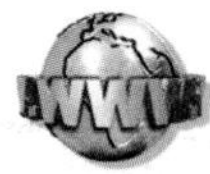

Down Syndrome Resources and Support

Evaluation

The expected outcomes of nursing care depend on the child's needs and developmental level. Early in the diagnostic phase, desired outcomes may involve the family's understanding of the diagnosis and the child's special needs. Later outcomes may focus on the child's communication of self-help skills. Outcomes related to cognitive performance and adaptive skills may be developed during childhood.

COMMUNITY CARE

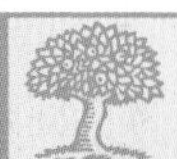

Some classes and community agencies offer transitional classes when children who are mentally retarded reach adolescence and young adulthood. These services help to teach self-care skills that may enable some youth to live in group homes or other community settings. Families receive help in planning for the child's future as parents look toward retirement. Information is provided on living options, health insurance, work opportunities, and other needs. This can also provide respite services for parents and other family members who have spent much time with the child for many years.

SCHIZOPHRENIA

Schizophrenia is a psychotic disorder that is relatively rare in young children and adolescents, although it can occur in children as young as 5 years of age. The prevalence of schizophrenia increases after puberty and reaches adult levels by late adolescence. About 1 in 10,000 children develop schizophrenia (Lambert, 2001).

The cause of schizophrenia is unknown, but genetic predisposition or a neurovirus during pregnancy may play a role in its occurrence (Lambert, 2001). The brain is altered in the disease, with progressively enlarged ventricles and nervous system arousal. Impaired glucose metabolism is often present. The disorder most often manifests between 15 and 20 years of age. Onset is usually slow with increasing intensity over time. Most often the child demonstrates restlessness, poor appetite, and social withdrawal over a period of several weeks to months. Behavioral problems, slowed development, and minor neurologic symptoms may occur.

The clinical manifestations of schizophrenia are the same in children as in adults. Characteristic behaviors of the schizophrenic individual include social withdrawal, impaired social relationships, flat **affect** (outward appearance of feeling or emotion), regression, loose associations (thought characterized by speech in which ideas shift from one subject to another that is unrelated), poor judgment and problem solving, anxiety, delusions, and hallucinations. Motor abnormalities may include rocking and arm flapping.

During adolescence, acute schizophrenia can occur suddenly while the teenager is making plans to leave home to attend college, marry, or work in another area. Onset of symptoms may be triggered by an important loss (death of a significant other, parent, child, or friend).

Clinical therapy for childhood schizophrenia is multifaceted, including individual psychotherapy, family therapy, and various psychotropic medications (antipsychotics such as haloperidol [Haldol], antianxiety agents such as lorazepam [Ativan], antidepressants such as imipramine [Tofranil], and newer antipsychotics such as dozapine, olanzapine, and risperidone). Drugs are only moderately effective at controlling hallucinations and delusions, responses vary considerably among individuals, and children may have different responses than adults. Side effects will determine what drugs are used and their duration. Antipsychotic medication is continued for at least 4 to 6 weeks before effectiveness can be determined. Medications often must be continued for several months or years after recovery from an acute schizophrenic episode, although medication-free trials may be attempted in children who have shown an absence of symptoms for 6 to 12 months (American Academy of Child and Adolescent Psychiatry, 2001, Bryden, Carrey, & Kutcher, 2001).

Often, episodes of acute schizophrenia require inpatient hospitalization on a psychiatric unit for thorough diagnosis and beginning management. Treatment may include an intensive school-based program in a structured, supervised setting with specially trained professionals. The goal of initial treatment is to reduce or control psychotic episodes and provide a safe, structured environment for the child or adolescent, enabling the child to live each day at an optimal level of functioning. Outpatient care is provided following initial diagnosis and establishment of treatment regimen.

Most children require long-term treatment, including intermittent periods of hospitalization. Children or adolescents whose symptoms are difficult to control and who present a safety risk to themselves or others may require long-term residential treatment. Earlier age at diagnosis and delay in treatment lead to poorer prognosis.

Nursing Management

The nurse may encounter the child or adolescent with schizophrenia during hospitalization for an acute episode, for treatment of another problem, or while working with the individual in the community. Nursing care centers on providing for physical safety and psychologic care, and normal growth and development for the child.

Family education and involvement in the treatment plan are essential. The family is taught to monitor the child's symptoms and progression. Educating the child and parents about the risk of recurrence and methods to alleviate side effects of prescribed medications may increase compliance with the treatment plan. The nurse performs assessments of the child for common medication side effects. For example, when excess weight is a potential side effect, frequent growth measurements are made. Neurological assessment and laboratory studies may be needed with some medications.

The family is assisted in establishing educational plans for the child and for integration within the school system. The nurse communicates with school personnel to ensure understanding of the child's condition and ongoing management of the individualized education plan.

NURSING ALERT

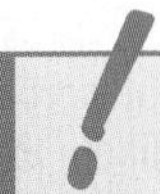

There is a lack of clear information about the effects of many psychiatric drugs in children. It is known that some drugs can have extrapyramidal side effects such as dystonia, Parkinson-like movement, and akathesia. Careful neurological examinations must be done on children who are receiving psychotrophic medications.

MOOD DISORDERS

DEPRESSION

Depression is psychological distress that can range from mild to severe. Only in recent years has depression in children been recognized as a clinical condition. Many children referred to child guidance centers and mental health professionals because of behavioral difficulties or poor achievement actually suffer from depression. The incidence of major depression is estimated to be about 5% in prepubertal children and about 10% to 20% in adolescents (Castiglia, 2000; Moldenhauer & Melnyk, 1999). Before puberty, depression is more common in boys than girls. Incidence of depressive symptoms and disorders increase with age, as does the female to male ratio.

GROWTH & DEVELOPMENT

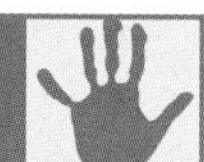

Symptoms of depression in children vary according to their developmental levels. Infants may fail to eat and grow, toddlers can show regressive behaviors in toileting and other activities, and school children may show a decrease in academic performance, increased or decreased activity, somatic complaints, and loss of friends. The adolescent can have a wide array of symptoms such as anxiety, decreased social contact, poor school performance, lack of prior involvement in activities, poor self-care, difficulty with parents and teachers, or focus on violence.

Etiology and Pathophysiology

Many theories have been proposed to explain the cause of depression in children and adolescents. Depression may be biologic in origin or a result of learned helplessness, cognitive distortion, social skills deficit, or family dysfunction. Childhood depression sometimes occurs secondary to parental depression, because the parent deprives the child of effective parenting. Abuse and neglect predispose children to depression, especially very young children. In about half of all children with depression, at least one other psychiatric diagnosis is made; these include conditions such as ADHD, anxiety disorder, or another personality disorder. Depressive disorders may contribute to other mental illness such as disturbed relationships, substance abuse, and suicide (Lyon & Morgan-Judge, 2000).

Clinical Manifestations

Characteristic findings of major depression in children and adolescents include declining school performance; withdrawal from social activities; sleep disturbance (either too much or too little); appetite disturbance (too much or too little); multiple somatic complaints, especially headaches and stomachaches; decreased energy; difficulty concentrating and making decisions; low self-esteem; and feelings of hopelessness. There is much variation among children in the symptoms displayed, and they often have some but not all of the major criteria (Williamson, Birmaher, & Brent, et al., 2000).

Clinical Therapy

Initial assessment is performed by a child psychologist or child psychiatrist. A variety of scales and techniques are used; however, very little guidance is available relating to evaluation of children under 6 years of age. Examples of useful tools are the Children's Depression Inventory and the Revised Children's Manifest Anxiety Scale.

SAFETY PRECAUTIONS

Serotonin syndrome, the serious and life-threatening side effect of SSRIs, is caused by overstimulation of serotonin receptors. It is more likely to develop when the child or adolescent is also taking St. John's Wort, other antidepressants, alcohol, diet pills, or abuse drugs such as ecstasy and LSD (Lyon & Morgan-Judge, 2000). Be certain to ask questions in a nonjudgmental way about intake of any alternative therapies, other medications, or substance use to identify those most at risk.

Treatment may include psychotherapy in combination with psychotropic medication. Often a combination of individual, family, and group therapy provides the greatest benefits for young children and adolescents. Involving parents and other family members in the treatment plan is essential. Group therapy is an effective treatment measure for adolescents because of the importance of peer group relationships during the teenage years. Cognitive therapy may be used with adolescents, and play therapy with younger children, as demonstrated in the case of Cassandra in the opening scenario (see discussion of play therapy earlier in this chapter).

Antidepressant medications, most commonly the selective serotonin reuptake inhibitors (SSRIs), imipramine (Tofranil), desipramine (Norpramin), and amitriptyline (Elavil), may be prescribed. The SSRIs act to block reuptake of serotonin in the synapse, so that serotonin levels (which influences mood) increase. Although the SSRIs are generally considered safer than some other types of antidepressants, their use in children has been limited, so side effects must be monitored. The major serious side effect is serotonin syndrome. This condition is characterized by agitation, muscle twitching, gastric upset, chills, fever, confusion, and dizziness. Generally the child is started with a low dose and it is increased slowly to minimize chance of side effects.

MEDICATIONS USED TO TREAT DEPRESSION

■ ***Selective Serotonin Reuptake Inhibitor (SSRI) Drugs Used to Treat Depression***

Medication	Pediatric Dose	Adolescent Dose	Selected Side Effects
Fluoxetine (Prozac)	5–40 mg qd	10–60 mg qd	Restlessness, headaches, akathesia
Sertraline (Zoloft)	25–125 mg qd	50–200 mg qd	Dry mouth, gastric upset
Paroxetine (Paxil)	5–40 mg qd	20–40 mg pd	Dry mouth, weight gain
Fluvoxamine (Luvox)	25–125 mg bid	200–300 mg qd	Dry mouth, gastric upset
Citalopram (Celexa)	Little data available	20–40 mg qd	Dry mouth, nausea, sleep disturbance

Note: Adapted from Labellarte, M. J., Walkup, J. T., & Riddle, M. A. (1998). The new antidepressants: Selective serotonin reuptake inhibitors. *Pediatric Clinics of North America, 45*, 1137–1155; and Lyon, D. E., & Morgan-Judge, T. (2000). Childhood depressive disorders. *Journal of School Nursing, 16*(3), 29–31.

NURSING MANAGEMENT

Nursing Assessment and Diagnosis

A thorough history and physical examination, including observation of behavior, are obtained at the time of admission. Assess the child for common risk factors for depression (Table 24-8).

Several nursing diagnoses that may be appropriate for the child or adolescent hospitalized with depression are included in the accompanying nursing care plan. Other diagnoses may include the following:

- *Altered nutrition: More than body requirements,* related to eating in response to internal cues other than hunger
- *Powerlessness,* related to sense of helplessness
- *Low self-esteem,* related to negative self-evaluation

TABLE 24-8

Risk Factors for Depression and Anxiety in Children and Adolescents

Parental neglect, abuse, or loss
Stressful social relationships
Academic pressures and underachievement
Dysfunctional family relationships
Family history of depression, suicide, substance abuse, alcoholism, or other psychopathology
Chronic illness and frequent hospitalization

Planning and Implementation

Nursing care of the child or adolescent hospitalized for depression includes administering medications and other therapy, and providing supportive care. Monitor vital signs of youth receiving antidepressant medications. Watch for common side effects of the agent(s) used. Carefully monitor for serious side effects of SSRIs and be aware that lower doses are used at initiation with doses increasing slowly to desired level. Monitor cardiovascular status, including hypertension and tachycardia, observe motor movement, and record dietary intake. Help parents to evaluate inpatient settings to be certain the care provided will best meet the needs of the child or adolescent. Refer to the nursing care plan for specific nursing interventions for the child or adolescent hospitalized with depression.

Discharge Planning and Home Care Teaching

When the child has been hospitalized and is returning home, teach parents to recognize signs and symptoms of worsening depression. Parents should also be taught dosages and side effects of any prescribed medications. Refer the family to appropriate health care professionals and to support groups for family members dealing with depression.

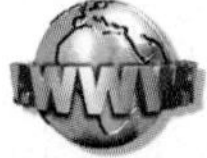

Depression Resources and Support

Care in the Community

Most children with depression are cared for in the community. Maintain regular contact with family members through their health care visits to outpatient agencies and by making

FAMILIES WANT TO KNOW

Selecting Residential and Inpatient Care for the Child with Mental Illness

Families need guidelines to assist them in evaluating inpatient facilities when a child with a mental disorder must be placed in an institution. They can be referred to the National Alliance for the Mentally Ill website. Nurses can provide questions for the families to ask:

- What is the staff to youth ratio?
- What are the guidelines for chemical and physical restraint?
- Are children isolated alone when behaviors are inappropriate?
- Are children constantly monitored visually when in restraint or when potentially dangerous to self or others?
- Does the child have a full physical and psychological evaluation by a specialist within 24 hours of entry to the facility?
- What professionals review the plan of care and how often?
- To whom can the family speak for regular updates on the child?
- How often can the family visit?
- What services will be covered by insurance?
- What subjective feelings does the family member have when visiting the unit and facility?
- What services will be offered on an ongoing basis upon discharge?

NURSING CARE PLAN The Child or Adolescent Hospitalized with Depression

GOAL	INTERVENTION	RATIONALE	EXPECTED OUTCOME
1. Hopelessness related to long-term stress			
	NIC Priority Intervention: **Hope Instillation:** Facilitation of the development of a positive outlook.		NOC Suggested: Outcome: **Hope:** Presence of internal state of optimism that is personally satisfying and life supporting.
The child or adolescent will discuss feelings of hopelessness.	■ Encourage open expression of feelings. Explore hopeless, sad, or lonely feelings. Point out the connection between feelings and behavior. Assess the child or adolescent to identify the precipitating event when feelings of sadness arose. ■ Encourage the child or adolescent to take part in self-care and unit activities. Use routines to establish feelings of control. ■ Medicate as ordered and document results.	■ Expressing feelings may help to relieve sadness, loneliness, despair, and hopelessness. An accepting and nonjudgmental attitude must be maintained regarding any feelings expressed by the child. ■ An active role in self-care and treatment helps the child or adolescent to feel more in control. ■ Antidepressants modify mood to a more hopeful outlook.	By discharge, the child or adolescent expresses an interest in the future.
2. Ineffective Individual Coping related to inadequate social support or disturbance in pattern of appraisal of threat			
	NIC Priority Intervention: **Coping Enhancement:** Assisting a patient to adapt to perceived stressors, changes, or threats which interfere with meeting life demands and roles.		NOC Suggested Outcome: **Coping:** Actions to manage stressors that tax an individual's resources.
The child or adolescent will use effective coping skills.	■ Teach positive, effective coping strategies such as guided imagery and relaxation. Assist the child or adolescent to focus on strengths rather than weaknesses. ■ Assist the child or adolescent to identify friends, family members, and others who are positive and supportive.	■ Therapeutic techniques can help the child or adolescent to replace negative thoughts and images with more positive and effective beliefs and images. These interventions foster resilience. ■ Helps the child or adolescent to become aware that people can be caring and supportive (thus validating self-esteem).	The child or adolescent verbalizes and demonstrates ability to cope appropriately for his or her age.

(continued)

home visits. Monitor the child's affect, activity, and food intake. School teachers and counselors often are aware of the child's ability to perform in the school setting. Have the family schedule after-school care so young children are not left at home alone for extended periods. Assist the family in finding support for financial and emotional needs related to managing the child's depression.

Major expected outcomes for nursing care of the child with depression are found on the accompanying nursing care plan.

BIPOLAR DISORDER (MANIC DEPRESSION)

Bipolar disorder is a mental illness in which extreme changes in affect and energy are manifested. Moods most often alter between mania and depression. Children often present with irritability or hyperactivity. About 1.5% of the total population suffers from bipolar illness, although diagnosis and accurate numbers are difficult to obtain due to the frequency of accompanying additional mental illness (St. Dennis & Synoground, 1998). About 10% to 20% of individuals with bipolar illness commit suicide. The average age for children to demon-

NURSING CARE PLAN The Child or Adolescent Hospitalized with Depression (continued)

GOAL	INTERVENTION	RATIONALE	EXPECTED OUTCOME
3. Impaired Social Interaction related to self concept disturbance			
	NIC Intervention: **Socialization Enhancement:** Facilitation of ability to interact with others.		NOC Outcome: **Social Interaction Skills:** An individual's use of effective interaction behaviors.
The child or adolescent will participate in and initiate activities and conversation.	■ Assist the child or adolescent to identify topics and activities of interest. ■ Encourage interaction with peers and staff. ■ Facilitate visits from family and friends. ■ Provide guidance to family regarding interaction that promotes self-esteem.	■ The more the child or adolescent focuses on areas of interest, the less he or she will focus on internal anxiety and depression. ■ Each positive interaction reinforces feelings of success. Each success reinforces the desire for future social interaction. ■ Reinforces positive and rewarding relationships. ■ The family's existing interaction style is often negative.	By discharge, the child or adolescent initiates conversation and activities with staff and peers.
4. Altered Nutrition: Less Than Body Requirements related to loss of appetite secondary to depression			
	NIC Intervention: **Nutrition Management:** Assistance with or provision of a balanced dietary intake of foods and fluids.		NOC Outcome: **Nutritional Status:** Amount of food and fluid taken into the body over a 24-hour period.
The child or adolescent's daily intake will be adequate to maintain optimal nutritional status.	■ Offer nutritious finger foods, sandwiches, and high-calorie liquid supplements frequently throughout the day. ■ Offer easy-to-carry drinks that are high in vitamins, minerals, and calories. ■ Encourage daily vigorous physical activity of at least 30 minutes.	■ Convenient easy-to-eat foods encourage the child or adolescent to eat and maintain nutritional status. ■ These are a convenient method for meeting hydration and electrolyte needs. ■ Physical activity stimulates appetite.	The child or adolescent's daily intake will be adequate to maintain optimal nutritional status by discharge.

strate bipolar disorder is 11 years. Children may show mainly depressive symptoms, and then develop mania in adolescence, or may have episodes of both mania and depression in the same day (Jellinek & Snyder, 1998).

The manic phase of bipolar illness is characterized by hyperactivity and high energy, irritability, aggression, and sometimes hallucinations. In the depressive phase, the child is sad, has alterations in sleep and eating patterns, and is socially withdrawn, similar to any depressive illness.

Diagnosis and treatment of bipolar disorder should be performed by mental health specialists. Use of alcohol or illegal drugs should be ruled out as a cause of symptoms, even in children. Since the manic phase is often manifested by hyperactivity, the child may incorrectly be treated with stimulants (see discussion of ADHD earlier in this chapter), and the disease can be worsened. The treatment of bipolar disease involves a variety of drugs used to stabilize mood. Nurses are instrumental in identifying children with the disorder, providing information to families, and monitoring the drugs and psychotherapy for the child.

GROWTH & DEVELOPMENT

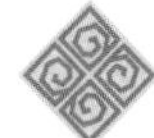

The separation anxiety experienced by a 2-year-old differs from the psychiatric disorder in age appropriateness, duration, and severity. Separation anxiety disorder affects children of preschool age or older, lasts for at least 2 weeks, and is characterized by excessive anxiety. In contrast, the separation anxiety experienced by the 2-year-old involves a single episode of separation from a familiar caretaker and is a characteristic response in toddlers.

ANXIETY AND RELATED DISORDERS

GENERALIZED ANXIETY

Anxiety is a subjective feeling of uncertainty and helplessness, usually accompanied by CNS signs, including restlessness, trembling, perspiration, and rapid pulse. Anxiety is second to only substance abuse (see Chapter 7) in incidence for mental disorders and is a common mental disorder among children (Smoller, Finn, & White, 2000). Anxiety disorders are strongly linked to familial and genetic factors.

Separation anxiety disorder is characterized by an extreme state of uneasiness when in unfamiliar surroundings and often by refusal to visit friends' homes or attend school for at least 2 weeks. Approximately 75% of children with separation anxiety disorder refuse to attend school (see School Phobia, to follow). This disorder occurs in approximately 4% to 5% of children and in twice as many girls as boys (Masi, Mucci, & Millepiedi, 2001).

Children with separation anxiety disorder tend to be perfectionistic, overly compliant, and eager to please. They appear to cling to the parent or caretaker. They may use physical complaints such as headaches, abdominal pain, nausea, and vomiting in an attempt to avoid being away from the parent. Depression frequently accompanies separation anxiety disorder. The resulting avoidant behaviors can interfere with personal growth and development, academic achievement, and social functioning.

Anxiety disorders are best treated by behavioral, family, and individual therapy. For children with significant or long-lasting impairment in functioning, drugs such as the SSRIs or other antidepressants may be tried.

Nursing care centers on educating parents about the disorder and management techniques. Encourage attendance at therapy sessions. Children with separation anxiety disorder benefit from a predictable routine and environment. Advise children in advance of any expected changes in routine. Help parents to plan consistent and reassuring contacts for the child after school and during activities. Instruct about medication administration and side effects if this therapy is used.

PANIC

Panic disorder is the presence of recurrent, unexpected panic attacks. These attacks are periods of intense fear and discomfort in the absence of real danger. The risk of panic disorder ranges from 1.5% to 3.5% of the population (Smoller et al., 2000), with adolescence a common age for the onset of symptoms. The risk of panic disorder is 20 times more likely when there is a family history of the disorder (American Psychiatric Association, 2000).

Examples of the physical symptoms experienced are palpitations, sweating, chills, hot flashes, shaking, shortness of breath, choking, chest pain, nausea, and dizziness. The person describes feelings of danger or doom. There may be accompanying agoraphobia in some people. **Agoraphobia** is an anxiety of being in places or situations from which escape may be difficult or embarrassing, or in which help may not be available. The attacks may be continuous or episodic, but generally are chronic in nature.

Similar to anxiety, treatment may involve individual and family therapy, with use of medication in some cases. Nurses can help to identify the disorder, refer for evaluation, and provide care in the community so that the child attends therapy sessions and takes medication when ordered (Carson, 2000).

RESEARCH

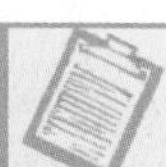

A connection has been observed between neuropsychiatric abnormalities and people who have acute rheumatic fever (a disease caused by *Streptococcus*). Some types of obsessive-compulsive and tic disorders may worsen after infections such as strep throat; this connection has been called pediatric autoimmune neuropsychiatric disorders associated with streptococcus (PANDAS). Current federal research is investigating the treatment of PANDAS with plasma exchange treatments and antibiotics (Kaplan, 2000).

OBSESSIVE-COMPULSIVE DISORDER

Individuals with obsessive-compulsive disorder may be mildly or severely affected. One in about 200 children is affected, and there may be associated conditions such as tic disorders or attention deficit hyperactivity (Leonard, Freeman, & Barcia, et al., 2001). Affected children have recurrent ritualistic thoughts or actions; these obsessions or compulsions interfere with daily life. Examples of behaviors and concerns are obsessions about dirt or germs, worries about harm, and sexual thoughts. Common behaviors are excessive handwashing, counting objects, and hoarding substances. These practices may take 1 or more hours each day.

The basal ganglia of the brain are affected and a genetic link is observed. Poststreptococcal autoimmune disorder may be a cause in some cases. Treatment may involve cognitive-behavioral therapy, where the feared occurrence is presented and the person learns that no harm will occur. Medications, particularly SSRIs, are effective in most children. Nurses can identify cases and refer for psychiatric evaluation. Families need instruction about medications and potential side effects.

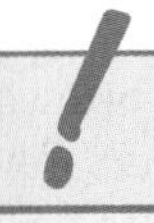

NURSING ALERT

Females have a greater incidence of the mental disorders anxiety, depression, and posttraumatic stress disorder. What relationship do you see between the high rate of sexual abuse experienced by females (see Chapter 7) and the incidence of these disorders? When a history of child abuse is known, be alert for signs of PTSD and other mental health disorders.

SCHOOL PHOBIA

School phobia (also called school avoidance or school refusal) is a persistent, irrational, or excessive fear of attending school. The child may fear being harmed or losing control. School phobia is common in children between 5 and 12 years of age, but can occur in children up to 16 years. The child's avoidance of school is often a manifestation of fear of leaving the parent or primary caretaker. Children commonly report that teachers and peers "pick on" them. Somatic complaints are similar to those in children with separation anxiety disorder. Characteristically, symptoms are present only on school days and not on weekends or holidays.

Treatment includes the family and child, and establishes firm limits for behavioral expectations and consequences. Antidepressant medications may sometimes be needed to help the child feel comfortable. The longer a child is out of school, the greater the likelihood that a chronic, treatment-resistant condition will result. Referral for psychiatric evaluation is indicated for persistent symptoms.

POSTTRAUMATIC STRESS DISORDER

Posttraumatic stress disorder (PTSD) victims have experienced or witnessed a life-threatening event with death or severe injury (Meltzer-Brody, Hidalgo, & Connor, et al., 2000). Although accurate statistics are not available on children, about 1% to 2% of children are probably affected, with increasing numbers as more children are exposed to war and other violence (Kessler, 2000). The child or adolescent with the disorder has feelings of fear, terror, and helplessness, and may relive the event frequently in thought and nightmares. The child may become emotionally numb in a subconscious attempt to protect the self, but may have a persistently increased state of arousal (Kent, Sullivan, & Rauch, 2000). Examples of events that are associated with posttraumatic stress include sexual or other child abuse, rape, car crash, fire, witnessing violence, and having experience in war. The events which occured in the United States on September 11, 2001, are

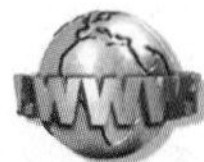

PTSD Resources and Support

FAMILIES WANT TO KNOW

Talking with Children About Traumatic Events

Whether a child or adolescent experiences trauma from a car crash, abuse, or environmental event, parents can help to decrease the effects of the stress and prevent the appearance of posttraumatic stress disorder by doing the following:

- Be sure children feel comfortable asking parents, teachers, or others about the events and their feelings.
- Assure children that their feelings are normal and may return over time.
- Be honest and open in responses, without overloading the child with more details than they need.
- Be prepared to repeat answers and discuss the same topics many times.
- Get help from counselors who can suggest how to talk with the child.
- Use communication methods appropriate at various ages, such as reading books, doing art projects, or drawing.
- Show children that they are loved by spending time and planning activities with them.
- Limit the television and other media time where the child is exposed to violence and traumatic events.
- Restore a sense of normal routines into the child's life.
- Be alert for increasing signs of distress and seek care from a professional if they occur.

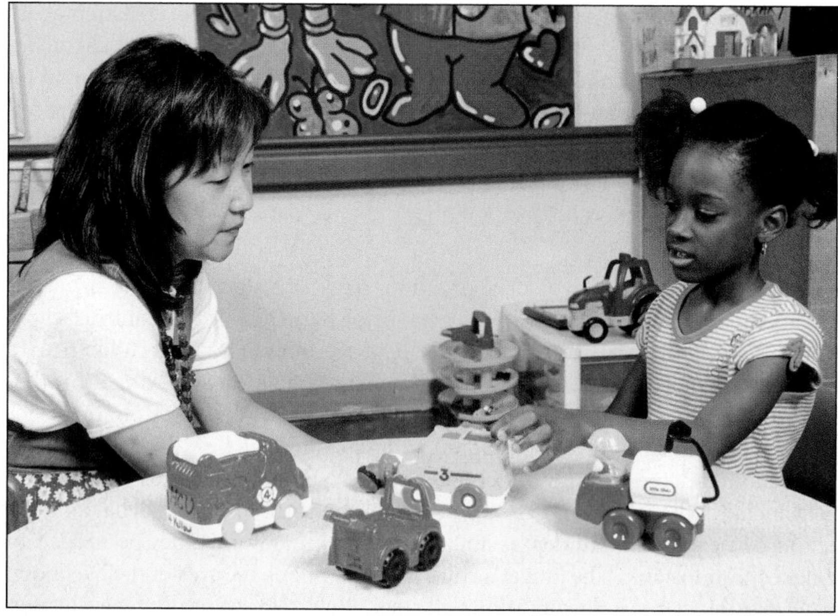

FIGURE 24-6 ◆
The psychologist uses play therapy to help Cassandra reenact her car crash. This helps her gain control over the event so that it is not so frightening.

potential causes of posttraumatic stress in children who either had a family member involved, lived near the events, or in some other way were profoundly affected.

Cassandra, described in the opening scenario, was experiencing PTSD due to a frightening car crash as she was driven to school. She was too young to describe her feelings verbally to her mother or school personnel; however, she manifested the sleep abnormalities and other complaints common in the disorder (Figure 24-6 ◆). Even children of Holocaust victims experience PTSD, leading mental health professionals to believe that the condition can be transmitted from parent to child (Yehud, Hallig, & Grossman, 2001). There is a relatively high incidence of PTSD among incarcerated youth (Lamberg, 2001).

The disorder involves both a traumatic event and the child's reaction to this event. It is believed that brain changes occur in trauma, leading to neurobiological alterations that cause dysfunction of memory. Females, those with other psychiatric disorders, a family history of psychiatric illness, and severe or lengthy trauma are all risk factors. The incidence ranges from 1% to 9% (Meltzer-Brody et al., 2000).

A variety of antidepressants and SSRIs are used for pharmacologic treatment. Counseling and other mechanisms of care can assist the victim in dealing with the events. Cassandra had visits to a clinical psychologist who used play therapy to help her to communicate her fears related to a car crash. Once the fears are clearly communicated, they often lose their power over the person, so that normal behaviors can resume. Nurses often help to identify PTSD victims so that care can be obtained. Mental health nurses may conduct group therapy sessions. All nurses should recognize that they are at risk for the disorder when their jobs present them with frequent traumatic events. They should seek assistance from counselors and use various resources to deal with the trauma.

CONVERSION REACTION

Conversion reaction is a disorder in which a disturbance or loss of sensory, motor, or other physical functions suggests neurologic or other somatic disease. The disturbance or loss cannot be explained by any known pathophysiologic mechanism. Instead, psychologic factors are involved. About 3% of the population experiences conversion reactions at some time (American Psychiatric Association, 2000). Adolescence and early adulthood are common times for the onset to occur.

Conversion reactions develop in response to a catastrophic event such as threat, loss, or harm. Clinical manifestations include altered sensations such as blindness or deafness; paralysis or ataxia, including inability to stand or walk and loss of ability to speak (aphonia); involuntary movements, such as pseudoepileptic convulsions; and constant complaints of pain with no physical basis (psychogenic pain). Children under 10 years usually present with gait abnormalities or seizures. The onset of conversion symptoms is usually dramatic and sudden. Symptoms often appear to be neurologic, but on careful examination obvious discrepancies are found. The person is usually calm about the symptoms even though they are serious. Often the child or family members appear indifferent or unconcerned over what health care providers consider an overwhelming physical disability.

Children suspected of having a conversion reaction require a complete physical and neurologic evaluation to rule out any possible physiologic basis for the symptoms. Individual and family therapy is usually necessary to identify the source of the psychologic conflict, pain, or need resulting in the conversion symptoms.

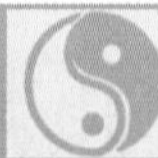

CULTURE

Some ethnic groups have a high rate of suicide. For example, Native Americans have a rate of suicide at 1.5 times the national average. Many youth in this group are suicide victims; it is the third major cause of death in Native American youth. The historic pain experienced by this ethnic group and lack of opportunities for many youth may be some of the reasons for a high suicide rate. Healthy People 2010 goals focus on eliminating such health disparities by finding the causes, setting up prevention programs, and providing more support and opportunities for native populations.

SUICIDE

Suicide is the third leading cause of death in adolescents between 15 and 19 years of age. Over the past 40 years, teenage suicide has nearly tripled (Fish, 2000; National Strategy for Suicide Prevention, 2001). Suicide accounts for about 16% of deaths in teens. Nine percent of teens and 1% of prepubertal children have attempted suicide (Jellinek & Snyder, 1998).

Boys die as a result of suicide 4 times more often than girls. This statistic is reversed for suicide attempts, perhaps because boys use lethal methods such as guns, hanging, and jumping more often than girls, who more commonly use drug overdose and wrist cutting. It is not unusual for health care professionals and parents to label suicide attempts by children and adolescents as accidents. Up to half of childhood suicides may be recorded as accidents; suicide data for children under age 10 years are not maintained. Adults may have difficulty believing that young children, in particular, would have any reason to want to end their lives. For this reason, many children who are brought to the emergency department with indications of a suicide attempt are often classified as unintentional injury victims and released without arrangements for appropriate follow-up care.

Many risk factors for suicide exist in children and adolescents (Table 24-9). The most common precursor to adolescent suicide is depression (see previous discussion). Common signs or symptoms of an underlying depression that could lead to suicide include boredom, restlessness, problems with concentration, irritability, lethargy, intentional misbehavior, preoccupation with one's own body or health, and excessive dependence on or isolation from others (especially adults or caregivers).

The child or adolescent found to be at high risk for suicide may be admitted to a psychiatric unit for care or cared for in a community mental health facility. Treatment may include individual, group, or family therapy. Negotiating a no-suicide contract is one method that may be used with a suicidal youth. In the contract, the child agrees not to attempt suicide during a specified time period. When a suicide attempt is made, the child or adolescent may be hospitalized for 24 hours, kept in a short-term monitoring unit, or sent home under close observation to ensure adequate assessment and monitoring. It is important to provide crisis intervention at the time of the suicide attempt to minimize the opportunity for repeat attempts and begin a therapeutic treatment plan.

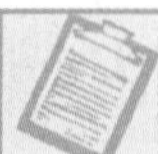

RESEARCH

Research has demonstrated that there may be different triggers for suicide in female and male adolescents. Female adolescents consider suicide more frequently when their situations are unstable, and it is often an impulsive act. Male adolescents think of suicide when they are depressed and when their social environment is unsatisfactory (Rohde, Seeley, & Mace, 1997).

NURSING MANAGEMENT

The major nursing role is in prevention of suicide. Most suicides are committed with firearms present in the home. Ask at each health care visit if the family has firearms. Encourage them to keep them unloaded, with ammunition and firearms locked in separate locations. Be sure that children and adolescents do not have access to the keys for the locked firearms.

Education in all school settings is appropriate to assist children in knowing about resources of help when needed and in identifying peers at risk. Be alert for children and adolescents at risk for suicide in any setting. Assess children and adolescents in schools, outpatient settings, and emergency rooms for the possibility of suicidal behavior. Report threats of suicide and depressive behavior. Recognize that when one suicide has occurred, there may be an increased risk for friends of the victim. Teach students to report to teachers, nurses, or counselors about friends who have threatened suicide or seem depressed or display behaviors different than usual. Nurses often plan with mental health specialists to implement suicide prevention programs in schools and communities. Provide supportive services to family and friends when suicide occurs.

TABLE 24-9

Risk Factors for Suicide in Children and Adolescents

School problems
Pregnancy
Drug use or abuse
Problems with a romantic relationship
Feelings of anxiety
History of chronic family problems
Chronic illness
Physical, emotional, or sexual abuse
History of suicide in a family member
History of depression
Chronic low self-esteem

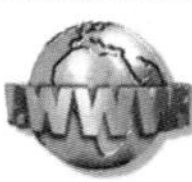

NURSING ALERT

If an adolescent or child persists in threatening suicide after the health care provider attempts to negotiate a no-suicide contract, hospitalization is necessary to ensure the child's safety. All suicide threats must be taken seriously.

Suicide Prevention

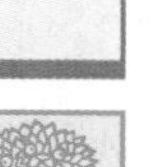

NURSING ALERT

Never underestimate the abilities or resourcefulness of a suicidal child or adolescent, regardless of age, IQ, or physical abilities.

COMMUNITY CARE

Children with Tourette's syndrome may initially be diagnosed with ADHD due to their increased activity. If they are medicated with a drug such as methylphenidate (Ritalin, Concerta), their activity will worsen. Monitor symptoms carefully after the child begins taking medication and be sure the child is seen regularly for ongoing care.

Nursing care centers on taking appropriate precautions to ensure the child's safety. Both the child and the hospital environment are monitored for any object that could be used for self-harm. All potentially harmful objects, such as shoestrings, belts, pantyhose, and hair ribbons, are removed. All personal care items (including toothbrush and shampoo) are kept locked at the nursing station and monitored constantly when used by the child.

Children or adolescents who are considered at high risk for suicidal behaviors are attended by a nursing staff member at all times, including while using the bathroom and sleeping. It may be necessary for the child to dress in a plain hospital gown, be kept in a visually monitored seclusion room, or (if seriously impaired and self-abusive) be medicated for restraint for a period of time. Restraints are used only when ordered by the physician and interdisciplinary team caring for the youth. Physical restraint is only a short-term approach to provide immediate safety if necessary. Chemical (medication) restraint may need to be used to prevent self-injury by the suicidal person. See page 927 for information to help families consider when choosing care for their suicidal child.

Hospitalization continues as long as the child's behavior is self-destructive. Children are referred for intensive individual and family therapy. Encourage parents to keep follow-up clinic appointments, to watch for self-destructive behaviors, and to administer any prescribed medications according to the treatment schedule. Arrange home visits and other community resources for families.

TIC DISORDERS AND TOURETTE'S SYNDROME

Tics are sudden, rapid, recurrent, nonrhythmic and brief motor movements or vocalizations. They may involve movement of the head or upper body, blinking of eyes, or a variety of verbal noises. They may be worse during periods of stress or tiredness. Severe motor tics accompanied by verbal utterances are known as Tourette's syndrome. The syndrome is often accompanied by other diagnoses such as attention deficit and learning disabilities (Kurlan, McDermott, & Deeley, et al., 2001). Many children have mild motor tics at some time which gradually disappear with no intervention. When the tics are severe or last over 1 year, they are considered chronic and may require attention from a mental health provider. This disorder is believed to be caused by dopamine abnormalities in the brain and can be successfully treated by haloperidol or other psychotropic medications. Nursing care involves supporting parents and encouraging normal developmental progression for the child. Stress should be minimized and relaxation techniques taught.

Chapter Highlights

- Major treatment modes for children with mental health disorders include individual therapy, family therapy, and group therapy.
- Therapeutic strategies for treatment of children and adolescents with mental health disorders include play therapy, art therapy, behavior therapy, visualization, and hypnosis.
- Families often attempt to treat mental health conditions with use of alternative and complementary therapy; nurses can provide information to assist families in evaluating the results of these therapies.
- Nurses are involved in conducting mental health assessments, preventing disorders when possible, participating in intervention to treat disorders, and evaluating success of treatments.
- Autistic spectrum disorder is the major type of pervasive developmental disorder, and is manifested by abnormal behavior, social interaction, and communication.
- Attention deficit disorder (ADD) and attention deficit hyperactivity disorder (ADHD) are characterized by developmentally inappropriate behaviors involving inattention, and sometimes hyperactivity.
- ADD and ADHD must be diagnosed using recommended criteria and are commonly treated with a combination of behavioral, environmental, and medication therapies.
- Mental retardation is a subaverage intellectual and adaptive functioning, and is caused by chromosomal, genetic, or environmental factors.

- Nurses identify children with possible mental retardation by careful evaluation of development.
- A multidisciplinary team plans the care for children with mental retardation and periodically evaluates the child's progress and the family's needs.
- Schizophrenia is a psychotic disorder manifested by social withdrawal, delusions, and hallucinations.
- Mood disorders in childhood and adolescents are commonly manifested as depression or manic depression (bipolar disorder).
- Several anxiety disorders occur in children and adolescents, most notably anxiety, panic, obsessive-compulsive disorder, and school phobia.
- Behavioral therapy and selective serotonin reuptake inhibitors (SSRIs) are used in treatment of anxiety disorders.
- Posttraumatic stress disorder may occur as victims relive the terror of traumatic events.
- Suicide is a frequent cause of death among youth.
- Nurses are key heath professionals in identifying youth at risk of suicide, instituting suicide prevention programs, and counseling family and friends of suicide victims.
- Children may experience tic disorders which impair development and social interactions; medications are helpful in treatment of these disorders.
- Nurses play a vital role in maintaining the mental health of children, identifying children at risk of mental health disorders, and providing care or referring families for mental health services.

EXPLORE MediaLink

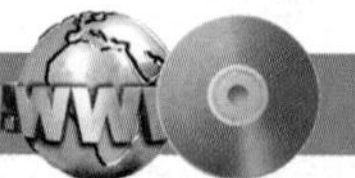

- NCLEX review, case studies, and other interactive resources for this chapter can be found on the Companion Website at **http://www.prenhall.com/ball.** Click on Chapter 24 to select the activities for this chapter.
- For animations, more NCLEX review questions, and an audio glossary, access the accompanying CD-ROM in this textbook.

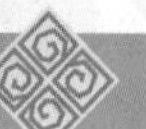

References

1. American Academy of Child and Adolescent Psychiatry. (2001). The practice parameter for the assessment and treatment of children and adolescents with schizophrenia. *Journal of the American Academy of Child & Adolescent Psychiatry, 40*(7), 4S–23S.
2. American Academy of Pediatrics, Committee on Quality Improvement, Subcommittee on Attention-Deficit/Hyperactivity Disorder. (2000). Diagnosis and evaluation of the child with attention-deficit/hyperactivity disorder. *Pediatrics, 105,* 1158–1170.
3. American Academy of Pediatrics. (2001a). Diagnosis and management of autistic spectrum disorder. *Pediatrics, 107,* 1221–1226.
4. American Academy of Pediatrics, Committee on Quality Improvement, Subcommittee on Attention-Deficit/Hyperactivity Disorder. (2001b). Clinical practice guideline: Treatment of the school-aged child with attention-deficit/hyperactivity disorder. *Pediatrics, 108,* 1033–1044.
5. American Academy of Pediatrics, Committee on Genetics. (2001c). Health supervision for children with down syndrome. *Pediatrics, 107,* 442–449.
6. Bailey, D.B., Roberts, J.E., Mirrett, P., & Hatton, D.D. (2001). Identifying infants and toddlers with fragile X syndrome: Issues and recommendations. *Infants and Young Children, 14,* 24–33.
7. Baird, G., Charman, T., Cox, A., Baron-Cohen, S., Swettenham, J., Wheelwright, S., & Drew, A. (2001). Screening and surveillance for autism and pervasive developmental disorders. *Archives of Disease in Childhood, 84,* 468–475.
8. Baralle, D. (2001). Chromosomal aberrations, subtelomeric defects, and mental retardation. *Lancet, 358,* 7–8.
9. Baumgaertel, A. (1999). Alternative and controversial treatments for attention-deficit/hyperactivity disorder. *Pediatric Clinics of North America, 46,* 977–992.
10. Blondis, T. A. (1999). Motor disorders and attention-deficit/hyperactivity disorder. *Pediatric Clinics of North America, 46,* 899–914.
11. Bryden, K. E., Carrey, N. J., & Kutcher, S. P. (2001). Update and recommendations for the use of antipsychotics in early-onset psychosis. *Journal of Child and Adolescent Psycho-Pharmacology, 11,* 113–130.
12. Cade, M., & Tidwell, S. (2001). Autism and the school nurse. *Journal of School Health, 71,* 96–100.
13. Carson, V. B. (2000). *Mental health nursing,* (2nd ed.). Philadelphia: WB Saunders.
14. Castiglia, P. T. (2000). Depression in children. *Journal of Pediatric Health Care, 14,* 73–75.
15. Dales, L., Hammer, S. J., & Smith, N. J. (2001). Time trends in autism and in MMR immunization coverage in California. *Journal of the American Medical Association, 285,* 1183.
16. Department of Health and Human Services. (2000). *Report of the surgeon general's conference on children's mental health: A national action agenda.* Washington, DC: U.S. Department of Health and Human Services.
17. *Diagnostic and Statistical Manual of Mental Disorders, Fourth Edition, Text Revision.* (2000). Washington, DC, American Psychiatric Association.
18. Fish, K. B. (2000). Suicide awareness at the elementary school level. *Journal of Psychosocial Nursing, 38,* 20–23.
19. Fletcher, J. M., Shaywitz, S. E., & Shaywitz, B. A. (1999). Comorbidity of learning and attention disorders: Separate but equal. *Pediatric Clinics of North America, 46,* 885–898.
20. Frederic, D. W., & Williams, S. L. (1998). New definition of mental retardation for the American Association of Mental Retardation. *Image, 30,* 53–56.

21. Hoagwood, K., Burns, B. J., Kiser, L., Rindeisen, H., & Schoenwald, S. K. (2001). Evidence-based practice in child and adolescent mental health services. *Psychiatric Services, 52,* 1179–1189.

22. Hunt, R. D., Paguin, A., & Payton, K. (2001). An update on assessment and treatment of complex attention-deficit hyperactivity disorder. *Pediatric Annals, 30,* 162–172.

23. Hyman, S. L., & Levy, S. E. (2000). Autistic spectrum disorders: When traditional medicine is not enough. *Contemporary Pediatrics, 17,* 101–116.

24. Jellinek, M. S., & Snyder, J. B. (1998). Depression and suicide in children and adolescents. *Pediatrics in Review, 19,* 255–263.

25. Kaplan, E. L. (2000). PANDAS? Or PAND? Or both? Or neither? *Contemporary Pediatrics, 17,* 81–96.

26. Kent, J. M., Sullivan, G. M., & Rauch, S. L. (2000). The neurobiology of fear: Relevance to panic disorder and posttraumatic stress disorder. *Psychiatric Annals, 30,* 733–742.

27. Kessler, R. C. (2000). Posttraumatic stress disorder. *Journal of Clinical Psychiatry, 61* (Suppl. 15), 4–12.

28. Koenig, K. (1998). Pervasive developmental disorders: Diagnosis, intervention and education. *American Journal for Nurse Practitioners, 2*(8), 15–28.

29. Kurlan, R., McDermott, M. P., Deeley, C., Como, P. G., Brower, C., Eapen, S., Adresen, E. M., & Miller, E. M. (2001). Prevalence of tics in school children and adolescents associated with placement in special education. *Neurology, 57,* 1383–1388.

30. Lamberg, L. (2001). Psychiatrists explore the legacy of traumatic stress in early life. *Journal of the American Medical Association, 286,* 523–526.

31. Lambert, L. T. (2001). Identification and management of schizophrenia in childhood. *Journal of Child and Adolescent Psychiatric Nursing, 14,* 73–80.

32. Leonard, H. L., Freeman, J., Barcia, A., Garvey, M., Snider, L., & Swedo, S. E. (2001). Obsessive-compulsive disorder and related conditions. *Pediatric Annals, 30,* 154–160.

33. Lyon, D. E., & Morgan-Judge, T. (2000). Childhood depressive disorders. *Journal of School Nursing, 16*(3), 29–31.

34. Masi, G., Mucci, M., & Millepiedi, S. (2001). Separation anxiety disorder in children and adolescents: Epidemiology, diagnosis and management. *CNS Drugs, 15,* 93–104.

35. Meltzer-Brody, S., Hidalgo, R., Connor, K. M., & Davidson, J. R. T. (2000). Posttraumatic stress disorder: Prevalence, health care use and costs, and pharmacologic considerations. *Psychiatric Annals, 30,* 722–730.

36. Moldenhauer, Z., & Melnyk, B. M. (1999). Use of antidepressants in the treatment of child and adolescent depression: Are they effective? *Pediatric Nursing, 25,* 643–645.

37. National Strategy for Suicide Prevention. (2001). *www.mentalhealth.org/suicideprevention.* Retrieved November 5, 2001, from the World Wide Web.

38. Navon, M., Nelson, D., Pagano, M., & Murphy, M. (2001). Use of the pediatric symptom checklist in strategies to improve preventive behavioral health care. *Psychiatric Services, 52,* 800–804.

39. Rohde, P., Seeley, J. R., & Mace, D. E. (1997). Correlates of suicidal behavior in a juvenile detention center. *Suicide and Life-Threatening Behavior, 27,* 164–175.

40. Smoller, J. W., Finn, C., & White, C. (2000). The genetics of anxiety disorders: An overview. *Psychiatry Annals, 30,* 745–753.

41. St. Dennis, C., & Synoground, G. (1998). Medications for early onset bipolar illness: New drug update. *Journal of School Nursing, 14*(5), 29–41.

42. Van Riper, M., & Cohen, W. I. (2001). Caring for children with down syndrome and their families. *Journal of Pediatric Health Care, 15,* 123–131.

43. Williams, P. G., Dalrymple, N., & Neal, J. (2000). Eating habits of children with autism. *Pediatric Nursing, 26,* 259–264.

44. Williamson, D. E., Birmaher, B., Brent, D. A., Bolach, L., Dahl, R. E., & Ryan, N. D. (2000). Atypical symptoms of depression in a sample of depressed child and adolescent outpatients. *Journal of the American Academy of Child and Adolescent Psychiatry, 39,* 1253–1259.

45. Yehud, R., Hallig, S. L., & Grossman, R. (2001). Childhood trauma and risk for PTSD: Relationship to intergenerational effects of trauma, parental PTSD, and cortisol excretion. *Developmental Psychopathology, 13,* 733–753.

46. Zickler, C. F., Morrow, J. D., & Bull, M. J. (1998). Infants with down syndrome: A look at temperament. *Journal of Pediatric Health Care, 12,* 111–117.

APPENDIX A: PHYSICAL GROWTH CHARTS

FIGURE A-1 ◆
Physical growth percentiles for length and weight—boys: birth to 36 months.
From CDC, 2001. *www.cdc.gov/growthcharts*

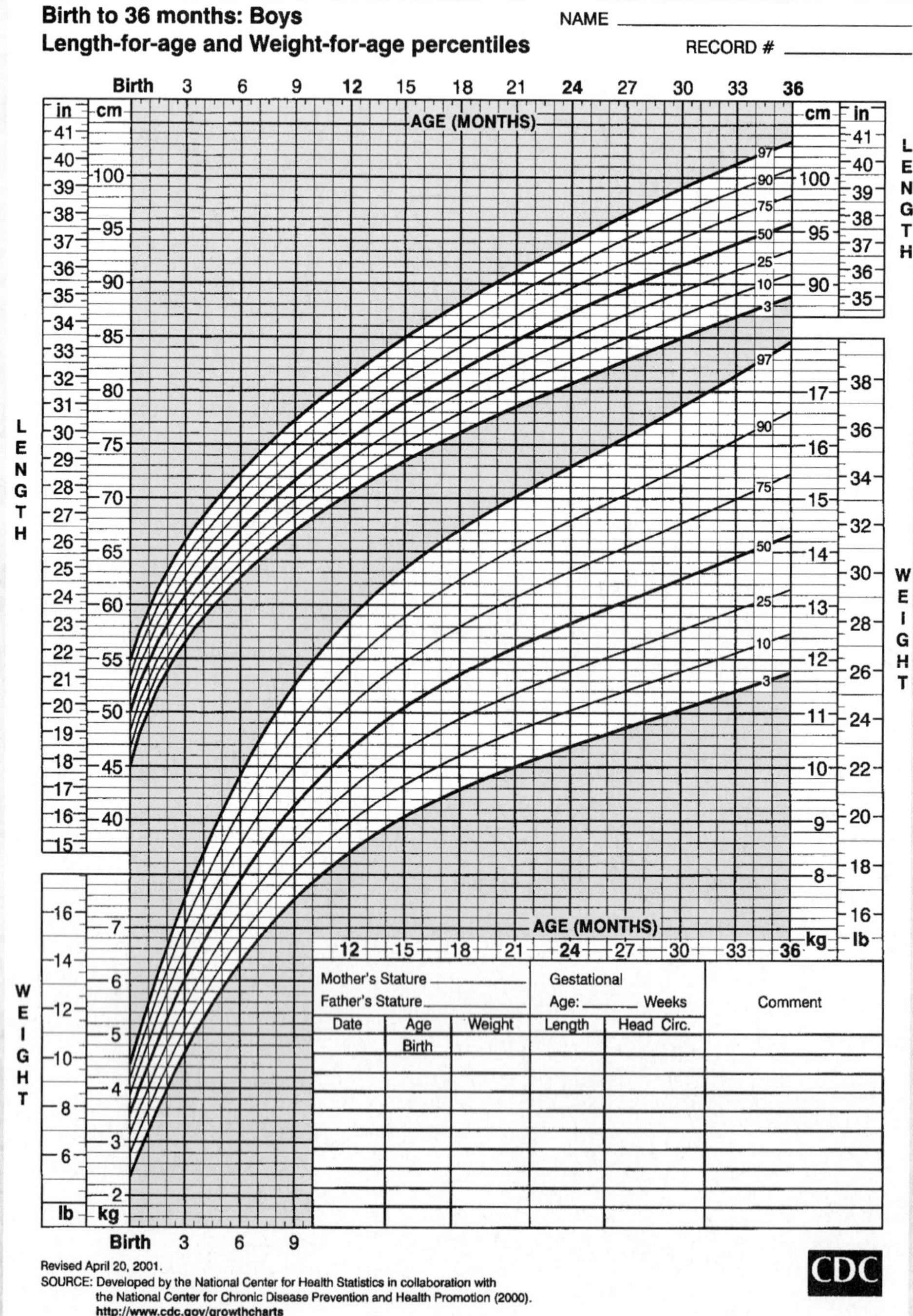

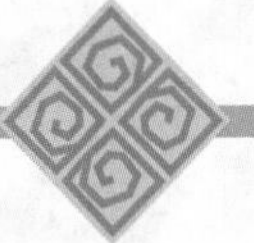
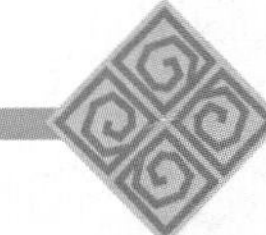

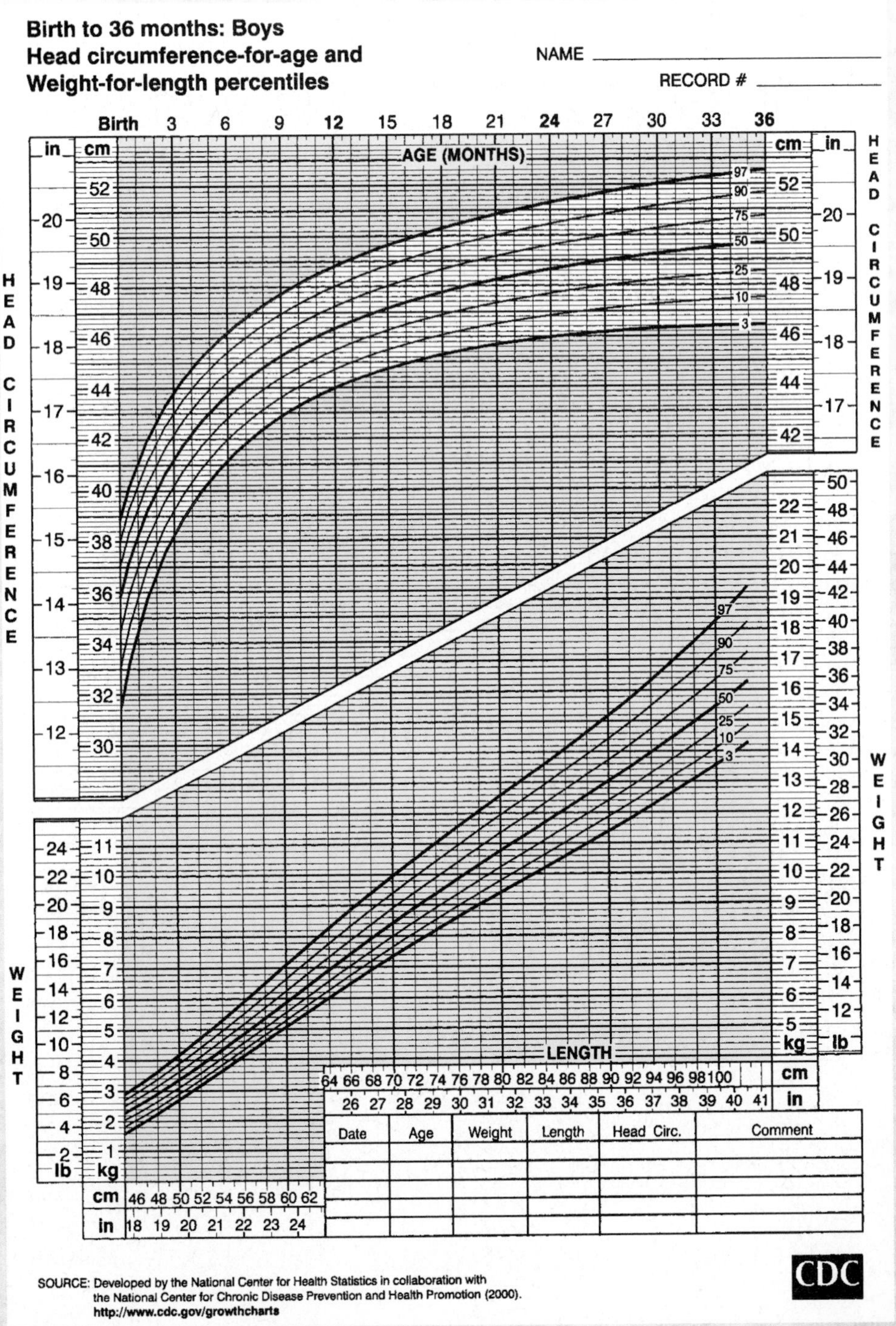

FIGURE A-2 ◆

Physical growth percentiles for head circumference, weight for length—boys: birth to 36 months.
From CDC, 2001. *www.cdc.gov/growthcharts*

Birth to 36 months: Boys
Head circumference-for-age and
Weight-for-length percentiles

NAME ______________________

RECORD # __________________

Birth 3 6 9 12 15 18 21 24 27 30 33 36

AGE (MONTHS)

HEAD CIRCUMFERENCE

WEIGHT

LENGTH

Date	Age	Weight	Length	Head Circ.	Comment

SOURCE: Developed by the National Center for Health Statistics in collaboration with the National Center for Chronic Disease Prevention and Health Promotion (2000). http://www.cdc.gov/growthcharts

CDC

FIGURE A-3 ◆

Physical growth percentiles for length and weight—girls: birth to 36 months. From CDC, 2001. *www.cdc.gov/growthcharts*

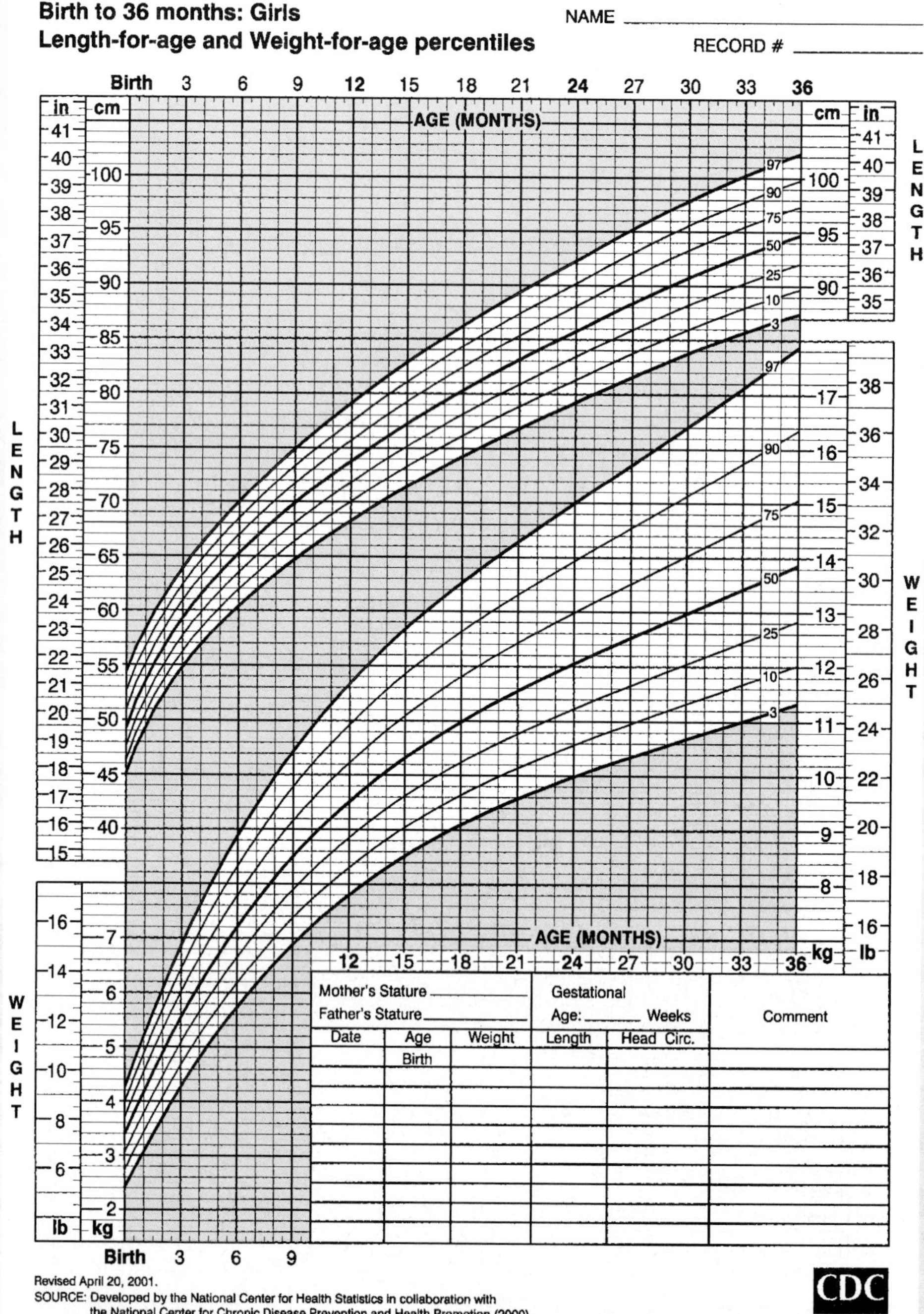

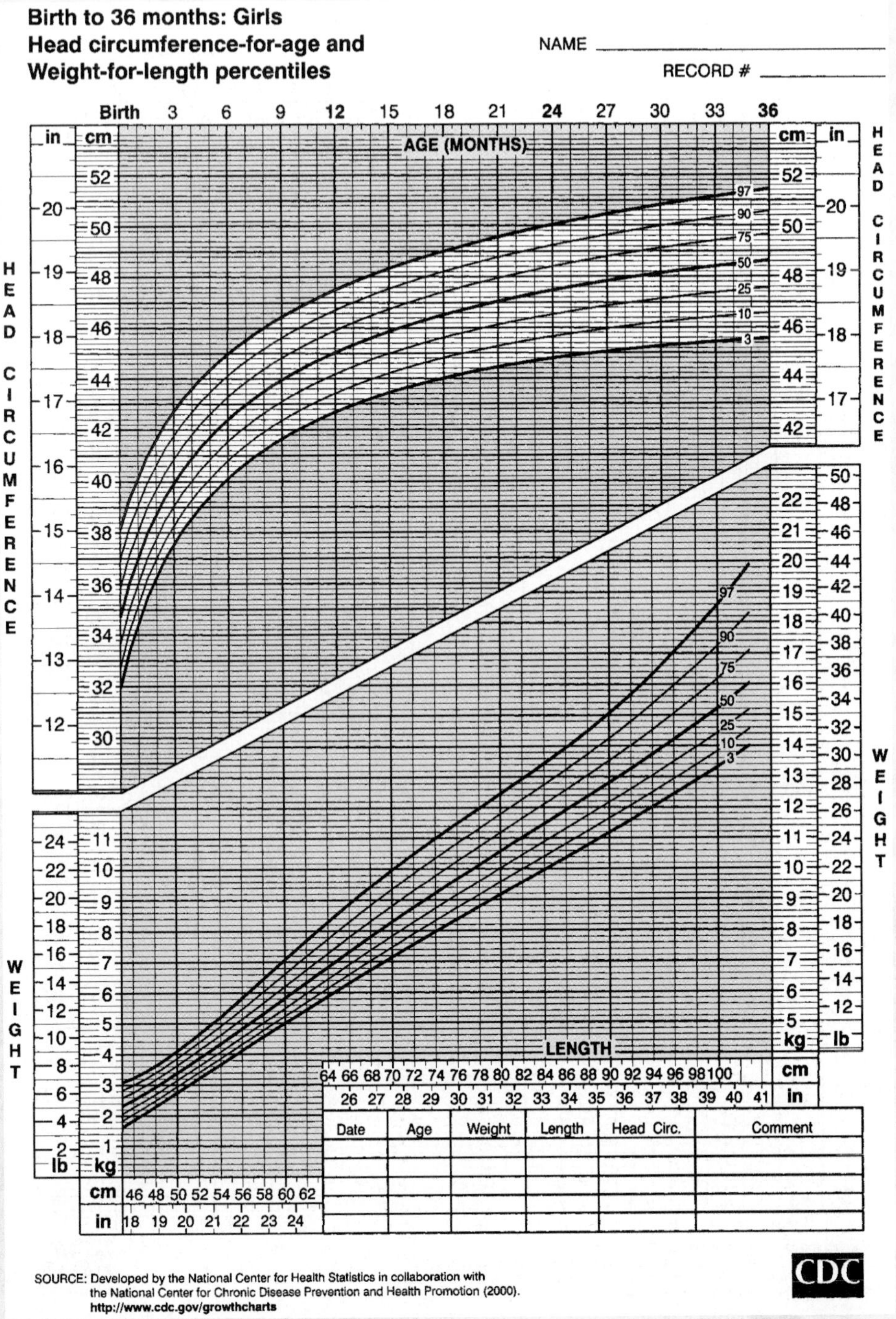

Birth to 36 months: Girls
Head circumference-for-age and
Weight-for-length percentiles

NAME ______________________

RECORD # ____________

Birth 3 6 9 12 15 18 21 24 27 30 33 36

AGE (MONTHS)

HEAD CIRCUMFERENCE

in: 12 13 14 15 16 17 18 19 20

cm: 30 32 34 36 38 40 42 44 46 48 50 52

Percentiles: 97 90 75 50 25 10 3

WEIGHT

kg: 1 2 3 4 5 6 7 8 9 10 11 12 13 14 15 16 17 18 19 20 21 22

lb: 2 4 6 8 10 12 14 16 18 20 22 24 26 28 30 32 34 36 38 40 42 44 46 48 50

LENGTH

cm: 46 48 50 52 54 56 58 60 62 64 66 68 70 72 74 76 78 80 82 84 86 88 90 92 94 96 98 100

in: 18 19 20 21 22 23 24 25 26 27 28 29 30 31 32 33 34 35 36 37 38 39 40 41

Date	Age	Weight	Length	Head Circ.	Comment

SOURCE: Developed by the National Center for Health Statistics in collaboration with the National Center for Chronic Disease Prevention and Health Promotion (2000). http://www.cdc.gov/growthcharts

CDC

FIGURE A-4 ◆

Physical growth percentiles for head circumference, weight for length—girls: birth to 36 months.

From CDC, 2001. *www.cdc.gov/growthcharts*

FIGURE A-5 ◆

Physical growth percentiles for stature and weight according to age—boys: 2 to 20 years.

From CDC, 2001. *www.cdc.gov/growthcharts*

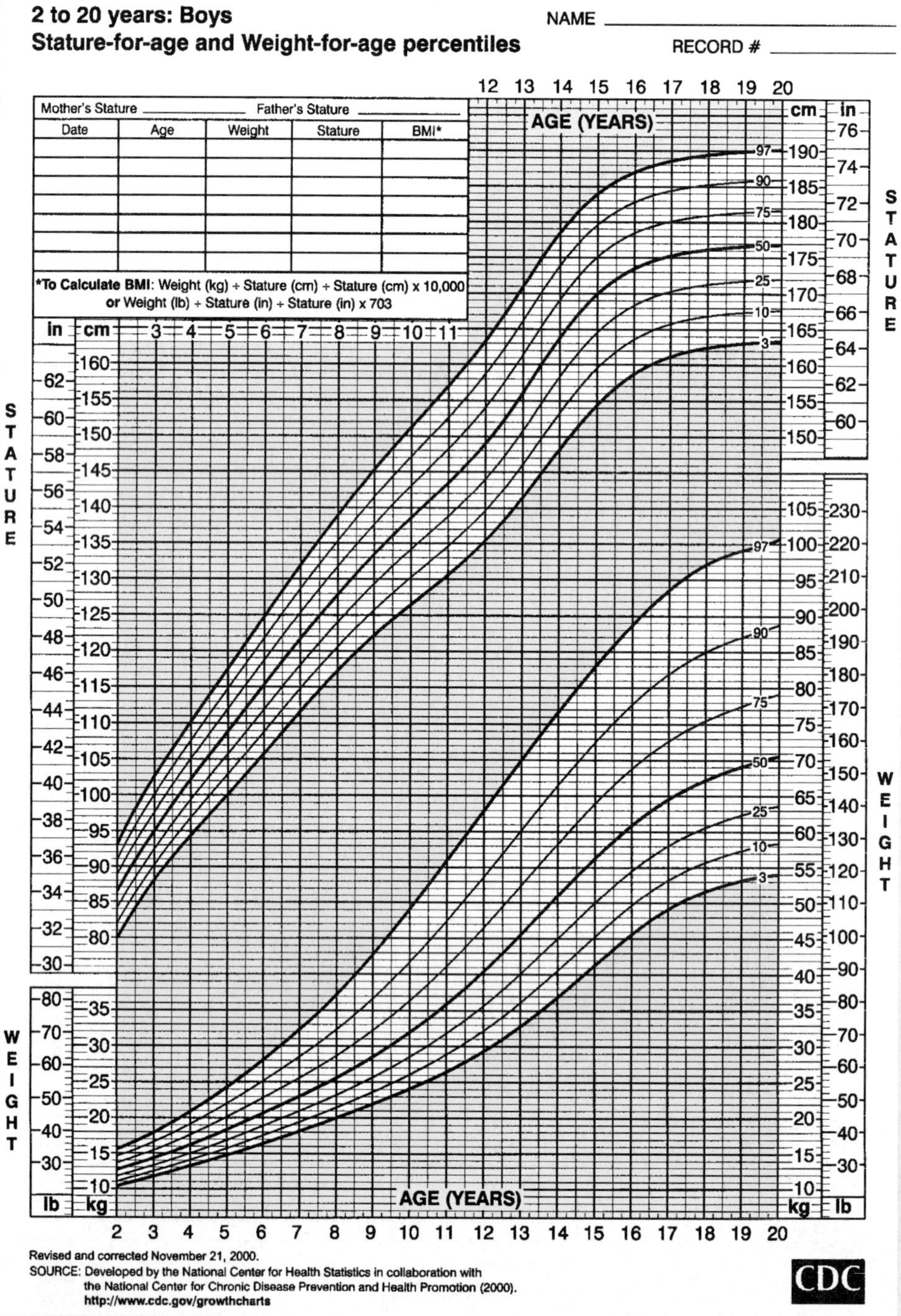

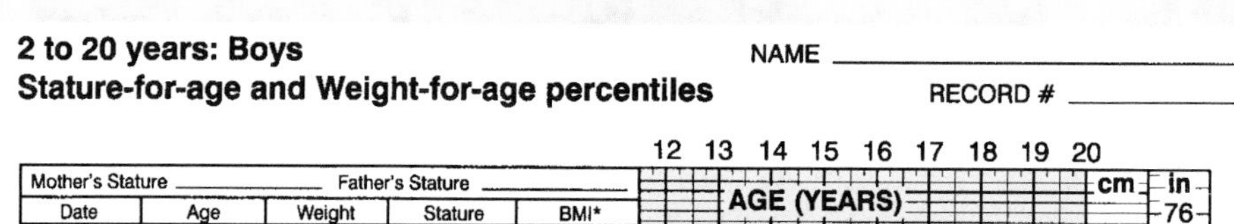

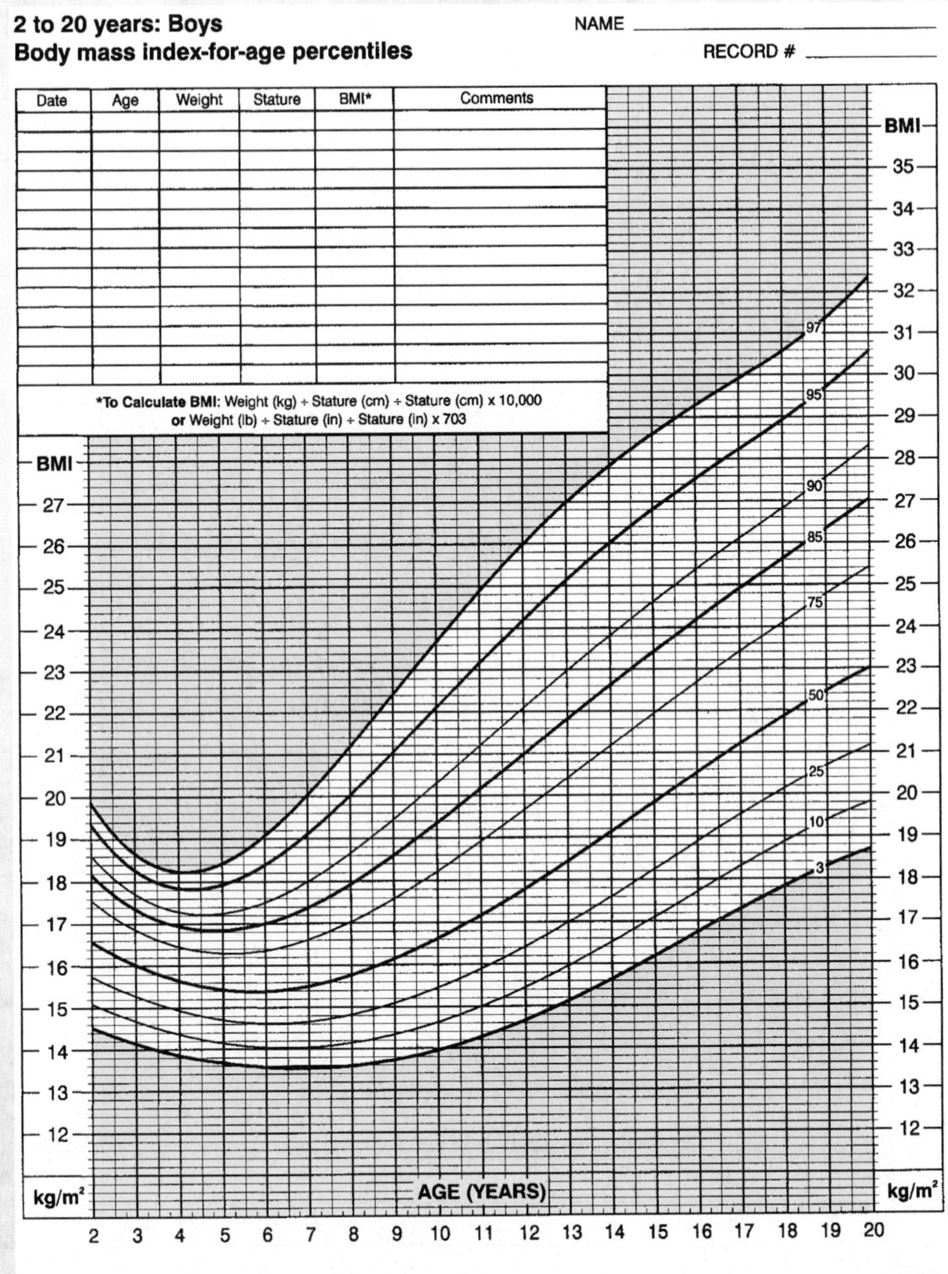

FIGURE A-6 ◆

Physical growth percentiles for body mass index according to age—boys: 2 to 20 years.

From CDC, 2001. *www.cdc.gov/growthcharts*

FIGURE A-7 ◆

Physical growth percentiles for weight for stature—boys: 2 to 20 years.
From CDC, 2001. *www.cdc.gov/growthcharts*

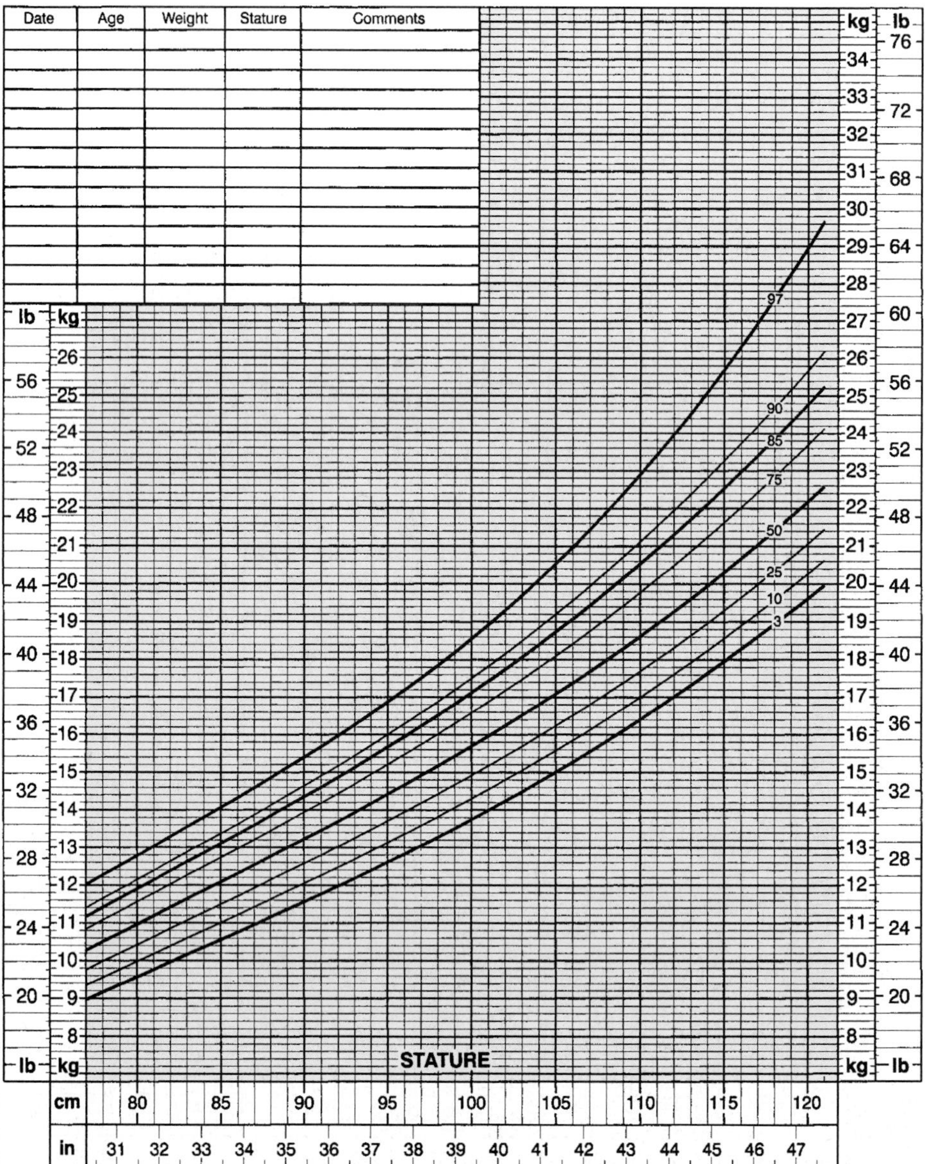

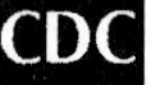

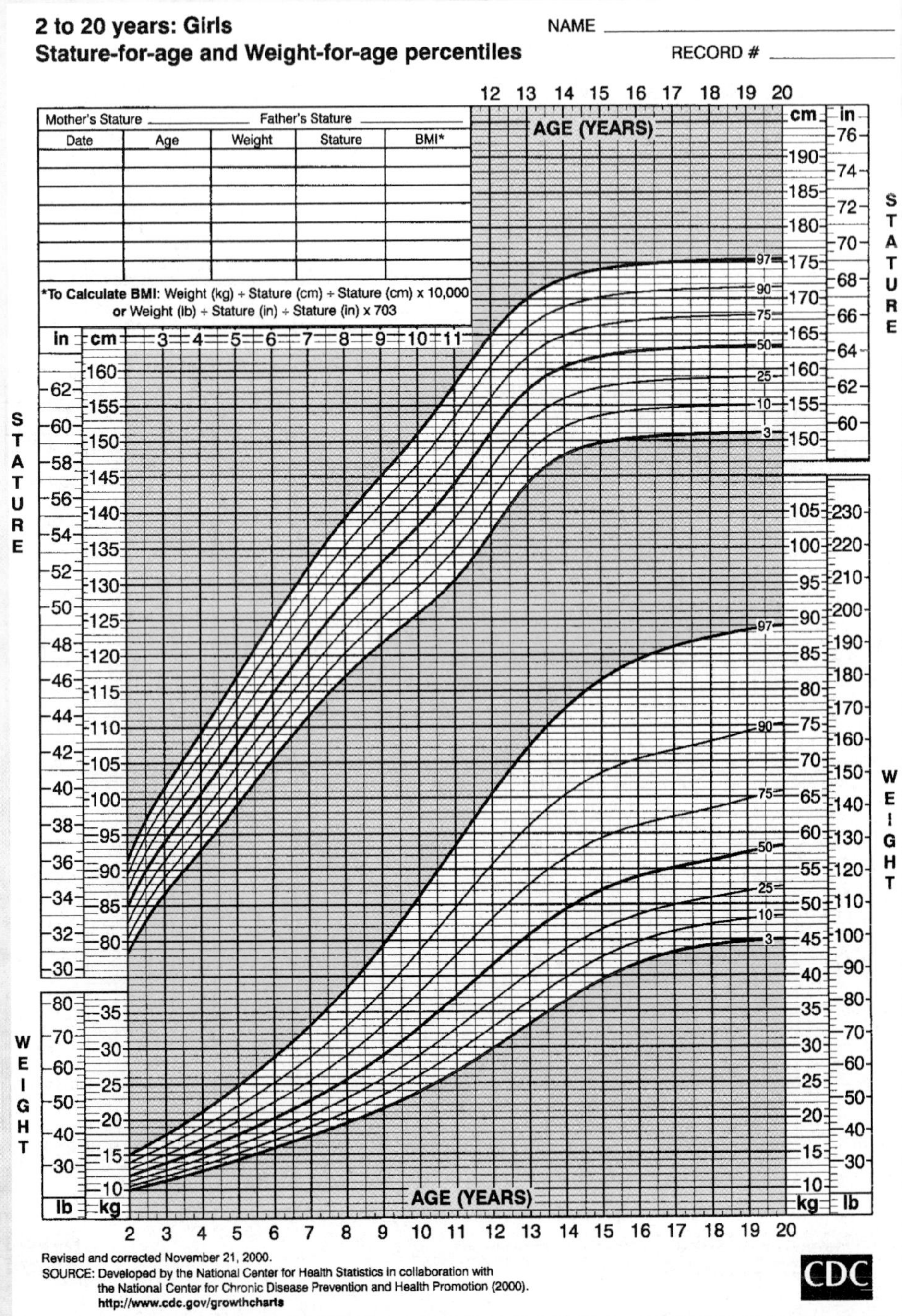

FIGURE A-8 ◆

Physical growth percentiles for stature and weight according to age—girls: 2 to 20 years.

From CDC, 2001. *www.cdc.gov/growthcharts*

FIGURE A-9 ◆
Physical growth percentiles for body mass index according to age—girls: 2 to 20 years.
From CDC, 2001. *www.cdc.gov/growthcharts*

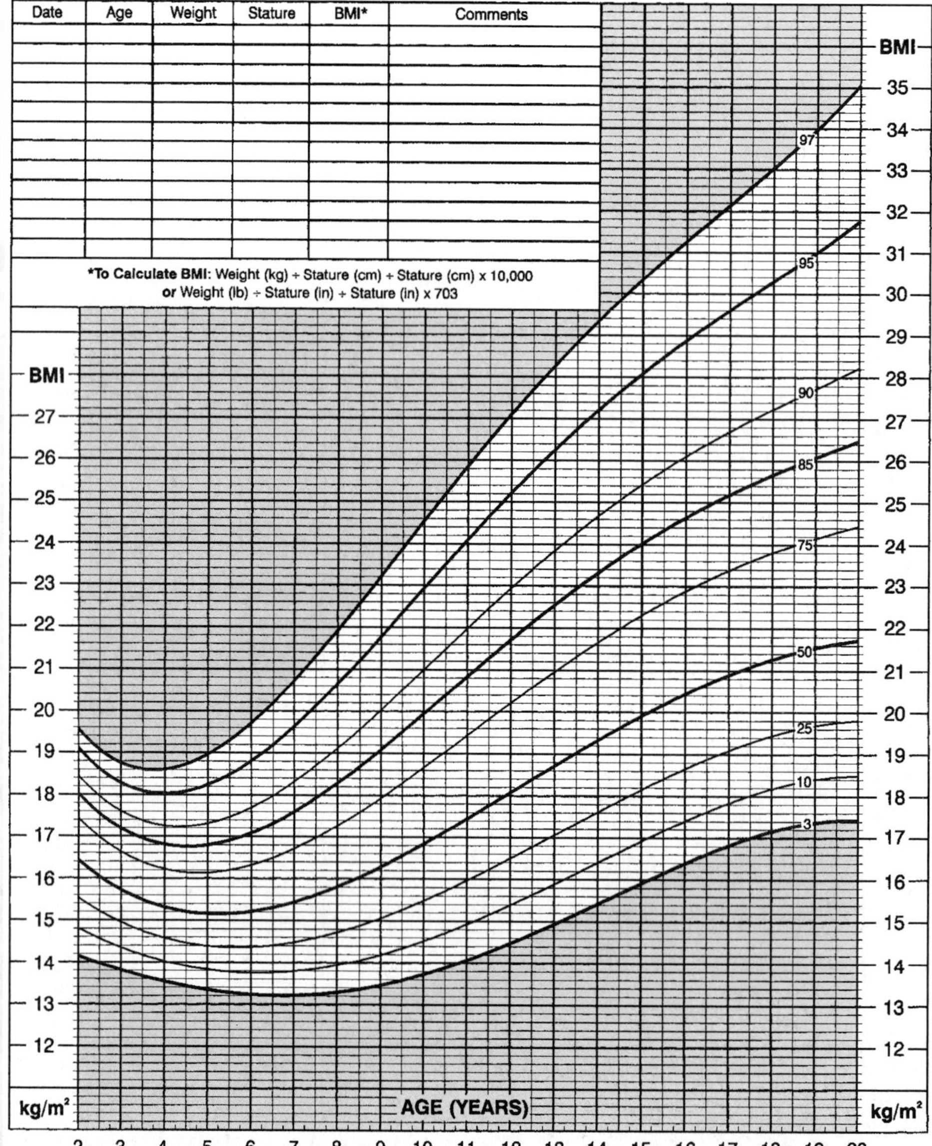

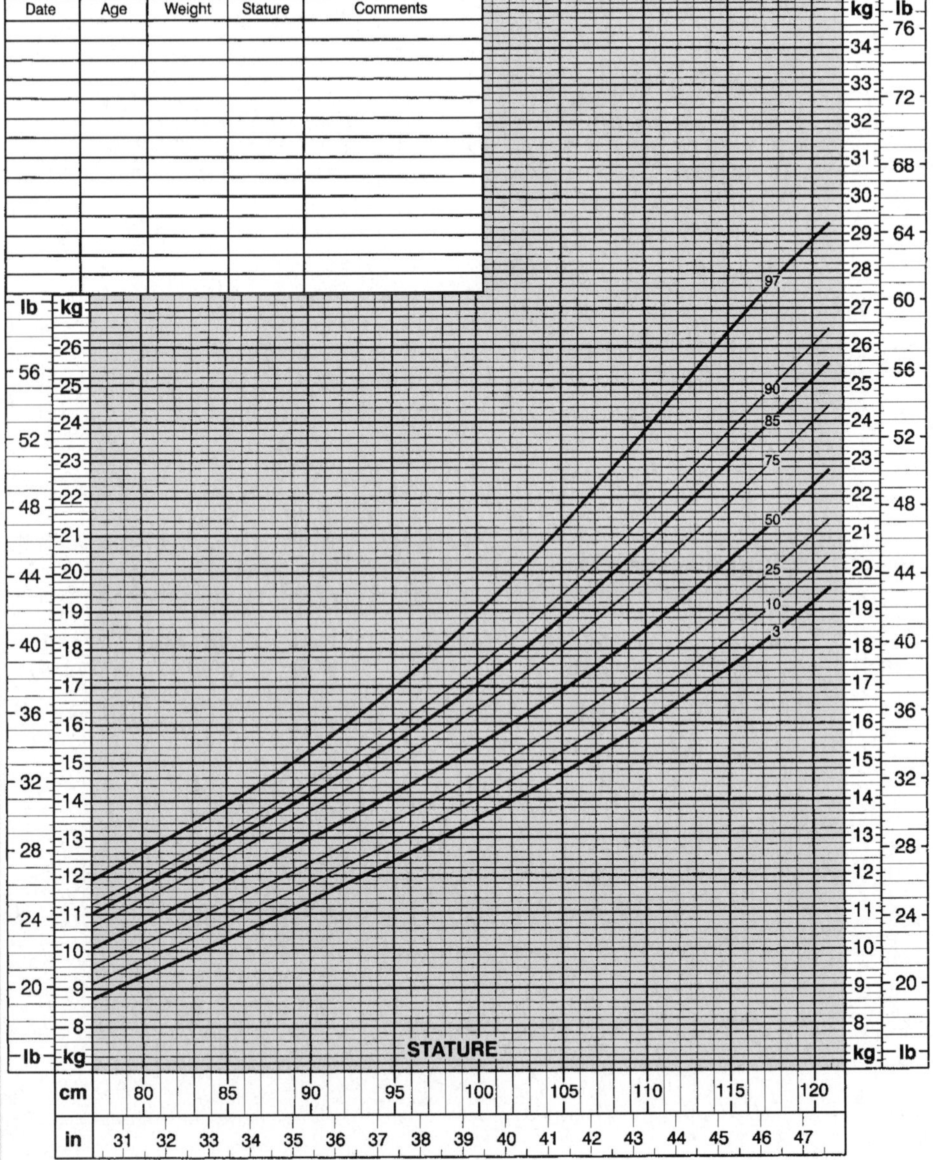

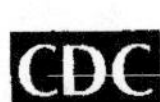

FIGURE A-10 ◆

Physical growth percentiles for weight for stature—girls: 2 to 20 years.

From CDC, 2001. *www.cdc.gov/growthcharts*

APPENDIX B: RECOMMENDED DIETARY ALLOWANCES

APPENDIX B Recommended Dietary Allowances

	AGE	VITAMIN A (μg/d)	VITAMIN D (μg/d)	VITAMIN E (mg/d α-tocopherol)	VITAMIN K (μg/d)	VITAMIN C (mg/d)	THIAMIN (mg/d)	RIBOFLAVIN (mg/d)	NIACIN (mg/d)
Infants	0–6 months	400*	5*	4*	2.0*	40*	0.2*	0.3*	~0.2*
	7–12 months	500*	5*	5*	2.5*	50*	0.3*	0.4*	~0.4*
Children	1–3 years	300	5*	6	30*	15	0.5	0.5	6
	4–8 years	400	5*	7	55*	25	0.6	0.6	8
Males	9–13 years	600	5*	11	60*	45	0.9	0.9	12
	14–18 years	900	5*	15	75*	75	1.2	1.3	16
Females	9–13 years	600	5*	11	60*	45	0.9	0.9	12
	14–18 years	700	5*	15	75*	65	1.0	1.0	14

*Values are Adequate Intakes (AI) rather than Recommended Dietary Allowances (RDAs). All other values on chart are RDAs. See Chapter 3 for a discussion of nutrient requirements.

Note: All data from Institute of Medicine. (1997–2001). *Dietary reference intakes.* Washington DC: National Academy Press. Available also at *http://www.nas.edu/iom*

VITAMIN B_6 (mg/d)	FOLATE (μg/d)	VITAMIN B_{12} (μg/d)	CALCIUM (mg/d)	PHOSPHORUS (mg/d)	MAGNESIUM (mg/d)	IRON (mg/d)	ZINC (mg/d)	IODINE (μg/d)	SELENIUM (μg/d)
0.1*	65*	0.4*	210*	100*	30*	0.27*	2.0*	110*	15*
0.3*	80*	0.5*	270*	275*	75*	11	3	130*	20*
0.5	150	0.9	500*	460	80	7	3	90	20
0.6	200	1.2	800*	500	130	10	5	90	30
1.0	300	1.8	1300*	1250	240	8	8	120	40
1.3	400	2.4	1300*	1250	240	11	11	150	55
1.0	300	1.8	1300*	1250	410	8	8	120	40
1.2	400	2.4	1300*	1250	360	15	9	150	55

APPENDIX C: NORMAL LABORATORY VALUES

All laboratory values listed are approximate. Consult your local laboratory for guidelines as to normal values for the specific testing procedures used.

NORMAL VALUES: BLOOD

ALBUMIN (S)[1]

Newborn: 2.6–3.6 g/dL
1–3 years: 3.4–4.2 g/dL
4–6 years: 3.5–5.2 g/dL
7–9 years: 3.7–5.6 g/dL
10–19 years: 3.7–5.6 g/dL

ALDOLASE (S)[1]

10–24 months: 3.4–11.8 U/L
2–7 years: 1.2–8.8 U/L
Adults: 1.7–4.9 U/L

ALDOSTERONE (S)[1]

6–9 years: 1–24 ng/dL
10–11 years: 2–15 ng/dL
12–14 years: 1–22 ng/dL
15–17 years: 1–32 ng/dL

ALKALINE PHOSPHATASE (S)[2]

Values in IU/L at 37°C (98.6°F) using *p*-nitrophenol phosphate buffered with AMP (kinetic).

AGE	MALES	FEMALES
Newborns (1–3 days)	95–368	95–368
2–24 months	115–460	115–460
2–5 years	115–391	115–391
6–7 years	115–460	115–460
8–9 years	115–345	115–345
10–11 years	115–336	115–437
12–13 years	127–403	92–336
14–15 years	79–446	78–212
16–18 years	58–331	35–124
Adults	41–137	39–118

α_1 ANTITRYPSIN (S)[1]

Newborn: 143–440 mg/dL
1–3 years: 147–244 mg/dL
4–9 years: 160–245 mg/dL
10–13 years: 166–267 mg/dL
14–19 years: 152–317 mg/dL

AMMONIA (P)[1]

Newborns: <50 mmol/L
Thereafter: 0–35 mmol/L

BASE EXCESS (B)[1]

Newborn: −10 to −2 mmol/L
Infant: −7 to −1 mmol/L
Child: −4 to +2 mmol/L
Thereafter: −3 to +3 mmol/L

Note: Modified from:
[1]Soldin, S.J., Brugnara, C., & Hicks, J.M. (1999). *Pediatric reference ranges* (3rd ed.). Washington, DC: AACC Press.
[2]Hay, W.W., Hayward, A.R., Levin, M.J., Sondheimer, J.M. (2000). *Current pediatric diagnosis and treatment* (15th ed.). New York: Lange Medical Books/McGraw Hill.
[3]Barone, M.A. (1999). Laboratory values. In J.A. McMillan, C.D. DeAngelis, R.D. Feigin, & J.B. Warshaw. *Oski's pediatrics: Principles and practice* (3rd ed., pp. 2216–2225). Philadelphia: Lippincott Williams & Wilkins.
S, serum; **B,** whole blood; **P,** plasma; **RBC,** red blood cells

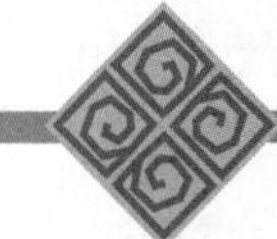

BICARBONATE, ACTUAL (P)

Calculated from pH and Pa_{CO_2}
Newborns: 17.2–23.6 mmol/L
2 months–2 years: 19–24 mmol/L
Children: 18–25 mmol/L
Adult males: 20.1–28.9 mmol/L
Adult females: 18.4–28.8 mmol/L

BILIRUBIN, CONJUGATED (S)[1]

Neonates: <10 μmol/L
Neonate: <2 μmol/L
Preterm (1–6 days): <10 μmol/L

BLEEDING TIME (SIMPLATE)[2]

2–9 min.

BLOOD VOLUME[2]

Premature infants: 98 mL/kg
At 1 year: 86 mL/kg (range, 69–112 mL/kg)
Older children: 70 mL/kg (range, 51–86 mL/kg)

CALCIUM (S)

Premature infants (first week): 3.5–4.5 mEq/L (1.7–2.3 mmol/L)
Full-term infants (first week): 4.0–5.0 mEq/L (2.0–2.5 mmol/L)
Thereafter: 4.4–5.3 mEq/L (2.2–2.7 mmol/L)

CARBON DIOXIDE, PARTIAL PRESSURE (P_{CO_2}) (B)[1]

Newborn: 27–40 mmHg (3.6–5.5 kPa)
Infant: 27–41 mmHg (3.6–5.5 kPa)
Children: 32–48 mmHg (4.3–6.4 kPa)

CARBON DIOXIDE, TOTAL (P)[1]

Cord blood: 13–29 mmol/L
<1 year: 17–31 mmol/L
Adults: 24–30 mmol/L

CHLORIDE (S, P)

<1 year: 96–110 mmol/L
1–17 years: 102–112 mmol/L
Adults: 100–108 mmol/L

CHOLESTEROL, HIGH-DENSITY LIPOPROTEIN (S)[1]

1–9 years: 35–82 mg/dL (0.91–2.12 mmol/L)
10–13 years: 36–84 mg/dL (0.93–2.17 mmol/L)
14–19 years: 35–65 mg/dL (0.91–1.68 mmol/L)

CHOLESTEROL, LOW-DENSITY LIPOPROTEIN (S)[1]

5–9 years: 63–140 mg/dL (1.63–3.63 mmol/L)
10–14 years: 64–136 mg/dL (1.66–3.52 mmol/L)
15–19 years: 59–137 mg/dL (1.53–3.55 mmol/L)

CHOLESTEROL, TOTAL (S, P)[2]

1–3 years: 44–181 mg/dL (1.15–4.70 mmol/L)
4–6 years: 108–187 mg/dL (2.80–4.80 mmol/L)
7–9 years: 112–247 mg/dL (2.90–6.40 mmol/L)
10–13 years: 125–244 mg/dL (3.25–6.30 mmol/L)
14–19 years: 106–224 mg/dL (2.75–5.80 mmol/L)

COMPLEMENT (S)[2]

C_3: 96–195 mg/dL
C_4: 15–20 mg/dL

CREATINE KINASE (S, P)[2]

Newborns (1–3 days): 40–474 IU/L at 37°C (98.6°F)
Adult males: 30–210 IU/L at 37°C (98°F)
Adult females: 20–128 IU/L at 37°C (98.6°F)

CREATININE (S, P)[2]

Values in mg/dL (μmol/L)

AGE	MALES	FEMALES
1–3 days[a]	0.2–1.0 (17.7–88.4)	0.2–1.0 (17.7–88.4)
1 year	0.2–0.6 (17.7–53.0)	0.2–0.5 (17.7–44.2)
2–3 years	0.2–0.7 (17.7–61.9)	0.3–0.6 (26.5–53.0)
4–7 years	0.2–0.8 (17.7–70.7)	0.2–0.7 (17.7–61.9)
8–10 years	0.3–0.9 (26.5–79.6)	0.3–0.8 (26.5–70.7)
11–12 years	0.3–1.0 (26.5–88.4)	0.3–0.9 (26.5–79.6)
13–17 years	0.3–1.2 (26.5–106.1)	0.3–1.1 (26.5–97.2)
18–20 years	0.5–1.3 (44.2–115.0)	0.3–1.1 (26.5–97.2)

[a]Values may be higher in premature newborns.

CREATININE CLEARANCE[2]

Values show great variability and depend on specificity of analytical methods used.

Newborns (1 day): 5–50 mL/min/1.73 m^2 (mean, 18 mL/min/1.73 m^2)

Newborns (6 days): 15–90 mL/min/1.73 m^2 (mean, 36 mL/min/1.73 m^2)

Adult males: 85–125 mL/min/1.73 m^2

Adult females: 75–115 mL/min/1.73 m^2

C-REACTIVE PROTEIN (S)[1]

Cord blood: 10–350 μg/L

Adult: 68–8,200 μg/L

FASTING INSULIN LEVEL

1.8–24.6 mU/L[3]

FIBRINOGEN (P)[2]

200–500 mg/dL (5.9–14.7 μmol/L)

GALACTOSE (S, P)[2]

1.1–2.1 mg/dL (0.06–0.12 mmol/L)

GALACTOSE-1-PHOSPHATE (RBC)

Normal: 1 mg/dL of packed erythrocyte lysate; slightly higher in cord blood.

Infants with congenital galactosemia on a milk-free diet: <2 mg/dL.

Infants with congenital galactosemia taking milk: 9–20 mg/dL.

GALACTOSE-1-PHOSPHATE URIDYL TRANSFERASE (RBC)[2]

Normal: 308–475 mIU/g of hemoglobin.

Heterozygous for Duarte variant: 225–308 mIU/g of hemoglobin.

Homozygous for Duarte variant: 142–225 mIU/g of hemoglobin.

Heterozygous for congenital galactosemia: 142–225 mIU/g of hemoglobin.

Homozygous for congenital galactosemia: <8 mIU/g of hemoglobin.

GLUCOSE (S,P)[2]

Premature infants: 20–80 mg/dL (1.11–4.44 mmol/L)

Full-term infants: 30–100 mg/dL (1.67–5.56 mmol/L)

Children and adults (fasting): 60–105 mg/dL (3.33–5.88 mmol/L)

GLUCOSE 6-PHOSPHATE DEHYDROGENASE (RBC)[2]

150–215 units/dL

GLUCOSE TOLERANCE TEST RESULTS IN SERUM[a2]

	GLUCOSE		INSULIN	
TIME	mg/dL	mmol/L	μU/mL	pmol/L
Fasting	59–96	3.11–5.33	5–40	36–287
30 min	91–185	5.05–10.27	36–110	258–789
60 min	66–164	3.66–9.10	22–124	158–890
90 min	68–148	3.77–8.22	17–105	122–753
2 hr	66–122	3.66–6.77	6–84	43–603
3 hr	47–99	2.61–5.49	2–46	14–330
4 hr	61–93	3.39–5.16	3–32	21–230
5 hr	63–86	3.50–4.77	5–37	36–265

[a]Normal levels based on results in 13 normal children given glucose, 1.75 g/kg orally in one dose, after 2 weeks on a high-carbohydrate diet.

GLYCOSYLATED HEMOGLOBIN (HEMOGLOBIN A_1)(B)[1]

Normal: 4–7% of total hemoglobin

Diabetic patients in good control of their condition: 8–10%

Diabetic patients in poor control: 8–18%

Pregnant Women: 5%–8%

Values tend to vary with testing technique.

Note: These values reflect total Hemoglobin A_1 levels. When Hemoglobin A_{1c} is computed, values are usually 2–4% lower.

GROWTH HORMONE (S)[2]

After infancy (fasting specimen): 0–5 ng/mL
In response to natural and artificial provocation (e.g., sleep, arginine, insulin, hypoglycemia): >8 ng/mL
During the newborn period (fasting specimen): GH levels are high (15–40 ng/mL) and responses to provocation variable

HEMATOCRIT (B)[1]

AGE	MALES (%)	FEMALES (%)
Newborns	43.4–56.1	37.4–55.9
6 months–2 years	30.9–37.0	31.2–37.2
2–6 years	31.7–37.7	32.0–37.1
6–12 years	32.7–39.3	33.0–39.6
12–18 years	34.8–43.9	34.0–40.7
>18 years	33.4–46.2	33.0–41.0

HEMOGLOBIN (B)[1]

AGE	MALES (g/dL)	FEMALES (g/dL)
Newborns	14.7–18.6	12.7–18.3
6 months–2 years	10.3–12.4	10.4–12.4
2–6 years	10.5–12.7	10.7–12.7
6–12 years	11.0–13.3	10.9–13.3
12–18 years	11.5–14.8	11.2–13.6
>18 years	10.9–15.7	10.7–13.5

HEMOGLOBIN A_{1C}

See Glycosylated Hemoglobin.

HEMOGLOBIN ELECTROPHORESIS (B)[2]

A_1 hemoglobin: 96%–98.5% of total hemoglobin
A_2 hemoglobin: 1.5%–4% of total hemoglobin

HEMOGLOBIN, FETAL (B)[2]

At birth: 50%–85% of total hemoglobin
At 1 year: <15% of total hemoglobin
Up to 2 years: ≤5% of total hemoglobin
Thereafter: <2% of total hemoglobin

IMMUNOGLOBULINS (S)[1]

AGE	IGG (mg/dL)	IGA (mg/dL)	IGM (mg/dL)
1–30 days	221–1031	1–19	12–117
1–6 months	195–794	1–59	9–212
7–12 months	184–974	9–107	4–216
1–3 years	507–1407	18–171	63–298
4–6 years	571–1550	47–231	64–298
7–9 years	589–1717	41–252	49–270
10–12 years	705–1871	61–269	58–340
13–15 years	709–1907	42–304	57–361
16–18 years	632–2108	89–322	59–360

IMMUNOGLOBULIN D (S)[1]

Newborn: 0 mg/dL
Thereafter: 0–8 mg/dL

IMMUNOGLOBULIN E (S,P)[1]

0–12 months	<1 KIU/L
1–3 years	<90 KIU/L
4–10 years	<193 KIU/L
11–18 years	<398 KIU/L

IRON (S, P)[2]

Newborns: 20–157 μg/dL (3.6–28.1 μmol/L)
6 weeks–3 years: 20–115 μg/dL (3.6–20.6 μmol/L)
3–9 years: 20–141 μg/dL (3.6–25.2 μmol/L)
9–14 years: 21–151 μg/dL (3.8–27 μmol/L)
14–16 years: 20–181 μg/dL (3.6–32.4 μmol/L)
Adults: 44–196 μg/dL (7.2–31.3 μmol/L)

IRON-BINDING CAPACITY (S, P)[2]

Newborns: 59–175 μg/dL (10.6–31.3 μmol/L)
Children and adults: 275–458 μg/dL (45–72 μmol/L)

LACTATE DEHYDROGENASE (LDH)(S, P)[2]

Values using lactate substrate (kinetic).
1–3 days: 40–348 IU/L at 37°C (98.6°F)
1 month–5 years: 150–360 IU/L at 37°C (98.6°F)
5–8 years: 150–300 IU/L at 37°C (98.6°F)
8–12 years: 130–300 IU/L at 37°C (98.6°F)
12–14 years: 130–280 IU/L at 37°C (98.6°F)
14–16 years: 130–230 IU/L at 37°C (98.6°F)
Adult males: 70–178 IU/L at 37°C (98.6°F)
Adult females: 42–166 IU/L at 37°C (98.6°F)

LEAD (B)[1]

0–15 years <10 μg/dL (<0.48 μmol/L)

MAGNESIUM (P)[1]

Values in mg/dL (mmol/L)

AGE	MALES	FEMALES
1–30 days	1.7–2.4 (0.70–0.99)	1.7–2.5 (0.70–1.03)
31–365 days	1.6–2.5 (0.66–1.03)	1.9–2.4 (0.78–0.99)
1–3 years	1.7–2.4 (0.70–0.99)	1.7–2.4 (0.70–0.99)
4–9 years	1.7–2.4 (0.70–0.99)	1.6–2.3 (0.66–0.95)
10–15 years	1.6–2.2 (0.66–0.91)	1.6–2.2 (0.66–0.91)
16–18 years	1.5–2.2 (0.62–0.91)	1.5–2.2 (0.62–0.91)

OSMOLALITY (S)[1]

Birth–1 month: 275–305 mOsm/kg
Adults: 282–300 mOsm/kg

OXYGEN, PARTIAL PRESSURE (PO_2) (B)[1]

Birth:	8–24 mmHg	1.1–3.2 kPa
>1 hour:	55–80 mmHg	7.3–10.6 kPa
>1 day:	83–108 mmHg	11.0–14.4 kPa

OXYGEN SATURATION (B)[1]

Newborns: 85%–90%
Thereafter: 95%–99%

PARTIAL THROMBOPLASTIN TIME (P)[2]

Children: 42–54 sec

PH (B)[1]

0–6 months	7.18–7.50
6–12 months	7.27–7.49

PHENYLALANINE (S, P)[2]

0.7–3.5 mg/dL (0.04–0.21 mmol/L)

PHOSPHORUS, INORGANIC (S, P)[2]

Newborns: 5.0–7.8 mg/dL (1.61–2.52 mmol/L)
1 year: 3.8–6.2 mg/dL (1.23–2.0 mmol/L)
10 years: 3.6–5.6 mg/dL (1.16–1.81 mmol/L)
Adults: 3.1–5.1 mg/dL (1.0–1.65 mmol/L)

PLATELET COUNT (RBC)[1]

Value × 10^3/μL. (μL = mm^3)

AGE	MALES	FEMALES
Newborns	164–351	234–346
1–2 months	275–567	295–615
2–6 months	275–566	288–598
6 months–2 years	219–452	229–465
2–6 years	204–405	204–402
6–12 years	194–364	183–369
12–18 years	165–332	185–335
>18 years	143–320	171–326

POTASSIUM (S, P)[2]

Premature infants: 4.5–7.2 mmol/L
Full-term infants: 3.7–5.2 mmol/L
Children: 3.5–5.8 mmol/L
Adults: 3.5–5.5 mmol/L

PROTEINS IN SERUM[A2]

AGE	TOTAL PROTEIN	α_1-GLOBULIN	α_2-GLOBULIN
At birth	4.6–7.0	0.1–0.3	0.2–0.3
3 months	4.5–6.5	0.1–0.3	0.3–0.7
1 year	5.4–7.5	0.1–0.3	0.5–1.1
>4 years	5.9–8.0	0.1–0.3	0.4–0.8

AGE	β-GLOBULIN	λ-GLOBULIN
At birth	0.3–0.6	0.6–1.2
3 months	0.3–0.7	0.2–0.7
1 year	0.4–1.0	0.2–0.9
>4 years	0.5–1.0	0.4–1.3

[a]Values are for cellulose acetate electrophoresis and are in g/dL. SI conversion factor: g/dL × 10 = g/L.

PROTHROMBIN TIME (P)[2]

Children: 11–15 sec

PROTOPORPHYRIN, "FREE" (FEP, ZPP)(B)[2]

Values for free erythrocyte protoporphyrin (FEP) and zinc protoporphyrin (ZPP) are 1.2–2.7 μg/g of hemoglobin.

RED BLOOD CELL COUNT (B)[1]

Values × $10^6/\mu L$. ($\mu L = mm^3$)

AGE	MALES	FEMALES
Newborns–6 months	4.2–5.5	3.4–5.4
6 months–2 years	4.1–5.0	4.1–4.9
2–12 years	4.0–4.9	4.0–4.9
12–18 years	4.2–5.3	4.0–4.9
>18 years	3.8–5.4	3.8–4.8

SEDIMENTATION RATE (MICRO) (B)[2]

<2 years: 1–5 mm/hr
>2 years: 1–8 mm/hr

SODIUM (P)[1]

Newborns: 133–146 mmol/L
Children and adults: 135–148 mmol/L

THROMBIN TIME (P)[2]

Children: 12–16 sec

THYROID-STIMULATING HORMONE (TSH) (P, S)[1]

Values in mU/mL.

AGE	MALES	FEMALES
1–30 days	0.52–16.00	0.72–13.10
1 month–5 years	0.55–7.10	0.46–8.10
6–18 years	0.37–6.00	0.36–5.80

THYROXINE (T4) (S, P)[1]

Values in μg/dL (nmol/L).

AGE	MALES	FEMALES
1–30 days	5.9–21.5 (76–276)	6.3–21.5 (81–276)
1–12 months	6.4–13.9 (82–179)	4.9–13.7 (63–176)
1–3 years	7.0–13.1 (90–169)	7.1–14.1 (91–180)
4–6 years	6.1–12.6 (79–162)	7.2–14.0 (93–180)
7–12 years	6.7–13.4 (86–172)	6.1–12.1 (79–156)
13–15 years	4.8–11.5 (62–148)	5.8–11.2 (75–144)
16–18 years	5.9–11.5 (76–148)	5.2–13.2 (67–170)

THROXINE, "FREE" (FREE T4)(S, P)[1]

Newborns: 0.80–2.78 ng/dL (10–36 pmol/L)
1–12 months: 0.76–2.00 ng/dL (10–26 pmol/L)
1–5 years: 0.90–1.72 ng/dL (12–22 pmol/L)
6–10 years: 0.81–1.68 ng/dL (10–22 pmol/L)
11–15 years: 0.79–1.57 ng/dL (10–20 pmol/L)
16–18 years: 0.83–1.53 ng/dL (11–20 pmol/L)

THROXINE-BINDING GLOBULIN (TBG) (P)[1]

1–12 months: 16.2–32.9 mg/L
1–3 years: 16.4–33.8 mg/L
4–6 years: 16.6–30.8 mg/L
7–12 years: 15.0–29.2 mg/L
13–18 years: 13.4–28.7 mg/L

TRIGLYCERIDES (S)[1]

Values in mg/dL (mmol/L)

AGE	MALES	FEMALES
1–3 years	27–125 (0.31–1.41)	27–125 (0.31–1.41)
4–6 years	32–116 (0.36–1.31)	32–116 (0.36–1.31)
7–9 years	28–129 (0.32–1.46)	28–129 (0.32–1.46)
10–11 years	24–137 (0.27–1.55)	39–140 (0.44–1.58)
12–13 years	24–145 (0.27–1.64)	37–130 (0.42–1.47)
14–15 years	34–165 (0.38–1.86)	38–135 (0.43–1.52)
16–19 years	34–140 (0.38–1.58)	37–140 (0.42–1.58)

TRIIODOTHYRONINE (T3) (S, P)[1]

1–30 days	15–210 ng/dL
1–12 months	50–275 ng/dL
1–5 years	80–258 ng/dL
6–10 years	96–232 ng/dL
11–15 years	73–211 ng/dL
16–18 years	69–201 ng/dL

UREA CLEARANCE[2]

Premature infants: 3.5–17.3 mL/min/1.73 m^2
Newborns: 8.7–33 mL/min/1.73 m^2
2–12 months: 40–95 mL/min/1.73 m^2
=2 years: >52 mL/min/1.73 m^2

UREA NITROGEN (P)[1]

1–3 years	5–17 mg/dL (1.8–6.0 mmol/L)
4–13 years	7–17 mg/dL (2.5–6.0 mmol/L)
14–19 years	8–21 mg/dL (2.9–7.5 mmol/L)

URIC ACID (S, P)[2]

Males:

0–14 years: 2–7 mg/dL (119–416 μmol/L)
>14 years: 3–8 mg/dL (178–476 μmol/L)

Females:

All ages: 2–7 mg/dL (119–416 μmol/L)

WHITE BLOOD CELL COUNT (B)[1]

Values × $10^3/\mu L$. ($\mu L = mm^3$)

AGE	MALES	FEMALES
Newborns	6.8–13.3	8.0–14.3
6 months–2 years	6.2–14.5	6.4–15.0
2–6 years	5.3–11.5	5.3–11.5
6–12 years	4.5–10.5	4.7–10.3
12–18 years	4.5–10.0	4.8–10.1
>18 years	4.4–10.2	4.9–10.0

NORMAL VALUES: URINE

ADDIS COUNT[2]

Red cells (12-hr specimen): <1 million
White cells (12-hr specimen): <2 million
Casts (12-hr specimen): <10,000
Protein (12-hr specimen): <55 mg

ALBUMIN[2]

First month: 1–100 mg/L
Second month: 0.2–34 mg/L
2–12 months: 0.5–19 mg/L

AMMONIA[2]

2–12 months: 4–20 mEq/min/m^2
1–16 years: 6–16 mEq/min/m^2

CALCIUM[2]

4–12 years: 4–8 mEq/L (2–4 mmol/L)

CATECHOLAMINES (NOREPINEPHRINE, EPINEPHRINE)[2]

Values in µg/24 hr (nmol/24 hr).

AGE	TOTAL CATE-CHOLAMINES	NOREPI-NEPHRINE	EPINEPHRINE
<1 year	20	5.4–15.9 (32–94)	0.1–4.3 (0.5–23.5)
1–5 years	40	8.1–30.8 (48–182)	0.8–9.1 (4.4–49.7)
6–15 years	80	19.0–71.1 (112–421)	1.3–10.5 (7.1–57.3)
>15 years	100	34.4–87.0 (203–514)	3.5–13.2 (19.1–72.1)

CHLORIDE[2]

Infants: 1.7–8.5 mmol/24 hr
Children: 17–34 mmol/24 hr
Adults: 140–240 mmol/24 hr

CORTICOSTEROIDS (17-HYDROXYCORTICOSTEROIDS)[1]

0–2 years: 2–4 mg/24 hr (5.5–11 mmol)
2–6 years: 3–6 mg/24 hr (8.3–16.6 mmol)
6–10 years: 6–8 mg/24 hr (16.6–22.1 mmol)
10–14 years: 8–10 mg/24 hr (22.1–27.6 mmol)

CREATINE[2]

18–58 mg/L (1.37–4.42 mmol/L)

CREATININE[2]

Newborns: 7–10 mg/kg/24 hr
Children: 20–30 mg/kg/24 hr
Adult males: 21–26 mg/kg/24 hr
Adult females: 16–22 mg/kg/24 hr

GROWTH HORMONE[1]

2.2–13.3 years (Tanner 1):
0.4–6.3 ng/24 hr (0.9–12.3 ng/g creatinine)
10.3–14.6 years (Tanner 2):
0.8–12.0 ng/24 hr (1.0–14.1 ng/g creatinine)
11.5–15.3 years (Tanner 3):
1.7–20.4 ng/24 hr (1.9–17.0 ng/g creatinine)
12.7–17.1 years (Tanner 4):
1.5–18.2 ng/24 hr (1.3–14.4 ng/g creatinine)
13.5–19.9 years (Tanner 5):
1.2–14.5 ng/24 hr (0.8–11.0 ng/g creatinine)

HOMOVANILLIC ACID[2]

Children: 3–16 µg/mg of creatinine
Adults: 2–4 µg/mg of creatinine

MUCOPOLYSACCHARIDES[2]

Acid mucopolysaccharide screen should yield negative results. Positive results after dialysis of the urine should be followed up with a thin-layer chromatogram for evaluation of the acid mucopolysaccharide excretion pattern.

OSMOLALITY[2]

Infants: 50–600 mosm/L
Older children: 50–1400 mosm/L

PHOSPHORUS, TUBULAR REABSORPTION

78%–97%.

PORPHYRINS[2]

δ-Aminolevulinic acid: 0–7 mg/24 hr (0–53.4 μmol/24 hr)
Porphobilinogen: 0–2 mg/24 hr (0–8.8 μmol/24 hr)
Coproporphyrin: 0–160 mg/24 hr (0–244 μmol/24 hr)
Uroporphyrin: 0–26 mg/24 hr (0–31 μmol/24 hr)

POTASSIUM[2]

26–123 mmol/L

SODIUM[2]

Infants: 0.3–3.5 mmol/24 hr (6–10 mmol/m^2)
Children and adults: 5.6–17 mmol/24 hr

SPECIFIC GRAVITY

1.010–1.030

UROBILINOGEN[2]

<3 mg/24 hr (<5.1 μmol/24 hr)

VANILLYMANDELIC ACID (VMA)[2]

Because of the difficulty in obtaining an accurately timed 24-hour collection, values based on microgram per milligram of creatinine are the most reliable indications of VMA excretion in young children.
1–12 months: 1–35 μg/mg of creatinine (31–135 mg/kg/24 hr)
1–2 years: 1–30 μg/mg of creatinine
2–5 years: 1–15 μg/mg of creatinine
5–10 years: 1–14 μg/mg of creatinine
10–15 years: 1–10 μg/mg of creatinine (1–7 mg/24 hr; 5–35 mmol/24hr)
Adults: 1–7 μg/mg of creatinine (1–7 mg/24 hr; 5–35 mmol/24 hr)

NORMAL VALUES: FECES

FAT, TOTAL[2]

2–6 months: 0.3–1.3 g/d
6 months–1 year: <4 g/d
Children: <3 g/d
Adolescents: <5 g/d
Adults: <7 g/d

NORMAL VALUES: SWEAT

ELECTROLYTES[2]

Normal: <40 mmol/L for both sodium and chloride.
Patients with cystic fibrosis: >60 mmol/L for both sodium and chloride.

NORMAL VALUES: CEREBROSPINAL FLUID

PROTEIN[1]

Newborns: 40–120 mg/dL
<1 month: 20–80 mg/dL
>1 month: 15–45 mg/dL

GLUCOSE[1]

All ages: 60%–80% of blood glucose

APPENDIX D: WEST NOMOGRAM-BODY SURFACE AREA

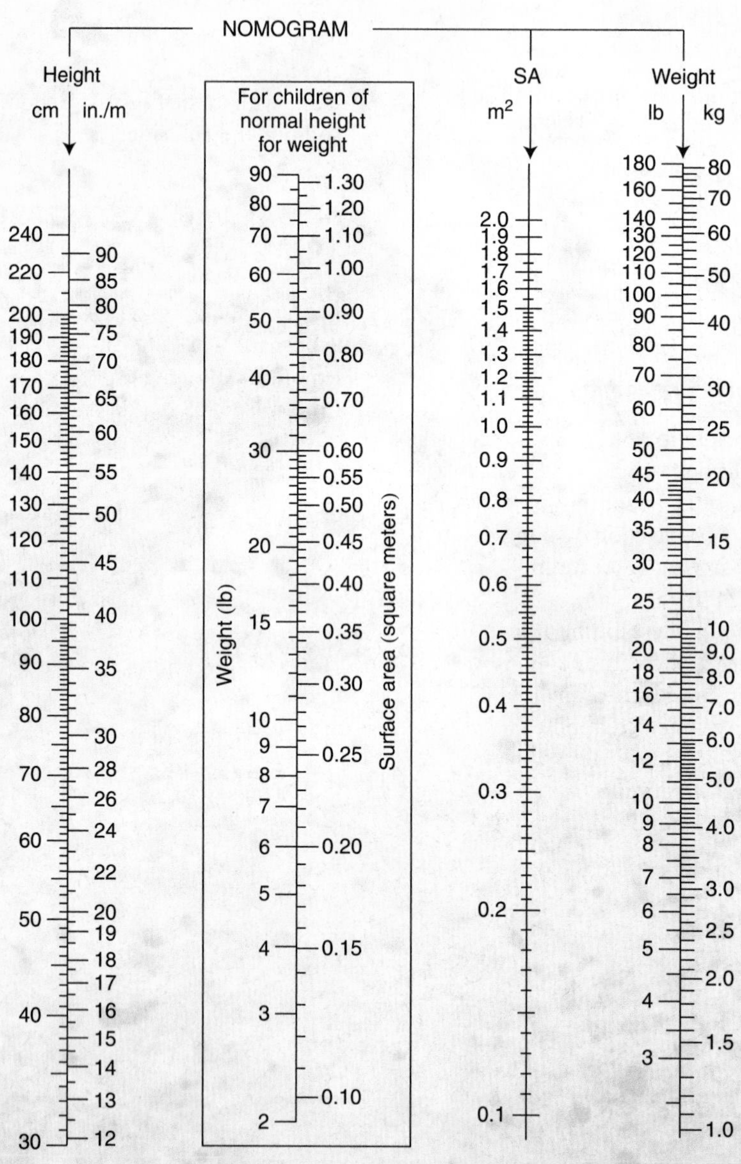

Note: *Nomogram modified from data of E. Boyd by C.D. West; from Behrman, R.E., Kliegman, R.M., & Jenson, H.B. (eds.). (2000).* Nelson textbook of pediatrics *(16th ed.). Philadelphia: W.B. Saunders.*

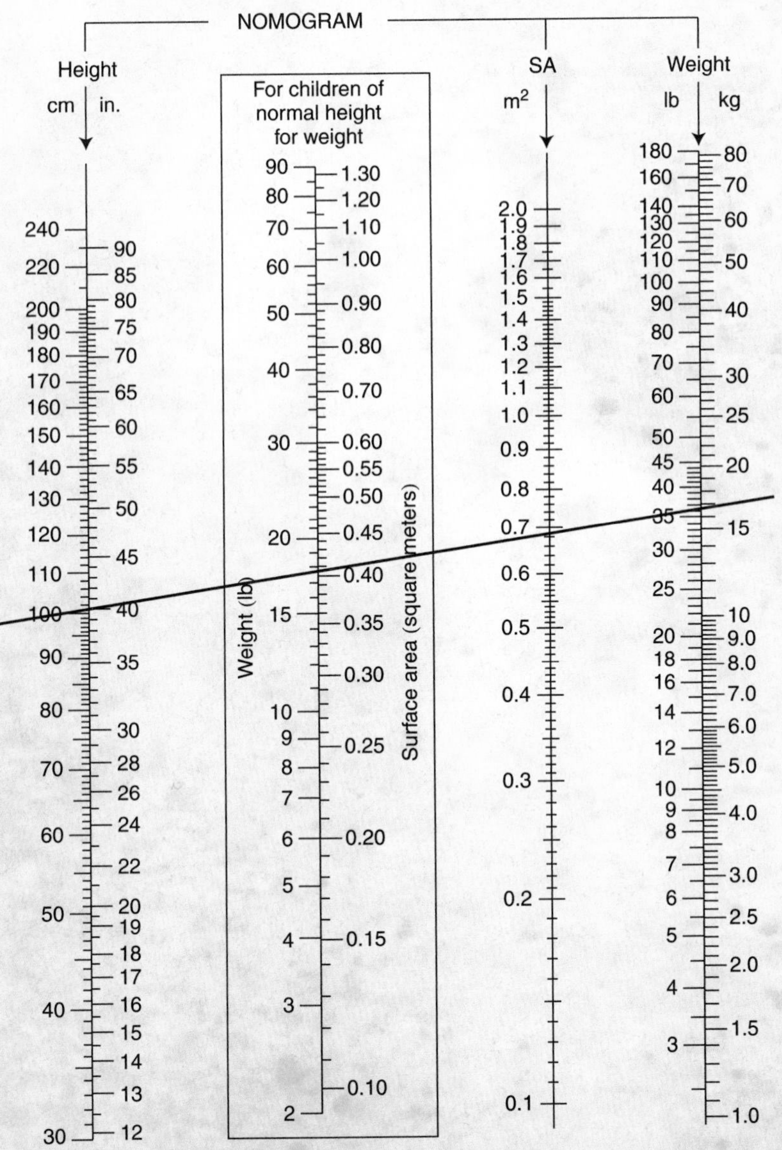

Pediatric doses of medications are generally based on body surface area (BSA) or weight. To calculate a child's BSA, draw a straight line from the height (in the left-hand column) to the weight (in the right-hand column). The point at which the line intersects the surface area (SA) column is the BSA (measured in square meters [m^2]). If the child is of roughly normal proportion, BSA can be calculated from the weight alone (in the enclosed area).

INDEX

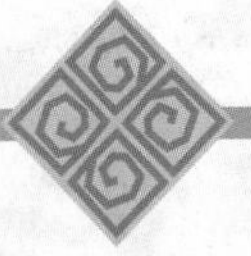
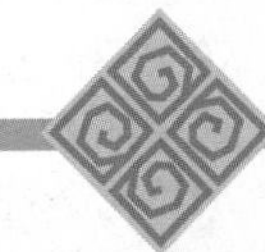

Page numbers set in bold indicate tables and figures.

B

J

K

L

M

SINGLE PC LICENSE AGREEMENT AND LIMITED WARRANTY

READ THIS LICENSE CAREFULLY BEFORE OPENING THIS PACKAGE. BY OPENING THIS PACKAGE, YOU ARE AGREEING TO THE TERMS AND CONDITIONS OF THIS LICENSE. IF YOU DO NOT AGREE, DO NOT OPEN THE PACKAGE. PROMPTLY RETURN THE UNOPENED PACKAGE AND ALL ACCOMPANYING ITEMS TO THE PLACE YOU OBTAINED THEM. ***THESE TERMS APPLY TO ALL LICENSED SOFTWARE ON THE DISK EXCEPT THAT THE TERMS FOR USE OF ANY SHAREWARE OR FREEWARE ON THE DISKETTES ARE AS SET FORTH IN THE ELECTRONIC LICENSE LOCATED ON THE DISK:***

1. GRANT OF LICENSE and OWNERSHIP: The enclosed computer programs and data ("Software") are licensed, not sold, to you by Pearson Education, Inc. ("We" or the "Company") and in consideration of your purchase or adoption of the accompanying Company textbooks and/or other materials, and your agreement to these terms. We reserve any rights not granted to you. You own only the disk(s) but we and/or our licensors own the Software itself. This license allows you to use and display your copy of the Software on a single computer (i.e., with a single CPU) at a single location for academic use only, so long as you comply with the terms of this Agreement. You may make one copy for back up, or transfer your copy to another CPU, provided that the Software is usable on only one computer.

2. RESTRICTIONS: You may not transfer or distribute the Software or documentation to anyone else. Except for backup, you may not copy the documentation or the Software. You may not network the Software or otherwise use it on more than one computer or computer terminal at the same time. You may not reverse engineer, disassemble, decompile, modify, adapt, translate, or create derivative works based on the Software or the Documentation. You may be held legally responsible for any copying or copyright infringement which is caused by your failure to abide by the terms of these restrictions.

3. TERMINATION: This license is effective until terminated. This license will terminate automatically without notice from the Company if you fail to comply with any provisions or limitations of this license. Upon termination, you shall destroy the Documentation and all copies of the Software. All provisions of this Agreement as to limitation and disclaimer of warranties, limitation of liability, remedies or damages, and our ownership rights shall survive termination.

4. LIMITED WARRANTY AND DISCLAIMER OF WARRANTY: Company warrants that for a period of 60 days from the date you purchase this SOFTWARE (or purchase or adopt the accompanying textbook), the Software, when properly installed and used in accordance with the Documentation, will operate in substantial conformity with the description of the Software set forth in the Documentation, and that for a period of 30 days the disk(s) on which the Software is delivered shall be free from defects in materials and workmanship under normal use. The Company does not warrant that the Software will meet your requirements or that the operation of the Software will be uninterrupted or error-free. Your only remedy and the Company's only obligation under these limited warranties is, at the Company's option, return of the disk for a refund of any amounts paid for it by you or replacement of the disk. THIS LIMITED WARRANTY IS THE ONLY WARRANTY PROVIDED BY THE COMPANY AND ITS LICENSORS, AND THE COMPANY AND ITS LICENSORS DISCLAIM ALL OTHER WARRANTIES, EXPRESS OR IMPLIED, INCLUDING WITHOUT LIMITATION, THE IMPLIED WARRANTIES OF MERCHANTABILITY AND FITNESS FOR A PARTICULAR PURPOSE. THE COMPANY DOES NOT WARRANT, GUARANTEE OR MAKE ANY REPRESENTATION REGARDING THE ACCURACY, RELIABILITY, CURRENTNESS, USE, OR RESULTS OF USE, OF THE SOFTWARE.

5. LIMITATION OF REMEDIES AND DAMAGES: IN NO EVENT, SHALL THE COMPANY OR ITS EMPLOYEES, AGENTS, LICENSORS, OR CONTRACTORS BE LIABLE FOR ANY INCIDENTAL, INDIRECT, SPECIAL, OR CONSEQUENTIAL DAMAGES ARISING OUT OF OR IN CONNECTION WITH THIS LICENSE OR THE SOFTWARE, INCLUDING FOR LOSS OF USE, LOSS OF DATA, LOSS OF INCOME OR PROFIT, OR OTHER LOSSES, SUSTAINED AS A RESULT OF INJURY TO ANY PERSON, OR LOSS OF OR DAMAGE TO PROPERTY, OR CLAIMS OF THIRD PARTIES, EVEN IF THE COMPANY OR AN AUTHORIZED REPRESENTATIVE OF THE COMPANY HAS BEEN ADVISED OF THE POSSIBILITY OF SUCH DAMAGES. IN NO EVENT SHALL THE LIABILITY OF THE COMPANY FOR DAMAGES WITH RESPECT TO THE SOFTWARE EXCEED THE AMOUNTS ACTUALLY PAID BY YOU, IF ANY, FOR THE SOFTWARE OR THE ACCOMPANYING TEXTBOOK. BECAUSE SOME JURISDICTIONS DO NOT ALLOW THE LIMITATION OF LIABILITY IN CERTAIN CIRCUMSTANCES, THE ABOVE LIMITATIONS MAY NOT ALWAYS APPLY TO YOU.

6. GENERAL: THIS AGREEMENT SHALL BE CONSTRUED IN ACCORDANCE WITH THE LAWS OF THE UNITED STATES OF AMERICA AND THE STATE OF NEW YORK, APPLICABLE TO CONTRACTS MADE IN NEW YORK, AND SHALL BENEFIT THE COMPANY, ITS AFFILIATES AND ASSIGNEES. HIS AGREEMENT IS THE COMPLETE AND EXCLUSIVE STATEMENT OF THE AGREEMENT BETWEEN YOU AND THE COMPANY AND SUPERSEDES ALL PROPOSALS OR PRIOR AGREEMENTS, ORAL, OR WRITTEN, AND ANY OTHER COMMUNICATIONS BETWEEN YOU AND THE COMPANY OR ANY REPRESENTATIVE OF THE COMPANY RELATING TO THE SUBJECT MATTER OF THIS AGREEMENT. If you are a U.S. Government user, this Software is licensed with "restricted rights" as set forth in subparagraphs (a)-(d) of the Commercial Computer-Restricted Rights clause at FAR 52.227-19 or in subparagraphs (c)(1)(ii) of the Rights in Technical Data and Computer Software clause at DFARS 252.227-7013, and similar clauses, as applicable.

Should you have any questions concerning this agreement or if you wish to contact the Company for any reason, please contact in writing: Prentice-Hall, New Media Department, One Lake Street, Upper Saddle River, NJ 07458.